MANAGEMENT
OF SPINAL
CORD INJURY

The Jones and Bartlett Series in Nursing

MANAGEMENT OF SPINAL CORD INJURY

SECOND EDITION

Cynthia Perry Zejdlik, R.N.

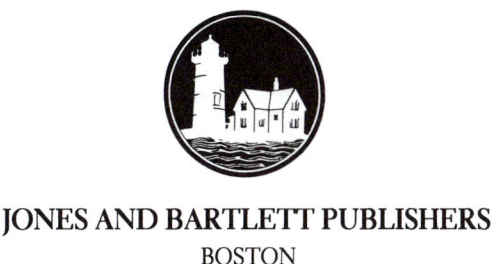

JONES AND BARTLETT PUBLISHERS

BOSTON

Editorial, Sales, and Customer Service Offices

Jones and Bartlett Publishers
20 Park Plaza
Boston, MA 02116

Library of Congress Cataloging-in-Publication Data

Zejdlik, Cynthia Perry.
    Management of spinal cord injury /
Cynthia Perry Zejdlik. — 2nd ed.
        p.   cm.
    Includes bibliographical references and index.
    ISBN 0-86720-438-9
    1. Spinal cord—Wounds and injuries.
    2. Physically handicapped— Rehabilitation.
    [1. Spinal Cord Injuries—rehabilitation.]
    I. Title.
        [DNLM: WL 400 Z48m]
    RD 594.3Z44   1991
    617.4′82044—dc20
    DNLM/DLC
    for Library of Congress   91-20889
                                                    CIP

Sponsoring Editor: James Keating
Manuscript Editor: Susan Lundgren
Production Editor and Designer:
    Joni Hopkins McDonald
Cover Design: Lina Haddad
Typesetting: *Omegatype*
Editorial–Production Service: *Wordsworth Associates*,
    Grace Sheldrick, Manager

Printed in the United States of America
95 94 93 92 91   10 9 8 7 6 5 4 3 2 1

PHOTO CREDITS

The thoughtful photographs have been provided courtesy of:

Joel Benard and University Hospital, Shaughnessy Site, Vancouver, BC: p. 592

British Columbia Paraplegic Association, Vancouver, BC: pp. 254, 640, 690

British Columbia Rehabilitation Society, Vancouver, BC: pp. 18, 287, 288, 293, 294, 295, 330, 336, 348, 391, 480, 481, 482, 483, 484, 485, 486, 491, 492, 504, 506, 512

California Medical Products, Long Beach, CA: p. 99

Casa Colina Centers for Rehabilitation, Pomona, CA: pp. 537, 538, 539, 540, 541, 542, 543, 544

Catholic Twin Circle, National Weekly Magazine, Studio City, CA: p. 30

Courage Center, Golden Valley, MN: pp. 240, 470, 522

Craig Hospital, Englewood, CO: pp. 435, 440L, 432, 433, 462, 465, 466, 478

K. Crawford, Chantilly, VA: p. 128

P. Eriksson, Edmonton, Alberta: pp. 527, 528, 532, 533

Hal's Pals, Winter Park, CO: p. 567

I.D.C. Medical Equipment, Inc., Folcroft, PA: p. 566

Independent Living Research Utilization project (ILRU), Houston, TX: pp. 136, 146, 396, 450, 634, 635, 637

J. Johnson, Options Independent Living Center, East Grand Forks, MN/Wilderness Inquiry, Minneapolis, MN: p. 630

Mr. and Mrs. G. Johnson and Johanna, Vancouver, BC: pp. 546, 642

Kashi Photographer, Berkeley, CA: pp. 144, 174, 582, 602, 660

James S. Keene, M.D.: p. 447

Life Support Products, Irvine, CA: p. 102

Robert R. Menter, M.D.: p. 683

PMT Corporation, Chanhassen, MN: p. 430

Rand-Scot, Inc., Fort Collins, CO: p. 487

Samaritan Rehabilitation Institute, Good Samaritan Medical Center, Phoenix, AZ: pp. xxviii, 2, 418, 420, 548, 628

Sigmedics, Inc., Northfield, IL: p. 503

University Hospital, Shaughnessy Site, Vancouver, BC: pp. 50, 52, 82, 104, 118, 202, 212, 228, 256, 270, 271, 272, 276, 304, 313, 319, 320, 352, 408, 425, 429, 431, 436, 437, 438, 440R, 441, 442, 459, 460, 474, 480, 487, 504, 570, 672

University of Michigan Medical Center, Ann Arbor, MI: p. 102

Vancouver Sun Newspaper, Vancouver, BC: pp. 86, 474

Ken Wright Supplies, Inc., Tulsa, OK: p. 467

Cynthia Perry Zejdlik, Bellingham, WA: p. 597

Roger Zejdlik, Bellingham, WA: pp. 91, 92, 349, 350, 378, 390, 443, 497, 498, 499, 500

Illustrations: Barbara Haynes; and Precision Graphics, Champaign, IL

To Roger, Gina, Karl, and my Mother.

*And to Douglas L. Mowat, C.M., A.R.W.,
M.L.A., Executive Director, British Columbia
Paraplegic Association, who was injured the year I
was born. With affection and respect, I salute his
inspirational achievements.*

Contents in Brief

Contents in Detail

FOREWORD

Life for most of us is a matter of adjusting to change. Yet few of us are prepared to adjust to all the changes in life caused by a spinal cord injury (SCI). Even under the best of circumstances successful adaptation to the results of SCI requires courage, perseverance, faith, support from family and friends, and quality rehabilitation.

Given advances in trauma care, improvements in the physical environment and in public attitudes about disability, more supportive services throughout the community, and great leaps in technology, it is now possible for people with the most severe disabilities caused by SCI, as well as other catastrophic impairments, to lead fulfilling, rewarding, and productive lives. Now, more than ever before, people with disabilities are working and living comparatively independent lives.

With the passage of new civil rights legislation such as the Americans with Disabilities Act, more and more people will be able to find opportunities in the workplace and in community life generally. Many communities are already beginning to adapt more appropriately to the varying needs of people with disabilities.

However, in order to reach the point at which relatively successful adaptation to SCI can become a realistic goal, one must have good rehabilitation, including adequate instruction and practice in doing or directing self-care. Few, if any, of us have the knowledge or ability to adapt to the challenge of SCI without considerable assistance from the health care community and from our families. Even professionals working in the health care and social service fields are inadequately prepared fully to assist someone who is severely spinal cord injured in adjusting most efficaciously to the challenges inherent in living with a disability.

Management of Spinal Cord Injury is a multidimensional, multiuse tool. As a person with SCI, I have used it as a reference tool. As a medical school faculty member, I have used it as a textbook and teaching aid. As a rehabilitation program administrator, I have used it as a program guide and management source book.

Management of Spinal Cord Injury is unique in terms of its broad-based perspective. By effectively integrating contributions from a distinguished array of authors with practical knowledge and expertise in virtually every aspect of SCI,

Cynthia Zejdlik has created the ultimate resource for everyone concerned—professionals, family members, and people with SCI.

Although *Management of Spinal Cord Injury* was originally conceived as a nursing textbook, it has become an interdisciplinary guidebook for all people involved in the treatment and care of people with SCI. This second edition has many new chapters that provide comprehensive background on such issues as prevention, case management, sports and recreation, SCI in children, brain injury, and attendant management skills. It is easily readable, with many tables and functional references, and it is abundantly informative, full of factual data and practical suggestions. Each chapter of *Management of Spinal Cord Injury* adds to the development of a functional knowledge base by focusing on the interaction between the person providing care and the person receiving the care.

Regardless of the reader's primary orientation and background, *Management of Spinal Cord Injury* will most assuredly enlighten and inform. While updating and supplementing the original material that made the first edition of *Management of Spinal Cord Injury* known and used throughout the world, this second edition uses a refined approach to organization that more clearly emphasizes current approaches to management and information utilization. The second edition of *Management of Spinal Cord Injury* will quickly become a useful and dependable resource for everyone involved in dealing with SCI and its effects. It will very likely become a standard text and reference tool for nursing education and rehabilitation education programs throughout the world. Adaptation to SCI is a difficult and challenging process. *Management of Spinal Cord Injury* facilitates the process of adaptation as well as any reference or educational tool can.

Lex Frieden
Senior Vice-President
The Institute for Rehabilitation
   and Research (TIRR)
Assistant Professor
Baylor College of Medicine
Houston, TX

PREFACE

To accomplish the goals of trauma rehabilitation, individuals and their families must make tremendous adjustments to cope with effects of disability. They require a great deal of support and assistance. The majority of persons enter the world of SCI with little or no idea of what their capabilities are and how they will manage. Immediately following injury, health care professionals ideally assume the role of experts, and individuals and families are largely recipients of knowledge and expertise. As rehabilitation progresses, with professional and peer facilitation, a transition toward regaining autonomy is experienced.

Few injuries are as devastating to people as spinal cord injury (SCI). Although the achievements of facilities worldwide and the collective expertise of interdisciplinary professionals continue to improve the quality of health care services, many people consider the problems SCI creates as insoluble. However, injured people themselves are often not of that opinion, and their positive beliefs have gradually but significantly influenced the health care system. Their needs are overwhelming, but together, people with SCI and interdisciplinary professionals have alleviated some of the major physical, psychological, social, and economic problems experienced by injured people, their families, and the communities in which they live.

The impact of trauma never ceases. As Dr. B. Halliday, Chairperson, House of Commons, Parliamentary Standing Committee on Human Rights and the Status of Disabled Persons, Canada, expressed when speaking of people with disabling injuries, "They have made it quite clear that their most urgent and pressing problems have little to do with their disabilities. Their concerns are focused on the social, physical and economic barriers which keep them outside of the Canadian mainstream" (Disabled Forestry Workers Foundation of Canada 1991: v).* Worldwide goals of trauma rehabilitation will never truly be met until practical solutions are implemented to secure social and economic reintegration. Questions should not be limited to who will take care of this person,

who will pay, and how much, but rather should emphasize a collective effort to overcome society's lack of awareness; to clear the maze of disincentives and bureaucratic mud puddles; and to plan overall use of resources so that all citizens have both the right and the means to participate fully in life, including the world of work. Health care professionals are well positioned to play important roles as allies with consumers, business, and governments toward improving the quality of life for people with traumatic injuries.

From the valued perspective of Gerald Bush, Ph.D.—a former senior vice-president of Gulf Oil, director of the Masters in Management of Human Services Program, Brandeis University, a founding member and former chairman of the National Head Injury Foundation, and the father of Patrick, who sustained a severe outcome from a traumatic brain injury—we must learn that

> trauma rehabilitation is ultimately *not* about management models, neurological or family systems research, outcome studies, or professions or laws. It is about the self-esteem of human beings whose lives have been disrupted, whose self-image has been set back. It is about human liberation and creative interventions and a positive advocacy and growth for everyone.
>
> For the world will never know true rehabilitation until the persons who have experienced the trauma are as much the heroes as the persons who give speeches, make policy, do research and lead associations. For it is true, that
>> Those who cannot count—count a great deal; and
>> Those who cannot speak—have much to say; and,
>> Those who cannot walk—must make the journey.
>> We must all make the journey together. (Bush 1991: 14)**

Management of Spinal Cord Injury, second edition, is based on this philosophy and provides a unique resource to both professionals and consumers. The book offers a complete, readable guide to the varied consequences of SCI, never losing sight of the importance of self-esteem in maintaining health and wellness.

---

*Disabled Forestry Workers Foundation of Canada. 1991. *Effective Strategies for the 90's: The Role of Employees, Unions, Governments and Consumers in Partnership*. Port Alberni, BC: Author

**Bush, G. 1990. *Self-Esteem: The First Step to Empowerment: Towards a Conceptual Base for Rehabilitation and Advocacy: A Working Paper*. Waltham, MA: Heller Graduate School, Brandeis University. Adapted with permission.

The roles of health care professionals are expanding in many challenging ways. Professionals need to understand the functions of many disciplines, and how they can collaborate with each other and how facility-based and community-based services can work together to provide an integrated approach—a complicated process. Nurses, physical and occupational therapists, social workers, psychologists, physicians, and others will find information useful for achieving interrelated health care goals. College and university students of varied disciplines and interests, from law to physical education, will find this an effective learning aid. The text offers practical guidelines for effectively coordinating services for people with SCI. The role of the nurse in the process of trauma rehabilitation and continuing health care is highlighted, particularly because other professionals rely on nurses to provide continuity throughout the variety of interventions and services.

Management of Spinal Cord Injury, second edition, considers each human need and examines the consequences that follow spinal cord injury. Management is detailed in a solid example of the uninterrupted continuum of care necessary from the moment of injury throughout life. The purpose of this approach—as opposed to presenting separate stages of acute, intermediate, and finally rehabilitative care as if isolated—is twofold:

1. To enhance awareness of how assessment and interventions rest on fundamental principles that apply throughout life. Interventions may require modification, but quality management, jointly with consumers and families, is needed to maintain health and prevent secondary disabilities as a result of SCI.

2. To gain an appreciation of other professionals' contributions, strengths, and limitations in the continuum of care and thus to facilitate planning, integration, coordination, and development of health service systems.

Part I of the book expresses a philosophical base for comprehensive care and describes current trends. Concerns about access to quality health care beyond the formal rehabilitation phase are presented in terms of a health care research capacity to maintain wellness and prevent secondary disabilities. The concept of and strategic planning for primary prevention of trauma, specifically SCI, are emphasized as major public health concerns.

Part II examines the priorities of life-saving techniques and concentrates on skilled assessment and management to prevent further neurological deficit and secondary complications. The current state of regeneration research is explained, as well as advancements and limitations experienced in attempts to cure paralysis, to help individuals and families grasp the implications of SCI. Legal intervention to protect injured persons is vital, and the benefits of early consultation are stressed in an effort to minimize future disadvantages.

Part III explores the psychosocial, sexual, and educational aspects of injury, including ways to incorporate effective interdisciplinary approaches. Promoting self-esteem is the crucial first step in the rehabilitation journey and beyond, and as such is explored early in the book to stress the singular importance of creating a positive and therapeutic environment. Without achieving this, individuals and families will not secure optimal benefits from other rehabilitation activities and be able to rebuild their lives. Included are case management services and preparation of individuals and families ultimately to become their own case managers.

Part IV describes specialized knowledge and skills essential to maintaining physiological well-being. It focuses on cardiopulmonary, gastrointestinal, and urinary function following injury.

Part V describes the momentum involved in regaining strength, reestablishing mobility, and achieving independence with daily living skills. Technology to enhance functional abilities and the introduction of sports to promote enjoyment and fitness are included, with information relevant to athletes preparing for competition.

Part VI presents complex issues requiring special considerations. It describes the unique needs of children with SCI and their parents and of people living with high quadriplegia. Current approaches to deal with the long-term difficulties experienced with chronic pain and spasticity are detailed.

Part VII is devoted to the highly relevant processes of discharge and reintegration into the community. "Is there life after rehabilitation?" is a question posed and answered by people with SCI. Their direct involvement will not merely effect immediate changes in the health care system, but will extend for the future a promise that a good life is possible.

To facilitate transition back into the real world, people need to be informed about interpersonal and social aspects of disability, with concrete, practical suggestions about what to do to feel comfortable. Staff are continually at the interface between people with SCI and the social environment, and reacting in appropriate, therapeutic ways is of great value. Many times and in many ways, it is expressed that physical limitations create disabilities, but that social barriers create the true handicaps. Related management skills to interact with the people who provide personal, ongoing care are important during rehabilitation to prepare for successful and full integration into community living.

Maintaining health and wellness and coping with ongoing needs are paramount for people living with SCI. Follow-up and related health care services are discussed, with special focuses on aging and on the need for health care professionals to develop sensitivity and adopt responsive attitudes to cope best with relatively unexplored challenges facing people who are living with SCI.

The 33 chapters in *Management of Spinal Cord Injury*, second edition, are organized to present:

- Learning objectives to be achieved.
- Interdisciplinary goals of health care.
- Assessment guides. Assessment sections include a review of normal anatomy and physiology and highlight neural functions. Anticipated dysfunctions are then correlated to the levels of SCI, which enables better preparation for emergencies, specific directions for prevention of complications, and accuracy in planning future rehabilitation.
- Intervention guides. Intervention sections include preventive and restorative measures.
- Specific interventions for potential complications. In the event of complications, a problem-solving approach presents a statement of the problem, goals of care, implementation of selected treatment, and outcome criteria to facilitate evaluation.
- Procedures to make selected assessment and intervention techniques easily accessible. Each procedure explains the purpose of the technique, details the recommended actions, and describes rationale to support those actions.
- Health education and self-care skills. This plan provides guidelines for education of individuals and families, an integral part of all care.
- Long-term implications. These concluding sections consider the effects of permanent disability and give information to adjust assessment data, redefine goals, and make decisions about consultation and referral.
- References for chapters and a resource section at the end of the book to help direct further learning and research.

Consumers and professionals who have expertise and communicate effectively can strengthen joint efforts to enhance positive outcomes of the rehabilitation process. *Management of Spinal Cord Injury*, second edition, promotes the principles Gerald Bush advocates that ultimately improve the quality of life that is saved.

Cynthia Perry Zejdlik

ABOUT THE AUTHOR

Cynthia Perry Zejdlik has spent 20 years in every phase of trauma rehabilitation, from prevention to advocacy for independent living. *Management of Spinal Cord Injury*, second edition, is based on that experience.

Cynthia Perry Zejdlik graduated from Vancouver General Hospital School of Nursing, British Columbia, and completed postgraduate studies at the Montreal Neurological Institute affiliated with McGill University in Montreal. Following an initial critical care focus, her interests in people living with severe disabilities developed into recreational and community-based work with the Alberta Rehabilitation Council for the Disabled, and rehabilitation counseling for the Canadian Paraplegic Association. She also served as nurse coordinator of the Developmental Clinic, Diagnostic Assessment and Treatment Centre, Alberta Children's Hospital.

In 1975, as the founding nurse clinician on the Acute SCI Unit at University Hospital, Shaughnessy Site, in Vancouver, BC, Ms. Zejdlik implemented rehabilitation philosophy beginning from the moment of injury and including early peer counseling.

As a private consultant, her projects have included interdisciplinary endeavors from the Rehabilitation Hospital of the Pacific in Hawaii to the remote Island of St. Helena in the South Atlantic Ocean. Currently, Ms. Zejdlik is the Research Project Director for the British Columbia Rehabilitation Society/British Columbia Paraplegic Association, studying life-time needs and development of health care delivery systems. She also provides consultation for Sigmedics, Inc. (Rehabilitation Technology for the Spinal Cord Injured) Northfield, IL; serves on the National Advisory Committee and provides technical assistance for the Robert Wood Johnson Foundation *Improving Service Systems for People with Disabilities* grant project; participated in the National Invitational Conference on *Developing a Comprehensive Health Services Research Capacity in Physical Disability and Rehabilitation* (National Institute on Disability and Rehabilitation Research); serves on the International Committee for the *World at Work* (government, labor, corporate, and advocate partners for economic independence, from Australia, Canada, Germany, and the United States), Independence 92 World Congress in Vancouver, BC; and also serves on the editorial board of the *SCI Nursing Journal*.

ACKNOWLEDGMENTS

Many people are involved with a project of the scope of *Management of Spinal Cord Injury*, second edition. Crosscutting issues associated with the trauma of spinal cord injury (SCI) affect every aspect of health care. Many different health care professionals, co-workers, and consumers require information that is fully integrated to address effectively the diverse needs of people who sustain SCI. To provide a comprehensive resource, *Management of Spinal Cord Injury*, second edition, blends multiple perspectives to communicate clearly what is known about SCI and what needs further investigation and implementation. I extend my sincere appreciation and thanks to everyone who assisted in many ways, and especially to

- All contributors for their willingness to impart professional expertise and permit flexibility in shaping their contributions to benefit an overall approach.
- Each person with SCI who shared a personal viewpoint to add unique insight into the world of living with a disability, and also to the professionals who shared their personal experiences.
- Susan Lundgren, White Lilac Press, Providence, RI, for her personal interest and extraordinary energies and editing skills, always with readers in mind. And to Grace Sheldrick, Wordsworth Associates, Editorial Services, Wellesley, MA, for her coordination of the entire project. Their concern and talents have greatly influenced the organization and style of this book.

Facilities, organizations, and associations by and for people with disabilities extended support and made available valuable network opportunities and resources. Thank you to

- American Association of Spinal Cord Injury Nurses, New York, NY, facilitated by Mary Lee Lynch, R.N., M.S.N., C.S., Chairperson, Program Committee, for their individual and group enthusiasm, guidance, and support. Ms. Lynch also reviewed the many psychosocial and ethical aspects presented throughout the text.
- American Trauma Society, Landover, MD, facilitated by Robert Sulsameda, R.N., M.N., Board of Directors.
- British Columbia Rehabilitation Society (G. F. Strong Rehabilitation Centre and Pearson Centre) under the leadership of William Fraser, President, for their generous sharing of time and wealth of interdisciplinary expertise and assistance.
- Canadian Paraplegic Association (CPA), in particular the British Columbia Division, facilitated by Norman Haw, A.R.W., Director, Rehabilitation Services, and Mary Lou Takasaki, Administrative Director. I wish to thank extensively Doug Mowat, Executive Director, whose first job paid $2.00 a day when taxi fare cost $1.00 each way; who has nurtured CPA into a dynamic resource for people with disabilities; who is recognized as a Member of the Order of Canada; and who, since 1983, has been elected to the Provincial Government of British Columbia as a Member of the Legislative Assembly. The opportunities, encouragement, and laughter he shares so freely with all of us is treasured.
- Georgetown University Child Development Center, Washington, DC, facilitated by Mary Deacon.
- Justice Institute of British Columbia, Emergency Health Services Academy, facilitated by Derek White, B.Sc., Program Director, Vancouver, BC.
- Member facilities of the Model SCI Systems for sharing educational information; especially to Craig Hospital, Englewood, CO, for generous donations of art and procedural materials used throughout the text; and to the University of Michigan Medical Center, Ann Arbor, MI, facilitated by Russ Waggoner, R.N., C.E.N., A.E.M.T., Flight Nurse Specialist, for assistance in developing prehospital and critical care aspects.
- National Spinal Cord Injury Association, Woburn, MA, and especially the SCI Network of Metropolitan Washington, Inc., Rockville, MD, for their endless contacts.
- National Rehabilitation Information Center, Silver Spring, MD, facilitated by Mark Odum, Director.
- National Rehabilitation Hospital, Washington, DC, facilitated by John Toerge, D.O., Director, SCI Service, and John Hudson, M.S.W., Director, Social

Services, for their welcoming spirit and sharing of clinical materials. As a strong consumer advocate, Mr. Hudson provided valuable input to many chapters throughout the text. Dr. Toerge skillfully assisted with updating many aspects of functional management and outcomes.

- The New South Wales College of Nursing, Glebe, N.S.W., Australia, facilitated by John Gale, Coordinator, Spinal Injuries Course, for contributions to international resources.
- To my colleagues with the Robert Wood Johnson Foundation/Independent Living Research Utilization (Houston, TX) *Improving Service Systems for People with Disabilities* project, for enriching my knowledge and for reaffirming the value of nurses in maintaining health throughout life for people with disabilities.
- Paralyzed Veterans of America, Washington, DC, for their appreciation of my efforts and access to resources.
- University Hospital, Shaughnessy Site, Vancouver, BC, and the interdisciplinary staff and patients on the Acute SCI Unit, who continued to share their energies and expertise on which the first edition was largely based. Also Kathy Fukuyama, R.N., B.S.N. M.Ed., Education Services, for never-tiring assistance with research.

To the reviewers for their time, dedication, and abilities to advise, add, and clarify information:

Part I

J. Paul Thomas, Ph.D., National Institute on Disability and Rehabilitation and Research, U.S. Department of Education. As Director of Medical Sciences Program that oversees the Model SCI Systems, Dr. Thomas interpreted the role and influence of the systems approach in depth.

Part II

Skender Adzijaj, E.M.T.
  Emergency Health Care Services
  Vancouver, BC

Lise Belanger, R.N., Critical Care Instructor
Charles Dyson, L.P.N.
Jan Taylor, R.N., B.S.N., Critical Care Instructor
Sara John Taylor, R.N., Head Nurse
Constance Yu, M.D., Radiologist
William Yu, M.D., Orthopedic Surgeon, and the
  interdisciplinary staff of the Acute SCI Unit,
  University Hospital, Shaughnessy Site, Vancouver, BC

Dianne Coen, R.N., C.N.S.
  Former Head Nurse

Acute Spine Injury Center
Northwestern Memorial Hospital
Chicago, IL

Lise McMullen Casady, R.N., B.S.N., C.R.R.N.
  Acute SCI Coordinator
  Tampa General Hospital
  Tampa, FL

Part III

Edward J. Desjardins, C.M., LL.D., Consultant
Bert Forman, M.S.W., Director, and
Penny Hicks, M.S.W.
  Social Services
Fran McKay, R.N., B.S.N.
  Director of Nursing
  British Columbia Rehabilitation Society, Vancouver, BC

Wendy Lawrence, R.N., B.S.N.
  Former Clinical Nurse Specialist
  University Hospital
  Vancouver, BC

Part IV

Caroline Alterman, B.S.N., M.S.N.
  Clinical Nurse Specialist
Marlon Finley, C.R.T.T., E.M.T.–C.T.
  Education Coordinator of Respiratory Care
Robert Mathews, R.R.T.
  Director of Respiratory Care
Donna Schachtel, R.N., B.S.
  Director of Education
  Shepherd Spinal Center, Atlanta, GA

Dr. J. Berezowskyj, Anesthesiologist
  University Hospital
  Vancouver, BC

Pat Corington, R.N.
  Head Nurse and
Susan Yob, R.N.
  Nurse Practitioner
  SCI Service
  National Rehabilitation Hospital
  Washington, DC

Nel Kirby, R.N., M.N., C.R.R.N.
  Assistant Professor, Division of Rehabilitation Medicine
  The Johns Hopkins University
  Baltimore, MD

Dr. J. R. Ledsome and J. Sharpe, R.N.
  Department of Physiology Research
  University of British Columbia
  Vancouver, BC

Dr. P. Maloney
Former Head, Department of Urology
University Hospital, Vancouver, BC

Dr. A. Santos
Veterans Administration Medical Center
Loma Linda, CA

Part V

Raymond Fulford, M.S.
Rehabilitation Engineer
Courage Center
Golden Valley, MN

Hilary Jebson, P.T.
Acute SCI Unit
and
Richard Ross, C.O.
Chief Orthotist
University Hospital
Vancouver, BC

Flora Thompson, O.T.
Rehabilitation Instructor
British Columbia Rehabilitation Society, and
Residents
Creekview 202 Independent Living Project
Vancouver, BC

Part VI

Donald E. Austin, R.N.
Nursing Unit Manager
Pearson Centre
Vancouver, BC

Kathleen DeSilva, J.D., The Institute for Rehabilitation
and Research, Houston, TX, and Johanna Johnson
and Mr. and Mrs. Gary Johnson (both nurses),
Vancouver, BC, for reviewing and sharing personal
perspectives about living with high quadriplegia

Julie Montgomery, R.N., M.S.N.
Clinical Nurse Specialist
National Rehabilitation Hospital
Washington, DC

Heather Naka, R.N., B.S.N.
Former Head Nurse
British Columbia Children's Hospital
Vancouver, BC

Part VII

Judy Kelly, R.N., B.S.N., M.Ed.
Director, Long-Term Care

Public Health Department
Burnaby, BC

Laura Williams
Deputy Project Director
Independent Living Research Utilization/Robert
Wood Johnson Foundation, *Improving Service Systems
for People with Disabilities*, Houston, TX

My grateful acknowledgement is extended to all of the
people who generously provided wonderful photographs,
especially to

- Individuals and families for personal photographs,
  and to Kirby Crawford, Chantilly, VA, for restoring
  and developing these photographs for production
- British Columbia Rehabilitation Center, Vancouver,
  BC, Phil Goodis, photographer
- Casa Colina Centers for Rehabilitation, Pomona,
  CA, courtesy of Julie Madorsky, M.D. (sports photog-
  raphy)
- Courage Center, Golden Valley, MN, courtesy of
  Gerald Michaelson, chairman of the Board of Direc-
  tors, and Terry Poehls, photographer
- Independent Living Research Utilization/The Insti-
  tute for Rehabilitation and Research, Houston, TX
- Kashi Photography, Berkeley, CA, courtesy of Ed
  Kashi
- Samaritan Rehabilitation Institute, Good Samaritan
  Hospital, Phoenix, AZ, courtesy of Shirley Benda,
  R.N., M.S., Assistant Program Director
- University Hospital, courtesy of Sara John Taylor,
  Acute SCI Unit, and the Biomedical Communica-
  tions Department, Vancouver, BC

My appreciation is also extended to the people involved
in the production services. Their orchestrated efforts resulted in the fine quality of this book. Thanks to Paula
Carroll and Joni McDonald of Jones and Bartlett Publishers, Boston; to Omegatype Typography, Champaign, IL;
and again to Susan Lundgren and Grace Sheldrick.

To my family and friends who have repeatedly juggled
their schedules to provide the impossible I extend my warm-
est thanks, and especially to my children, who find all of
this writing "very boring, Mom." I am deeply grateful to my
husband, Roger, for his economic support and patience
with the unbelievable time demands for the five long years
in preparation of the first edition and the three subsequent
years devoted to the second edition.

Thanks also to E. DesJardins, L. Casady, N. Haw, J.
Hudson, W. Lawrence, L. Williams, and the residents of
Creekview 202, who reviewed the manuscript with the
additional perspective of personal experience with SCI.

CONTRIBUTORS

Andrew I. Batavia, J.D., M.S. *(ch. 2)*

White House Fellow
Associate Director for Health
  Services Research
National Rehabilitation Hospital
  Research Center
Washington, DC

D. Sue Briggs, R.N., M.S.N., C.R.R.N. *(ch. 21)*

Assistant Director of Nursing
Craig Hospital
Englewood, CO

Lester Butt, Ph. D. *(chs. 9, 29)*

Clinical Psychologist
Craig Hospital
Englewood, CO

Kathleen Cain, A.C.S.W. *(ch. 3)*

Director, Office of Injury Control
Missouri Department of Health
Jefferson City, MO

Rosemary Cox, R.D., L.D. *(ch. 17)*

Nutrition/Wellness Coordinator
INTELSAT
Washington, DC

Dennis Crowley, M.D. *(ch. 22)*

Acting Chief
Physical Medicine Service
Tripler Army Medical Center
Honolulu, HI

Alfred H. DeGraffe, M.S., S.E.A. *(ch. 32)*

Author and Publisher
Fort Collins, CO

Gerben DeJong, Ph.D. *(ch. 2)*

Director of Rehabilitation Research
National Rehabilitation Research
  Center
Washington, DC
Professor, Department of School
  and Family Medicine
Georgetown University School of
  Medicine
Washington, DC

William Donovan, M.D. *(ch. 15)*

Director, Spinal Cord Injury
  Service
The Institute for Rehabilitation and
  Research
Houston, TX

Michael Dunn, Ph.D. *(chs. 13, 31)*

Spinal Cord Injury Center
Veterans Administration Medical
  Center
Palo Alto, CA

Peter Eriksson, B.Sc. *(ch. 24)*

Rick Hansen Centre
Department of Physical Education
  and Sports Studies
University of Alberta
Edmonton, Alberta, Canada

David F. Fairholm, M.D., F.R.C.S.C. *(ch. 28)*

Division of Neurosurgery
Vancouver General Hospital
Vancouver, British Columbia,
  Canada

Robert E. Falcone, M.D., F.A.C.S. *(ch. 5)*

Director of Trauma Services
Grant Medical Center
Clinical Assistant Professor of
  Surgery
Ohio State University
Columbus, OH

Lex Frieden *(ch. 30)*

Senior Vice-President
The Institute for Rehabilitation and
  Research, and
Assistant Professor
Baylor College of Medicine
Houston, TX

Hank Gambina, M.S., L.M.F.C.C. *(ch. 13)*

Spinal Cord Injury Center
Veterans Administration Medical
  Center
Palo Alto, CA

Michael Grossman, R.N. *(ch. 25)*

Director of Nursing
Shriners Hospitals for Crippled
  Children
Philadelphia, PA

Tim Gust, Ph.D. *(ch. 14)*

Rehabilitation Counselor and
  Neuropsychologist
Vallejo, CA

Karen H. Hildebrand, R.N. *(ch. 26)*

Outpatient Coordinator
Craig Hospital
Englewood, CO

Shayna Hornstein, P.T. *(ch. 23)*

Neil Squire Foundation
Deep Cove, British Columbia,
Canada

**Fina Canave Jiminez, R.N.,
M.Ed.** *(chs. 15, 29)*

Nursing Instructor
British Columbia Rehabilitation
Society
Vancouver, British Columbia,
Canada

James S. Keene, M.D. *(chs. 4, 20)*

Associate Professor of Orthopedics
Co-Director Spine Injury Center
University of Wisconsin
Madison, WI

**Corrine Koehler, R.N., B.S.N.,
C.C.R.N.** *(ch. 20)*

Radiology Coordinator
Craig Hospital
Englewood, CO

Daniel P. Lammertse, M.D.
(ch. 27)

Medical Director
Craig Hospital
Englewood, CO

Sarah Layman, C.R.N.P. *(ch. 25)*

Department of Neurosurgery
University of Washington
Seattle, WA

**Mary Lee Lynch, R.N., M.S.N.,
C.S.** *(ch. 9)*

Psychiatric Clinical Specialist
Veterans Administration Medical
Center
Long Beach, CA

Arthur G. Madorsky, M.D.
(ch. 24)

Clinical Professor, Internal
Medicine
College of Osteopathic Medicine of
the Pacific
Pomona, CA

Julie G. Madorsky, M.D. *(ch. 24)*

Medical Director, Spinal Cord
Injury Program
Casa Colina Hospital for
Rehabilitation Medicine
Pomona, CA

**Sam Maddox, author and
publisher** *(Epilogue)*

Spinal Network
Boulder, CO

Katrina McKay, O.T. *(ch. 23)*

Neil Squire Foundation
Deep Cove, British Columbia,
Canada

**Louise Bouscaren McKnew,
LL.D.** *(ch. 8)*

Attorney-at-Law
Bethesda, MD

**Audrey Nelson, R.N., M.N.,
Ph.D.** *(ch. 12)*

Rehabilitation Nursing Care
Coordinator
James A. Haley Veterans Hospital
Tampa, FL

Robert R. Menter, M.D. *(ch. 33)*

Medical Director
Spinal Cord Injury Service
Craig Hospital
Englewood, CO

George Richardson, M.R.C.
(ch. 33)

Director of Follow-Up Services
Craig Hospital
Englewood, CO

Eileen Rosenfeld, R.N. *(ch. 25)*

Spinal Cord Injury Clinical Nurse
Specialist
Shriners Hospital for Crippled
Children
Philadelphia, PA

**Sandra Schaefer, R.N., M.S.,
C.C.R.N., C.N.A.** *(ch. 6)*

Nurse Manager
Surgical Intensive Care Unit
James A. Haley Veterans Hospital
Tampa, FL

**Lois A. Schaetzle, R.N., M.S.,
C.R.R.N.** *(ch. 21)*

Nursing Education Coordinator
Craig Hospital
Englewood, CO

Noreen Sommer, R.N., M.S.N.
(ch. 13)

Spinal Cord Injury Center
Veterans Administration Medical
Center
Palo Alto, CA

George Szasz, M.D. *(ch. 10)*

Professor, Department of Psychiatry
University of British Columbia
Director, Sexual Health Services
University Hospital, Shaughnessy
Site, and
Director, Sexual Health Services
British Columbia Rehabilitation
Society
Vancouver, British Columbia,
Canada

**Charles H. Tator, M.D., Ph.D.,
F.R.C.S.(C)** *(ch. 7)*

Professor and Chairman, Division
of Neurosurgery
University of Toronto
Director, Canadian Paraplegic
Association
Spinal Cord Injury Research
Laboratory
Toronto Western Hospital,
University of Toronto
Toronto, Ontario, Canada

Susan S. Thomason, R.N., M.N.
(ch. 6)

Clinical Nurse Specialist
Spinal Cord Injury Service
James A. Haley Veterans Hospital
Tampa, FL

Linda J. Todd, R.N., C.R.R.N.
(ch. 21)

Patient Education Specialist
Craig Hospital
Englewood, CO

Kelly Cox Watkins, R.N., M.N. *(ch. 21)*

Nurse Manager, Spinal Injury
  Service
Craig Hospital
Englewood, CO

Stacey Phaneuf Wasko, P.T. *(ch. 22)*

Director of Rehabilitation
Ballard Comprehensive Care
Seattle, WA

Alan H. Weintraub, M.D. *(ch. 26)*

Medical Director
Head Injury Treatment Program
Craig Hospital
Englewood, CO

**Peter C. Wing, M.D., M.B.,
Ch.B., M.Sc., F.R.C.S.(C)** *(ch. 3)*

Clinical Associate Professor
University of British Columbia
Head, Department of Orthopedic
  Surgery
University Hospital, Shaughnessy
  Site
Vancouver, British Columbia,
  Canada

James E. Wilberger, M.D. *(ch. 25)*

Vice-Chairman, Department of
  Neurosurgery
Allegheny General Hospital
Pittsburgh, PA

Thomas A. Zdeblick, M.D. *(chs. 4, 20)*

Assistant Professor of Orthopedics
Director, Spine Surgery Service
University of Wisconsin
Madison, WI

Wolfgang Zimmermann *(ch. 3)*

Executive Director
Disabled Forestry Workers of
  Canada
Port Alberni, British Columbia,
  Canada

A. Batavia, M. Dunn, A. De-
Graffe, L. Frieden, L. McKnew, and
W. Zimmermann are professionals
who have the additional perspective
of personally experiencing spinal
cord injury.

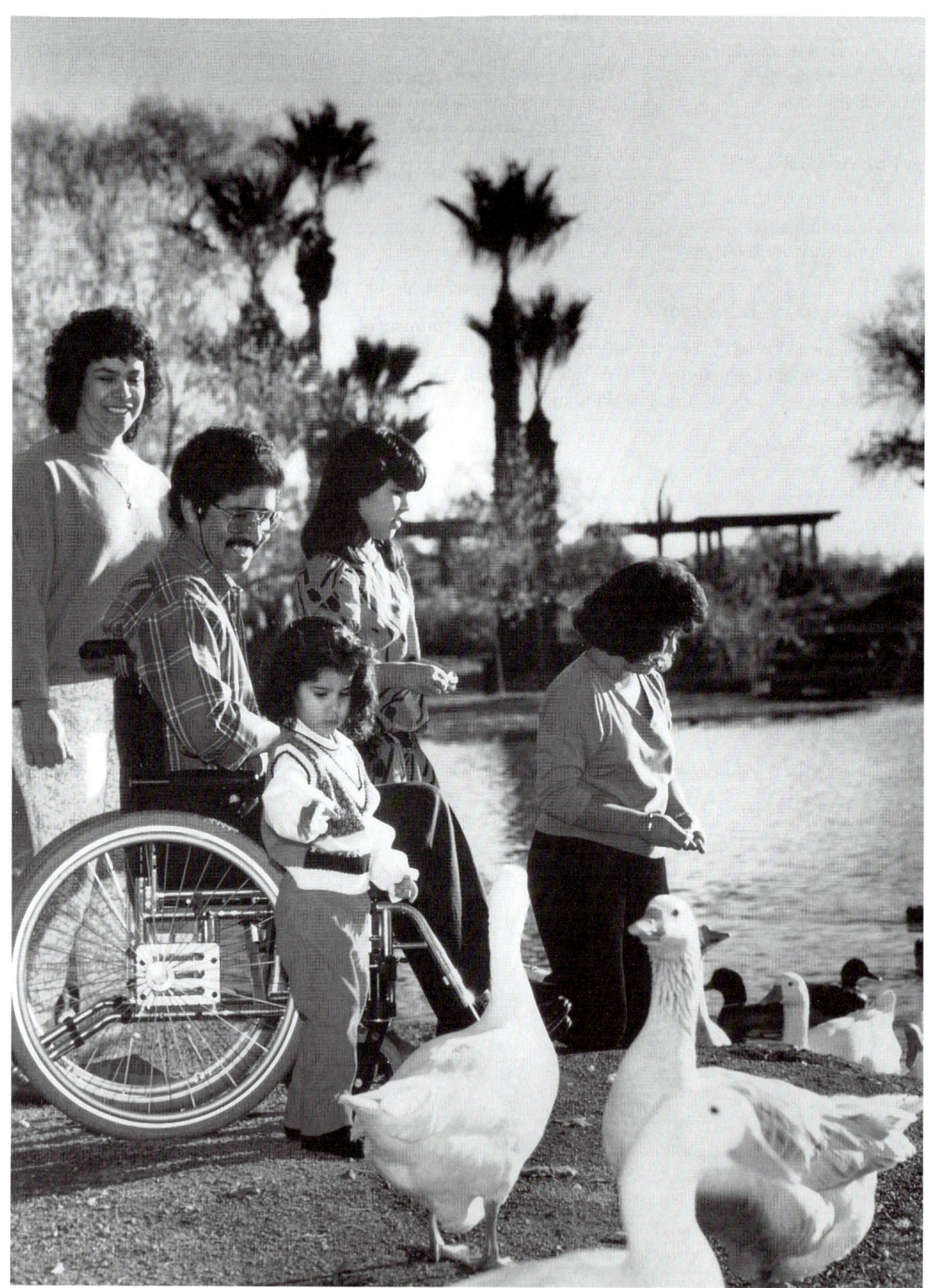

PART
— I —

PERSPECTIVES ON SPINAL CORD INJURY

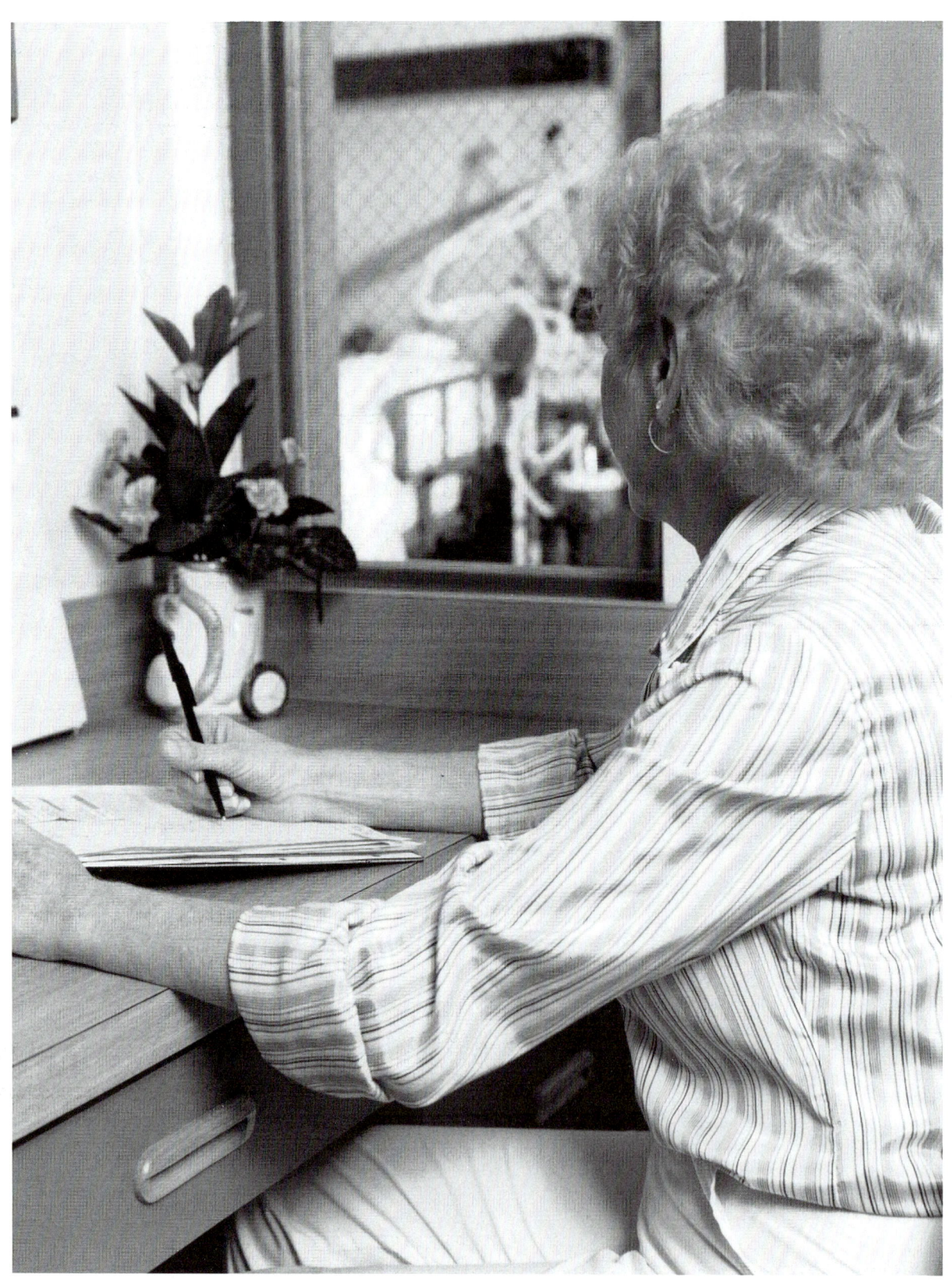

CHAPTER
— 1 —

Health Care Concepts and Spinal Cord Injury

Chapter Outline

Objectives

- To define spinal cord injury (SCI) and the implications of severe physical disability
- To gain perspective on the impact of SCI and its meaning to individuals, families, the health care system, and the community at large
- To identify steps of goal-oriented rehabilitative care
- To identify ways, beyond providing optimal professional care, to help secure a life of independence for people with SCI

Spinal cord injury (SCI), if complete, causes permanent motor paralysis below the level of the injury with corresponding loss of sensation. However, as emphasized by the National Spinal Cord Injury Foundation (1981: 26):

> The catastrophic nature of spinal cord injury is much more complex than loss of feeling and inability to move. Individuals who experience damage to their spinal cords also contend with impairment of bladder, bowel, and sexual function. Added to this are the psychological effects of adjustments that must be made to social, economic, and emotional ramifications of spinal cord injury.

Paraplegia refers to paralysis of the lower portion of the body, which includes the legs and may include the trunk. Paraplegia occurs with injury to the second thoracic segment (T_2) or below. *High paraplegia* refers to SCI from T_2 to T_6; *low paraplegia* generally refers to SCI at T_7 and below. Because upper body strength is preserved, a paraplegic person has the potential physical ability to become independent in all aspects of personal care and wheelchair mobility; ambulation, with or without orthotics, crutches, and canes, is possible.

Quadriplegia, or *tetraplegia*, refers to paralysis of the lower and upper portions of the body including partial or complete involvement of the arms and hands. Quadriplegia occurs with injury to the first thoracic segment (T_1) or above. Physical rehabilitation is much more complex. Abilities and independence potential for personal care and wheelchair mobility are dramatically affected by the level of injury. In addition, the autonomic nervous system, coordinated from higher centers, does not function normally. Quadriplegia also poses a significant threat of respiratory insufficiency.

High quadriplegia, or *pentaplegia*, are terms used for extremely high cord injury in which paralysis extends to the muscles of the neck and the back of the head and the breathing muscles, primarily the diaphragm. A person with injury at C_4 and above requires a lifelong respiratory support system and total assistance with personal care. Power wheelchairs and environmental control systems, such as electronic devices to operate lights or a radio (described in Chapter 23), are options available to promote independence.

See Chapter 4 for a complete discussion of consequences of SCI. Also, Table 22–7 gives an overview of levels of functioning for people with SCI.

HISTORICAL BACKGROUND

Spinal injury with paralysis has been recorded throughout civilization. Ancient Greek and Egyptian medical records; accounts of historical figures, such as Lord Nelson, who suffered spinal cord injuries; and horrific tales from the battlefields of World War I consistently depict the victims of spinal cord injury as doomed to death. Survivors were wracked with infections, contractures, bedsores, and mental anguish—surely one of the most depressing pictures in medicine. Only recently has this gloomy picture begun to brighten.

Health care concepts of SCI remained virtually the same until the twentieth century. The major turning point occurred when great numbers of World War II veterans returned home. Although combat injuries cause a relatively small percentage of spinal cord injuries, veterans' needs have often inspired worldwide movements to improve comprehensive health care.

By 1945, the health sciences were sufficiently advanced and public attitudes sufficiently receptive to allow appropriate attention to the total rehabilitative need of people with SCI. After World War II, Sir Ludwig Guttman, working at Stoke-Mandeville Hospital in England, virtually revolutionized the concept of health care for people with spinal cord injuries (1976). He emphasized centralized, comprehensive services for the *total spinal person*, as opposed to institutionalized custodial care for *cripples*. Guttman developed an integrated, interprofessional team; improved and interrelated acute and long-term care facilities; and provided social and vocational counseling and after-care services. This model inspired other countries to adopt a similar approach.

The belief that the spinal cord injured individual is a physically disabled but healthy person, with a productive future in society, is now a fundamental concept of health care in most modern nations. In support of this approach, Schweigel and Peerless (1971: 2–4) write:

> It is generally agreed that intensive medical/rehabilitative care must begin as soon as possible after the spinal cord injury. The dramatic improvement in the morbidity and mortality statistics in countries where centers were established years ago, for example, in Great Britain in the 1940s, Australia in the 1950s, and South Africa in the 1960s, has clearly shown the desirability for such centers for the management of the spinal injured. . . . However, a fragmentary and haphazard approach to this problem currently exists.
>
> *It is sometimes said that a patient with spinal cord injury is too ill to be moved to a major center. Actually those individuals are too sick to be safely managed in small hospitals or in large hospitals where fragmentation of services and specialty groups prevent the overall view of their complex problems.* The care of these severely disabled patients includes the prevention of the complicating manifestations; as well, the psychological, physical, social, and vocational rehabilitative measures require a highly sophisticated team approach in which each team member contributes within the realm of their expertise. Over and above the humane factor, favorable prognosis as to the life expectancy and stability of neuromuscular disability justifies a considerable investment of time, money, and effort

Here's Looking at You, Kid: From the Other Side of the Sheets
A Patient's View of the Professional's Role

Try to see me as an individual. I need you to see me as the unique person I used to be before I became a patient under these sheets. It doesn't feel good to be so dependent on you. You rule here. And I need you so much it hurts. I need your care, but I also need you to have patience with me. You are my bridge to tomorrow, a guide across this terrible abyss in my life's journey. Please try to see me as the unique and worthwhile person I am. Remind me that I am still the person of the past evolving into someone with different yet equal potential for life. Help me keep faith with myself out of your faith that life can still be worthwhile, even after this devastating injury.

Our first encounter with the medical world is unbalanced: you are strong, we are weak. You are in control, we are not. You are trained for an encounter we would never have chosen. It is not surprising that our relationship does not always proceed smoothly. Yet our mutual battle to mend and rebuild a ruptured life can best be won when there is a sense of trust and respect.

Traumas that would have killed our parents now merely limit our functioning. Medical science prolongs our lives. Various disabilities, including SCI, will bring more and more of us into the modern hospital to be patched up and returned to our communities, equipped to continue our lives as fulfilled and productive individuals.

Although my neurological wiring and physiological responses may be fitted into neat diagnostic charts, other factors make me unique. There are no uniform answers to every clinical question. Not only my body, but also my mind and spirit have been injured. Everyone has been socialized to pity so-called crippled invalids, and we who are injured are thus devastated when we find ourselves joining their ranks.

It hurts when you dismiss our attempts to be taken seriously. Once I asked a particular professional to let me participate in my own treatment. I told her about some needs she hadn't been considering. I was scared because if she got mad at me, she could make my life even more uncomfortable. The sarcastic tone cut even before the words brought tears of humiliation: "I haven't noticed that anyone has authorized you to run this show, so I'd suggest you just lie back and try to be a little more appreciative!" Her response blocked my efforts at recovery for a time. I withdrew from the struggle toward improvement. Passive resistance seemed the only way to assert my independence. Finally, however, I realized that I harmed myself more than her with my lack of enthusiasm to get better. In fact, I'm sure she never even noticed my relapse! Yet I still cringe when I think of her.

As the injured self-image is slowly prepared for return to the community, the person exchanges the role of patient for a role with more power and dignity. That process of moving from being controlled by professional care givers to taking back responsibility for one's self is rather like the pain of adolescence. When those of us who have graduated from rehabilitation share impressions of this transition, we usually vie over who can top the last horror story of miscommunication and misunderstanding. In retrospect, the complexity of the experience emerges: most former patients remember their hospital experience as a love/hate relationship. The experience saved our lives, but we wonder if there had to be so many demeaning factors.

We should all become more sophisticated and knowledgeable about developing civil rights protections for the handicapped and learn how to assist people with SCI to return to managing their own lives. Then we will be better equipped to defuse our natural fear of human vulnerability. It is unfortunate that people with SCI who have prevailed in the battle for independence so seldom return to tell health care professionals about the lessons they have learned after rehabilitation. Life does go on after injury, and every day new recruits in the army of survivors are proving that paralyzed bodies cannot defeat the human spirit's desire for self-determination.

The independent living movement that came of age in the late 1960s and early 1970s altered the way disabled people see themselves. However, popular opinion and social attitudes still have not caught up. Our society still views physical flaws as detracting from the value of the whole person. We all—including the newly injured and care givers—have a burden of negative stereotypes to overcome. We all grew up thinking of spinal cord injured persons as "cripples." It is easy to set up categories and classifications. We try to base them on scientific observation, but our charts and graphs are imperfect and can obscure certain possibilities from our notice. Although tables of function and clinical prediction are essential, too great reliance on

(Box continues)

them can prevent us from seeing possibilities that lie beyond rigid charts or organizational categories.

In her book *Mindfulness*, Harvard professor Ellen Langer reports on 15 years of research into how to think beyond the "routinized conformity" of our traditional training patterns. When we think only in those categories we learned in school, we are processing the world "mindlessly," failing to make maximum use of all our senses. Sometimes we are saved from the pain of interaction by such routine behavior, but those of us with disabilities need you to view us beyond those limitations. We need you to feel the freedom to respond to us improvisationally. Those persons who have moved beyond the hospital walls have learned that life with physical impairments is based on a balance of careful planning and a willingness to be open to the possibilities inherent in each moment and each new situation

and challenge. Professor Langer suggests, "Those who can free themselves of mindsets, open themselves to new information and surprise, play with perspective and context, and focus on process rather than outcome are likely to be creative, whether they are scientists, artists, or cooks." That certainly applies to health care professionals, and particularly those who must meet the challenges of diverse patients who happen to have injured their spines.

The sheet between us is very thin. "Here's looking at you, kid"—with affection.

Mary Jane Owen, M.S.W.
Executive Director
Disability Focus, Inc.
Washington, DC

required to rehabilitate the patient with a spinal cord injury.

The complexity of the many intrinsic and extrinsic factors encountered in the care and rehabilitation process of these patients demands the full cooperation of a large number of health professionals and nonmedical personnel, ranging from the ambulance driver to the future employer of the patient, characteristically exemplifying the so-called team approach.

From the moment of injury, extending beyond rehabilitation, people need comprehensive health care service systems in order to maintain health and successfully manage the effects of SCI over the life-span.

CURRENT HEALTH CARE SYSTEMS IN THE UNITED STATES

In the United States, health care for people with spinal cord injuries is currently delivered in three distinct systems: those using the model systems concept; Department of Veterans Affairs (Veterans Administration) spinal cord injury centers; and community facilities (Trieschmann 1980).

The Model Systems Concept: A Categorical Care Approach

The Model Spinal Cord Injury Systems were begun in 1970 under the management of the National Institute on Disability and Rehabilitation Research (NIDRR) of the U.S. De-

partment of Education. Although membership in the model systems remains fairly consistent, grants are awarded on an annual basis. See the Resources section at the end of this book for a complete listing. The model systems embody an interdisciplinary concept of comprehensive care from the moment of injury through acute care, rehabilitation, community integration, and long-term follow-up. The concept encourages the acquisition of clinical knowledge and the development, demonstration, and evaluation of related approaches, techniques, and equipment to improve care. Registry, research, and prevention are also emphasized. The comprehensive data base maintained at the Spinal Cord Injury Statistical Center at the University of Alabama-Birmingham is one of the model systems' projects.

In an extensive research project report supported by the National Spinal Cord Injury Foundation to determine cost-effectiveness of specialized treatment centers, Matlack (1974) summarizes the economic and clinical issues surrounding comprehensive care for spinal cord injured persons. He found that leaders unanimously prefer coordinated, comprehensive, concurrent care by all the related health care professionals from the onset of injury, through rehabilitation, to discharge, with ongoing specialized services for the disabled person in the community. Yet, as a federal government representative notes,

> Despite the fact that there is every reason to believe that the . . . model systems approach to spinal cord injury care is appropriate, beneficial in rehabilitation outcomes, and significantly cost-effective over all other alternatives; and that alternatively, there is every likelihood that there will be unsatisfactory patient-client outcomes, catastrophic medical complications, incredibly high costs for hospital and nursing home care, and a tremendous drain on per-

sonal, private, and public resources; *only about 15 percent of all newly injured patients receive care under this concept.* [Humphreys 1978: 3–5]

If the model systems concept is superior, why has it not been more widely adopted in North America? Matlack and others concluded that medical apathy, characterized by parochialism and institutional rigidity, is one problem but that financial concerns are probably the main reason. However, the conclusions of Matlack's cost-effectiveness study invalidate these concerns. Analyzing direct costs (primarily for hospitalization and lifelong nursing and medical costs) and indirect costs (primarily for lost earnings) and comparing the costs for patients who were cared for in specialized centers with the costs for patients who were not, he writes:

> There are no competing economic or medical costs to compare—all are on the side of spinal cord injury center treatment. . . . The parameters of the model suggest norms for the length of hospitalization and treatment outcomes. Since prolonged treatment is often due to preventable complications, cost control and quality control reinforce each other. At least in the case of spinal cord injury, the best quality treatment is also the least costly for the patient, for third-party payers, and for society. [Matlack 1974: 20]

Today the quest is virtually unchanged. The federal government cannot underwrite the costs of SCI care for everyone, and it cannot dictate to individuals or state governments how to provide certain types of services. However, through the model systems demonstration projects, the government sets an example, educates, and disseminates information.

Department of Veterans Affairs (VA) Spinal Cord Injury Centers

The VA centers have also been at the forefront of these endeavors, laying much of the groundwork. The Vietnam War caused a sudden and disproportionate increase in the incidence of SCI among young Americans. Not only has this group significantly increased public awareness, they and health care professionals have strengthened and advanced the interdisciplinary concept to improve comprehensive services from the acute stage, during rehabilitation, and indeed, continuing throughout life.

The VA has expertise in dealing with issues of lifetime care and aging with a disability. Specialized SCI centers are strategically located in VA hospitals throughout the country.

Veterans injured either in active service or during inactive duty qualify for care at a specialized center within a VA hospital. However, this is a relatively small percentage of the total SCI population; the majority of patients receive care in community facilities.

Community Facilities

Between 50% and 70% of the people with new spinal cord injuries probably receive their acute management and rehabilitation at a local facility. Only persons with complicated cases of high quadriplegia are likely to be referred to a specialized center.

The decision to refer people with SCI to a specialized center depends largely on the consulting physician and the preference of the patient and family. However, it is doubtful that most individuals get appropriate or adequate information about the health care delivery options available, both from a clinical and economic point of view. In the emotional turmoil surrounding the initial injury, patients and families must have objective help so that they can make a well-informed choice from the available alternatives. Yet some professionals may not give assistance. Solutions may depend on collaboration with a third party, such as the patient's family physician, a personal attorney (Chapter 8), and increasingly, case managers representing third-party payers (Chapter 14). The National Spinal Cord Injury Hotline can also help. See Resources.

SPINAL CORD INJURIES: SOME STATISTICS

The purpose of the Spinal Cord Injury Statistical Center at the University of Alabama-Birmingham has these objectives (Young 1978: 9–12):

- To acquire sufficient data and develop information that will lead to the upgrading of the quality and availability of health care for the spinal cord injured.
- To help define the most cost-effective method of supplying this care.
- To direct ongoing study to supplying answers to questions pertaining to the care and treatment of spinal cord injured persons. Many of those questions are epidemiological in nature, relating not only to the injury but also to the disability created by the injury.
- To discover specifically what type of person gets hurt? What is the etiology of injury? What is the specific nature of injuries? What associated injuries do they have? Are there psychological and social components associated with the etiology of the accident?

The following information is based on accumulated data from 1973 through 1985. *Spinal Cord Injury, The Facts and Figures* (Stover and Fine 1986) represents the long-awaited answers to earlier questions summarized in Table 1–1. Data characterizing the SCI population document (Stover and Fine 1986: ix):

- The systems' continually increasing national capture rate

- Reduced time between injury and admission to the system
- Reduced lengths of stay
- Cost-containment efforts
- Reduced complication rates
- Reduced mortality statistics
- Changes in extensiveness of neurologic involvement patterns
- Changes in domestic and vocational patterns following SCI

SCI occurs predominately in the young male population (82% male versus 18% female); 57% of the victims possess at least a high school education; and most of them were either working (59.9%) or were full-time students (19.7%)

TABLE 1–1   SCI Research Issues

Nature of Disability

We need information pertaining to the nature of the disability in its broadest sense: medical, psychological, and social. We must be interested not only in what happens to the individual but also to family members.

We need to know what compounds the disability. What is contributed by the attitudes of the family and friends, the attitudes of society and such things as architectural barriers limiting function of the spinal cord injured person in the environment?

We are also interested in negative motivational factors compounding disability. Included in these are the effects of benefits and awards given to handicapped persons that may tend to perpetuate their disability.

Health Service Delivery

Of paramount interest to the project is the identification of present methods for delivery of health services to the spinal cord injured. What services are given? What is the time sequence of delivery? What is the pattern of delivery? Is it a systematized approach? Lastly, what is the Optimal System?

Medical Care

We will investigate ongoing spinal cord injury medical care. What recurrent medical complications do spinal cord injured people have? What is their life expectancy? What are the causes of death? In addition to the medical end product, we must define the social end product. How well do spinal cord injured people live? What should society expect from them and what should they expect and receive from society? What is the cost of medical treatment, rehabilitation, health maintenance, and loss of productivity? Last, to what extent can the cost of spinal cord injury be offset by containment of personal cost and productive employment?

Questions such as these require multivariate analysis and correlation for they represent the summated effects of many variables. As a consequence, large numbers of cases are required to produce meaningful information.

Young 1978:8

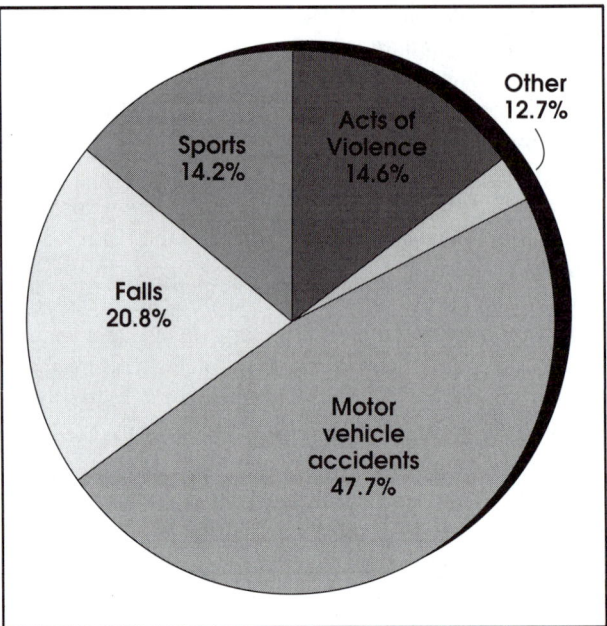

FIGURE 1–1   Distribution of SCI by etiology (Stover and Fine 1986: 15).

at the moment of injury. The highest incidence of SCI occurs in July, the lowest in January and February.

As shown in Figure 1–1, motor vehicle accidents account for most of the injuries (47.7%) followed by falls (20.8%), acts of violence (14.6%) and sports (14.2%) Causes vary in different groups depending on such characteristics as age of onset, sex, and racial or ethnic background. For example, motor vehicle accidents and sports injuries had a high occurrence in the 15- to 30-year-old group, whereas older people (over 60) were more likely to be injured by falls, a trend on the increase as this segment of the population increases.

Violence is on the increase, dramatically so in the 16- to 30-year-old group. Overall, spinal cord injuries in the cervical vertebrae account for slightly more than one-half of all new injuries; thoracic vertebrae injuries account for more than one-third; and lumbar and sacral vertebrae injuries account for the remaining tenth. The same percentage of quadriplegia and paraplegia resulted from motor vehicle accidents. However, paraplegia occurs more with penetrating wounds (which are more likely to be received in the back than in the small area of the neck), and quadriplegia occurs more with sports injuries. Contact sports and diving accidents are the main sports causes of quadriplegia, accounting for approximately 10% of all injuries. See Chapter 3 for more information about the factors contributing to and the prevention of injury.

The causes of injury in different racial or ethnic groups vary, and among given communities there are likely to be differences in etiology of injury. Although most spinal cord injured people are white, the incidence rate is somewhat higher among nonwhites. Among whites the leading cause of injury is the motor vehicle accident, whereas violence is more prevalent in nonwhite groups. Green notes that there is a 1 in 12 risk of dying of a handgun wound for the black urban male under age 40 (Green et al. 1987). This contrasts with the Canadian experience, where sports and work injuries are more likely causes of injury than acts of violence (Boyd and Schweigel 1985; Tator and Edmonds 1986). Gun control in Canada probably accounts for some of these differences. SCI primarily affects young adults 16 to 30 years old. See Figure 1–2. Trieschmann (1980) notes that it is a low-incidence but high-cost disability that makes tremendous changes in a person's life-style.

People with spinal cord injuries who were admitted immediately postinjury to specialized centers usually spend 3 to 5 months for initial treatment and rehabilitation. Ironically, as the trend toward shorter hospital stays increases, costs continue to escalate.

The combination of early onset of severe disability coupled with achievements in health sciences that allow almost a full life expectancy yields a catastrophe in terms of human disability and social economics. A realistic estimate of expenses for lifetime care may well exceed $1 million for each person (McKnew pers. com. 1991). The economic consequences of injury are staggering; hidden costs and lost potential are explored by Mackenzie (1990); and methods to predict the costs for an individual's lifetime are skillfully presented by Bush (1990). Stripling (1991) conducted a nationwide probability sample of economic costs for the entire SCI population, but some of the aggregate costs have been seriously questioned.

In the past, lifelong institutional care was common; today, more than 90% of persons return home. When this does not occur, medical complications, inability of families to cope, or lack of personal or financial resources, rather than the severity of injury, seem to be the deciding factors.

Because of the youthful age of this population, most people are single when injured. It is difficult to predict marital opportunities, but SCI reduces the statistical chance of marriage and increases the chance of divorce (78% were still married at the end of a 5-year period, compared with 89% for the general population). Marital problems peak at the second and third year postinjury (Stover and Fine 1986).

The opportunity to work is a great concern for the majority of disabled people. Five years postinjury, employment rates ranged from 27.6% for people with incomplete paraplegia down to 13.6% for people with complete quadriplegia. The labor shortage predicted for this decade and the passage of the Americans with Disabilities Act (see Chapter 8) may provide mainstreaming opportunities for all physically disabled persons, including people with SCI. Vocational and financial uncertainty unfairly plague many people with spinal cord injuries and their families. How-

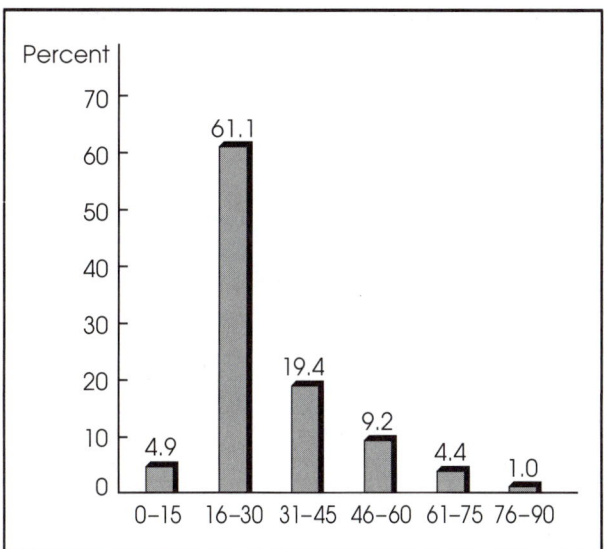

FIGURE 1–2 Age at injury (1986). Average mean age is 29.7 years and the most frequently occuring age at injury (mode) is 19 years (Stover and Fine 1986: 14).

ever, as Justin Dart, chairman of the President's Committee on Employment of People with Disabilities, cautions, "We must not assume that equality will occur automatically. . . . We must create attitudes and environments that will enable all people with disabilities to be fully equal and fully productive not only in law, but also in everyday life" (National Association of Rehabilitation Facilities [NARF] 1990: 1).

Disability management in the workplace is becoming more widespread. Efforts to improve employment rates of people with disabling injuries in Australia are particularly worth noting. In 1988, the Australian federal government established Comcare, an integrated prevention, rehabilitation, and compensation approach that helps people with disabilities return to work. Comcare's approach seeks to prevent illness and injury at work. It provides incentives to employers to improve occupational health and safety, rehabilitation programs to speed up return to work, and a new package of compensation benefits. An accompanying box in this chapter gives further information.

Employers in the United States and Canada are also becoming more involved in improving opportunities for disabled workers. Chapter 3 discusses this as well as employee associations' responsibilities to their members.

The predominantly young, typically male spinal cord injured population is at critical juncture in planning for adult life. Analysis of statistics helps direct efforts in prevention, health care planning, reducing complications, educational/vocational capacity, and, ultimately, community integration. Comparison of specialized versus nonspecialized care underlines the significant benefits of the former and encourages the extension of specialized services for *all*, instead of the few.

An Integrated Approach to Prevention, Rehabilitation, Compensation: The Comcare Plan in Australia

Who Is Covered:

525,000 federal employees in 160 departments, including Australian Airlines, federal police, defense forces, Australian National Railways, and all government departments and agencies.

What Comcare Provides:

Workplace-based illness and injury prevention programs, incentives to employers to improve occupational health and safety, employer-coordinated rehabilitation programs, and adequate compensation.

Prevention

The 1988 Act mandated that Comcare cooperate with other organizations to reduce the number of injuries to employees, conduct and promote research on injury prevention, and disseminate information on occupational health and safety trends.

As part of its prevention strategy, Comcare identifies risk areas by examining compensation claims. Health and safety committees in each state also report on causes of injuries. These efforts have already resulted in changes to workplaces.

Rehabilitation

Comcare's responsibilities: Comcare trains the case managers and monitors all case management plans for the first 12 months. It also approves accredited rehabilitation service providers and monitors them to ensure that they achieve, do not overservice, and comply with Comcare standards. Service providers are on 12-month contracts. Employees may appeal to Comcare for reconsideration of a plan's content if disagreement arises, and may thereafter resort to external appeal mechanisms. Comcare also assists in the difficult job of redeployment between agencies. Its return-to-work policy priorities are:

1. Same job, same workplace
2. Modified job, same workplace
3. Different job, same workplace
4. Modified job, new workplace
5. Different job, new workplace

Employer responsibilities:

- Submit a *rehabilitation policy and procedure statement* to Comcare. Unions and staff associations can consult in the development and implementation of their agencies' statement.

- Develop a *rehabilitation program* when an injured worker has missed 28 days of work. The employer is the best one to coordinate rehabilitation because:
  - Knows the employee and the workplace
  - Can assess the reasons for accidents and quickly implement remedies
  - Knows what retraining and redeployment are possible
  - Knows the work history and job skills of the injured worker
  - Wants to keep compensation costs to a minimum

- Appoint a *case manager* from the workplace to:
  - Develop a *case management plan*, essentially a return-to-work program designed by the case manager and an appropriate rehabilitation service provider. The plan lists objectives of actions necessary to achieve the goal, who implements the actions (medical practitioner, therapist, etc.), time frame, cost, and who is responsible. The plan and the employee's rights are explained to the employee. Employee and case manager both sign so that everyone knows exactly what should happen when, especially the return-to-work date. The plan is reviewed quarterly or as necessary, and also if the estimated costs increase by more than 10%.
  - Contact an injured employee's doctors, surgeons, physical and occupational therapists, and other care givers as necessary.
  - Coordinate workplace supervisors, other workers, and unions.
  - Develop a relationship with the injured employee.
  - If a return to work is not possible, find the best possible social outcome for the injured employee and family.

Premiums are based on the agency's size, risk profile, cost of salaries, and duration and number of past claims. Premiums average 2.8% of the cost of wages and include Comcare's administrative costs. Premiums are adjusted annually to reflect an employer's safety record and performance, thus providing incentive to improve workplace safety and to implement effective rehabilitation and redeployment programs.

(Box continues)

An Integrated Approach to Prevention, Rehabilitation, Compensation:
The Comcare Plan in Australia   (continued)

Compensation Benefits

Benefits are related to income rather than based on a flat statutory rate. Payment for the initial period of incapacity is up to 45 weeks on normal weekly earnings (NWE). After 45 weeks, 75% of NWE is payable if the injured person cannot return to work. This is subject to a minimum and maximum rate payable. Persons who return to work are paid as follows:

- Hours worked are 25% or less of normal hours: 80% of NWE.
- Hours worked are more than 25% but less than 50% of normal hours: 85% of NWE.
- Hours worked are more than 75% but less than 100% of normal hours: 95% of NWE.
- Hours worked are 100% of normal hours: 100% NWE. This is particularly applicable when the person returns to a lower-paying job than the one previously held.

No-fault lump sums (in addition to weekly benefits) may be for *permanent impairment* (of more than 10% of whole person) up to A$86,160 and *pain and suffering* (noneconomic loss) up to A$32,310. An injured employee may alternatively go to court to pursue payment for permanent impairment and/or pain and suffering up to a maximum of A$110,000.

Household and attendant care services are covered up to A$215.40 per week each for attendant care and for 50% of household costs.

Results

Comcare has established a data bank that provides a national picture for monitoring and developing programs. In this program, significantly more people have returned to work, the average length of time off work decreased, and the injury rate dramatically declined.

Jean Sherrell
State Manager, Queensland
Comcare
Brisbane,
Australia

A PHILOSOPHICAL APPROACH TO CARING FOR PEOPLE WITH SPINAL CORD INJURIES

In 1975 the United Nations Assembly published a *Declaration on the Rights of Disabled Persons* that calls for national and international action to protect the human rights of disabled people. The following rights are particularly relevant to the care of people with SCI and serve as the basis for a theoretical approach to care.

- The term *disabled person* means any person unable to ensure by himself or herself, wholly or partly, the necessities of a normal individual and/or social life, as a result of a deficiency, either congenital or not, in his or her physical or mental capabilities.
- Disabled persons shall enjoy all the rights set forth in this Declaration. These rights shall be granted to all disabled persons without any exception whatsoever and without distinction or discrimination on the basis of race, color, sex, language, religion, political or other opinions, national or social origin, state of wealth, birth, or any other situation applying either to the disabled person himself or herself or to his or her family.

- Disabled persons have the inherent right to respect for their human dignity. Disabled persons, whatever the origin, nature, and seriousness of their handicaps and disabilities, have the same fundamental rights as their fellow citizens of the same age, which implies first and foremost the right to enjoy a decent life, as normal and full as possible.
- Disabled persons are entitled to the measures designed to enable them to become as self-reliant as possible.
- Disabled persons have the right to medical, psychological, and functional treatment, including prosthetic and orthotic appliances, to medical and social rehabilitation, education, vocational training and rehabilitation, aid, counseling, placement services, and other services which will enable them to develop their capabilities and skills to the maximum and will hasten the process of their social integration or reintegration.
- Organizations of disabled persons may be usefully consulted in all matters regarding the rights of disabled persons.
- Disabled persons, their families, and communities shall be fully informed, by all appropriate means, of the rights contained in this Declaration. [United Nations 1975: n.p.]

Individuals must adapt to disability as total people. Health care professionals can facilitate this process by recognizing that all human needs are interwoven and that

TABLE 1–2 Correlating Philosophy with Goals of Care for Spinal Cord Injured Patients

Philosophy	Goals	Role Emphasized
1. Patients suffering from SCI are entitled to receive optimum care to meet their complex clinical, psychosocial, and economic needs.	To provide or secure the best health care possible for patients suffering from SCI	Practitioner/advocate
2. Patients should be assisted to achieve and maintain an optimal level of physical and mental health and retain a sense of spiritual and social well-being.	To ensure that patients are cared for with respect as individuals and to help them reestablish their autonomy	Partner/counselor/educator
3. Families (or significant others) constitute an integral part of patients' lives and should be included in comprehensive health care for spinal cord injured patients.	To provide psychosocial support to families and include them in assessing and meeting patients' rehabilitative needs	Partner/counselor/educator
4. Nurses should develop expertise to apply a problem-solving process of assessment and diagnosis, goal setting, implementation, and evaluation skillfully and systematically to ensure individualized total patient care.	To promote physical and psychological well-being by minimizing risk factors, practicing preventive measures when possible, recognizing onset of complications early, initiating immediate action, within the scope of nursing practice and policies, and evaluating care given	Practitioner/partner
5. Patient and family health education is an integral part of rehabilitation and must begin the moment of injury. Provision of an environment in which patients, families, and nurses can use their education, judgment, and individuality (creativity) is most conducive to a successful rehabilitation experience.	To provide a teaching/learning rehabilitation experience that actively involves patients (and families when appropriate) as participants and resource persons in the decision-making process, through which they can experience personal growth and independence	Partner/educator
6. Acute and concurrent rehabilitative care requires a skilled, well-integrated, interdisciplinary team.	To devise collaborative goals and provide coordinated care in a helpful, tolerable sequence for patients and families	Collaborator/coordinator
7. Nurses should coordinate and secure continuity of health care to facilitate transition (relocation) periods, especially on return to the community.	To determine patients' readiness for discharge and to initiate appropriate continuing health services	Coordinator/practitioner
8. Nurses should take responsibility for assessing and improving personal knowledge, attitude, and skills and should maintain awareness of current developments in the health care field.	To plan and participate in ongoing educational activities on a regular basis	Practitioner/advocate
9. Nurses must join forces with disabled people fighting to live independently in the community.	To participate in overcoming barriers—personal, social, financial—and obtain access to quality health care	Facilitator/supporter/advocate

people fulfill their needs in highly individual ways (Mahoney 1979). To attain the goals of rehabilitation, health care professionals must fulfill multifaceted roles. Providing or securing optimal health care not only challenges our roles as expert practitioners, but also as coordinators, counselors, educators, advocates, and most of all, partners. Frequently this involves the defense of the rights of the disabled person: always it requires seeing things from the patient's point of view, which further enhances personal and professional growth and development.

Philosophical beliefs are correlated with nursing practice and roles in Table 1–2. The interdisciplinary team approach empowers and expands the nurse's role: nursing is accountable 24 hours per day for coordinating the rehabilitation program. Collaboration ensures that the physical, social, vocational, spiritual, psychological, and economic needs of individuals are addressed (American Spinal Injury Association [ASIA] 1985).

Many factors affect the quality of care delivered, not the least of which are the personal attributes of each profes-

What Is Rehabilitation Nursing?

I came into SCI nursing through the back door. I began my professional life as a teacher and coach and never planned to become a nurse. However, I had kept a poster for several years that shows a little girl. The caption in her handwriting reads, "When I grow up I want to be a nurse." In retrospect, I now feel that my varied experiences enabled me to grow enough to become a nurse. Rehabilitation nursing is much more than technical or medical knowledge.

My introduction to rehabilitation was as a recreation therapist (RT). I was choreographing a local opera in Birmingham, AL, when the costume mistress told of a job opening at Lakeshore Rehabilitation Hospital for a RT. I went for an interview and much to my surprise (and later, concern), I was hired. The RT job required taking young, male spinal cord injured patients into the community for reentry training. I felt increasingly distressed as the first day of work approached—I had never worked with a disabled person nor had I ever known someone with SCI.

For the first 3 weeks I feared saying or doing something offensive. I didn't know a wheelchair from a leg bag! I tried to be everywhere and do everything for everyone. Fortunately, however, I discovered three important things:

1. I had a great group of clients who taught me everything I needed to know.
2. My clients were handicapped not by their physical disabilities, but by my trying to do everything for them.
3. Most important, there is no difference between teaching nondisabled and disabled persons. Rehabilitation is merely teaching a different method of doing things. As my education continued in the capable hands of my clients, I soon forgot they were in wheelchairs.

I became director of the recreation department after 6 months and began developing a wheelchair sports program. I knew nothing about wheelchair sports, but I did know that people with new spinal cord injuries need something to challenge them. I had seen this work with able-bodied students in search of self-discipline, self-respect, and their own success.

Unable to find any books, articles, or suggested workout schedules for disabled athletes I turned to books on regular workouts. During the first year of competitions, my team of four people with quadriplegia and four people with paraplegia did quite well. We developed their technique together by common sense and by applying common principles of *athletic* training to wheelchair sports.

We soon realized that the men with quadriplegia would have to become more independent in their daily living skills and transfers if we were to get everyone on the track (or road) in time to race. It is amazing how a person who cannot transfer suddenly learns when it means going from an everyday wheelchair to a racer.

Because of my nonmedical background, I didn't know what was *supposedly* impossible. I assumed that a person could find a way to do almost anything if the desire and commitment are there. Imagine my surprise when, 5 years later in nursing school, I was told that patients with quadriplegia at the C_{5-6} level could not dress, drive, and certainly not catheterize themselves or hope to live independently. I had already traveled to Hawaii and all over the United States with independently functioning guys with quadriplegia. I have now worked 5 years as an RN with spinal cord injured people. Although attitudes regarding the potential for independence have improved in many centers, I still often hear these same kinds of limiting statements.

As nurses, we wish to help and nurture, but we are vulnerable to pitying our patients. We often become frustrated and angry when our patients do not do what we know is best. We label them noncompliant, troublemakers, and manipulators. However, manipulators cannot manipulate unless someone lets them. Noncompliance may mean, "I've tried that way and it doesn't work for me." We must allow our students to make choices and also to accept the responsibility for those choices.

Nurses should think of themselves as *partners*. After spinal cord injured *patients* are medically stable and no longer ill, they become *clients*, individuals who must learn to live in a different way. Medical professionals themselves must experience the *real world* by venturing from the hospital into the field so that their teaching will truly prepare clients for living in the world. Some of our sacred cows must be sacrificed. For instance, a Foley catheter might be recommended if it would allow a person to live independently. I know of a 19-year-old who was independent in all skills except catheterization. He lived in a nursing home! Medical

(Box continues)

sional. Caring for patients with severe physical disability demands interest, dedication, and an openness to develop a positive attitude toward severe physical disability. The work is both physically and mentally difficult, but the rewards are great: it is not depressing work as many people tend to think. Desirable qualities in any team member include: sound professional judgment, knowledge, and skills; ability to work enthusiastically and relate continually with other team members in a variety of situations in a close setting; willingness to learn from and to teach others; endless patience for exacting work; and a good sense of humor! Working together is explored further in Chapter 13.

As advanced prehospital and critical care save people with increasing degrees of disability, the demands on the health care profession escalate. The challenge is to share expertise as practitioners, researchers, change agents, educators, and partners. Professionals have a responsibility at personal, local, national, and international levels to defend the rights of disabled people and help secure the resources they need to fulfill their potential.

THE PROCESS OF GOAL-ORIENTED REHABILITATIVE CARE

Goal-oriented rehabilitative care requires skillful problem-solving. This continuous educational process involves the interrelated steps of assessment and diagnosis, goal setting, implementation, and evaluation. Throughout this section, the nursing profession is used as an example, but this approach is fundamental for all health care professionals and is emphasized throughout this book.

Despite theories and conceptual frameworks, certain themes are common to the evolving profession of nursing (Kozier and Erb 1991: 5). Nursing is:

- Caring for and about people
- Adapted to individual needs
- Taking a holistic view of the person when planning care

- Teaching
- Involved in health and illness with individuals, families, and the community
- Involved with health promotion, health maintenance, health restoration, and care of the dying
- Critical thinking

Assessment and Diagnosis

A major premise of this book is that *many complications are entirely preventable or can be minimized if recognized early*. Therefore, comprehensive *assessment* is the cornerstone on which to plan, implement, and evaluate care. Assessment can directly enhance or limit the quality of total patient care. It focuses on the patient's current clinical status and on collected background information.

Data pertaining to physical and psychological health are obtained from numerous sources: direct patient observation and contact; the medical record; diagnostic tests; monitoring devices; communication with other health team members; and consultation with significant people in the patient's life. The patient's *health history* is of vital importance. Factors such as associated injury and preexisting health and illness (both from a physical and a psychological viewpoint) profoundly influence how and to what extent each individual experiences the effects of SCI.

Diagnosis outlines the patient's (and family's) actual and potential health problems (Kozier and Erb 1991: 5).

Goal Setting and Implementation

Planning and implementing goal-oriented care is a progressive, step-by-step process. For example, in rehabilitation staff must lead patients to take responsibility for managing the effects of their disabilities and maintaining optimal health. Patients must participate in personal care, initially as informed observers and gradually as active performers.

Another major premise of this book is that *rehabilitation is a process that begins at the moment of injury*. Health care objectives, from an interdisciplinary perspective, are presented in each chapter to facilitate care planning.

Evaluation

Evaluation is necessary to determine the effectiveness of all the previous steps. Evaluation also is a continuous process, not a final step. Such continuous evaluation ensures flexibility and gives direction to care planning. To facilitate evaluation, chapters on physiological function describe ideal outcome criteria that can be expected following SCI.

LIFE AFTER
REHABILITATION ——————————

Fully achieving rehabilitation goals demands more than average commitment. When people with disabilities join forces with health care professionals, policy makers, and other interest groups, progress toward these goals can build momentum that enables people with SCI to sustain throughout their lives the level of functioning achieved during rehabilitation (Public Service Information International 1983). Such dynamic interaction requires sensitivity and courage. The course is uncharted, and professionals must become comfortable in a world where people living with disabilities are the true experts.

The physical prognosis for a person with SCI depends on the level and completeness of injury (Chapter 4). However, the ability to live independently has less to do with the actual physical outcome of injury than with personal attitudes. Architectural, educational, vocational, economic, and social barriers exist, reflecting society's low expectations for people with disabilities. Nevertheless, despite these barriers and their own disabling conditions, many people not only have overcome—or at least dealt with—these obstacles successfully, but also have established organizations that assist others in achieving and maintaining an independent life-style (ILRU 1991). Chapter 30 explores the independent living concept in detail.

Rehabilitation professionals all too often hear from former patients, "We were never truly prepared for the real world." This type of feedback would be less frequent if the disabled community were involved in sharing its substantial survival expertise. This community has been a largely untapped resource for rehabilitation program development, although this situation is changing. An example of health care professionals and independent living specialists working together with spinal cord injured people is *Hospital to Community: A Collaborative Program for Independent Living and Medical Rehabilitation* (University of Michigan 1989). This effort on the part of the University of Michigan, Department of Physical Education and Rehabilitation, and the Ann Arbor Center for Independent Living, is designed for both consumers and professionals from many disciplines. The program manual reflects the independent living paradigm as well as the medical rehabilitation paradigm.

The program can be completed during 8 weeks in a comprehensive rehabilitation setting and complements established traditional programs.

The key concepts combining independent living and personal skills development address mobility, transportation, communication, self-determination, adjustment to disability, recreation and leisure, problem-solving skills, advocacy, rights and benefits, personal care assistance, housing options, technology, vocational options, and employment.

A national crisis exists regarding these and other issues. The lack of comprehensive health care and related services to meet the needs of the disabled population in the community is overwhelming. Recognizing the impact of this crisis on the daily lives of disabled people, the Robert Wood Johnson Foundation has established an $8.4 million grant program, Improving Service Systems for People with Disabilities. Its aim is to strengthen community-based resources that are run for and by people with disabilities. This program should produce several viable approaches that can be replicated throughout the country. It emphasizes financial diversification strategies to overcome episodic public and charitable financing.

To bring about communitywide changes that improve opportunities for independent living, grantees must

1. Identify unmet needs.
2. Help coordinate and integrate existing and new services into supportive systems.
3. Coordinate, integrate, and create payment systems.
4. Increase the numbers of people with disabilities who have access to and use health and support services, and their financing systems.

Grantees work together with health care professionals to develop these informational and educational strategies.

As Corcoran (1984) stresses, although acute care is the high priority in health care today, the price of surviving SCI is permanent disability that requires ongoing services. Corcoran urges an examination of the effects of medical progress and health policy changes on *independence*, rather than on survival rates from trauma. When "power failures, strikes, and natural disasters periodically remind us how pervasive our dependence is on human and mechanical assistance," we may then view *independence*, for both disabled and nondisabled as "having access to, and utilizing the necessary mechanical devices and human helpers to perform ordinary mobility, communication, and daily living activities" (Corcoran 1984: 6). When we can all accept this, independent living for people with disabilities will have a better chance of becoming a widespread reality.

In addition, better education of health professionals responsible for providing continuing care is needed to prevent secondary disabilities associated with SCI and to care for primary health problems unrelated to the disability. The effects of aging, thought to be accelerated with SCI, must also be considered. See Chapter 33. Reliable access to quality health care is essential for maintaining a healthy and independent life-style.

"To those of us who are researchers or academicians, application of the concept of independence to people with disabilities is intellectually stimulating and challenging. To those of us who are practitioners in the field of rehabilitation or in other areas of human service, the idea of independent living by people with disabilities is imaginative and promising. Finally, to those of us who are disabled, independence is a goal that we believe is justifiable and worth making great sacrifices to achieve" (Frieden 1984: n.p.).

REFERENCES

American Spinal Injury Association. 1985. *Spinal Cord Injury Nursing: A Task Force Report*. Atlanta: Author.

Boyd, M. C., and Schweigel, J. F. 1985. Diving-related spinal injuries in British Columbia. *British Columbia Medical Journal* 27 (6): 391–394.

Bush, G. 1990. Calculating the cost for long term living: A four-step process. *The Journal of Head Trauma Rehabilitation* 5 (1).

Corcoran, P. J. 1984. *The Health Care Dilemma*. Research and Training Center on Independent Living (RTC/IL), Monographs on Independent Living. Lawrence, KA: University of Kansas.

Frieden, L. 1984 Introduction. In P. J. Corcoran. *The Health Care Dilemma*. RTC/IL Monographs on Independent Living. Lawrence, KA: University of Kansas.

Green, B. A., Eismont, F. J., O'Heir, J. T. 1987. Spinal cord injury—A systems approach: Prevention, emergency medical services, and emergency room management. *Critical Care Clinics* 3: 471–493.

Guttman, L. 1976. *Spinal Cord Injuries Comprehensive Management and Research*. 2d ed. London: Blackwell Scientific Publications. *A classic, multifaceted reference text on spinal cord injuries. Includes historical background information; general statistics; legal aspects; detailed anatomy and neuropathology of cord trauma and resulting effects on all body systems; regeneration; fractures and dislocations, gunshot injuries and stab wounds; and neurophysiological and clinical management aspects. Extensive bibliography.*

Humphreys, R. R. 1978. Role of Rehabilitation Services Administration in the Improvement of Spinal Cord Injury Services. *Proceedings of the National Spinal Cord Injury Model Systems Conference*, Phoenix, AZ: April, pp. 3–5. *Overview of federal government concerns.*

ILRU (Independent Living Research Utilization). 1991. Brochure. ILRU. Texas Institute for Rehabilitation and Research.

Kozier, B., and Erb, G. 1991. *Fundamentals of Nursing Concepts and Procedures*. 4th ed. Menlo Park, CA: Addison-Wesley. *An excellent text, contemporary in approach and content, with emphasis on increasing responsibility, accountability, and autonomy of nurses. Offers indepth and updated review material for nurses. Explains expanded roles of nurses in a wide variety of settings.*

Langer, Ellen. 1989. *Mindfulness*. Reading, MA: Addison–Wesley.

Mackenzie, E. 1990. *The Cost of Injury: A Report To Congress*. Baltimore, MD: Johns Hopkins Research and Development Center.

McKnew, L. 1991. Personal communication to author.

Mahoney, K. E. 1979. A philosophical approach to nursing education. In *Current Perspectives in Rehabilitation Nursing*, Eds. R. Murray and J. L. Kijeck. St. Louis: C. V. Mosby, pp. 27–31. *Presents philosophical principles of rehabilitation, to help meet the ever-changing needs in society and thus in health care.*

Matlack, D. R. 1974. *Cost-effectiveness of Spinal Cord Injury Center Treatment*. Chicago, IL: National Spinal Cord Injury Foundation. *Careful and specific documentation of financial savings to society when comprehensive and system care programs are made available. Cost savings analysis presented to stimulate expansion of other spinal cord systems throughout the United States. Highly recommended.*

National Association of Rehabilitation Facilities. 1990. Americans with Disabilities Act (ADA). *Rehabilitation Review* 7 (31).

National Spinal Cord Injury Foundation. What is spinal cord injury? And what can we do about it? 1981. Chicago, IL. *National Spinal Cord Injury Foundation Convention Journal. Defines spinal cord injury and goals of the foundation. Includes implications for both health professionals and the general public.*

Public Services Information International. 1983. *Rehab Brief* 6 (3). *Bringing research into effective focus.*

Schweigel, J., and Peerless, S. 1971. A proposal for a spinal cord injury unit at Shaughnessy Hospital. Preliminary research review for Canadian Paraplegic Association, Vancouver, BC. *Summary of historical developments and current local developments to stimulate development of specialized services.*

Stover, S. L., and Fine, P. 1986. *Spinal Cord Injury: The Facts and Figures*. Birmingham, AL: National Spinal Cord Injury Research Data Center, University of Alabama.

Stripling, T. 1991. *Economic Costs of Traumatic Spinal Cord Injury* (Health Studies and Analyses). Washington, DC: Paralyzed Veterans of America (PVA).

Tator, C. H., and Edmonds, V. E. 1986. Sports and recreation are a rising cause of spinal cord injury. *The Physician and Sports Medicine* 14 (5): 157–167.

Trieschmann, R. 1980. *Spinal Cord Injuries, Psychological, Social and Vocational Adjustment*. New York: Pergamon Press. *Only existing work exclusively devoted to the psychosocial impact of spinal cord injuries on both disabled people and their families. Includes an exhaustive critique of the literature with a view to dispelling myths and stimulating research.*

United Nations. 1975. *Declaration on the Rights of Disabled Persons*, n.p.

University of Michigan. 1989. *Hospital to Community: A Collaborative Program for Independent Living and Medical Rehabilitation*. Ann Arbor: Author.

Young, J. S. 1978. National Spinal Cord Injury Data Research Center. *Proceedings of the National Spinal Cord Injury Model Systems Conference*, Phoenix, AZ: April, pp. 9–12. *Statement of objectives and services.*

Young, J. S., and Northrup, N. E. 1979. *Statistical Information Pertaining to Some of the Most Commonly Asked Questions About Spinal Cord Injury.* National Spinal Cord Injury Data Research Center, Phoenix, AZ. *Data collected from 1973 through 1978. Analyzes etiology, hospitalization time and costs, and some postdischarge factors. Ready reference in question/answer format, for example, what is the life expectancy of persons with spinal cord injury? Subheadings include demography, etiology, length of hospital stay, cost of hospitalization, use of ongoing services, social and vocational achievements, and life expectancy.*

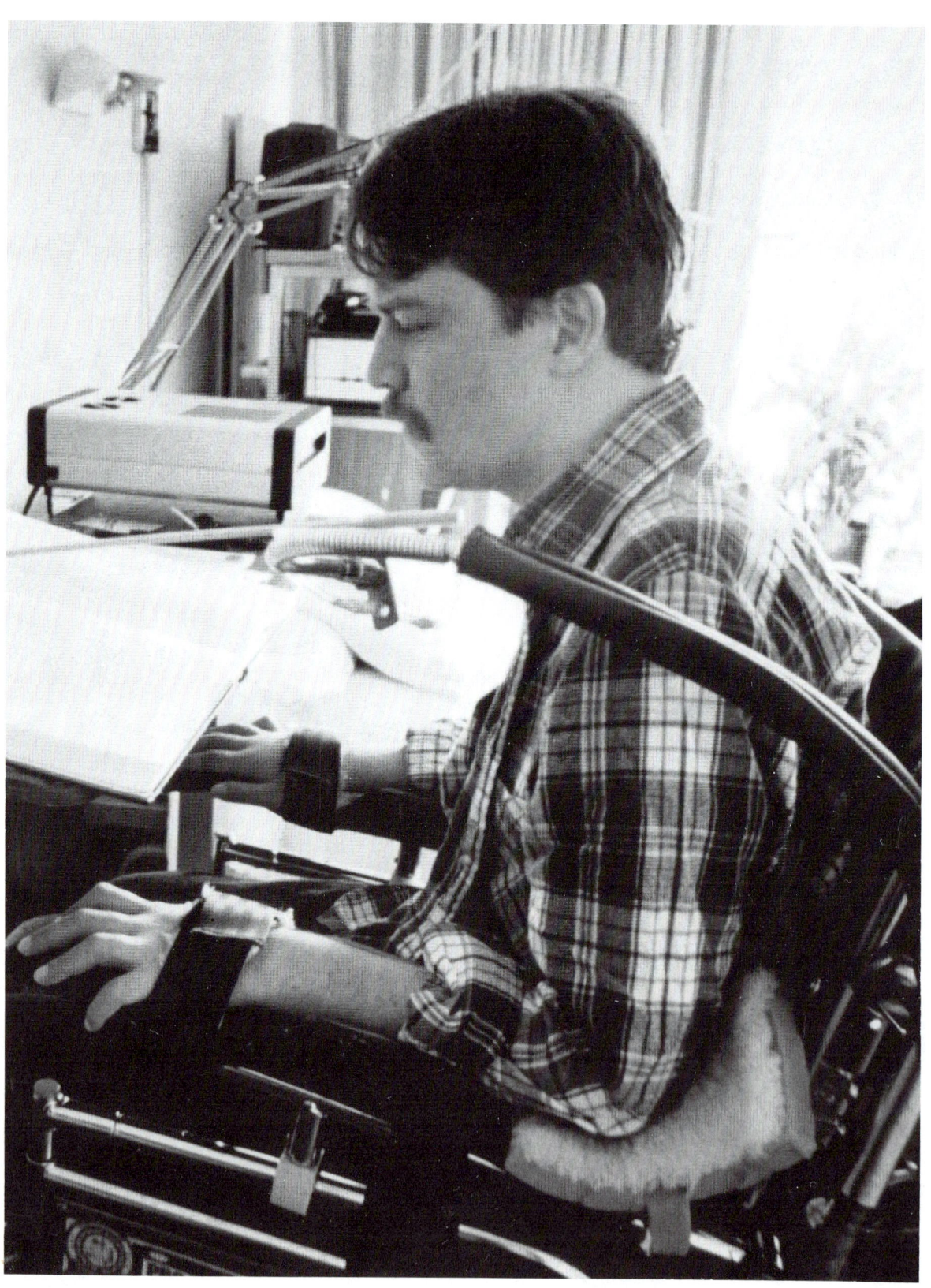

CHAPTER
— 2 —

Toward a Health Services Research Capacity in Spinal Cord Injury

Gerben DeJong, Ph.D., and Andrew I. Batavia, J.D., M.S.

Chapter Outline

Objectives

- To define health services research
- To be aware of current health services research in SCI
- To become involved in removing long-term disability-related barriers and in securing lifelong quality health care services for persons with disabilities
- To suggest strategies to stimulate research and development of services for postrehabilitation health care and personal assistance needs

From Gerben DeJong and Andrew I. Batavia. "Toward a Health Services Research Capacity in Spinal Cord Injury." *Paraplegia* (in press) by permission of Churchill Livingstone.

INTRODUCTION

Each year an estimated 8,000 individuals or more incur a traumatic spinal cord injury (SCI) in the United States alone. Almost 50% of these injuries result from motor vehicle accidents. The prevalence of persons with SCI in the United States—the number of persons with a physical disability resulting from SCI at any given time—is estimated at 700 to 800 per 1 million population.

These statistics convey the number of people who have sustained SCI in the United States, but they do not convey the challenges facing persons with SCI or the issues affecting these individuals and their families, providers, payers, and others. Substantial physiological, psychosocial, and environmental factors affect the spinal cord injured person's chances for long-term survival and prospects for living an independent and productive life. These factors require a broadened research agenda.

Because persons with SCI now are living longer than ever before, it is no longer sufficient to focus research primarily on health care provided to save their lives at the time of injury or to restore their functional capacity shortly after injury. We must develop a broad research capacity to evaluate not only trauma care and medical rehabilitation, but also the ongoing health care needs of spinal cord injured persons well after their rehabilitation. In other words, we need to develop a comprehensive health services research (HSR) capacity on SCI. Persons with SCI have a specific constellation of ongoing health problems that are not being addressed by the mainstream of the U.S. health care system, and that demand the attention of the HSR community.

This chapter focuses on health services research on SCI conducted in the United States—in particular, on building the capacity for conducting such research. Actually many of the problems highlighted in this chapter concern persons with SCI throughout the world, but because the United States currently has one of the most highly developed capacities for HSR, the issues presented here are probably even greater problems in other countries (see the Box on p. 21).

HEALTH SERVICES RESEARCH AND SPINAL CORD INJURY

Health services research seeks to examine systematically the organization, provision, and financing of health care services. This research draws on the skills of many disciplines and professions, such as biostatistics, health care economics, epidemiology, health care finance, health law, medicine and allied professions, political science, and medical sociology. Health services researchers commonly consider issues of cost, access, quality, and effectiveness of health care services (Flook and Sanazaro 1973).

At present, there is only a rudimentary HSR capacity in the area of spinal cord injury management and its related discipline of medical rehabilitation (Fuhrer 1988; DeJong, Batavia, and Griss 1989; Batavia and DeJong 1990). The research community in the SCI and medical rehabilitation fields is comprised largely of physicians, allied health professionals, and persons trained in the behavioral sciences such as psychology. Notably in short supply are SCI and rehabilitation researchers who are trained in HSR disciplines (DeJong, Batavia, and Griss 1989; Batavia and DeJong 1990).

Similarly, the HSR field has almost completely ignored the health care needs of persons with SCI and the field of medical rehabilitation. The HSR literature includes few articles that address the organization, provision, or financing of services for people with physical disabilities. Yet this literature has addressed the concerns of various other subpopulations with special needs, such as elderly people, indigent people, and people living in underserved geographic areas. The HSR community must now focus its efforts on the needs of people with such physical disabilities as SCI (DeJong, Batavia, and Griss 1989; Batavia and DeJong 1990).

The development of a HSR capacity in SCI is particularly timely: in the past two decades, the clinical management of SCI, the expectations of persons with SCI, and the financing and provision of health care services have changed markedly. These changes have nurtured creative new ideas on how to meet the needs of persons with SCI. Collectively these changes provide an important perspective on why a HSR capacity in spinal cord injury is long overdue.

Changes in the Clinical Management of Spinal Cord Injury

To understand the health care needs of persons with SCI today, it is valuable to have a historical perspective on the clinical management of SCI. Before the 1940s, the main issue in SCI management was mere survival. Persons who sustained a SCI often would survive the original trauma but would later die because of such secondary complications as urinary and respiratory tract infections that could not be arrested. When sulfa drugs were introduced in the late 1930s followed by penicillin, modern medicine dramatically improved the ability to control complications. The medical specialties of physical medicine and rehabilitation, established in the late 1940s, reduced the functional limitations of persons with physical disabilities and increased their capacities to live independently and productively.

However, even in the 1950s, most spinal cord injured rehabilitation patients were discharged to highly restrictive

SHARING EXPERTISE INTERNATIONALLY:
SETTING UP A SPINAL CORD INJURY REHABILITATION UNIT IN ARMENIA

During the earthquake that shook Armenia in 1988, 219 persons suffered spinal cord injuries. Because no rehabilitation facilities existed in Armenia or the Soviet Union for these victims, a spinal cord injury rehabilitation unit was established by an international team of specialists to treat them and to teach Armenian health professionals to become experts in spinal cord injury rehabilitation.

The patients arrived malnourished, with contractures, bladder and bowel complications, and horrendous pressure sores. All of these conditions, of course, resulted in moderate to severe degrees of sepsis. It was obvious that only the strong had survived, as the team saw only 45 spinal cord injury earthquake victims during the first 9 months of the project. An additional 22 acutely injured persons were admitted and hundreds of outpatients seen.

During the first 3 months, the team concentrated on caring for the general well-being of this very sick patient population. They relied heavily on family help to administer basic care. A family member was always with each patient and, even so, it took a full month for the nursing staff to earn the patients' and families' trust so that the families would sleep away from the patient's bedside. We recognized that these people had lost everything, and everyone lost family members. They were fighting hard not to lose anything or anyone else. Therefore, the obvious solution was to sell this community on the concepts of rehabilitation and independence and to involve them in the plan for care. This was difficult because disabled persons are rarely seen in public in the Soviet Union. They remain in the patient role and are cared for in the home by family members. Nothing in the community is wheelchair accessible.

One barrier to teaching SCI management and rehabilitation was acquiring Armenian personnel to do it. It was immediately obvious that trained nurses were not interested in becoming trainees in our program. Soviet nurses do not actually provide hands-on patient care—family members do—and the 2-year nurse-training program actually trains nurses to assist doctors, little more. However, with the help of the Minister of Health for Armenia, we acquired 20 trainee nurses from the medical college in Yerevan. This group of bright, 19-year-old women had never seen a naked male body,

let alone entertained thoughts of caring for one in such intimate detail. Teaching was a long and often frustrating process because of lack of basic knowledge and skills, and problems with interpretation and overcoming cultural differences. Yet whenever a concept was grasped or an idea took hold, our program took a giant step forward.

After the first 3 months, we made progress on rehabilitation. Teaching patients intermittent self-catheterization was smooth, but actually getting them to do it was a battle of wits. Soon, however, the patients were telling the team how to do it. Patients showed great expertise on the unit but, again, trying to get them to take an outing was a challenge. They were different and thought they would be isolated. But after the first few times, they were unequalled heroes in the community, and the team found it difficult to keep up with their excursions to sporting events and concerts. As the community saw what they could do, they recognized their capabilities.

When the patients were discharged, the team made home visits, helped acquire temporary housing for patients and their families, ran outpatient and follow-up clinics, and established a home visiting program. We initiated teaching local personnel in the smaller towns spinal cord injury management skills. We also recognized a great need for the care of the acutely injured and regularly visited acute care hospitals to follow such patients.

What began as a 6-month mission by the League of Red Cross and Red Crescent Societies to service the spinal cord injury victims of the Armenian earthquake evolved into a project of more than 2 years. The facility we established is the first of its kind in the Soviet Union. The international team was extremely proud to be a part of this history-making project, but history is really being made by the Armenian people themselves.

Sara John Taylor, R.N.
Acute SCI Unit
University Hospital
Shaughnessy Site
Vancouver, B.C., Canada

long-term care institutions that limited their opportunities for independent and productive lives. The development of specialized SCI centers within the U.S. Department of Veterans Affairs (VA) and of regional spinal cord injury systems within the civilian sector finally changed this dependency-producing outcome. These specialized systems produced a new cadre of professionals with clinical and research expertise that extended knowledge of the long-term consequences of SCI and brought a sharpened clinical focus to the ongoing needs of persons with SCI.

Changes in Expectations for People with Spinal Cord Injury

Perhaps more than any other factor, the independent living (IL) movement of the 1970s radically altered expectations about the opportunities available to persons with disabilities. This movement was initiated by disabled persons in the United States who sought to remove environmental barriers that reduced their capacity for self-direction, independence, and productivity (DeJong 1979). It gave persons with SCI (and persons with other disabilities) a vision of how they could direct their own lives. In so doing, the IL movement also reshaped the relationships between physician and patient and between rehabilitation professional and disabled consumer. Persons with SCI served notice that they wanted to direct and manage their health care on their own terms (DeJong 1981).

With respect to postrehabilitation health services delivery, persons with SCI have sought to manage their own primary health care connected to large medical centers. This has often proved difficult, however, because relatively few primary care providers are familiar with the health care needs of persons with physical disabilities. Many disabled veterans testify that they must rely on the expertise of a VA SCI service to meet their ongoing primary care needs because they cannot locate such expertise in their own communities. Likewise, many nonveterans seek out the expertise of rehabilitation hospital outpatient clinics because they have difficulty locating primary care providers who understand disability-related problems.

Changes in Health Care Finance and Delivery

During the past decade, the financing and delivery of American health care has also changed substantially. These changes fall into two categories: experimentation in the payment of health care services and new health care delivery systems. Experimental payment concepts include (Batavia 1988):

- *Capitation payment*, paying a health care provider a prespecified payment per patient for a set period of time (typically 1 year) to provide a comprehensive set of health care services, as needed, to the patient during that period.
- *Diagnostic related groups* (DRGs), payment groups in which patients are classified primarily on diagnosis. DRGs are the basis for payment of inpatient hospital care under the Medicare *prospective payment system* (PPS).
- *Preferred provider arrangements* (PPA), contracting relationships between payers and providers in which the provider agrees to accept discounted fees for its services and the payer agrees to provide incentives for its enrollees to use the preferred provider.

New health care delivery systems include *health maintenance organizations* (HMOs) that provide managed care financed with prepaid capitation payments, and *preferred provider organizations* (PPOs) that use preferred provider arrangements and conform to certain additional agreements with payers such as utilization review by payers (Batavia, DeJong, Burns, Smith, Melus, and Butler 1989). Many old assumptions about financing and delivering health care— for example, cost-based reimbursement systems—are clearly on the decline, and some providers have had to reposition themselves in a more competitive health care economy (Batavia 1988; Batavia 1989).

The past 10 years have clearly witnessed much innovation and experimentation in health care. The challenge for SCI is now: How can we take advantage of these changes to accommodate the health care needs and expectations of persons with SCI? We must evaluate how different models of health care delivery and financing meet the needs and expectations of persons with disabilities. Approaches that appear promising should be tested before new political and economic constraints begin to limit the options available to persons with SCI. The present holds historic opportunities not to be missed.

HEALTH SERVICES RESEARCH IN SPINAL CORD INJURY TODAY

Researchers have not yet been drawn in substantial numbers to HSR issues concerning persons with SCI or other physical disabilities. One reason for this neglect is that persons with physical disabilities have been a devalued population in our society. Until recently, they have not been considered worthy of serious research, but fortunately this negative attitude is changing, due in part to the successes of the IL movement (DeJong, Batavia, and Griss 1989).

To the extent that a HSR capacity in SCI exists, it is largely a result of data collected by the regional spinal cord injury systems and compiled in the National Spinal Cord

Injury Database. Health services researchers in SCI concentrated mainly on trauma care, posttrauma acute care, and rehabilitative care, which are discussed in the following sections.

The National Spinal Cord Injury Database

An integrated system of SCI management, beginning with trauma care, is essential to favorable outcomes. Discontinuities in care can severely compromise the road to medical stability and successful rehabilitation. Early prevention of medical complications, such as pressure sores and urinary tract infections, expedites the rehabilitation process and improves the disabled individual's prospects for returning to the community. This wisdom is the cornerstone of the regional spinal cord injury centers throughout the United States.

The regional SCI centers have long recognized that a good national data base is essential for conducting empirical research on SCI, and particularly for documenting the effectiveness of an integrated approach to SCI management. The *National SCI Database* is now located at the National SCI Statistical Center (NSCISC) in Birmingham, Alabama.

The National SCI Database has a mixed history. On the one hand, it has compiled a rich source of uniform data to serve the research needs of its affiliates. The resources of the Database may represent the nation's most advanced capacity for HSR in SCI. It has data on more than 10,000 individuals collected over a decade or more. Some individual records include longitudinal data spanning more than 10 years, which provide an excellent basis for methodologically sound empirical studies in HSR. The SCI research community, therefore, is very fortunate to have the resources of the National SCI Database.

On the other hand, the National SCI Database experienced limitations in its ability to service the information needs of the model systems and to support a broadened HSR agenda. Although the Database represents one of the best data bases in the field of medical rehabilitation today, its capacity has not been exploited fully for research purposes. We believe that the National SCI Database could support a fairly broad HSR agenda if it were not for two factors.

First and foremost, some of the participants in the National SCI Database system perceive their primary mission to be analyses that will strengthen the merits of the regional SCI systems approach. Although postrehabilitation data are acquired by the National SCI Database, these data are evaluated primarily in terms of how they reflect on the efficacy of the original trauma and rehabilitation interventions. Discontinuities in postrehabilitation health care that result in rehospitalizations receive some attention, but it is insufficient relative to the scope of the problem. Moreover,

such problems may be viewed by some of the participants as reflecting negatively on the regional systems approach, although the problems actually are widespread and are not specific to the model systems.

Second, participants in the National SCI Database have not adequately exploited the Database's potential for HSR research among third-party investigators. The Database needs to be made more accessible to investigators outside the model SCI system network. Of course, there would have to be safeguards for maintaining patient and institutional confidentiality.

Trauma and Posttrauma Acute Care Research

Newly injured persons enter the health care system through some form of trauma care, whether it be at a small rural hospital or at a highly triaged Level I trauma center in a large urban medical complex. In recent years, traumatology has emerged as a recognized discipline with a budding research capacity. Trauma researchers have developed a variety of tools for measuring the severity of an injury, such as the Injury Severity Score (Baker, O'Neill, Haddon, and Long 1974) and the Revised Trauma Score (Champion, Sacco, Carnazzo, Copes, and Fouty 1981). However, in evaluating the outcomes of trauma care, researchers seldom look beyond discharge from an acute care setting. Moreover, trauma researchers typically limit their outcome analysis simply to whether the patient lived or died.

Nevertheless, it is important to look beyond mere survival. Trauma researchers have yet to examine how trauma care affects residual disabilities and functional losses. Thus, the impact of trauma care should next be evaluated in terms of:

1. How advances in emergency medical management and trauma care are changing the chances of survival for a person with SCI for a given level of injury severity
2. How trauma care is affecting the degree of residual disability among survivors, especially among new survivors with high-level injuries (who earlier would have died)
3. How trauma care is altering the mix of patients with SCI seen by medical rehabilitation, such as the proportion of patients who require permanent use of a ventilator
4. How trauma care may be reshaping the postrehabilitation health care needs of selected survivors

To answer these kinds of questions, it is important that health services researchers in the field of rehabilitation collaborate with researchers in the field of trauma care. Each will benefit from the other's tools. For example, trauma researchers are largely unfamiliar with the functional status measures commonly used in rehabilitation research. Likewise, most rehabilitation researchers are unfamiliar with injury severity measures used in trauma research.

Medical Rehabilitation Research

Since the demise of polio in the 1950s, SCI has been the model disability in the field of medical rehabilitation. Only recently has SCI's preeminent role in medical rehabilitation been challenged by the compelling needs of persons with brain injury (DeJong and Batavia 1989). By serving as medical rehabilitation's benchmark disability, SCI has received a disproportionate amount of the resources available for rehabilitation research. As a result, the SCI research literature is perhaps the most extensive of any medical rehabilitation research.

Stated simply, research related to physical restoration and to psychosocial rehabilitation dominates the research literature in SCI rehabilitation. Thus, although much rehabilitation research has focused on SCI, relatively little of it has concerned HSR (Batavia 1988). These few efforts at HSR have been limited largely to issues of costs and cost-effectiveness. Their findings, however, have not been conclusive (Johnston and Keith 1983).

Many other HSR issues concerning the medical rehabilitation of persons with SCI, largely overlooked or simply unfunded (Fuhrer 1988), include access to rehabilitative care, the effects of payment mechanisms on rehabilitation utilization and outcome, the relative effectiveness of various outpatient modalities, and the impact of health maintenance education on subsequent health care use (Batavia 1988). A HSR capability in the medical rehabilitation phase of SCI requires the following:

1. A core group of researchers trained in several HSR-related disciplines (such as those cited) and committed to disability issues
2. Longitudinal data bases that can track patient resource use, patient progress, functional status, and patient outcome well into the postrehabilitation period
3. Lots of money

Longitudinal studies are labor intensive, and therefore very expensive, despite advances in computer-supported data base management.

Although the core group of researchers is largely nonexistent, longitudinal data bases are present to one degree or another. We have already noted the role of the National SCI Database. In addition, two factors have motivated medical rehabilitation providers to develop longitudinal data bases. The first is the requirements of the Commission on Accreditation of Rehabilitation Facilities (CARF) for a program evaluation capability that can assess patient outcomes in functional terms. The second is the requirements of changes emerging in the economics and financing of health care. As the health care market becomes more competitive, providers will be motivated to assemble data on patient outcomes and resource use to convince payers that

it is in their interest to cover the medical rehabilitation costs of their enrollees. These two factors have also led to the recent development of other data bases such as the Uniform Data System (UDS) for Medical Rehabilitation located at the State University of New York at Buffalo. UDS serves as a repository for medical rehabilitation outcome data and includes data on persons with SCI.

AN AGENDA FOR FUTURE HEALTH SERVICES RESEARCH IN SPINAL CORD INJURY

Among the most neglected health care needs of persons with SCI are those that surface after discharge from rehabilitation. At present, there is no system of primary care that is responsive to the particular constellation of health care problems commonly experienced by persons with SCI. Spinal cord injured persons become virtual orphans—their ongoing care is not the province of any medical discipline (Batavia, DeJong, Halstead, and Smith 1988). One reason for this is that there are only about 700 to 800 persons with SCI per 1 million population—hardly enough to interest providers who might otherwise wish to specialize in this market niche. Potential providers may not realize, however, that persons with SCI use a disproportionately large share of health care resources, and thus can fill excess capacity in their practices. Providers may also fear that patients with SCI will require a disproportionate share of their time and that third-party payers will not compensate them for the additional time required.

The provision of postrehabilitation health care services has lagged behind the progress made by persons with SCI in living independently and becoming informed consumers of health care services. When persons with SCI remained primarily in institutional settings, the person's health care needs were addressed in the framework of the institution. No comparable mechanism meets the health care needs of persons with SCI now that they are living routinely in community settings.

Three health service issues dominate the SCI population following rehabilitation:

1. the very high rate of unscheduled rehospitalizations
2. the lack of access to primary care
3. the development of new health problems as a result of aging with a disability

These health service problems require the consideration of new health service delivery models that are targeted more carefully to the needs of persons with SCI. Finally, there is also the problem of access to long-term care, especially the availability of user-directed, community-based, long-term care services (that is, attendant care services).

Avert Rehospitalization

Persons with SCI are not necessarily sick by virtue of their disability. In fact, they must be medically stable even to participate in a rigorous medical rehabilitation program. Yet, it is known that a person with SCI has a very narrow margin of health that must be maintained scrupulously. Spinal cord injured persons are highly vulnerable to a variety of acute conditions, such as respiratory tract infections. One of the primary goals of medical rehabilitation is to teach the patient the health maintenance skills needed after rehabilitation to avoid complications.

However, research has shown repeatedly that many persons with SCI do not maintain their vital margin of health. Spinal cord injured persons experience a high rate of post-rehabilitation rehospitalization. Young and Northup (1979) analyzed data on 383 persons with SCI who were discharged from model regional spinal cord injury centers. They report that about 50% had at least one rehospitalization episode in their second year after discharge. Zook, Savickis, and Moore (1980), in their study of rehospitalization among persons discharged from six Boston-area hospitals, report that persons with SCI had the highest rate of rehospitalization of any diagnostic group. They report that, of the 86 persons discharged from a VA SCI center, 70% were rehospitalized within a 1-year period.

DeJong (1981) performed secondary data analysis on a sample of 111 persons with SCI discharged from 10 comprehensive medical rehabilitation centers. He reports that 55% were rehospitalized within a 12-month period approximately 2 to 3 years after discharge from medical rehabilitation. Young, Burns, Bowen, and McCuthchen (1982) report that, among persons represented in the National SCI Database, those persons with complete quadriplegia had the highest rates of rehospitalization. The rehospitalization rate ranged from a high of 61% in the second year following discharge to 32% in the sixth year. Meyers and associates (1985) conducted a health care use study of 96 postrehabilitation persons with SCI in eastern Massachusetts. They found that 57% percent were rehospitalized in a 12-month period.

The length of stay among spinal cord injured persons who have been rehospitalized is also striking. Young and Northup (1979) report a mean of 34 days once rehospitalized. DeJong (1981) reports a mean of 55 days. Meyers and associates (1985) report a mean of 45 days in their 12-month study period. Drawing on data from the National SCI Database, Stover and Fine (1986) report a mean of 33 days of rehospitalization in the first year and 28 days in the tenth year postdischarge.

Finally, Batavia and associates (1989) surveyed more than 600 persons living in the Washington, DC, area who had at least 1 of 10 specified conditions (amputation, cerebral palsy, cystic fibrosis, head injury, muscular dystrophy, multiple sclerosis, SCI, spina bifida, postpolio, and stroke [Batavia et al. 1989]), and found that persons with SCI had the highest rate of hospitalization (34% in the previous year). The study, which was not limited to persons recently discharged from rehabilitation, found that 54% of persons with SCI (n = 41) admitted in the previous year were hospitalized for a week or more in their most recent admission.

Although these studies have consistently reported the seriousness of the problem, they have not clearly identified the causes and predictors of rehospitalization. In the Meyers and associates (1985) study, younger persons with low self-assessments of health and those who did not leave their residence at least once a day had higher rehospitalization rates. In an earlier study of 70 persons with cervical level injuries, Burnside and Cook (1976) report that age and occupational status were significantly related to readmission. Younger patients who had worked in predominantly manual occupations exhibited higher rehospitalization rates. They suggest that low intelligence (and inability to follow preventive routines) may promote rehospitalization.

Other researchers such as DeJong (1981) and DeJong and associates (1987) are more reluctant to blame the victim. After two major studies, DeJong, Osberg, McGinnis, Seward, Branch, and Campion (1987) did not uncover any systematic predictors of rehospitalization or identify a consistent profile of the individual at greatest risk of rehospitalization. However, DeJong and his team refuse to accept rehospitalization as a random event, and suggest that more careful attention be paid to the responsiveness of the health care system to the particular needs of people with SCI as an explanatory factor.

Hospital costs comprise the single largest component of health care costs. Furthermore, Zook and Moore (1980) estimate that rehospitalizations (in all diagnostic categories) account for 60% of all hospital costs. An understanding of the rehospitalization phenomenon thus may significantly contribute to the development of improved cost-management strategies in SCI health care.

Aside from the economic factors, rehospitalization also exacts a high personal toll. Prolonged rehospitalizations disrupt a person's ability to live independently and productively. They result in absences from work, school, and family life. Disabled individuals' personal control over their lives diminishes, and they must rely on others to make decisions during rehospitalization. Finally, rehospitalizations can result in extended bedrest that can compromise many functional gains.

We know which conditions are most likely to precipitate rehospitalization—urinary tract infections, pressure sores, and lower respiratory tract problems. The great tragedy is that those conditions are largely preventable. Thus far, researchers have failed to find clear demographic or behavioral explanations for the problem. We must therefore look beyond the individual to the health care system, and particularly to the availability of timely primary health care.

Provide Access to Primary Care

The conditions that precipitate rehospitalization episodes usually start as relatively minor health problems that rapidly escalate into major medical crises if not detected and treated in a timely manner. Thus, timely access to primary care is essential. Yet many persons with SCI indicate that, after their injuries, they could no longer use their customary source of primary care for common health problems. A recurring complaint among persons with SCI is that they must constantly educate their primary care physicians about the idiosyncracies of their impairments and how they affect prescribing treatment (Batavia et al. 1988; Batavia et al. 1989; DeJong, Batavia, and Griss 1989).

The family physician, the local internist, or the obstetrician/gynecologist is generally unaccustomed to treating patients with a major physical impairment. For the practitioner, the disability, not the common complaint, becomes the more important health issue. Providers therefore tend to refer these patients to specialists. As a result, persons with SCI are likely to be sent to a urologist; a neurologist; a specialty, hospital-based outpatient clinic; or an emergency room. In turn, the unfortunate outcome is unnecessary hospitalization or delayed attention to an emerging health problem that will ultimately require hospitalization (Batavia et al. 1989).

These shortcomings in the U.S. primary health care system often lead persons with SCI to seek out a local physiatrist (a specialist in rehabilitation medicine) who is acquainted with the person's impairment and its implications for health management. Alternatively, persons with SCI may turn to the physiatrists they knew during their rehabilitation in a distant city. Although rehabilitation medicine has not viewed itself as a primary care specialty, some physiatrists are known to provide primary care services willingly to persons with SCI because of shortcomings elsewhere in the health care system (Batavia et al. 1988).

The irony about the undersupply of knowledgeable physicians is that in many urban areas there is an oversupply of primary care physicians who could be addressing these unmet needs (Batavia et al. 1988). Although persons with SCI represent a very small part of the health care market, many other groups with physical disabilities experience similar problems with access to appropriate primary care (Batavia et al. 1989; DeJong, Batavia, and Griss 1989).

Understand Aging with a Disability

The life expectancy of SCI survivors now approximates that of the general population. However, even though persons with SCI are likely to experience the common chronic health conditions that everyone experiences with advancing age—for example, arthritis, heart disease, and cancer (Mahoney, Estes, and Heumann 1986; Trieschmann 1987)—several qualifications must be noted.

First, persons with SCI cannot undertake many of the same preventive measures available to the general population. For example, paralyzed limbs limit the spinal cord injured person's capacity for aerobic exercise. Most adaptive devices for aerobic exercise have serious practical limitations. Persons with high cervical injuries cannot even exercise their arms. The use of a bicycle ergometer powered by electrically stimulated leg muscles requires expensive equipment and tedious set-up, and is difficult to integrate into the daily routine of a person with SCI. Moreover, we do not know the long-term effects of such exercise.

Second, persons with SCI may experience the onset of some chronic health conditions earlier in life than nondisabled persons. Although earlier onset is not certain, prolonged physical immobility and the use of compensatory muscles may aggravate certain body systems and thus precipitate an earlier manifestation of certain health conditions.

Third, persons with SCI may be at risk of unknown new health problems. For example, the long-term effects of regular urinary tract infections and long-term exposure to antibiotics are not known (Ohry, Schemesh, and Rozin 1983). As Trieschmann (1987: n.p.) observes, "the true experts are those who have survived a disability . . . or injury for 30, 40, or 50 years."

Fourth, persons with SCI are likely to experience secondary functional losses because of a chronic health condition. For example, the presence of arthritis in the fingers is likely to compromise what little dexterity remains. The onset of angina may limit the person's willingness to exert himself or herself physically when facing certain architectural barriers.

In responding to these needs, the health care system must take into account specific complicating factors of spinal cord injury:

- Early detection may be difficult because persons with SCI do not experience pain in many body regions.
- Secondary prevention may be difficult because of functional limitations.
- Various kinds of therapy may be difficult because the disabled person may not be able to participate actively.

At present, the health care system is not equipped to respond to these needs and limitations as persons with SCI become older. New ways must be found in which primary care disciplines, rehabilitation medicine, and other specialty disciplines can work together on behalf of the patient. The challenges of aging with a disability are already evident at the VA, which serves a population of spinal cord injured veterans of World War II and the Korean War. Vietnam veterans are also reaching middle age. There are also many veterans with nonservice-connected spinal cord injuries. The VA is thus in an excellent position to develop innovative ways to meet the needs of older persons with SCI.

Develop New Models of Health Care Delivery

The unresponsiveness of the present health care system to the needs of persons with SCI and to persons with other physical disabilities compels us to search for more responsive models of health care delivery. These new models must avert unnecessary rehospitalization, offer access to timely primary care, and respond to new health needs as persons with SCI become older.

One major shortcoming of the U.S. health care system is how it pays for health care. For example, rehabilitation providers have no direct financial incentive to improve postrehabilitation outcomes, such as unscheduled rehospitalizations (Batavia 1988). Likewise, third-party payers often are not willing to cover certain types of durable medical equipment because they fear this will attract high-cost disabled persons to their policies, or if their financial liability for the patient's care will soon end (Batavia 1989). The present health care financing system does not reward providers and payers who make the up-front investments needed to avert long-term medical problems (Batavia 1988).

Because of increased competition, however, some new approaches are being tried that provide managed care using an innovative financing mechanism. In San Francisco, the On Lok Senior Health Services program has been providing managed health care services to the frail elderly population since 1979. Since 1983, the On Lok program has been funded on a capitation basis under Medicare and Medicaid (Zawadski, Shen, Yordi, and Hansen 1985). In Boston, the Urban Medical Group conducted a pilot project to evaluate the merits of a capitation-financed program for persons served by the Boston Center for Independent Living, many of whom had a spinal cord injury (Meyers et al. 1987; Meyers et al. 1988).

In Washington, DC, the National Rehabilitation Hospital (NRH) conducted a feasibility study funded by The Robert Wood Johnson Foundation. This study determined that a managed health care plan for working age (18 to 65) disabled persons in the metropolitan Washington, DC, area should be developed and implemented (Batavia et al. 1989). The NRH health plan includes case management services (see Chapter 14) and home visits by nurse practitioners in an effort to prevent unnecessary hospitalizations. The results of these projects must be monitored carefully in order to evaluate their implications for the health management of persons with SCI. Nurse practitioners usually have advanced clinical nursing preparation and can exercise judgment more independently than is permitted in most settings. They are skilled at making physical assessments, counseling, and teaching and are most valuable in treating (together with the physician) people with long-term, stable conditions such as physical disability. Their role functions are health maintenance, evaluation and management of symptoms, and appropriate referrals (McGrath 1990; Kozier and Erb 1991). Career opportunities in lifetime health care for people with disabilities are more attractive to many nurses with a background in rehabilitation than traditional inpatient/outpatient care.

Provide Attendant Services

Immediately following discharge from a rehabilitation facility, many persons with SCI must find affordable and reliable attendants to assist them in personal care and various other activities. The only alternative for many people would be institutional care. Accordingly, attendant care is the premier long-term care issue for people with SCI (DeJong and Wenker 1983; Litvak, Zukas, and Heumann 1987).

The terms *attendant care* and *attendant services* refer to a specific model of in-home services. In the attendant care model, the users of the service (persons with SCI) manage and direct their own attendant care employment relationships. Attendants are accountable to the consumers of the services, not to an outside agency as in the case of home health care. Attendants are not an extension of a home health agency that is usually managed by nurses who direct care in keeping with a physician's plan of treatment. Attendants are, in a sense, extensions of disabled persons and do what the disabled persons ordinarily would do for themselves (DeJong and Wenker 1983; Litvak, Zukas, and Heumann 1987).

This conception appears to place attendant services outside the boundaries of health care and thus beyond the scope of HSR. However, attendant care is very much a long-term health services issue because it is an alternative to institutional care. Attendant care is often financed by health-related payment systems such as Medicaid. An attendant also helps the user carry out health maintenance regimes and detect health problems early. Thus, attendant care is an important adjunct to the user's overall program of health maintenance.

Despite the rather straightforward nature and scope of attendant services, the United States (and the vast majority of other developed countries) has yet to develop a coherent attendant services policy that can address the varied needs of potential users such as persons with SCI. Instead, we have a needlessly complex patchwork of programs—extensions of other health and social service programs that are not responsive to consumer needs. In some states, disabled persons have no access to attendant services unless they can afford to purchase their own attendant services. In a national study on publicly funded in-home service programs conducted by the World Institute on Disability (Litvak, Zukas, and Heumann 1987), investigators found that

- 44% exclude certain disabling conditions
- 42% do not cover both personal and domestic services
- 22% do not cover services 7 days per week
- 50% do not serve persons with incomes above the poverty level
- 67% do not allow attendants to assist in personal care involving medications, catheters, suppositories, or menstrual needs

These findings indicate how unresponsive most in-home service programs are to the attendant care needs of persons with SCI.

A major obstacle in the development of a coherent national attendant services policy is the absence of a good research base. The development of this policy requires an aggressive HSR agenda that can effectively define the parameters of the debate with respect to the future of attendant services by asking such questions as:

1. How many and what types of persons both need and want user-directed attendant services?
2. Can a user-directed model of attendant services foster a more independent and productive life-style?
3. Do user-directed models of attendant services foster health maintenance behaviors that help avert complications leading to hospitalizations?
4. Can user-defined criteria be developed by which the quality of attendant service programs can be evaluated and alternative models can be critiqued?
5. How do eligibility and income requirements for attendant services create disincentives for work, and how can such disincentives be averted?
6. How should attendant services be financed? For example, should they be financed within the framework of a health maintenance plan?
7. How much will a national attendant care program cost?

The VA has had its own attendant care program in the form of the aids and attendants allowance (Batavia 1989). This program is viewed widely as an entitlement. There are no earned income restrictions for service-connected veterans. This long-standing program should be evaluated in terms of its implications for the nonveteran population. The availability of affordable attendant care is the quintessential requirement for independent living. Without it, persons with SCI are relegated to an often destructive dependence on family members or on institutional care. Moreover, the ability of spinal cord injured persons to maintain dependable sources of personal care is an important determinant of their long-term health prospects.

IN CLOSING

Some elements of a core HSR capacity in SCI already exist in the United States. There are various longitudinal data bases, primarily the National SCI Database. In addition, various medical rehabilitation facilities have emerging data bases within the scope of their respective program evaluation systems. The critical element—and the one most frequently missing—is the acquisition of postdischarge outcome and health use data. Other elements of a HSR capacity in SCI are in very short supply. These include researchers trained in HSR disciplines and HSR programs dedicated specifically to issues concerning SCI and physical disability.

The HSR issues in SCI and related disabilities are compelling. The knowledge gained by researchers in this field affects the assumptions and conclusions underlying federal and state legislation that allocates millions of dollars and affects thousands of lives. We believe that once exposed to these issues, investigators will develop an enduring commitment to address them. Of course, these researchers will need to obtain financial support for pursuing their research agendas. They must find an institutional and academic home in which to base their research. Therefore, it is important that federal, state, and local government; the philanthropic community; and the nonprofit provider community develop strategies to foster this research.

Trained personnel are needed in such fields as biostatistics, health economics, epidemiology, health care finance, health policy, health law, medical sociology, political science, and social psychology. With respect to research funding sources, large grants for longitudinal research projects are less important than significant grants for individual dissertations, postdoctoral fellowships, research fellowships, visiting senior scientist awards, and other awards for individual investigators. These grants should be awarded to investigators trained in the aforementioned disciplines and should be designed to bring new researchers into the field. The Mary E. Switzer Research Fellowship Program of the U.S. National Institute on Disability and Rehabilitation Research (NIDRR) is one example of such a program. In addition, however, investigators attracted to the field must be reasonably sure of continued funding if they are to make a sustained commitment.

The involvement of persons with SCI (and persons with other disabilities) in HSR issues that directly affect their lives is particularly important. Thus, the disbursement of investigator awards should take into account the person's disability status as one relevant indicator of expertise. Moreover, financial support should be offered specifically to encourage persons with SCI (and other disabilities) to pursue HSR careers. Dissertation support for spinal cord injured persons in the most needed disciplines is one way to foster the intellectual commitment required to make a significant contribution to the issues identified in this chapter.

Many of the HSR needs of the SCI population resulted from our medical successes in prolonging their lives and enhancing their functional capacities. However, success brings with it new responsibilities and new problems. As more and more persons with SCI live independently in the community, new health care needs surface that have yet to be recognized fully. Health service researchers must conduct studies to document these new needs, and to shape the agenda for meeting them.

REFERENCES

Baker, S. P., O'Neill, B., Haddon, W., and Long, W. B. 1974. The Injury Severity Score: A method for describing patients with multiple injuries and evaluating emergency care. *The Journal of Trauma* 14: 3.

Batavia, A. I. 1988. *The Payment of Medical Rehabilitation Services: Current Mechanisms and Potential Models.* Chicago: American Hospital Association.

Batavia, A. I. 1989. *The Payors of Medical Rehabilitation: Eligibility, Coverage, and Payment Policies.* Washington, DC: National Association of Rehabilitation Facilities.

Batavia, A. I., and DeJong, G. 1990. Developing a comprehensive health services research capacity in physical disability and rehabilitation. *Journal of Disability Policy Studies* 1 (1): 37–61.

Batavia, A. I., DeJong, G., Burns, T. J., Smith, Q. W., Melus, S., and Butler, D. 1989. *A Managed Care Program for Working-Age Persons with Physical Disabilities: A Feasibility Study.* Washington, DC: National Rehabilitation Hospital Office of Research.

Batavia, A. I., DeJong, G., Halstead, L., and Smith, Q. W. 1988. The primary medical needs of people with disabilities. *American Rehabilitation* 14 (4): 9–12.

Burnside, I. D., and Cook, J. B. 1976. Factors influencing readmission to hospital. *Paraplegia* 14: 220–224.

Champion, H. S., Sacco, W. J., Carnazzo, A. J., Copes, W. S., and Fouty, W. J. 1981. Trauma Score. *Critical Care Medicine* 9: 9.

DeJong, G. 1979. Independent living: From social movement to analytic paradigm. *Archives of Physical Medicine and Rehabilitation* 60: 435–446.

DeJong, G. 1981. *Environmental Accessibility and Independent Living Outcomes: Directions for Disability Policy and Research.* East Lansing, MI: Michigan State University, University Center for International Rehabilitation.

DeJong, G., and Batavia, A. I. 1989. Societal duty and resource allocation for persons with severe traumatic brain injury. *Journal of Head Trauma Rehabilitation* 4 (1): 1–12.

DeJong, G., Batavia, A. I., and Griss, R. 1989. America's neglected health minority: Working-age persons with disabilities. *The Milbank Quarterly*, 67 Suppl. 2, Pt. 2.

DeJong, G., Osberg, J. S., McGinnis, G. E., Seward, M. L., Branch, L. G., and Campion, L. G. 1987. Rehospitalization following rehabilitation, Part II: Findings and analysis. Based on a paper presented at the Annual Meetings of the American Congress of Rehabilitation, Baltimore, MD. October 20, 1986.

DeJong, G., and Wenker, T. 1983. Attendant care as a prototype independent living service. *Caring* 2 (2) : 26–30.

Flook, E. E., and Sanazaro, P. J. (editors). 1973. *Health Services Research and R & D In Perspective.* Ann Arbor, MI: Health Administration Press.

Fuhrer, M. J. 1988. Rehabilitation research in the 1980s. In *Advances in Clinical Rehabilitation. Vol. II.* Eds. M. G. Eisenberg and R. C. Grzesiak. New York: Springer Publishing.

Johnston, M., and Keith, R. A. 1983. Cost-benefits of medical rehabilitation: Review and critique. *Archives of Physical Medicine and Rehabilitation* 64: 147–154.

Kozier, B., and Erb, G. 1991. *Fundamentals of Nursing Concepts and Procedures.* 4th ed. Menlo Park, CA: Addison-Wesley.

Litvak, S., Zukas, H., and Heumann, J. E. 1987. *Attending to America: Personal Assistance for Independent Living.* Berkeley, CA: World Institute on Disability.

McGrath, S. 1990. The cost-effectiveness of nurse practitioners. *Nurse Practitioner* 15 (7): 40–42.

Meyers, A. R., Cupples, A., Lederman, R. I., Branch, L. G., Feltin, M., Master, R. J., Nicastro, D., Glover, M., and Kress, D. 1987. A prospective evaluation of the effect of managed care on medical care utilization among severely disabled independently living adults. *Medical Care* 25 (11): 1057–1068.

Meyers, A. R., Cupples, A., Lederman, R. I., Branch, L. G., Feltin, M., Master, R. J., Nicastro, D., Glover, M., and Kress, D. 1988. The epidemiology of medical care utilization by severely disabled independently living adults. *Journal of Clinical Epidemiology* 41 (2): 163–172.

Meyers, A. R., Feltin, M., Masters, R. J., Nicastro, D., Cupples, A., Lederman, R. I., and Branch, L. G. 1985. Rehospitalization and spinal cord injury: Cross-sectional survey of adults living independently. *Archives of Physical Medicine and Rehabilitation* 66: 704–708.

Mahoney, C. W., Estes, C. L., and Heumann, J. E. 1986. *Toward A Unified Agenda: Proceedings of a National Conference on Disability and Aging.* San Francisco: Institute For Health and Aging, University of California at San Francisco.

Ohry, A., Schemesh, Y., and Rozin, R. 1983. Are chronic spinal cord injured patients prone to pre-mature aging? *Medical Hypotheses* 11: 467–469.

Stover, S. L., and Fine, P. 1986. *Spinal Cord Injury: The Facts and Figures.* Birmingham, AL: National Spinal Cord Injury Data Research Center, University of Alabama.

Trieschmann, R. B. 1987. *Aging With A Disability.* New York: Demos Publications.

Young, J. S., Burns, P. E., Bowen, A. M., and McCuthchen. 1982. *Spinal Cord Injury Statistics: Experience of the Regional Model Spinal Cord Injury Systems.* Phoenix, AZ: Good Samaritan Medical Center. National Spinal Cord Injury Data Research Center.

Young, J. S., and Northup, N. E. 1979. Rehospitalization in years two and three following spinal cord injury. *SCI Digest* 1: 21–26.

Zawadski, R., Shen, J., Yordi, C., and Hansen, J. C. 1985. On Lok's community care organization for dependent adults: Research and development project—Final Report (1978–1983) San Francisco: On Lok Senior Health Services.

Zook, C. J., and Moore, F. D. 1980. High cost users of medical care. *The New England Journal of Medicine* 302: 996–1002.

Zook, C. J., Savickis, S. F., and Moore, F. D. 1980. Repeated hospitalized for the same disease: A multiplier of national health costs. *Milbank Memorial Fund Quarterly* 58 (3): 454–471.

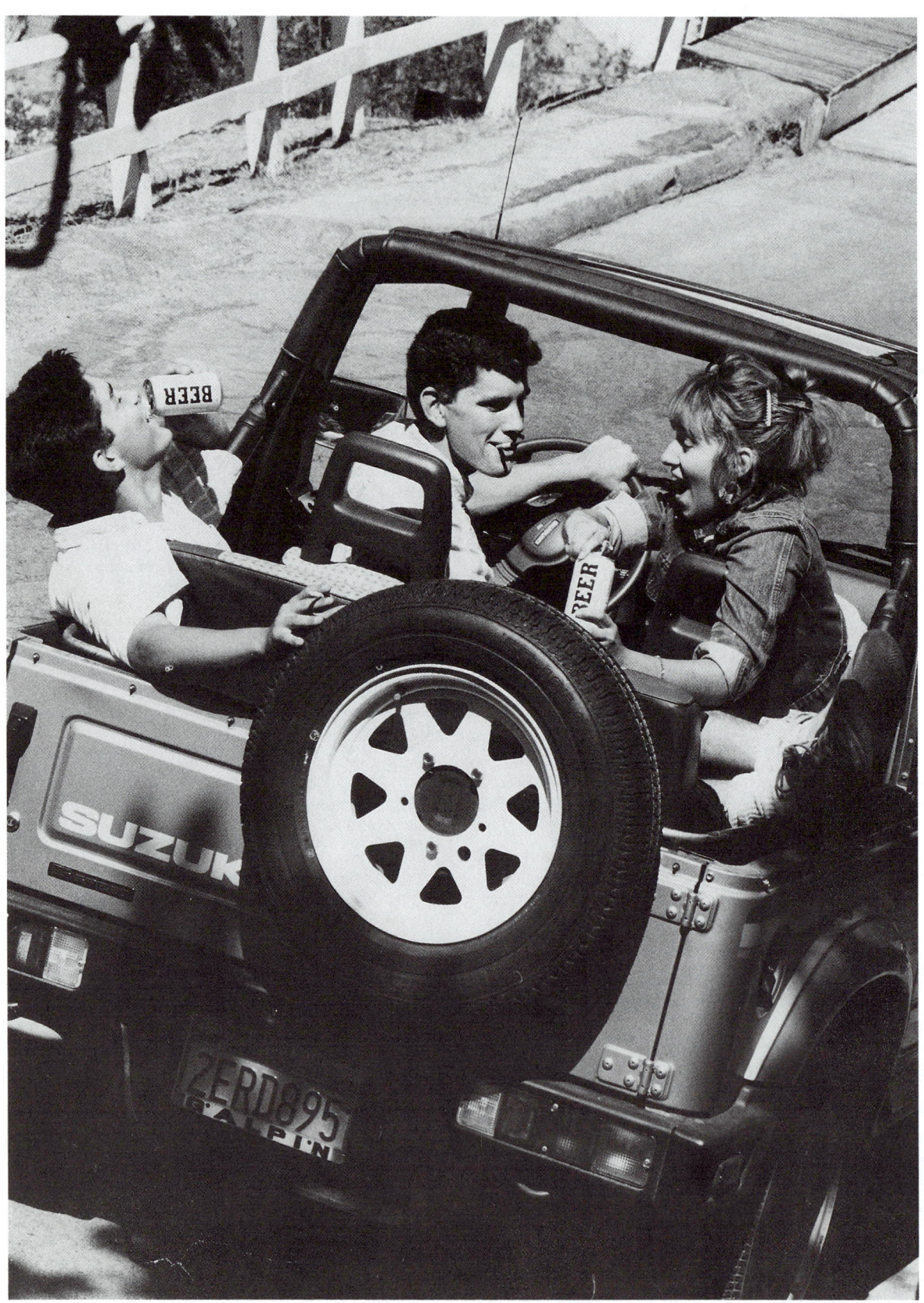

CHAPTER
— 3 —

Spinal Cord Injury Prevention

Peter C. Wing, M.B., Ch.B., M.Sc., F.R.C.S.(C.), and Kathleen Cain, A.C.S.W.

Chapter Outline

CONCEPT OF INJURY PREVENTION
  Injury as a Preventable Disease
  Spinal Cord Injury Surveillance
PREVENTABLE ASPECTS OF SPINAL CORD INJURY
  Risk Taking
  Substance Abuse
  Violence
  Motor Vehicle Accidents
    On-road motor vehicles: automobiles and
    motorcycles
    Off-road, all-terrain vehicles
  Diving Injuries
    Mechanics of diving
    Diving in the natural environment
    Water slides
    Responsibility for diving accidents
  Work-Related Injuries
    The role of government in worker safety
    Health care professionals and worker safety
DEVELOPMENT OF PREVENTION PROGRAMS
ORGANIZING A PREVENTION PROGRAM
REFERENCES

Health Care Objectives

• To explain injury prevention
• To analyze different injury types
• To describe effective and innovative injury prevention programs
• To direct the design of a spinal cord injury prevention program

The help of Elizabeth Matheson is acknowledged.

CONCEPT OF INJURY PREVENTION

Spinal cord injury (SCI) is a potentially preventable disease. Injury has only recently been considered an epidemic that might warrant a preventive approach, and SCI has only recently been receiving the careful attention that may reduce the incidence. During a lifetime, a person has more than a 50/50 chance of being injured in a car crash. If other activities such as biking, skiing, diving, and sports are included, the chance of being injured is much higher. These injuries are, after all, tragedies that everyone wishes to see reduced, avoided, eliminated. Surely, we should do something to prevent the next young persons from diving into a life so different from the ones they would have chosen.

Public health measures have a major effect on the quality of life in today's society. From malnutrition to the diarrheal diseases, from smallpox and tuberculosis to AIDS, methodical application of preventive methods has paralleled or exceeded the advances in therapy of the diseases. Prevention can modify various parts of the disease process: the host, the agent or its vector, or the environment.

Life-style factors—such as continued exposure to harmful bacteria, toxins, or physical insults—are important in the development of a certain group of diseases. Examples include diseases in which exposure to sunlight or alcohol, tobacco, or drugs play a role. Risk of these diseases can be reduced through education, legislation, and economic incentives. An approach to SCI prevention shares tactics common to several of these disease-control programs.

Injury as a Preventable Disease

"Most injuries to people—and nearly all injuries to children—*can* be predicted and *can* be prevented." (Koop n.d.). *Injury in America* (Foege et al. 1985) is essential reading for anyone working in the field of injury prevention. In the summary, the authors point out that:

- Each year, more than 140,000 Americans die from injuries, and one person in three suffers a nonfatal injury. Alcohol is often a causative factor. (Risk taking is another [National Committee on Injury Prevention 1989].)
- Injury is the last major plague of youth, killing more people aged 1 to 34 than all other diseases. It is the leading cause of death up to the age of 44.
- Because its victims are young, injury produces a relatively greater loss of productive years than do cancer or heart disease.
- One of every eight hospital beds is occupied by an injured patient.

- Every year more than 80,000 people in the United States become permanently disabled due to injury of the brain or spinal cord.
- Injury is one of the most expensive and devastating health problems.

Young and others state that SCI is one of the most expensive injuries found in our society (Young, Burns, and Wilt, 1982).

Spinal Cord Injury Surveillance

Spinal cord injury is a disease of low frequency but great cost to the individual and to society. Nevertheless, the total number of injuries and their cost are high enough to warrant detailed national and regional surveillance, the ongoing monitoring process whereby incidence trends are established. Chapter 1 summarizes data gathered by the National SCI Database and published by Stover and Fine (1986).

Several agencies monitor SCI regionally and nationally. The statistics generated vary in purpose and completeness. The Centers for Disease Control in Atlanta have made SCI the first noninfectious disease to be the subject of a surveillance program. Centers participate either on a mandatory or voluntary basis and presently include nine states collecting information on central nervous system trauma and 10 collecting on spinal cord injury only. In 1988, the Centers for Disease Control established five Injury Prevention Research Centers (National Committee on Injury Prevention 1989). A number of other data bases exist or are in development throughout the world. Some are national, some regional or local. Compliance may be mandatory or voluntary. The major question to be asked of each data base is: are all cases of SCI within a given population included so that the data base provides reliable incidence figures?

PREVENTABLE ASPECTS OF SPINAL CORD INJURY

The relative importance of preventable causes varies from region to region (Stover and Fine 1986). Also spinal cord injuries caused by motor vehicle accidents, falls and jumps, firearms, pedestrian and bicycle accidents, diving, or motorcycle accidents each have a different frequency pattern in terms of the level and type of the cord injury (Fife and Kraus 1986).

In general, causative factors are factors that predispose to any injury (age, risk taking, alcohol) or that lead directly to a specific injury (motor vehicle accident or shallow-water dive).

Risk Taking

Youth may take risks partly as the natural outcome of a developmental stage and partly because they fail to perceive the dangers of injury resulting from a particular activity. This can lead to a "risk behavior syndrome" (Jonah 1989; Jessor and Jessor 1977). Jonah showed that the risk behavior adopted by young drivers aged 20 to 24 is greater than for those aged 16 to 19, especially with respect to drinking, drinking and driving, and nonuse of seat belts (Jonah 1989).

Substance Abuse

Substance abuse has received much attention as a cause of injury from motor vehicle accidents (MVAs). The risk of being involved in a crash rises with the amount consumed. There is evidence in the survivors of MVAs that injury severity may be higher in people with higher blood alcohol concentrations than in those people with lower levels (Kraus, Morgenstern, Fife, Conroy, and Nourjah 1989).

Violence

Violence by one person against another is part of the larger spectrum of violence in our society—particularly among adolescents (Tonkin 1981 and 1987). In injury statistics, the term refers to assaults, either as a method of conflict resolution or as incidental to the commission of some other crime—typically drug or gang-related conflicts. Little is published with respect to violent crime as a cause of SCI; refer to details of the Violence Prevention Program in Detroit described in Table 3–1. Also review the appropriate section in *Injury Prevention, Meeting the Challenge* (National Committee on Injury Prevention 1989).

Motor Vehicle Accidents

On-Road Motor Vehicles: Automobiles and Motorcycles

Automobile accidents are a major cause of SCI. Rimel and associates (1982) described 1331 patients with central nervous system trauma admitted to the University of Virginia Medical Center during a 20-month period. Of the total 1331 patients admitted, 80% had head injuries, 12% had spinal cord injuries, and 8% had combined head and spinal injuries.

The accidents leading to SCI have features in common with those causing head injuries or fatalities. Mercer has shown that accidents causing SCI more closely resemble fatality-producing traffic accidents than accidents causing other kinds of injuries (Mercer 1987). Such accidents typically occur on a rural, high-speed road in the dark on a weekend. They involve a single vehicle that either fails to negotiate a curve or simply runs off the side of a straight road. If a second vehicle is involved, there is often a head-on collision. The most frequent contributing factors are excessive speed and/or alcohol (Mercer 1987; Canadian Medical Association Review 1989).

The design of automobiles affects injury rates. Kraus showed that SCI crash rates are higher in pre-1968 passenger cars than for cars produced from 1968 to 1971 (Kraus, Franti, and Riggins 1982). (In 1968 U.S. federal standards were enacted on door latches, interior padding, energy-absorbing steering wheels and other occupant protection features.) Because safety-related features in cars and buses are expensive, legislation has often been necessary to ensure their development and introduction.

To identify general trends in MVAs, a review was done of case files in British Columbia comprising all claims for a 2-year period (1986 and 1987) involving SCI. In all but one out of 55 cases, the driver of the car in which an occupant was injured was held to be at fault; in 75% loss of control was the cause of the accident. Alcohol use seemed to be a factor in 40%. When seat belt usage was identified, two-thirds of persons with SCI were unrestrained (Mercer 1988).

The severity of a neck injury in a MVA is related to the type of crash (Huelke et al. 1981). More occupants sustain severe neck injuries in frontal or side impacts, but the rate of such injuries is highest in roll-over accidents. Almost all of the more serious neck injuries are sustained by occupants not wearing seat belts (97%). Those persons suffering more serious cervical injuries while wearing a lap or lap-shoulder belt are all in extremely severe crashes.

When comparing the number of vehicles involved in SCI crashes with the number of vehicles registered, Kraus found crash involvement rates to be highest for motorcyles and large trucks (Kraus et al. 1982). An association between helmet use and cervical spine injury due to motorcycle accidents is not clear. One group (Carr, Brandt, and Swanson 1981) found no association. Another researcher (Yeo 1979) reported that the type of helmet was a factor in the occurrence of SCI, and that full face helmets were more protective than an open face design.

The contributing factors to single-vehicle, casualty-causing motorcycle accidents are similar to those for single-vehicle nonmotorcycle accidents (alcohol, driving without due care, and unsafe speed). However, inexperience is more often a factor in motorcycle than automobile accidents. Weather is less a factor in motorcycle accidents compared to other vehicles (Mercer 1988).

Off-Road, All-Terrain Vehicles

All-terrain vehicles (ATVs) were first introduced in the early 1970s. Sales of ATVs jumped by more than 300% from 1980 to 1983 (Sneed et al. 1986), and the incidence of injury related to these vehicles has increased concomitantly (Wiley 1986).

Larger ATVs can attain speeds of up to 100 km/hr. The three-wheel ATV is unstable because of the lack of a rear-wheel differential, the absence of independent suspension, and the high center of gravity. Low-pressure tires on ATVs can also create problems when the terrain changes suddenly. The four-wheel ATV has more stability, but it also readily tips over.

Losing control and falling from the vehicle is the most common injury sequence (Wiley et al. 1989). Loss of control is frequently related to movement into or out of a ditch, turning suddenly, or losing control of the vehicle over irregular terrain. Some drivers are struck by their own vehicles. Pyper and Black (1988) reviewed 233 children with musculoskeletal injuries due to off-road vehicles. One hundred and eighty-nine children were driving the vehicle when they were injured, 31 were passengers, and 8 were bystanders.

Despite these dangers, advertisements for ATVs depicted the "sport" of driving over rough terrain inclines, hills, or sand dunes, even though these machines can easily go out of control in such environments (Sneed et al. 1986). The researchers obtained manufacturers' advertising brochures on three- and four-wheel ATVs and found that some models were promoted as being "built for youngsters." This review of brochures showed that little or no information was provided on the top speeds that ATVs can attain, perhaps leading parents to think they are suitable for children.

Regulations controlling the use of ATVs and insurance provisions covering their operation vary widely from one jurisdiction to another. It is important for people involved in injury prevention to ascertain the regulations in their own regions. The American Academy of Pediatrics has effectively brought pressure to bear on federal regulatory bodies to improve safety standards with respect to ATVs.

Diving Injuries

In 1985, the National Swimming Pool Safety Commission was set up by the U.S. Consumer Product Safety Commission and the National Spa and Pool Institute to address child drowning and diving accidents (National Swimming Pool Safety Commission 1986). A subcommittee was charged with reviewing research on the incidence of child drowning and diving accidents and with recommending future directions for study.

The subcommittee found that diving produces a significant proportion of all spinal cord injuries. There is a high fatality rate, and injuries sustained from diving accidents are more likely to result in quadriplegia than paraplegia. Boyd and Schweigel (1985) have shown that the most common spinal level involved is C_5 (35%), with 78% involving C_4 to C_6.

Many injuries occur in private pools, although the Canadian experience is that approximately 50% occur in lakes, rivers, or the ocean (Boyd and Schweigel 1985; Tator and Palm 1981). Alcohol is a factor in 20% to 40% of diving accidents.

The subcommittee did not find sufficient data to document the effectiveness of different kinds of warnings posted around pools. No one can design a pool to account for all imprudent behaviors or unintentional errors on the part of the diver; regardless of pool design there will be a need for diving education. The subcommittee pointed out the need for research to determine which factors influence accidents. For example, it suggested observation of typical diving activities that do *not* result in accidents.

Mechanics of Diving

The height, weight, center of gravity, and body proportion of the diver all affect performance, as will general athletic ability, diving skill and experience, and psychological condition.

Gabrielson (1985) collected detailed data on more than 300 spinal cord injuries due to diving in the United States, of which 200 occurred in pools. Gabrielson's research combined medical chart reviews, review of rescue squad reports, newspaper accounts, and litigation documents. He also visited 90% of the accident sites and interviewed 80% of the diving injured persons. He showed that inexperienced divers from springboards and high platforms typically dive in a different manner than experienced divers and put themselves at greater risk of injury. The inexperienced diver often runs in the approach, has a longer, faster hurdle jump, and is propelled a considerable distance from the end of the board. This is dangerous if the upward slope of the pool bottom from the diving well to the shallow end is not forward enough from the board. Inexperienced divers also tend to go off-line as they leave the board, which can be dangerous.

Gabrielson also described the typical profile of the person injured while diving:

- Male, between 18 and 31 years of age (none below the age of 12) who is close to 6 feet in height and weighs more than 175 pounds.
- Not intoxicated, but in 40% to 50% of cases had consumed some alcohol, usually beer.
- Had little or no training in diving and was visiting the pool for the first time. The dive made was the first one in that pool.
- Not warned, either verbally or by any signs, not to dive in that spot. Had witnessed other people diving before diving.
- Removed from the pool by friends who were not aware of a fractured neck. No spine board was used.
- Not aware of the risk of breaking the neck by making a dive in that spot.
- Quadriplegia resulted in 88% of the accidents. The most vulnerable vertebra was C_5 (29% of injuries); next was C_5-C_6 (27%).

The design and construction of a springboard can influence diving performance, as well as the height of the board from the water and the distance the board extends over the edge of the pool. In one study of diving injuries *all* springboard accidents had occurred in pools with spoon- or hopper-shaped bottoms.

Many more people dive from the deck of a pool than from a springboard (the ratio is estimated to be as high as 50 to 1), and the vast majority of such diving takes place in shallow water. Dives from starting blocks (usually mounted at the shallow end of pools with a water depth of only 3.5 to 4 feet) have become increasingly dangerous due to a trend to adopt a jackknife position (rather than the traditional flat dive) in competitive swimming starts. The swimmers are instructed to jackknife in the air to achieve an entry angle of almost 40 degrees, and then immediately steer up to surface. Failure to steer up properly, however, can cause contact with the pool floor.

A person diving from a deck into water 3.5 feet deep with an entry angle of 45 degrees has little time to correct a diving mistake or move arms into position for protection. Experienced divers usually enter the water with hands together and arms clamped on the sides of the head with the elbows locked. The untrained diver typically has the arms spread and bent at the elbows, which greatly diminishes the protection that arms can give to the head if the diver hits the bottom. Another common fault is that untrained divers tend to pull their arms back after entering water (leaving the head completely unprotected), or to surface too quickly by raising the head and arching the back.

The heavier the person the greater the loading on the spine will be if the head comes into contact with the bottom. However, relatively little impact on the pool bottom is required to cause spinal cord injuries, and most injured persons do not have noticeable abrasions or contusions to the head.

Pool design is an important factor in SCI (Gabrielson 1985). The point of transition, water depths, or the bottom of the pool are rarely marked, and thus are rarely apparent to the diver. Other important factors are poor lighting of the pool at night or a hopper-shaped bottom.

Diving thus involves the interaction of numerous factors, and accomplishment in this sport requires considerable training. Inexperienced divers believe themselves to be in control of their dive; in fact, they are not. Divers who have not had training require more, not less, area and depth in which to dive because their dives are unpredictable.

Diving in the Natural Environment

Gabrielson further discussed diving injuries that occurred in the natural environment (Gabrielson 1986). He identified 15 different types of locations for 71 injuries. The most frequent locations of accidents were docks and piers bordering lakes and rivers, and the beach or shore when running dives into the surf or lake were taken.

In the United States, diving injuries that occur in natural bodies of water can result in litigation, raising concern among those who manage land designated for recreational use. The dilemma becomes how to warn the public adequately of potential hazards without interfering with the enjoyment and beauty of the setting. This issue is far from resolved.

Water Slides

The only safe way to use a water slide is sitting in a head-up position with the back slightly arched and the palms up and forward. Most water slide injuries occur when the person goes down the slide in a head-first position. The factors influencing velocity are the overall height of the slide, the vertical height of the chute exit from the water surface, the angle and curvature of the slide bed, and the friction of the slide chute surface. The depth of water immediately under the chute exit is important, but of equal significance is the depth of the pool at a horizontal distance of 6 feet to 8 feet in front of the chute.

Responsibility for Diving Accidents

It is unreasonable to place full responsibility on divers for their own safety, as this would assume they have the training and experience to make sound judgments on the many complex factors that influence diving performance. For this reason, it is also wrong to assume that a person who is severely or fatally injured as a result of a diving accident has been fooling around or doing something wrong. Given the low level of public knowledge about the mechanics and hazards of diving, and the minimal effort that has gone into safe design of most private swimming pools, it is clear that the injured person simply was not able to recognize or evaluate the risks involved in the situation.

In the case of the natural setting, it is often best to avoid diving completely as it is impossible to monitor the wilderness and impractical to clear it of hazards.

Work-Related Injuries*

Every 11 minutes during the average 40-hour work week, an American worker is killed on the job. Every 4 seconds an American worker is disabled on the job, requiring time off work to recover. In 1986, these industrial accidents imposed a $34.8 billion burden on society, a tragic and unnecessary cost. Yet although this is a horrendous sum, it pales in comparison to the heartbreak, pain, and suffering associated with many of these accidents (National Safety Council 1986).

*This section is contributed by Wolfgang Zimmerman, Executive Director, Disabled Forestry Workers Foundation of Canada, Port Alberni, BC, Canada.

INJURED WORKER'S VIEWPOINT

Wolfgang Zimmerman was injured in an industrial logging accident in June 1977. He had worked as a faller for less than 5 days when the accident occurred and had not been adequately trained for the job. He suffered a SCI at the T_{12}–L_1 level.

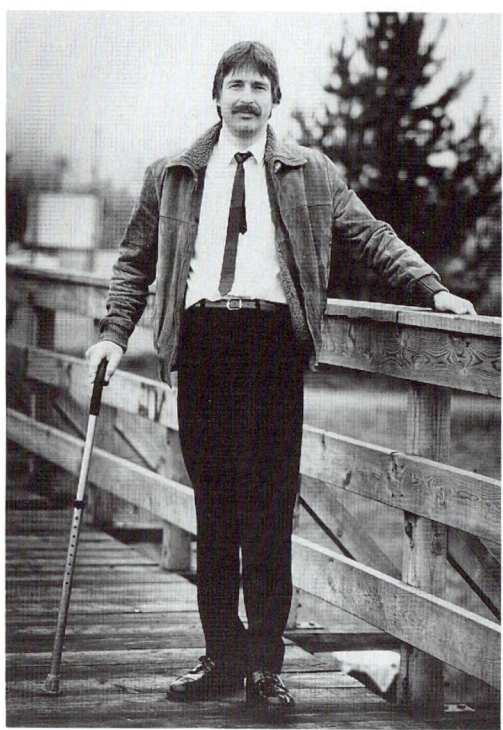

Wolfgang refused to settle for a wheelchair, and instead worked to ambulate with forearm crutches and leg braces. He continued with physical therapy for the next 5 years, progressing from the crutches to canes. Today he walks with the help of one cane and two light-weight, below-knee braces.

Wolfgang had earned a diploma in civil engineering and forest engineering that allowed him to return to work 6 months after the accident in an administrative capacity in the company's forestry division. However, 4 years later, the company, Canada's largest forest products corporation, terminated him and all the other disabled individuals at the same major division. The workers fought this decision with an extensive political and public relations campaign, and in so doing, they also exposed Canada's serious deficiencies in effective legislative policies regarding disabled people. Wolfgang and his colleagues won their case, and today, after retraining and earning a business administration diploma, he works as an accountant for the same company.

Personal Viewpoint

I enjoy working on home construction projects, having completed our house in stages. At the time of the accident, the house was not even roughly framed, and the intense frustration from not being able to continue without outside assistance—in fact being scarcely able to move on the construction site—was perhaps the most important factor in my desire to become mobile again. A strong desire to do the things I used to do—including social activities such as dancing, which I very much enjoy—inspired my drive to recover as much physical ability as possible.

A positive attitude, an uncompromising belief in the future, and physical effort cannot be sustained without a holistic support system that includes the patients' family, friends, employers, unions, and various medical professionals. I had been married for less than a year when the accident occurred, and I was fortunate to have a loving, caring wife on my side at all times, an employer who was willing to ensure my return to work, and a wonderful nurse named Cynthia Perry, whose compassion, dedication, and concern for my physical and mental well-being went well beyond her professional duties.

A comprehensive support system and a belief in a worthwhile yet realistic future are keys to maintaining a creative spirit, a hopeful soul, and a healthy body. All too often, when we hear of individuals who have attained their dreams, we only admire the achievement and fail to realize that without tremendous outside support, most of these individuals would not have succeeded.

Wolfgang Zimmerman

Occupational safety and health issues account for approximately 20% of total annual trauma even though this area has the greatest concentration of prevention efforts and initiatives. Nevertheless, these prevention efforts are highly developed and organized and have the greatest potential for reaching the greatest number of individuals on a cost-effectiveness scale.

Intensive industrial accident prevention programs began in the early part of the 20th century, the result of the often acrimonious accident compensation process of that time.

Accident compensation itself resulted from legal proceedings that required the plaintiff—either the injured worker or the company—conclusively to prove negligence, on the part of the defendant, that led to either injury, damage, or both. This process was highly unsatisfactory, expensive, and often traumatic. A sizable settlement could bankrupt a company, and the injured worker faced a physical disability compounded by severe financial difficulties. In turn, a no-fault insurance system was established, financed by employers, with employees' surrendering the right to civil tort action in exchange for certain guaranteed financial compensation.

Many variations of this system now exist throughout the world. Although these systems may be flawed, they nevertheless have provided an important basis for the development of sound, comprehensive, and innovative accident prevention systems. One important program is the Australian government's Comcare plan, which is described in Chapter 1. This workplace-based disability management program integrates prevention, rehabilitation, and compensation.

Although not typically included in SCI-specific prevention efforts, general promotion of safety at the workplace, including getting there and home again, encompasses similar prevention strategies to those presented in this chapter. Encouraging employees to be cautious can benefit the entire family, particularly when one or two corporations dominate community life. The National Head Injury Foundation (NHIF) offers corporations and businesses some of the most effective employee education programs for increasing seat belt use, both on and off the job (NHIF 1991). The same programs that aim to reduce head injury can be applied to SCI.

Coming to work with a clear mind and keeping it focused on getting the job done safely involves, among other things, staying off alcohol and drugs. Lack of concentration can disable and kill. Personal problems get in the way of concentration, too. Employee assistance programs can provide confidential, unbiased help, and participation needs to be encouraged.

Almost exclusively, Workers' Compensation plans are funded by employers. Contributions are based on a company's business type—for example, manufacturing, logging, or mining—and on the company's accident record. Thus, accident prevention is now a viable means for reducing business expenses. The effectiveness of this incentive varies among individual jurisdictions, depending on the assessment, penalty, and rating systems used by various compensation boards.

Apart from financial considerations concerning various forms of employer-funded insurance plans, industries in general have a major stake in a safe work environment: not only does this contribute to a more motivated, productive, and satisfied work force, but also, and more important, a poor safety performance can lead to deteriorating public relations, image, and credibility, with subsequent legal investigations and possible closure, license withdrawal, or bankruptcy.

The Role of Government in Worker Safety

Beginning with the first Workers' Compensation programs, state and federal governments have been concerned with accident prevention, primarily because of the substantial expense associated with accidents. Governments are subject to various pressures from a diverse range of interest groups. Industries often see elaborate safety regulations as a major expense, controlled exclusively by government.

Accident prevention programs and Workers' Compensation benefit payments can seriously affect a corporation's financial performance. Thus, industry tends to use its financial resources to reduce the size, format, and extent of these rules and regulations. On the other hand, when corporations show little regard for the trauma suffered by accident victims, the public and employee associations can be the balancing force to ensure a safe work environment for all employees. See "Responsibilities of Employee Associations" box in this chapter.

State and federal governments are under constant pressure for reduced occupational safety and health regulations. Therefore, public pressure must be exercised to guarantee a safe, healthy, and responsible work environment particularly in times of difficult economic circumstances when companies are tempted to reduce safety efforts and compliance as a means of cost reduction and improved financial performance.

Health Care Professionals and Worker Safety

Today health care is faced with ever-increasing demands for treatment, escalating costs, rising government deficits and ever-growing public pressure to reduce costs. These conditions are not confined to any one state, province, or country—they are universal. We can conceive of developing and implementing ideal approaches that could result in both optimum care and optimum return in terms of continued societal contribution by the injured person. However, these ideals are in stark contrast to today's realities.

All health care professionals should be encouraged to become active through professional organizations, political activities, and increased advocacy work. Such activism will build effective, compassionate, and caring support for people with disabilities and prevent additional injuries.

Human error causes 95% of all accidents (Disabled Forestry Workers of BC, 1990). The sawmill operator who fails to install safety guards around a moving blade and the powerboat driver running at night without lights can cause injuries that could have been avoided. Despite knowledge of basic safety rules and ongoing prevention programs, terrible tragedies happen. Health care professionals have great potential for effective, lasting, and direct impact. They, and people with disabilities, can illustrate from firsthand experience the effect of severe injuries and the disastrous results and impact on an individual's life much more effectively than textbook safety rules and presentations by so-called safety experts. Health care professionals have credibility that can persuade people to change their attitudes and actions.

DEVELOPMENT OF PREVENTION PROGRAMS

Injury prevention programs can be implemented at any of three levels (National Committee on Injury Prevention 1989):

Primary injury prevention includes those measures directed at prevention of the single episode referred to as an accident. By changing the behavior of a risk group, events (accidents) leading to injury are less likely to happen. Prevention education is an example.

Secondary prevention measures reduce the severity of injury once such an event happens. Examples would be changes in vehicle design, or the use of seat belts or air bags to minimize harm to the occupant in an automobile crash.

Tertiary preventive measures are designed to prevent or minimize the consequences of such an injury. Skilled and efficient ambulance services that prevent death from hemorrhage, acute care that prevents pressure sores, or aseptic urinary care to prevent urinary infections are examples of tertiary preventive measures.

Many SCI prevention programs exist, funded by various levels of government, the insurance industry, and automobile or liquor manufacturers. Some programs are included in workplace safety. Businesses may become involved because of impending legislation, for risk and cost containment, or as part of a public relations campaign. Most programs include education to increase the use of seat belts and to reduce alcohol consumption. No prevention program should ignore the major role of alcohol in events leading to injury.

Although most primary prevention program models concern smoking cessation and prevention of heart disease, prevention programs that identify risk factors related to injury are now being developed. A recent report discusses the National Adolescent Student Health Survey, conducted in 1987. This "is the first national survey since the 1960s to assess both the extent to which adolescent students in the United States may be at risk for several important health problems and their perceptions of these risks" (*Morbidity and Mortality Weekly Report* 1989). Publications such as this are valuable resources for developing new prevention strategies.

To raise public awareness that alcohol and risk activities do not mix safely, educational programs can target specific

Personal Viewpoint:
The Toney Lineberry Story

Toney Lineberry was a young champion wrestler obsessed with the sport, but on an icy winter night an automobile accident changed his life forever. He was not wearing a seat belt and lost the use of his hands and legs.

Yet Toney did not lose his heart and courage. He acquired a new obsession. Passionately studying highway safety, he was determined to find out how his accident could have been prevented. His story, *Twice a Champion* (available from 570 Seay Road, Manakin-Sabot, VA 23103), is devoted to preventing other people from enduring the tragic fate of spinal cord injury. It describes Toney's struggle to get back on top and truly discover what it means to be a champion. The photo album powerfully captures the momentum that builds through rehabilitation and into living with disability.

This book is endorsed by the National Highway Traffic Safety Administration. Toney's efforts are heart warming and full of inspirational, preventive insight for parents, teenagers, and health care professionals alike.

groups such as young drivers. Legislation can also reduce the association of alcohol with risk activities by, for example, lowering the legally acceptable blood alcohol level for motorists. Enforcement methods have included random roadside sobriety checkpoints. People who serve alcohol can be required not to serve alcohol to those who may drive and to limit the amount consumed by patrons; they may be held liable for the conduct of an intoxicated patron or guest (Canadian Medical Association Review 1989). In Vermont, drink calculators were given away at licensed alcohol outlets as part of an educational program encouraging self-regulation (Worden, Flynn, Merrill, Waller, and Haugh 1989). This self-regulation approach in association with media messages was shown to be effective in reducing alcohol use as measured by roadside checks. TV spots alone were found to be less effective (Worden et al. 1989). Nevertheless, such community interventions require careful evaluation (Graitcer 1989).

Drug and alcohol education introduced at an appropriate age in the school curriculum may encourage the development of positive lifelong social skills that will reduce the use of alcohol. Risk taking can be introduced as a concept into the school curriculum, so that the developing adult can become aware of the possibility of negative con-

sequences of an act. Conflict resolution skills may be taught to reduce the tendency to resort to violence, as is done in the Detroit program. See Table 3–1. This may be combined with legislation to reduce the availability of firearms.

If alcohol is a major factor in causing accidents, the compulsory use of seat belts is the single most important measure in reducing the number of deaths and injuries on the road, especially in frontal impacts. Some studies suggest that there should be no medical exemptions to the use of the seat belt (Dooley 1987), and others have shown that lives can be saved by making seat belt laws all-inclusive (Wells, Williams, and Fields 1989). On the other hand, it is difficult to ensure the consistent use of seat belts. Foss (1989) found that the compliance rate is affected by enforcement, although the rate remains variable despite educational and incentive programs. He also identified the extreme difficulty in (and importance of) reaching the preschool-aged child, and he indicated the need to understand the parent-child interactions that influence the use of seat belts by young children.

The educational approach to SCI prevention has received attention in most programs. The target group is young people in school who are approaching the age with the highest incidence of injury and have the most to lose if hurt. Prevention programs have also developed public service announcements (PSAs) and, occasionally, full media campaigns to reach the community at large.

Evaluation of the efficacy of programs is essential. Many early programs were not evaluated at all, some programs were evaluated poorly, and only a few were done well. Evaluation is vital because it is related to funding: a program will not be funded if no connection can be demonstrated between the program and a reduced injury rate. The best motivated exhortations to avoid injury are difficult to justify if the injury rate is unaffected. On the other hand, demonstrably successful programs can be replicated, to the benefit of the entire community.

Legislative changes may affect safety; many programs have joined coalitions to lobby for seat belts laws, for instance.

For an extensive review of current prevention programs, refer to *Resources: A National Directory of Spinal Cord Injury Prevention Programs* (University of Alabama-Birmingham 1990). A few of the better-known programs are summarized in Tables 3–1 and 3–2. These programs were innovators, providing either a different type of approach or an important contribution toward the difficult task of evaluation.

Other state and federal agencies and private organizations interested in injury prevention are listed in Table 3–3. These groups include state health, education, and natural resource departments, the National Park Service, the Centers for Disease Control, and the National Safety Council. Several programs stress the risks of diving into shallow or

TABLE 3–1   Spinal Cord Injury Prevention Programs

Program	General Information	Media Campaign	Special Features
United States:			
Head and Spinal Cord Injury Prevention Programs, Health Sciences Center, University of Missouri Columbia, MO	One of the earliest SCI prevention programs in the U.S. A model for other programs Sponsored by several key state agencies involved in public safety programs and policies including the Missouri departments of Public Safety, Highway Safety, Health, Coalition for Safety Belt Use, and the General Assembly	PSA's on TV concerning diving safety Program with poster distributed through Missouri's park services	Large assemblies in schools. See Table 3–2 Consultant to Ozark National Scenic Riverways staff. Trains new park personnel River area scouted to locate potential landing sites for air evacuation of injured persons National park literature for the public on hazards of diving and jumping Program for youthful speeding offenders that includes a day of instruction by hospital neurosurgery and rehabilitation personnel Workshops with Missouri Highway Patrol about enforcing Missouri seat belt law
Feet First First Time Also Known as "Think First" Hollywood, FL	Cost/benefit analysis by Florida Department of Health and Rehabilitative Services showed that the 2 districts with full prevention programs had a 6% reduction in SCI while the other 9 had an 11% increase.	Extensive media campaign Art work signs carved with the "Feet First First Time" posted at potentially hazardous diving areas	50–minute program in driver or physical education classes in high schools. Model for school presentations regarding spinal cord injuries. See Table 3-2
Play it Safe Pittsburgh, PA	Keystone Regional SCI System comprehensive prevention program Program based on private market research firm's survey of young adults' knowledge of factors related to SCI. Survey found: • Ignorance of effects of SCI • Overwhelmingly negative view of the life of an injured person • 95% knew of the dangers of drug and alcohol abuse (received mostly from schools)	Direct mail Year-round billboards PSAs at holidays and graduation season News releases about seasonal prevention tips	Kits, distributed to all grades, include brochures, diving posters, coloring books, parent guidelines 40–50 minute school presentations. See Table 3–2 Health fairs Presentations at public libraries, recreational facilities, area camps, youth group meetings Seminars for coaches and trainers
Spinal Cord Injury Prevention Program Fishersville, VA Shepherd Spinal Center Atlanta, GA	Founded in the 1980s at the Woodrow Wilson Rehabilitation Center		Presents to 62% of all state schools, especially senior high schools (and sometimes grades 8 and 9). See Table 3–2 Developed 2 videos: "The Time It Takes" on automobile injuries, and "Chances" on diving injuries Set up speakers bureau of volunteers, including persons with spinal cord injuries. Trains them to give informal talks to small audiences such as health or physical education classes

(Table continues)

TABLE 3–1   Spinal Cord Injury Prevention Programs (continued)

Program	General Information	Media Campaign	Special Features
United States:			
Violence Prevention Program	Sponsored by Southeastern Michigan Spinal Cord Injury System	Bumper stickers, buttons	Poster contest in schools
Detroit, MI	Focuses primarily on gunshot wounds, the primary cause of spinal cord injury in the region	Videotape of students with spinal cord injuries shown on CBS and cable networks	Students brought to the SCI unit in a hospital. Patients impressed students most
	Based on public health model of disease occurrence: violence is a complicated interaction among the environment, the host or victim, and the agent (a gun in the hand of an assailant)	Poster with slogan "One gunshot turned a participator into a spectator"	Produced videotape of students with spinal cord injuries describing how they were shot and what they might have done to avoid the incident
	Identifies predisposing behaviors: particularly risk taking in the host in arguments, fights, play with guns, association with known drug users or dealers		
Head and Spinal Cord Injury Prevention Program	Begun in 1987		Large assemblies presented in schools
Portland, OR	Sponsored by the Oregon Neurosurgical Society (See Nunwelt, Coe, Wilkinson, and Avolio 1989)		Evaluated by comparing schools that had assemblies with a control group of schools that did not have assemblies. See Table 3–2
Canada:			
Alberta Prevention and Research Foundation	Publishes newsletter		"Tagged for Life" program. Exposes drivers whose licenses have been suspended to the results of injury in a hospital setting
Edmonton, Alberta			"HEROES: A Program for Teenagers." A 1-hour audiovisual presentation on spinal cord injury and its consequences for high school audiences. Will include an evaluation component
Spinal Cord Injury Prevention Program (SCIP)	Established in 1987 to prevent injury through research, education, technical development, and enforcement	Speakers on radio and TV shows	Distributes educational materials from a variety of sources
Vancouver, BC	Sponsored by University Hospital (Shaughnessy Site) and the BC Paraplegic Association		Stresses community cooperation. Works with other education programs by sharing information, ideas, and funding sources
	Has a 5-member steering committee, 25-member advisory panel, and program manager		Speakers bureau of young spinal cord injured persons, supported by a local foundation, a large logging corporation, and governments
	Receives financial support from governments, corporations, community groups, health organizations, and private donations		Speaker training helps these young people in seeking employment. Speaker training kits available
			Extensively researched program that focuses on reduction of serious injuries, especially SCI and injuries to the head

(Table continues)

TABLE 3–1   Spinal Cord Injury Prevention Programs (continued)

Program	General Information	Media Campaign	Special Features
Canada:			
Royal Ottawa Rehabilitation Centre Ottawa, Quebec	Coordinated by a committee that includes the Red Cross, the Royal Lifesaving Society, and the Canadian Amateur Diving Association	Yearly media campaign that includes press releases and an audio PSA with the theme, "Dive Only from a Diving Board"	Information kit for pool owners that includes the B.C. Red Cross's "Safe Diving" brochure, the Royal Lifesaving Society's "It's Your Neck" brochure, the Ontario government's "It Doesn't Hurt to Help" brochure (which discusses liability laws concerning assistance at the scene of an accident). Distributed through local pool chemical suppliers Distributed the Red Cross's "My Boyfriend's Back" poster and the film "Harm's Way" to schools

unknown waters depending on the region targeted, although some programs focus only on aquatic risks for a specific target group.

ORGANIZING A PREVENTION PROGRAM

Procedure 3–1 describes how to start an injury prevention program. Developing prevention programs requires research. For instance, if the program goal is to increase the use of seat belts, it is important to search the literature on the subject. The program developers would read a report such as Maron and colleagues (1986), which examined the psychosocial and behavioral correlates of seat belt use among tenth graders in selected California high schools. Maron and associates (1986: 621) discovered that

> failure to wear seat belts was associated with a higher use of alcohol, cigarettes, marijuana, and cocaine; more tolerance for speeding and drinking while driving; less exercise; and preference for fat in the diet. Our findings attest to the power of parent and peer influence in shaping seat belt use by adolescents and suggests that not wearing seat belts can be conceptualized as one facet of general risk taking behavior.

Findings such as this are highly important in deciding on any educational intervention regarding seat belts.

Another consideration in organizing a program is understanding how problem behaviors are acquired and how they are maintained. For example, the reasons people begin to smoke may be quite different from the reasons (such as addiction) that they continue to smoke. In the case of risk factors involving injury, it may be important to understand whether prevention strategies should be directed at preventing the acquisition of undesirable behaviors or at modifying

factors that maintain undesirable behaviors (Chassin, Presson, and Sherman 1985: 615).

Educational approaches can be discussed in terms of routes, techniques, and materials.

Educational assemblies are one kind of *route* as are PSAs, which may be the best way to reach large numbers of people on a seasonal basis. Local radio and TV stations are often happy to include this material in their programming, and local newspapers may include verbatim copy sent to them. Every prevention group needs a person skilled and/or experienced in working with the media. However, PSAs alone have not been shown to change behavior.

Techniques include educational theory. Seek advice about how to teach, how often to repeat the message, and when to teach for the best effect. Although people with SCI provide the most effective voice in established programs, these people must be trained; the training and experience will be of benefit not only to the prevention program, but also to these individuals as a future job skill. An honorarium will usually be necessary.

Materials produced can be simple brochures or expensive videos. Local students may be willing and able to produce a video at cost if there is a special need in the region not met in currently available material.

Set realistic objectives. Recognize the group's limitations when starting out. Some educational interventions may be only a beginning, merely calling public attention to a serious problem such as SCI. Programs that will measurably reduce these devastating injuries may require the commitment of massive resources and time. Resources should become more available when the public and decision makers become more aware of the devastating impact of SCI on those people affected. According to Pless and Arsenault (1987: 102).

> In general, it appears programs based on social learning principles are more successful than those relying on traditional approaches. Overall, the most successful are programs that combine education with legislative change or

TABLE 3–2 Sample Prevention Programs for School Assemblies (continued)

Program	Speakers	Assembly Schedule and Content	Evaluation
Head and Spinal Cord Injury Prevention Programs Columbia, MO	Young spinal cord injured person Paramedic	• Show film "Harm's Way" • Lecture about SCI • Discussion led by a young person with SCI • Discussion of secondary injuries • Demonstration by a paramedic of how to handle an injured person and how to get emergency help • Students try a wheelchair obstacle course	Follow-up study of students who attended assembly showed significant retention of safety information 3 years later. They used seat belts more frequently; were less likely to ride with friends who had been drinking; and knew more about how to prevent injuries than a control group.
Feet First First Time Hollywood, FL	Registered nurse Vocational rehabilitation counselor Person with SCI, usually of the same age and community as the audience Sometimes includes emergency medical personnel or physicians	(50–minute program, given in driver or physical education classes.) • Distribute brochures (5 minutes), and ask students to write questions throughout the presentation for later discussion • Describe SCI (10 minutes): slides and lecture by nurse • Show film "Harm's Way" • SCI speaker (10 minutes): emphasis on permanence of SCI • Q&A (15 minutes). Students discuss how SCI affects daily activities; emotional impact of injury • Summary: first student to answer a review question correctly wins a T-shirt	
Play it Safe Pittsburgh, PA	Spinal cord injured person sometimes speaks	(40–50 minute program) • Lecture with slides on understanding SCI, its causes, and the life of a person with paraplegia or quadriplegia; learning how to prevent accidents and participate safely in high-risk activities • 10–minute film ("Consequences") • Q&A session • Students given brochures about seat belt use, drinking and driving, diving, and football at end of presentation	Questionnaires sent before and after presentation, with testing of some students 3 months later. Knowledge was retained longer and increased more than attitudes were changed. Males did not retain the information on the follow-up test.
Spinal Cord Injury Prevention Program Fishersville, VA	Two speakers, one of whom is a young person with SCI. Speakers are trained to work as a team.	(Presentations during assembly, physical education or health education classes) • Introduction of speakers. Spinal cord injured person talks (5–10 minutes), first about high school experience and then about the injury and its consequences • Film (10 minutes), either "Consequences" or "Harm's Way" • Slide show (10 minutes) gives statistics of incidence of SCI, alcohol use, seat belt use, and MVAs • Spinal cord anatomy demonstration using a model of the spinal column (5 minutes) • Q&A (15–20 minutes) • Conclusion (5 minutes): Short film from Chrysler "Seat Belts Save Lives" • Brochures distributed with a picture of spinal cord, a description of its function, and statistics	Questionnaires given to schools to distribute to participating students after presentation.

(Table continues)

TABLE 3–2 Sample Prevention Programs for School Assemblies (continued)

Program	Speakers	Assembly Schedule and Content	Evaluation
Head and Spinal Cord Injury Prevention Program Portland, OR (Begun in 1987 by the Oregon Neurological Society)	Young spinal cord injured persons Paramedic	(Large assembly format) • Film about causes and results of head and spinal cord injuries • Young speaker who has had such an injury • Paramedic presentation about what bystanders should do • Wheelchair obstacle course Reinforcement activities being considered as a way to strengthen impact	Students' knowledge significantly improved in 3 of the 4 experimental schools, but no difference was reported in attitude and behavior measures (observing shoulder-belt use in school parking lot 2 weeks before and after assembly) between the group of schools with assemblies and the control group of schools. See Neuwelt et al. 1989.

modifications in regulations. The policy implication of these findings is that heavy investment in health education of the traditional kind, if used in isolation, will have only limited success. Instead, strategies that use health education along with other preventive strategies are most likely to achieve the goal of reducing the frequency of severity of nonintentional injuries to children.

Table 3–2 highlights the features of several school assembly programs. Some programs are given to small groups—for instance a health education class—and other programs are designed for large assemblies. Schools in the Head and Spinal Cord Injury Prevention Program in Portland, Oregon, did not want to use the assembly format. They argued that material would have greater impact in smaller groups; that students were required to be in the classroom for a specified number of hours each year; that students had poor behavior during assemblies; and that assemblies are disruptive to regular classroom schedules. However, four schools agreed to feature the program. Three other schools were selected to act as controls. See Table 3–2 for the evaluation of the assembly program format. Students were well behaved even in very large assemblies but possibly there were too many topics in too short a time to bring about specific behavioral change. The cost of the program is modest, however, and even the slight increase in knowledge is considered sufficient reason to continue the program.

Many professional and advocacy organizations play an active role in prevention; it is important for each group to identify a specific role and collaborate with others to avoid duplication and maximize efforts. However, each group should promote safety messages relevant to their local injury pattern or target group and provide guidance in techniques and educational materials. Concerned individuals are necessary instigators; many important prevention activities began when someone cared enough to get involved. The National Committee on Injury Prevention (1989) recommends these guidelines:

• Do not try to reinvent the wheel; build on other people's efforts.
• It takes a long time to make a difference.
• Individuals make a difference.

National Trauma Awareness Month

Since 1988, the American Trauma Society has sponsored National Trauma Awareness Month (NTAM) in May. An extensive media campaign for NTAM includes billboard signs, information exhibits in shopping malls, community awareness days or health fairs, state and local proclamations, bike rodeos and other activities to promote SAFE KIDS Week (also in May), local news conferences, student contests (essay, trauma awareness, poster), safety lectures to high schools, trauma room and helicopter tours for the public, rescue demonstrations, and safety messages inserted with employee paychecks. The ATS sponsors national media PSAs and encourages its grass-roots organization to produce newsletters and to seek radio and TV coverage of local events.

The ATS requests a congressional proclamation for NTAM each year. It distributes to local groups sample promotional packets that include media tip sheets, sample news releases and PSAs, questions and answers for talk shows, a resource list and order forms, and an evaluation form. It sponsors news conferences on trauma prevention legislation that generate national coverage in newsletters and newspapers, and on TV and radio.

TABLE 3–3 Selected Organizations and Agencies Interested in Safety Issues

Prevention Programs of State and Federal Agencies (U.S.)

Centers for Disease Control/Centers for Injury Control	The Centers for Disease Control encourage state health departments to declare injury a priority and have funded five demonstration projects on injury control in health departments and universities.
National Park Service	Administers the national parks, recreational sites for large numbers of people. The headquarters in Washington, DC, has a safety office, and the parks themselves have staff designated to address safety issues. The national parks collect data on all incidents that occur within their boundaries. Some national parks are very receptive to collaborative efforts to provide safety messages to the public, especially about diving.
State Education Departments	Can be powerful allies in disseminating messages to school children about head and spinal injuries.
State Health Departments	State health departments may establish trauma registries or registries for head injuries, spinal cord injuries, or both and collect other data to evaluate the effectiveness of injury prevention programs. County and local health agents can be valuable allies in reinforcing safety messages. They may assist in follow-up and evaluation of programs, or incorporate materials of other prevention programs in their own outreach efforts.
State Natural Resources Departments	These departments may disseminate information about diving safety and such specialty recreation activities as the use of ATVs. They may have jurisdiction over state land used for recreational pursuits.

Private Organizations and Special Projects

United States:

American Academy of Pediatrics	The Injury Prevention Program (TIPP) provides materials for providing anticipatory guidance to parents and children.
American Farm Bureau Federation	Local chapters of this federation have extensive outreach potential in rural communities.
American Public Health Association	This group and the National Environmental Health Association develop standards and regulations pertaining to diving for pools and swimming areas.
American Spinal Injury Association (ASIA)	Along with other organizations such as the American Association of SCI Nurses and the National Coordinating Council on SCI, ASIA encourages members to initiate and participate in prevention activities and endorses and supports selected programs.
American Trauma Society (ATS)	Nationwide voluntary health organization of individuals, institutions, and businesses founded in 1967 to improve emergency care. A national clearinghouse on trauma information, ATS cooperates with other organizations such as SAFE KIDS, National Buckle-Up Week, and National Drunk and Drugged Driving Awareness Week. It sponsors National Trauma Awareness Month each May, and it uses a grass-roots network to stimulate support of appropriate federal legislation. Also see National Trauma Awareness Month box in this chapter. ATS has a grass-roots network of trauma-care professionals and lay persons who educate their communities on trauma prevention. It has produced many educational materials describing trauma and its effects and presents trauma experts in radio, TV, and print media.
Aquatic Injury Safety Foundation (AISF)	Makes presentations at various conferences and committee hearings to press for better safety standards for pools and pool equipment and better enforcement of standards. AISF produces warning signs for swimming areas and a small handout, "Safe Diving Rules," which was distributed through the school system and paid for by an insurance company. The group also encourages media coverage of court cases involving diving accidents and acts as a general clearinghouse for information. It is working to have either insurance companies or municipal governments do mandatory checks on backyard swimming pools.
Consumer Product Safety Commission	Consumer alerts from this commission offer valuable information regarding safety.
Mothers Against Drunk Driving (MADD)	Activities focus on prevention of alcohol-related MVAs. Also has a victim assistance program (1–800–GET–MADD).

(Table continues)

TABLE 3–3   Selected Organizations and Agencies Interested in Safety Issues (continued)

Private Organizations and Special Projects

National Head and Spinal Cord Injury Prevention Program (NHSCIP)	Sponsored by the American Association of Neurological Surgeons and the Congress of Neurological Surgeons and based on programs in Missouri and Florida (described in Table 3–1). NHSCIP provides a detailed instruction guide/syllabus and other materials to assist people interested in launching similar programs in their own regions. Interested persons may also attend a school presentation and meet with program personnel to discuss budgets and administration. NHSCIP sponsored the film, "Harm's Way," which features 26 young people with head and spinal cord injuries.
National SAFE KIDS Campaign Washington, DC	Interested in the five areas of greatest risk for preteens. SAFE KIDS is a collaborative project of Children's Hospital in Washington, DC, Johnson & Johnson, and the National Safety Council. The campaign sponsors SAFE KIDS Week in May and grass-roots coalitions in communities throughout the United States. It also sponsors PSAs and provides materials for children and parents. It can provide many ideas regarding how to conduct local safety campaigns.
National Safety Council	Provides comprehensive information about most safety programs in the United States. Call the council (1–800–848–5588) for phone numbers of other private organizations listed in this Table.
National SCI Association	Provides a national information line (1–800–962–9629) and has an active SCI prevention committee. Various educational materials and national resource directory available.
National Spa and Pool Institute (NSPI)	The institute's materials stress the responsibility of divers to learn how to "steer up" on entering the water, thus avoiding injury. It produced a brochure, "Learning How To Dive," and a film, "Learning How To Dive Safely." NSPI provides a four-page booklet, "The Sensible Way To Enjoy Your Pool," in cooperation with the U.S. Consumer Product Safety Commission.
National Swimming Pool Safety Commission	Established in 1985 by the U.S. Consumer Product Safety Commission and the NSPI to address child drowning and diving accidents.
Canada:	
Canadian Paraplegic Association	Coordinates national SCI prevention program to reduce injury rate. Develops school curricula, works with government agencies, police forces, health professionals, insurance groups, and nonprofit organizations. Aims to establish a national data base for injury surveillance. Excellent coordinating resource (1–604–324–3611, BC Division).
Canadian Red Cross B.C./Yukon Division	Has had a Spinal Injury Prevention Education Project for several years. In 1986–1987 this group developed a "Safe Diving" brochure and miniposter, and a full-size, full-color poster with the slogan, "My Boyfriend's Back." It also produced a supplement to the Red Cross Instructor's Guide and Reference Manual, used by instructors across Canada. The supplement provides water safety instructors with information regarding the prevention of spinal injuries.
Canadian Sports Spine and Head Injuries Research Centre, Toronto Western Hospital	Focuses on preventing hockey and diving accidents. It has hosted international conferences on catastrophic head and spinal cord injury resulting from sports. The center has collaborated with the Canadian Amateur Hockey Association to have rules for amateur hockey changed so that checks from behind (which can send players head first into the boards) are prohibited. The center has also developed a brochure on neck and spine conditioning exercises to prevent injuries among hockey players.

Procedure 3–1 Starting a Prevention Program

Action	Rationale
1. Read and gather information. Obtain materials referenced at the end of this chapter and in the Resources section at the end of this book.	Self-education improves the ability to interpret information and apply benefits to the community.
• Review the videos	Videotapes are especially good motivators.
• Call other people who have successful programs	Other programs are usually glad to share tips on how to achieve success and avoid failure.

(Procedure continues)

Procedure 3–1 Starting a Prevention Program (continued)

Action	Rationale
2. Define and quantify the problem of SCI in your community. • Obtain regional statistics • Identify causes (including risk behaviors) • Identify significant trends related to injury	The causes and seasonal timing of SCI vary from region to region. Knowledge of local causes is especially important when seeking funding for a particular program and planning strategies to combat the causes.
3. Link with other interested local, state, and/or national groups; role models for the target group (teachers or coaches, for example); media experts.	Document information and make resources available to other groups that may be interested in similar activities. A coalition of groups representing a number of interests can be very effective in the injury prevention field. See Table 3–3 for suggestions of appropriate groups.
4. Define regional priorities.	Funding may restrict an ambitious program, requiring a more realistic compromise.
5. Define the target groups. Is it school-aged children? Recreational users of water resources? Off-road vehicle users?	
6. Identify the target group's risk factors and problem behaviors. This will probably require research.	It is important to offer low-risk or no-risk alternatives to high-risk behaviors and know what the target group should do differently after exposure to the program.
7. Study how problem behaviors are acquired. Distinguish between causative factors and factors that maintain undesirable behaviors.	It is important to understand whether prevention strategies should be directed at preventing the acquisition of undesirable behaviors or at modifying factors that maintain undesirable behaviors (Chassin, Presson, and Sherman 1985).
8. Develop corrective strategies, a mix of interventions. For instance: • Education to modify behavior • Legislation, which may require lobbying • Collaboration with other groups	
9. Make a plan and define priorities, which may include:	Most groups cannot do everything at the beginning. It is vital to the health and credibility of the program to take time to determine goals and mission, and to develop a systematic, long-range plan.
• Research: create retrospective and prospective data bases and participate in studies related to current trends, for example, drug and alcohol abuse	Data bases are an integral part of any prevention program. A data base manual with draft computer program is available (Wing 1991). Research fuels injury prevention strategies. Cooperative funding is usually necessary and results ultimately in more widespread effect.
• Education: presentation development and speaker training with the dominating theme, "Prevent injuries, take smart risks"	If people are trained and know their abilities, physical environment, and attitudes, they will be better able to avoid injury.
• Resource collection and/or production: videos, brochures, posters, etc.	Young people are used to seeing and respond well to high tech productions.
• Use existing programs	Purchasing materials saves time and effort.
• Public relations and media campaigns, PSAs	
• Enforcement of safety regulations and technical development	A prevention program can help by collecting briefing materials and data—for example, monitoring injury/death rates on a stretch of highway in order to improve roadways, or lobbying to change manufacturer warnings on ATVs.
10. Implement the project and enlist or employ a manager.	A creative and competent manager is essential for running a successful program.
11. Evaluate results.	Some form of evaluation should be a part of any prevention program. Surveillance can show incidence trends in the region by comparison of retrospective and prospective data bases, especially important if it can be shown that the injury rate is being reduced. Attitude, and preferably behavior change, should be monitored in the target group. See Table 3–2 for examples of evaluation procedures.
12. Develop financial plans for continued implementation and expansion of the program.	Working with such well-established organizations as departments of education helps to develop and secure long-term plans.

REFERENCES

Boyd, M. C., and Schweigel, J. F. 1985. Diving related spinal injuries in British Columbia. *British Columbia Medical Journal* 27 (6): 391–394.

Canadian Medical Association Review. 1989. Substance abuse and driving. *Canadian Association Journal* (June suppl.).

Carr, W. P., Brandt, D., and Swanson, K. 1981. Injury patterns and helmet effectiveness among hospitalized motorcyclists. *Minnesota Medicine* 64: 521–527.

Chassin, L. A., Presson, C. C., and Sherman, S. J. 1985. Stepping backward in order to step forward: An acquisition oriented approach to primary prevention. *Journal of Consulting and Clinical Psychology* 53: 612–622.

Disabled Forestry Workers of British Columbia. 1990. It Happens Every 12 Seconds. Brochure.

Dooley, B. J. 1987. Medical significance of occupant restraint on road-crash victims and the role of the medical profession. *Canadian Journal of Surgery* 30: 400–402.

Fife, D., and Kraus, J. 1986. Anatomic location of spinal cord injury—Relationship to the cause of injury. *Spine* 11 (1): 2–5.

Foege, W. H., et al. 1985. *Injury in America: A continuing public health problem*. Committee on Trauma Research, Commission on Life Sciences, National Research Council and the Institute of Medicine. Washington, DC: National Academy Press.

Foss, R. D. 1989. Evaluation of a communitywide incentive program to promote safety restraint use. *American Journal of Public Health* 79 (3): 304–306.

Gabrielson, M. A. 1985. How injuries occur and what approaches might be appropriate to reduce injuries. Paper presented to the National Pool and Spa Safety Association Conference, May 14, 1985.

Gabrielson, M. A. 1986. Diving injuries—A critical look at the problem. Paper presented to the National Aquatic Management School in Temple, Arizona, April 7, 1986.

Graitcer, P. L. 1989. Evaluating community interventions to reduce drunken driving. *American Journal of Public Health* 79 (3): 271.

Huelke, D. F., et al. 1981. Cervical injuries suffered in automobile crashes. *Journal of Neurosurgery* 54: 316–322.

Jessor, R., and Jessor, S. L. 1977. *Problem behavior and psychosocial development: A longitudinal study of youth*. New York: Academic Press.

Jonah, B. A. 1989, September. Age differences in risky driving. Paper presented at the Conference on Risk-Taking Behavior in Youth: Perspectives and Strategies. Toronto, Ontario, Canada.

Koop, C. E. n. d. Trauma is no accident. A brochure published by the American Trauma Society, Landover, Maryland.

Kraus, J. F., Morgenstern, H., Fife, D., Conroy, C., and Nourjah, P. 1989. Blood alcohol tests, prevalence of involvement, and outcome following brain injury. *American Journal of Public Health* 79 (3): 294–299.

Kraus, J. F., Frantin, C. E., and Riggins, R. S. Neurologic outcome and vehicle and crash factors in motor vehicle related spinal cord injuries. *Neuroepidemiology* 1: 223–238.

Maron, D. J., Telch, M. J., Killen, J. D., Vranizan, K. M., Saylor, K. E., and Robinson, T. N. 1986. Correlates of seat-belt use by adolescents: Implications for health promotion. *Preventive Medicine* 15: 614–623.

Mercer, G. W. 1988. *Motorcycle casualty traffic accidents: Trends, characteristics, persons involved, and consequences* (Counter Attack Research Papers). Victoria, BC: Ministry of the Attorney General.

Mercer, G. W. 1987. Fatality-producing vs. injury-only traffic accidents: Trends, characteristics, persons involved, and consequences (Counter Attack Research Papers). Victoria, BC: Ministry of the Attorney General.

Morbidity and Mortality Weekly Report. 1989. Results from the National adolescent student health survey. 38: 147–150.

National Committee on Injury Prevention. 1989. Injury prevention, meeting the challenge. Supplement to the *American Journal of Preventive Medicine* 5 (3). Oxford University Press. *Should be read by everyone seriously interested in the prevention field. An excellent introduction to the principles of injury prevention, with a chapter for each of several specific injury patterns and detailed recommendations for prevention based on research work to date.*

National Head Injury Foundation (NHIF). 1991. *Head Injury Prevention* (Corporate Safety Belt Program). Southborough, MA: Author.

National Safety Council. 1986. Brochure.

National Swimming Pool Safety Commission. 1986. Report of the Data Sub-Committee. October 10, 1986.

Neuwelt, E. A., Coe, M. F., Wilkinson, A. M., and Avolio, A. E. C. 1989. Oregon head and spinal cord injury prevention program and evaluation. *Neurosurgery* 24 (3): 453–458.

Pless, I. B., and Arsenault, L. 1987. The role of health education in the prevention of injuries to children. *Journal of Social Issues* 43: 87–103.

Pyper, A. J., and Black, B. G. 1988. Orthopaedic injuries in children associated with the use of off-road vehicles. *Journal of Bone and Joint Surgery* 70 (2): 275–281.

Rimel, R., et al. 1982, October. A prospective study of severity of cns trauma and vehicular accidents. 26th Annual Proceedings, American Association for Automotive Medicine, Ottawa, Ontario, Canada.

Sneed, R. C., et al. 1986. Spinal cord injury associated with all-terrain vehicle accidents. *Pediatrics* 77 (3): 271–274.

Stover, S. L., and Fine, P. 1986. *Spinal Cord Injury: The Facts and Figures*. Birmingham, AL: University of Alabama at Birmingham.

Tator, C. H., and Palm, J. 1981. Spinal injuries in diving: Incidence high and rising. *Ontario Medical Review* 48: 628–631.

Tonkin, R. S. 1981. Child Health Profile: Violence in adolescence (Child Health Profile Mini Series No 2). Vancouver, BC: Vancouver Public Health Department.

Tonkin, R. S. 1987. Adolescent risk-taking behavior. *Journal of Adolescent Health Care* 8 (2): 213–220.

University of Alabama-Birmingham, Department of Rehabilitation Medicine, Spain Rehabilitation Center. 1990. *Resources: A National Directory of Spinal Cord Injury Prevention Programs*. Birmingham, AL: Author. *A widely distributed directory to help minimize duplica-*

tion of efforts, increase awareness, and identify gaps in existing prevention materials. Sponsored by NIDRR.

Wells, J. K., Williams, A. F., and Fields, M. 1989. Coverage gaps in seat belt use laws. *American Journal of Public Health* 79 (3): 332–333.

Wiley, J. J. 1986. The dangers of off-road vehicles to young drivers. *Canadian Medical Association Journal* 135: 1345–1346.

Wiley, J. J., et al. 1989. Injuries associated with off-road vehicles among children. *Canadian Medical Association Journal* 135: 1365–1366.

Wing, P. C. 1991. SCIP Data Base Program. Unpublished manuscript, University Hospital, Shaughnessy Site, Vancouver, BC.

Worden, J. K., Flynn, B. S., Merrill, D. G., Waller, J. A., and Haugh, L. D. 1989. Preventing alcohol impaired driving through community self-regulation training. *American Journal of Public Health* 79 (3): 287–290.

Yeo, J. D. 1979. Five year review of spinal cord injuries in motorcyclists. *Medical Journal of Australia* 2: 381.

Young, J. S., Burns, P. E., and Wilt, G. A. 1982. Medical charges incurred by the spinal cord injured during the first six years following injury. *Spinal Cord Injury Digest* 4: 19–34.

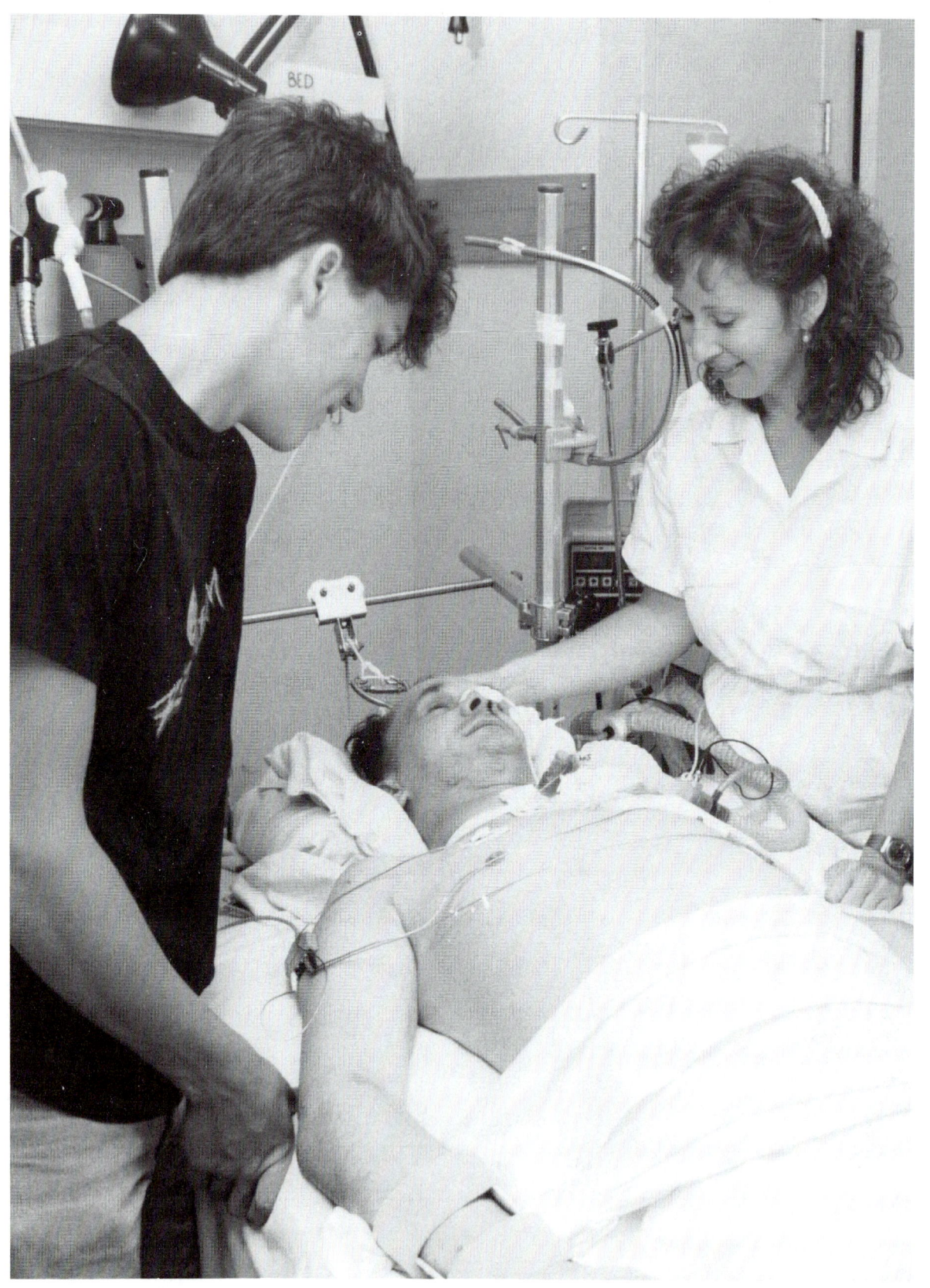

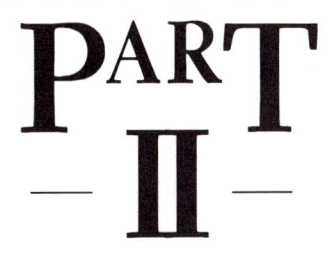

PART
II

CRITICAL DECISIONS: EARLY ASSESSMENT AND CARE

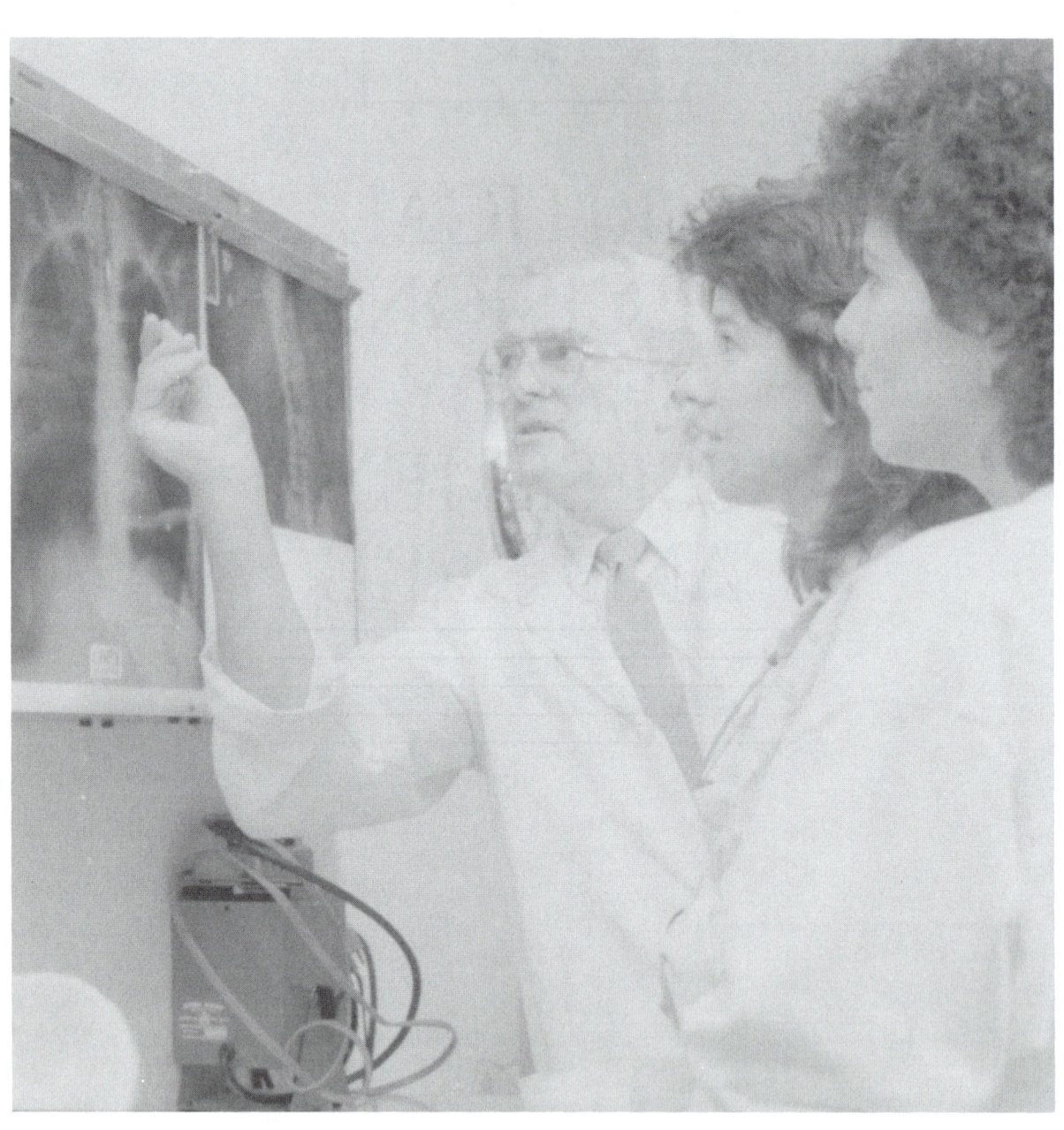

CHAPTER
— 4 —

Physiological Consequences and Assessment of Injury to the Spine and Spinal Cord*

Chapter Outline

*This chapter was developed with assistance from James S. Keene, M.D., and Thomas A. Zdeblick, M.D.

Health Care Objectives

- To understand the spine and factors that govern stability
- To understand the structure and function of the spinal cord, spinal nerves, and autonomic nervous system
- To anticipate dysfunctions following spinal cord trauma as related to the level of injury sustained
- To recognize factors that contribute to SCI

- To implement appropriate physical assessment techniques and diagnostic procedures
- To provide a correct and accurate diagnosis on which to initiate appropriate management
- To establish reliable baseline date with which all future physical assessments can be compared to determine improvement or deterioration and to evaluate progress
- To develop realistic goals for physical rehabilitation that will restore as much functional activity as possible

In order to deliver competent specialized care to the spinal cord injured person, it is essential to understand the spinal cord and its role in the integration of body function and movement. Closely related to the neurological assessment is assessment of vertebral column injury. A correct and accurate diagnosis of the physiological consequences of spinal cord injury (SCI) is the first fundamental step in delivery of comprehensive health care.

This chapter focuses on assessment skills and will help to identify immediate and potential problems; establish realis-

tic goals for physical rehabilitation; and offer reassurance, guidance, and health education for patients and families.

THE SPINE

The spine is composed of 33 individual and fused vertebrae, sharing certain common characteristics and grouped according to site and function. See Figure 4–1. There are 7 cervical, 12 thoracic, and 5 lumbar vertebrae; the sacral and

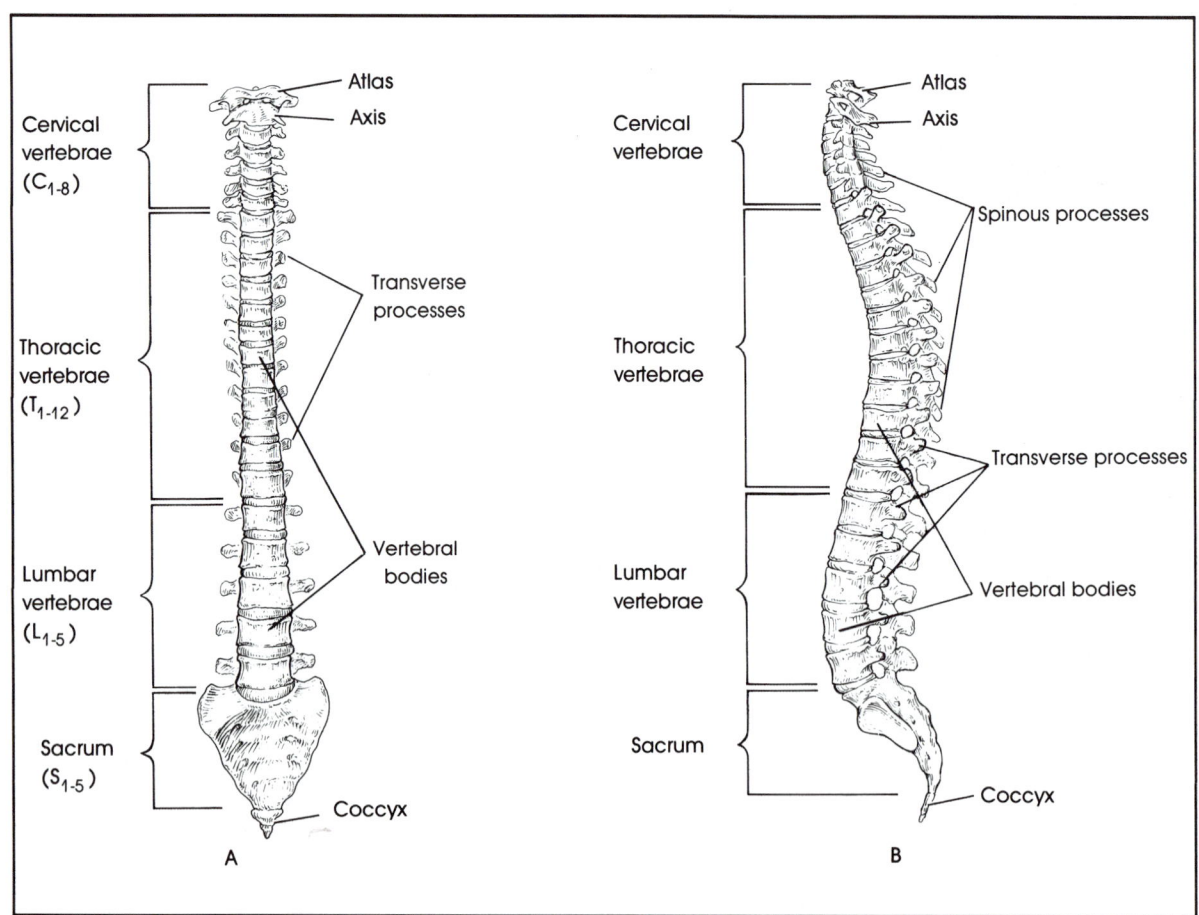

FIGURE 4–1   Anterior (A) and lateral (B) views of the vertebral column.

coccygeal vertebrae are fused in the adult to form the sacrum and coccyx or tail bone. The vertebral column is strong and flexible because it is composed of separate bones connected by tough, fibrous tissues called ligaments and cushioned by cartilaginous discs. Contributing to control and balance of the spinal column are the stabilizing rib cage, the superficial and deep trunk muscles, and the natural curvatures of the spine.

Vertebrae

All the vertebrae, with the exception of the first cervical vertebra, share general features but differ slightly according to their function and level in the body. Each vertebra consists of a body (anterior) and an arch (posterior). See Figure 4–2.

Each arch is composed of two paired *pedicles*, which attach the arch to the disc body; two paired *laminae*, which form the roof of the arch to complete the structure; and seven *processes* or bony protrusions—two above and two below (*superior* and *inferior facets*), two at the sides (*transverse processes*), and one behind (*spinous process*). These articulating surfaces form the *neural* (vertebral) *arch*. The spinal foramina of the vertebrae provide bony protection for the cord by forming the *spinal canal*. See Figure 4–3.

The vertebrae in different portions of the spine have different sizes and shapes and directions of processes. For example, the transverse processes in the lumbar area are large to accommodate the attachment of lower limb muscles; in the thoracic area they possess tubercles or stumps for rib attachments; and in the cervical area they have openings to admit the generous arterial blood supply.

Different vertebrae also have functional differences. The lumbar vertebrae allow for powerful flexion and some extension; the thoracic vertebrae limit movement, and, at the

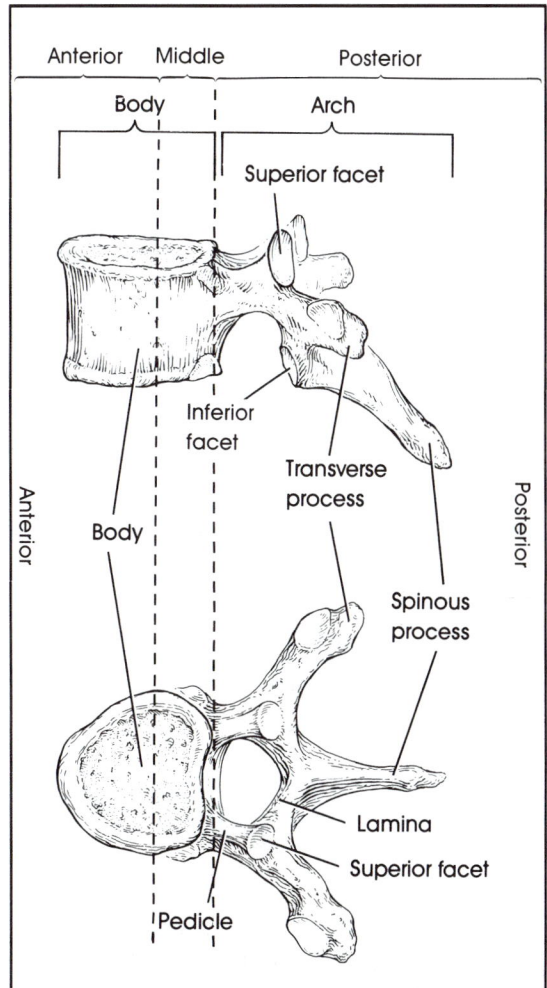

FIGURE 4–3 A lateral view and cross-section of a vertebra detailing the vertebral arch.

cervical level, the atlas (C_1) and the axis (C_2) are so formed as to allow flexion, extension, and rotation of the head. Vertebral bodies generally increase in size to bear additional weight as they descend. The sacrum unites the vertebral column with the pelvis.

Intervertebral Connections (Discs and Ligaments)

Vertebral bodies are joined by intervertebral cartilaginous discs. These discs are made of a tough outer shell and a soft, gelatinous center that acts as a shock absorber and weight-bearing structure. With age, the gelatinous nucleus becomes firmer, offering less protective cushioning of the spine.

Two major longitudinal ligaments run from the atlas to the sacrum on the front and back surfaces of the bodies and discs, holding them in alignment. See Figure 4–4.

Vertebral arches are joined to each other up and down the spinal column by short, dense ligaments. Ligamenta flava run between laminae, supraspinal and interspinal

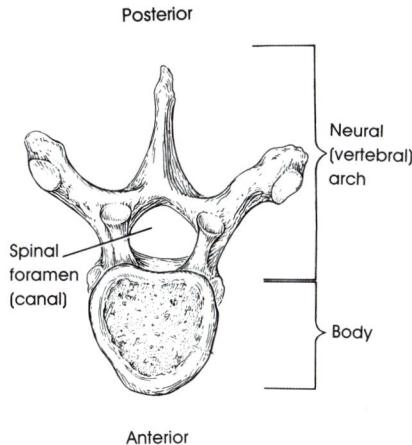

FIGURE 4–2 A simple cross-section of a vertebra.

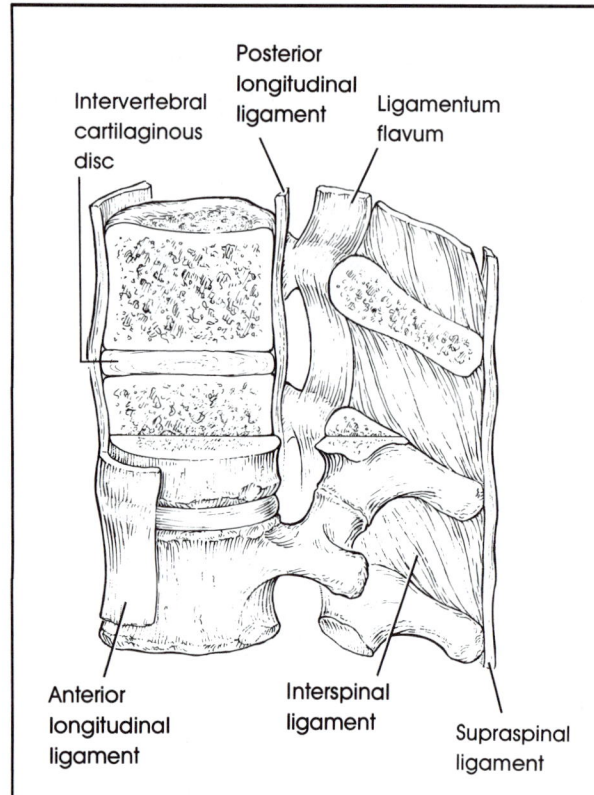

FIGURE 4–4 A median section through vertebrae illustrating the supporting ligaments.

ligaments run between spinous processes, and the inter-transverse ligaments run between the transverse processes. See Figure 4–5. These ligaments protect the spine against undesirable movement such as severe hyperextension or extreme flexion. Table 4–1 summarizes specific features of the vertebral column.

THE SPINAL CORD AND SPINAL NERVES

The *central nervous system* is composed of the brain and spinal cord. The spinal cord is essentially an extension or elongation of brain tissue, sharing similar functions and protective structures of bone, meninges (coverings), and cerebrospinal fluid.

The *systemic (peripheral) nervous system* is composed of the cranial and spinal nerves, which extend from the brain and spinal cord to branch out into many free nerve endings over the entire body. The basic structural and functional unit of the nervous system is the *neuron*, or nerve cell. The cell body, which contains the nucleus, is the vital center; any injury to this area results in degeneration of the distal segments. Typically in the spinal cord, the *motor* neuron has *dendrite* projections that extend off the cell bodies and

act as receptor membranes; a single, long, fibrous *axon* that originates in the cell body serves to conduct impulses away from the dendrite zone to various termination points. The axon acquires a *myelin sheath*, containing a protein-lipid complex required for nourishment and function. Today, much hope for regeneration research focuses on the isolation, identification, and synthetic reproduction of these proteins to help cure paralysis. Efforts to reproduce cell bodies from fetal cell transplants are ethically debatable and have not been successful to date.

The main properties that distinguish neurons from other types of cells are (Liebman 1979):

- Their specialization for conduction of impulses
- Their great sensitivity to oxygen deprivation
- Their importance for many vital functions
- The fact that they don't multiply or regenerate once destroyed (as would a broken bone or damaged skin)

This last fact is responsible for the irreversible damage caused by spinal cord injury.

The Spinal Cord

The spinal cord runs through the hollow canal (formed by the spinal foramina) in the center of the vertebral column and is a cylindrical, pliable structure that extends from the brain, starting at the foramen magnum and ending at the

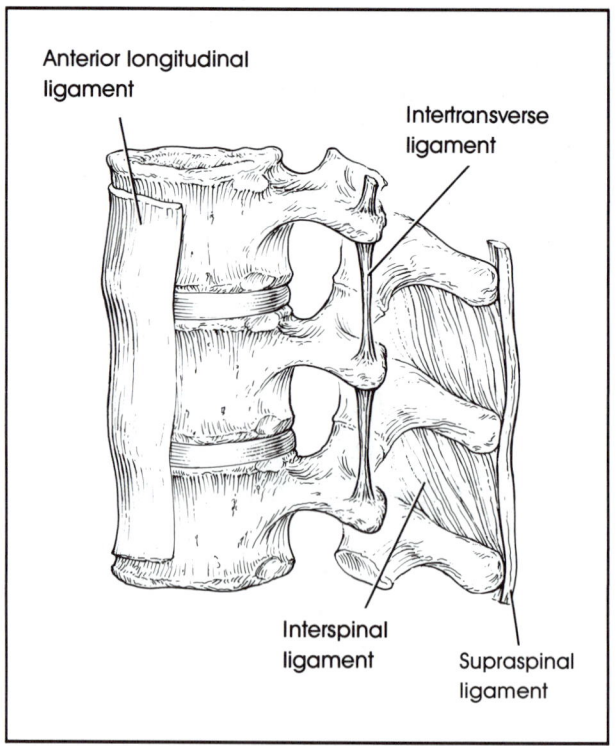

FIGURE 4–5 A lateral view of vertebrae illustrating the supporting ligaments.

TABLE 4-1   Characteristics of the Spinal Vertebrae and Intervertebral Connections

The 33 Vertebrae

C_1 (Atlas)

• Lacks a vertebral body; basically a ring-shaped arch on which the skull rests

  • Lateral masses articulate with the skull (occipital condyle)

  • Allows flexion, extension, and lateral movement; no rotation

C_2 (Axis)

• Mainly a vertebral body and a large, strong, odontoid process (rising perpendicularly from the midportion) to fit inside the C_1 ring

• Articulates with C_1 vertebra at dens-atlas joint and two lateral (almost flat) facet joints

  • Allows rotation; no flexion or extension

  • Movements controlled by alar and apical ligaments

Lower Cervical Vertebrae (C_{3-7}) [5]

• Articular facets oriented with superior facets facing posteriorly, slightly medially, and upwards

  • Small facet joints at each side of body

  • Allows flexion, extension, and rotation

Thoracic Vertebrae (T_{1-12}) [12]

• Articular facets oriented with superior facets facing posteriorly, almost vertical, and slightly laterally

• Joints for head of ribs on transverse processes and vertebral bodies

  • Increase in size from above downward

  • Allows flexion and rotation of trunk

Lumber Vertebrae (L_{1-5}) [5]

• Articular facets oriented with superior facets facing medially, posteriorly, and almost vertically

  • Transverse processes large for lower body muscle attachment

  • Vertebrae are large and massive for their weight-bearing function; lumbar curve is convex anteriorly for mobility

  • Movements mostly flexion and extension

The Sacrum (S_{1-5}) [5 fused vertebrae]

• Fused vertebrae in a solid triangular block; articulates with the fifth lumbar vertebra, the coccyx, and the two hip bones

• Foramina allow for exit of lower lumbar and sacral spinal nerves

• Unites the vertebral column with the pelvis (forms the posterior wall of the pelvis)

The Coccyx [4 rudimentary vertebrae]

• Articulates with the sacrum superiorly and diminishes in size until it reaches the lowest portion (apex) commonly called the tailbone

• Accommodates a division of the fifth sacral nerve

Intervertebral Connections

Intervertebral Discs

• Cartilaginous joints between discs with soft gelatinous substance (nucleus pulposus) forming the center, surrounded by a tough fibrous annulus that conforms to the size of discs between which they lie; extend from the axis to the sacrum

• Mainly function as a cushion between vertebrae to absorb stress although allow for greater mobility at the cervical and lumbar regions of the spine

Ligaments   See Figures 4-4 and 4-5.

• Strong fibrous bands that surrounded the vertebral column, holding it together

• Vary in width and strength depending on function performed; form various fusions and interconnections to enhance functions

• Anterior and posterior longitudinal ligaments extend entire length of the spinal column

  • Ligamenta flava run between laminae

  • Supraspinal and interspinal ligaments join the spinous processes

  • Ligaments of the sacrum and coccyx form a rich network to stabilize the pelvis and strengthen lower body stability and movement

---

first or second lumbar vertebra. It acts as a two-way communication cable, carrying motor messages from the brain to the systemic nervous system and carrying sensory messages from the peripheral nervous system back to the brain.

The cord is divided into cervical, thoracic, lumbar, and sacral segments. The cord enlarges in the cervical and lumbar areas to receive additional nerves from the upper and lower limbs. Because the cervical and lumbar areas of the spine are most mobile, these areas of the cord are most vulnerable to injury. The cord terminates in a tapered cone shape called the *conus medullaris*. This area contains major reflex centers for bowel, bladder, and sexual functions. Figure 4–6 details this information.

The main blood supply for the spinal cord is provided by two major vessels:

1.   The anterior spinal artery supplies the front two-thirds of the cord.
2.   The posterior spinal arteries supply the back one-third of the cord.

In addition, many smaller vessels (radicular arteries) supply the outer circumference of the cord at various levels. See Figure 4–7. Interruption of this vital blood supply can cause necrosis (cell death) and permanent cord damage, which can result in specific clinical patterns of pathophysiology.

Throughout the central nervous system, *cell bodies* of neurons group together to form gray matter. Nerve fibers of neurons that are insulated or myelinated group together to form white matter.

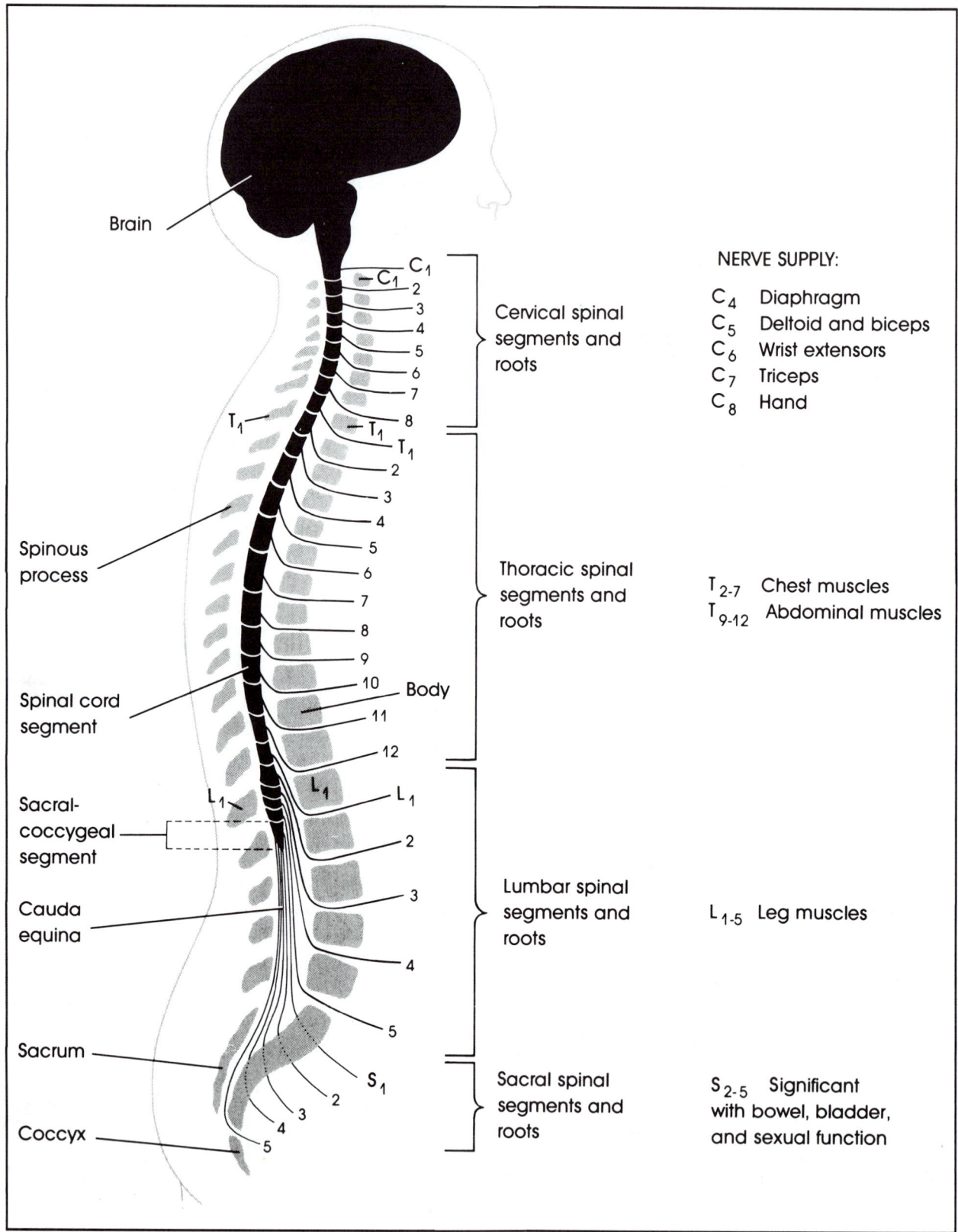

NERVE SUPPLY:

C_4 Diaphragm
C_5 Deltoid and biceps
C_6 Wrist extensors
C_7 Triceps
C_8 Hand

T_{2-7} Chest muscles
T_{9-12} Abdominal muscles

L_{1-5} Leg muscles

S_{2-5} Significant with bowel, bladder, and sexual function

FIGURE 4–6   The spinal cord and spinal nerves.

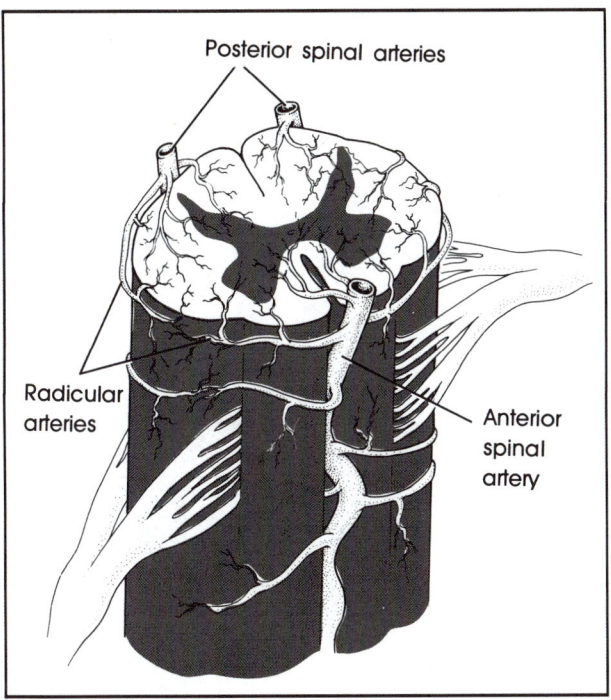

FIGURE 4–7   The blood supply to the spinal cord.

Gray Matter

In the spinal cord, gray matter is composed of groups of cell bodies in a centrally located **H** or butterfly shape. This shape varies at different levels of the cord:

- *Anterior columns* or *horns* compose the front portion or legs of the **H** and contain motor cells to transmit messages of movement from the brain out through the anterior root.
- *Posterior (dorsal) columns* or *horns* compose the back portion or legs of the **H** and contain sensory "relay cells" to transmit incoming messages received through the posterior root from the body to the brain.
- *Intermediate* or *lateral columns* contain a number of intermediate cell bodies and in the thoracic section, give rise to the sympathetic nervous system.

White Matter

White matter is composed of ascending and descending nerve fibers that are insulated or myelinated and surround the central gray matter. Tracts, or bundles, of these nerve fibers (*axons*) are organized within the spinal cord according to function and act as transmission cables, sharing a common origin and common destination. For example, all fibers carrying motor messages travel together, as do all fibers carrying pain messages. See Figure 4–8.

Tracts have specific and complicated names, but the beginning of the word usually describes the origin; and the ending, the destination. All tracts are bilateral for control of each side of the body. There are three major tracts:

1. The *corticospinal tract* or *voluntary motor pathway* originates in the motor cortex of the brain and descends through the brain stem (where it crosses over to innervate the opposite side of the body), to the spinal cord.

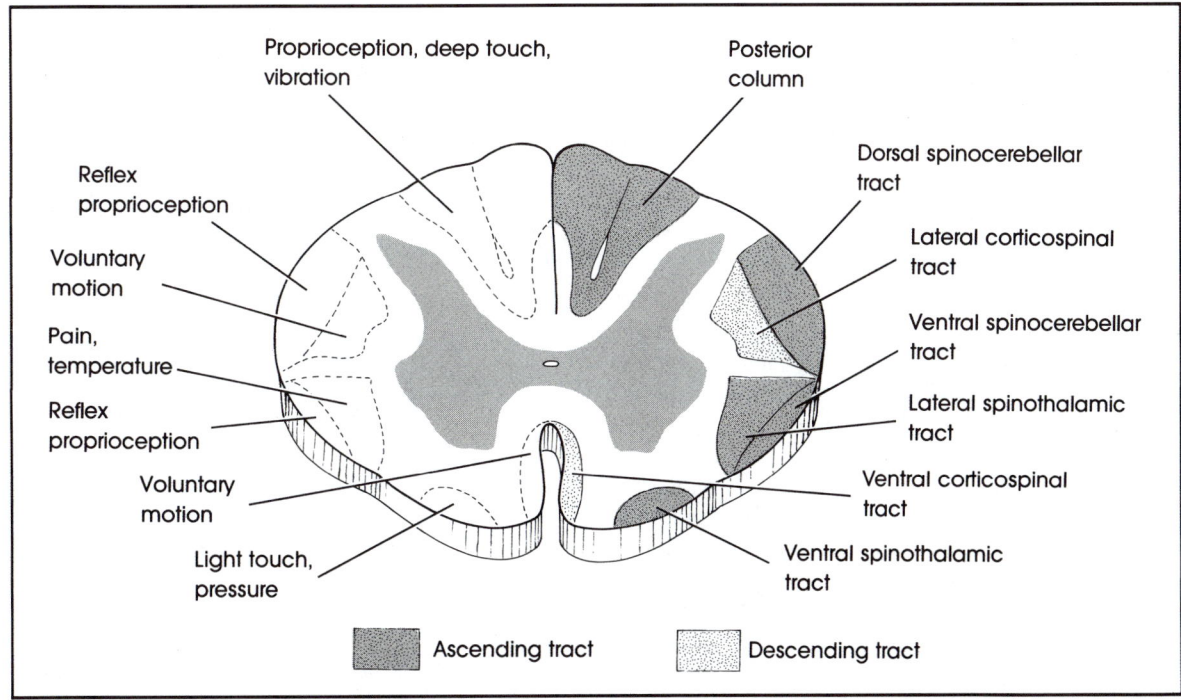

FIGURE 4–8   A cross-section of the spinal cord detailing major motor and sensory tracts and their functions.

2. The *spinothalamic tract* originates in the spinal cord and ascends to the thalamus in the brain. Sensations of pain and temperature enter the cord from the opposite side of the body.

3. The *posterior columns* are composed of sensory pathways for touch, vibration, and position sense. They are composed of several tracts.

The Spinal Nerves

The *spinal nerves* (Figure 4–6) provide common pathways for controlled movement, sensory input, and reflex responses. *Efferent fibers* carry outgoing motor messages from the brain through the cord to various parts of the body. *Afferent fibers* carry incoming sensory messages to the cord where they are relayed to the brain. Reflex responses occur within a reflex arc. See Figure 4–9.

The spinal nerves occur in pairs and correspond to the 31 segments or divisions of the cord. Each nerve is attached to the cord by an *anterior (ventral)* and *posterior (dorsal) root*. The two roots join in a common sleeve before exiting through openings at vertebral levels to branch out to almost all parts of the body (Figure 4–9).

Some of the spinal nerves join in complex networks outside the spinal cord to form a *plexus* to innervate certain body parts. For example, the brachial plexus controls most of the arm and hand. Some spinal nerves have important functions and are given specific names. For example, the phrenic nerve innervates the diaphragm.

The *cauda equina*, which literally translated means the "horse's tail," is so named because of its appearance and is formed from the lowest nerve roots fanning out from the end of the cord. Injury to this area has some potential for recovery.

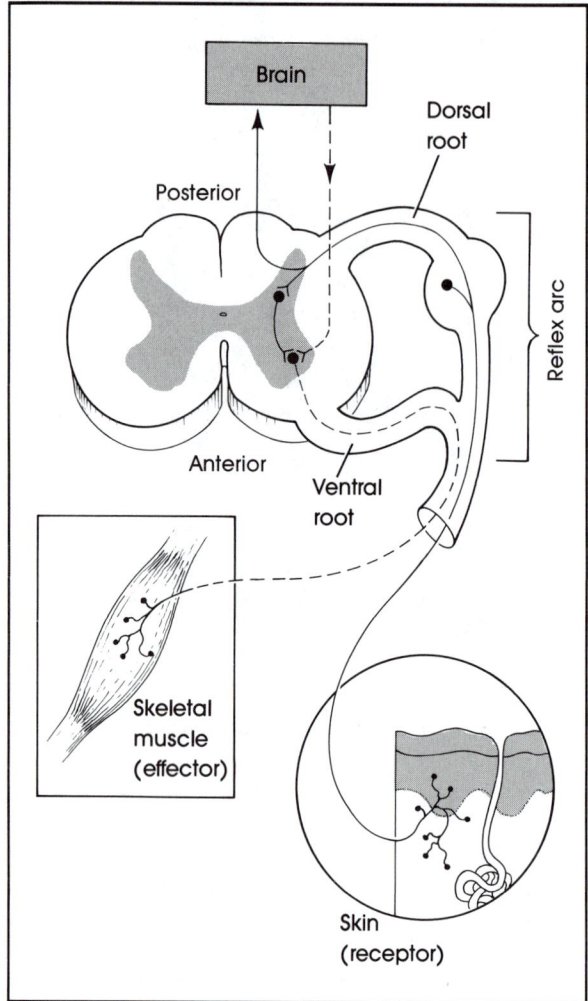

FIGURE 4–9   A cross-section of the spinal cord detailing the attached spinal nerve.

THE AUTONOMIC NERVOUS SYSTEM

The *autonomic nervous system* is composed of complex nerves outside the brain and spinal cord that can be severely affected by spinal cord injury. The autonomic nervous system provides automatic control, at a subconscious or involuntary level, of such vital functions as blood pressure, heart rate, body temperature control, appetite, fluid balance, bladder emptying, gastrointestinal motility, carbohydrate and fat metabolism, sleep, and sexual functioning.

Governing the autonomic nervous system is a function of the *hypothalamus*, located deep within the brain, and, to a certain extent, of local reflex activity. From the hypothalamus, neurons descend through the brain stem and spinal cord to terminate in three groups:

- One group clustered near certain cranial nerve roots in the brain stem (cranial outflow)

- Another group located between the first thoracic and first lumbar segments of the spinal cord (thoracolumbar outflow)
- A group centered between the second and fourth sacral segments of the cord (sacral outflow)

The *thoracolumbar outflow* gives rise to the *sympathetic* division of the autonomic nervous system (see Figure 4–10A), and the *craniosacral outflow* gives rise to the *parasympathetic* division (see Figure 4–10B). These autonomic nerve fibers then share various common pathways with cranial and spinal nerves and blood vessels to arrive at their destination in muscles, organs, and glands.

The division of the autonomic nervous system into *sympathetic* and *parasympathetic* sections is based on differences not only in structure but also in function. The sympathetic and parasympathetic systems are functional opposites, thus maintaining a stable internal environment. Most muscles and organs receive stimulation from both systems. For example, the sympathetic system will speed the heart rate, whereas the parasympathetic will slow it down. The balance can be changed in two ways: by increasing the amount of stimulus to either division or by decreasing (blocking) the amount of discharge from either division. This very important principle forms the basis for many neurologically active drugs, which in SCI are used to manage both acute reactions and long-term complications.

The Sympathetic Division

Function

The sympathetic division allows for maximum energy expenditure for stress response (*fight or flight* mechanism). Stimulation to this system provides a generalized response from the body because of the widespread network of nerves to the entire body. See Figure 4–11.

To prepare the body for stress response, the sympathetic nervous system will:

- Increase heart rate and respirations and shunt blood from less-important areas to cardiopulmonary circulation
- Decrease gastrointestinal, urinary, and other less-important functions
- Release red blood cells from storage in the spleen for additional energy
- Stimulate the adrenal gland above the kidney to release epinephrine

Structure

The dorsal and ventral roots attach each spinal nerve to the spinal cord. At the point where these roots join in a common sleeve, nerve fibers extend both upward and downward to establish communication with a sympathetic ganglion. A sympathetic ganglion is simply a mass of sympathetic nervous tissue clustered or grouped around each side of the thoracic and lumbar cord. These ganglia are then linked together to form a chainlike structure that extends bilaterally from the base of the cranium to the coccyx just outside the vertebral column and innervates the entire body.

The chemical transmitter between the sympathetic fibers and the structures they innervate is epinephrine (or norepinephrine). Drugs that mimic this effect are known as *adrenergic* or *sympathomimetic* agents.

The Parasympathetic Division

Function

The parasympathetic division plays a greater role in nonstress, everyday body functioning. See Figure 4–12. It initiates such functions as digestion or elimination and conserves body energy. Stimulation to this system produces more specific responses than are produced in the sympathetic system, for example, increased intestinal motility to aid elimination or increased contractions of the bladder wall to accomplish voiding.

Structure

Long nerve fibers extend from their *craniosacral* origin in a direct pathway to reach the muscle or organ innervated by the parasympathetic nervous system. Stimulation is most abundant in the head and abdominal area. Parasympathetic stimulation is not extended to certain muscles and organs, which allows the sympathetic influence complete control in stressful situations. Receiving sympathetic stimulation only are the voluntary muscles, skin, sweat glands, adrenal gland, and spleen.

The chemical transmitter between the parasympathetic fibers and the structures they innervate is *acetylcholine*. Drugs that mimic this effect are known as *cholinergic* or *parasympathomimetic* agents; thus such a drug's reaction resembles parasympathetic discharge.

CONSEQUENCES OF INJURY ——————

Vertebral Column Injuries

Mechanisms of Injury

Several factors can contribute to SCI. Most important, the forces or stresses producing injury, called *mechanisms of injury*, must be identified.

Blunt injury, by far the more common kind, involves a number of forces that often occur in combination:

- Forced flexion (anterior), or flexion with rotation
- Forced extension (hyperextension)
- Vertical compression (axial loading)

Penetrating injury, such as gunshot or knife wounds, may also cause SCI. Although not as common, the incidence of such injuries is on the rise with the increase of violence in our society.

The common sites of injury are the most mobile parts of the spine: the cervical area and the thoracolumbar junction. The severity of bony injury does not always correspond to the extent of neurological impairment. Gross fractures may cause little or no motor or sensory loss, and minor fractures may result in extensive paralysis. Table 4–2 illustrates some common mechanisms of injury apparent at the accident scene, and the spine and spinal cord injuries that may result.

Kinds of Fractures

Fractures can occur to any portion of the vertebral body or arch (Figure 4–3) but generally occur in combination. Fractures also differ in severity and may or may not result in trauma to the spinal cord: varying degrees and syndromes

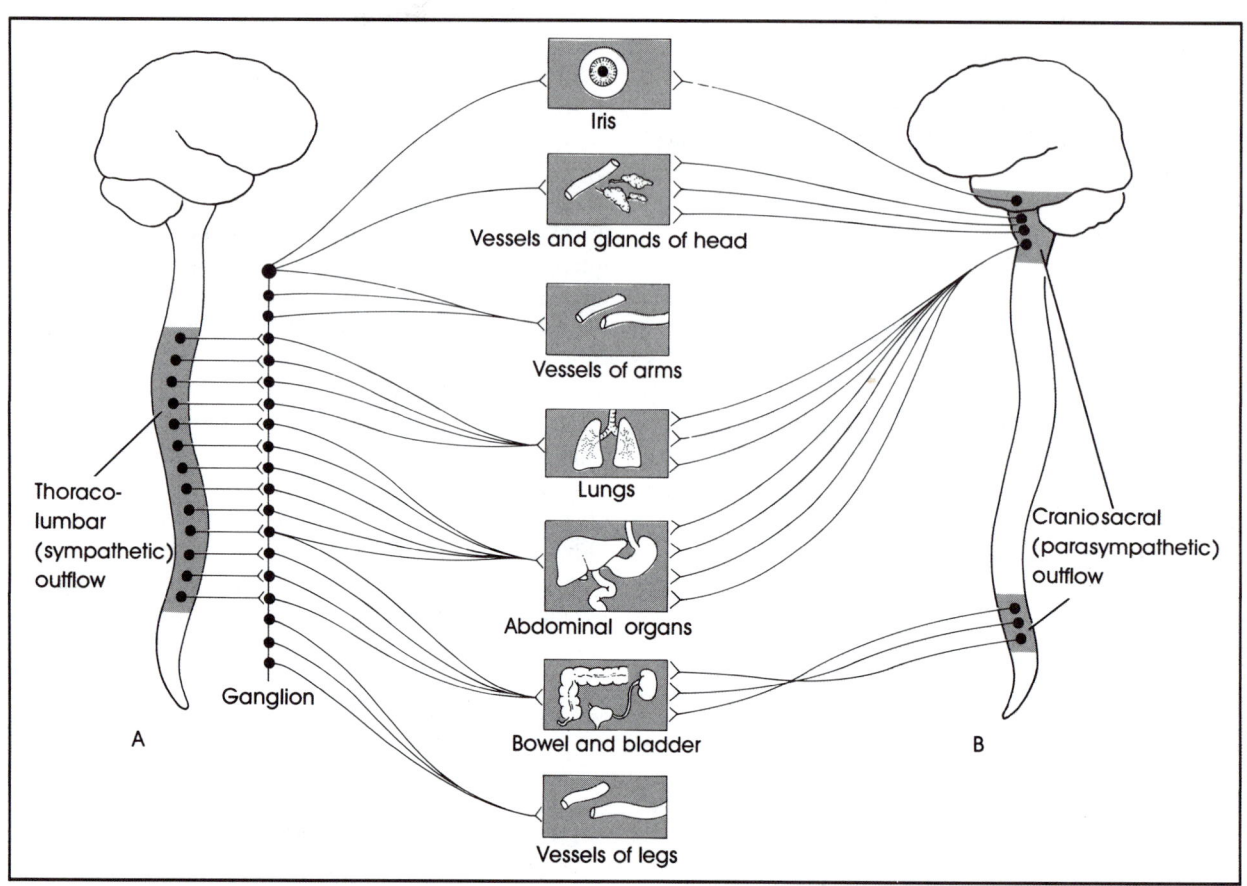

FIGURE 4–10 A symbolic diagram of the sympathetic nervous system, composed from the thoracolumbar outflow (**A**), and of the parasympathetic nervous system, composed from the craniosacral outflow (**B**).

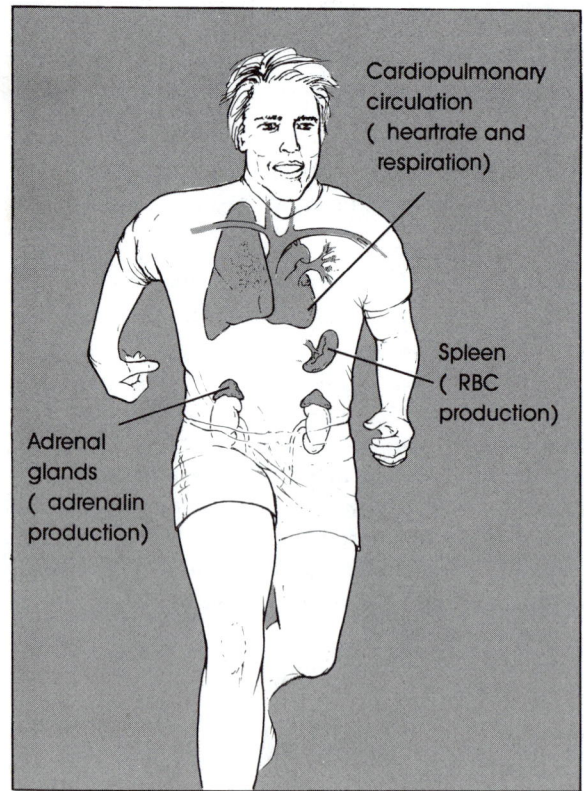

FIGURE 4–11 The sympathetic division activates the body for stress response.

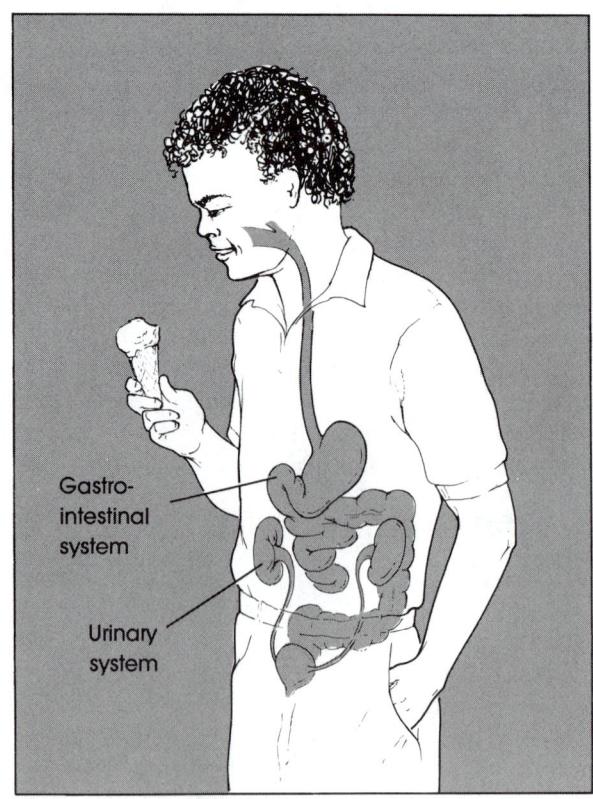

FIGURE 4–12 The parasympathetic division mediates nonstress responses to create an internal homeostasis.

TABLE 4-2   Some Common Mechanisms of Injury and Examples of Resultant Trauma to the Vertebral Column and Spinal Cord

Forward Flexion Injury

Flexion injuries to the cervical spine may result from a motor vehicle accident, typically a head-on collision, when the victim's head is first hyperextended then thrown violently forward from the arrested momentum. Similar flexion injuries can result when the head is struck from behind or the victim falls and strikes the back of his head. In the cervical region extensive tearing of the posterior ligamentous complex may result in severe forward dislocation.

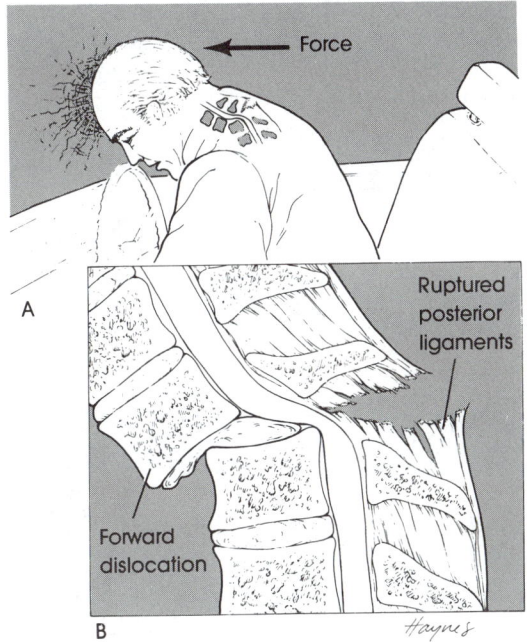

Flexion-Axial Compression Injury

In the thoracic or lumbar region flexion injuries can be caused by a fall onto the buttocks. Typically the vertebral bodies are wedged and compressed as a result of a pure flexion injury.

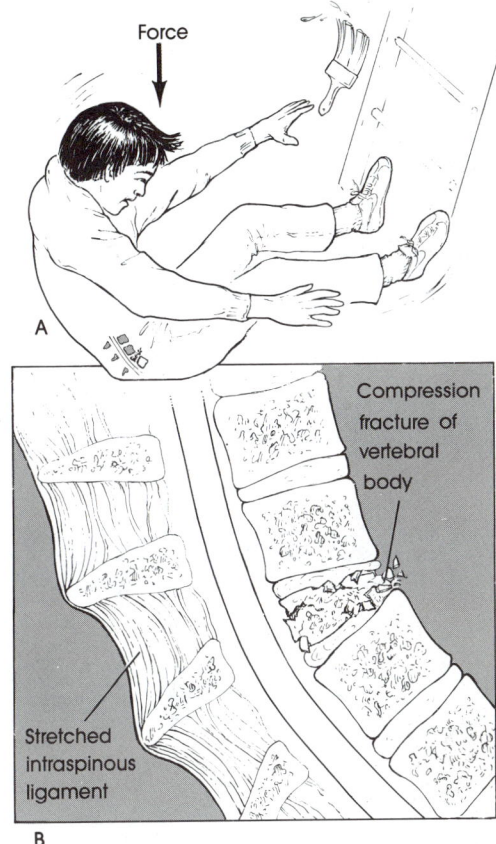

(Table continues)

---

of neurological deficits can result. Table 4–3 describes several kinds of vertebral fractures.

Stable and Unstable Injuries

Vertebral column injuries are also defined in terms of clinical stability, that is, *stable* or *unstable* injuries. The distinction between stable and unstable situations cannot be made without clinical expertise and radiological diagnosis because a mixture of mechanical, symptomatic, and neurological features are involved.

An unstable situation exists when vertebral and ligamentous structures are not able to support or protect the injured area. Inexpert movement can cause increased pressure with resultant damage to the spinal cord from displacement of the bony structures at the injury site. SCI is considered stable when the bony and/or ligamentous structures support the injured area sufficiently to prevent progression of neurological deficit and prevent body deformity. If the posterior

supporting complex—consisting of the ligaments that run between the neural arches and the articulating facet joints—survive, the spinal injury is considered stable.

A three-column concept of the spine, advocated by Mc-Afee, Hansen, Fredrickson, et al. (1983) and by Denis (1978), has fostered the most manageable, yet accurate classification scheme for delineating stable from unstable injuries. For this evaluation system, the spine is divided into *anterior*, *middle*, and *posterior columns* (Figures 4–3, 4–4, and 4–5):

- The anatomic structures of the anterior column include the anterior longitudinal ligament and the anterior two-thirds of the vertebral body and intervertebral disc.
- The middle column is formed by the posterior longitudinal ligament, posterior one-third of the intervertebral disc, and the posterior wall (one-third) of the vertebral body.

TABLE 4-2 Some Common Mechanisms of Injury and Examples of Resultant Trauma to the Vertebral Column and Spinal Cord (continued)

Flexion with Rotation (Distraction)

Flexion and rotational forces occurring concurrently are particularly potent and are associated with fracture dislocations at any level of the spinal column. Typically the posterior ligamentous complex is ruptured accompanied by vertebral body fracture(s) rendering this injury highly unstable. Causes may be related to any number of accidents.

Forced Extension (Hyperextension)

Forced extension (hyperextension) injuries are typically seen in elderly persons, when degenerative changes have narrowed the spinal canal. Injuries, usually at the cervical level, are often related to falls in which chin or face is struck, causing violent extension of the neck.

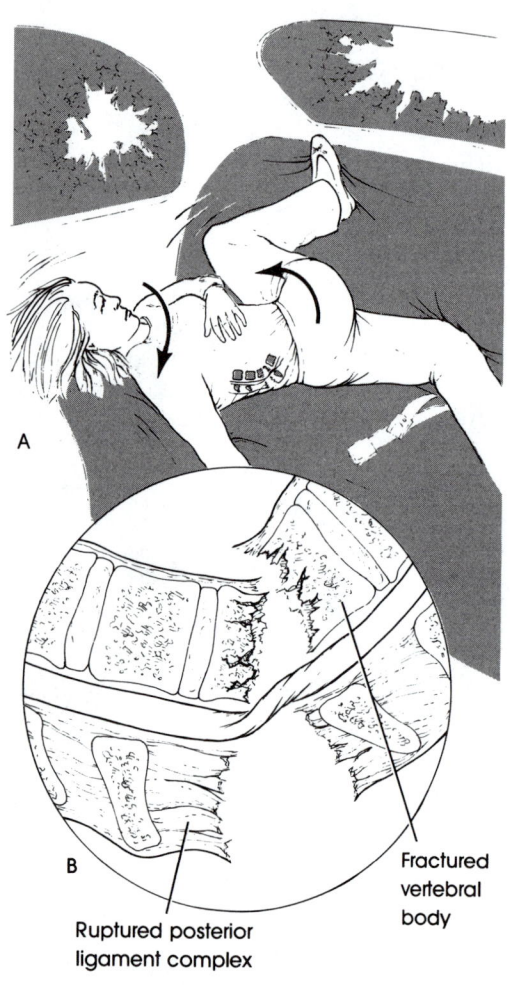

B Ruptured posterior ligament complex

Fractured vertebral body

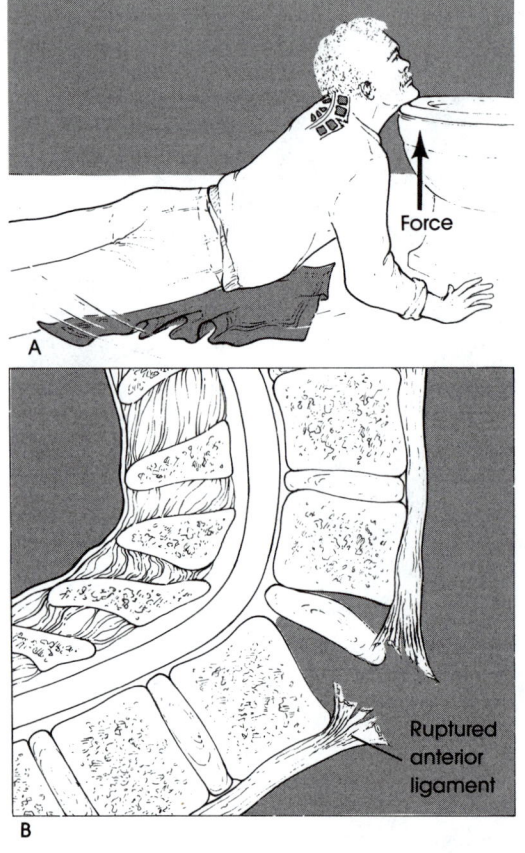

Force

Ruptured anterior ligament

(Table continues)

- The posterior column is composed of the neural arch (lamina, pedicles, and ligamentum flavum), the articular processes and facet-joint capsules, and the spinous processes, and the interspinal ligaments.

Based on this three-column concept, there are four major categories of spinal injuries (Denis 1978; McAfee et al. 1983):

- Forward flexion injuries (anterior compression fractures)
- Flexion-axial compression injuries (burst fractures)
- Flexion-distraction injuries (seat-belt injuries and chance fractures)

- Fracture-dislocation (sheer injuries that cause sagittal or coronal plane translation of the spinal column)

Spinal injuries in which there is disruption of all three columns are considered to be unstable. See Table 4–4.

Fractures of the cervical spine are differentiated into fractures that occur in the atlas or axis, that is, C_1 or C_2, and fractures located in the subaxial cervical spine (C_{3-7}). Fractures of C_1, or the atlas, are most commonly axial-load injuries in which a blow to the top of the head or a fall on the top of the head causes disruption of the ring of C_1. This is known as a *Jefferson's fracture*. Fractures of C_2 (the axis)

TABLE 4-2   Some Common Mechanisms of Injury and Examples of Resultant Trauma to the Vertebral Column and Spinal Cord (continued)

Vertical Compression (Flexion-Axial Compression)

Fractures resulting from vertical compression typically occur at the cervical and sometimes thoracolumbar areas of the spine. A high-velocity blow to the top of the head can cause a shattered vertebral body to burst into the spinal cord.

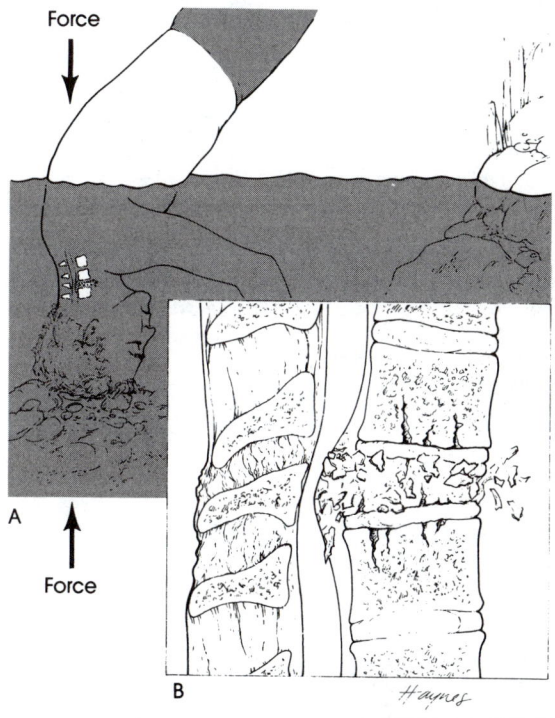

TABLE 4-3   Kinds of Vertebral Fractures

Simple Fracture—Generally involves elements of the neural arch (the spinous or transverse process) without injury to the spinal cord.

Compression or Wedge Fracture—Anterior compressed injury to the vertebral body.

Comminuted or Burst Fracture—A shattering injury to the vertebral body with the likelihood of fragments impinging on the spinal cord with resultant severe damage.

Teardrop Fracture—A small fragment chipped from the vertebra becomes free to lodge in spinal canal. Generally associated with posterior dislocation of the vertebral body and neurological deficit. Surgical intervention required for removal of bone fragment.

Dislocation—Occurs when one vertebra overrides another and unilateral or bilateral facet dislocations lock and prevent correct alignment of the vertebral column.

Subluxation—A partial or incomplete dislocation of one vertebra over another.

Fracture-Dislocation—A commonly used term to describe a fracture and a dislocation often associated with ligament and cord injury.

Adapted from Hickey (1986).

most commonly involve the odontoid process or posterior elements. This is caused by a flexion injury and is usually treated with either a halo brace or with a fusion of the C_1 and C_2 vertebrae. The *hangman's fracture* is a fracture through the posterior elements of C_2 due to forced hyperextension. This type of fracture is the typical result of a judicial hanging. Most of these fractures do not cause neurologic deficit and can be treated in a halo brace.

Fractures from C_{3-7} (subaxial cervical spine fractures) are most commonly axial-load flexion fractures with a burst type injury of the vertebral body, or flexion-distraction injuries with dislocations of one vertebra on another. With these latter injuries, there are either bilateral or unilateral facet dislocations depending on the amount of rotation present at the time of injury. Fractures of the subaxial spine (C_{3-7}) often result in injury to the spinal cord, particularly with complete dislocations or burst fractures. These fractures, due to disruption of the vertebral body and the posterior elements, are classified as unstable injuries. Table 4–5 summarizes common injuries at various levels of the spine.

Neurological Impairment

Following the moment of trauma to the spinal cord, several mechanisms become operative that cause progressive neurological damage. Progressive damage can be related to mechanical insult, biochemical responses, and hemodynamic changes often associated with multiple

TABLE 4–4 Major Categories of Injuries to the Spine and the Types of Injuries Sustained by Each (Anterior, Middle, Posterior) Column of the Spine

Category	Mechanism of Injury	Anterior	Middle	Posterior
Anterior Compression Fractures				
Stable	Forward flexion	Compression (50%)	None	None
Unstable	Forward flexion	Compression (50%) or contiguous fracture	None	Ligaments torn
Burst Fractures				
Stable	Flexion-axial Compression	Compression	Axial compression Displaced fragment	Vertical laminar fracture
Unstable	Flexion-axial Compression	Compression	Axial compression Displaced fragment	Facet-joint Disruption
Flexion-Distraction Injuries				
Stable (e.g., chance fracture)	Flexion and distraction	Compression (30%) transverse fracture	Distraction, transverse fracture	Distraction
Unstable	Flexion and distraction	Compression (50%)	Distraction, disc separation	Distraction ligaments torn joints dislocated
Fracture-Dislocation				
Stable* (T_1–T_5)	Translational (sheer) forces	Compression and translation	Compression and translation	Translation and facet fractures
Unstable (T_6–L_5)	Translational (sheer) forces	Compression and translation	Compression, distraction, and translation	Translation and facet fractures

*Sternum intact

James S. Keene, M.D., University of Wisconsin Spine Injury Center.

trauma. See Table 7–2. The primary pathological changes are related to subsequent bleeding and swelling directly at the site of injury causing severe central necrosis of the gray matter. Secondary associated biochemical and hemodynamic changes also alter physiological response to injury. Changes in systemic blood flow and oxygen tension, either as a result of impaired autonomic nervous system function and/or systemic blood loss, are believed to compromise the delicate cord structure further and to cause progressive destruction resulting in extension of the initial neurological insult.

Neurological impairments are described as either *complete* or *incomplete*. A complete injury is loss of all conscious motor and/or sensory function below the level of injury. An incomplete injury preserves (or spares) some motor or sensory function. This includes several particular syndromes or distinct patterns of neurological deficit. Incomplete injury is significant because there is potential for recovery. Sometimes, however, preserved sensory functions are not very helpful; they may cause feelings of painful nerve irritation or build false hopes. Sometimes a person can feel an unpleasant sensation of "pins and needles" or numbness in a limb. This is referred to as *paresthesia*. Even more painful is *hyperesthesia* when touch is grossly exaggerated. For example, when a bed sheet touches a limb, it may be described as "nails driving into the skin." Unpleasant sensations may be caused by root irritation. At other times, preserved sensation can be helpful in alerting the person to a full bladder or to the position of legs in the wheelchair.

Complete Syndrome

Complete transverse syndrome. This syndrome causes loss of all motor and sensory nerve transmission to areas below the level of the injury. See Figure 4–13. Complete paraplegia or quadriplegia occurs. Causes are:

TABLE 4–5 Common Types of Injuries at Various Levels of the Spine

CERVICAL SPINE

C₁ (Atlas)

Jefferson Fracture

- A vertical load produces a burst fracture, splitting the arch of the atlas ring
- Frequently no neurological deficit because the fracture actually enlarges the upper spinal canal.

C₂ (Axis)

- Odontoid process (dens) fractures and dislocations frequently occur from axial-loading (vertical), or flexion and extension forces that fracture the odontoid across the base.
- May cause sudden death, but often minimal displacement does not cause neurological deficit.

Hangman's Fracture

- Severe hyperextension forces produce fracture across posterior arch of the axis with or without subluxation of C₂ on C₃.
- Often not associated with neurological injury except in judicial hanging when force is prolonged.

LOWER CERVICAL VERTEBRAE (C₃₋₇)

- Various Dislocations* and Subluxations can occur with common flexion-rotation types of injury.
- If facet(s) ride up over each other they may interlock and prevent the vertebrae from rotating back into position (often associated wtih severe flexion injuries and quadriplegia).
- Subluxation and relocation without fracture may damage the cord without producing any damage visible on X ray as is often seen with hyperextension injuries.*
- Neurological deficits occur when displacement is sufficient to compromise the cord.

- Fracture Dislocations* are produced by multiple mechanisms of injury (either extension, flexion, or vertical forces [axial loading and/or axial rotation] often in combination).
- The body of the vertebra is crushed, usually anteriorly with subluxation.
- Caused by penetrating wounds, such as gunshot and knife wounds.

THORACIC VERTEBRAE

- Usually Fracture or Fracture Dislocations*
- Mechanisms of injury vary but often include axial-loading and flexion forces with a rotational factor.
- Usually anterior compression fracture with a variable degree of posterior protrusion.

THORACOLUMBAR JUNCTION

- Susceptible area for spinal injury because it is an area of stress and increased mobility, and it is located beneath the rigid rib cage.
- Associated with flexion and rotational forces.
- Often causing conus and/or cauda equina damage.
- Fractures, usually compression, often caused by falls.*

LUMBAR AND SACRAL SPINE

- Similar to thoracolumbar injuries.

Chance Fracture

- A lap-belt injury unique to the lumbar spine due to severe flexion and rotation around a fixed axis (the pelvis secured by the lap belt), resulting in bony and ligamentous disruption to the lumbar spine.
- Commonly associated with internal abdominal injuries.

*Illustrated in Table 4–2

- Complete severance of the cord.
- Complete breakage of nerve fibers by stretching of the cord. Coverings may still be intact and the cord may still look normal.
- Complete ischemia of the cord by interruption of the total blood supply.

Incomplete Syndromes

Central cord syndrome. Central cord syndrome is caused by damage to the central portion of the cervical cord. See Figure 4–14.

Corticospinal tract fibers are organized with those controlling the arms located most centrally, the trunk intermediately, and the legs laterally. Fibers located most centrally are damaged and fibers located most laterally are spared. Some distal nerve transmission is still intact. Therefore, arm movement is affected, but leg movement may not be.

Anterior artery syndrome or sparing of posterior columns. Anterior artery syndrome is usually caused by damage due to infarction from the main anterior artery; the resulting loss of blood supply damages the anterior two-thirds of the cord. The posterior third of the cord is unaffected. See Figure 4–15.

The effects include:

- Loss of function below the level of injury of the portion of the cord that controls voluntary motor pathways and major sensory tracts
- Sparing of the posterior columns as the vascular supply is obtained from a different source
- Preservation of position, vibration, and touch sense

Brown-Séquard's syndrome. This syndrome is caused by damage to one side of the cord only. See Figure 4–16.

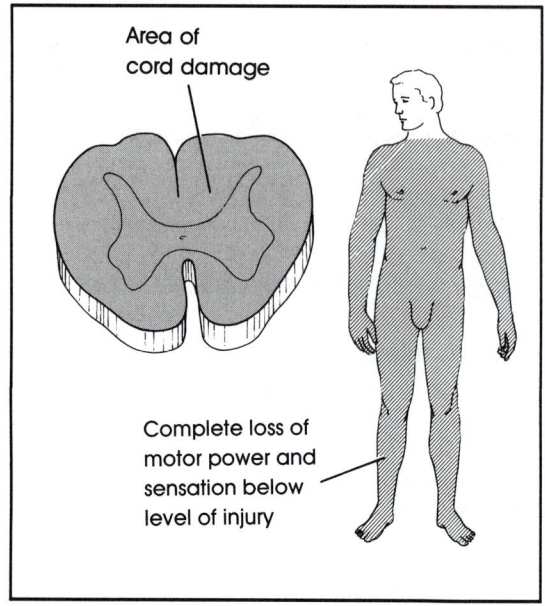

FIGURE 4–13   Spinal cord damage causing a complete transverse syndrome.

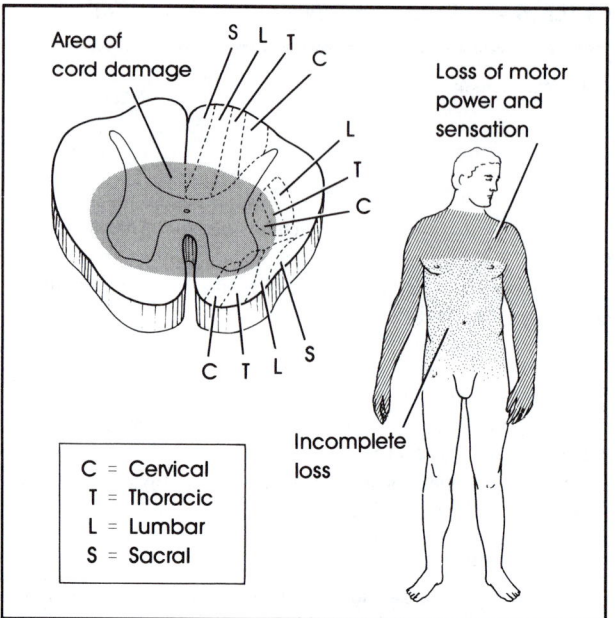

FIGURE 4–14   A cross-section of the spinal cord depicting damage that causes a central cord syndrome.

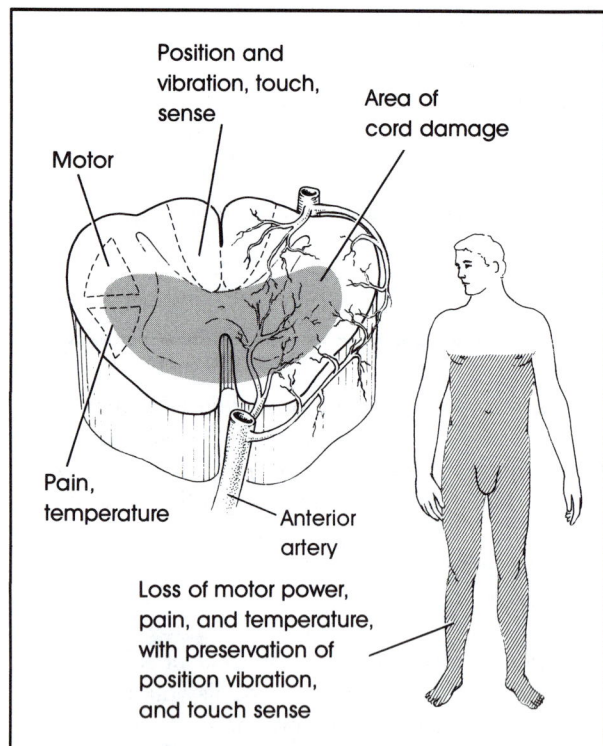

FIGURE 4–15   A cross-section of the spinal cord depicting damage that causes an anterior artery syndrome (or sparing of the posterior columns).

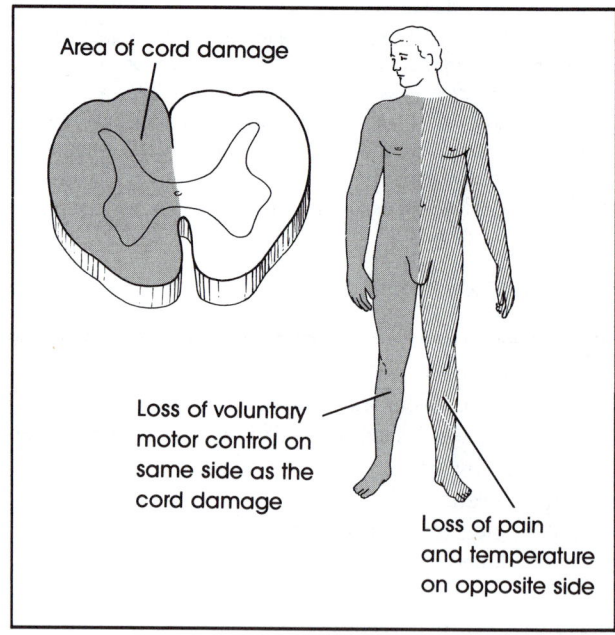

FIGURE 4–16   A cross-section of the spinal cord depicting damage that causes a Brown-Séquard syndrome.

The effect is loss of function below the level of the injury of the portion of the cord that controls voluntary motor pathways on the same side of the body and pain and temperature on the opposite side of the body.

Conus and cauda equina injuries. These injuries involve damage to the conus medullaris or spinal nerves forming the cauda equina (see Figure 4–17). Common effects are:

- Loss of motor function (leaving sensory function not markedly impaired).
- An extremely variable pattern with asymmetrical involvement. Roots have some recovery potential, so outlook is often favorable.
- Lower motor neuron (flaccid) involvement of bowel, bladder, and sexual functioning because those reflex centers are located in the conus.

Sacral sparing. In this syndrome there is damage to the major part of the cord and/or blood supply, but radicular arteries preserve the outer circumference of the cord. See Figure 4–18. Therefore, sensation of the sacral area is preserved in an otherwise paralyzed patient.

Upper Motor Neuron and Lower Motor Neuron Lesions

To understand the many neurological aspects of rehabilitation, it is essential to grasp the concept of *upper motor neuron* and *lower motor neuron lesions.* Spinal cord injury can result in damage to upper motor neurons, lower motor neurons, or a combination of both. Particularly when the sacral portion of the cord is injured, differentiating between upper motor neuron and lower motor neuron involvement is essential to determine the nature and extent of bladder, bowel, and sexual dysfunction.

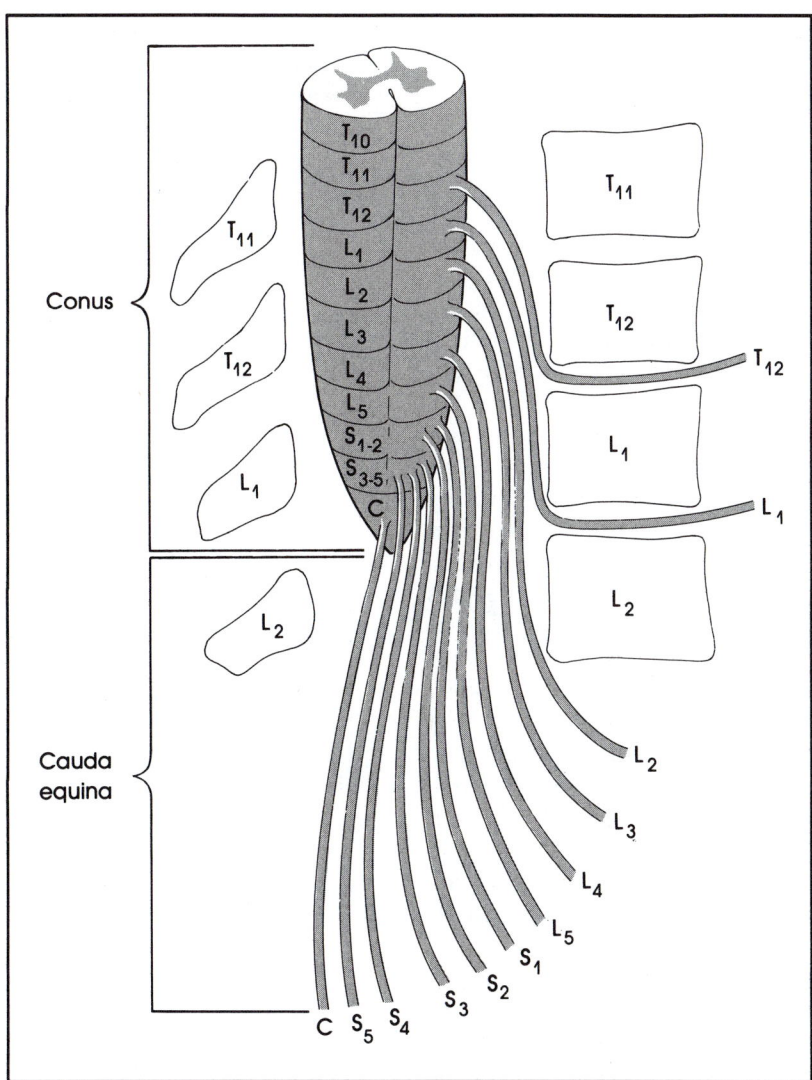

FIGURE 4–17 The conus and cauda equina in relation to the thoracolumbar junction of the spine.

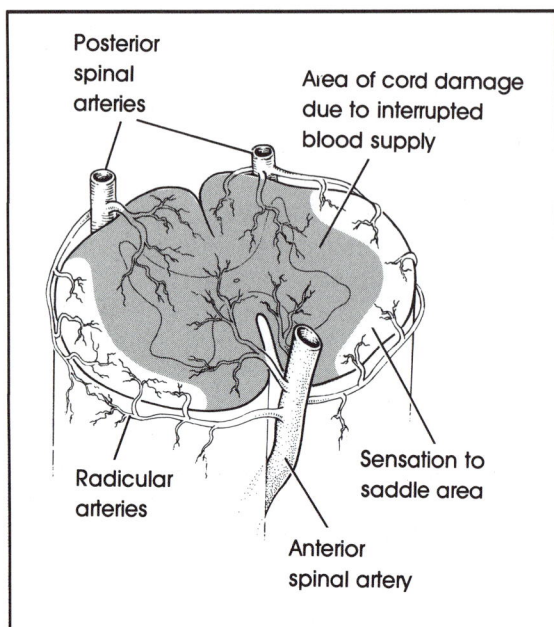

FIGURE 4–18 A cross-section of the spinal cord illustrating damage that allows sacral sparing.

Upper motor neurons. Upper motor neurons are long neurons that originate in the brain and travel in bundles or tracts within the spinal cord. The cell bodies of these neurons are located in the motor strip of the cerebral cortex and the brain stem with the axons extending down through the spinal cord. These ascending and descending tracts resemble transmission cables. Upper motor neurons terminate at each segmental level throughout the entire length of the spinal cord to *synapse* (transmit a nerve impulse) with lower motor neurons, which arise in the spinal cord and connect to a muscle or organ. See Figure 4–19. The brain, via the upper motor neurons, suppresses or inhibits the lower motor neurons so that they do not become hyperactive to local stimuli. Any injury that damages upper motor neurons destroys cerebral influence or control over lower motor neurons and is termed an *upper motor neuron lesion*.

An *upper motor neuron* or *spastic paralysis* results when damage to the upper motor neuron pathways causes loss of coordinated and integrated cerebral control over all reflex activity below the level of injury. Patients experience spasticity of limbs and of bowel and bladder functioning. Men experience reflex erections. However, spasticity is not all undesirable, and rehabilitation includes training these abnormal movements to assist with mobility and management of body functions.

Lower motor neurons. Lower motor neurons originate in the spinal cord and travel outside the central nervous system to form the spinal nerves and subsequent branches of the systemic nervous system. The cell bodies of these neurons are located in the central gray matter throughout the entire length of the spinal cord. The axons extend out

through the spinal nerve roots and peripheral nerve branches to muscle fibers throughout the body. A lower motor neuron may be thought of as a wishbone, with the joint inserted into the spinal cord. A lower motor neuron may transmit stimulation from a muscle or organ to the spinal cord where it synapses with another lower motor neuron, which carries the response back to the muscle or organ. This pathway is known as a *reflex arc* and must be intact to create an involuntary response, such as jerking a finger away from a hot stove. See Figure 4–20. Although simultaneously the painful sensation is appreciated, the reflex action is innervated by the spinal cord and not controlled by the brain. Any damage to the lower motor neuron is termed a *lower motor neuron lesion*.

A *lower motor neuron* or *flaccid paralysis* results when damage to the lower motor neuron pathways causes destruction of the reflex arc and breaks pathways of communication to the intact upper motor neurons. Although lower motor neuron damage can occur at any segment of the cord, significant clinical manifestations clearly result from damage to the sacral portion of the cord. When injuries occur to the sacral portion of the cord where lower motor neurons have a vital role in controlling major body functions (such as bowel, bladder, and sexual responses), the implications are very obvious and serious. Patients experience "floppy"

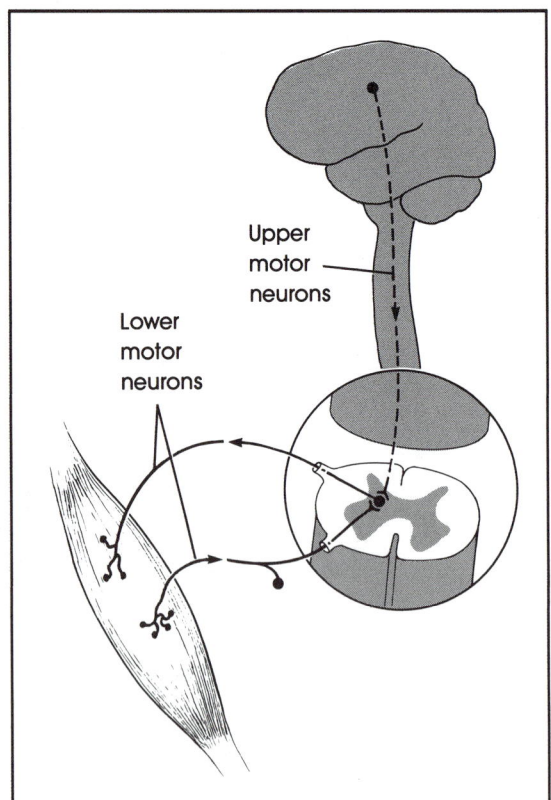

FIGURE 4–19 Diagram depicting upper motor neuron and lower motor neuron pathways.

paralysis of lower limbs, loss of bowel and bladder tone, and eventual muscle atrophy or wasting. Reflex erections are not possible. Circulatory problems tend to be more serious due to chronic passive vasodilation and lack of muscle tone. Retention of stool tends to be more of a problem; thus, bowel programs are more difficult to regulate.

The sacral segments of the cord correspond to the T_{12} vertebra. Fractures at or above this level usually cause a general spastic paralysis. However, many injuries near this level can result in a *mixed* upper motor neuron/lower motor neuron picture that particularly complicates bladder management problems.

Sexual, bladder, and bowel management are discussed in Chapters 10, 18, and 19, respectively.

Autonomic Nervous System Dysfunctions

Because maintaining homeostasis within the body is largely a function of the autonomic nervous system, internal stability is threatened when intricate communications with the central nervous system are interrupted. Generally, the higher the level of SCI, the more profound the effects become, as a greater portion of the body is involved.

Instability of the cardiovascular system and inability to regulate body temperature are particular problems for the patient with neurological injury at the T_6 level or above. A lowered pulse, a lowered blood pressure, postural hypotension, and a tendency to assume the temperature of the environment are symptoms. See Chapter 16.

Spinal shock (Chapter 6), an immediate complication, and *autonomic dysreflexia* or *hyperreflexia* (Chapter 16), a later complication, are two predominant autonomic nervous system dysfunctions associated with SCI.

ASSESSMENT OF SPINE INJURY

Other Factors Contributing to the Diagnosis of Spinal Cord Injury

Preexisting conditions or disease—and even the normal aging process—may predispose a person to initial injury and/or contribute to the severity of consequences experienced. Certainly general preinjury health and any conditions that would limit movement or impair sensation must be included in assessment data.

Preexisting Conditions or Disease
Any condition or disease process compromising the spine places a person at increased risk of SCI. Sequelae that cause

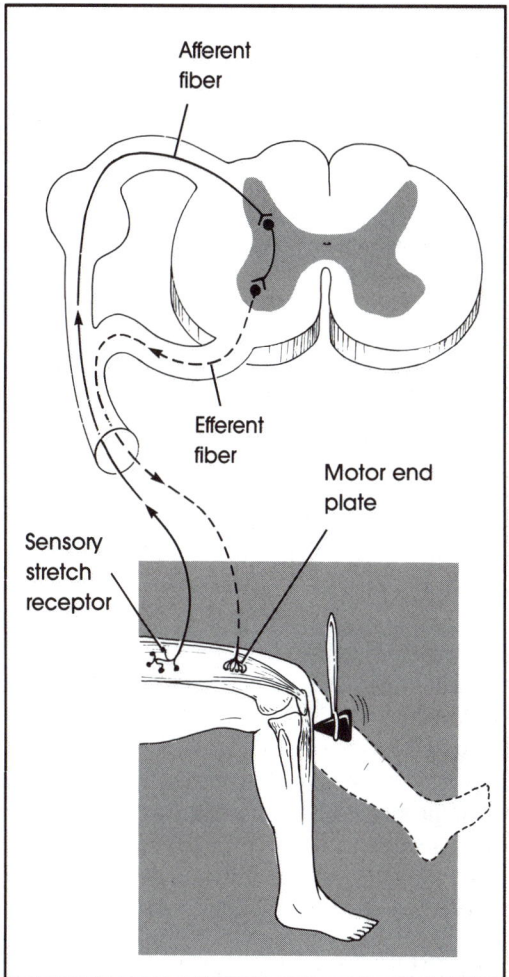

FIGURE 4–20 Pathway of the lower motor neuron or reflex arc.

stenosis (a narrowing of the spinal canal) increase the risk of serious injury from relatively minor trauma. Some of the more common conditions include:

- *Ankylosing spondylitis*, a disease affecting the spinal column characterized by calcification and ossification of soft tissues and ligaments, converts the spine into a rigid structure. When the shock-absorbing qualities of the spine are lost, particularly in the cervical area, severe cord damage can result from minor trauma to the spine.
- *Rheumatoid arthritis*, a chronic inflammatory condition, may attack the spine, causing osteoporosis and mobility impairments that increase vulnerability to injury.

Space-occupying lesions—primarily cancer—and such *infective processes* as an epidural abscess may also lead to disc degeneration or collapse, pathological fractures, and *compression* of the spinal cord with interruption of cord blood supply (infarction).

The spine is rarely a primary site for *cancer*. Metastasis to the spinal cord is present in approximately 10% of all people with cancer and is often associated with lymphomas (Yarbro 1987) and multiple myelomas. Spinal cord compression is a dreaded complication, not only because of paralysis but also because of extreme pain. Progressive back pain may be present for months before neurological deficit is detected. Weakness, paresthesias, bladder and bowel dysfunctions, and gait disturbances are associated. Favorable outcome depends on early diagnosis. Rehabilitation to enhance functional and psychosocial abilities, although perhaps modified for the person living with cancer, can greatly improve the quality of life (Groenwald and Thaney 1987: 757). The principles of management presented throughout this text are applicable.

The Normal Aging Process

As the age of the general population increases, more older people are suffering SCI. In the course of normal aging, muscles, bones, and articulations undergo changes that affect their physiological function and physical appearance. Degenerative and osteoporotic changes in the spine are referred to collectively as *cervical lordosis of aging*. The back may be rounded, the shoulders stooped, and the head tilted backward to compensate. Hyperextension injuries of the cervical spine due to a blow to the face or forehead are often caused by a simple fall. This kind of injury results in the classic central cord syndrome with minimal or no body damage from cervical spine injuries (Burke and Murray 1975).

Physical Examination of the Spine

The Neck and Back

The spine is the main axial support of the body and functions with the skin, major muscles and muscle groups, and supporting bony structures to hold the head erect and the body in an upright position. Natural slight curvatures of the vertebral column—the cervical curve (convex anteriorly), the thoracic curve (concave anteriorly), and the lumbar curve (convex anteriorly)—enhance this strength. Any exaggeration of these curves or lateral deviations are abnormal: for example, an excessive thoracic curve (*kyphosis* or hunchback); an excessive lumbar curve (*lordosis* or swayback); a lateral curve (*scoliosis*). Abnormal shape of the back or unusual bony protuberances or prominences may be caused by congenital deformity or disease or the initial trauma. Spinal curvatures may also be postinjury complications associated with inadequate early immobilization and stabilization.

The Fracture Site

Examine the fracture site for surrounding edema, open areas, or entry wounds in gunshot or stabbing cases. Compound spinal fractures are rare. A *gibbous* deformity—a humped protuberance or sharp angulation of the spine—may occur immediately as a result of vertebral injury. When there is any abnormality in the shape of the neck or back or at the fracture site, anticipate modifications to turning, positioning, and skin care measures.

Assessment of Neurological Function

Neurological assessment involves examination of *movement*, *sensation*, and *reflex activity* and is essential to determine realistic physiological and functional goals. Note especially Table 22–7, which correlates neurological status and function. Chapter 20 also discusses the spine.

The key to neurological assessment is using consistent methods and terms to define the level and nature of the injury and comparison of serial data to detect any deterioration or improvement. When describing the vertebrae or cord segments, abbreviations of letters and numbers are used for convenience. For example, the fourth cervical vertebra and segment are labeled C_4; the seventh thoracic vertebra and segment are labeled T_7; and so on.

The number of the vertebra does not necessarily correspond to the number of the adjacent cord segment. Review Figure 4–6. In the cervical region the spinal roots extend almost laterally, and there is little difference between the cord segments and the vertebral body levels. From C_8 down, the spinal roots travel varying distances in the spinal canal before exiting through the vertebral column. In the fetus, the cord extends the full length of the vertebral canal, but later the canal grows longer than the cord, thus causing the appearance of cord shrinkage and the downward projections of roots into the canal. This can become confusing when trying to relate the vertebral fracture level to the injured spinal cord segment (Burke 1979). For example, a T_{12} fracture may cause S_2 cord damage.

Diagnosis describes both the level of the vertebral fracture and the extent of neurological deficit, to the last normal functioning segment of the spinal cord. For example, the diagnosis "fractured C_5 with C_5 quadriplegia complete" means that the C_5 segment and nerve root are functioning normally, and C_6 and below are damaged. If the injury is incomplete, it is described in more detail such as "incomplete below C_5" and "complete below C_7." Involvement may differ between the right and left sides. This would also be described.

Motor Function

Examination of functional movements helps determine motor power. Individuals vary widely in strength due to sex, age, hand dominance, and general preinjury fitness. Assessment of motor function is critical during the initial postinjury period, primarily to detect deterioration in neurological status. Continual assessment is used throughout the rehabilitation period.

Figure 4–21 presents an assessment tool, suitable for critical care use, that includes the international five-point scale for grading muscle strength. (American Spinal Injury Association [ASIA] 1989). See Procedure 4–1 for illustrated test instructions. ASIA further recommends a method for scoring key muscle segments to simplify and facilitate communication and comparison of the functional effects of SCI. The muscle groups were selected for functional significance related to SCI. See Table 4–6.

Sensory Function

Detailed sensory testing is also used to detect changes in neurological function. Sensation may be described as simple or crude, such as appreciation of light touch, pain, or temperature, or as more sophisticated or discriminative, such as position sense, or appreciating where limbs are in space, and vibration sense. For ease of examination, sensory testing can be confined to testing for pain with a pinprick (indicator of posterior column sensory tract function) and for light touch with the aid of a cotton swab (indicator of spinothalamic sensory tract function). See Procedure 4–2. General appreciation of basic touch by placing hands on the patient and asking for a verbal response can also be used. It is important to correlate the level of injury to the actual body surface area that is without sensation or has impaired sensation. Again, the most important clinical aspect is to know the exact point or level on the patient where normal sensation is present.

Sensory distribution to the entire skin surface of the body is organized in dermatomes. A *dermatome* is a section or area of cutaneous distribution innervated by a cranial or spinal nerve. Arrangement of dermatomes is more easily understood if an individual is first considered in the quadruped (crouched) position (Figure 4–22).

Sensation may be described as normal, impaired, or absent. Sometimes the terms *anesthesia* (sensation of touch absent); *analgesia* (sensation of pain absent); *hypoesthesia* (reduced sensation) or *hyperesthesia* (exaggerated sensation) are used. Figure 4–23 presents illustrations for a detailed sensory test.

Reflex Activity

Be aware of the presence or absence of general reflex activity below the level of injury, particularly the perineal reflexes. For example, during care, the beginning of reflex penile erections or extremity spasms may be noticed. Knowing the status of reflex activity will help formulate diagnosis and prognosis and help plan interventions, specifically bladder and bowel management.

Useful reflexes are the *deep tendon reflexes* of the biceps (C_5), supinator (C_6), and triceps (C_7) in the upper extremities; and the knee (L_3) and the ankle (S_1) in the lower extremities. If a patient presents soon after injury with deep tendon reflexes below the level of injury, it can be a good prognostic sign of an incomplete neurological injury (Burke 1979). However, following acute trauma to the spinal cord, most patients experience temporary physiological disorganization of cord function (spinal shock) characterized by a flaccid paralysis with depressed or no reflex activity below the level of the injury. The presence of the bulbocavernosus reflex and the anal wink reflex are the first indications that cord function reorganization is occurring. The presence or absence of these reflexes helps differentiate between an upper motor neuron lesion and a lower motor neuron lesion involving the conus or cauda equina. The presence of these reflexes suggests upper motor neuron dysfunction; their absence suggests lower motor neuron dysfunction. The status of these reflexes becomes the main indicator of the physiological basis for bladder, bowel, and sexual dysfunction.

The *bulbocavernosus* reflex can be elicited by placing a gloved finger in the patient's rectum and squeezing the glans penis in the male or clitoris in the female or by tugging on the Foley catheter. A positive reflex will cause a sharp, distinct rectal sphincter contraction. The *anal wink* is another cord reflex. A pinprick in the perianal skin will cause a visual external anal sphincter contraction.

Injury to the spinal cord may result in reduced or absent reflexes, or alternatively, hyperactive reflexes. Activity is recorded as follows:

- Absent   0
- Decreased   +
- Normal   + +
- Increased   + + +

Diagnostic Procedures

Neuroradiological and neurophysiological techniques are becoming increasingly sophisticated adjuncts to clinical assessment and are improving the accuracy of diagnosis, particularly in the acute phase of injury. See Figure 4–24. State-of-the-art equipment and noninvasive techniques, minimizing the need for movement of the patient with an unstable spine injury, have reduced the risk of further neurological injury.

General patient preparation for diagnostic procedures includes explanation of the procedure, its purpose, and informed consent; descriptions of the equipment; preanalgesia for comfort; and early completion of routine bladder and bowel care before examination to promote comfort. Throughout the procedure, especially when procedures are prolonged, the patient's general tolerance, particularly if cardiopulmonary status is impaired, must be carefully and continuously monitored. Examination tables must be padded with a foam sheet or sheepskin to protect sensitive areas from pressure whenever possible.

Addressograph
Information

| | | DATE: | | | | | | | |

| | | TIME: | | | | | | | |

| | | INITIALS: | | | | | | | |

upper extremities

	Function	Key Muscle	Level	left right					
Elbow	Flexion	Biceps	C_5						
	Extension	Triceps	C_7						
Wrist	Flexion		C_6						
	Extension		C_6						
Fingers	Thumb-index pinch		C_8–T_1						

lower extremities

	Function	Key Muscle	Level						
Hip	Adduction	Illiopsoas	L_2						
Knee	Flexion	Hamstrings	L_5						
	Extension	Quadriceps	L_3						
Ankle	Plantar flexion		S_1						
	Dorsiflexion		L_4						

*Motor Grading Scale
0—Absent   Total paralysis
1—Trace   Palpable or visible contraction
2—Poor   Active movement through full ROM with gravity eliminated
3—Fair   Active movement through full ROM against gravity
4—Good   Active movement through full ROM against resistance
5—Normal

Note: ASIA (1989) recommends the use of sensory testing (Procedure 4–2) for levels $C_{1–3}$ (C_4 diaphragm), T_2–L_1, and S_2–S_5.

FIGURE 4–21   Motor assessment flow sheet. (Adapted from University Hospital, Shaughnessy Site, Vancouver, BC)

Procedure 4–1   Techniques for Examining Motor Power

Purpose:

To test motor function

Action	Rationale
1. Collaborate with physical therapist to review goals and process (including individual responses) and determine frequency of testing (Rinehart 1990).	A complete motor assessment is recommended every 8 hours during the first 72 hours with rechecks of the last normal functioning level every 2 hours. Patients demonstrating deterioration will need more diligent observation. Building interdisciplinary rapport promotes optimal management of priorities. Limitations of time, other diagnostic tests and care requirements need to be coordinated. See Chapter 6.
2. Ensure patient is comfortable and warm and explain procedure.	To maximize cooperation necessary to obtain reliable and consistent results (especially when there is no appreciable improvement in function).
3. Position supine.	The supine position, although a difficult position in which to test, allows for consistency in the initial postinjury period.
4. Test upper and then lower extremities (as in Figure 4–21). When testing extremities near the fracture site (that is, upper extremities of cervical injured patients and lower extremities of thoracolumbar injured patients), apply resistance with caution and stop if causing neck or back pain. Protect weak or paralyzed extremities from falling, either on the patient or off the bed during testing.	Test one side of the body and then the other. It may be necessary to recheck a movement to compare the right and left side accurately.
5. Move joint passively through full range of motion first. Exception is hip flexion (never beyond 45°) for low thoracolumbar injured patients.	Helps to evaluate tone and range as well as demonstrate the required movement to the patient.
6. Position limbs in opposition to the movement being tested. For example, place wrist in full flexion if extension is being tested.	
7. Ask patient for an active movement. If the response is weak, *palpate* over the belly of the muscle and *look* for any movement. If the response is strong, stabilize the joint (at the proximal point) and apply resistance (immediately distal); repeat request.	The muscle should always be at full mechanical advantage against resistance.

8. Grade muscle strength on a five-point scale and record response (Figure 4–21). Test as illustrated.

Upper Extremities	Lower Extremities
• Elbow	• Hip
• Wrist	• Knee
• Fingers	• Ankle

ELBOW: Flexion (A) starting position, (B) against resistance

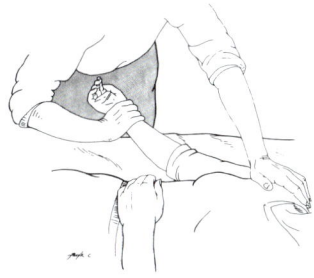
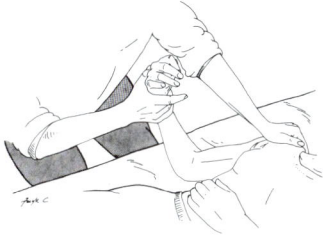

(Procedure continues)

L. Belanger, R.N. Critical Care Instructor, University
Hospital, Vancouver, BC.

Procedure 4–1   Techniques for Examining Motor Power (continued)

Extension (A) starting position against gravity, (B) against resistance

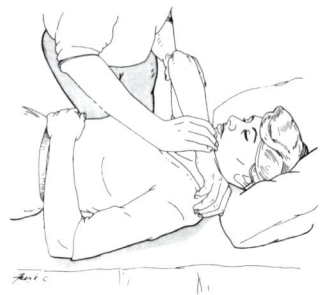
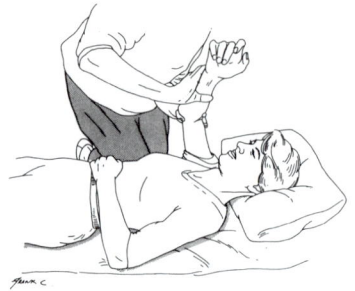

WRIST: Flexion (A) starting position with gravity eliminated, (B) full range with gravity eliminated, (C) starting position against gravity, (D) full range against gravity

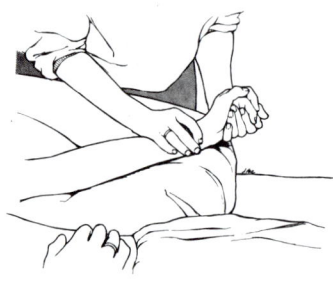
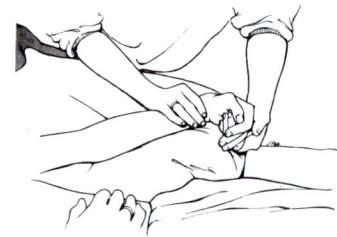

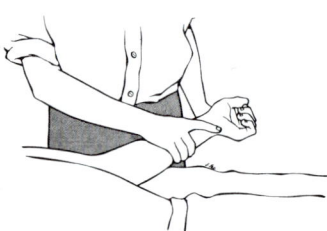
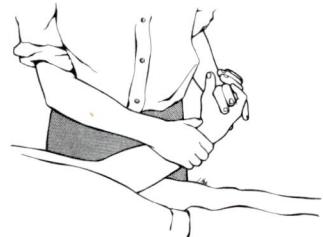

Extension (A) starting position with gravity eliminated, (B) full range with gravity eliminated, (C) starting position against gravity, (D) full range against gravity.

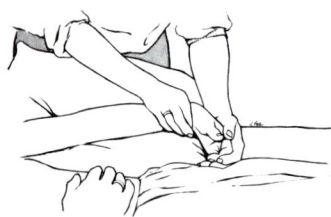
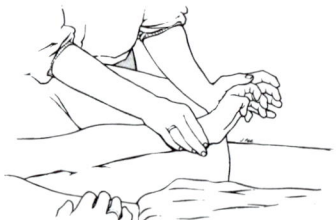

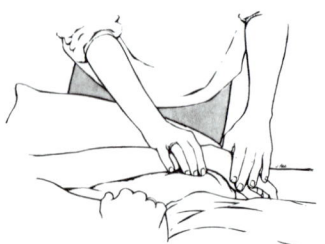
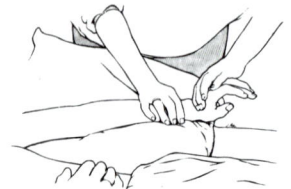

(Procedure continues)

Procedure 4–1   Techniques for Examining Motor Power (continued)

HAND: Opponents (thumb-index opposition) (A) starting position,
(B) full range against gravity, (C) full range against resistance

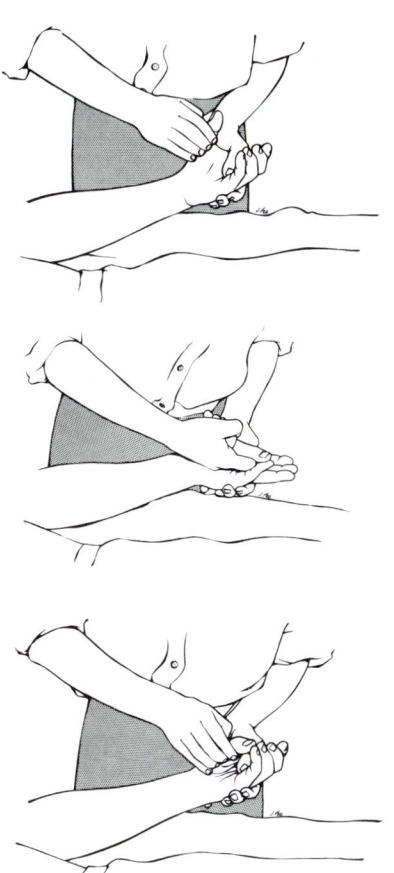

LOWER EXTREMITIES: Hip: Adduction   (A) starting position, (B) full range (note opposite hip
does not rise off the bed)

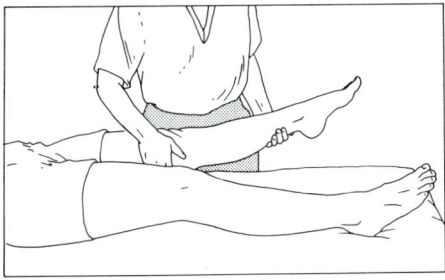 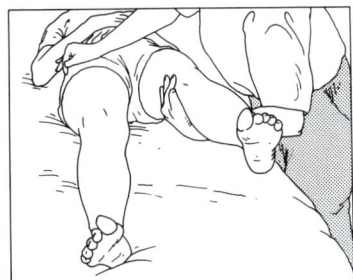

(Procedure continues)

Procedure 4–1   Techniques for Examining Motor Power (continued)

Knee: Flexion   (A) starting position (never flex hip greater than 45°), (B) full range

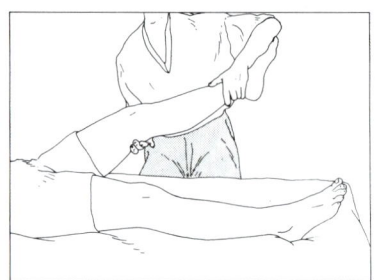 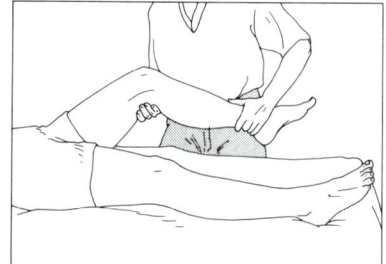

Extension   (A) starting position, (B) full range against gravity

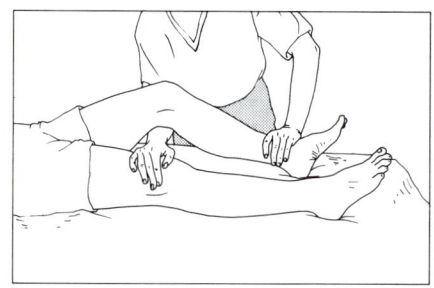 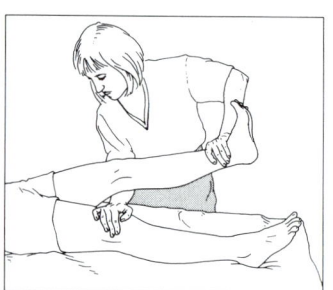

Ankle: Pantar flexion   (A) starting position, (B) almost full range against gravity

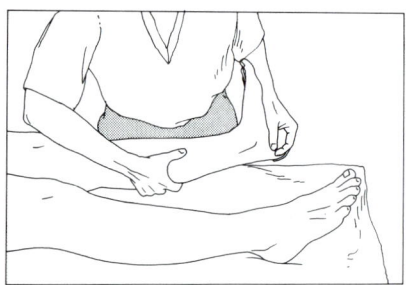 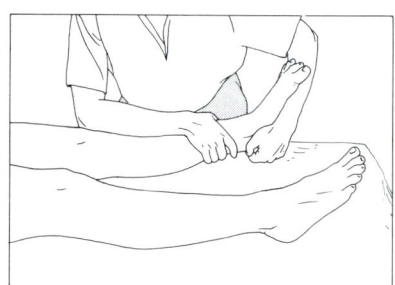

Dorsiflexion   (A) starting position, (B) full range against gravity

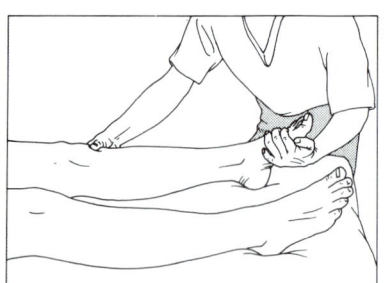 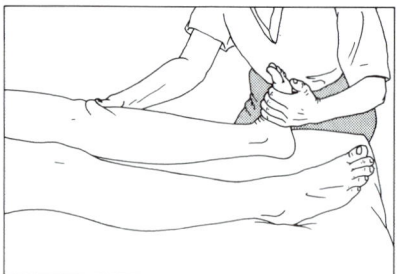

Radiographic Assessment of Spine Fractures

Management of spinal trauma is predicated on thorough clinical evaluations and radiographic assessment. The goals of radiographic assessment are to:

- Document the level of injury
- Demonstrate bone and soft tissue injury
- Provide information necessary to determine stability of the injury

Radiographic assessment does not necessarily capture the extent of bony displacement at the moment of injury if the injured vertebra(e) has returned to normal alignment. Neurological deficit may well occur without radiographic evidence of damage to the vertebral column, particularly in children and the elderly.

Standard radiography can accurately demonstrate the level of bony injury and the amount of anterior compression of a vertebral body (Figure 4–25). *Cone-down views* of the injured vertebral segment often provide greater clarity of fracture lines and vertebral body translation. If the standard radiograph demonstrates a fracture at one level, lateral films of the entire spine from the craniocervical to the lumbosacral junction should be obtained to determine if *noncontiguous* fractures (occurring at separate levels of the spine, specifically, two fractures separated by a normal segment of the spine) have occurred. The reported incidence of noncontiguous fractures ranges from 5% to 7%, and in one study the delay in diagnosis of the second fracture averaged 53 days (Calenoff, Chessare, Rogers, et al. 1978). Thus it appears that a second or third level of injury to the spine is

TABLE 4-6 Motor Index Score. (The motor index score provides a numerical rating system to document changes in motor functions. Each of the key muscles is graded according to the 0 to 5 point motor grading scale [detailed in Figure 4–21]. The scale and the scoring of a normal exam are illustrated below.)

Right	Key Muscle Segment	Left
5	C5	5
5	C6	5
5	C7	5
5	C8	5
5	T1	5
5	L2	5
5	L3	5
5	L4	5
5	L5	5
5	S1	5
50		50

Total Score 100 (Maximum Score Possible)

From ASIA 1989.

Procedure 4–2 Sensory Testing

Purpose:

To detect changes in neurological function especially during the initial 72 hours postinjury.

Action	Rationale
1. Explain procedure and ask patient to close eyes.	Reduces chances of "wishful thinking" that might lead to an inappropriate response.
2. Position in basic anatomical alignment.	
3. Select pin, cotton swab, or light touch of hand for examination.	
4. Systematically test dermatomes, working upward on the body from area of impaired sensation to normal zones.	Easier for patient to first concentrate and then give exact verbal response
5. Conduct testing of the trunk in the midaxillary line, progress to the arms, and then to the hands.	Without inclusion of the arms, T_2 borders on C_4 on the anterior chest; C_{6-8} dermatomes are represented on the hands.
6. Lightly mark patient's skin where normal sensation is present.	Ensures continuity and accuracy of comparing serial data.
7. Compare data bilaterally.	
8. Draw on sensory chart.	

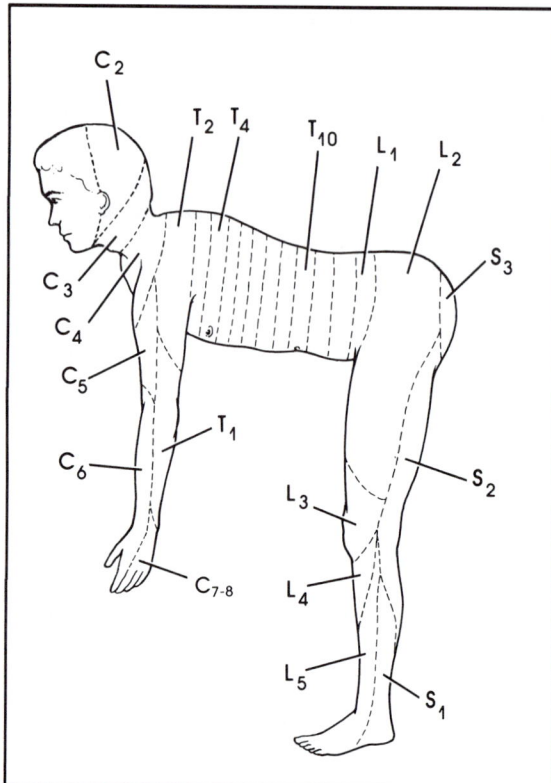

FIGURE 4–22 Arrangement of dermatomes is more easily understood when an individual is considered in quadruped (crouched) position. It is important to correlate the level of injury with the area of the body surface that is affected (dermatome).

often not diagnosed. Table 4–7 details a complete radiographic examination of the spine.

Standard films do not consistently permit an accurate assessment of the posterior elements of the neural canal (Keene, Goletz, and Lilleas 1982). Therefore when posterior element injury or compromise of the neural canal is suspected, standard films should be augmented by an ancillary radiographic method (polytomography, computed tomography, and magnetic resonance imaging) that will demonstrate these injuries.

Repeated radiologic examinations evaluate treatment, determining if correct alignment and, eventually, stability have been achieved. For example, during closed reduction attempts, when progressive traction (added weights) is increased, serial X rays indicate whether satisfactory reduction has been achieved. Postoperative films are used to ascertain correct alignment.

Computerized Axial Tomography (CAT) Scanning

Computerized axial tomography (CAT) scanning outlines the spine and perispinal structures clearly. Computerized scans accurately assess the middle column of the spine, the

key column in determining stability. Review Figure 4–3. CAT scanning accurately demonstrates the amount of neural canal impingement (NCI), the posterior element injuries and the concomitant soft tissue injuries (Figure 4–26), but it is insufficient for evaluating the level of injury and the amount of anterior vertebral body compression (Keene, Goletz, and Lilleas 1982; Keene 1984). CAT (as compared with conventional tomography) offers the additional benefits of:

- Supine (versus lateral) positioning throughout the procedure, precluding risk of injury to patients with unstable fractures
- Less average radiation exposure (10 times less than for conventional tomography)
- Demonstrating injuries to other organ systems

CAT scanning uses computer-reconstructed images from multiple X-ray absorption (density) measurements, expressed in Hounsfield units (named after the British physicist who researched the technique). The technique uses a thin, concentrated X-ray beam rather than the scattered radiation used in conventional X rays. The major components consist of the scanner itself; the computer necessary for data processing, computer printouts, and visual displays; and a controller's console and monitor.

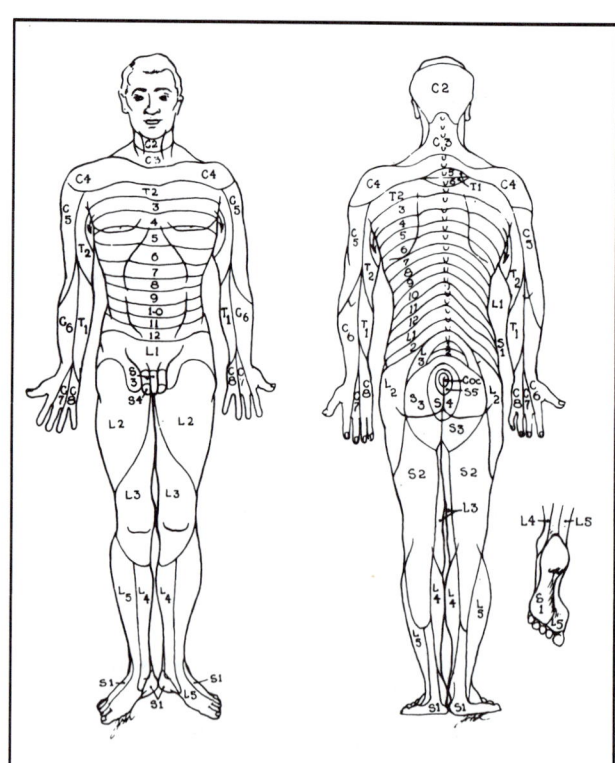

FIGURE 4–23 Sensory dermatomes. Make assessments at desired intervals and chart progression/ regression over a period of time. Tools may be adapted from this illustration to monitor sensory status. Shaded areas indicate landmark dematomes. (From Klose and Goldberg 1980.)

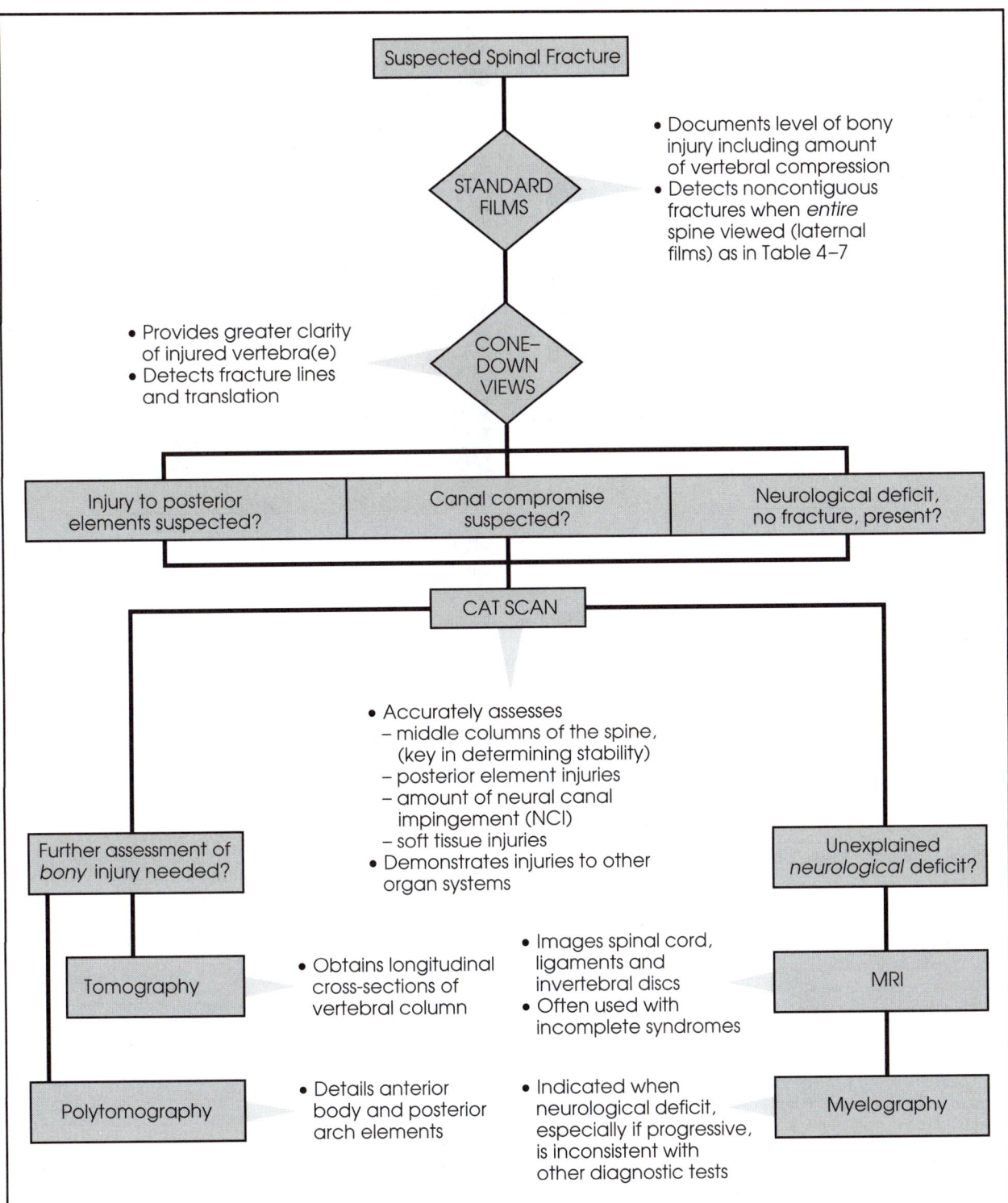

FIGURE 4–24   Algorithm for diagnostic procedure evaluation. (J. Keene, M.D., University of Wisconsin Spine Center)

A CAT scan is a noninvasive, painless procedure lasting about 30 minutes. Contrast enhancement, administered via spinal puncture, may occasionally be required. If contrast material is used, preparation and postprocedure care are similar to that for a myelogram.

Tomography

Although rapidly being replaced by CAT scanning, tomography or polytomography is still useful to evaluate the extent of bony injury. Tomography can obtain longitudinal cross-sections of the vertebral column, especially help-

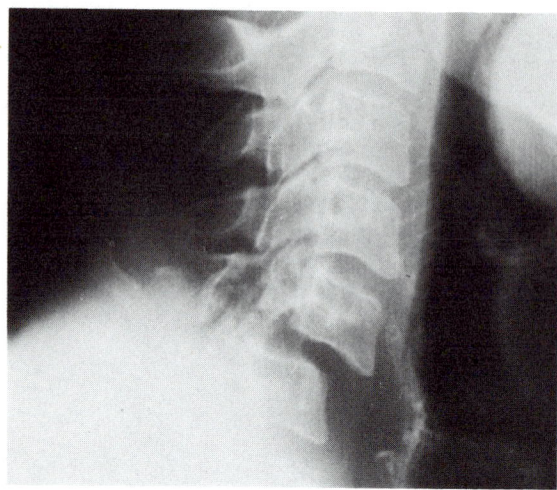

FIGURE 4–25 C₆ bilateral facet dislocation.

ful for visualizing transverse and interarticular fractures. X rays are taken at various levels, or *cuts*, by a large X-ray arm that swings back and forth overhead. Equipment that is capable of taking lateral tomograms while the patient remains supine is particularly desirable for patients with SCI.

Conventional polytomography accurately demonstrates the amount of anterior body compression and injuries to the

TABLE 4-7 Complete Radiography of the Spine

A full series of initial radiographic studies* of the spine includes:

Cervical spine films
• A cross-table lateral view with all 7 cervical vertebrae viewed. Complete visualization may be facilitated by gently applying traction (pulling) on the arms to lower the shoulders. If this is not possible, a "swimmer's view," taken through the axilla with the arm abducted, may help visualize C₇–T₁.
• The anteroposterior view helps to evaluate lateral displacements and dislocations caused by rotational forces.
• The odontoid view taken through an open mouth, which can be obtained only in a conscious patient, visualizes the odontoid process and demonstrates the atlantoaxial (C₁₋₂) articulations.

Thoracic spine films
• Lateral and anteroposterior views of all 12 vertebrae

Lumbosacral spine films
• Lateral and anteroposterior views of all 5 lumbar vertebrae and the sacrum

*A chest radiograph (a supine anteroposterior view) is included with initial assessment to rule out associated chest trauma.

University of Michigan Hospitals 1990.

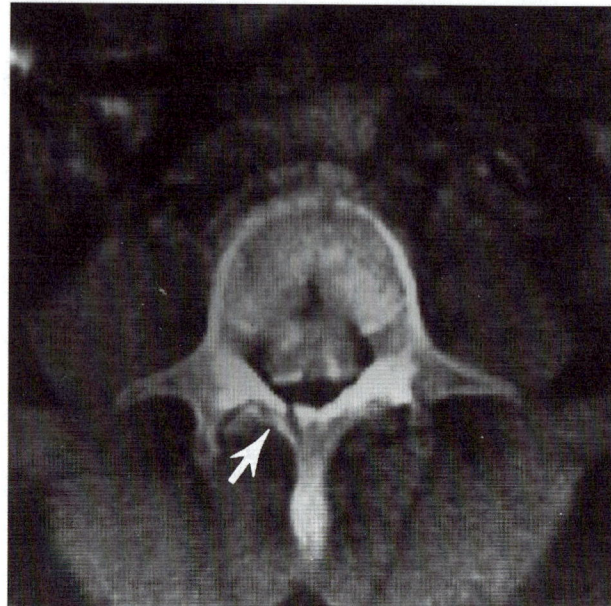

FIGURE 4–26 A CAT scan of a stable burst fracture of the fourth lumbar vertebra demonstrating 75% compromise of the neural canal, and a vertical undisplaced fracture (arrow) of the lamina.

posterior elements, but it is not accurate for determining the level of injury or the percentage of neural canal compromise, particularly if only anteroposterior tomograms are obtained.

Magnetic Resonance Imaging (MRI)

MRI is an imaging modality most helpful for assessing both the amount of spinal cord compression and the type of injury that the spinal cord has sustained (that is, either edema or hemorrhage). MRI can provide direct imaging of the soft tissues, namely the spinal cord, ligaments, and intervertebral discs, whereas CAT scanning gives better images of bony structure. Advantages include:

• More accurate than CAT or myelogram in demonstrating the relationship of fracture fragments or disc to the neural canal and spinal cord
• Noninvasive, without the use of contrast medium or radiation
• Patient manipulation not required, minimizing risk to the unstable fracture site

Skull tongs and halo rings have been developed to be compatible with the MRI.

Disadvantages are that the MRI cannot be used in patients on life-support systems, with cardiac pacemakers, or loose ferromagnetic objects within the body. MRI is also not universally available, but in time, it should replace the use of myelography. It is probably most indicated in patients with incomplete cord injury who may need surgery.

Myelography

With the advent of MRI, the indications for myelography are less clear. See the Box, "Research Note," for comments on recent comparative studies. Myelography should be used when:

- The bony injury demonstrated on the CAT is inconsistent with neurological (clinical) findings.
- The neurological deficit is rapidly progressive.
- A neural injury that has shown improvement suddenly reaches a plateau.

Based on these criteria, myelography is seldom indicated.

Myelography is an invasive procedure. A water-soluble, nontoxic contrast is injected into the arachnoid space via spinal puncture (at the C_{1-2} interspace for persons with cervical injuries or the lumbar spine for persons with thoracolumbar injuries, although the thoracic spine cannot be viewed well). The patient is tilted in various directions to exert gravitational forces on the contrast while serial X rays are taken. Because of the inherent danger in manipulating the patient with an unstable spine fracture, myelography is considered a high-risk procedure.

After the procedure, tilt the bed up 30 to 45 degrees, if possible, to exert gravitational forces on the unremoved contrast and thus minimize cerebral irritation. To dilute the contrast, increase fluid intake for a 12-hour period, if not contraindicated. Analgesics and antiemetics may be required.

Somatosensory-evoked Potentials

Recording of somatosensory-evoked potentials is done mainly to establish a prognosis. The test is done by stimu-

---

Research Note
Neural Canal Impingement

Magnetic resonance imaging clearly delineates injuries to the spinal cord and surrounding soft tissue structures. Cotler and associates (1988) evaluated patients with thoracolumbar fractures and SCI and found three patterns of injury to the spinal cord. In type 1, MRI demonstrated decreased signal intensity consistent with acute intraspinal hemorrhage. MR images of type 2 injuries had increased signal intensity, consistent with acute cord edema, and type 3 had a mixed signal of hypointensity centrally, and hyperintensity peripherally, consistent with cord contusion. They noted that patients with the type 1 pattern showed no improvement in their neurological status, but patients with type 2 and 3 patterns showed significant neurological recovery. A comparison of CAT and MRI by Kitchel and associates (1988) found that CAT demonstrated fractures and spinal malalignment best. However, MRI demonstrates spinal cord compression, intra- and extramedullary hemorrhage, and intrinsic spinal cord edema that were not evident on the CAT scans. The study concluded that MRI should be obtained in patients with incomplete SCI and in those patients with SCI who have no demonstrable fracture.

One remaining question is the significance of acute posttraumatic bony encroachment of the neural canal. In a recent study, the relationship between acute, posttraumatic neural canal impingement (NCI) and the immediate postinjury neurological status of the patient were examined (Keene, Fischer, Vanderby, et al. 1989). Eighty consecutive patients were evaluated and the amount of NCI demonstrated on CAT scans was correlated with each patient's neurological status, level of injury, and type of fracture. Results indicated that average NCI was 62%, 55%, and 27% in patients with complete injuries, incomplete injuries, and no deficit, respectively. However, although average NCI was significantly higher in the 34 patients with neurological deficits, the range of NCI (complete lesions 0–100%, incomplete injuries 0–94%, no deficit 0–85%) was similar to that observed in the 46 patients with no deficits. Burst fractures and fractures in the lumbar spine had the highest average NCI (52% and 58%, respectively), but the lowest percentage of patients with neurological deficits. The study documented that with all types of injuries, and at all levels of injury (thoracic, thoracolumbar, and lumbar), there was no simple, direct relationship between a patient's *initial* neurological impairment and the percent of posttraumatic, bony encroachment of the neural canal demonstrated by CAT.

In the cervical spine, however, preexisting spinal stenosis does seem to have some affect on neurologic outcome. It appears that people having a stenotic spinal canal suffered a greater degree of neurologic loss than those with a large spinal canal. Torg and associates (1986), in a study of college and professional football players, have shown that cervical spinal stenosis does predispose these athletes to transient quadraparesis. They then developed a simple ratio of the vertebral body depth compared to the width of the spinal canal, which may be helpful in delineating those athletes at higher risk for cervical spinal cord injuries.

lating a peripheral nerve in the arm or leg (below the level of injury) and recording the neurological response (evoked potential) from the cerebral cortex through scalp electrodes (similar to those used in electroencephalography). This is a noninvasive procedure and can be done in the emergency or operating room, because a small portable computer is used to summate the responses.

When the injury is complete, somatosensory-evoked potentials are absent; when the injury is incomplete, a marked alteration in response is noted. The test has been valuable in the assessment of prognosis and response to treatment (Tator and Rowed 1979). Early persistence and progressive normalization of evoked potentials precedes the clinical evidence of improvement and is therefore a favorable prognostic sign.

Undetected Complications

The immediate consequences of spine fractures causing SCI are readily apparent. However, there are several problems that may not be immediately evident. These include genitourinary dysfunction in patients who otherwise have no neurological deficit, and late complications of chronic instability, including those of undetected noncontiguous fractures, and syringomyelia. Although bladder dysfunction is usually present in patients with vertebral fractures

and abnormal sacral sensation and rectal tone, this dysfunction often goes undetected in patients with these injuries in whom sacral sensation and rectal tone are normal. Late complications are discussed in Chapter 20.

Complaints of incomplete emptying, urgency, and impotence are dysfunctional. Because clinical examination alone does not rule out genitourinary dysfunction, and significant renal destruction can ensue, patients with fresh fractures should be evaluated for residual urine volumes immediately following voiding. If volumes are greater than 60 ml, evaluation by a urologist is indicated. With late onset of symptoms, urological investigation is similar.

Management of individuals with spinal fractures depends on expert clinical examination and carefully selected use of diagnostic procedures to evaluate injury. Lateral radiographs of the entire spine cannot be overstressed. Of the ancillary radiographic studies, CAT scanning is the best noninvasive modality for classifying the injury and determining stability by assessing the middle column of the spine, which is the key to stability. MRI may have the most prognostic value for patients with incomplete syndromes. Problems can remain unrecognized after injury to the spine. With awareness of these conditions and assessment that includes salient diagnostic tests, these problems will not go undetected.

REFERENCES

ASIA. 1989. Standards for Neurological Classification for SCI. ASIA, 2020 Peachtree Road, NW, Atlanta, GA 30309

Burke, D. C. 1979. The neurological examination (spinal). *Australian Family Physician* 8 (Feb.): 119–128. *Excellent guide to accurate diagnosis of SCI; simplified guide to some traps and subtleties of diagnosis. Highly recommended.*

Burke, D. L., and Murray, D. D. 1975. *Handbook of Spinal Cord Medicine.* London and Basingstoke: MacMillan Press. *Concise review of functional anatomy and injuries to the spinal column and spinal cord in Chapters 2, 3, and 4.*

Calenoff, L., Chessare, J. W., Rogers, L. F., et al. 1978. Multiple level spine injuries: Importance of early recognition. *American Journal of Roentology* 130: 665–669.

Cotler, H. B., Kulkarni, M. V., Bondurant, F. J., et al. 1988. Magnetic resonance imaging in acute spinal cord injury. Presented at the American Spinal Cord Injury Association Annual Meeting, May 2–4, 1988, San Diego, CA.

Denis, F. 1978. The three-column spine and its significance in the classification of acute thoracolumbar injuries. *Spine* 8: 160–166.

Groenwald, S. L., and Thaney, K. 1987. In *Cancer Nursing Principles and Practice.* Ed. S. Groenwald. Boston: Jones and Bartlett.

Hickey, J. 1986. *The Clinical Practice of Neurological and Neurosurgical Nursing.* Philadelphia: J. B. Lippincott Company.

Keene, J. S. 1984. Radiographic evaluation of thoracolumbar fractures. *Clinical Orthopedics* 189: 58–64.

Keene, J. S., Goletz, T. H., Lilleas, F. 1982. Diagnosis of vertebral fractures. A comparison of conventional radiography, conventional tomography, and computed tomography. *Journal of Bone and Joint Surgery* 64A: 586–595.

Keene, J. S., Fischer, S. P., Vanderby, R., Jr., et al. 1989. Significance of acute post-traumatic bony encroachment of the neural canal. *Spine* 14(8): 799–802.

Kitchel, S. H., Eismont, F. J., Quencer, R. A., et al. 1988. Evaluation of acute thoracolumbar fractures with MR imaging. Paper presented at the American Spinal Cord Injury Association Annual Meeting, May 2–4, 1988, San Diego, CA.

Klose, K. J., and Goldberg, M. L. 1980. Neurological change following spinal cord injury: an assessment technique and preliminary results. *Spinal Cord Injury Digest* 2 (Summer): 35–42. *Description of a quantitative tool: the University of Miami Neurospinal Index (UMNI), which consists of the sensory scale and the motor scale. Scale scores are indicators of overall spinal cord functional capacity within the sensory and motor modalities.*

Liebman, M. 1979. *Neuroanatomy Made Easy and Understandable.* Baltimore: University Park Press. *Presents fundamental basis for neuroanatomy, neurophysiology, neuropharmacology, physical diagnosis, and neurology. Helpful sections on spinal pathways and the auto-*

nomic nervous system. Valuable glossary relating Latin origins to everyday language.

McAfee, P. C., Hansen, A. Y., Fredrickson, B. E., et al. 1983. The value of tomography in complicated thoracolumbar fractures: An analysis of 100 consecutive cases and a new classification. *Journal of Bone and Joint Surgery* 65A: 461–473.

Rinehart, M. E. 1990. Early mobilization in acute SCI. *Critical Care Nursing in North America* 2: 399–405.

Tator, C. H., and Rowed, D. W. 1979. Current concepts in the immediate management of acute spinal cord injuries. *Canadian Medical Association Journal* 121 (Dec.): 1453–1464. *Excellent review of updated care: describes sophisticated diagnostic tests, treatment methods,*

and related nursing care to minimize secondary pathological processes following initial trauma. Extensive bibliography. Highly recommended.

Torg, J. S., Pavlov, H., Genuario, S. E., Sennett, B., Wisneski, R. J., Robie, B. H., and Jahre, C. 1986. Neuropraxia of the cervical spinal cord with transient quadriplegia. *Journal of Bone and Joint Surgery* 68A: 1354–1370.

University of Michigan Hospitals. 1990. *Spinal Cord Injury Protocol.* Ann Arbor: University of Michigan Spinal Cord Injury Center.

Yarbro, C. H. 1987. In *Cancer Nursing Principles and Practice.* Ed. S. Groenwald. Boston: Jones and Bartlett.

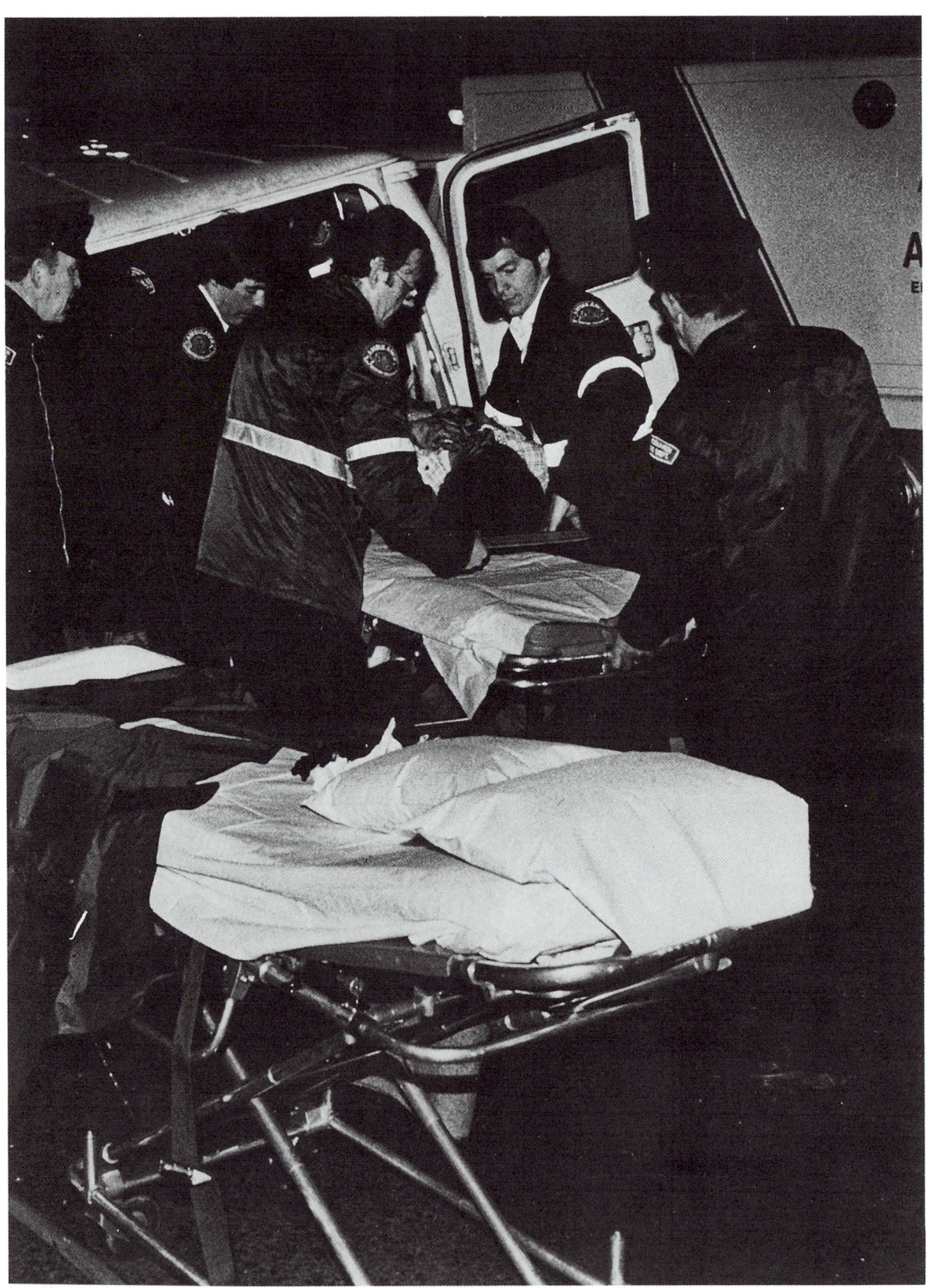

CHAPTER
— 5 —

Prehospital Care for People with Spinal Cord Injuries[*]

Chapter Outline

Health Care Objectives

- To anticipate spinal injury based on mechanism
- To assess the patient and initiate appropriate lifesaving interventions oriented toward the possibility of SCI
- To prevent further neurological injury through immobilization and other techniques
- To understand basic triage considerations
- To transport to the nearest appropriate facility
- To manage associated complications appropriately

*This Chapter was developed with the assistance of Robert Ξ. Falcone, M.D.

There are few injuries whose ultimate outcome is as dependent on prehospital care as spinal cord injury (SCI). Correct management at the scene of the injury may make the difference between recovery or lifelong paralysis. A clear understanding of the potential for injury, expert rescue, rapid and appropriate transport, and careful coordination with inpatient receiving facilities are essential. The first person who provides care at the scene of injury begins the rehabilitation process.

Before initiating active intervention or moving the patient, always suspect SCI. The type of accident (which indicates the mechanism of injury) is the most important clue to the possibility of spinal injury.

APPROACHING THE SCENE: SECURING A SAFE ENVIRONMENT

The prehospital providers' first responsibility is to ensure a safe environment for themselves in which to work. Burning buildings, unsecured heights, downed power lines, explosive materials, and noxious chemicals are typical examples of environmental hazards. Dangerous environmental situations should be secured by trained fire and police personnel before rescue is attempted. Note environmental factors—for example, heat and cold—that play a role in preparing the patient for eventual transport. Figure 5–1 outlines appropriate actions for the first persons (who are probably not trained in emergency procedure) to come on the scene.

ANTICIPATING THE POSSIBILITY OF SPINAL CORD INJURY: MECHANISMS OF INJURY

The scene should be quickly evaluated for mechanism(s) of injury, the number of injured people, and potential problems in extrication and transport. Victims in hazardous areas should be moved to safety before interventions are initiated.

The most common cause of SCI is the motor vehicle accident. Falls (especially head first or from heights), diving and sporting injuries, and penetrating injuries to the neck or back may also lead to spinal damage. It is not uncommon for alcohol and drug abuse to be a contributing factor. *The unconscious or unreliable patient is especially vulnerable to missed injury and should always be assumed to have a spinal injury until proven otherwise.* See Chapter 1 for detailed

information on causes and Table 4–2 for mechanisms of spinal cord injury.

ASSESSMENT AND INTERVENTIONS IN PREHOSPITAL CARE

Primary Survey

In addition to anticipating SCI, complete a *primary survey* —a rapid assessment of *airway, breathing, and circulation (ABCs)*. Decisions can then be made as to the urgency of extrication and transport. A person in cardiopulmonary arrest must be moved with more urgency than one who is awake, alert, and relatively comfortable. Priorities always remain the ABCs. However, *some patients can never be stabilized in the prehospital setting and are best rapidly transported to the nearest appropriate facility.* When the patient is stabilized, conduct a secondary head-to-toe survey that includes a brief history. See Figure 5–2.

Airway and Breathing

Rapid assessment and management of the airway are the first priority, but they must be adapted to the possibility of spinal injury. Airway compromise can be due to a variety of factors. In the unconscious patient, aspiration, foreign bodies, and the patient's own tongue are common causes of airway obstruction. Direct injury to the face and its bony structure can also cause mechanical airway compromise. With cervical spine injury neurological control of breathing is impaired. People sustaining injury to C_4 and above cannot breathe spontaneously.

Remember:

- Recognize
- Protect
- Provide

The first step to successful airway management is to recognize airway compromise:

- *Think.* Always suspect airway compromise in people who are unconscious or intoxicated, have head and facial injuries, or have inhaled smoke or toxic gas or nearly drowned. In people with cervical spine injuries, if the respiratory rate is approaching 35 breaths per minute consider immediate ventilatory assistance to avoid impending decompensation (University of Michigan Hospitals 1990).
- *Look* for evidence of breathing difficulty or agitation, signs of hypoxia (a lack of blood oxygenation). With *diaphragmatic or paradoxical breathing* the chest does not rise and fall with respiration. Instead there is a more exaggerated movement of the abdomen (dia-

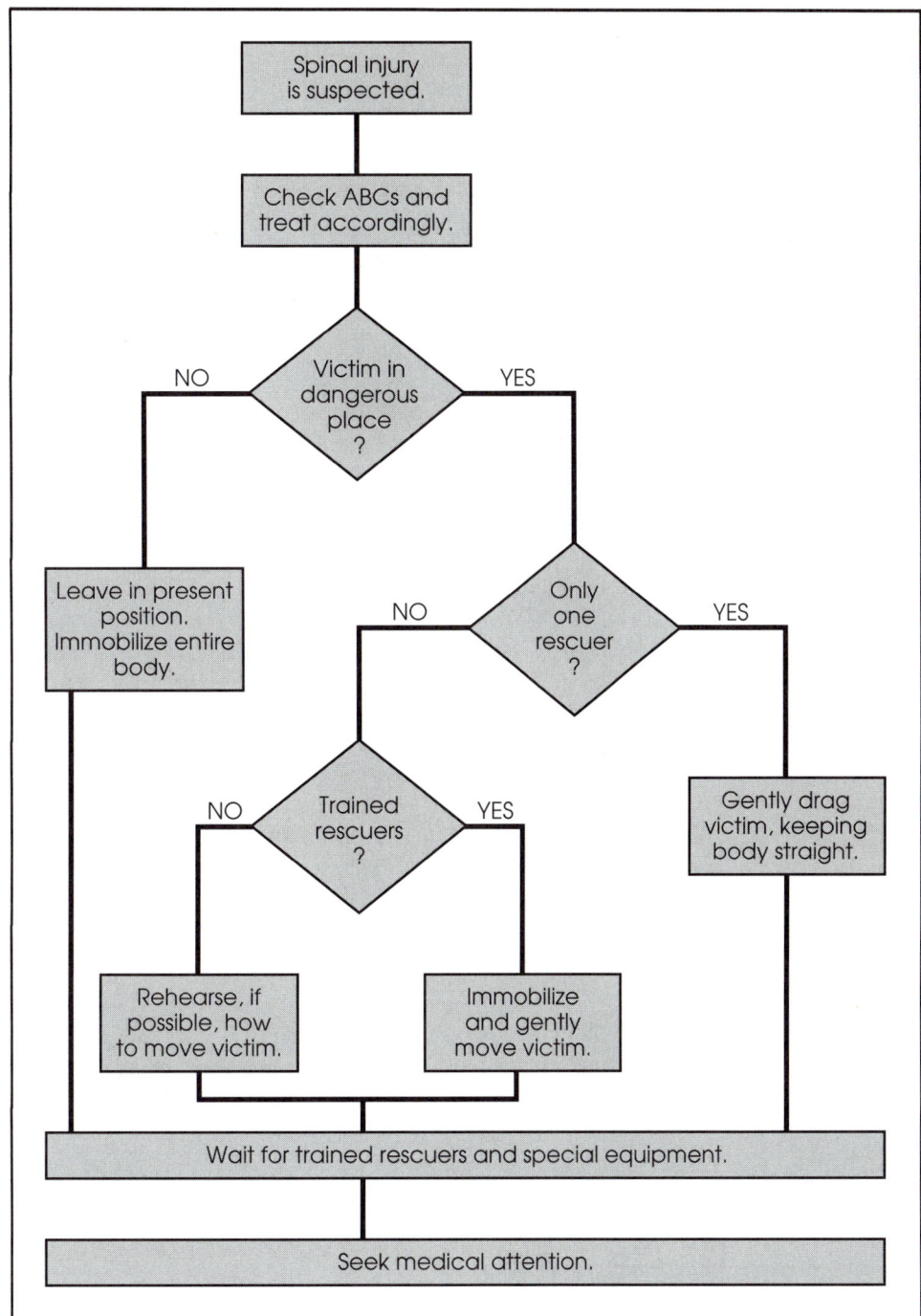

FIGURE 5–1 Spinal injury: Appropriate actions for the first responder. (Thygerson 1987: 4).

phragm) just below the rib cage. Respirations tend to be shallow and rapid.

- *Listen* for evidence of airway compromise such as hoarseness, gurgling.
- *Feel* for air exchange, trachial deformity, or foreign bodies in the mouth or throat.

Protect the threatened airway with the least manipulation of the neck possible to do the job. Victims are found in many awkward positions (Table 4–2). Return the person to the supine position and the neck to the neutral position as in Procedure 5–1. Many times simply restoring this position will be enough to reestablish the airway.

If breathing and a noiseless exchange of air are not restored, clear the mouth and open the airway by using a jaw thrust maneuver or a chin lift maneuver (Procedure 5–2) to lift the tongue off the back of the throat with minimal movement of the neck. Administer 100% oxygen.

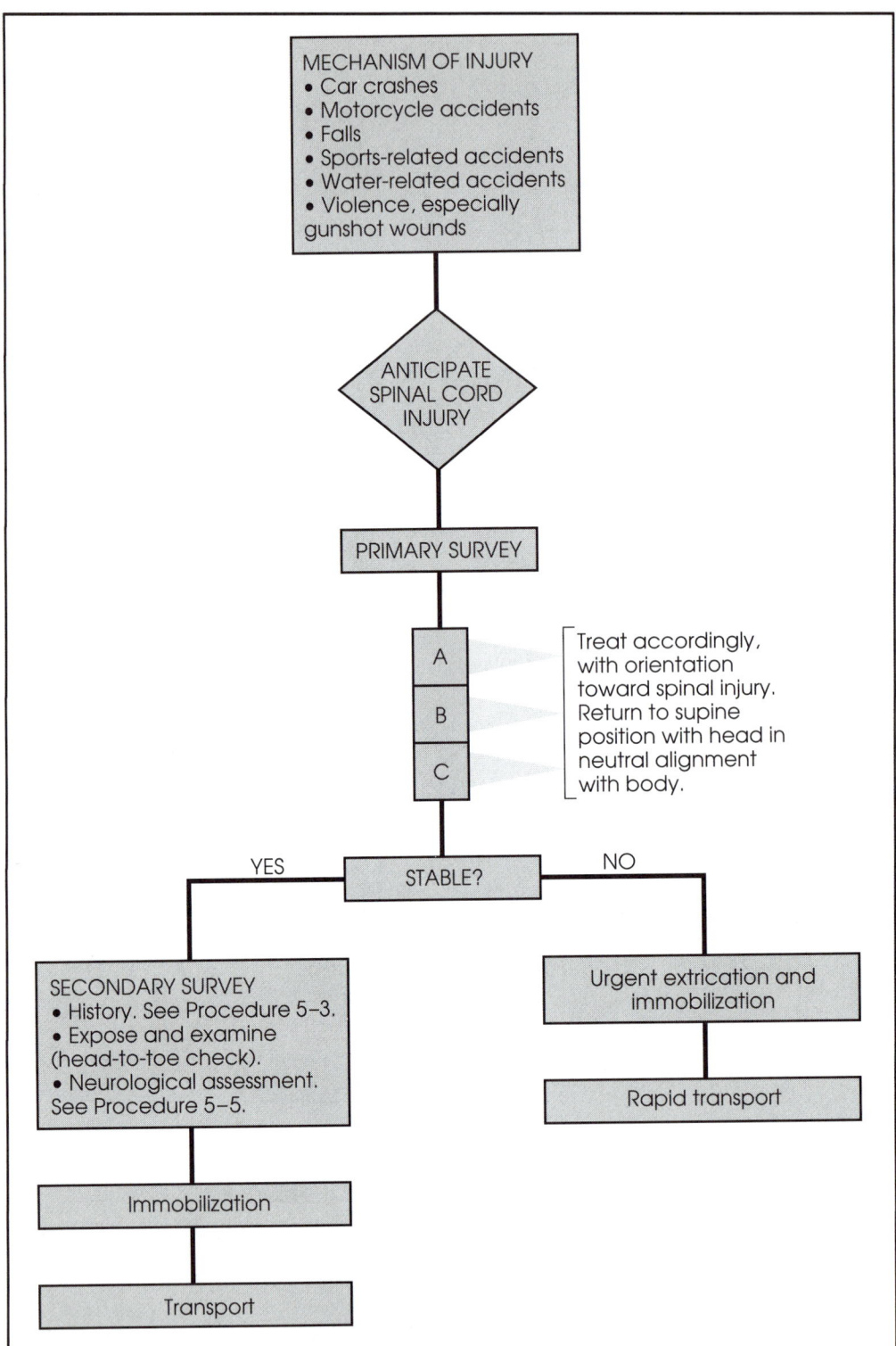

FIGURE 5–2 Prehospital care demands critical decisions.

If needed, an oropharyngeal airway (in the unconscious person) or nasopharyngeal airway (in the responsive person) can be placed to keep the tongue off of the pharynx and protect the airway during transport. If the patient is moving some air, *nasotrachial intubation is the route of choice* because it can be consistently accomplished with minimal manipulation of the cervical spine. Failure of nasotrachial intubation or the presence of apnea mandates orotrachial intubation. Surgical airways such as cricothyrotomy for adults and needle cricothyrotomy for children can readily

Procedure 5–1   The Delicate Spine: Returning to a Neutral Position

Purpose:

To protect the cervical cord from further injury by aligning the neck with the body in the supine position

Action

1. To establish level of consciousness and to reassure and instruct the patient, first rescuer should say, "Hello, can you hear me? Don't move."

2. Secure a stable position for yourself before attempting to stabilize the patient.

3. First return the patient's neck to the neutral position (in line with the body) before attempting to position the body.

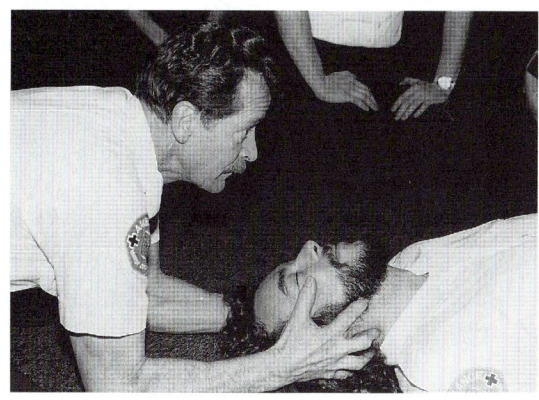

4. If the person is found in the sitting position, approach the victim from behind, if possible. Stabilize your elbows to perform this maneuver.

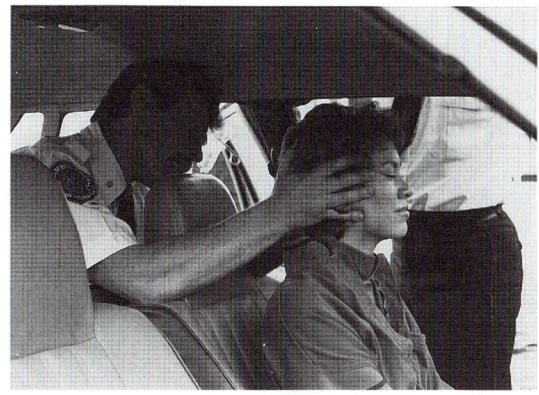

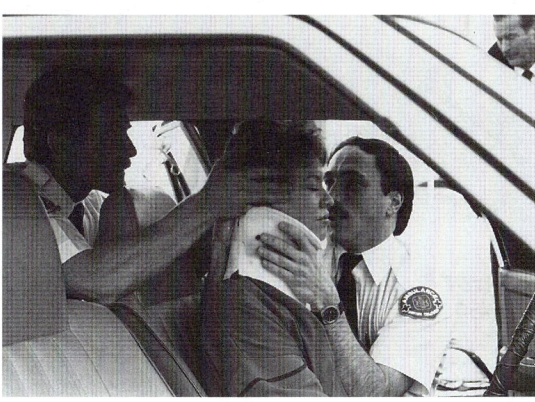

5. If the patient is found in the prone position with the head to the side:

   • Think ahead to be ahead. Most often there is time to stabilize the patient carefully before attempting extrication. Remember to talk to your partner. Make sure the other rescuer has a good grip to maintain alignment before you let go.

   • The first rescuer must support the head, while the second rescuer(s) turns the body.

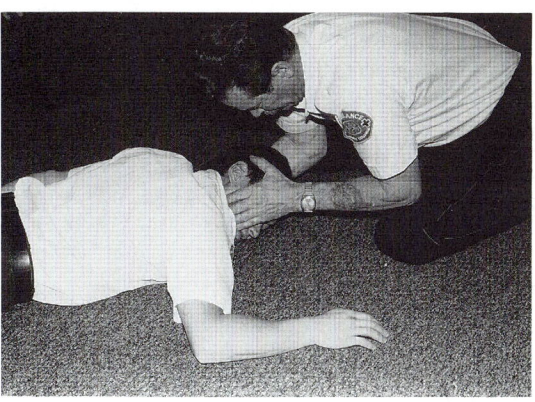

(Procedure continues)

Procedure 5–1   The Delicate Spine: Returning to a Neutral Position (continued)

• The second rescuer must then assume the responsibility for holding the neck in line while the first rescuer repositions hands to resume control of the head and realign the spine.

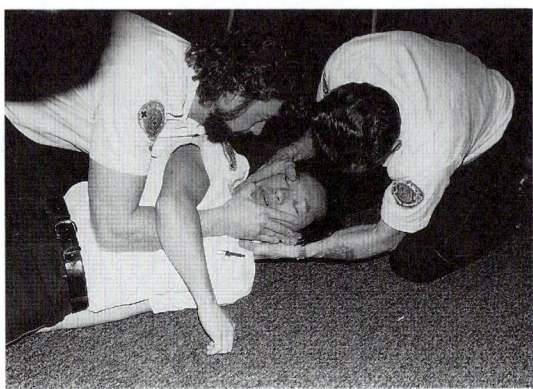

6. Many rescuers find it helpful to splint the head to the body. A "full trap" may be used to secure the neck and minimize risk of movement. This involves a vice-grip action with the forearms placed on the chest and back. In a modified version of this procedure, forearm action on one side and a hand on the other guide the head.

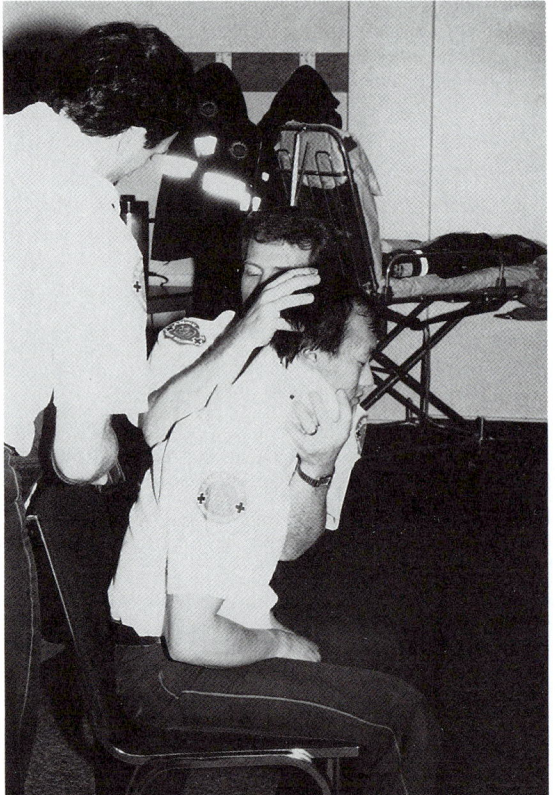

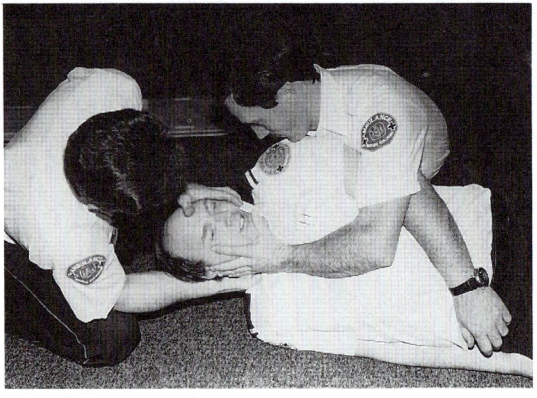

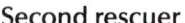

7. Hold the patient's head firmly, pushing up slightly to immobilize the cervical spine.

Second rescuer

8. Apply rigid or semirigid collar and secure with Velcro closures or tape. If there is resistance—for instance, extreme pain at the fracture site—and the rescuer is unable to achieve the desired position, apply a soft collar as a last resort.

9. Immobilize and extricate the patient.

Adapted from Paramedic Academy, 1991.

Procedure 5–2   Maneuvers to Open the Airway with Cervical Spine Injury

Purpose:

To avoid hyperextension of the neck, which is the standard maneuver, by minimizing neck movement when opening the upper airway

Action	Rationale

The Jaw Thrust Maneuver

1. Be sure that the neck is in the netural position and the patient is supine.

2. Stand or kneel behind the patient's head if possible; place hands on either side of the patient's head. Work from a stable position.

   To maintain the head and neck in a fixed, neutral position without hyperextension or tilting from side to side.

3. Open mouth.

4. Grasp the angles of the patient's lower jaw with fingers, place thumbs carefully on patient's cheekbones.

   Positioning of thumbs also provides an opposing point to gain momentum with lifting movement.

5. Using the thumbs to provide a focal point for opposing pressure, thrust (displace) the jaw forward with a lifting movement.

   This thrust unlocks the jaw and avoids inadvertent movement of the head.

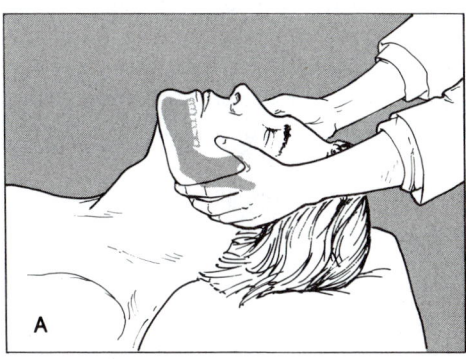
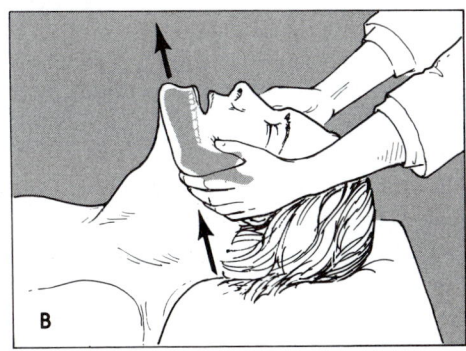

6. If the lips close, quickly move one thumb to retract the lower lip.

7. If this is unsuccessful, tilt the head slightly backward and make another attempt to open the airway or proceed with the chin life maneuver.

   Establishing an open airway takes priority over treatment of the spinal cord injury.

The Chin Lift Maneuver

1. Using one hand, place your thumb in the patient's mouth with the thumbnail between the patient's teeth; grasp the patient under the chin with your fingers.

   If the patient's mouth closes, the teeth will strike your thumbnail.

2. Lift the patient's chin.

   Establishing an open airway takes priority over treatment of the spinal cord injury.

3. Observe for elevation of the chest to indicate air entry.

---

be adapted to the prehospital setting. However, these procedures generally require training and experience beyond typical paramedical skills.

After an airway has been established, deliver 100% oxygen via a nonrebreather mask with gas flow of 12 to 15 liters per minute. If the respiratory rate is not adequate for age (see Table 5–1 for guidelines), assist ventilation with a bag mask resuscitator. Inability to ventilate after appropriate airway management requires rechecking of the airway for foreign bodies, accumulated blood, or secretions. Endotrachial tubes can kink or clog with blood and secretions.

TABLE 5–1 Normal Vital Signs

Age	Weight Range	Pulse Range	Mean Respiration	Lower Limit Systolic BP
Infant 0–2 years	0–12kg	120–160	40	70
Preschool 2–6 years	12–25kg	110–140	30	70
School age 6–14	25–45kg	80–120	20	80
Adult 15	45kg	60–100	16	90

Adapted from the American College of Surgeons (1986).

Other common mechanical impediments to ventilation include *tension pneumothorax, open pneumothorax, massive hemothorax,* and a *flail chest,* which are detailed in Table 5–2. Chest trauma is not uncommon with thoracic spine injuries: a force violent enough to fracture the strong thoracic spine will often crush the chest also.

Circulation
Check the patient's color and the carotid and peripheral pulses. Good color and a strong regular pulse, especially in an arm or leg, implies good *perfusion* (tissue circulation). Pale or ashen color with weak, rapid, or absent pulses suggests poor perfusion (shock). The patient in severe shock will have a low blood pressure for age (see Table 5–1 for guidelines). *Hypovolemic (hemorrhagic) shock* is common in trauma patients. *

However, the patient with SCI also sustains hypotension (low blood pressure) as a result of *spinal (neurogenic) shock.* Spinal shock occurs as a result of autonomic nervous system changes that decrease vascular resistance causing blood to pool in the extremities. Patients experiencing spinal shock will generally have good perfusion when lying supine (unlike persons with hypovolemic shock), and have warm, dry skin. Differentiating between spinal and hypovolemic shock is critical in estimating the nature and volume of fluid replacement. Especially high volumes of intravenous fluids given to compensate for low blood pressure, when caused from spinal shock, will overload the patient and cause serious complications. Chapter 6 explains the complication of spinal shock in more detail.

Trauma Arrest
Cardiopulmonary arrest secondary to drugs, illness, or cardiac dysrhythmias may often be successfully reversed in the

External bleeding should be controlled with direct pressure. Shock management is aimed at restoring normal circulating blood volume.

field by cardiac life support measures. However, cardiopulmonary arrest as a result of trauma poses a different problem. Airway disruption, hypovolemia, and cardiac tamponade often make CPR ineffective.

Survival in trauma arrest is unusual. Those patients who do survive either have an isolated problem that is easy to remedy (such as a respiratory arrest in the patient with cervical SCI), or are transported to definitive care rapidly enough to have more complex problems addressed.

Although prolonged field management of arrest due to illness may be successful, arrest due to trauma is uniformly fatal. Trauma patients who do not achieve palpable pulses and visible chest excursion with CPR have a mechanical problem until proven otherwise. They will only survive if rapidly transported, ideally to a trauma center if minutes away, otherwise to the nearest emergency facility.

Secondary Survey

History
Recording the mechanism of injury at the accident as accurately as possible can aid in the diagnosis of injury and initial hospital management. If the patient is conscious, obtain a name and address, a brief list of complaints, previous illnesses, allergies, and current medications. In the unconscious patient, identification bracelets, and medical alert cards, friends, relatives, and bystanders can often be of help. Refer to Procedure 5–3.

Expose and Examine (Head-to-Toe Check)
The prehospital secondary survey should include a rapid head-to-toe evaluation of the injured patient in light of the mechanism of injury. Ideally this should be done in an organized and thorough fashion. However, the seriously injured person should not be kept at the scene to examine trivial injuries. Most of the survey should be done during transport. It is difficult to examine through clothing, which should be carefully removed when possible.

The removal of protective helmets in the field remains controversial, but it should be left to people trained in helmet removal, who are usually the prehospital providers, *not* the emergency department personnel. Procedure 5–4 presents some guidelines.

Look, listen, and feel, starting at the head and working down the body. Injury hurts, and the alert patient will normally complain of pain and tenderness to touch at the site of injury; below that level sensation (including pain) is lost. Chest injury will often be associated with respiratory difficulties and abnormal breath sounds. Abdominal injury will often be associated with distension but typically is not felt. Most bony injuries will show evidence of bruising and deformity.

Level of consciousness is the most sensitive indicator of central nervous system injury, but this can be altered by

TABLE 5–2 Airway Complications Requiring Rapid Transport

Complication	Explanation	Symptoms	Field Treatment
Tension Pneumothorax	Due to air leaking into the pleural cavity and accumulating under pressure because of an injury. As tension develops, the movable midline chest structures (heart, vessels, trachea) begin to shift to the opposite chest leading to respiratory distress and cardiovascular collapse (from a decreasing venous return).	• Rapidly escalating respiratory distress with a patent upper airway • Progressive hypovolemic shock • Diminished breath sounds of involved side of chest with hyperresonance (a hollow drumlike sound if tapped with the finger) • Decreased respiratory motion • Distended veins in the neck • Tracheal deviation away from the involved side	• Needle decompression with flutter valve of the involved chest (by protocol for those providers trained to do so) • Rapid transport
Open Pneumothorax (Sucking Chest Wound)	Direct communication between the pleural cavity and the environment created by trauma. May severely impair ventilation because of altered pulmonary mechanics.	• Progressive respiratory impairment	• Cover the defect with a sterile, partially occlusive dressing such as a patch taped on three sides, that allows air to leak out with expiration, but prevents air from being sucked in during inspiration. Improves ventilatory mechanics. • Rapid transport
Massive Hemothorax	Massive bleeding into the chest	• Respiratory distress • Hypovolemic shock • External evidence of chest injury • Decreased breath sounds, but with diminished resonance (chest makes a dull sound if tapped—in contrast to tension pneumothorax) • Neck veins flat	• General supportive measures • Shock management • Rapid transport
Flail Chest	Caused by multiple rib fractures that can lead to a segment of chest wall moving independently on ventilation. Paradoxical movement with inspiration and expiration is mechanically disadvantageous. More important, however, an injury forceful enough to cause a flail chest will cause a serious underlying pulmonary contusion (lung bruise). A contused lung not only fails to oxygenate blood, but allows unoxygenated blood to return to the central circulation (shunt) leading to a decrease in total body oxygenation.	• Progressive respiratory impairment/distress	• Supplemental oxygen Note: Standard measures such as splinting the flail segment with sandbags or positioning the patient on the affected side may be dangerous for people with spinal injury. • Immobilize patient securely on spine board first, then tip toward affected side • Rapid transport

R. Falcone, M.D., Grant Medical Center, Ohio

Procedure 5–3 Secondary Survey: Taking a History During Prehospital Care

Purpose:

To determine how the injury was sustained (mechanism of injury) and if any other medical factors require emergency intervention

Action

If the patient is conscious:

1. Ask if there is any neck or back pain.

2. Ask what bothers the patient the most (isolation of chief complaint).

3. Note details concerning mechanism of injury.

4. Ask if patient has any medical problems, for instance, chronic illnesses or allergies; is on any medication; has taken any alcohol or drugs.

5. Ask name, age, address, next of kin.

If the patient is unconscious or unable to provide reliable information:

Ask a witness (a relative if possible) these same questions.

Rationale

Patient will likely have severe pain at the injury site, which will localize level of injury.

Isolation of chief complaint gives direction to further questioning. If, for example, patient complains of difficulty in breathing, the nature of the complaint must be clarified. Checking medical history for such problems as cardiac insufficiency or asthma helps determine whether difficulty breathing is a direct result of cord injury.

To determine force of mechanism(s) ask questions like how fast the car was going or what the road conditions were. Note height of fall, and describe other contributing factors.

Procedure 5–4 Helmet Removal When Cervical Spine Injury Is Suspected

Action

1. Rescuer #1 applies in-line neutral traction by placing hands on each side of the helmet. (Approach patient from the top of patient's head.)

2. Rescuer #2 secures the jaw with one hand and applies pressure to the back of the neck (occiput) with the other. (Approach the patient from the patient's chest.)

3. Rescuer #1 removes the helmet, taking care to cut straps, and expand and tilt gently as necessary to clear face and ears.

4. After the helmet is removed, Rescuer #1 places palms of hands over ears and secures the occiput and jaw with fingers to maintain in-line position.

Rescuer #2 is now responsible for maintaining the in-line neutral position of the neck.

Rescuer #1 becomes responsible for maintaining immobilization of the neck.

Third person

5. Rescuer #2 then applies cervical collar.

Adapted from Paramedic Academy (1990).

drugs, intoxication, metabolic imbalance, and hypotension. The AVPU method provides a simple means of quantifying level of consciousness:

- A—alert
- V—responsive to voice
- P—responsive to pain or
- U—unresponsive

Also important is the symmetry of response and pupillary symmetry; asymmetry in either may be a sign of intracranial mass lesion. The Glasgow Coma Scale (GCS), frequently used in the hospital setting, is infrequently used in the prehospital setting. Table 5–3 roughly correlates GCS to AVPU for field estimation.

Recognition of SCI includes evaluation for paralysis and loss of sensation (below the level of injury), pain, lacerations or contusions at the fracture site, characteristic diaphragmatic breathing, loss of bladder and bowel function, and the presence of spinal shock. Performing an assessment to detect injury to the spinal cord is detailed in Procedure 5–5.

TABLE 5–3 Correlation Between Glasgow Coma Scale and Level of Consciousness

Glasgow Coma Scale				AVPU	
Eye Opening Response					
Spontaneous	4 points				
To speech	3 points	A	GCS	13–15
To pain	2 points				
None	1 point	V	GCS	9–12
Best Motor Response		P	GCS	4–8
Obeys command	6 points				
Localizes	5 points	U	GCS	3
Withdraws	4 points				
Decorticate	3 points				
Decerebrate	2 points				
None	1 point				
Verbal Response					
Oriented	5 points				
Confused	4 points				
Inappropriate	3 points				
Incomprehensible	2 points				
None	1 point				

A Glasgow Coma Scale (GCS) is the sum of the best score in eye opening, best motor, and verbal responses. GCS ranges from 3 to 15 with 15 being essentially normal, and a score of less than 8 classified as coma. The AVPU mnemonic scale, developed by the American College of Surgeons, stands for A—alert, V—responds to voice, P—responds to pain, U—unresponsive.

R. Falcone, M.D.

Immobilization of the Spine

The cardinal principle in moving a patient with suspected SCI is to prevent any further damage to the spinal column, cord, and nerve roots. Proper extrication and immobilization prevent undesirable movement and minimize the potential for further injury.

To stabilize the neck, one rescuer must apply gentle (but firm) manual immobilization to the head while another applies a rigid cervical collar and secures it. The collar must fit snugly to immobilize the neck adequately. The Stifneck collar is the most widely used (Figure 5–3), and manufacturer's guidelines include instructions for using your fingers to measure the neck quickly and determine the correct size.

Once the neck is secured, immobilize the rest of the spine (neck, chest, abdomen, pelvis, and lower extremities). Victims found lying flat must be logrolled onto a long backboard using techniques to ensure the spine is kept motionless (Procedure 5–6). When possible, victims found in a sitting position should be immobilized with a short backboard (Procedure 5–7) before extrication and transfer to a long board.

The Kendricks Extrication Device (KED) may be used as an alternative to the short backboard. Horizontal flexibility is designed for use in confined spaces or awkward positions. Vertical rigidity is achieved by battens inserted in this jacketlike device pictured in Figure 5–4. Principles of extrication that apply to the use of the short backboard apply to the KED. Immobilization of the injured cervical spine must be secured first and maintained throughout. Handles on the device do allow for lifting the patient independently if necessary for extrication, but resting on the backboard for additional support is recommended as soon as is possible. A long board with an advanced design is illustrated in Figure 5–5. Extrication from the water requires adaptation of techniques already described. See Procedure 5–8.

TRANSPORT

Triage

The concept of *trauma centers*, although medically accepted, is politically still in the early stages of development. Ideally, each region should establish protocols and definitions for trauma center development and criteria for patient selection and transport (triage).* The American College of Surgeons (1986) field criteria for transfer to a trauma center are reasonable and provide guidelines for regional

*For more information on the development of trauma systems, educational materials, including public awareness and prevention, and legislative and other issues that impact trauma care, contact the *American Trauma Society (ATS), 1400 Mercantile Lane, Suite 188, Landover, MD 20785. (800)556-7890, (301)925-8811.*

Procedure 5–5   Secondary Survey: A Focus on Neurological Assessment

Purpose:

To detect injury to the spinal cord

Action	Rationale
1. Measure and record vital signs (pulse, respirations, and blood pressure).	Anticipate spinal shock; rule out hypovolemia.
2. Look for lacerations, contusions, or puncture wounds along the spinal column. Deformity is rare.	
3. Assess pain at the injury site. Gently palpate along the spinal column noting tenderness.	
4. Assess motor strength in upper and lower extremities:	
• Ask if there is any paralysis or weakness in arms or legs; note any numbness, tingling, "feeling weird"	SCI must be suspected if the patient has any difficulty in moving extremities on command. If patient shows any obvious weakness, assume there is injury to the spinal cord. Paralysis is obvious.
• Ask patient to wiggle fingers of both hands. If this is achieved, have patient raise arms, one at a time. Then ask patient to squeeze your fingers with both hands.	Movement of the upper extremity is undertaken if no obvious fractures are present. The strength of patient's grasp should be similar in both hands. If patient cannot move fingers and arms, or has obvious weakness, there probably is spinal cord damage in the neck, whereas failure of only the lower extremities to respond indicates injury to the lower back.
• Ask patient to wiggle toes. If toes of both feet can wiggle, ask patient to raise legs slightly, one at a time.	
5. Perform sensory examination:	The presence of a sensory deficit confirms the suspicion of cord injury. If your touch is felt, spinal cord damage is not probable. If your touch is not felt in one or more places, or if there is numbness or tingling, spinal cord damage is likely.
• Ask if there is any numbness in arms or legs.	
• Touch patient's ankles and wrists and ask if your touch is felt.	
6. Check the condition of the unconscious patient who is a victim of trauma:	The unconscious patient who is a victim of trauma shold be suspected of having SCI because the forces necessary to produce a brain injury are also in the range of those that cause cervical injuries.
• Observe for *diaphragmatic breathing*.	The presence of diaphragmatic breathing in an unconscious patient is the most obvious sign of SCI.
• Prick the fingertips of each hand and soles of the feet or skin of the ankles with a sharp object, such as a pin.	If there is no spinal cord damage, the painful stimulus triggers an involuntary muscular reflex and the extremity will move. If the cord is damaged, there will be no reflex reaction. Lack of response to a pinprick in the upper extremities indicates damage to the spinal cord in the neck, whereas failure of only the lower extremities to respond indicates injury in the spinal cord of the back.
• Note facial grimace without limb movement in response to painful stimuli.	
7. Note incontinence of urine and possibly feces. Urinary retention is also common. Note priapism (a persistent penile erection).	Initial urinary incontinence and involuntary defecation are often followed by retention. Priapism is extremely rare, but if present, is a sure sign of SCI.

adaptation. Ideally, transfer anyone suspected of an injury to the spine, with or without neurological impairment, to a trauma center for optimal management. The concept of initial air transport remains more controversial. Patients within 20 minutes of definitive care by ground should be transported by ground. Generally, if the distance is greater than 60 miles (97 km), air evacuation is indicated; otherwise, ground transport is usually reasonable. Helicopter transport can provide an advantage to those patients who must be transported over a long distance, whose transport has already been delayed because of prolonged extrication, or who bypass local facilities for trauma centers (note guidelines in Table 5–4, p. 103). The major advantage for air transport is in the rural environment where distances may be great and providers may not see trauma often enough to maintain needed skills. Fixed-wing aircraft are generally reserved for interhospital transfer of stable patients over long distances.

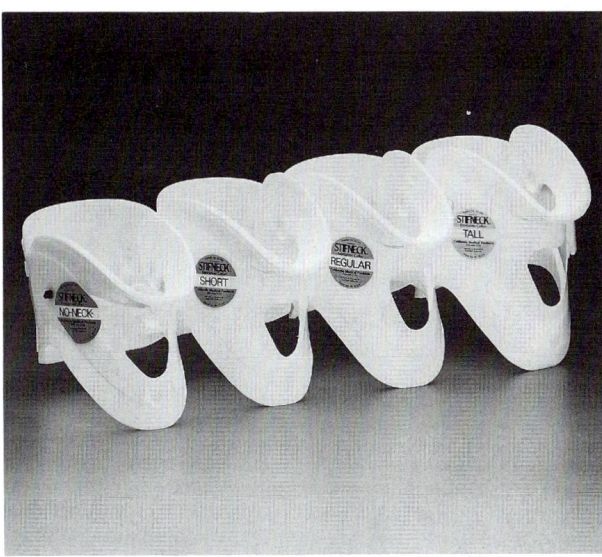

FIGURE 5–3 The Stifneck collar, in a variety of sizes, is available from California Medical Products, 2841 East 19th Street, Long Beach, CA 90804.

Communications

Prehospital care givers should inform the hospital base station of the following:

- Patient's age and sex
- Mechanism of injury
- Patient's condition—vital signs and level of consciousness
- Brief history
- Pertinent information including neurologic exam
- Summary of injuries
- Treatment given
- Estimated time of arrival
- Information about family members

Anticipating Complications

Patients with SCI may present unique problems during transport that need to be anticipated.

Injury to the cervical spine can lead to *impaired respiration*. Just as a runner tires, the patient's diaphragm becomes fatigued and respiratory insufficiency advances. Inadequate air exchange from impaired respiration may not only lead to hypoxia, but can also cause carbon dioxide to build up in the blood (hypercapnia). Hypoxia can cause further damage to the oxygen-sensitive spinal cord; hypercapnia can increase brain and spinal cord swelling, compounding the effects of injury. Management must be directed at continuous and astute assessment of respiratory status (dangerous if rate increases over 30 per minute),

---

Procedure 5–6   Use of the Long Backboard

Purpose:

To immobilize the victim's spine in preparation for transport. Patients are secured in such a manner that they may be positioned laterally, turned to the side to facilitate vomiting or drainage of secretions, or rotated or raised vertically without experiencing significant movement. Unless the clamshell is available, this procedure requires four or five people. If necessary, bystanders may need to be recruited.

Equipment Needed

- Clamshell stretcher (ideal adjunct but optional)
- Long backboard
- Two 7–8 foot (2.5 meter) straps
- Two rolled (bathsize) towels or foam pieces
- Bandaging materials

Action

If a clamshell stretcher is available:

1. Position the patient supine. Ensure the cervical injured patient has a collar on. Then place patient on the clamshell stretcher.

2. Place the patient, in the clamshell stretcher, on top of a long backboard.

3. Proceed to secure the patient to the long backboard with straps and implement steps 9–11.

Rationale

The stretcher clamps together underneath the patient with minimal movement of the spine.

(Procedure continues)

Procedure 5–6   Use of the Long Backboard (continued)

Action	Rationale
If a long backboard only is available:	

1. Position the long backboard alongside the patient.

2. Place padding on the backboard for the buttocks, the knees, and the ankles. Pad areas where pressure may cause a problem.

3. Position one rescuer at the patient's head, one at the chest, one at the hip, and one at the lower leg.

The rescuer positioned at head leads the transfer.

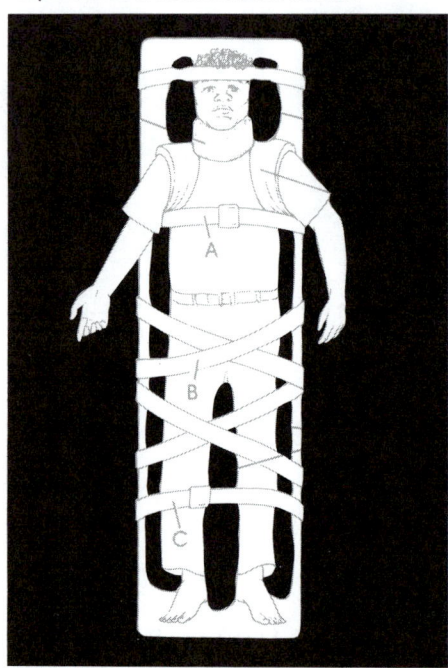

4. While the first rescuer supports the head and neck, the others reach across the patient's body. On a signal from the first rescuer at the patient's head they logroll the patient, as a unit, toward themselves.

5. Instruct another rescuer to slide the backboard under the patient. Tilt the backboard upward to center the patient on the backboard as it is lowered.

6. On a signal from the first rescuer at the patient's head, lower the patient onto the backboard.

7. Place foam pieces or rolled towels on each side of the patient's head and tape into place. Alternatively improvise with clothing.

8. If the patient is smaller than the backboard, add extra padding between the patient's legs and along each side of the body.

9. Secure the patient to the backboard with straps:

   • Place strap over the patient's chest, midsternum above the nipple line, and attach under axillae and secure shoulders (A).

   The lower chest and upper abdomen are left free of restrictive straps to facilitate impaired breathing. Also the chest is accessible for resuscitation.

   • Place additional straps in a criss-cross manner over the iliac crests, lower abdomen, pelvic region (B), and below the patient's knees (C).

   Diagonal straps best minimize the momentum of body movement in any direction. Movement of the body can cause a dragging or a compression force on the neck.

10. Immobilize the patient's head to the board with bandages. Do not wrap too tightly.

    The chin is left free to facilitate drainage of vomitus or secretions.

11. Immobilize the arms by tying wrists together. Do not place the arms under a strap.

    The arms are left free to monitor blood pressure and to start intravenous therapy, if necessary.

---

airway control, supplemental oxygen, and assisted ventilation.

Spinal shock causes misleading symptoms because perfusion is usually adequate even in the presence of mild hypotension. As cord injury disrupts the autonomic nervous system control of the heart rate and blood pressure, the patient sustains hypotension (80–100mmHg/50–60mmHg) and relative bradycardia (around 60 beats/minute). Although spinal shock may or may not require treatment (such as vasopressors), prehospital therapy should try to exclude true hypovolemia (secondary to blood loss) and *judiciously* replace fluids—*by protocol*—to avoid fluid overload. Careful application of pneumatic antishock garments will usually improve the blood pressure and central circulation temporarily. Slightly elevating the foot of the spine board will also help.

Nausea and vomiting can lead to aspiration of stomach contents. Airway compromise in patients unable to cough from muscular paralysis and the resulting pneumonia can be devastating. Keep suction equipment handy and be ready

Procedure 5–7 Use of the Short Backboard

Purpose:

To immobilize the spine of a victim found in a sitting position

Equipment Needed

Short backboard; straps to secure head, neck, torso, groin, and legs and arms

Action	Rationale

First Rescuer

1. Stabilize the patient's head, neck, and shoulders, and continue to do so throughout the procedure.

Second Rescuer

2. Apply rigid or semirigid cervical collar.

3. Slide the short backboard behind the patient; squeeze the bottom end of the backboard in place between the lower back and the car seat.

4. Pivot backboard to its normal upright position.

5. Once in place, tilt forward against the patient's back, centering the patient's head on the headpiece.

6. As a unit tilt victim and the backboard back to rest on the seat of the car.

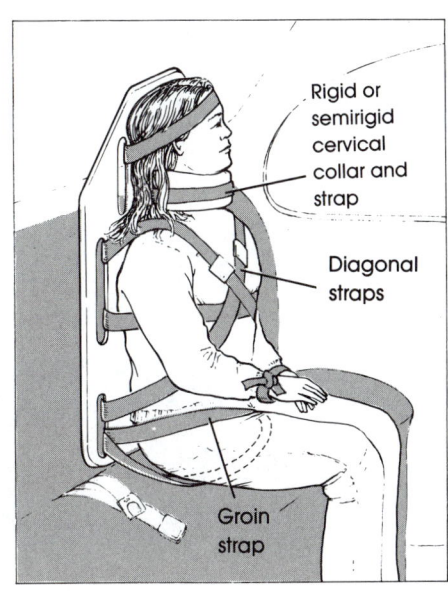

Rigid or semirigid cervical collar and strap

Diagonal straps

Groin strap

7. Secure the patient to backboard with straps:

 • Attach across forehead and across the collar.

 • Attach diagonally across torso, across chest under axillae, and across abdomen.

 • Attach around each thigh, as close to the groin as possible, and tie to lower corners of backboard.

 • Immobilize legs with straps around the knees and ankles.

 • Immobilize arms with a strap at the wrists.

Both Rescuers

8. With one hand under the patient's hip and one hand behind the short backboard, raise the patient or depress the seat sufficiently to permit another person to slide the foot of the long backboard under the patient

9. With the patient sitting on the long backboard, pivot and tilt the patient to the supine position. Then slide the patient as a unit onto the upper part of the long backboard.

10. Place the patient on backboards on the ground. Secure the short backboard to the long one with straps across upper chest and lower abdomen. Untie the legs, and place flat on the long backboard; resecure them.

Rationale column:

The chin is left free to protect the airway.

This prevents the patient from slipping sideways.

This anchors patient to the backboard and prevents slipping down and out of head straps.

Padding between legs may also be added for protection from pressure.

This prevents arms from slipping, becoming trapped, or being injured.

The priority is to maintain alignment from the head to the hips. The legs can be bent and moved with caution.

Use additional rescuer as needed to manage the long backboard.

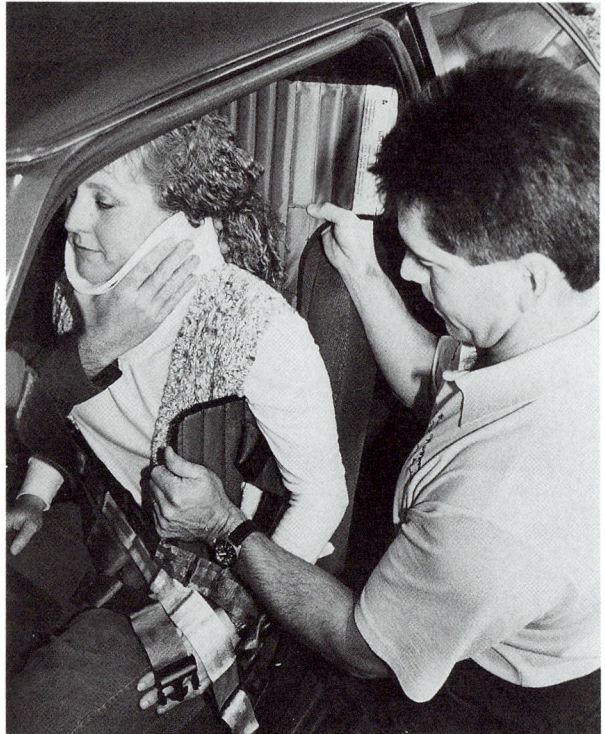

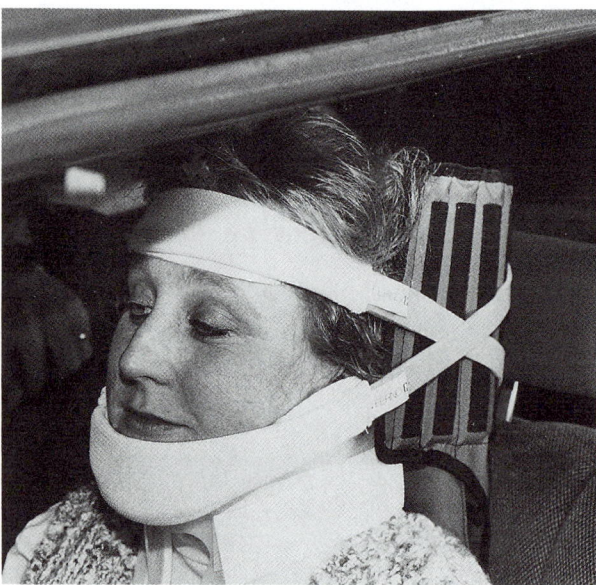

FIGURE 5-4 Kendricks Extrication Device (KED). After immobilizing the cervical spine, the KED is positioned well down behind the hips; chest supports need to fit snugly under the armpits to secure the torso; and leg straps (not shown) anchor the device (A). An adjustable neck pad allows positioning of the head before securing the head with the chin and forehead straps (B). Ideally, proceed to swivel the patient and extrication device as a unit onto a backboard to remove from the car.

to logroll patients (spine board and all) onto their sides if emesis becomes a problem.

The loss of ability to regulate body temperature is a problem also related to autonomic nervous system dysfunction

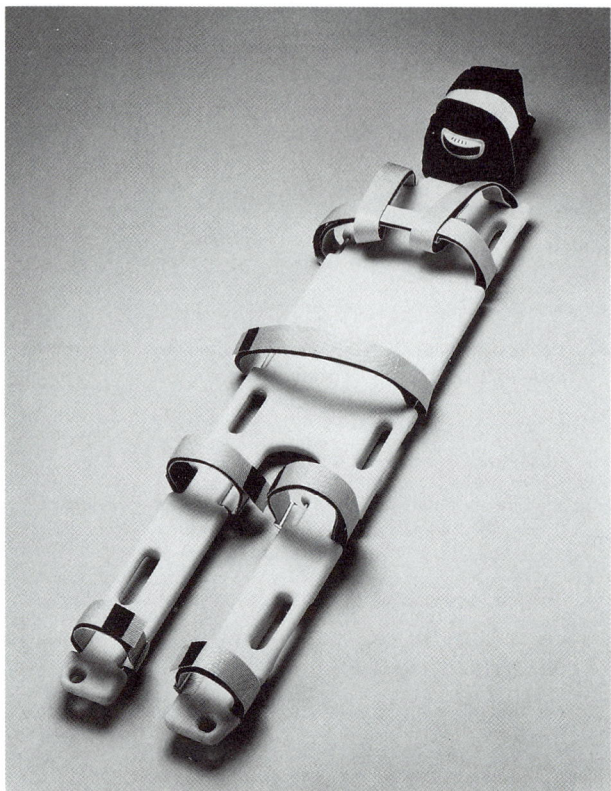

FIGURE 5-5 The Miller Full Body Splint/Litter is a versatile spine immobilization board and litter with a full, adjustable head and body harness. This harness system allows secure side positioning for airway management or to effect a difficult extrication without jeopardizing a spinal immobilization position. It is manufactured from a lightweight, high-visibility yellow resin, resistant to gasoline and other chemicals. A foam core renders the board strong and buoyant: it will float for hazardous water rescues and is compatible with standard basket litters to accommodate vertical lift and rough terrain rescues. The U.S. Coast Guard and the military use this device. The Miller Splint/Litter is X-ray compatible, and the split-leg design allows each leg to be treated separately. Available from Life Support Products, Inc., P.O. Box 19569, Irvine, CA 92713. (714) 727-2000.

leading to a dilation of skin capillaries and the loss of normal sweating mechanisms below the level of injury. The patient will rapidly assume the temperature of the environment. In an environment cooler than body temperature this can lead to *hypothermia* (initially more common); in an environment warmer than body temperature, *hyperthermia*. Cover or cool the patient accordingly.

Pressure areas on the skin overlying body prominences can develop rapidly on transports longer than 1 hour and add immeasurable barriers to recovery. Vulnerable areas include the *sacrum*, *back of head*, *elbows*, and *heels*. Adequate padding, tilting the spine board slightly every 15 minutes, and gently slipping a hand in to rub the sacrum (being careful not to compromise immobilization) will especially help.

TABLE 5–4 Indications for Helicopter Transport*

Site
  Inaccessible sites
  Impassible roads
  Ground transport 20 minutes
  Prolonged extrication

Severity
  Need to bypass local facilities for trauma center
  Multiple victims requiring trauma center triage
  Disaster

Skill
  Need for life support during rescue
  Need for life support during transport
  Search and rescue

*Modify according to local conditions, availability, and medical control.

RESEARCH NOTE

In recent breakthrough research, the commonly used drug *methylprednisolone (Solu-Medrol)* was found to decrease neurological impairment significantly following SCI, without serious negative side effects. To be effective, administration of large doses must begin immediately postinjury (within 8 hours). Undoubtedly use by paramedical personnel will become more widespread. The dosage recommended is methylprednisolone 30mg/kg IV over 15 minutes initially, then 5.4mg/kg IV every hour for the next 23 hours (Apple 1990). This research is discussed further in Chapter 6.

Procedure 5–8 Extrication of a Patient from the Water

Purpose:

To establish an airway and adequate ventilation while immobilizing the spine

Equipment Needed

Long backboard or substitute, such as a door or any object that provides a rigid, flat surface

Action

1. If the patient is found floating face up in the water, maintain in straight position. If the patient is found floating face down in the water, support the head and neck while turning victim over.

First Rescuer

• Position yourself at patient's head. Grasp shoulders and stabilize the neck and head between your arms.

Second Rescuer

• Start mouth-to-mouth ventilation, if necessary.

2. Position patient on a long backboard (or substitute) before removing victim from water.

First Rescuer

Hold head, neck, and shoulders firmly in alignment.

Second Rescuer

Slide long backboard under the patient. Float the board to the edge of the water and gently lift the patient and the board out of the water *with additional rescuers*.

3. Secure patient to long backboard in preparation for transport.

REFERENCES

American College of Surgeons, Committee on Trauma. 1986. *Prehospital Advanced Trauma Life Support Manual*. Chicago: Author.

Apple, D. 1990. Medical Director, Shepherd Spinal Center, Atlanta, GA. Personal communication.

Paramedic Academy, Justice Institute of British Columbia. 1990. *Emergency Medical Technician: Spinal Injuries Training Manual*. Vancouver, BC: Author.

Thygerson, A. L. 1987. *First Aid and Emergency Care Workbook*. Boston: Jones and Bartlett Publishers. Produced in cooperation with the National Safety Council.

University of Michigan Hospitals. 1990. *Spinal Cord Injury Transport Protocol*. Ann Arbor: University of Michigan Spinal Cord Injury Center.

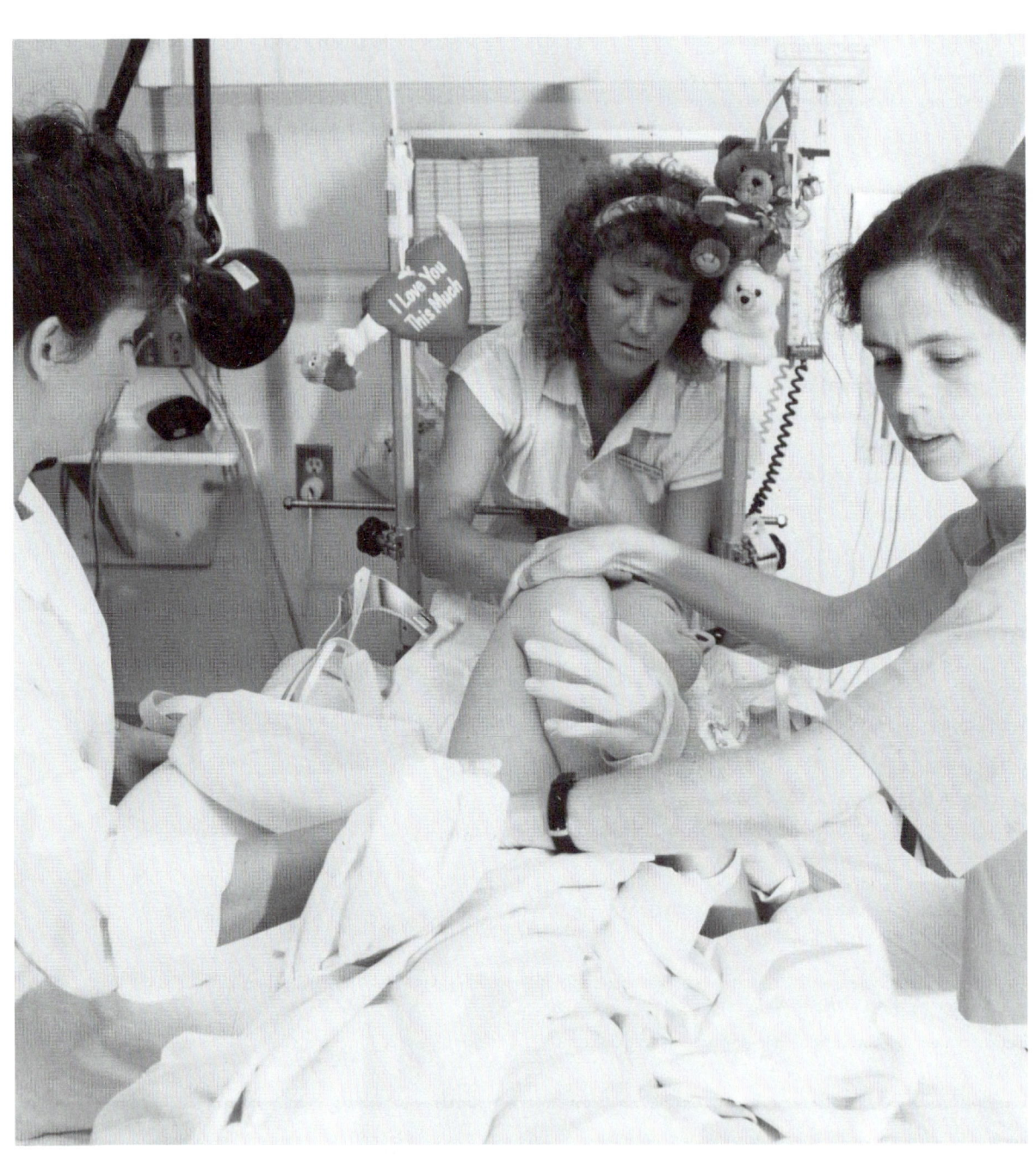

CHAPTER
— 6 —

Critical Care:
A Rehabilitative Focus*

Chapter Outline

Health Care Objectives

- To assess accurately and manage appropriately concurrent trauma complications in the presence of SCI
- To prevent further neurological damage
- To prevent or control secondary complications
- To promote optimal function, which will contribute to successful rehabilitation
- To provide psychosocial support and health education for patients and families
- To describe the rehabilitation role of the interdisciplinary critical care team

*This chapter was developed with the assistance of Susan S. Thomason, RN., M.N., and Sandra Schaefer, R.N., M.S., C.C.R.N., C.N.A.

CRITICAL CARE IN A REHABILITATIVE PERSPECTIVE

Rehabilitation is a continuous process beginning at the moment of injury and is an integral part of critical care. If critical and rehabilitative care are not combined, people with spinal cord injuries (SCI) are subject to serious clinical and economic consequences that could otherwise have been prevented (Oakes 1990). The critical care team profoundly influences the outcome of the rehabilitative process.

Intensive care has decreased mortality and morbidity significantly in the last decade. However, the impact that critical care has on rehabilitation has not been significantly emphasized. Only the collective expertise of an interdisciplinary team can identify the many actual and potential complications of SCI during critical care. Expert management to maximize physical and psychosocial strengths and minimize deterioration greatly shortens the rehabilitative process. An interdisciplinary team must be cohesive. It must deal with many problems simultaneously and provide continuous care by communicating with everyone involved: patients, families, and the health care professionals themselves all benefit from the combined expertise of a coordinated approach. To improve coordination in trauma care, the American Trauma Society (ATS) emphasizes the influential role of the Trauma Nurse Coordinator (ATS 1990). This person's leadership role involves coordinating interdisciplinary professionals and participating in research, education, and liaison activities with rehabilitation specialists and community resources (Sulsameda and McBride 1986). Preparation of interdisciplinary protocols and evaluation of interdisciplinary services are other important aspects of the role.

Viewing rehabilitation as a continuum emphasizes the significance of functional gains despite paralysis. It also highlights the profound psychosocial needs of patients and families, how they perceive the implications of disabling injury, and whether staff understand their reactions.

This chapter describes priorities of care during the initial postinjury period, generally considered to be the first 72 hours. This time frame may be extended considerably for patients with unstable conditions. Many patients with quadriplegia and/or multiple trauma, especially those requiring ventilator support, experience a prolonged stay in the critical care environment. In these situations, the varied physical and psychological responses to SCI become increasingly complex. To further address these issues, cross-references to other chapters of the text are provided.

ADMISSION MANAGEMENT

The priorities of initial care are to establish ventilation and hemodynamic stability while protecting the spine to prevent further cord injury. Simply put, **ABCs** are oriented toward **D** (delicate spine). In varying degrees, patients have unstable vital signs, experience an abnormal cardiovascular response to associated trauma, and cannot feel normal pain below the level of injury. Therefore, in the immediate aftermath of SCI, management with the assistance of established interdisciplinary protocols is highly recommended (Meyer 1989; and Davidoff 1987). Table 6–1 highlights important aspects of admissions management.

A preadmission data base (Figure 6–1) and the initial clinical assessment outlined in Procedure 6–1 establish accurate and complete baseline information. Serial assessments will be compared to this information during acute care and throughout rehabilitation to detect deterioration or improvement. Document carefully. Because of the unpredictability of neurological sequelae minutes to hours after injury, and the severe and permanent nature of SCI, these records have serious legal significance. See Chapter 8 for further explanation of legal ramifications.

When life-threatening situations have been stabilized, complete a patient history data form such as shown in Figure 6–2. An interdisciplinary information sheet facilitates team communication for continuity of care.

PROMOTING OPTIMAL RESPIRATORY FUNCTION

Respiratory insufficiency tends to be difficult to detect and can progress rapidly. Consequently a skilled interdisciplinary team approach, guided by a pulmonary medical specialist, is needed to ensure successful outcomes and avoid respiratory failure (Meyer 1989; Dollfus and Gschaedler 1987).

Chapter 14 describes detailed procedures for physical assessment; diagnostic procedures including arterial blood gas analysis, pulmonary gas analysis, and X-ray techniques; and specific preventive and restorative management including bronchial hygiene techniques; respiratory support systems; and management of pulmonary complications.

Hypoventilation, caused by paralysis of the muscles of breathing, limits chest expansion/recoil with implications for both inspiration and forced expiration (coughing). Secretions tend to accumulate and be retained, leading to atelectasis and pneumonia.

TABLE 6–1 Admission Management Summary

1. Prepare the environment:
   - Establish interdisciplinary protocols.
   - Prepare equipment for cardiopulmonary support and skeletal immobilization (stretcher or specialized beds and traction systems with weights).
   - Obtain preadmission data (Figure 6–1) from transferring personnel.

2. Perform admission assessment and prioritize interventions as for prehospital care. See Chapter 5.
   - Establish level of consciousness: Glasgow coma scale (Table 5–3).
   - Orient **ABC**s toward **D,** protection of the delicate spine.
   - Use sensory level to localize lowest normal neurological segment quickly.
   - Perform a head-to-toe check searching for associated injuries.
   - Continue to immobilize neck and back with prehospital equipment until permanent alternatives are secure.

3. Manage airway and breathing impairment.
   - Clear obstructed airways with cervical spine injury:
     - Secure supine position, align neck in neutral position and immobilize with rigid collar if not already in place.
     - Insert oral airway.
     - Bag and mask ventilation with 100% oxygen (12 to 15 liters/minute).
     - Nasoendotrachial intubation preferred (if necessary).
   - Administer 100% oxygen
   - Perform immediate chest assessment:
     - Obtain chest X ray
     - Manage hemopneumothorax with insertion of 28/32 chest tube connected to low pressure suction (Pleur-evac or water bottle system).
   - Monitor for progressive signs of respiratory dysfunction:
     - Clinical assessment for ineffective airway clearance and ineffective breathing pattern.
     - Serial arterial blood gases, pulmonary gases, and vital capacity
   - Consult with respiratory specialist for all patients with quadriplegia, high paraplegia, and/or associated chest trauma or preexisting conditions.
   - Provide ventilator support if indicated by rapid, shallow, ineffective respirations greater than 30 to 35/minute; drug or alcohol intoxication; hypoventilation (hypoxemia, hypercapnia and/or respiratory acidosis); and vital capacity falling below 1000–1200 ml.

4. Establish hemodynamic stability (circulation).
   - Administer cardiopulmonary resuscitation (CPR) for absent pulse.
   - Obtain CBC with differential, SMA–6 and SMA–12, coagulation studies, type and crossmatch, and arterial blood gases.
   - Anticipate hypotension and bradycardia:
     - Establish IV line (14 to 18 gauge for potential resuscitation fluids and medications).
     - Infuse lactated Ringer's solution or normal (0.5%) saline judiciously. (Do not overload.)

- Establish central venous pressure (CVP) line (Swan-Gantz catheter) if cardiovascular status is questionable.
- Give humidified oxygen (approximately 12 l/min).
- Consult with cardiologist as needed.
- Administer appropriate pressor agents as needed for hypotension (dopamine 2–5/kg/minute or similar drug).
- Obtain a 12-lead electrocardiogram regardless of age.
- Provide continuous monitoring for patients with multiple trauma and over 40 years of age.
- Administer Atropine (0.5 to 1.0 mg as necessary up to 2.0 mg/hour) to combat bradycardia.
- Use warmed blankets to combat hypothermia.
   - Detect hemorrhage from associated injuries:
     - Respond to hypotension unresponsive to pressor agents; an unexplained fall in hematocrit; urinary output is less than 30cc/hour; altered level of consciousness (unrelated to head injury).
     - Determine hemorrhage site.
     - Take measures to arrest bleeding.
     - Replace blood loss.
     - Consult with various specialists as needed.

5. Prevent further neurological damage.
   - Immobilize spine (Chapter 20):
     - Apply traction system to stabilize the fractured cervical spine. Generally prepare 5 lbs weight per level of injury (for example, a C_6 injury requires 6 × 5 lbs = 30 lbs).
     - Prepare for repeated lateral X ray after increased weights are added to evaluate reduction attempts.
     - Maintain spinal alignment for thoracic, lumbar, and sacral injuries. Logrolling on regular or stretcher beds or turning frames are used. Surgery is generally indicated.
     - Administer methylprednisolone (Solu-Medrol) 30 mg/kg IV over 15 minutes within 8 hours of injury initially, then 5.4 mg/kg IV every hour for 23 hours.

6. Maintain gastrointestinal function (Chapters 17 and 19).
   - Insert nasogastric tube and connect to low suction.
   - Monitor amount of gastric returns and note any blood, which requires immediate investigation.
   - Monitor abdominal distention.
   - Obtain diagnostic tests when intraabdominal injuries are suspected including ultrasound and scan procedures, peritoneal lavage, and minilaparotomy.
   - Collaborate with nutritional team or dietitian to initiate nutritional supplements within 72 hours.

7. Maintain urinary function (Chapter 18).
   - Insert indwelling catheter for continuous drainage.
   - Monitor output.
   - Note hematuria, which requires immediate investigation.
   - Consult urologist within 24 hours.

(Table continues)

TABLE 6–1   Admission Management Summary (continued)

8. Promote musculoskeletal integrity (Chapter 20).
   - Apply traction system for cervical injured patients.
   - Immobilize the spine of thoracic, lumbar, and sacral injured patients.
   - Splint and control bleeding of extremity fractures.
   - Initiate turning and positioning schedule (Chapters 20 and 21). Note arm and hand positioning modifications for cervical injured patients (Figure 6–4).
   - Collaborate with physical and occupational therapists within 24 hours to promote functional activities.

9. Protect the skin (Chapter 21).
   - Completely visualize the sacrum and other bony prominences. Inspect for reddened and/or open areas.
   - Relieve pressure by turning and correct positioning every 2 hours or as indicated when on specialized beds.
   - Disperse the effects of pressure with padding.

10. Provide psychosocial support for patients and families.
   - Offer and repeat simple explanations. A calm, confident, empathetic manner is soothing.
   - Consult with social worker for family support and others if indicated.
   - Complete neuropsychological testing within 5 days.

11. Complete a detailed assessment.
   - Give a full neurological examination:
     - Identify level of neurological injury by checking sensation, motor power, and reflexes.
     - Check for *changes* in symptomatology since injury.

   - Give a physical examination.
   - Obtain spine X rays:
     - The *entire* spine needs to be visualized to detect noncontiguous fractures. (See Table 4–7)
     - Obtain cross-table lateral views first, then AP views. Depress shoulders by pulling arms toward feet to visualize all 7 cervical vertebrae.
     - Include open-mouth view to visualize the odontoid process in the conscious patient with cervical injury.
   - Confirm suspected associated fractures with X rays.

12. Expedite transfer to appropriate facility as necessary.
   - Obtain physician referral required.
   - Arrange air transport if greater than 60 miles from specialized center; generally ground transport if less than 60 miles.

13. Prepare patient for safe transport. Ensure:
   - Immobilization of spine is adequate and secure. Nongravitational traction systems are recommended during transport.
   - Airway is clear and "guaranteed."
   - Ventilation (spontaneous or assisted) is satisfactory.
   - Blood pressure and pulse are stable.
   - IV lifeline is patent.
   - Nasogastric tube is draining freely.
   - Indwelling urinary catheter is draining freely.
   - Sacrum and heels are well padded.
   - All records (with prehospital information) including neurological assessments, total intake and output records, lab results, and X rays are sent with the patient.

*This information is based on Davidoff (1987: 70), Meyer (1989), and University of Michigan Hospitals (1990).

For most patients with quadriplegia, paralysis of the intercostal and abdominal musculature leaves the diaphragm as the primary source of respiration (with minimal assistance from the accessory muscles in the neck and shoulders). In patients with C_{1-4} injuries, however, phrenic nerve impairment results in the loss of diaphragmatic function; spontaneous respiration is lost necessitating ventilatory support, which may be required for the remainder of the person's life.

The major muscles involved in forced expiration are the abdominal muscles, innervated by the lower thoracic cord (T6–10). Therefore, patients with thoracic injuries also have difficulty coughing and clearing secretions effectively. See Table 15–1.

Progressive respiratory insufficiency is a constant danger throughout the initial postinjury period and beyond, especially for the patient with quadriplegia. Although the patient may not be in severe, or even obvious, distress initially, there is a high risk of deterioration because of accumulative *fatigue*. Tiring of the remaining muscles of breathing takes

a heavy toll and often does not peak until the third or fourth day postinjury. The effect is similar to an untrained runner participating in a marathon. Occasionally, progressive ascending edema or hemorrhage at the injury site may also contribute to respiratory insufficiency.

Anxiety, sedation, drugs or alcohol, advanced age, and other preexisting conditions significantly affect pulmonary function. Associated trauma may further compromise pulmonary function particularly if systemic hemorrhage decreases oxygen-carrying capacity. Unconscious patients and those who have nearly drowned are at risk for *aspiration pneumonia*. Pulmonary contusions and chest wall fractures are almost inevitable with fractures of the upper thoracic spine. A *hemopneumothorax* and fractured ribs are very often associated.

Paralytic ileus, aspiration of vomitus, and *pulmonary edema*, as a result of fluid overload to compensate mistakenly for neurogenic shock, are other possible major complications. To detect progressive respiratory dysfunction monitor for:

PREADMISSION DATA

Name _____   Date _____

Address _____   Telephone number _____

_____   Next of kin _____

Person giving report _____ Title _____

Prehospital provider/facility _____ Address _____

Telephone number _____   _____

Time/date of injury _____   Age _____

Level of injury _____   Height _____

Cause of injury _____   Weight _____

Method of stabilization _____   Allergies _____

SYSTEMS STATUS REVIEW
Neurological:
 LOC
 Head injury _____ yes _____ no
 Motor loss _____ level _____ (if known)
 Sensory loss _____ level _____ (if known)

Respiratory:
 Respirations _____ rate _____ character
 Airway _____ tracheostomy _____ endotracheal tube
 Secretions _____ frequency of suctioning _____
 Ventilator-tidal volume _____ ABGS-Sat. _____

            FIO_2 _____ $PaPO_2$ _____
            Rate _____   pH _____
            PEEP _____ $Paco_2$ _____

Cardiovascular:
 Rhythm _____
 Vital signs _____ pulse _____ BP _____ temp _____

Gastrointestinal:
 NG tube _____ type of drainage _____

Genitourinary:
 Indwelling catheter _____ yes _____ no
 Urine output _____

Other injuries:
 Type _____   Treatment _____

 _____

 _____

Medications: _____ IV fluids _____ Total intake _____

Preexisting conditions: _____

Other comments: _____

_____

Mode of transport: _____   Expected time of arrival _____

_____ Person taking report/title

FIGURE 6–1 Preadmission data.

PATIENT HISTORY
REHABILITATIVE PROCESS*

Patient's name _____ Age _____
Date of injury _____

A. History of Present Illness/Injury
   Diagnosis _____
   _____

   Chief complaint _____
   _____
   _____

   History present illness/injury _____
   _____
   _____
   _____
   _____
   _____

   Date onset _____

B. History of Previous Illnesses/Injuries
   Previous illnesses/injuries _____
   _____
   _____
   _____
   _____

   Previous hospitalizations _____
   _____
   _____
   _____

   Medications taken before admission _____
   _____
   _____

C. Sociocultural Background
   Marital status _____ Spouse's name _____
   Children _____
   Family/significant others: _____
   _____

   Occupation _____
   Education _____

   Languages spoken _____
   Religious affiliation _____
   Significant cultural practices _____
   _____
   _____

FIGURE 6–2   Patient history for the rehabilitative process.

D. Activities of Daily Living
   Personal hygiene   Shower _____
                       Bath   _____
                       Time   _____
                       Mouth care _____
                       Time   _____
                       Dentures/partials _____

   Sleeping pattern
   Bedtime _____ Time of awakening _____
   Naps _____ Quality of sleep _____

   Nutrition
   Food allergies _____
   Likes _____
   Dislikes _____
   Eating habits _____
   _____
   _____

   Recreation _____
   _____

   Sexuality _____
   _____

   Drugs/alcohol/smoking _____
   _____

E. Body Systems—Patient History before Hospitalization
   General (weakness, fatigue, change in weight, appetite, chills, fever, night
   sweats) _____
   _____
   _____

   Cardiovascular (chest pain, varicose veins, edema, heart murmur, palpitations,
   BP, cool extremities) _____
   _____
   _____

   Respiratory (cough, sputum, shortness of breath, preexisting conditions,
   infections) _____
   _____
   _____

   Neurological (tingling, numbness, headache, paralysis/paresis, tremor, ataxia,
   vertigo, syncope) _____
   _____
   _____

   Gastrointestinal (BM frequency, time of day, use of laxatives, abdominal pain,
   diarrhea, constipation) _____
   _____
   _____
   _____

FIGURE 6–2   Patient history for the rehabilitative process.

Urinary (dysuria, hematuria, polyuria, urgency, hesitancy, incontinence, calculi, nocturia, infections) _____

_____

_____

_____

Genitoreproductive (menstruation, pregnancy, leukorrhea, penile discharge, lesions, infertility) _____

_____

_____

_____

Musculoskeletal (pain, stiffness, deformity, limitation of movement, fractures, sprains) _____

_____

_____

_____

Integument (color changes, pruritus, infections, tumors, hair or nail changes, lesions, rashes) _____

_____

_____

_____

Audiovisual (eyeglasses, near-sighted, far-sighted, blurred vision, hearing aid, tinnitus, deafness) _____

_____

_____

_____

Psychological (nervousness, depression, anxiety, hallucinations, apprehension, nightmares) _____

_____

_____

F. Psychosocial Self-Assessment
   Perception of illness/injury _____

_____

   Personal concerns _____

_____

_____

_____

   Previous coping abilities _____

_____

_____

Source of Database _____

Relationship to Patient _____

Interviewer's Comments _____

_____

_____

_____

Interviewer _____   Date _____

*To be completed 72 hours postadmission to ICU

FIGURE 6-2   Patient history for the rehabilitative process.

Personal Viewpoint

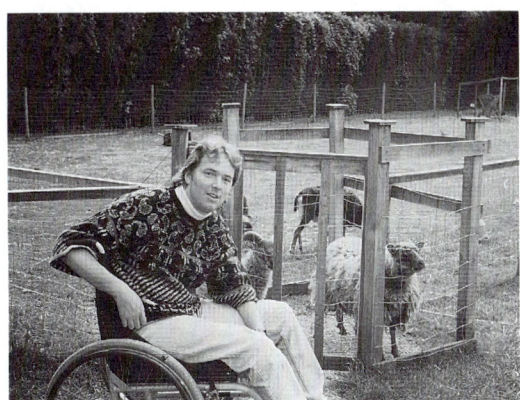

My name is Steve Hartley, I am 24 years old and have C_5 quadriplegia. Six years ago I sustained a spinal cord injury while diving into a swimming pool. I am paralyzed from the shoulders down with some use of my arms. Although it was a painful and traumatic experience, I came away from the accident focusing on the positive aspects of my injury. At first, it was hard to understand how anything positive might result from SCI, but being able to take something good from something so terrible is the first sign of acceptance so that you can carry on your life. The word *acceptance* does not imply that you are giving up: to accept that you might not walk again is not giving up hope but is the first stage of recovery.

My rehabilitation and recovery was the most incredible time of my life. (I use the word *recovery* to describe my attitude.) I felt every emotion from the deepest anger to love. My preinjury life was nothing to be proud of; I was involved in crime and drugs, and I didn't really care about other people. Suddenly my life was trans-

formed, and the world seemed to change. Like most people with SCI, I divide my life in two—before and after my accident. Feelings of invincibility and superiority were replaced with childlike emotions; I cried, I felt enormously vulnerable and helpless. I had difficulty with these feelings which compounded my anger. "Real men" aren't supposed to cry so I would hold back the tears. I felt I had to be brave so as not to scare my family and friends. But it just made me feel alone.

I knew my neck was broken from the second my head hit the bottom of the pool. My biggest problem for the first 6 weeks was breathing. I had been under water for at least 3 minutes, during which time I aspirated vomitus. I spent several weeks with physical therapists perched on my stomach, pushing for all their worth on my diaphragm. I could not imagine spending the rest of my life like this. Some sensation remained on the bottom of my feet so the doctors decided not to operate and destroy chances for any nerve recovery. My family dangled this hope like a carrot to keep me going, but it proved false, highlighting what I would never have.

After ICU, I shared a ward with various people—a grandmother, an athlete, a minister from Kenya. They had character and somehow we drew energy from each other. The staff and our friends and families would leave the hospital for at least a few hours each night but we had to stay, often for months, day in, day out. Still, I felt that I was the only one who was suffering and felt cheated that they could go home and escape this horrible nightmare. My sole escape was sleep. Although I acknowledged my family's pain at the time, it was only once I truly accepted the disability that I could fully appreciate how they were ripped apart.

- Increase in rapid, shallow respirations (greater than 30–35 per minute)*
- Labored paradoxical breathing (diaphragmatic movement in the abdomen unaccompanied by chest expansion)
- Increased use of the accessory muscles of respiration (exaggerated shoulder movements to assist breathing)
- Inability to cough up secretions despite repeated attempts
- Altered consciousness (associated with anxiety, irritability, and restlessness in early onset)
- Pale color progressing to cyanosis

*Important indicators that ventilator assistance is needed to minimize risk of respiratory arrest.

- Progressive loss of motor and/or sensory function on neurological assessment
- Drug or alcohol intoxication*
- Hypoxemia (PaO_2 less than 60 mmHg or SaO_2 less than 40%); hypercapnia (elevated $PaCO_2$ over 40 mmHg); respiratory acidosis (pH less than 7.3)*
- Vital capacity (VC) below 1000 to 1200 ml*

The VC, which can be readily obtained with a simple spirometer at the bedside, is the most useful measure of pulmonary function to indicate deep breathing capacity and ability to cough effectively. The higher the level of injury, the greater the degree of respiratory impairment and the lower the VC. See Table 15–1 for anticipated acute and long-term values.

Late complications may ensue. The incidence of *pulmonary embolism* peaks at approximately 11 to 14 days and lasts for 12 weeks. See Chapter 16. This complication, which may or may not occur with obvious peripheral thrombosis, must be ruled out whenever respiratory dysfunction deteriorates without evidence of atelectasis or pneumonia (McCagg 1986). One other possible complication experienced by people with quadriplegia is *central alveolar hypotension* or *sleep apnea*, breathing cessation during sleep, which may lead to cardiopulmonary distress.

The main *goals* of acute respiratory management are to maintain or reestablish ventilation, pulmonary gas exchange, and gas transport and to prevent retention of secretions. Bruised or edematous cord tissue surrounding the injury site is especially sensitive to low oxygen tension levels. Irreversible damage to cord tissue due to oxygen deprivation can progress rapidly even in the absence of clinical signs of hypoxemia. Whatever combination of preventive, restorative, and/or respiratory support systems are selected, arterial blood gases should be stabilized within an acceptable range of PaO_2 80 to 100mmHg, $PaCO_2$ 35 to 40 mmHg, and a pH greater than 7.3 to avoid increasing the severity of SCI.

If respiratory dysfunction progresses to respiratory arrest, emergency intubation poses major additional risks to the patient with quadriplegia. Resuscitation techniques must be modified to avoid unnecessary manipulation and hyperextension of the fractured neck, which could compromise vascular supply to the cord or further compromise the nerve roots or the cord itself, resulting in progressive neurological damage. For nasal or oral airway insertion and endotracheal intubation use the jaw thrust maneuver (Procedure 5–2). Nasal intubation is preferred to oral intubation because less manipulation of the neck is required.

Maintaining bronchial hygiene, exercising, and early mobilization are important elements of acute respiratory management of the spinal cord injured patient. Bronchial hygiene techniques must be used aggressively to ensure adequate pulmonary function in the presence of paralysis of the muscles of breathing (Gilbert 1987). Preventive measures to promote air entry and combat retention of secretions should be employed *before* clinical signs of retained secretions become evident.

Because it strengthens the muscles used in breathing and prevents complications, respiratory therapy significantly contributes to the rehabilitation process. Patients need increased endurance and an efficient pulmonary system to undertake other rehabilitation activities. Active physical therapy to unaffected muscle groups—for example, exercising with arm pulleys while on bedrest—also enhances cardiopulmonary reserve and indirectly strengthens the muscles of breathing that remain intact.

Application of fitness training principles gradually increases the quantity and quality of exercise. However, rest is prescribed as carefully as exercise to permit recuperation and nourishment at a cellular level. See Chapter 24. Incentive spirometry and ventilatory muscle training (VMT), which strengthen respiratory capacity (Chapter 15), are often the first rehabilitation activities in which patients experience successful outcomes.

Skilled respiratory management facilitates good pulmonary hygiene, prevents complications, and decreases the risk factors for mechanical ventilation. Inadequate, inconsistent management not only slows recovery during the acute stage but inevitably prolongs and complicates future rehabilitation.

PROMOTING OPTIMAL CARDIOVASCULAR AND THERMOREGULATORY FUNCTIONS

Of great concern following trauma that causes SCI is the maintenance of the vital functions of the heart, brain, and kidneys—functions critically dependent on cardiac output. Due to secondary autonomic nervous system dysfunction following SCI, disturbances in regulation of blood pressure, heart rate, and systemic vascular resistance decrease cardiac output. In the critical hours following trauma, the spinal cord itself is immensely sensitive to blood oxygen levels needed for immediate response and for enhancing potential recovery.

The cardiovascular system remains severely unstable for several days immediately after injury. Abnormalities, namely hypotension, supraventricular dysrhythmias, and primary cardiac arrest, do occur during the initial weeks postinjury, a period in which life-threatening disturbances must be anticipated. Lingering cardiovascular complications can be quite critical and are now the leading cause of death in the SCI population (Le and Price 1982), as for the general population. However, risks tend to peak and then gradually decline within 2 to 6 weeks.

Spinal Shock

Below the level of cord injury, superimposed on either temporary or permanent neurological loss, is the transient depression of all reflex activity, *spinal shock*. Initially a brief period of hyperreflexia occurs followed by a flaccid paralysis below the level of cord injury. Effects are extreme in the initial postinjury period primarily because of impaired blood flow, but spinal shock eventually passes as explained in Chapter 16.

Casady and Zinszner (1989) distinguish between *spinal shock*, strictly speaking, the interruption of the sympathetic nervous system (SNS), and *neurogenic shock*, the body's reaction to the sudden interruption of central nervous system (CNS) control. (Review anatomy and physiology of the nervous systems in Chapter 4.) Throughout this text, *spinal shock* refers to both spinal and neurogenic shock because they commonly occur together.

Spinal shock is characterized by a classical triad of signs that include (Figure 6–3):

- *Hypotension*, low blood pressure (70–100/50–60 mmHg), is caused by the passive vasodilation of the systemic vascular network below the level of injury, which significantly diminishes the circulating blood volume and decreases cardiac output.
-]*Bradycardia*, a slow pulse rate of 60—often 50—beats per minute, is due to the unopposed effects of the vagus nerve—parasympathetic nervous system (PNS)—which is unbalanced by the sympathetic nervous system. A most dangerous phenomenon, *abnormal vasovagal response*, may occur during this time. Stimulation, such as rapid changes of body position when turning or tracheal suctioning, is believed to trigger this response.
- *Hypothermia*, body temperature instability secondary to the lack of vasomotor control, hampers the body's ability to conserve body heat. Through the passively dilated cutaneous vascular bed, the body loses heat and assumes the temperature of the environment, which is generally lower than normal body temperature.

Generally, the higher the level of cord injury the greater the body area involved and the more profound the effect. The patient with a high thoracic lesion (T_{1-6}) may experience these signs to a lesser degree. The patient with a lower thoracolumbar lesion should not demonstrate these signs because the sympathetic nervous system is intact.

Hypovolemic Shock

In the patient with multiple trauma, spinal and hypovolemic shock can, and often do, coexist. Hypovolemic shock is due to reduction in blood volume. The most frequent sites of associated trauma are (Meyer 1989: 27): head and face (26.2%); chest (16.1%); intraabdominal injuries (10%); and fractures of the long bones and pelvis (8.5%). The latter two injuries cause the most blood loss. Patients involved in high-velocity accidents, such as motor vehicle accidents or falls from significant heights, are at greatest risk of hemorrhagic injury. Thoracolumbar injury is particularly associated with abdominal trauma.

Detection of internal bleeding is made more difficult by the lack of normal sensation below the level of injury. Pain and tenderness to palpation cannot be felt or are impaired. Table 6–1 outlines assessment parameters.

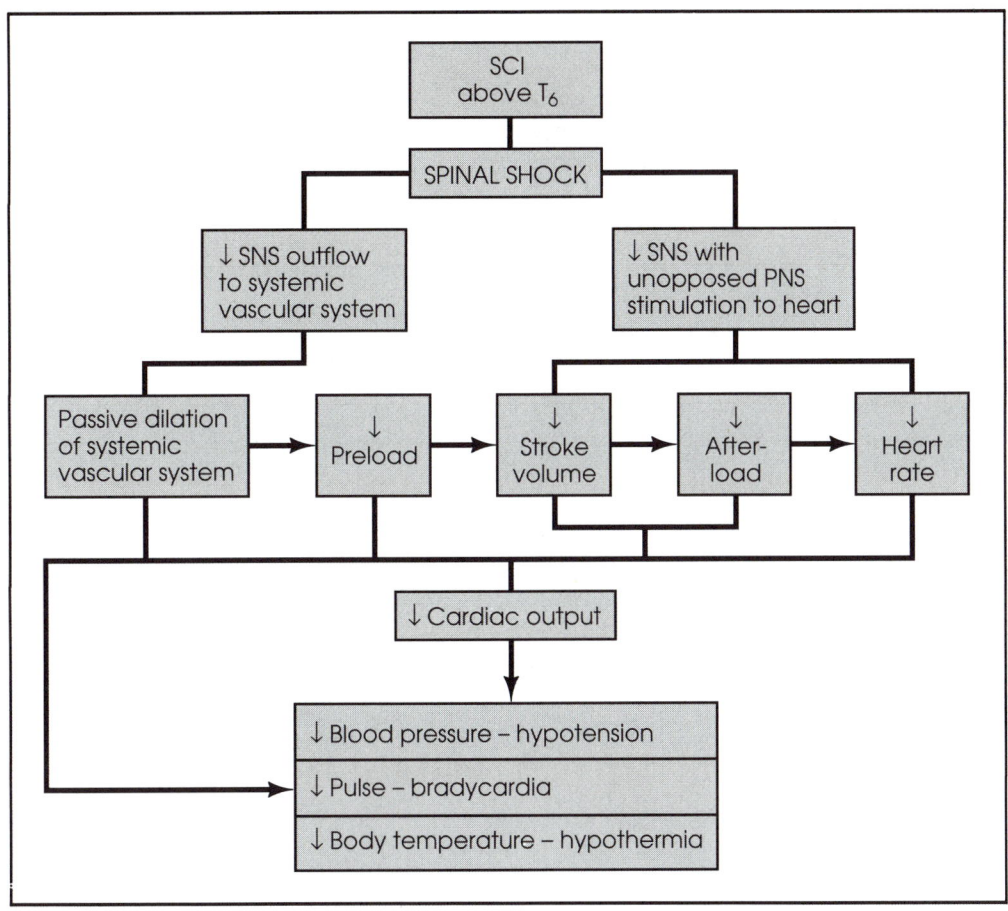

FIGURE 6–3   Mechanisms involved in spinal shock. (Based on L. Belange, SCI Unit, Shaughnessy Site, Vancouver, BC, unpublished material.)

It is imperative to understand that the vital signs of multiple-trauma patients with SCI do not match the extent of their trauma (Meyer 1989: 40). Spinal shock exacerbates the effects of hypovolemic shock by disabling normal neurologic reflexes, that is, vasoconstriction and tachycardia, that ordinarily preserve blood flow to vital organs. Goals in the initial postinjury period focus on regulating blood pressure, heart rate, and body temperature complicated by spinal shock and/or hypovolemic shock. Assessment and management of cardiovascular consequences and thermoregulatory difficulties are fully described in Chapter 16.

To stabilize *hypotension* due to spinal shock, do not seek to overcompensate for a low blood pressure. Acute respiratory distress syndrome (ARDS) or noncardiogenic pulmonary edema results from overhydration. Judiciously replace prescribed fluids as follows (University of Michigan Hospitals 1990; Meyer 1989):

- Establish intravenous lines (preferably 14 to 16 gauge for potential resuscitation fluids and medications).
- Administer intravenous fluids cautiously to maintain urinary output above 30 ml per hour (indicator of end organ perfusion) and a systolic blood pressure around 90 mmHg. *The maintenance of tissue perfusion cannot be overemphasized, as spinal cord ischemia due to hypotension (either from spinal or hypovolemic shock) can extend the neurological deficit.*
- Lactated Ringer's solution or normal (0.5%) saline is recommended. Avoid fluids unable to carry oxygen. Use whole blood to replace blood loss. Initial volume challenge is considered 2 liters plus an infusion rate of 100 to 150 ml per hour (for a total of 3 liters per 24 hours). If the patient requires transport, generally 50 to 100 ml per hour is sufficient.

Pressor agents are rarely necessary, but if indicated, administer dopamine 2 to 5 kg per minute or similar drug to increase the blood pressure. Intractable hypotension with end organ failure (less than 30 ml per hour) suggests the possibility of hemorrhage injury.

Bradycardia associated with spinal shock does not require specific treatment. However, nodal or ventricular escape rhythms may emerge which can be corrected with Atropine (0.5–1.0 mg) administered as necessary up to 2.0 mg per hour.

Bradycardia may progress to profound limits if stimulation of an abnormal vasovagal response is great enough to cause cardiac arrest. Suctioning or inserting a nasogastric tube typically elicits such a response, but simple manipulation of an endotrachial tube during mouth care or rapid change of body position can also be the cause. In most situations cessation of the cause allows the heart to return to the previous rate. To minimize risk or control progression toward profound bradycardia:

- Keep Atropine 1 mg IV on hand, perhaps taped to the head of the bed, for emergency administration.

- Hyperoxygenate the patient before and after suctioning to prevent hypoxia and reduce risk (McCagg 1986).
- Hyperventilate with a manual resuscitator before suctioning to increase the heart rate above baseline. Then when vagal stimulation occurs, the heart rate will drop back to baseline if suctioning is completed quickly.
- For very sensitive patients, complete suctioning within 10 seconds in a single pass of the catheter.
- For patients sensitive to vagal stimuli, give Atropine as prescribed before such procedures as nasogastric tube insertion.
- Avoid sudden position changes.

Use warmed blankets to treat *hypothermia* associated with spinal shock. Initially stabilize body temperature above 96.5°F. Never use electrical heating devices or hot water bottles for patients without sensation. A slight degree of hypothermia to decrease oxygen requirements may be beneficial during the initial postinjury period when hypoxia is most likely to occur.

Although previous measures take priority, an important adjunct is *promotion of blood flow in paralyzed limbs.* Tissue perfusion when the vascular bed is passively dilated is enhanced by

- Regular turning
- Correct positioning to prevent gravitational edema (including elevation of limbs)
- Passive range of motion exercises, especially ankle-pumping exercises
- Application of antiembolitic stockings with/without sequential compression devices.
- Protection of blood vessels from localized trauma

Immediate physical therapy composed of active and passive exercises preserves existing muscle function, minimizes risks associated with inactivity, and enhances cardiopulmonary reserve. Early mobilization, with posture changes, helps to minimize complications such as orthostatic hypotension. Exercise promotes health for this predominantly young group of people.

THE DELICATE SPINE AND SPINAL CORD: PREVENTING FURTHER NEUROLOGICAL DAMAGE

Immobilizing the Spine

A most important aspect of caring for the spinal cord injured patient is the prevention of further neurological deficit. Emergency treatment must be oriented toward minimal movement of the delicate spine. Stability of the fractured site must then be achieved.

A primary goal of early treatment is to decompress the spinal cord by realignment of the spinal canal. The spine must be kept immobilized until definitive treatment is accomplished. Ideally, closed reduction of a cervical fracture can be accomplished promptly with skeletal traction. However, surgical reduction is frequently required for other spine fractures.

The health care team must select a total treatment approach that accommodates the patient's general condition, stabilizes the fracture site, and facilitates any potential neurological recovery. In North America, treatment often favors early intervention to achieve internal skeletal stability and prevent other hazards of immobility. Chapter 4 describes assessment of vertebral column injuries, factors that influence spinal stability, and neurological consequences. Treatment of spinal injury, including surgery, is discussed in Chapter 20.

Naturally, great care is needed whenever the patient is moved to prevent risks of damaging the unstable spine and spinal cord. The design of radiolucent fracture boards and the features of specialized beds eliminate movement of patients from one surface to another, especially for purposes of X rays. The *mobilizer stretcher* is also useful. Patient movement is minimized because its base remains stable while the narrow, flat, supporting surface extends by roller mechanisms to slip beneath the patient. Otherwise, several people are required to lift the patient and manage the move so that the spine is kept in alignment (Procedure 6–1). Methods for immobilizing the spine, including the halo brace, are presented in Chapter 20.

Long-term consequences of inadequate immobilization during acute management contribute to late postoperative instability, spinal curvatures, chronic pain, and progressive loss of function. Prolonged immobilization is associated with numerous cardiopulmonary complications and loss of bone calcium.

Promoting Neurological Function

The initial neurological assessment establishes the level and completeness of cord injury. Motor, sensory, and reflex responses must be examined and clearly documented to facilitate future assessments. Serial comparison is the key to determining deterioration or progression of neurological involvement. Assessment procedures and recording tools, designed for critical care use, are presented in Chapter 4. Potential functional status as correlated with the level of injury is detailed in Table 22–7.

Accurate neurological assessment is complicated by concurrent head injury, anticipated with cervical spine trauma. Level of consciousness is frequently assessed by the Glasgow coma scale (Table 5–3). The acute postinjury course in

traumatic brain injured patients is complicated by a more prolonged period of unconsciousness and posttraumatic amnesia. Consequently, brain injury becomes a major factor in care and treatment. Because traumatic brain injury results in an array of cognitive disturbances that affect the SCI rehabilitation process, it is important to recognize those patients early and set up appropriate interventional strategies. Chapter 26 discusses combined traumatic brain and spinal cord injury.

Trauma to the cord seems to produce an autodestructive process that progressively slows spinal cord blood flow. A major research breakthrough, announced in March 1990, established that the drug *methylprednisolone (Solu-Medrol)*, if begun within 8 hours of injury, could reduce the effects of neurological sequelae without untoward side effects. The drug is FDA approved and is widely used for a variety of reasons, albeit in much smaller doses than for SCI. The recommended dosage is: Methylprednisolone 30 mg/kg IV over 15 minutes initially within 8 hours of injury; then 5.4 mg/kg every hour for 23 hours (Bracken et al. 1990). Other therapies, such as cord hypothermia or hyperbaric oxygen, to achieve optimal local cord effects, may also be implemented immediately but only in specialized centers familiar with their application. Researchers disagree about the efficacy of these methods. Further research is discussed in Chapter 7; it is important to become familiar with trends to answer questions that patients and families often ask soon after injury.

CARING FOR PHYSIOLOGICAL NEEDS

Early mobilization significantly contributes to promotion of physiological function and prevention of the diverse hazards of immobility. Loss of motor control and lack of sensation over much of the body, complicated by the transient loss of reflex activity (spinal shock), demands an integrated interdisciplinary approach. Maintaining optimal physiological functions and protecting existing muscular tone in the presence of spinal shock, which imposes loss of tone, incorporates rehabilitative concepts into initial care. Although effects are less readily apparent than in the cardiovascular system, spinal shock permeates all body systems below the level of injury. When spinal shock resolves, the well-maintained body can better respond to future rehabilitation interventions.

Maintaining Gastrointestinal Function

The nature and extent of gastrointestinal dysfunction is directly related to the level of injury. The patient with a

PROCEDURE 6–1 Safely Transferring a Patient (A Four-Person Lift)

Purpose:

To maintain alignment of the spinal column and to prevent any movement at an unstable fracture site that can further damage the cord

Action

1. Assess strength and experience of four assistants. Select five assistants for taller, heavier patients.

2. Assign one assistant to manage the head and neck and three assistants, standing on the same side of the patient, to lift the body. Assign the strongest assistant to lift the heavier midsection of the patient.

3. Explain the planned procedure to prepare the patient.

4. Instruct the patient to fold arms on chest if possible. Secure or tie paralyzed arms together.

5. Try to maintain direct eye contact throughout.

6. Whenever possible, plan to relocate the stretcher and bed, not the patient. Allow ample space to move beds quickly (perhaps most convenient in the hallway); remove any obstacles on the floor; and remove armboards and footboards from the bed. When the lift is performed, have other assistants remove the stretcher and then position an immobilization bed directly underneath the patient. See Figure A.

Rationale

A typical critical care unit is cramped for space. Clearing the area, except for those directly involved with the actual transfer, will eliminate confusion.

Patients feel tense and fear pain on movement.

It is important for the patient not to attempt to hold on to the assistants and cause twisting of the spine.

This reassures the patient and ensures relaxation during the transfer. Because neck immobility restricts the visual field, the person situated at the patient's head usually maintains eye contact.

This eliminates those lifting the patient from actually walking while trying to maintain skeletal alignment.

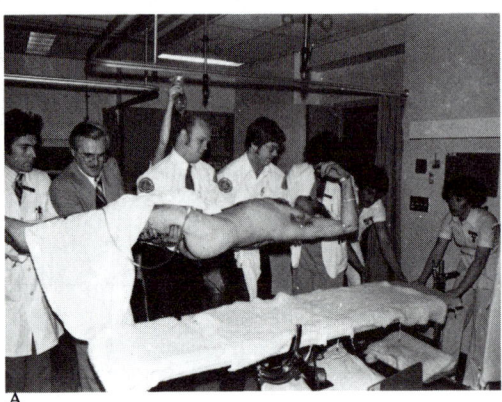

A

7. Have the person at the patient's head immobilize the neck by placing the inner forearms against the side of the head and firmly grasping the patient's shoulders. See Figure B.

8. Clearly communicate the plan of action:
   - Delegate "positions" for lifting
   - Assign additional duties, such as managing intravenous or respiratory equipment.
   - Clarify any questions.

9. Instruct the assistant at the head to count "1, 2, 3" when ready.

10. Move the patient on the count of "3."

This helps avoid inadvertent flexion of the head while lifting and is possible with a neck collar or skull tongs in place.

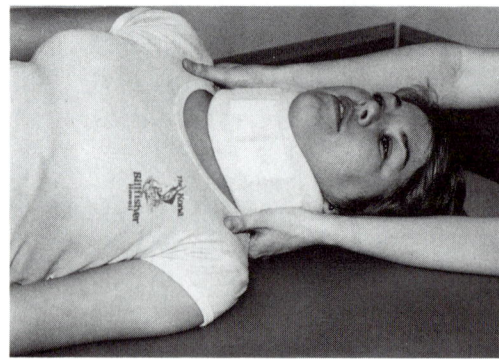

B

cervical cord injury runs the greatest risk of developing gastrointestinal difficulties that can progress to fatal complications. Also, patients involved in high-velocity accidents are at risk of associated abdominal injuries including the gastrointestinal system, which can cause significant blood loss. Traumatic pancreatitis is not uncommon.

Paralytic ileus is a likely consequence of SCI. Onset tends to be immediate for those with thoracolumbar lesions; delayed 24 hours for those with high thoracic lesions; and delayed 48 hours for those with cervical lesions. If unchecked, paralytic ileus can lead to aspiration of vomitus and subsequent respiratory arrest. This is also true of acute gastric dilation from any cause.

Ileus is characterized by loss of bowel sounds and is frequently accompanied by visible abdominal distension. Diagnosis may be confirmed by abdominal X ray, ultrasound examination, and CAT scans.

Oral intake must be withheld. Management focuses on decompression of the stomach by insertion of a nasogastric sump tube with continuous low-pressure nasogastric suction (approximately 20 mmHg) applied. As nasogastric returns decrease and bowel sounds slowly return, the sump tube may be removed. When strong bowel sounds have returned, with the passing of flatus and possibly stool, gradually advance from oral fluids to diet as tolerated. A minimum fluid intake of 2000 ml per day is recommended. Oral intake is usually possible on the second or third day after injury unless paralytic ileus is prolonged or other complications have set in.

Acute stress ulceration is a related potential complication during the initial 7- to 14-day postinjury period and, if unchecked, can present as an acute gastrointestinal bleed. To minimize risk of bleeding combine the interventions described for treatment of ileus with these prophylactic measures: frequent checks for blood in the nasogastric returns; monitoring of gastric acidity; titrating an antacid regimen to maintain a pH above 4.5 (Davidoff 1987: 84); and administering histamine receptor (H_2) antagonists as prescribed.

Malnutrition during the acute phase is increasingly recognized as a major barrier to rehabilitation. Life-threatening situations often overshadow nutritional needs, but maintaining optimal nutrition is vital to cardiopulmonary and hemodynamic stability. Inadequate nutritional support contributes to fatigue, poor wound healing, skin breakdown, and generally longer rehabilitation.

Energy needs must be determined as accurately as possible, taking into account disuse of paralyzed muscles, which decreases demands, and stress and trauma, which increase nutritional requirements. Overall, nutritional and metabolic responses after SCI indicate that caloric requirements decrease from the moment of injury, to approximately 80% of normal for patients with quadriplegia. Both overfeeding and underfeeding must be avoided. Critically ill patients frequently have altered fuel metabolic mechanisms, and as such, cannot compensate for excessive quantities of any nutritional substrates—more is not necessarily better. Overfeeding can increase oxygen requirements to aid in digestion and subsequently elevate the $PaCO_2$. Respiratory failure and congestive heart failure may ensue in patients with marginal cardiopulmonary reserve. Underfeeding, on the other hand, produces complications of malnutrition, particularly problematic when weaning from a mechanical ventilator, for example. Metabolic alkalosis may also occur.

Immediately consult a registered dietitian or nutritional support team as soon as possible (within 24 hours) postinjury to complete a nutritional assessment, determine calorie and protein requirements, and set a time frame (within 48 to 72 hours) of starting oral, enteral, or parenteral nutritional support. This will prevent or minimize complications before substantial malnutrition occurs.

Early swallowing is difficult for patients with cervical injuries, especially with traction in place. Eating in a side-lying position seems to be easiest—certainly safest, should airway obstruction occur. For patients on turning frames, the prone position is recommended. Following application of the halo-thoracic brace, difficulty swallowing occurs with too much neck hyperextension. Minor adjustment is usually sufficient to alleviate this problem. Naturally, soft foods are easier to manage.

Chapter 17 fully addresses the assessment and management of the complications of ileus, stress ulceration, and malnutrition during the critically ill phase. Practical guidelines to facilitate continued difficulty swallowing, for example, when on mechanical ventilation, are also included.

Almost all patients will experience partial or complete loss of voluntary bowel control on a permanent basis. Correct techniques for evacuating the bowel during the acute period contribute to maintenance of bowel tone, regularity, and ease in developing a reliable bowel program.

Initially after injury, a small-volume enema may be used to ensure an evacuated bowel; thereafter enemas should be avoided because they overstretch the bowel and endanger future bowel management.

Due to lack of oral intake, frequent paralytic ileus, and immobilization, it is not unusual for a patient to be without a substantial bowel movement for 5 to 7 days. Procedure 19–3 outlines certain measures, which, if initiated early, can avert serious problems.

Stool softeners, which may be added to enteral solutions, facilitate stool evacuation. During spinal shock, however, laxatives, suppositories, and enemas tend to be less effective. Gentle manual extraction of stool from a flaccid bowel is more effective and may need to be done daily at first.

Accurate and comprehensive recording of bowel program results is often difficult in an acute care setting. Standard clinical records provide only a small space to check whether bowel movements have occurred, and descriptive data frequently become lost when charted in other

Personal Viewpoint

I was injured in a parachuting accident (my first jump) at age 23 and received a T_{12} spinal cord injury. This resulted in complete paralysis below that level, but I still have some preserved sensation. Now I attend the university and live in an apartment in Vancouver's West Side. I am able to walk with the aid of short leg braces and arm crutches but use my wheelchair most of the time around home, on campus, and when shopping.

On looking back, the nurses at the Acute Spinal Cord Injury Unit at Shaughnessy Hospital played the most important role of all in helping me maintain my self-esteem and regain my independence.

During the early days when I depended on them for everything, they were never patronizing. Since many of them were my own age, they treated me like one of their peers. They related to the part of me that was whole and like them, not the part of me that had changed. They reassured me about my future by portraying their own positive attitude. At the same time they educated me about my body. They allowed me to participate in my care—first as an informed observer, then as a guided participant—until finally I was independent.

I will always remember the sensitivity that was used to help me accept my bowel and bladder routines. (We spent many long hours locked in the bathroom together!) The warmth and understanding that was shown to me by these special nurses will always be a treasured memory.

Colleen Smith

notes. To meet this need, a clinical flow sheet from a rehabilitation setting may be adapted.

Dependency on other people for bowel elimination can be a most unpleasant and degrading experience. To maximize independence, establishing a *reliable* routine is essential, not only for physical health but for emotional comfort to begin dealing with adaptation to disability. When the patient's general condition stabilizes, question the patient about preinjury habits, nutritional and fluid intake, reaction to loss of bowel control, and any associated injuries that may negatively affect reestablishment of bowel control.

The patient will have to continue a routine throughout life. If a reliable bowel program is not established, the patient will live in fear of bowel accidents and tend to be isolated socially. It creates a major barrier to community reintegration. See Chapter 19 for a complete discussion of bowel management.

Maintaining Urinary Function

Neurogenic bladder management is of paramount importance because genitourinary complications can develop throughout the life span. Prevention must begin at the moment of injury. Abdominal trauma, even rupture of the bladder itself, can be associated with high-velocity accidents, fractures of the thoracic spine, and sometimes seatbelt injuries. Any hematuria, or other signs of abdominal trauma, requires immediate investigation. Accurate hourly measurements are needed when urine output is low, as with spinal and/or hypovolemic shock, or abnormally high, as is seen with posttraumatic diuresis. Acute tubular necrosis of the kidney can be associated with hypotension resulting in poor tissue perfusion with low urine output (less than 30 ml/hour).

The relation of intake to output is critical to detect and treat fluid imbalances. Be sure to include and record the kind and total amount of fluid intake and output *during transport* and look for evidence of fluid overload. Overcompensation for hypotension associated with spinal shock is not unusual.

Initially an indwelling catheter is necessary to prevent overdistension and ureterovesical reflux while monitoring for adequate urine output. During spinal shock, the pressure of the catheter in the urethra can produce ischemia and lead to formation of an abscess or fistula. Suprapubic catheterization to reduce the incidence of urethral complications is an alternative in both acute and long-term management, although some people suggest the increased risk of late bladder cancer is significant. However, a suprapubic route is usually preferred to manage direct trauma to or complications of the urethra and bladder.

Early removal of an indwelling catheter is desirable to reduce the chance of infection. An intermittent catheterization regimen is recommended to maintain reduction of infection and preserve the upper urinary tracts. The recovery time for the patient to become catheter free is shortened (O'Donnell 1987). However, the regimen should include a fluid restriction of approximately 2000 cc per 24 hours. Initially, this may be difficult, as fluid intake may be required to maintain cardiovascular status and other physiological parameters (Nemeth and Kiljanczyk 1988).

Early mobilization promotes urinary function by combatting urinary stasis. Also, immobilization can lead to hypercalcemia and predisposes the patient to development of calculi (McVicar and Luce 1986).

Detailed urinary assessment and management is discussed in Chapter 18. Physical assessment, diagnostic tests, criteria for selection and evaluation of various alternatives, including an intermittent catheterization regimen (method of choice), and complications such as infection and calculi formation are among topics in that chapter. Initiating an appropriate bladder program is essential to promote independence, and it is important to include these retraining parameters in the early plan of care for the rehabilitation process.

Promoting Musculoskeletal System Integrity

The entire philosophy of maintaining musculoskeletal integrity and reestablishing physical activity in SCI rests on preventing further neurological damage, facilitating return of potentially weak muscles, and promoting maximum activity of unaffected muscles. An optimal interdisciplinary approach in critical care encompasses immediate collaboration with physical and occupational therapists and consultation with nurses specialized in rehabilitation. All care is directed toward functional ability, that is, preventing deterioration and complications, and developing useful movements that will eventually help the disabled person with everyday living.

Regular turning and correct positioning cannot be overstressed. Specialized immobilization beds may facilitate this process. For example, the RotoRest Treatment Table provides a continuous, slow turning and is used for multiple-trauma patients. However, even in specialized centers, diligent care for patients on regular beds is often preferred. Turning is required every 2 hours. Minor, more frequent changes of position are often necessary for comfort. Turning (logrolling) and methods to achieve correct side-lying, supine, and prone positions, including modifications for patients in cervical traction, are detailed in Chapter 21. Avoid actually scheduling periods to be in the supine position. Patients are on their backs enough for various treatments and procedures. To help maintain functional alignment, Multipodis boots or high-top tennis shoes (larger than normal size) are helpful. These and other aids are also described.

Active and passive range of motion exercises, begun immediately, will prevent loss of muscle tone and range. As spinal shock passes, pain and spasticity, with specific patterns of contractures associated with muscle paralysis, are aggravated by immobilization. Contractures hinder functional ability. For example, flexion contractures of the hip or knee limit future ability to sit in a wheelchair.

Many clinicians feel that the long-term outlook for spasticity and related complications in a given individual is determined during the early course of management postinjury. If patients are properly positioned, receive range of motion exercises, and can avoid medical complications, severe spasticity may be avoided. Although there are benefits to spasticity and it need not be treated unless it interferes with functional abilities, spasticity can also contribute to the formation of pressure areas and contractures. (Chapters 27 and 28 explore spasticity and pain management.)

Protection of upper extremity function is vital to potential independence. For example, a full range of shoulder motion is needed to propel a wheelchair (Ozer 1988: 66). Thus shoulder contractures, with subsequent capsulitis, are devastating for the patient with quadriplegia (McCagg 1986; Egerton et al. 1986). Position arms as illustrated in Figure 6–4 to avoid this complication. (Consistent arm positioning is probably more effective than inconsistent range of motion

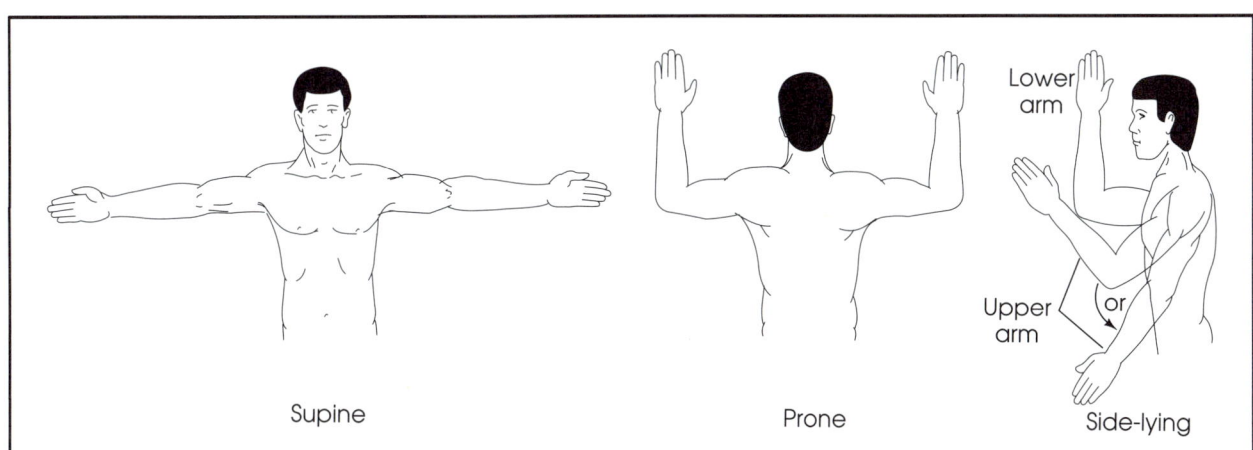

FIGURE 6–4 Position of arms for a patient with quadriplegia to prevent shoulder contractions and subsequent capsulitis. Positions also help to relieve pain associated with the fractured cervical spine. (Based on Egerton et al., 1986.)

exercises.) Correct arm positioning will also greatly relieve acute shoulder pain.

To maintain a functional hand position, immediate splinting is essential to support tenodesis. A natural tenodesis grip, the automatic finger flexion that is activated when the wrist is hyperextended, is widely used later for the gripping action involved in many daily living activities (Chapter 22).

The incidence of *associated skeletal injuries* has been reported as high as 56% (Meinecke 1973). Although some fractures are obvious, many are not, particularly if sustained in an area of the body that is without sensation. Lack of sensory warning mechanisms also hampers conventional treatments, such as casts or braces, due to the high risk of skin breakdown.

If conservative management is needed, pillow splints, thick padded bandages (made of cotton batting, wadding, and elastic tensor bandages), or individualized splints lined with foam rubber should be used. Difficult turning and frequent (daily) removal of supports for skin care often render these stabilization measures insufficient for fixation.

Surgical intervention to achieve early stabilization is warranted to avoid skin problems and prevent other hazards of immobility. Callus begins to form very soon in paralyzed patients, thus, operations may become more difficult later on. If fractures are left untreated the patient may develop complications, such as osteomyelitis, soft tissue damage, muscle contractures, loss of joint mobility, and malalignment. *It is just as important to restore skeletal function for the disabled patient as for the nondisabled.* Even though limbs are paralyzed they maintain a supporting function in skills of daily living such as transferring or even eating.

Improved options for maintaining spinal alignment now permit early mobilization of the paralyzed patient. With the introduction of the halo-thoracic brace to immobilize the cervical spine, patients with quadriplegia can now enter into active rehabilitation shortly after injury. Improved technology to enhance surgical interventions and the development of sturdy, light-weight orthotics have offered people with thoracolumbar injuries more security for earlier rehabilitation participation.

Hypercalcemia, reabsorption of bone distal to the injury, and *heterotopic bone formation*, abnormal bone deposits in paralyzed joints, are specific examples of skeletal complications associated with immobility. Early weight-bearing exercises using a tilt table help to reduce risk and severity (McCagg 1986). Skeletal complications and gradual increase in physical activity are addressed in Chapters 20 and 22.

Protecting the Skin

Lack of sensation, inability to move freely, and circulatory changes predispose patients with SCI to skin breakdown. Once the skin has broken down, even though it heals, it never regains its full resistance to the effects of pressure.

During spinal shock, capillary pressure is greatly reduced. This reduction is accentuated by hypotension, hypoxia, and/or anemia, factors that render the integumentary system even more susceptible to the effects of pressure during the immediate postinjury period.

Linares, Mawson, Suarex, and Buindo (1987) studied the association between pressure sore development and immobilization in the immediate postinjury period. They identified a high correlation between patients who developed pressure sores and patients who were immobilized for 2 hours or more before reaching an acute care unit. Therefore, consider backboard time: thorough inspection of the skin immediately on admission is critical to prevention. Continued skin inspection must be performed following each turn.

Successful management of the immobilized, acutely ill patient involves understanding the effects of pressure as a primary cause of skin breakdown and determining secondary factors that contribute to skin breakdown.

Even minor cuts, typically from gravel or glass, will not heal normally during spinal shock. Thorough cleansing and application of topical antibiotics along with protecting these areas from pressure are usually successful.

Most health care professionals have seen large, open, pressure ulcers, mostly caused by neglect, but most patients have not. Health education begins almost from the moment of injury by explaining actions to combat the effects of pressure that will become an important, integral part of a daily routine.

As the largest organ of the body, the skin is also perhaps the most vulnerable to damage as a consequence of SCI. Pressure areas and other integumentary problems notoriously slow the rehabilitation process (Keppler 1987). Inability to sit in a wheelchair, progressive infections, and surgical repair are costly complications in every sense. Recurrence becomes increasingly difficult to avoid. Skin breakdown itself is disabling. It detracts from self-esteem, impinges on family and social relationships, and creates barriers for both vocational and avocational pursuits. See Chapter 21.

PROVIDING PSYCHOSOCIAL SUPPORT

The many life-threatening complications surrounding the initial trauma of SCI often overshadow the emotional needs of patients and families. However, care givers must understand the intensity and effects of the fear and anxiety that patients and families experience.

Overwhelming fears of death and pain, both physically and psychologically, dominate. The higher the level of anxiety, the less patients and families comprehend. The

---

Personal Viewpoint

The emotional trauma of being in a fishbowl, typical of the intensive care setting, can frighten anyone, particularly the spinal cord injured patient who may not only be paralyzed, but also intubated and unable to call for help. These feelings are best described by a patient:

When I woke up, I felt lost. Then I realized I had no control over my own body. I couldn't talk because of my trache; it was hard telling anybody anything about how I felt and my discomfort.

I went through almost every emotion. I was scared and didn't think I was going to live. Once there was a storm and the power went out in the ICU. They transferred over to the generators, but not before everybody's alarms went off. They immediately came and let everyone know everything was all right. It was scary; but then it was all scary.

At first, some therapists would come in and work with the machines, but they would never talk to me. People would explain things to me, but I would usually have to ask. Eventually they started encouraging me—first the doctors, and then the nurses followed through.

---

patient frequently is in an *impaired conscious state* that blocks information, and even simple explanations must be repeated again and again. Additionally, forced dependency leads to feelings of powerlessness and inadequacy that can diminish self-worth.

Concerns regarding sexuality linked with body image can sometimes occur sooner than professionals anticipate, and acting out through sexual innuendos by the patient should be dealt with openly, preferably by people who are most comfortable and willing to speak honestly and give needed and correct information.

Chapter 10 suggests sexual health approaches for use in both specialized and nonspecialized settings. Family abilities, strengths, and resources must be assessed, not assumed (Richmond and Craig 1986). In the critical care environment, counseling professionals are able to provide formal, uninterrupted opportunities for assessment and expression of grief and concerns, especially for families, whereas nurses often form closer relationships with patients during direct care. Just as shared interdisciplinary knowledge and skills enhance physical rehabilitation, cooperative approaches offer optimal psychosocial support. Collective expertise better facilitates support and better secures the involvement of the family, whose cooperation is paramount in the rehabilitation process.

Goals or acute psychosocial interventions focus on helping patients and families:

- To receive accurate and complete information about the consequences of SCI at a rate tolerable to them.
- To adopt coping mechanisms so they can deal with the crisis imposed by losses from trauma. This includes incorporating disability into changed body image; feeling in control, experiencing successes, and regaining esteem; and dealing with role changes and altered family communications and activities, very often dominated by economic concerns.
- To recognize and express personal strengths and resources.
- To identify benefits of and participate in rehabilitation.

Good management incorporates all these processes while assisting patients and families to participate fully in the various stages of rehabilitation. Although the pace of physical rehabilitation is accelerating with modern health and technological advancements, psychosocial adaptation is a slower process. Furthermore, although theoretical and descriptive generalizations are possible, recent research indicates that responses to losses such as disability are so highly individualized that so-called normal responses almost escape definition.

Expect discouragement when setbacks occur and progress is slow, typically experienced when stays in critical care areas are prolonged. This truly represents a crisis situation, and all support systems must be utilized to support those in the grieving process. Patients often experience a wide range of emotions and, understandably, may become very demanding. Families often experience similar emotions, and/or may be the target of patients' behavior. Be prepared to set limits and explore other helping strategies presented in Chapter 9.

In a supportive milieu, patients, families, and staff can benefit by clarifying concerns, eliciting information regarding the patients' and families' preinjury coping abilities, and determining long-range plans of care to promote psychosocial well-being. The critical care unit is the initial setting to promote trusting relationships among patients, families, and the interdisciplinary team.

HEALTH EDUCATION

The educational process for patients and families also facilitates the adjustment process. The rationale for focusing on health education in the acute phase of SCI is expressed in the following objectives (Fukuyama et al. 1977):

- To increase patient and family knowledge and understanding of the effects of SCI on physical, vocational, social, and psychological functioning

The Prognosis

When and how to discuss a prognosis in the early stages is difficult. Most people gently approach the subject early but other care givers wait until patients and families actually ask.

Because patients can be extremely ill at this time, explanations need to be simple with further information communicated in a timely manner. Explanations need to include what SCI is and its general implications; limitations of current research in terms of regenerating the spinal cord; the patient's level and completeness of injury; potential outcomes; and the positive aspects of rehabilitation which will increase function despite disability. McCagg (1986) emphasizes that patients and families need frequent opportunities to ask questions as they become more able to tolerate the answers.

Then staff must deal with such questions or statements as: "What do you think?" "What does that doctor know anyway?" "Why didn't they just let me die? I wish I were dead." These times are stressful even for the most skilled and experienced care givers.

In retrospect, many people with SCI remember expressing such feelings and say now they mostly appreciated the staff just being physically present. It was reassuring to know they could cry and express grief without fear of being abandoned. However, a pessimistic attitude or lack of positive feedback on what the future can hold has the potential of creating even more negativity. Coming from an able-bodied person, responses such as "I understand how you must feel" or "You owe it to your family to live" tend to arouse more anger and frustration. It is more helpful to say something like: "I am trying hard to imagine how you must feel. It must be overwhelming, but I do know of people who have a similar injury to yours who are enjoying life" (and then give an example). The latter response conveys messages not only of concern but also of realistic hope.

Although the earlier literature reflects the importance of staff continually revealing the bleak prognosis so the patient and family can set realistic goals, this particular aspect of intervention is being reevaluated. More than one author has suggested that "denial" can be helpful in reaching maximum rehabilitation potential (Dillingham 1988). It is best to avoid confrontations that create tension and tend to be futile anyway.

- To increase the participation of family members in the patient's rehabilitation program and decrease feelings of isolation, hopelessness, and anxiety
- To maintain or reestablish communication channels among family members and enhance mutual support in emotionally dealing with disability
- To direct the patient and family toward discharge and planning for an independent future

The Critical Care Foundation, affiliated with the American Association of Critical Care Nurses and the Society of Critical Care Medicine, is a national nonprofit organization dedicated to improving and humanizing care for the critically ill and injured. One goal is to improve informational and emotional support for families. A handbook, *The Waiting Room Survival Guide*, written by critical care professionals with family members of former critical care patients, encourages the role of family members as support persons, spokespersons, and advocates for patients. Suggestions for getting and giving information, communicating with the critical care team, visiting, and taking care of themselves, as well as a glossary, are included.

Before becoming active participants in rehabilitative activities, patients and families need to be informed observers. To ease patients and families from illness into wellness, continually share knowledge, set appropriate expectations, and communicate the message, "I am going to care for this now, but in the future you will be able and responsible for completing or supervising this task yourself." This type of involvement conveys messages of concern, recognition of the patient's and family's abilities and importance, and prepares the way for future participation in the rehabilitation process.

A complete educational introduction for SCI patients and families, prepared by acute care nurses and educational specialists, is available (Shaughnessy Site 1988). A flipchart format was specifically chosen for convenience and flexibility required for individual teaching at the bedside. Further information on educational strategies, program development, and resource materials is presented in Chapter 11.

SECURING AN OPTIMAL CRITICAL CARE ENVIRONMENT

Securing an optimal critical care environment for the person with SCI demands not only integrity within the immediate critical care environment but also efforts beyond delivery of quality professional services. Personal feelings and attitudes toward disability enter into professionals' relationships with patients and families.

The Immediate Critical Care Environment

Bourdon (1986) has described the enormous sequelae to which the neurotrauma patient is initially subjected. The crisis-oriented care is compounded by the increased number of staff, frightening environment, excessive auditory stimulation, and multiple procedures. Thus, the interdisciplinary team must minimize the stimulation to which the patient is exposed.

Measures to relieve pain and anxiety and minimize environmental factors that contribute to stress include:

- Planning and coordinating interdisciplinary care at a tolerable rate for the patient. Group activities and treatments to coincide with peak periods of pain relief and small, frequent doses of narcotic analgesics, given intravenously, are most effective.
- Allowing for as much uninterrupted rest as possible.
- Planning with the family for the most desirable visiting times.
- Providing calm and simple explanations of the many procedures required. The patient may seem to understand what is said, but information may have to be frequently repeated.
- Frequently orienting the person to time and place and always alerting the person before performing care. Due to limited field of vision imposed by immobilization, orientation devices such as calendars and pictures can be placed on the ceiling.
- Establishing some means of communication when verbal response is not possible. Inability to communicate verbally is a problem for all ventilated patients, but in addition, patients with quadriplegia are unable to move their hands and arms to attract attention or write a simple message. A bell, pillow, or bulb type of call light, which is innervated by slight pressure from head or shoulder movements, must be accessible to establish some sense of control. A simple alphabet chart, using eye movements, is described in Chapter 15. Also, consultation with occupational and/or speech therapists will help explore the more sophisticated boards and communication devices now available on the commercial market. Minimize the terror felt by people unable to communicate: *immediate*, rather than delayed, collaboration is urged.

Personal Attitudes and Professional Development

Even in the critical care arena, an overly sympathetic, nonobjective attitude can convey feelings of hopelessness to patients and families. Sympathy is a natural human reaction, but the professionals who empathize will acknowledge these feelings and move on to develop more positive attitudes about the quality of life for people with spinal cord injuries. The best, and perhaps the only, way to develop positive attitudes is to include rehabilitated disabled persons into orientation and ongoing educational programs for the interdisciplinary critical care team. When people who continually care for patients and families in the early stages of adaptation to disability are unable to see a spinal cord injured person coping well and enjoying life, they may well perceive their efforts as futile and experience feelings of hopelessness themselves.

A highly successful, long-term model for this kind of educational partnership exists at the Acute Spinal Cord Injury Unit, Shaughnessy Site, Vancouver, BC. Spinal cord injured rehabilitation counselors from the British Columbia Paraplegic Association provide peer consultant services to newly injured patients and families, and the role modeling and support they provide for the interdisciplinary staff cannot be surpassed. Social functions are a highlight.

The physical prognosis for a person with SCI depends on the level and completeness of injury (Chapter 4). However, the ability to live independently has less to do with the actual physical outcome of injury than with attitudes. Architectural, educational, vocational, economic, and social barriers exist, reflecting society's low expectations for people with disabilities. Nevertheless, despite these barriers and their own disabling conditions, many people not only have overcome—or at least dealt with—these obstacles successfully but also have established organizations that assist others in

---

Personal Viewpoint

During the early days of acute treatment I remember some terrible nights when the medications and my physical condition resulted in hallucinations and extreme discomfort. I remember a nurse on nights who showed her concern by taking extra time, sitting near my bed when she could. It certainly decreased my anxieties and enabled me to sleep more easily. I don't remember what she said or even her name, but I do remember her obvious concern. I certainly agree that the acute care nurse has a lot of extra stress and that the realization of the kinds of life experiences their patients can look forward to may help.

Tom Parker
Executive Director
Alberta Paraplegic Association
Edmonton, Alberta, Canada

achieving and maintaining an independent life-style. To develop professionally, it is important to become familiar with the philosophy of independent living. Contact spinal cord injured persons who live in the community through local chapters of the National Spinal Cord Injury Association, The Canadian Paraplegic Association, or Independent Living Centers. Chapter 30 gives further information. However achieved, it is crucial for the staff to develop helpful attitudes because they set the tone for the entire rehabilitation process.

REFERENCES

American Trauma Society. 1990. *The Trauma Nurse Coordinator—A Position Paper.* Washington, DC: Author.

Bracken, M., et al. 1990. A randomized controlled trial of Methylprednisolone and Naloxone in the treatment of acute spinal cord injury. *New England Journal of Medicine* 322: 1405–1411.

Bourdon, S. E. 1986. Psychological impact of neurotrauma in the acute care setting. *Nursing Clinics of North America* 21 (4): 629–640. *Excellent section regarding the psychological reactions of the spinal cord injured patient and staff.*

Critical Care Foundation. 1988. *The Waiting Room Survival Guide.* Washington, DC: Author.

Casady, L., and Zinszner, K. 1989. The recognition and management of spinal shock. Proceedings of the American Association of Spinal Cord Injury Nurses, Las Vegas. *In-depth and clearly presented update of spinal shock available on cassette tape.*

Davidoff, R. A. (Ed.) 1987. *Congenital Disorders and Trauma.* Vol. 4. *Infections and Cancer.* Vol. 5. *Handbook of the Spinal Cord.* New York: Marcel Dekker. *Very readable series offering a broad and comprehensive survey of state-of-the-art knowledge about the spinal cord, both from a clinical and research-oriented viewpoint.*

Dillingham, T. R. 1988. Prevention of complications during acute management of the spinal cord-injured patient: First step in the rehabilitation process. *Critical Care Nursing Quarterly* 11 (2): 71–77. *Addresses the responses of the body systems to SCI and management in the acute care setting.*

Dollfus, P., and Gschaedler, R. 1987. Initial hospital care of spinal cord injured patients. *Paraplegia* 25: 241–243.

Egerton et al. 1986. ABC of spinal cord injury. *British Medical Journal* 292 (Feb.): 325–329. *Provides a nursing focus on initial management with emphasis on positioning, lifts, and turns.*

Fukuyama, K., Kelly, J., and Little, J. 1977. Unpublished material. *A group of staff nurses present rationale for establishing a formal health education program on an acute SCI unit.*

Gilbert, J. 1987. Critical care management of the patient with acute spinal cord injury. *Critical Care Clinics* 3 (3): 549–567. *Comprehensive management of the cardiopulmonary system is emphasized.*

Keppler, J. P. 1987. Rehabilitation in spinal cord injury. *Critical Care Clinics* 3 (3): 637–654. *Concise presentation of the neurological levels of SCI and the functional expectations.*

Le, C. T., and Price, M. 1982. Survival from spinal cord injury. *Journal of Chronic Disabilities* 35 (6): 487–492. *Spinal cord injured persons are living increasingly longer lives. The leading causes of death were related to the cardiovascular system, respiratory system, suicide, and urinary tract.*

Linares, H. A., Mawson, A. R., Suarex, S., and Buindo, L., et al. 1987. Association between pressure sores and immobilization in the immediate postinjury period. *Orthopedics* 10 (4): 571–573. *Almost all patients without evidence of pressure sores said they were turned within 2 hours of injury by a nurse. Whereas most of those without sores took 2 hours or less to reach a specialized SCI unit, those who later developed pressure sores took 3 hours or more to be transported.*

McCagg, C. 1986. Postoperative management and acute rehabilitation of patients with spinal cord injuries. *Orthopedic Clinics of North America* 17 (1): 171–182. *Describes assessment and rehabilitative interventions of the spinal cord injured patient by body systems.*

McVicar, J. P., and Luce, J. M. 1986. Management of spinal cord injury in critical care. *Critical Care Clinics* 2 (4): 747–758. *An interesting article on the effects of SCI on the major body systems.*

Meinecke, F. 1973. Pelvis and limb injuries in patients with recent spinal cord injuries. *Proceedings Veterans Administration Spinal Cord Injury Conference* 19 (Oct.): 205–212. *Incidence and rationale for prompt treatment of associated fractures to facilitate later rehabilitation.*

Meyer, P. R. 1989. *Surgery of Spine Trauma.* New York: Churchill Livingstone. *Liberally illustrated guide to retrieval and assessment, anatomy, specialty management areas, and general surgical management of spinal fractures. Outstanding and comprehensive medical resource of interdisciplinary interest.*

Nemeth, L., and Kiljanczyk, H. R. 1988. Intensive care of the spinal cord-injured patient: Focus on early rehabilitation. *Critical Care Nursing Quarterly* 11 (2): 79–84. *Concentrates on the rehabilitative aspects of nursing care in the spinal cord injured patient in the acute care setting using nursing diagnoses as a framework.*

Oakes, D. 1990. Benefits of an early admission to a comprehensive trauma center for patients with SCI. *Archives of Physical Medicine Rehabilitation* 72 (9): 637–643. *Concludes that patients do benefit from early admission to comprehensive treatment. Prevention of complications and more expertise in the timing and type of surgery were dominating factors in reduction of length of stay. Calculated to save $50,000 for each patient with quadriplegia.*

O'Donnell, W. F. 1987. Urological management in the patient with acute spinal cord injury. *Critical Care Clinics* 3 (3): 599–617. *Covers the acute and recovery phases of urological management, including surgical interventions.*

Ozer, M. N. 1988. *The Management of Persons with Spinal Cord Injury.* New York: Demos Publications. *Excellent handbook for interdisciplinary reference with emphasis on rehabilitation and continuing care needs.*

Richmond, T. S., and Craig, M. 1986. Family-centered care for the neurotrauma patient. *Nursing Clinics of North America* 21 (4): 641–651. *Uses a theoretical systems framework to provide psychosocial care for the patient with neurotrauma.*

Shaughnessy Site Education Services. 1988. *Spinal Cord Injury Flip Chart Learning Series.* Vancouver, BC: Author. *Designed by specialist nurses and therapists (in a critical and acute SCI care setting) in consultation with educational specialists, this series is excellent for early patient and family health education. Plasticized, color-coded flip charts are durable and tailored specifically for individual bedside use during recovery from trauma. Topics include understanding SCI, skin care, respiratory function, bowel and bladder management, hand function, and range of motion exercises. Complete with interdisciplinary teaching flow chart for patients and families. Provides a solid introduction and rationale for rehabilitation activities. Highly recommended.*

Sulsameda, R., and McBride, E. 1986. Linking trauma and rehabilitation services. *American Archives of Rehabilitation Therapy* (Winter): 32–34.

Trieschmann, R. 1980. *Spinal Cord Injuries, Psychological, Social and Vocational Adjustment.* New York: Pergamon Press. *Addresses the psychosocial impact of SCI on both people with disabilities and their families. Includes an exhaustive critique of the literature with a view to dispelling myths and stimulating research.*

University of Michigan Hospitals. 1990. *Spinal Cord Injury Transport Protocol.* Ann Arbor: University of Michigan Spinal Cord Injury Center.

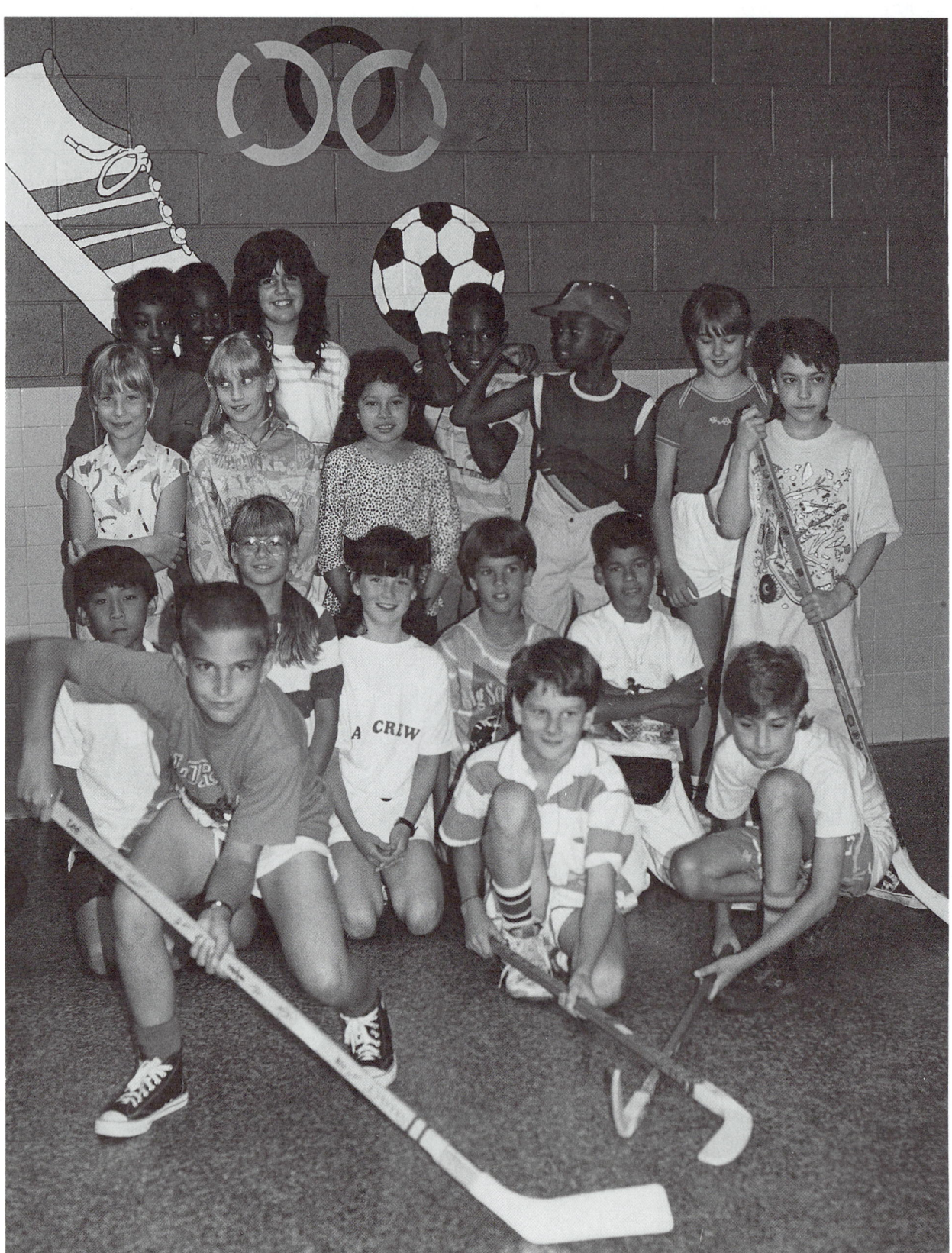

Regeneration Research: Hope for the Future

Charles H. Tator, M.D., Ph.D.

Chapter Outline

Health Care Objectives

- To survey research into spinal cord recovery and regeneration
- To gain knowledge of the barriers and of the hopes related to SCI research and, in turn, communicate this to individuals and families

Recent evidence suggests that the axons or message-carrying fibers of the neurons in the spinal cord can recover some of their function after major injury, or in some circumstances, can even regenerate after having been severed (Richardson, McGuinness, and Aguayo 1980; Aguayo, David, Richardson, and Bray 1982). Although clinicians always knew that the axons could recover some function after minor injury, it is now known that they can recover even after major injury. An example of axonal recovery after minor injury is spinal cord concussion in which a patient may lose motor and sensory function for a brief time, such as for one hour after injury, and then quickly regains that function. An example of recovery after a major injury is the patient who continues to regain small amounts of function below the site of the spinal cord injury (SCI) even 3 or 4 years after a major, incomplete injury. This late return of function most likely represents regeneration of transected axons or sprouting of new axons from nontransected axons adjacent to the injury site. It is now known from laboratory examination of the spinal cords of victims who did not survive their injuries (mainly those with multiple trauma) that the spinal cord is rarely completely transected (Kakulas 1988). All of this new information stimulates researchers to discover better methods for promoting the recovery of nontransected fibers and the regeneration of transected fibers (Tator, Linden, and Fehlings 1987).

Indeed, basic laboratory research has shown very hopeful results (Collins 1983; De La Torre 1981) and has confirmed the clinical findings. For example, after certain injuries, especially incomplete cord injuries with some preservation of motor or sensory function below the level of the injury, axonal recovery can occur and can be promoted by several types of experimental therapeutic measures. Furthermore, basic research indicates that even completely transected axons can be stimulated to regenerate under specific experimental conditions. Thus, there is hope that further research will increase the effectiveness and prove the safety of many of these treatments, so that they can be used in patients.

Due to lack of research funds, only about a dozen major laboratories in the world are concentrating on the study of acute SCI. In comparison with other diseases, governments, private foundations, and individuals have contributed relatively little money for SCI research.

There has been excellent communication among SCI researchers by means of journal publications, visits, meetings, and symposia so that all the major laboratories can quickly make use of advances in knowledge. This has prevented needless duplication, although some duplication is essential in order to confirm experimental results.

LABORATORY MODELS OF ACUTE SPINAL CORD INJURY

Since the early 1900s, various techniques have been developed to standardize a laboratory model of SCI in animals. For example, dropping a known weight from a known distance on the spinal cords of dogs results in SCI very similar to some injuries experienced by people. The weight-dropping injury technique has been most commonly used, yielding a great deal of useful information. Other techniques, primarily cuff, clip, and balloon compressions, have been developed for use in small-animal models of SCI such as ferrets, rabbits, and rats.

An extradural clip technique in the rat model has the major advantages of closely simulating the main kind of human SCI in which there is a circumferential compression-impact injury followed by persisting compression of the cord (Rivlin and Tator 1978). This model simulates the most common type of SCI in humans, which produces an initial compression impact of the cord due to impingement by fracture-dislocation of the spine, burst fracture of a vertebral body, or disc rupture, with subsequent persisting compression of the cord by bone or disc (Tator 1983). The rat model also allows researchers to use sufficient numbers of animals for statistically reliable results. The rats are colony bred for research, and are of reasonably low cost.

Models that involve actual fractures or dislocations of the spine have also been developed, but they are less useful because they are difficult to reproduce exactly in a series of animals. Transection of the cord is also a useful model for some experiments, but this must be done with precision so that the researcher can consistently interrupt a specific segment of the cord or totally transect the cord. For example, if a few fibers are left intact when the intention was to perform a complete transection, the results can be very misleading.

The development of these laboratory models has been an essential step in the evolution of SCI research into reliable, scientific work. Unfortunately, SCI researchers did not have these consistent models until recently, and many unsubstantiated, so-called breakthroughs were announced, creating false hope and disappointment. Every SCI researcher is aware that there will be a Nobel Prize awaiting the scientist who discovers the true breakthrough. With such a large incentive, there is the possibility of bias in the design of experiments or the interpretation of results. Thus, rigorously scientific design and objective interpretation of results are mandatory in all SCI experiments.

Of course, it would be highly desirable to avoid animal experimentation. However, to examine precisely the microscopic and biochemical changes in the cord and to develop treatments to counteract these changes, researchers must be able to study a model of the human situation. The long-term goal is to learn enough from the animal models so that research on isolated cells in glass containers would suffice, but knowledge has not yet accrued sufficiently to eliminate the animal models.

OUTCOME MEASURES USED IN SPINAL CORD INJURY RESEARCH

Objective, quantifiable measures of outcome are also essential for determining the consistency and reliability of an experimental SCI model and whether a treatment has improved recovery or made matters worse. Many consistent, reliable tests have been developed over the past few years. See Table 7–1. In general, to avoid observer bias, these tests must be applied blindly, so that the researcher does not know how a given animal has been treated until all the results are recorded.

The clinical, neurological examination can be assessed and coded according to a preestablished scale of functioning, but simple functional scales can only be applied to higher animals such as monkeys because animals such as rats can appear to walk even when the spinal cord has been

TABLE 7–1 Scientific Tests Used in Experiments on Spinal Cord Injury

1. Functional Tests
   Functional scale
   Inclined plane

2. Anatomical Tests
   Computerized image analysis
   Axon counts
   Axon tracers and labeled cell counts

3. Neurophysiological Tests
   Spinal-evoked potentials
   Somatosensory-evoked potentials
   Motor-evoked potentials

4. Blood Flow Analysis
   Hydrogen clearance

5. Biochemical Tests
   Chemical assays
   Magnetic resonance spectroscopy
   Microdialysis of cord

6. Imaging Tests
   Magnetic resonance imaging

completely transected. Occasionally, researchers have used these simple scales to evaluate lower animals and have obtained misleading results. To avoid misinterpretation, researchers have developed specific tests of behavioral tasks such as the inclined plane test, which assesses an animal's ability to maintain itself on an inclined plane of increasing angle. It has gained wide acceptance because of its objectivity, repeatability, reliability, ease of application, and low cost (Rivlin and Tator 1977).

Many excellent anatomical tests of the cord have been developed in the last 10 years. Some can be automated to assess by computerized image analysis the extent of cord injury, while others require the painstaking counting of all the intact axons at the injury site (Blight and Decrescito 1986). For example, the normal rat spinal cord in the cervical region contains about 400,000 axons, and it takes more than a full day to count designated samples of these axons by hand. Axons can transport certain tracers either toward or away from the nerve cell body from which the axon originates. These tracers can then be used to assess the intactness or integrity of the nervous pathways in the spinal cord. With one such tracer, a precise method for quantifying the number of intact axons in specific tracts crossing the site of injury has been developed (Midha, Fehlings, Tator, Saint-Cyr, and Guha 1987).

There are several methods of assessing the function of the pathways in the spinal cord. These neurophysiological tests can provide information about the functional integrity of various sensory or motor pathways in the spinal cord. For example, a nerve can be stimulated in the leg and the resulting impulse can be detected when it reaches a higher level in the cord or brain. Similarly, the brain can be stimulated and the response recorded downstream in the cord, peripheral nerve, or muscle. These tests have greatly improved our ability to assess the amount of damage from a certain degree of injury, and the amount of recovery after a treatment is applied. Similar tests have also been applied to patients because many can be performed with stimulating and recording electrodes placed on the surface of the skin. Indeed, there is now a method of stimulating the nervous system with magnetic energy that is completely noninvasive and does not elicit any discomfort.

Precise methods have been developed to measure spinal cord blood flow. One of the most frequently used is the hydrogen electrode technique, which has the major advantage of allowing repeated studies in the same animal. Thus, this test can be performed before and after injury, and then again, before and after treatment (Guha, Tator, and Rochon 1989).

A variety of biochemical tests assess the effects on the spinal cord of injury or treatment. Most of these require assay of excised segments of the spinal cord. However, newer techniques can be performed on the intact cord, such as *microdialysis*, which requires the insertion of fine catheters into the cord, or magnetic resonance spectroscopy, which is done with external detectors.

Finally, it is now possible with magnetic resonance imaging (MRI) to obtain repeatable, anatomical images of the cord in the living animal in order to assess the degree of injury and the response to treatment.

Thus, researchers can now accurately assess the functional anatomical, biochemical, and physiological effects of trauma and therapy. Indeed, in most current research, several of these scientific outcome measures are used in the same experiment to improve knowledge of SCI.

THE DAMAGING EFFECTS OF ACUTE SPINAL CORD INJURY

Acute SCI causes numerous widespread (systemic) damaging changes in the body, and a multitude of deleterious local changes in the cord. These mechanisms of damage have been intensively researched, an essential step in developing specific treatment modalities to counteract these damaging mechanisms (Tator 1982).

The higher the injury in the cord, and the more severe it is, the more profound the systemic hemodynamic changes (Guha and Tator 1988). Also see Chapter 6.

The physical or mechanical injury to the cord is known as the *primary* injury and may take the form of contusion (bruising), laceration (tearing), traction (stretching), or, rarely, complete transection. No matter how this primary injury occurs, it incites a multitude of damaging, *secondary* injuries in the cord. See Table 7–2. These secondary injuries include damage to the blood vessels, electrolytes, and numerous biochemical components of the cord. Researchers have worked extensively to understand these secondary injury mechanisms, how to counteract them in order to promote recovery and regeneration of the cord.

One of the most important secondary mechanisms is damage to the blood vessels of the spinal cord, both at the site of injury and for a considerable distance into adjacent segments of the cord. These vascular effects begin to occur during the first few hours after injury and include hemorrhages—predominantly in the central gray matter, but also extending out into the surrounding white matter. Both in the hemorrhagic zones and in the cord tissue surrounding the hemorrhages there is a progressive loss of the small blood vessels and a progressive decline in the amount of blood flowing in the spinal cord. If the loss of blood flow persists, there may be death of spinal cord tissue. These processes are known as posttraumatic ischemia (loss of blood supply). The exact cause of the loss of blood supply is unknown, but one hypothesis suggests it may be due to spasm of the blood vessels (vasospasm) or vascular thrombosis (clotting) due to one or more of the biochemical changes outlined below.

TABLE 7–2 Primary and Secondary Mechanisms of Acute Spinal Cord Injury

Primary Injury to the Cord
- Physical, Mechanical Disruption
  - Contusion, laceration, traction, transection

Secondary Mechanisms of Injury
- Systemic Hemodynamic Changes
  - Hypotension
  - Reduction of cardiac output
- Microvascular Changes in the Cord
  - Central hemorrhages
  - Loss of small blood vessels
  - Reduction in blood flow
  - Posttraumatic infarction
- Spinal Cord Edema (swelling)
- Electrolyte Shifts
  - Increased intracellular calcium
  - Loss of intracellular potassium
- Free Radical Release
  - From lipid peroxidation
  - Arachidonic acid
- Excitotoxic Amino Acid Release (vasospasm)
  - Glutamate, aspartate

Edema or swelling of the spinal cord also occurs after injury, although currently this is not thought to be one of the major secondary mechanisms of injury. Of more importance are numerous biochemical abnormalities in the traumatized spinal cord. For example, major changes in the cord electrolytes occur after injury, especially an increase in total tissue calcium, a reduction in extracellular calcium, and an increase in intracellular calcium. Increased intracellular calcium may cause further damage to the blood vessels and axons of the cord. There is also a major loss of potassium from the injured cells of the cord. Indeed, leakage of potassium from the inside to the outside of the cells may cause a block in the conduction of impulses by the spinal cord.

The membranes of the spinal cord are rich in *phospholipids*, which undergo chemical breakdown following trauma and then produce other chemicals capable of inducing secondary damage. It has been postulated that these injurious chemicals result in the production of further damaging agents known as *free radicals*. These free radicals can attack any remaining tissue, rendering it functionless. Another class of damaging chemicals has only recently been identified: a group of agents known as *excitotoxic amino acids*, specifically glutamate and aspartate. These agents have been shown to be present in injured tissue in much higher quantities than in normal tissue. Certain of these damaging substances may in turn cause vasospasm, one of the first mechanisms of secondary injury to be postulated, although this mechanism remains unproven.

EXPERIMENTAL TREATMENT OF ACUTE SPINAL CORD INJURY

During the past 15 years, research laboratories around the world have made much progress in discovering methods to counteract secondary mechanisms of SCI in the acute stage.

Rapid treatment of any compromise of airway, breathing, or circulation (the ABC priority list of trauma management described in Chapter 5) is essential for the general survival of the spinal cord injured victim.

Recently laboratory methods for counteracting the loss of blood supply to the cord, including drugs such as calcium channel blockers (Guha, Tator, and Piper 1985) combined with dextran, a blood volume expander, have been successful. This combination not only improved posttraumatic blood flow, but also restored function as shown by evoked potentials in research animals. Steroids and other agents have been used extensively to counteract edema, but consistent restoration of function after major cord injury had not been shown convincingly until 1990.

The results were announced of a multicenter trial in the United Sates of the acute administration of large doses of the steroid drug methylprednisolone. The study was very carefully performed and involved more than 400 patients (Bracken et al. 1990). The researchers found that if the drug was administered within the first few hours of injury, there was better neurological recovery in both complete and incomplete cases than in those who received Naloxone or a placebo. This study confirmed the previous results of studies of steroids in experimental models of acute SCI and may point the way toward finding even better agents to administer in the acute stages of the condition. Although not formally tested, it is very unlikely that methylprednisolone would be of any value for patients months or years after injury.

One recent therapeutic strategy counteracts the production of free radicals by using a new class of steroids with specific antioxidant properties. This group of drugs known as 21-aminosteroids has shown promising results, although it is too early to determine their ultimate role in the management of spinal cord injury (Hall 1988). The same applies to another new group of drugs of which MK-801 is an example. These drugs are designed to block the glutamate receptor, which is the site of action of this toxic amino acid whose concentration is markedly increased in damaged spinal cords (Faden and Simon 1987, 1988). Current research on drugs designed to counteract free radicals or excitotoxic amino acids is promising.

Decompression of the spinal cord is controversial among clinicians, but two convincing studies show that early, versus late, external decompression improves recovery (Guha, Tator, Endrenyi, and Piper 1987; and Dolan, Tator, and Endrenyi, 1980).

Surgeons have also attempted to perform an "internal" decompression of the cord by removing the dead, hemorrhagic tissue from the central regions of the cord in order to preserve the still viable surrounding tracts of the cord with minimal experimental evidence to support this concept.

Table 7–3 lists the main experimental strategies with some examples of agents tried. Virtually every agent in the table has given positive results in spinal cord injured animals in at least one laboratory. Unfortunately, many agents have subsequently proven useful only in animals with mild-to-moderate injuries. Some agents have been used in patients with discouraging results. Clinical trials have included patients with severe injuries because they usually obtain little or no spontaneous recovery. Some researchers have been reluctant to test agents in animals with severe injuries, for fear of missing a possibly beneficial effect.

EXPERIMENTAL TREATMENT TO PROMOTE AXONAL RECOVERY OR REGENERATION

Although the treatments in Table 7–3 are useful during the acute stage, many may also promote axonal recovery. Most of the therapeutic strategies listed in Table 7–4 are designed

TABLE 7–3 Experimental Treatment of Acute Spinal Cord Injury

1. To Counteract Posttraumatic Systemic Hypotension
     ABCs of trauma management
     Blood volume expansion
     Dopamine
     Vasopressors

2. To Counteract Posttraumatic Ischemia of the Spinal Cord
     Calcium channel blockers
     Glucocorticoids

3. To Counteract Spinal Cord Edema
     Glucocorticoids
     Diuretics

4. Decompression of the Spinal Cord
     External by removal of bone or disc or reduction of dislocation
     Internal by removal of damaged cord tissue

5. To Counteract Free Radicals
     21-aminosteroids

6. To Counteract Excitotoxic Amino Acids
     NMDA antagonists (e.g. MK-801)

TABLE 7–4 Experimental Treatment to Promote Axonal Recovery or Regeneration

1. Direct Current Fields

2. Thyroid Hormones

3. Growth Factors
   Nerve growth factor

4. Bridges
   Nonbiological
   Biological

5. Transplants
   Nerves
   Fetal cord or brain
   Cell suspensions

to be applied after the acute stage has passed or in animals with complete transection, and many have been applied to animals in the chronic stage.

Researchers have known for about 50 years that direct current fields affect the rate and direction of growth of axons in tissue culture. However, this modality has only recently been tried in spinal cord injury, first in the lamprey, an animal that can regenerate its traumatized cord, and then in guinea pigs and rats, animals that normally do not regenerate the axons of the spinal cord. A current field applied directly to the injured spinal cord of rats for 8 weeks can increase the inclined plane score and axon counts, (Wallace and Tator 1987; Fehlings, Tator, and Linden 1988). Furthermore, the function of the motor tracts was improved when the cathode or negative pole was placed caudal to the injury site. Although these results are encouraging, further work is needed to determine the safety of the technique and the minimum amount of current necessary to produce an effect before this technique could be applied to people.

There is research in several laboratories studying the issue of the *central pattern generator for locomotion*. There are groups of cells in the brainstem and spinal cord of experimental animals that when electrically or chemically stimulated, produce a reflex-patterned response of the legs similar to walking. It is possible that these reflex activities can be made to function in a useful way after SCI.

Several hormones including thyroid hormones are known to influence the growth of normal axons, and there is some evidence that these hormones can influence the recovery or regeneration of injured axons. Other biochemical agents have been shown conclusively to accelerate the growth of axons. However, neither nerve growth factor nor any of the other recently discovered growth factors has been effective in promoting recovery or regeneration following SCI. With the newly developed techniques of molecular

biology, researchers are now determining the nature of the molecules that can support or inhibit axonal growth. Modern molecular methods promise to accelerate the identification and production of growth-promoting agents for axons.

Researchers have implanted a multitude of biological and nonbiological bridges into the gap between the stumps of the transected spinal cord and have shown some growth of axons into the bridging material. One of the most exciting studies (Aguayo et al. 1982; Richardson et al. 1980) showed that axons of the spinal cord can grow into peripheral nerves that were previously grafted into the spinal cord. These researchers reasoned that the transected axons of peripheral nerves regrow readily because the environment in the peripheral nerve is a growth-promoting environment while that of the spinal cord is a hostile environment. Accordingly, supplying the spinal cord axon with a peripheral nerve environment should allow it to grow. Their hypothesis was correct because they showed that central axons in the rat spinal cord grew as much as several centimeters into the grafted peripheral nerves.

More recent experiments on the transected rat optic nerve show that axons from the retina of the eye grew into a grafted peripheral nerve and then back into the brain to form functional connections in the brain. Thus, transplanted peripheral nerves can possibly form useful bridges to carry axons across the injury site in the spinal cord. Maybe these axons can ultimately form useful connections on the other side; however, this has not yet been shown conclusively. Other tissues transplanted or grafted into the gap between the two stumps of the transected spinal cord include fetal brain or spinal cord, and suspensions of various types of cells from the brain or spinal cord. Although there has been remarkable axonal growth from the grafts into the spinal cord and vice versa, restoration of spinal cord function has not occurred. Nevertheless, the results to date with these biological bridges, grafts, and transplants hold promise.

IMPLICATIONS FOR INDIVIDUALS AND FAMILIES

Our knowledge of the effects of SCI has increased remarkably, and promising results have been achieved in the experimental setting. However, it is so very important to understand that these achievements are painstaking. It may take more than a decade to isolate one chemical when hundreds or more may play a role in regeneration. One researcher likened it to finding a person in New York City. We can get to New York easily from anywhere in the world but without further information, it is like looking for a needle in a haystack. But recent discoveries excite and hold promise for the future, and researchers feel they are on the threshold of important new developments in the field of SCI.

The science/time/money formula can be greatly influenced by individuals, families, and friends. Numerous associations devoted to SCI have specific research interests and need support, both monetarily and politically, to alter the present inadequate way SCI research is episodically funded. These associations also provide updated information on the status of current research in understandable terms. Use the Resource section in this text or contact the SCI Hotline for further details.

REFERENCES

Aguayo, A. J., David, S., Richardson, P., and Bray, G. M. 1982. Axonal elongation in peripheral and central nervous system transplants. In *Advances in Cellular Neurobiology*. Vol. 3. Eds. S. Federoff and L. Hertz. New York: Academic Press, 215–234.

Allen, A. R. 1911. Surgery of experimental lesions of spinal cord equivalent to crush injury of fracture-dislocation of spinal column. A preliminary report. *Journal of the American Medical Association* 57: 878–880.

Blight, A. R., and Decrescito, V. 1986. Morphometric analysis of experimental spinal cord injury in the cat: The relation of injury integrity to survival of myelinated axons. *Neuroscience* 19: 321–341.

Bracken. M., et al. 1990. A randomized controlled trial of Methylprednisolone and Naloxone in the treatment of acute spinal cord injury. *New England Journal of Medicine* 322: 1405–1411.

Collins, W. F. 1983. A review and update of experimental and clinical studies of spinal cord injury. *Paraplegia* 21: 204–219.

De La Torre, J. C. 1981. Spinal cord injury: Review of basic and applied research. *Spine* 6: 315–334.

Dolan, E. J., Tator, C. H., and Endrenyi, L. 1980. The value of decompression for acute experimental spinal cord compression injury. *Journal of Neurosurgery* 53: 749–755.

Faden, A. I., and Simon, R. P. 1987. N-methyl-D-aspartate receptor antagonist MK-801 improves outcome following experimental spinal cord injury in rats. *Neuroscience Abstracts* 13: 1031.

Faden, A. I., and Simon, R. P. 1988. A potential rule for excitotoxins in the pathophysiology of spinal cord injury. *Annals of Neurology* 23: 623–626.

Fehlings, M. G., Tator, C. H., and Linden, R. D. 1988. The effect of direct-current field on recovery from experimental spinal cord injury. *Journal of Neurosurgery* 68: 781–792.

Guha, A., and Tator, C. H. 1988. Acute cardiovascular effects of experimental spinal cord injury. *Journal of Trauma* 28: 481–490.

Guha, A., Tator, C. H., Endrenyi, L., and Piper, I. 1987. Decompression of the spinal cord improves recovery after acute experimental spinal cord compression injury. *Paraplegia* 25: 324–339.

Guha, A., Tator, C. H., and Piper, I. 1985. Increase in rat spinal cord blood flow with the calcium channel blocker, nimodipine. *Journal of Neurosurgery* 63: 250–259.

Guha, A., Tator, C. H., and Rochon, J. 1989. Spinal cord blood flow and systemic blood pressure after experimental spinal cord injury in rats. *Stroke* 20: 372–377.

Hall, E. D. 1988. Effects of the 21-aminosteroid u74006F on posttraumatic spinal cord ischaemia in cats. *Journal of Neurosurgery* 68: 462–465.

Kakulas, A. 1988. The applied neurobiology of human spinal cord injury: A review. *Paraplegia* 26: 371–379.

Midha, R., Fehlings, M. G., Tator, C. H., Saint-Cyr, J. A., and Guha, A. 1987. Assessment of spinal cord injury by counting corticospinal and rubrospinal neurons. *Brain Research* 410: 299–308.

Richardson, P. M., McGuinness, U. M., and Aguayo, A. J. 1980. Axons from CNS neurons regenerate into PNS grafts. *Nature* 284: 264–265.

Rivlin, A. S., and Tator, C. H. 1977. Objective clinical assessment of function after experimental spinal cord injury in the rat. *Journal of Neurosurgery* 47: 577–581.

Rivlin, A. S., and Tator, C. H. 1978. Effect of duration of acute spinal cord compression in a new acute cord injury model in the rat. *Surgical Neurology* 10: 39–43.

Tator, C. H. (Ed.). 1982. *Early Management of Acute Spinal Cord Injury*. New York: Raven Press, p. 444.

Tator, C. H. 1983. Spine-spinal cord relationships in spinal cord trauma. *Clinical Neurosurgery* 30: 479–494.

Tator, C. H., Linden, R. D., and Fehlings, M. G. 1987. Current status and future prospects for the neurosurgical management of acute spinal cord injuries. *Paraplegia* 25: 250–253.

Wallace, M. D., and Tator, C. H. 1987. Recovery of spinal cord function induced by direct current stimulation of the injured rat spinal cord. *Neurosurgery* 20: 878–884.

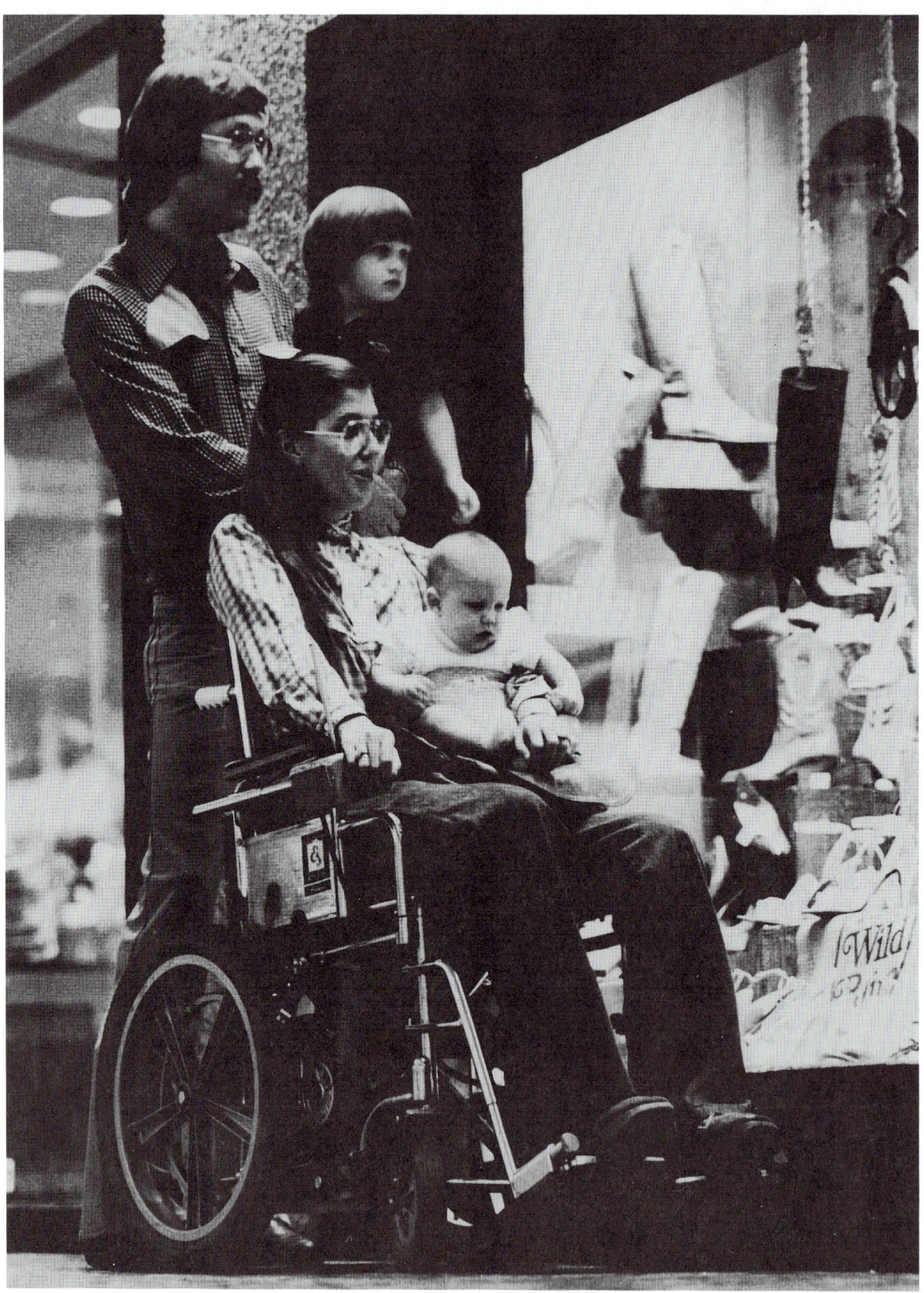

CHAPTER
— 8 —

Legal Considerations

Louise Bouscaren McKnew, Attorney at Law*

Chapter Outline

LEGAL GOALS
PROTECTIONS
HOW TO CHOOSE A LAWYER
CRITICAL QUESTIONS
INSURANCE
ADDITIONAL SOURCES OF SUPPORT
IN CLOSING

Health Care Objectives

- To understand the lawyer's vital role in protecting spinal cord injured patients during acute care and thereafter
- To incorporate legal considerations into health/life care planning for disabled persons and their families
- To provide practical information on legal matters for catastrophically injured persons and their families

*Louise Bouscaren McKnew is an attorney and an acknowledged expert in SCI, having immersed herself in the subject following the "accident" that paralyzed her son in 1978. She cofounded a national research program, established a SCI hotline, initiated national and local legislation, and produced an award-winning documentary. She writes, lectures, and testifies on the subject, serves on boards and task forces, and advises attorneys nationwide—all because of her dedication to people with SCI. She practices law in Bethesda, MD, and offers full advocacy services to people with catastrophic injuries.

LEGAL GOALS

What happened, who, where, why, when? What do we do now? These questions are always asked in pain, anger, and fear by newly injured patients and their families. The trauma of sudden, total physical devastation raises the issues of fault, responsibility, accountability, and cause. Unfortunately, these issues are often ignored, their resolution avoided or postponed, and their long-term implications overlooked in the rush to stabilize and manage the immediate medical consequences of paralysis.

Furthermore, the popular image of lawyers is not altogether complimentary, and medical practitioners do not usually refer patients to lawyers. Indeed, lawyers have not been included in management plans for spinal cord injury (SCI). Hospital and medical specialists often actively block what they see as interference by lawyers, claiming sole authority for the care of the newly injured.

The law's purpose, and the lawyer's goal, however, are not interference in the healing process but protection of the patient. An attorney can and should be an important part of the team working on behalf of the injured person, the family, the community, and the public at large during the immediate recovery period.

PROTECTIONS

SCI presents an extraordinarily complicated and demanding challenge to the medical profession. The stakes for all involved—the professionals, the patient, and family—require the best care. Without state-of-the-art medical expertise, technology, facilities, and personnel, there is no hope of restoring lost function or of adequate protection against additional physical and financial losses.

Although lawyers cannot participate in the health care itself, a good lawyer who specializes in catastrophic personal injury representation can assure that the client receives the best care available. Protection against poor, inadequate, or even negligent care can be initiated immediately after injury, thus preventing further unnecessary injury. Not all ambulance attendants are trained paramedics, not all emergency rooms offer catastrophic trauma services, not all hospitals specialize in, or can adequately treat, people with SCI, and not all rehabilitation hospitals aggressively pursue restoration of function. Hospitals or hospital employees rarely admit they are not sufficiently specialized, and if the patient has medical insurance, SCI is a source of enormous revenue. With no vested interest in the patient's choice of hospital or physician, a knowledgeable attorney can guide the client to the best health care available.

Treating a patient with SCI is exceedingly expensive, and a good attorney sometimes can protect against financial ruin. The decision as to who should be held responsible for the financial consequences often is based on legal principles. Even when fault cannot be legally assigned to another party, decisions as to who should pay the bills must still be made. Insurance coverage, social service programs, tax consequences, and employer, spousal, and parental obligations are all legally grounded. An attorney should address such questions as whether and how to collect, from whom, how much, and when.

Finally, the law has assumed a vital role in protecting the public at large from faulty products, negligent behavior, and unconscionable acts. Courts assess damages in many lawsuits partly to prevent additional injuries resulting from similar so-called accidents and to punish deliberate, unreasonably dangerous acts. Attorneys are pivotal in preserving this public interest role of the plaintiff's bar. Their work has contributed, for example, to requiring seat belts and air bags in cars, removing asbestos from buildings, and stopping the marketing of drugs known to be dangerous, to name just a few.

In short, the law's purpose is to help the injured person: to ease trauma, to restore losses, to prevent recurrences, and occasionally, to punish.

HOW TO CHOOSE A LAWYER

A person with SCI needs an attorney who specializes in personal injuries and has extensive experience specifically with SCI, head trauma, or another central nervous system injury. Such an attorney should be a member of the plaintiff's bar, a trial lawyer who represents people bringing lawsuits against someone alleged to have personally and/or physically caused them injury.

An attorney without this experience is not a good choice. The next-door neighbor who happens to be a lawyer, the attorney who drew up a will or settled the purchase of a house, or a relative who is an attorney—even a plaintiff's attorney—who has not specialized in this kind of injury cannot provide the best assistance. Spinal cord injuries are complicated: many possible causes, myriad consequences, and the risk of additional injury require an experienced attorney to determine how the injury occurred and to anticipate the patient's future needs.

A few, very visible lawyers who walk the line between ethical behavior and self-serving greed have led the public to question all trial lawyers' motives. Indeed, some lawyers are simply greedy, assessing potential cases solely by the probable fee they will receive. Nevertheless, many trial

Legal Checklist for the Spinal Cord Injured Person and Family

Consider your need for an attorney and begin a search for a good one. Meanwhile,

SIGN NOTHING

Sign nothing until you have read what you are asked to sign, and until you understand what you have read. If you do not understand what you are asked to sign, call an attorney.

FILE

File all bills, invoices, and receipts together in a safe place. Tally all costs and expenses incurred as a result of the injury.

LOG

Log all incoming and outgoing phone calls relevant to the injury. Note dates, times, persons, and purposes of calls, and results when relevant.

RECORD EVIDENCE

Record evidence as appropriate:

- *Witnesses:* Write down all names, addresses, work and home telephone numbers, and notes about any conversations.

- *Physical evidence:* Throw nothing out; preserve all relevant evidence concerning the injury including cars, helmets, clothing, and any other product involved. Take photographs, for instance, of skid marks or damaged property.

- *Police and accident reports:* Get copies of the initial police report written by the officer at the scene, the report the officer writes for his superior, and any other official report of the injury.

- *Insurance policies:* Find and carefully read insurance policies relevant to the injury—medical, home owner, automobile.

- *Medical personnel:* Write down the names, addresses, and telephone numbers of all medical personnel involved: ambulance drivers and attendants, emergency room physicians and nurses, and other specialists. Be sure to include the names and addresses of all hospitals involved.

NOTIFY

Notify your insurance company or agent. State the facts, but be careful not to offer opinions. Consult an attorney if possible. Also contact your employer, school personnel, or colleagues who should know of your absence from scheduled or routine appointments. Call the hospital social worker who can begin the process of securing state and county social services, of contacting agencies, and of collecting forms and applications.

THINK OF LIFE GOALS

Paralysis means long-term problems that require an attorney's help. Insurance companies will refuse payment for services they deem medically unnecessary, social service agencies will cut off benefits without due process, and employers will discriminate on the basis of handicap. The newly mandated civil rights of people with disabilities will be violated. Although these problems do not arise during the initial emergency period, they are nonetheless critical.

BE INFORMED

Every person with SCI should secure and read two publications before final discharge from the hospital:

The new *Americans with Disabilities Act* passed by Congress in 1989 details a civil rights code for all people with disabilities. See the brief summary of the act's requirements in this chapter and obtain a copy from the local office of your congressman or senator.

Paraplegia News, published monthly by the Paralyzed Veterans of America, is written for both veterans and civilians. It provides valuable information about research, products, legislation, travel, other organizations, and sources of support. An annual subscription is $12 (foreign, $20). Write to *Paraplegia News,* 5201 North 19th Avenue, Suite 111, Phoenix, AZ 85015.

lawyers are ethical, competent, and caring of the injured person's long-term welfare. Patients and their families should seek information and be cautious in choosing counsel. Talk with other injured people who have secured the services of a lawyer, consumer groups that collect information about attorneys who represent spinal cord injured persons, a local lawyer referral service provided by the American Trial Lawyers Association (headquartered in Washington, DC), or the local bar association. Advertisements by lawyers in telephone directories, although a risky source, have also helped some people find competent representation. The critical care team should know about local referral sources and guide newly injured patients to seek experienced legal counsel.

Interview the prospective lawyer thoroughly. Ask questions about training, values, and previous cases. The working relationship will be close: does the lawyer sound sensible and seem trustworthy? Are personal and professional qualifications acceptable? What does the attorney think of the situation—what are the priorities, the strong and weak points of the case? Are the attorney's intentions for proceeding reasonable, possible, and proper? Get references and call them. Remember, a client must trust the attorney. If the client believes it is no longer possible to work with the attorney, or if the attorney proves less than reliable, responsive, attentive, or knowledgeable, the attorney can be fired.

Ask how and when the lawyer expects to be paid *before* formal hiring. Unlike other legal specialists, plaintiff's lawyers ordinarily collect contingency fees if and when successful in generating funds on behalf of the client. Clients are usually not assessed hourly charges, up-front deposits, or prepaid expenses. Some lawyers offer to advance the costs of preparing a case, to be repaid by the client after settlement or a court award. Be sure all financial arrangements between attorney and client are in writing before proceeding with the case.

This method of recompense has several advantages. Contingency fee services are available despite poverty or ability to pay. It guarantees access to the judicial system, with capable counsel, for all citizens. This method also encourages both plaintiffs and lawyers to bring only those cases that warrant the time and expense involved, discouraging frivolous suits and expensive delays. Court time, investigative procedures, and paid expertise are kept to a reasonable minimum. Finally, when a large award or settlement is generated, attorneys sometimes make larger fees than would have resulted from an hourly fee system. This additional money permits attorneys to advance the up-front costs of the next case, to take less than perfect cases, to fight for more protection for the next person, and to cover the representation costs of a reasonable but unsuccessful lawsuit. Indeed, an attorney may be financially able to represent a spinal cord injured client only because of an award generated by the previous case.

Fees are usually set as a percentage of the award or settlement. They range from 20% to as high as 50% *after* deducting expenses. Both the attorney and the client must decide together what is fair and equitable. Some arrangements cap the total fee, regardless of the amount of the award; others set the fee on a sliding scale, depending on the amount of the award—for example, a certain percentage up to a certain amount, decreasing as the recovered amount increases. Fair apportionment should depend on the risks involved, the potential recovery, anticipated pretrial expenses, the attorney's resources, and the client's financial needs. Local bar associations have been known to sanction and punish attorneys who structure excessive fee arrangements.

Sometimes lawyers who take personal injury cases refer them to more experienced or specialized colleagues. If your attorney makes such an arrangement, be sure to discuss the role of each attorney and what their fee arrangements are.

All fee arrangements should be specified in a written agreement, signed by both attorney and client, that documents in detail why the client has retained the attorney.

CRITICAL QUESTIONS

Not all injuries are accidental. Purposeful omissions by manufacturers are not accidental, failures to exercise reasonable care are not accidental, commissions of illegal acts are not accidental. Sometimes people fall off poorly constructed ladders *because* the ladder was poorly constructed, crash into roadside barriers *because* the road was poorly designed or marked, or develop medical complications *because* of poor care.

The attorney focuses initially on what actually happened—where, when, why, how, and who. Theories of liability vary, and creative lawyers find ways either to fit the particular case into an existing theory or to invent a new one. Contract law, Uniform Commercial Code regulations, tort law, and legal precedents set by previous court cases provide the basis for recovery claims.

The attorney's initial inquiries are shaped by the need to support four claims. Each claim has further complications, but simply stated they are:

- *Duty:* There must be a legal duty owed by the injuring party to the injured party. Duties vary and may not be apparent to anyone except an experienced attorney. They may be contractual in nature, or found to exist, by law, without any written document.

- *Breach:* The injuring party must have failed to fulfill (breached) a duty to the injured party of care, contract, or some other legal obligation.

- *Injury:* The injured party must have sustained an injury.

- *Causation:* The breach of the duty must have caused the injury.

In addition, the lawyer must decide whether state or federal law should govern, which state or federal law applies if more than one is available, and the pros and cons of each option. For example, in Maryland and a few other states, any finding that the plaintiff was guilty of contributory negligence precludes recovery of damages. Other states' laws may permit recovery only if the plaintiff was less than 50% negligent; still others offer recovery based solely on a percentage of negligence. The attorney should discuss the applicable theory with the client.

Depending on where and under what circumstances the injury occurred, local laws and regulations may govern the appropriateness of a lawsuit. Workers' Compensation contracts exist to help employees recover medical costs and wages lost for injuries sustained on the job. However, Workers' Compensation may sometimes preclude additional legal proceedings. No-fault laws vary from state to state: some offer a range of options while others restrict the injured party's recovery routes.

The attorney must also consider which costs consequent to the injury are recoverable. Medical expenses, lost income, compensation for pain and suffering, and loss of consortium are among the most typical. Other costs may include punitive damages. The costs of going to trial, the adequacy of offers of settlement, the possibility of structured settlements, and the legal limitations (caps) on amount of pain and suffering awards are some other considerations both the attorney and client must discuss. Going to court is an expensive, painful, and extraordinarily time-consuming enterprise, and the client needs experienced and knowledgeable counsel to choose the best option.

Finally, the attorney must have evidence to back up all claims. Photographs, products, correspondence, bills and invoices, sales slips and contracts, notes on conversations, and information about witnesses must all be preserved. Names, addresses, and telephone numbers of everyone involved are essential. Throw away nothing and write down everything: what appears inconsequential may prove to be essential.

INSURANCE

Insurance companies are in business to make money. Spinal cord injuries cost a lot of money. Some insurance companies refuse to honor their commitments: the greater the costs, the more they may resist paying claims. However, if the injured person, the family, or employer paid premiums for medical, automobile, or other insurance coverage, there is a legally binding contract with the insurer and consequent financial rights depending on the specific coverage purchased. Read the policy and file claims promptly. For medical payments, get receipts from doctors and pharmacies.

Never take the insurance company's refusal as a final answer or decision. Always refile any denied claim. An attorney can help; often a note on the lawyer's stationery gets results. If the claim is reasonable and remains rejected by the insurer, consider a lawsuit. Too many people pay expenses that should have been paid by their insurance carriers because they believed the companies' rejections were legitimate.

Some social service programs serve as insurance policies for people who sustain catastrophic injuries. Congress has mandated Social Security entitlement programs that help pay for medical equipment, rehabilitation projects, education, prescriptions, vehicle adaptations, and more. Other programs can vary state to state. Additional county and local programs may also exist. Sometimes help is available depending on economic need or on degree of disability. Unfortunately, people are rarely told that help is available and thus do not receive benefits to which they are entitled. Furthermore, most benefits become available from the date or request, not from the date first needed.

Until good case management programs are in place, and until social workers, nurses, and doctors are in a position to assume responsibility for full service to their catastrophically injured patients, lawyers must assist people so that they receive the help these taxpayer-funded programs offer. Many injured people have legal rights to services they themselves have paid for through taxation. Attorneys can respond effectively to refusals to pay or denials of claims by the administrators of these publicly funded programs. Here again, the rule is never to take "no" as the final word. The government may owe a duty overlooked or ignored by an administrator, or the claimant may have a legal right that was taken away without cause, a hearing, or due process.

ADDITIONAL SOURCES OF SUPPORT

An attorney specializing in SCI should know about and refer the client to other legal, community, and private sources of assistance and information. Elected officials, community leaders, consumer groups, and SCI organizations can be especially helpful.

Inform elected officials at all levels of the existence of a new spinal cord injured person within their jurisdiction.

Americans with Disabilities Act (ADA) Fact Sheet

Employment

Employers may not discriminate against an individual with a disability in hiring or promotion if the person is otherwise qualified.

Employers can ask about one's ability to perform a job, but cannot inquire if someone has a disability or subject a person to tests that tend to screen out people with disabilities.

Employers will need to provide "reasonable accommodations" to individuals with disabilities. This includes steps such as job restructuring and modification of equipment.

Employers do not need to provide accommodations that impose an "undue hardship" on business operations.

Who needs to comply:

All employers with 25 or more employees must comply, effective July 26, 1992.

All employers with 15-24 employees must comply, effective July 26, 1994.

Transportation

New public transit buses ordered after August 26, 1990, must be accessible to individuals with disabilities.

Transit authorities must provide comparable paratransit or other special transportation services to individuals with disabilities who cannot use fixed route bus services, unless an undue burden would result.

Existing rail systems must have one accessible car per train by July 26, 1995.

New rail cars ordered after August 26, 1990, must be accessible.

New bus and train stations must be accessible.

Key stations in rapid, light and commuter rail systems must be made accessible by July 6, 1993, with extensions up to 20 years for commuter rail (30 years for rapid and light rail).

All existing Amtrak stations must be accessible by July 26, 2010.

Public Accommodations

Private entities such as restaurants, hotels, and retail stores may not discriminate against individuals with disabilities, effective January 26, 1992.

Auxiliary aids and services must be provided to individuals with vision or hearing impairments or other individuals with disabilities, unless an undue burden would result.

Physical barriers in existing facilities must be removed, if removal is readily achievable. If not, alternative methods of providing the services must be offered, if they are readily achievable.

All new construction and alterations of facilities must be accessible.

State and Local Government

State and local governments may not discriminate against individuals with disabilities.

All government facilities, services, and communications must be accessible consistent with the requirements of section 504 of the Rehabilitation Act of 1973.

Telecommunications

Companies offering telephone service to the general public must offer telephone relay services to individuals who use telecommunications devices for the deaf (TDD's) or similar devices.

Source: U.S. Department of Justice

Local representatives and members of Congress can be enormously helpful in cutting through red tape and bureaucratic barriers. School board members, city council leaders, the governor's office, and housing officials may know of special community programs. In fact, contacting such people may directly contribute to immediate and improved patient care—elected officials often know the best doctors and first-rate facilities and can get the patient into such care faster than the patient and family can.

School principals, teachers, ministers, priests, and rabbis also should be informed. Employers, work colleagues, and the local newspaper are other sources of potential support.

It may also be appropriate to inform consumer groups, public interest organizations, or consumer product reporters of a person with a new injury. However, take care because initial impressions of the injury may not be accurate. Early statements may inadvertently compromise a future lawsuit. Attorneys can advise.

Finally, several SCI groups around the country may be helpful and informative. However, be cautious—some organizations simply want money. Most groups will send a free sample publication and outline their priorities, services, programs, and costs. Attorneys specializing in SCI can identify the legitimate organizations.

IN CLOSING

Anyone who sustains SCI needs help—it is an awesome, painful, devastating trauma. No one profession or professional can offer all the help available, owed, or needed. Specialists from many disciplines must work together to minimize the physical, financial, psychological, and social destruction such an injury inflicts. An experienced attorney should be an integral part of the team. Without an attorney, the injured person remains unnecessarily vulnerable to further harm, and without adequate resources, further health and quality of life may be unnecessarily jeopardized. Engage an attorney—the sooner the better.

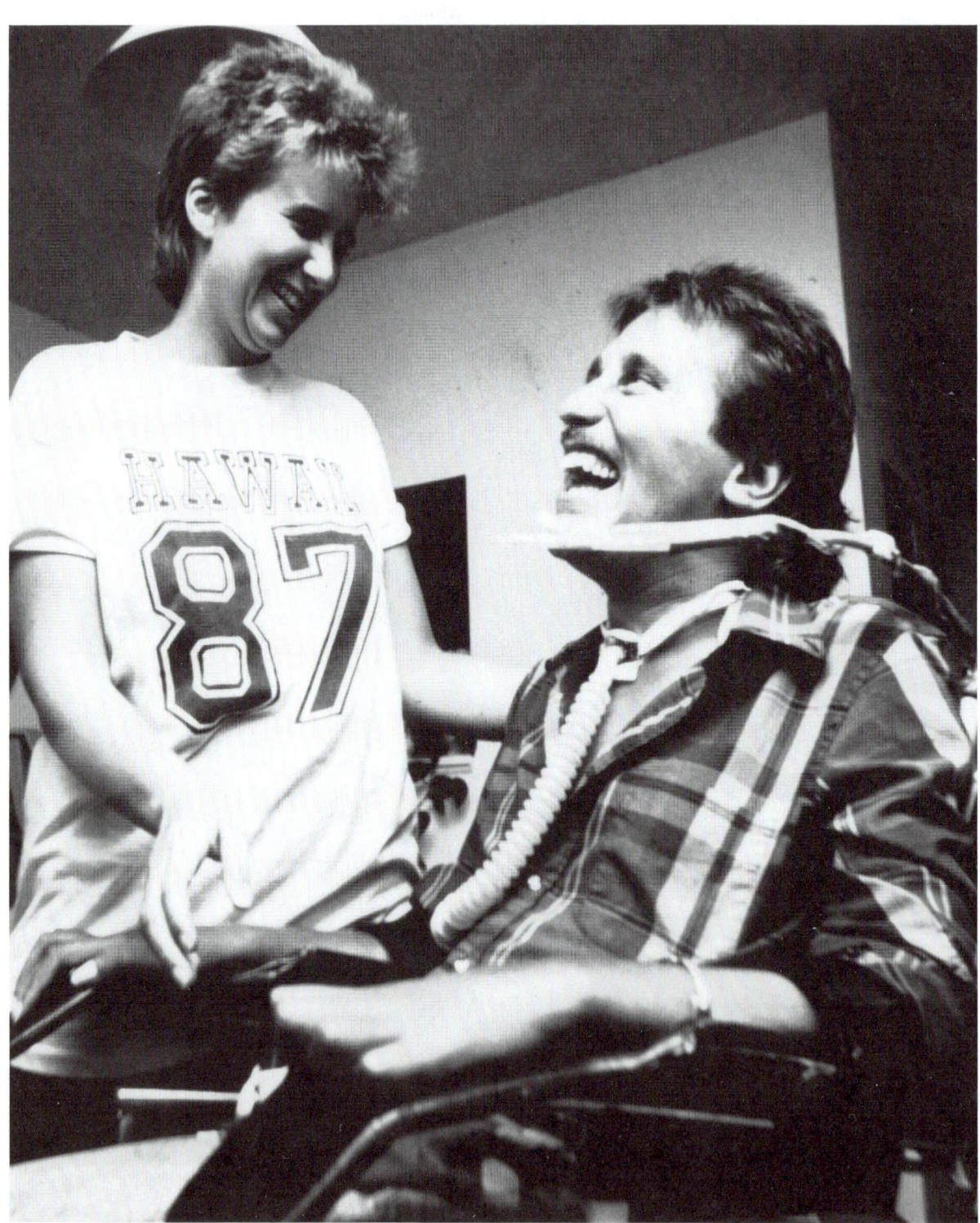

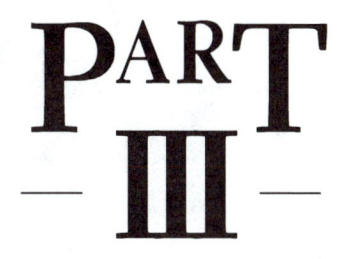

PART III

CREATING AN OPTIMAL REHABILITATION ENVIRONMENT: A COOPERATIVE EFFORT

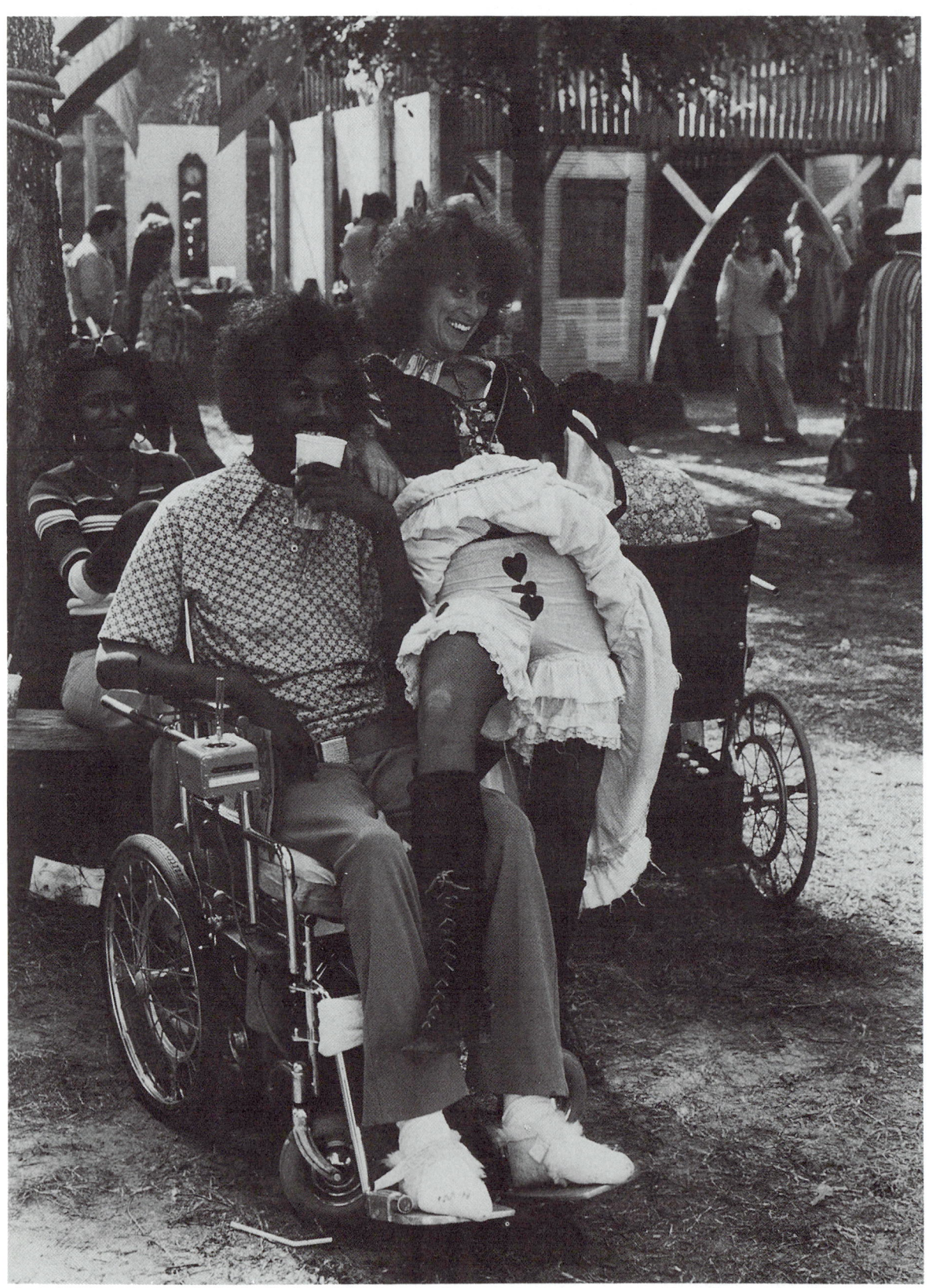

CHAPTER
— 9 —

Enhancing Feelings of Self-Worth*

Chapter Outline

*This chapter was developed with the assistance of Mary Lee Lynch, R.N., M.S.N., C.S.

Health Care Objectives

• To create a therapeutic rehabilitation environment
• To recognize and understand the significance of individual and family relationships, values, beliefs, and past coping mechanisms in relation to the rehabilitation process
• To understand how experiencing loss and crisis intervention techniques apply to rehabilitation

• To develop, in partnership with patients and families, an individualized plan of care that will help them to live with the disability within their own environment
• To recognize psychosocial problems that require additional professional help and refer appropriately
• To realize personal limitations and seek appropriate help from interdisciplinary team members
• To recognize the impact that personal attitudes have on individuals and families during rehabilitation

---

Medical science has developed sophisticated techniques to sustain and improve the quality of physical life for people with spinal cord injuries (SCI). In recent years, the overwhelming psychological needs of the SCI patient have been repeatedly recognized. Yet the current health care delivery system frequently fails to deal with these multiple psychosocial needs. Spinal cord injuries are as emotionally devastating as they are physically disabling.

Patients with SCI are confronted with complex changes such as limited mobility, increased dependence on others, chronic pain, loss of bowel and bladder control, and altered sexual functioning. They must cope with the loss or change of vocational goals, earning capacity, and disrupted family and social relations. Often they must bear the social stigma of being "different." All of these changes can lead to feelings of anger, resentment, fear, frustration, uselessness, or helplessness, and a loss of self-esteem.

Providing psychological support is a dramatic challenge for all health care professionals. Emotional distress experienced during hospitalization can be reduced by integrating appropriate psychosocial interventions into the plan of care. Given adequate psychological support, plus a healthy rehabilitation setting, the majority of patients with SCI can ultimately lead satisfying, meaningful and productive lives within the community.

FACTORS THAT AFFECT THE THERAPEUTIC ENVIRONMENT

The Philosophy of Rehabilitation Practice

The National Council on Rehabilitation defines *rehabilitation* as the restoration of individuals to the fullest physical, mental, social, vocational, and economic capacity of which each is capable. This process begins the moment an individual is disabled and continues throughout life. Each individual possesses certain strengths, as well as limitations, that influence the course of rehabilitation, the goal of which

should be to help the individual learn to live with disability. Thus rehabilitation does not end when the individual is discharged but actually begins when the disabled person practices and applies coping skills in the home and community. This learning encompasses health and physical aspects as well as activities that enrich and reward the disabled person's individuality and life-style.

All too often values and goals are determined for individuals without including them in the process. To develop a successful rehabilitation program, the person, family, and the rehabilitation team, must set realistic short- and long-term goals that are based on the abilities and priorities of the individual and the home environment. A rehabilitative philosophy provides vital concepts to believe in or strive for and a structure for rehabilitation practice. How the philosophy of rehabilitation is practiced within any one institution significantly affects the scope of personal interactions among the interdisciplinary team, patients, and families.

The Interdisciplinary Team

To help ensure that the definition of rehabilitation is not exclusively physical, counseling professionals trained in the behavioral sciences are becoming increasingly involved in interdisciplinary treatment. The primary role of these team members is to assist with the psychosocial aspects of rehabilitation. Some examples include sexual health counselors, educational and vocational counselors, leisure therapists, and people with SCI engaged in peer counseling.

The Social Worker

Social workers are an integral part of the treatment team, whose involvement encompasses the patient, the family, the interdisciplinary team, and the community at large. Social workers gather and interpret personal, family, financial, and environmental resource data to help patients and families cope with the many stressful psychosocial problems that sudden, severely disabling injuries bring.

Social workers are also concerned with the interactions between the patient and the social environment—staff, families, peer group, and the community, for example—

focusing on factors that affect the ability of the person to deal with life tasks. Social workers can alleviate distress, enhance personal ability to solve problems and cope, and help people realize hopes and goals. They conduct individual and group counseling and also provide links with systems (insurance companies and government agencies, for example) and resources (perhaps funding for equipment or securing attendant care) for ongoing concerns.

The Rehabilitation Psychologist

Psychologists take on the primary roles of therapists, counselors, behavior analysts, evaluators of the psychological strengths and assets of individuals with SCI, and researchers into the rehabilitation process. In addition, psychologists act as behavior consultants to interdisciplinary staff, provide education regarding psychosocial needs, and develop individual treatment plans.

Psychologists emphasize that rehabilitation is a learning process. The difficulty in coping with the everyday stress of learning to adjust to such a traumatic injury requires support and feedback. Psychologists are trained in principles of behavior, with a strong emphasis on the process of learning and adjustment. Psychologists thus can maximize benefits from the learning opportunities offered within a rehabilitation setting.

The Peer Counselor/Consultant

The disabled person living and coping well in the community is one of the most valuable, but frequently underused, resources that health care professionals have. Today, peer counseling and/or peer role modeling programs are increasingly integral parts of rehabilitation programs. Innovative facilities are inviting disabled people not only to serve as positive role models for individuals and families but also to serve as resource persons to team members. These persons encourage the growth of sensitive and helpful professional attitudes. See Chapter 30.

The Nurse: The Nature of Nursing and Significance of Attitudes

The very nature of nursing presents some unique difficulties that are not always given the thoughtful consideration or recognition they deserve, either by nurses or other members of an interdisciplinary team. The basic essentials of eating, bathing, getting up in the morning, and going to bed at night take place in the ward setting as they do in the home. The ward environment also provides opportunities to establish acceptable behavioral patterns and social skills. Finally, the ward is the place where patients return when they become too fatigued, too upset, or too "something" to function elsewhere in the therapeutic environment (Gunther 1980). Thus, the nursing service provides a combination of home base, school or workplace, and retreat from overwhelming feelings and activities of the day. For these reasons, patients often direct their feelings of hostility, frustration, and exhaustion toward nurses. Nurses may also be perceived as parentlike figures who monitor, control, reward, and punish.

Furthermore, nursing functions frequently involve exposing the patient for bathing and handling of intimate areas of the body for bladder and bowel procedures. The nature of these activities tends to heighten the patient's feelings of embarrassment, helplessness, dependence, and asexuality. Even self-care for these procedures tends to create rather than relieve frustration because it involves fine motor activity.

Nurses thus need specific preparation and ongoing support to deal with this turmoil. This is particularly true of the large numbers of nursing assistants, such as practical nurses, aides, and orderlies, who spend a great deal of time engaged in direct patient care and yet are not trained in behavioral sciences. Staff engaged in direct daily care are of paramount importance to the disabled person's socialization process. Therefore, so are their values and attitudes. As studies by Leinart (1979) and Sadlick and Penta (1975) point out, a positive attitude toward the rehabilitation outcome is essential to the success of the process.

Lack of positive feelings can and do block communication, and patients can begin to perceive themselves as helpless and less worthwhile. In addition, overly sympathetic attitudes can easily communicate feelings of helplessness to the patient and family. To overcome these feelings it is important to understand the human potential for adjustment to disability—an understanding appreciated on an emotional rather than an intellectual level. Unfortunately, health care professionals often fail to recognize the importance of this fundamental concept.

The Psychiatric Clinical Nurse Specialist

The psychiatric clinical nurse specialist represents an expanded role in professional nursing practice based on scientific theories of human behavior. Holistic nursing requires that psychiatric clinicians promote an understanding of the importance of sociocultural, interpersonal, and psychological factors as they help individuals, families and systems cope with SCI. Psychiatric nurse specialists function as consultants, clinicians, therapists, and educators to promote, maintain, or restore physical and mental health, prevent illness, and affect rehabilitation. These roles evolve naturally because of the many nurses and interdisciplinary staff who provide direct patient care in nonpsychiatric settings and require assistance in meeting the psychological challenges of patients and their families.

The psychiatric clinical nurse specialist can provide individual, group, or family therapy to selected patients; assist nursing staff in assessing, planning, implementing, and evaluating a plan of care to help meet the psychosocial needs of patients; participate as a member of the interdisciplinary team; and identify learning needs of staff, patients, and/or families, implementing formal as well as informal educational programs that explore the psychological responses to acute and chronic illness.

Psychosocial and Educational Implications for the Team

The impact of catastrophic injuries on the entire health care team can never be underestimated. All staff members must examine their beliefs about the quality of life remaining for the physically disabled person, and their role in it.

Because of the nature of accidents causing SCI and the physical demands of care, staff and patients are often in the same young-adult age range. The closer in age and life circumstances the staff member is to the patient, the closer and more threatening the identification. Staff beginning to care for patients with SCI may especially need the support of more experienced staff. Many of them must work through somewhat the same psychological processes as patients and families. It is important for them to verbalize feelings of *identification*, anger, and depression appropriately if they are to have the psychic energy to help others. Tucker (1980) warns that staff who care for people with SCI tend to be more chronically affected and troubled by their experiences than professionals who work with less severely compromised patients.

Thus, a total support program for staff should include psychosocial education and provide avenues for sharing ongoing concerns, frustrations, suggestions for change, and new methods of intervention. The task of putting all the pieces together to create a therapeutic milieu is an ongoing process. See Chapter 12.

Conflicts within the team can lead to each discipline feeling poorly understood, ineffectual, and frustrated. If, for example, counseling professionals cannot convey a feeling of empathy for nurses, who may be faced with outrageous behavioral situations, nurses feel unsupported and isolated. By the same token, if nurses become so emotionally entangled in the situation that they lose professional objectivity, *they lose the ability to be therapeutic with their patients.*

Each member of the interdisciplinary team possesses a unique personality, a specialized body of skills and knowledge, and a variety of professional assets and expectations. To develop a truly skilled interdisciplinary team, it is necessary to create a warm and respectful atmosphere in which the significance, expectations and limitations of each team member's role are recognized and understood, *and open communication is encouraged.* See Chapter 13.

Preparation and ongoing education is a multifaceted issue. A comprehensive orientation, ideally including direct participation from all disciplines, can ease team mem-

bers into the intricate care needed by the catastrophically injured and help develop harmonious interdisciplinary relationships. Veteran staff members also require support and educational opportunities to avert the problems of burnout. Educational activities and moral support can best be built around ongoing, informal meetings of small groups to discuss problems with self, patients, families, and fellow staff members (Gunther 1980). These groups are best led by an accepted member of the staff, who is aware of both the rehabilitative and the psychological implications of staff problems. The most beneficial techniques include eliciting feedback from more experienced staff members, facilitating peer support, and sharing of suggestions or coping techniques other staff members use (Roglitz 1978).

The pressures of this work demand a strong, supportive structure and personal stability and maturity. These circumstances require a strong working collaboration with professionals trained in the behavioral sciences and recognition that staff must support each other and often need help with their feelings. Interdisciplinary leaders must recognize staff needs and learn how to deal with them, seeking appropriate help when necessary.

FACTORS THAT AFFECT PSYCHOSOCIAL RESPONSES TO SPINAL CORD INJURY

Patient Concerns

SCI affects all aspects of an individual's life. It instantly imposes an overwhelming complex of losses: of mobility, control, independence, and wholeness (Weller and Miller 1977a). The person must face the loss of life as it was and find new ways to live. There may also be a temporary loss of future life expectations, such as marriage, parenthood, employment or career, and one's general place in the community. In addition, many patients are separated from families and loved ones when they are transported to and rehabilitated in a major center. Concerns about their families' reaction to disability, their ability to cope at home, sexuality, and economic pressures are also a burden. Generally, patients experiencing higher levels of life stress before injury have greater difficulty adjusting after injury, regardless of age (Frank and Elliot 1987; Frank et al. 1988). Most people find themselves reevaluating their lives in terms of how injury affects their future. Some thoughts and concerns (Virginia Spinal Cord Injury System 1988: 8) include:

- Am I a valuable person?
- Am I sexually attractive?
- Can I be a parent and/or can I be a good parent?

- Am I a burden to my family?
- Will my old friends accept me?
- Will I be able to make new friends?
- Will I be able to support myself or my family?
- Would it be better if I had died?
- Will I be able physically to protect myself and my family?
- What will I do if I have a bowel or bladder accident in public?
- Will I ever be able to work again?
- Can I enjoy life again?

Family Concerns

Family concerns closely reflect those of the patient. Initially families are concerned about the patient's survival, relief from pain, and adequate medical care. Adaptive changes required of families are in many ways equal in magnitude to the changes required of the patient. Families are often encouraged to participate in rehabilitation plans that do not take their own developmental needs into account (Steinglass 1982). They are deeply aware of shattered dreams or life expectations for a spouse, son or daughter, or other relative. Reactions to this loss include anger, disbelief, helplessness, and guilt. Overprotectiveness is a common reaction (Weller and Miller 1977b: 370). Some questions families may ask include:

- Will they live?
- Will they be crippled for life?
- Why did this happen to us?
- What can we do to help?
- How will they ever manage their lives?
- Will they always be depressed?
- Can they have sex again?
- How can we look after them at home?
- How will our friends react?
- Can they get a job?
- Will there be enough money?
- How can we protect them?
- How will we cope?

An effective family is a system of complex, mutually interdependent relationships. Inherent within the family are duties and responsibilities that are essential for its functioning, and constituting role behaviors that allow the family system to endure. When the family is thought of as a *system*, it may be described in terms of how close or distant members are from each other (Freeman and Trute 1981). Disability not only affects the injured member but also impacts the whole family. Family systems have an internal balance that tends to resist change: families that are more rigid in interactional style resist change more than families that are more flexible. Dysfunctional families may attempt to adapt by resisting acknowledgment of the disability, thereby retaining homeostasis (balance). These families usually see the patient as "the problem"; or the patient has the problems and the family has none. Staff must realize that the whole family is the client.

The rehabilitation team must also note family dynamics. Too often health professionals think of the family as a reliable support structure, somewhat like another health professional, without realizing the full impact of disability on the family system (Williams and Kay 1990). Even the strongest families can become exhausted during the process of rehabilitation. Coping with a disabled family member may create a number of internal problems: altered or even reversed roles (for example, the homemaker who must become the breadwinner); altered financial status; added responsibility for physical care tasks, especially bowel and bladder management, which may be awkward or even repulsive for both patient and family; and numerous other practical difficulties, such as caring for the children or the elderly within the home. Children of the disabled person seem to get lost in the shuffle, often without recognition or access to the support system they so badly need. Thus, skilled history taking, interviewing, and sensitivity in daily interpersonal interactions are essential to assess current patient and family strengths, resources, needs, and problems (Steinglass 1982).

Self-Concept and Self-Esteem

Self-concept is a combination of feelings and beliefs that people hold in regard to themselves. Both the physical and the personal are included in self-concept. Self-esteem is one's feeling of personal value or worth (Kozier and Erb 1990). Self-esteem is largely developed on feedback from others in our lives. The way in which we deal with feelings and expressions of anger and aggression, in particular, stems from the limitations imposed by others during our upbringing. Without such limitations we cannot learn the consequences of various behaviors and as adults may have difficulty setting limits or controlling our behavior.

Psychosocial development is a natural part of the maturational process. In past decades the original work of psychologists such as Erikson and Maslow stressed the ability to learn and to grow psychologically through life. Learning is a continual process that enables adaptation to new roles in life: intimate partner, parent, or leader, for example. Psychological growth also permits adaptation to crises such as injury leading to disability.

The way people feel about themselves affects the way in which they deal with their environment. People with high self-esteem deal more actively with their environment and feel secure. People with low self-esteem view the environment as negative and threatening (Roy 1976: 233).

Some common manifestations of low self-esteem include (Roy 1976: 236–237):

- Expressions of self-depreciation or self-dislike
- Sensitivity to criticism; self-consciousness
- Anorexia or overeating
- Tendency to be a listener rather than a participant
- Difficulty sleeping or oversleeping
- Withdrawal from activities
- Decreased motivation, interest, and concentration
- Seeing self as burden to others

These reactions involve withdrawal, but counteractive aggressive, verbose, overvaluing behavior is also common with problems of self-esteem.

Through assessment of a patient's self-concept, it is possible to predict potential problems the patient will have in reacting to and coping with SCI. Moreover, the health care team can promote the patient's adaptation to disability by capitalizing on strengths of self-concept and self-esteem.

In the aftermath of SCI, both patients and families are subject to a magnitude of psychosocial influences during and after the rehabilitation period. Strong psychosocial support from a variety of sources is essential to enhance all other aspects of the rehabilitation program and prepare for discharge (Figure 9–1).

Helplessness

Patients may feel powerless if they fail to realize the connection between behavior and control of environment. Initially patients are generally aroused by this threat to their freedom, but some patients gradually stop trying when they feel complete loss of control (Trieschmann 1980: 61). The person may then become apathetic, anxious, and depressed. The theory of *learned helplessness* states that uncontrollable failure leads to depression and feelings of helplessness, while self-controlled success fosters feelings of competence and industriousness.

Although not generally diagnosed as having a learned helplessness syndrome by rehabilitation counsellors, many spinal cord injured patients seem to demonstrate a learned helplessness response to their paralysis. Often these emotions, natural reactions to the initial trauma and early recovery period following spinal cord injury, become ingrained and, as with learned helplessness effects among other patient populations, they begin to influence the spinal cord patient's general life orientation. [Wool et al. 1980: 321]

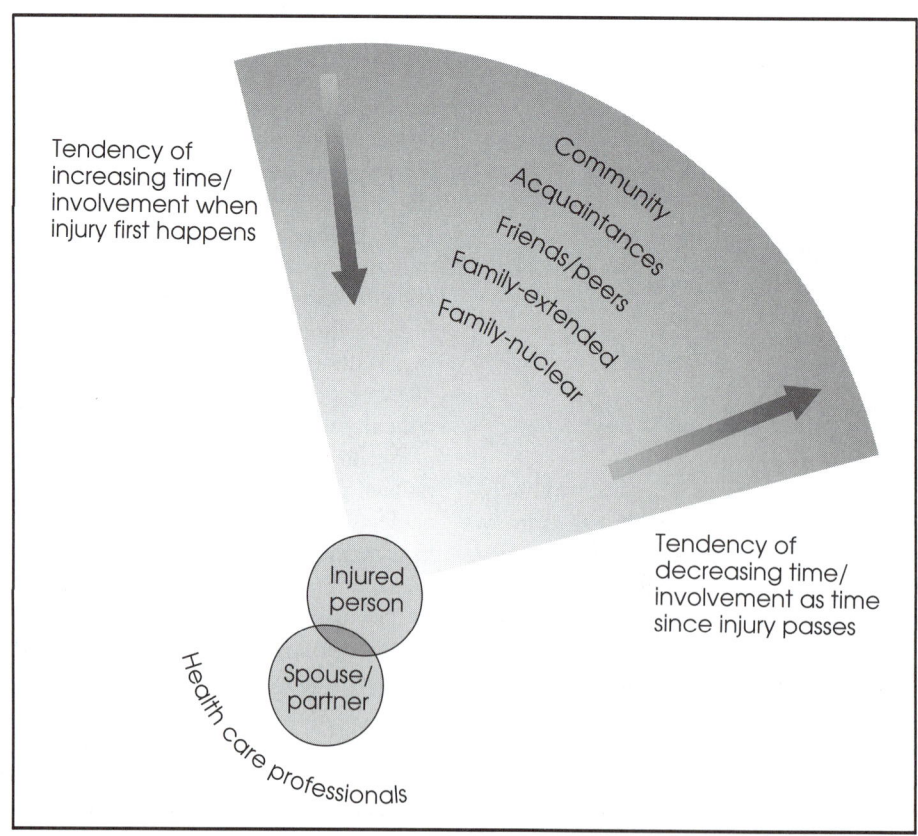

FIGURE 9–1 Circles of support and involvement for the person with a spinal cord injury. (Courtesy of Penny Hicks, M.S.W., G. F. Strong Rehabilitation Centre, Vancouver, BC)

Age and Developmental Stage

Age and developmental stage at onset of disability is an important factor affecting psychological adjustment. Individuals born with a disability, or who acquire one early in life, learn behavioral patterns appropriate to their degree of impairment while growing up; there is essentially no interruption or lack of congruence between old behaviors and new. Disabilities acquired later in life generally have a sudden onset, which precipitates a basic incongruence between old and expected new behaviors and initial difficulty in performing the new and different behaviors.

Young adults, for example, strive to separate from their families and to demonstrate to the community and themselves that they are socially and physically acceptable as adults. Developmental tasks for this maturational period can include establishing a home, getting started in a career, marrying and starting a family, and finding a congenial social group. The young adult with SCI is faced not only with achieving physical independence, but also with finding alternate ways to achieve appropriate maturational goals. The nature of the goals that have been interrupted and the extent to which the individual is able to set new goals that are congruent with an altered reality are important factors to consider in the rehabilitation process. The degree of flexibility in previous patterns of coping with stress influences the ability to set alternative roles. Older people frequently find this very difficult.

Acquisition of New Roles

Rehabilitation is a process of socialization during which people with SCI learn new roles. The extent to which disabled individuals successfully perform their roles may reflect the degree to which they are able to adapt to their disability.

Thomas (1966) describes characteristic roles for disabled people. The first of these, the "disabled patient role," is characterized by sick-role expectations extended and made enduring. The "helped person role" involves being on the receiving end of helping acts and adaptation to being an object of aid. The "disability co-manager role" is a role characterized by active participation of the disabled person in decisions attending impairment and rehabilitation. Finally, the "role of the public relations person" places a burden of explanation and interpretation of impairment on the disabled person. Learning these new roles is viewed as a resocialization process whereby new behaviors are learned and other behaviors no longer possible or appropriate are unlearned.

Adaptation to disability is an important intervening variable influencing role performance of the disabled person. The essence of acquiring these new behaviors is to enhance normal interactions with others. When disabled people feel comfortable with themselves they will communicate the feeling to others. In turn, when others feel more at ease, they will respond with more valid or normal behaviors.

Physical disability can be a stigma, particularly when as highly visible as SCI. In the sheltered social environment of the hospital, patients are somewhat protected, but in the world outside the hospital, the social stigma becomes readily apparent. Although the situation is improving, a disabled person can still be devalued in our society. To become successfully rehabilitated, people with SCI must learn the social skills necessary to project positive feelings of self-worth to reduce stigmatizing effects (MacLean 1981).

Physical Health and Functional Ability

Psychological health cannot be considered in isolation from physical health, mobility, and independence. In general, if physical health is poor or if methods to control body functions are unreliable, ability to deal with psychological adjustments is lowered. Therefore, throughout the rehabilitation period, physical needs must be assessed and managed carefully. *Never* underestimate how irritable or depressed a patient can be if suffering from chills, fever, nausea, pain, or spasticity.

A person's functional ability (level of injury) does *not* appear to be a significant factor in adapting to disability. People with quadriplegia seem just as capable as those with paraplegia in achieving psychological equilibrium (Orbaan 1986).

PSYCHOSOCIAL RESPONSES TO SPINAL CORD INJURY*

Impaired Conscious State

Following SCI, most people are initially aware of the trauma, loss of feeling and movement, and a rising anxiety. Then a variable period ensues in which they are unaware of what occurs around them. Even though individuals may be fully awake and responsive to questions and discussion (as described in Chapter 6), psychological defenses take over to protect them from too rapid a perception of the catastrophic disability.

Reverting to forms of behavior, feelings, or ways of thinking characteristic of an earlier stage of life is a coping mechanism that helps the injured person avoid inner feelings as well as external reality. Regression may take many

*This section was developed with the assistance of Lester Butt, Ph.D.

forms and in a moderate degree represents an understandable and useful adaptation to SCI. However, becoming self-centered, emphasizing physical sensations and symptoms, and relying extensively on staff and family for every need can frequently generate unrealistic expectations.

Understandably, patients may feel threatened by increased dependency and uncertain futures, or may lack a sense of trust in those who care for them, and thus need to exert their autonomy. Complaining or demanding behavior may be a way to exert control over personal environment. *Sensory deprivation*, which may develop immediatly in the complex, critical care environment (Chapter 6) or any time thereafter, may be severe and is also a contributing factor. Anger, and the frustration over the inability to communicate, particularly for the ventilator-dependent patient with a tracheostomy, frequently give way to intense anxiety that, if unchecked, can lead to panic.

Characteristic features of sensory deprivation include anxiety, tension, inability to concentrate and organize one's thoughts, depression, depersonalization, and perceptual distortion. In severe cases delusions and hallucinations may occur. The combination of factors such as sensory monotony of routines, sensory overload, sleep deprivation, pain, altered sensory input from the body, and restriction of movement and isolation in the hospital or house setting profoundly affect behavior and emotional responses.

Robert, a person with high quadraplegia, enjoyed a successful and active life before SCI. He vividly described his fear and terror after he had been routinely turned one night and the nursing assistants forgot to return his environmental control sip-and-puff straw. He had a tracheostomy and was frightened that if something happened to him he could not get help. His fear turned to panic and resulted in delusions and hallucinations. This person continued to have anxiety attacks, particularly at night, for the rest of his life.

Florence Stroebel-Kahn describes a difficult night when she thought the flowers on the overbed table were flowers on an altar at a funeral. She was lucky to be cared for by a nurse who responded to her distorted perception of reality. The nurse moved the bed as the patient asked her to and also called her mother, at the patient's request, who came to the hospital during the middle of the night and provided security, making the unbearable become bearable. The patient was able to drift into sleep (Aadalen and Stroebel-Kahn 1981).

Supportive psychological intervention is generally the most effective treatment and less dangerous than drug treatment. Most important is staff awareness of the terror the patient experiences when disoriented. Such awareness may soften staff annoyance and frustration when the patient asks redundant questions, becomes loud and anxious, or responds to hallucinations.

Appropriate interventions include giving patients factual information regarding equipment and procedures, repetition of information in a calm and reassuring manner, encouraging patients to discuss their feelings, and devising a system for the ventilator-dependent tracheostomy patient to communicate. Sleep should be given priority not only in the critically ill but also in all patients. It is a restorative process, and sleep deprivation not only impedes recovery but can alter mental status.

Changes in Body Image

A change in body image is an important psychosocial factor in response to SCI. Body image, an aspect of one's self-image, can be defined as the psychological experience of one's body. It is influenced by all the conscious and unconscious feelings and perceptions about one's body, including attitudes about its parts and functioning. The literature relating body image to SCI is limited but tends to focus on distortions of body perception and the relationship of body image to the adjustment process.

It is based not only on appearance, but on how one perceives intelligence, sexuality, physical strength, endurance, values, beliefs, and personal goals. Feedback from other people also plays an important role in determining the sense of self. Cultural and societal values additionally influence a person's body image. For instance, western societies value youth, beauty, and wholeness. Individual, family, and societal perceptions, values, and beliefs about people with disabilities are typically negative, create difficult barriers to overcome, and profoundly influence personal adjustment. Injured people may thus have difficulty accepting a changed body image.

The stress generated by SCI may precipitate any number of compensatory and self-protective behaviors in response to a threatened body image—anger and hostility; rebelliousness, such as refusing care or refusing to get up; refusal to socialize (fearing rejection, the person shuns others including family and friends); depersonalization; avoiding or disowning altered body parts; and refusal to participate in activities. While providing physical care, staff should deal with altered body image by talking about SCI in a gentle, straightforward manner. By identifying and reinforcing positive coping skills, acceptance of a changed body image becomes possible.

Theories of Adaptation

In addition to the medical situation, individuals with SCI experience psychological stresses fraught with acute anxieties. When faced with sudden disability, patients must absorb the traumatic effect of injury, physical shock, hospitalization, severe motor and sensory loss, and changes in body image and self-identity. They experience interactional changes within both their families and the community.

PERSONAL VIEWPOINT

Flo Kahn has a B.A. in Education, a B.S. in Nursing, and completed graduate work in pediatric nursing. In 1973, her life changed dramatically as the result of a car accident that left her with quadriplegia. The catastrophe not only cost her physical mobility; she lost her unborn child, a successful semiprofessional singing career, and later her husband through divorce. Flo's will to live and personal strength eventually brought her to Courage Center Residence, where she received rehabilitation and personal counseling. Today, she shares her apartment with her attendant and has a part-time teaching job in rehabilitation nursing, speaking engagements, and many challenging volunteer activities. In her free time she enjoys nature study, classical music, painting, and reading current novels and inspirational books.

Recently I gave an attitude awareness session to the staff of a rehabilitation facility. The title was: "Talk to me, not my disability." When I am out in the community, I find that people often look at my wheelchair, not me. They are uncomfortable. This session, therefore, explored the reasons for discomfort and the stereotypical attitudes that prevent people from connecting with the individual who happens to live with a disability.

My journey of adapting to the many changes SCI caused was not on any map, but in looking back at my journey thus far, I can see many bridges that nurses provided. As part of the rehabilitation team, nurses help people redefine themselves and learn about their disabilities so they can live full, healthy, balanced lives and not let society's messages devalue them. When I broke my neck, I became physically paralyzed; but I also became paralyzed as a whole person. The nurses I remember, helped at different times in different ways, caring for one part of me or all of me depending on the situation.

The journey to adjustment is not orderly, and the bridges that prepared me to live in society again were not built just before discharge. They were begun right away!

The first bridge occurred even before they met me. What expectations did they have for me? I think that professional staff can be most effective when they realize the journey to living with a disability happens one step at a time. The staff wanted me to move through rehabilitation and achieve goals, but I was the one

directing the pace of the journey. Sometimes I stood still, but other times I was "dancing" there were so many steps. One physiatrist told me, "Flo, give yourself 6 years." At the time, I had no idea what he meant! I know now, as I think of all the people and experiences I needed to achieve balance again.

The biggest obstacles to accepting being disabled were my attitudes toward people with disabilities. Attitudes hindered me; can inner attitudes hinder other nurses' expectations of a return to a full, meaningful, creative life? Nurses saw me at the toughest times in my journey and their inner attitudes can show through any action.

The second bridge was "talking to me." This began with the attitude each nurse projected: "Wherever you are, however you are, you are of value and I respect you!" During the first scary months when I needed continuous care, I would see that familiar nurse's face through my fog of anxiety and would relax. At times of intense physical crises, nurses still talked to me, listened to strange requests from nightmares, and told me what was happening. By involving me in my own care, they tapped into my inner strengths and faith to help me survive. When I was busy in rehabilitation activities or struggling at home, I was also slowly realizing all the physical functions, abilities, roles, and activities I had lost: finger movement, balance, walking, cooking, knitting, biking with my husband, rocking a sick child, on and on. Nurses "talked to me" by knowing how important this painful discovery process was. They didn't try to fix me, but acknowledged the internal sadness and fatigue without magic words of comfort. They were beside me in my pain. One nurse sat beside me and massaged my hands with lotion. Another would talk with me about my former hobbies, college, family, my day at O.T., or tell me crazy jokes.

I was in the process of grieving over all I had lost, but I didn't realize it! I would tell everyone, "I'm just fine," but I wasn't; I was depressed. Finally, at a transitional facility, I was ready for grief counseling and had a safe environment where I could begin to talk, cry, process all that was lost, and find the many valuable parts of me that remained. I regained my balance and was stretched psychologically and spiritually.

The nurses who cared about my emotions and spirit during those tough times were so helpful. One nurse gave me such joy one day when she placed two poodle

(Box continues)

PERSONAL VIEWPOINT (continued)

puppies on my chest! I have to say that this bridge was the most important to me as I struggled to find and redefine "Flo" with a disability and move forward as a valuable person living a meaningful life.

One other bridge was that of helping me learn about and live with my body, my disability. During the early weeks when I was numb with shock, nurses took excellent care of me physically so that I didn't go home with skin problems, and so on. Slowly, I began to learn to take responsibility for my new disabled body. I could not live in the community if I hadn't been taught. At first, I didn't want anything to do with the changes, especially bowel and bladder care. But after some crises, I began to hear what the nurses were telling me and pay attention. I remember asking, "Why am I sweating?" and not understanding anything about autonomic dysreflexia, but the nurse patiently explained

again. I was taught through classes and one-to-one teaching, but it took me years to understand my body systems—its weird signals and how to solve each problem situation—and I'm a nurse! I would follow the established regimes and procedures and then, as I experienced problems, change them to fit my body and life-style. Ultimately, however, I am the bridge. It is my personality, strengths, weaknesses, faith, and abilities that carry me through the piece-by-piece discovery of re-forming ME so I can live WITH SCI. Yet I didn't do it alone, and nurses were some of my most important bridge supports so that I could strive for rehabilitation goals with honest expectations.

Florence Stroebel-Kahn, R.N., B.S.N., B. Ed.
Minneapolis, MN

How can they deal with these changes? Much of the literature attempts to answer this question within the realm of mastering adaptation and coping techniques.

The most widely known, but now questionable, theories of how people adapt are the so-called stage theories that compare the reactions of persons facing disability to those facing death. However, death is a final stage, but living with a disability is not. Similarities include psychological transit through phases of shock, denial, depression, and adaptation. From the initial impact of SCI (psychological shock), through the defensive reaction of denial, individuals progress to eventual accommodation to injury. Although beneficial in the sense that these theories attempt to bring order and understanding to psychological chaos, the clinical difficulties lie in rigid application to people with SCI (Trieschmann 1980).

In a unique variant of the stage theorists, Vash (1981) proposed a model that involves the following three stages:

- *Recognition of the facts*, wherein the individual acknowledges the extent and implications of the disability, but disdains it
- *Acceptance of the implications*, when the changes caused by the disability are integrated into the lifestyle and viewed as an inconvenience
- *Embracing of the experience*, wherein disability is viewed, along with all other life experiences, as an opportunity for learning that is positively valued

Shontz (1975) views severe physical disability as a crisis, and adjustment to crisis as *a succession of approach-avoidance cycles*. In the early stages, cycles recur rapidly with high levels of emotional intensity. Later the cycles become less frequent, less intense, and gradually fade out. Shontz be-

lieves it is essential to go through the sequence of two phases: the impact phase (shock and encounter) and the postimpact phase (retreat and acknowledgment). Shock is described as a depersonalized emergency reaction; the characteristics of encounter are panic, disorganization, and helplessness as shock wears off. Because encounter is too intense the stage of retreat begins. Denial and isolation can be forms of retreat. Acknowledgment is the final stage in adaptation and consists of cycles of approach and avoidance. This cyclical approach denotes a dynamic and lengthy adaptation process through which patients must encounter and be forced to face different crises. Consequently they are permitted to get a feeling of themselves in new terms at their own pace.

Thompson and Lott (1980) relate the sequences of psychosocial events following SCI injury to the descriptions of Erikson's life span development stages. The most relevant concept is that people must continually *reprocess* past stages to deal with ordinary life development.

> Think of the severity, the intensity, the psychosocial trauma that is present when a person starts to reprocess these stages after intense body changes brought about by spinal cord injury. . . . To regain the balance in a positive direction means a redevelopment of trust, autonomy, initiative, industry, and identity, versus mistrust, shame, guilt, inferiority, and diffusion. [Thompson and Lott 1980: 43]

Hohmann (1975) postulates that a person experiences a number of feelings and attitudes similar to those that may be experienced with any severe loss—in other words "normal reactions to an abnormal situation." The first reaction is denial, which, when relinquished, allows depression to set in. The depressive phase may be characterized by withdrawal and internalized hostility, which is then externalized. After these reactions have been worked through, there will usually be a reconstitution of the person's preinjury personality. The stages of grieving are likened to phases of adjustment to disability and are often described as feelings of shock, denial, anger, depression, and finally adjustment. These feelings may also be thought of as periods of disorganization, reorganization, and resolution. However, the most striking observation is the variability of each individual's response.

Until recently, it was assumed that the inevitable psychological consequence to loss is depression. As a result, most professionals believe that depression is expected following SCI and tend to overestimate its occurrence (Ernst 1987). In the traditional vision of loss, secondary depression follows. In other words, the patient is either clinically depressed or is still in a state of denial. The most sophisticated studies to date are those of Lawson (1976) and more recently Wortman and Silver (1989) whose conclusions ran counter to traditional clinical inferences in that persons who manifest less depressive affect or loss during the course of rehabilitation had more successful outcomes.

Instead of overconcern about the failure to become depressed or the apparent denial of the implications of disability (which might actually be coping mechanisms or signs of resilience), focus on patient and family strengths, coping resources, and sources of support. Concentrate on minimizing the factors that induce stress (including the misconceptions imposed by staff as to what those factors are).

Additional research suggests that repression may be the way to a cure (Associated Press 1989). Holocaust survivors who do well have often successfully sealed away their traumas. Instead of dwelling on the trauma, they concentrate on the here and now, which may be the best healer. This may apply to treatment of posttraumatic stress syndrome accompanying SCI.

The outcome of SCI, either in terms of adaptation or maladaptation, is multifaceted. Outcome depends on:

- *Background/personality factors*, including age, intellectual capacity, philosophical and religious beliefs, emotional level, family structure, previous losses and coping abilities, academic background, quality of interpersonal relationships, and the symbolic and connotative meanings of SCI
- *Illness-related factors*, including type and location of the course of the trauma and potential complications, and coping abilities as influenced by physiological factors, immobility, and medications that may cause general disorientation and cloud thought processes for weeks
- *Physical/social environment*, including both the degree of afforded privacy and stimulation as well as the general ambiance of the treating institution.

As a result, it is impossible to speak of a predictable, uniform psychological course when discussing adjustment and accommodation to this kind of injury.

A Crisis Response to Stress

All individuals attempt to achieve a state of physical, social, and psychological equilibrium. Toward this end people use a variety of tactics to reduce stress and resolve problems. People usually can contend with daily life and can tolerate a reasonable level of frustration, resolve problems, and discharge accumulated tension. However, some situations can present difficulties that defy resolution. This constitutes a *crisis*—an emergency plus a sense of incapacity. If crisis is successfully managed it can improve the ability to cope; however, if it is not well managed, a crisis can reinforce maladaptive patterns. Crises thus have growth-promoting potential. An individual in crisis is searching for a solution in an attempt to regain balance. Again, this balance can represent a healthy adaptation that promotes growth or a maladaptive response that signifies psychological deterioration and decline.

Crisis theory is based on understanding *stress* (Hoff 1989). The word *stress* means different things to different people. Pain, fear, effort, fatigue, or even unexpected success can produce stress. The stress-producing factors, called *stressors*, are different, yet they elicit essentially the same biological stress response. Stress is the nonspecific response of the body to any demand made on it. Psychologically, reactions may cause individuals to feel disoriented, disorganized, angry, depressed, frustrated, helpless, apathetic, afraid, irritable, withdrawn, or unable to concentrate. If these symptoms are not dealt with they can lead to physical disorders such as ulcers, myocardial infarctions, and various emotional disorders such as depression, addiction, or psychosis. The fact that the same stressor can cause different responses in different individuals is the result of conditioning factors that can selectively enhance or inhibit one or the other stress effect. Conditioning may be internal, such as age, sex, genetic predispostion, or past experiences, or it can be external such as treatment with drugs or therapies. Stress inevitably evokes behavior, which may be an effort to deal with the threat (fight) or avoid facing up to the threat (flight). Individuals with SCI are confronted with an overwhelming array of problems that severely test their resources. Every aspect of daily living presents a challenge. The potential for crisis is therefore great.

Developing Coping Techniques

Adaptation to disability is highly individualized. It seldom progresses smoothly from beginning to end but is more like a series of encounters and reencounters with any number of events or setbacks that occur over time. This significant observation suggests that problems have to be faced again and again in different situations and with different degrees of intensity, rather than "worked through" once and for all. Chapter 12 discusses how people with SCI learn to cope.

It is unrealistic to expect that individuals with SCI must accept their disability and not at times feel frustrated, angry, and depressed by their condition. Nondisabled individuals experience similar feelings in dealing with the hassles of everyday living.

It is important to realize that although the rehabilitation process has a beginning and an end, the process of adaptation to disability may not. However, as most disabled people attest, it is possible to adapt to or cope with the effects of SCI. As one person with respiratory quadriplegia explains,

> I still get depressed but manage to keep it within working bounds. Personally, I believe that a disabled person never really accepts being the way they are. After all, every day you are working against nature. We are not meant to be like this. However, I know that with maturity and understanding one can work around it and live a constructive, meaningful life.

Given adequate psychological support and a healthy rehabilitation environment that sets the expectancy of living a meaningful, productive, and gratifying life, it is realistic to expect that most people will lead satisfying lives in the community or at least will cope adequately (Hohmann 1975). However, without appropriate interventions, some people do become overwhelmed by feelings of inadequacy and helplessness and will likely develop a lifetime pattern of maladaptive coping mechanisms.

A PROCESS TO PROMOTE PSYCHOSOCIAL ADAPTATION

Assessment

Psychosocial assessment of the patient and family encompasses two major components: comprehensive history taking and continuous observation of psychosocial strengths, weaknesses, and progress.

A Preinjury Profile
Understanding the patient's and family's background provides a basis on which to plan and offer psychosocial support. The patient is the same person after SCI as before. Therefore, if patient and family were harmonious, industrious, and satisfied before the disability, they are likely to resume that pattern. If there were major difficulties, however, the disability is likely to make the situation worse.

Counseling professionals make an in-depth assessment of the patient's preinjury personality and family support structures. They assess the strengths and resources of both patient and family and interpret them to the interdisciplinary team. Values and belief systems, religion, cultural influences, position or role in the family, interpersonal relationships, recent losses or difficulties, interests, educational and vocational background, and socioeconomic status must all be assessed with insight and expertise.

All patients experience varying degrees of stress in dealing with the effects of SCI. However, if preexisting psychosocial problems—chronic drug and alcohol abuse; recognized psychiatric illness; criminal behavior; or severe, unresolved family disruption—exist, the ability to adapt to permanent and dramatic changes in life-style is compounded. Extreme depression, suicide attempts (sometimes the cause of SCI), or a history of psychiatric illness are signs of the need for immediate psychiatric referral.

Continuous Psychosocial Assessment
Adaptation to a loss such as that incurred as a result of SCI occurs over time. The time interval since injury is a significant factor in the adjustment process to disability, particularly with regard to patients' ability to solve problems, to make decisions about their care, and to set realistic goals for themselves (MacLean 1981).

Psychosocial assessment is thus a continual, ongoing process. The emotional or psychological profiles of patients and families are gradually clarified for the staff during the weeks of hospitalization. Therefore, sensitivity in daily interpersonal interactions is essential to assess current strengths and progress, problems and needs. Listen, and get to know the perceptions and expectations of the disability and deal with the patients' concerns early (Richmond and Metcalf 1986).

Good assessment is actually good intervention because empathetic, attentive listening is therapeutic.

> It is important to recognize and respond to patients' and families' need for communication and to capitalize on a warm, trusting relationship with them to encourage expression of feelings and concerns. People feel good when they are listened to and their integrity as human beings is confirmed. This ultimately increases satisfaction with the care provided and cooperation with the recommended program of treatment. [Szasz 1980: 8]

Goal Setting

People with SCI comprise a truly heterogeneous population whose personalities and adjustment capabilities vary widely. However, factors that seem to aid in adjustment are youth, emotional maturity, good self-esteem, intact family supports, higher levels of education, and financial and job security. People whose work and leisure activities are more physical might find the onset of SCI more disruptive than people who are less physically inclined (Trieschmann 1980).

Many people with SCI are young, emotionally immature, and usually at an age when confusion about identity and developing intimate relationships can threaten and lower self-esteem and confidence. Young people are also at a crossroad where they must make the choice between employment and further education and are at a peak of physical prowess, which tends to outweigh intellectual interest (Weller and Miller 1977a). This crucial juncture in the lives of individuals who are severely injured obviously has a profound impact on their reaction to disability and to their ability to plan for their future. The problems of this group are compounded by all the ramifications of a society rapidly departing from traditional values about morality, work, family life, and spiritual beliefs, many of which seem to help people adjust to disability. Moreover, because of their developmental stage and difficulties controlling impulsive, verbally explosive behaviors, younger patients often require more support and assistance in setting limits on a day-to-day basis. Fortunately, most younger disabled individuals have a greater capacity to adjust and adapt to new situations than older individuals. Those who seem so difficult during rehabilitation may do very well in the long run.

Planning and implementing goal-oriented care during rehabilitation must lead the patient and family to take responsibility for managing the effects of disability and maintaining optimal physical and psychological health. Interdisciplinary staff must collaborate with the patient and family to devise concrete and attainable goals that are related to assessment data. For example, coping with the effects of disability requires consistent and positive behavioral changes. When an individual's background is unstable and strong support systems are not available, behavioral changes, though not impossible, are slow and difficult to achieve. Unrealistic expectations are both harmful and frustrating to patients, families, and staff members. Realistic goal setting must not be equated or confused with reducing standards of care. While patient input and involvement in determining goals increase the likelihood of attainment, in practice it is difficult to know just how and when this participation can be maximized. This difficulty is largely because rehabilitation is a dynamic process of evolvement and change.

The level or degree of patient and family participation is a reflection of the stage of the rehabilitation process. Therefore, accurate assessment of psychosocial readiness is important in the rehabilitation process. For example, highly anxious patients are unable to set long-term goals for themselves or carry out activities consistently without supervision. Others who are more self-directing need opportunities for greater input and involvement. Ideally, pro-fessional opinions are blended with personal choices in goal setting.

Implementation

Having established goals related to assessment data, it is important to implement an approach that will best help patients and families capitalize on strengths, resources, choices, and readiness to learn.

Establishing Effective Interpersonal Relationships

Building effective relationships with patients and families begins during the assessment phase. It is important to be sensitive and to recognize and respond to all fears and concerns throughout rehabilitation. Patients are dealing with pain and incapacitation, and learning to tolerate a rehabilitation environment and maintain adequate relationships with people who care for them. Remember that preserving an emotional balance and satisfactory self-image while maintaining a sense of mastery and competence are difficult under the circumstances.

Communication needs to be open and truthful without taking away all feelings of hope. Professionals sometimes feel helpless. They joke, perhaps to hide an undercurrent of anger, irritation, or frustration at their inability to change things, which brings them face to face with their own limitations—in a sense, a similar experience to that of the patient. Other times humor can be a powerful tool to help strengthen positive thinking.

Be sensitive to the patients' needs for social acceptance, especially in regard to sexuality (see Chapter 10), and the subtle ways in which this can be communicated. Former patients often recall casual interactions with staff as very significant. Encourage individuals to take responsibility for their recovery, reinforcing the belief that personal attitudes, interests, and abilities ultimately determine the degree of success in reaching life goals.

A special issue is that of emotional attachments. Although these feelings may be very real for the team member and the patient, there may be confusion about the roles of a care giver as opposed to a romantic partner. A similar situation occurs if a care giver and patient become "good buddies." Maintaining an appropriate professional relationship in these situations is almost impossible. Orientation should warn of the potential difficulties of close personal relationships and why such relationships are best discouraged until the patient is discharged, when the two adults involved are, of course, free to make their own choices.

Often team members feel obligated to patients, feeling that refusal to meet a request or arrange an outing may contribute to feelings of rejection or lowering of self-esteem. They may simply need help in explaining their role in order to avert complicated emotional situations during rehabilitation.

Providing Health Education

Patients and families need relevant, accurate and specific information regarding disability, treatments, procedures, and illness symptoms. Education must be complete if they are going to maintain health and manage the effects of the disability for life. See Chapter 11. Promoting active participation throughout rehabilitation promotes acquisition of independent living skills.

From the moment of injury, implementing general care with a preventive and restorative focus contributes to a sense of independence and helps minimize feelings of helplessness and loss of control. Encouraging self-care promotes self-esteem. Every small thing that patients can do increases their sense that independence may be possible. Structure, schedule, and simplify tasks so that patients will be successful and thereby receive positive reinforcement. It is important to use specialized knowledge and skills to find practical ways of applying this concept. Throughout the text specific guidelines are given on when and how patients can be expected to participate in their care. For example, participation in the intermittent catheterization program can begin within a few days of injury by self-regulation of fluid intake.

Thompson and Lott give a good example of the connection between self-care and self-esteem.

> A well-planned and early developed bowel program, and a reliable bladder training program commenced during the beginning of the rehabilitation phase can initiate a sense of independence; a *sense of autonomy* so that the patient does not have to dwell on shame and doubt. . . . *Success at physical and physiological tasks can blend into success at social reconditioning.* A night out with others—with a consistent control of bodily functions—can lead to the kind of self-certainty which fosters greater interactions in the future. [Emphasis added. Thompson and Lott 1980: 42]

On the other hand, so-called *denial* of injury can prevent a patient from engaging in self-care activities or a family from supporting educational programs. Initially, it is easier for a family to avoid the consequences of injury, since the physical changes are less obvious while the patient is still on bedrest. The realization comes when the patient is first mobilized to a wheelchair and still cannot move. The efforts of staff members as they lift or transfer the paralyzed patient emphasize the reality of the situation. True denial occurs infrequently, but sometimes hope of recovery or such statements as, "I am going to walk out of here," are confused with denial (Trieschmann 1988). As long as the patient is participating in the rehabilitation program, these statements are an understandable and natural reaction to sudden disability. Only if the avoidance of the effects of injury is obsessive and interferes with treatment does it become detrimental.

Many patients do not wish to participate in suggested activities and programs because, "I will walk again, so why bother?" Some physical recovery, or return of reflex activity when spinal shock subsides, strengthens beliefs that disability is not permanent. In the early stages of the rehabilitation program, patients must be convinced that working with the disability as it is today avoids deterioration of any muscle strength and is the best preparation for any return of function. No time is wasted. This approach does not shatter all hope but does not reinforce unrealistic expectations either. It usually helps both patients and families to resolve some inner turmoil. It is an honest and comfortable way to respond.

Above all, patients should participate in decision making as much as they can, so that they can take an active part in regaining health. When patients are not making good choices in relation to their physical care, ways must be found of making the educational content more meaningful and relevant so that patients will be more committed to it. Help patients realize that making good choices about physical care enhances their health and ensures greater freedom to pursue other activities of which they are still capable.

To reinforce these capabilities, creative collaboration, with counseling professionals in particular, can explore ways in which the patient's authority can be exercised. For example, if a telephone is available, businesspeople can still participate in handling finances, and teenagers can maintain peer contact. Computers make access to data possible, as well as providing games and recreation. Involving teenagers in decision making is infinitely more difficult. Learning to be self-directing or that one's behavior has certain consequences is a normal developmental task for teenagers, and they may not be ready to make decisions about their own care.

Many rehabilitation facilities have structured in-house patient groups involved with formal decision making about policies. These opportunities present patients with constructive outlets for their aggression and opportunities to exercise authority. In such settings peer counselors can be invaluable as role models to effect needed change, and in helping patients see the positive aspects of rehabilitation and benefit from the present opportunities to prepare for future productive activities in the community.

Applying Crisis Intervention Techniques in Rehabilitation

Developmental stages in a crisis are described by Caplan (1964):

- Tension initially rises as habitual problem-solving techniques are tried in response to hazardous event.

ANGER

Anger often surfaces during rehabilitation, and verbal abuse is a common outlet. Patients may project their anger on the staff who care for them. Families may also be targets, and may in turn displace their anger on staff.

Family and staff can find anger directed at them very hard to handle (Morant 1978). To the staff, the patient's anger may seem ungrateful, unreasonable, hurtful, and sometimes frightening. Some staff members take attacks personally, experiencing feelings of guilt, inadequacy or helplessness. Some return the patient's anger, sometimes inappropriately; some atone for their inner anger by forcing themselves to be especially nice; and some accept the criticisms and complaints at face value and wear themselves out trying to please someone who cannot be pleased. Family members also become confused and hurt by the patient's antagonism. Staff help by seeking explanations of these actions and helping patients and families to communicate and deal with their feelings.

Staff members need to recognize their own anger. Such feelings are not shameful in a "professional" person. If team members are assured that their anger is a normal response, uncomfortable feelings tend to recede. Staff may feel less anxious when they realize that patients' anger is partly their way of turning a festering rage at themselves outward rather than holding it in and aggravating their gloom.

No person can bear too much abuse, nor should one try. Patients' destructive energies must be channeled into learning and labor if they are to achieve their full potential for recovery. All concerned must have appropriate outlets for expression of feelings.

Providing Outlets. Limited opportunities for both physical and emotional releases of tension are very real problems for patients with SCI. Advanced medicosurgical techniques have contributed to earlier mobilization, and socialization opportunities are increasing, but significant difficulties still exist.

Gross motor activities provided by a physical therapy program tend to relieve physical tension. Manipulating heavy medicine balls, using punch bags, or wheeling around outside are some examples.

There must also be opportunities to vent frustration and anxieties verbally. One problem is lack of privacy in an institutional setting, particularly in acute care. Physical space for private discussions and relaxation is needed; simply drawing curtains does not provide a sound barrier. Some of the most meaningful conversations between the nurse and the patient inevitably take place in a bathroom! Counseling professionals spend a great deal of time working through anger with various techniques. Use them *early*.

Encouraging personal control. Personal control is a critical factor in coping effectiveness (Ferington 1986).

A visitor left some alcohol for a quadriplegic patient tucked between his legs and the wheelchair. When the nurse became aware of this, she took the alcohol from the patient without any preliminary discussion. Physically unable to stop her, the patient retaliated by running into her with his electric wheelchair.

This is outside control and its likely result.

In another situation a patient and visitor were drinking alcohol at the patient's bedside. The nurse approached them kindly but firmly, restated the regulations and reasons for alcohol control and requested cooperation. Typically the patient responded "Come on, don't you ever take a drink?" The nurse might respond "Yes, I do, but controlling when one drinks is important." The nurse realized the focus was not on her behavior but on the patient's and proceeded to remove the alcohol. Although presented with a choice, the patient felt embarrassed, belittled, and became very angry and shouted obscenities at the nurse. Later he apologized, and at this point the nurse and the patient were able to discuss more meaningfully how his behavior related to consequences and what other alternatives could be explored to increase his independence.

Here the nurse encouraged the patient to control his own behavior and acted as a helper in his efforts.

The critical point in the latter interaction was when the patient became angry. The nurse felt hurt and was moved to the point of tears, but with support from fellow staff members was able to regain composure. When the patient apologized, the nurse chose to confront the patient and said, "After all we have been through together, how could you talk to me like that? I realize that you are under a lot of stress, but wheelchair or not, you cannot expect to treat people like this without alienating them." In this way the nurse alerted the patient to his responsibility for the consequences of his actions. An honest response from the nurse is wonderful because it makes patients feel like "real" rather than "disabled" people. It also communicates

(Box continues)

ANGER *(continued)*

that the nurse is a caring person, an adult who can feel angry, express a feeling, and then let it go. It provides a role model to demonstrate dealing with anger before it becomes aggression.

Although seldom mentioned in professional literature, the feeling of *forgiveness* is also important in a situation like this (Buscaglia 1975). Forgiving demonstrates a willingness to carry on and communicates

confidence in the patient and hope for the future. If these everyday situations are managed well, the individual will have a better chance with others in the future.

At an appropriate time, acknowledging staff anger toward patients is therapeutic. If staff tend to avoid angry patients, outbursts will increase as patients attempt to get their needs met through negative behavior.

- Coping is unsuccessful, the stimulus continues, and discomfort increases.
- Further increase in tension stimulates an attempt to mobilize internal and external resources. Emergency problem-solving mechanisms are tried. The problem may be redefined, or the person may become resigned or give up certain aspects of goals as unattainable. There is a pervasive feeling of helplessness.
- If the problem continues and can neither be solved nor avoided, tension increases to a breaking point. Major disorganization of the individual occurs.

At each of these developmental stages, previous experience shapes what occurs. A current threat is often linked to long-standing difficulties, thus reactivating unresolved or partially resolved unconscious conflicts. The energy needed to maintain repression of the earlier unresolved problem may possibly be redirected to solve the current problem in a more appropriate, mature manner. The outcome will be determined by the choices made by the individual.

If the problem is viewed as a challenge, it is more likely to be met with energy and purposive problem-solving. The new pattern of coping to resolve the crisis may help the individual deal more realistically with future hazardous events.

Approaching difficult situations when behavior is negative using crisis intervention techniques emphasizes a more straightforward person-to-person approach rather than in-depth psychoanalytical counseling.

Several techniques can be applied to coping with a crisis situation. These include exploring how the individual has handled problems in the past and how strengths can be used in the present situation; listening actively and with concern; encouraging open expression of feelings; helping the patient to gain understanding of events that lead to crisis, to accept reality and to explore new ways of coping: experiencing varying degrees of control in planning care; linking the patient with social contacts and activities; and reinforcing the newly learned coping devices after resolution of the crisis. These techniques, some actually preventive, apply in everyday situations. Crisis intervention techniques are really a way of assessing and organizing concerns and helping the

person do something about them—a model for "putting it all together."

Families that are well integrated can provide support during times of stress and can help resolve stress through interfamily activities. However, the emotional needs of the family must also be addressed since difficulties will hinder the injured individual in adapting to the disability.

Mary, a 47-year-old homemaker, married with four children, was referred to a major center two weeks after being diagnosed as experiencing "hysterical" paralysis at a local hospital. Following neurological assessment, her injury was accurately diagnosed as a central cord injury at C_{5-6} cord segment (without bony injury). A comment by the nurse expressing how fortunate Mary was to have escaped a complete injury elicited a hostile response. Mary insulted the nurse's youth and appearance and accused her of being stupid because she had no idea of what life was all about. The nurse was able to look beyond this response and identify several events that culminated in this inappropriate behavior. Although Mary was able to walk and therefore did not "look" that disabled, upper limb and torso weakness rendered her dependent for many activities of daily living and personal hygiene. In addition, she had just experienced a negative relationship with local health professionals who did not believe her complaints, had a daughter who had just left home, and was worried about her husband being left alone with a young woman who was hired to care for the other children. The nurse perceived a severe threat to Mary's self-concept and self-esteem, and the social worker immediately initiated marital and family counseling. This enabled the entire interdisciplinary team to proceed with a more empathetic approach. The staff also took immediate steps to resolve some of Mary's hostility toward local health resources, because she would require their supportive services to return home as soon as possible.

The staff recognized that hostile, acting-out behavior is frequently a call for attention. Attentive listening, giving support and recognition, and consistent limit setting helped to decrease negative behavior.

Crises may arise for care givers when dealing with uncooperative, depressed, or angry patients during care essential to maintain physical integrity. Typically these situations are most pronounced during the evening or night, when reactions to significant experiences encountered during the day, or on return from passes, seem to surface. When this happens, it is extremely difficult to control inner feelings or even to begin to understand the underlying cause for the patient's behavior. It is normal to feel hurt and enraged, and care givers should be prepared to give themselves and their patients time to cool off.

Tony, a 17-year-old boy, and youngest of four children, was injured in an alcohol-related diving accident at a high school graduation party. He was diagnosed as having complete quadriplegia at C_7. Several weeks after injury, although still in a halo brace, he was able to go home on a weekend pass. He returned late on Sunday night, and the nurse was hurrying to get him into bed. Something went wrong and a very unpleasant scene followed. The nurse simply stated she was not prepared to deal with that type of behavior but would return before she went off. It is almost a natural reaction to tell the patient you can't stand this scene one more time but it is far more helpful to focus on the experiences of the day rather than dwelling on previous, similar negative reactions. Tony eventually explained that he had attended a family reunion and was overwhelmed by the reactions of others. Tony had remained silent only to explode later at the nurse.

Once the causes of the behavioral outbursts are identified (and this may be an ongoing process with several long-standing causes), the nurse can proceed with counseling professionals to encourage the patients to reflect on how to approach the same situation another time; to examine their feelings; and to think about what to do to get other people to react more positively toward them. Many different forms of therapy, including role playing and group interaction, can help establish these new coping techniques. This kind of experience points toward the need for assertiveness and social skills training during rehabilitation. See Chapter 31.

Be alert for drug and alcohol abuse that precipitates unmanageable behavior. Typically this problem increases as rehabilitation progresses.

Illicit use of alcohol and drugs, particularly among the more vulnerable youth population, is influenced by the need to be like their peers; curiosity; and the need to test and experiment, all of which are related to the age and stage of development. Factors that are related to the disability are primarily *boredom* and the *inability to deal with the reality of disability*. Mind-altering substances provide an escape. In conjunction with the more traditional psychological interventions, management of recreational and leisure time emerges as an important element in achieving productivity. Staff, particularly on evenings and weekends, have important roles to play in supporting this preventive therapy.

Reasonable policies with disciplinary action, such as administrative discharge following repeated offenses, only provide temporary solutions. Boyink and Strawn (1980) point out the necessity for clear-cut rules on how many infractions constitute a reason for disciplinary action. The policy must then be supported by all staff members and known to all patients. This encourages the patients to become more responsible for the consequences of their behavior. If policies are not enforced, continued use of alcohol and drugs is condoned implicitly and the staff feel angered and unsupported. Liaison with drug and alcohol abuse programs is helpful.

Crisis by its very nature is self-limiting. It cannot continue indefinitely as it is too painful. The emotional discomfort stemming from extreme anxiety forces a person to seek resolution of the problem and restore a sense of equilibrium. How a crisis is resolved significantly affects the future emotional health of an individual.

Evaluation

The outcome of rehabilitation is the result of the patient, the family, and all aspects of the therapeutic environment working together. The rehabilitation milieu must be flexible enough to meet individual needs as patients and families help to define these needs.

Evaluation encompasses such factors as feedback from the patient and family; ability to set realistic goals and solve problems; and effective or functional patterns of behavioral change. Achievement of patient and family health education goals also reflects the degree of psychosocial adaptation. In general, the more completely the patient and family meet educational goals, the greater the degree of adjustment. The ultimate success or failure of the rehabilitation process will eventually be determined by the ability of the person with SCI to enjoy life. Productivity may or may not include financial, vocational, and physical independence, but it must reflect personal satisfaction with one's own life-style.

SPECIFIC MANAGEMENT OF PSYCHOSOCIAL COMPLICATIONS*

Psychiatric Illness

Some patients with SCI may have a history of psychiatric problems before injury while others develop problems as a result of the overwhelming stresses and conflicts of disability. Initial assessment focuses on the individual's personality, how the patient has coped with past stress, and the

*This section was contributed by Mary Lee Lynch, R.N., M.S.N., C.S.

patient's current level of functioning. Collaboration with psychiatric professionals is imperative to:

- Understand patient behavior
- Initiate effective treatment plans
- Promote positive patient-staff relationships
- Develop appropriate as well as consistent staff intervention and evaluation techniques

Management with antidepressant and antipsychotic medications must be exercised cautiously for the patient with SCI because side effects may be particularly troublesome (Judd and Burrows 1986). Anticholinergic side effects may interfere with desired reflex voiding. Anti-adrenergic blockers may cause hypotension with sympathetic nervous system dysfunction with injury above T_4 (see Chapter 4). Newer generations of medications tend to cause fewer problems.

Depression

Situational reactions are often mistaken as depression. In this regard, it is important to distinguish between a predictable grief/mourning reaction in contrast to true clinical, reactive depression. See Table 9–1.

Mourning can appear similar to depression. For example, mourning presents with sensations of somatic distress, preoccupation with a former self-image, feelings of guilt, a tendency to respond with irritability and anger, and a change of behavior. Typically, grief or mourning reactions abate as the individual accommodates over time to the disability. However, there is an important distinction between mourning and depression. In a *grief/mourning reaction*, the emphasis is on the lost body part and the concomitant secondary emotional reactions. For example, the disabled individual would lament the compromised quality of life without independence and limbs. In a *reactive depression*, the emphasis is on the disability's implication as to who the person is. In other words, reactively depressed people would be self-critical and punitive. This could manifest itself in the form of believing themselves useless, worthless, or bad. The distinction is important in its implications for psychotropic medications, style of interaction regarding rehabilitation, and use of psychological/psychiatric consultations.

An important manifestation of reactive depression is characterized by *withdrawal* and feelings of worthlessness. Patients are uncommunicative, lying quietly in bed with the sheets drawn up over their heads.

A middle-aged quadriplegic man, injured in a skiing accident, became increasingly withdrawn approximately four weeks after injury. He began by refusing to get up in the wheelchair. Gradually he refused to eat, had difficulty sleeping, ceased to respond verbally, and finally passively resisted any verbal or physical contact. The psychiatrist began treatment with antidepressant medication in con-

TABLE 9–1   Distinguishing between Grief Response and Depressive Illness

	Grief Response	Depressive Illness
Long-term Effect	Reactions tend to lessen as time passes after injury	Symptomatology worsens over time
Sleep Disturbance	No regular pattern of difficulty sleeping	Fixed pattern of inability to sleep
Appetite Disturbance	Poor appetite comes and goes in waves; weight loss	Total distinterest in food; weight loss
General Physical Responses	Anxiety symptoms vary; tiredness, listlessness common but transient	Total lack of energy; sustained lowered ability to function
Psychosocial Responses	Complex emotional response to loss; feelings of despair and hopelessness lessen over time; usually feel minimal guilt; anger is expressed and directed outwardly; able to participate in rehabilitation activities	Preoccupied with sense of worthlessness; inappropriately laden with guilt; anger not expressed but may act in a hostile and demanding way or become withdrawn; self-neglectful; may be suicidal
Treatment Aims	Promotion of normal emotional responses; supported and encouraged expression of feelings; limit setting for angry outbursts; full participation in rehabilitation activities	Neuropharmaceutical treatment (antidepressant, antipsychotic medications); psychotherapy; individually planned management program; avoidance of preconceived negativity about patients with psychiatric problems in rehabilitation settings (Ostrow 1985)

Based on Judd, Burrows, and Brown 1986.

junction with psychotherapy. As all attempts to encourage participation in his care were futile, the psychiatrist suggested that the patient be allowed to regress to a fully dependent role to regain his strength before new activities were gradually introduced. The patient began to work through his numerous marital, family, and vocational problems that had existed before the injury. This approach met with relative success and the patient was finally able to participate in a rehabilitation program and return to his rural home. However, one year later family disruption and resultant problems were again evident.

This situation indicates the importance of seeing long-standing psychosocial problems not as "cured" but as processed and reprocessed. As the problem changes, the person may or may not need help to redefine and cope anew.

Suicidal Thoughts and Intent

People with SCI who feel that the future is bleak, that disability is insurmountable, and that they are unworthy of any intervention present a great suicidal risk. A common error in caring for suspected suicidal patients is not asking directly about their wishes and intentions regarding death and suicide. Never assume that because patients are disabled, they cannot commit suicide. Suicide is a significant cause of death in the disabled population.

If patients express suicidal thoughts, ask them to describe how they would carry out the act and if they have the means. Initiate suicidal precautions to protect the patient from self-destructive impulses, obtain a psychiatric consultation, and treat the underlying depression.

Continuation of intervention includes regular visits with the patient; active listening to what the patient has to say; allowing the patient to express feelings, and helping the patient to cope effectively. Also it is important to aid in maintaining hygiene, nutrition, and bowel and bladder programs while the individual is in this depressed state.

Other Psychiatric Disorders

Schizophrenia. Schizophrenia refers to a group of conditions characterized by disturbances of thought, affect, and behavior that lead eventually to social and emotional withdrawal, mood disturbances, periods of excitement and immobility, misinterpretations of reality, delusions, and hallucinations. Stress resulting from physiological and psychosocial problems associated with SCI may cause the patient to decompensate. In fact, some patients become spinal cord injured as a result of the schizophrenic process.

Communication and reality testing become problematic for the patient as well as the staff. In order for the staff to intervene appropriately, the differences between a *delusion*, a *hallucination*, and an *illusion* must be clear. Table 9–2 defines these terms and suggests some general therapeutic interventions.

Schizophrenic patients with SCI seem to respond reasonably well to the treatment program prescribed for all other patients as long as specific attention is also given to their particular psychiatric needs.

Neuroses. *Neuroses* are a group of syndromes characterized by anxiety. The original source of the anxiety relates to highly charged interpersonal situations that lead to unresolvable conflict. The individual experiences anxiety whenever stimulated by anything associated with the original conflict. For instance, a young child, whose mother does not fulfill dependency needs, becomes very self-sufficient so as not to need help from others. The problem may be unresolved even though the individual is functional.

All persons experience anxiety as a normal condition of everyday living. Neurotic anxiety differs from the usual transitory anxiety in that the nature of what threatens the individual is not clear or recognized. Also, people with neurotic anxiety tend to defend themselves against the perceived threats. The particular form of neurosis is labeled according to the defense mechanisms the individual uses to deal with the anxiety. Neurotic behavior may take several different forms as outlined in Table 9–3.

The spinal cord injured patient who presents with underlying neurotic behavior can be managed with appropriate general interventions:

- Establish a relationship of trust and confidence
- Provide reassurance particularly during acute anxiety attacks
- Teach relaxation techniques
- Explain interventions clearly and repeatedly and check that the patient understands (patients with heightened anxiety may not hear or retain explanations)
- Encourage and expect participation in the rehabilitation program
- Allow expression of feelings and concerns without focusing excessively on phobias or compulsive behavior
- Teach coping skills that enhance interpersonal relationships

It is necessary to assess and then to determine specific goals and interventions with individual patients. The judicious use of antianxiety medication may help.

Personality Disorders. *Personality disorders* are characterized by clusters of deeply ingrained traits, attitudes, and patterns of behavior that have been present since adolescence or earlier. These characteristics are inflexible and maladaptive, causing a degree of impairment in social or occupational functioning. Individuals with personality disorders are difficult to treat unless they become uncomfortable or dissatisfied with their maladaptive patterns of behavior. Perhaps a slightly larger proportion of preexisting personality disorders may be found among SCI individuals because their impulsive acts may involve them in situations that lead to initial injury (Hohmann 1975).

Under conditions of stress, such as SCI, features of personality disorder often become accentuated. Also, after formal rehabilitation individuals may seek help for incidental illness or for complications associated with their antisocial behavior such as alcohol or drug abuse, accidents, or trauma from fights. On occasion, individuals may seek medical help, while actually using health care professionals to obtain drugs or to avoid legal prosecution.

Patients with personality disorders may not be diagnosed as such but are readily identified by the staff as difficult, demanding, angry, impulsive, and at times violent, self-destructive, or threatening. Depression may alternate with anger. These patients are unable to sustain genuine reciprocal human interactions. They have a lonely inner void they try to fill with impulsive, self-destructive, acting-out behaviors, such as drug or alcohol abuse and physical abuse of their bodies.

Management must focus on the attitudes and behavioral characteristics of the individual.

- Make expectations clear to patients. Inform them of hospital rules and regulations, participation, and outcomes expected.
- Set limits and negotiate contractual agreements on behavior. All staff should enforce these limits consistently.
- Meet regularly with the team to provide staff support, consistent care, and sharing of patient response and progress.
- Communicate the plan of care to the patient and leave a copy of the plan at the bedside.
- Clarify patients' requests or complaints but do not be drawn into patients' attempts to split staff by flattery or derogatory comments.
- Allow patients choices where possible. Giving the same control and encouraging appropriate independence usually leads to greater compliance.
- Encourage constructive expression of angry feelings—perhaps athletic activity also. Listen to patients and attempt to clarify feelings and nonverbal cues.

TABLE 9–2 Perceptual Disorders: Some General Therapeutic Interventions

Delusions

An individual's judgment, beliefs, reasoning, and even perceptions are influenced to a degree by current emotions, and the stress of hospitalization—with its fears, forced dependency and loss of control—may elicit delusions. *Delusions* exist to satisfy emotional needs. They are unfounded or false beliefs that have little or no basis in reality and cannot be changed by reason or logic. Deluded people may think certain staff are spying on them, fear they are being controlled by other people or "outside forces," or believe thoughts are being inserted or withdrawn from their minds. General therapeutic interventions stress not to agree with patients regarding delusions and not to argue with them. Listen to the patients and respond to their feelings of fear, apprehension, or other concerns. Always let them know who you are and the reason for your interaction. Clearly explain treatments and procedures and do not whisper near the patients. Attempt to identify possible triggering events (such as medication or sensory deprivation). Do recognize that the patient is trying to tell you something.

Hallucinations

Hallucinations are false sensory perceptions that have no physical or environmental stimuli. They may involve any of the five senses but usually are auditory. Hallucinations are common in psychotic illnesses but can also be caused by certain drugs and poisons, local diseases of sensory organs, or from anxiety and unmet psychological needs. With any kind of overwhelming stress and conflict, an individual can revert to a lower level of functioning; thus hallucinations are seen as primitive or immature thought processes. It is generally felt that the contexts of these thoughts are related to the patient's past anxiety-provoking experiences and are therefore kept out of the conscious mind. A common difficulty is that speech does not follow the usual rules of logic and appears to be bizarre

and disconnected. Staff who care for hallucinating patients find that frequent visits are particularly valuable in help them maintain contact with reality. Other specific interventions include: keeping the patients' attention focused on outside realities such as occupational therapy, television programs, or recreational activities; acknowledging the patients' hallucinations but letting them know you are not experiencing it; exploring the content and nature of the hallucinations; not arguing or challenging patients regarding hallucinations; offering gentle reassurance, as the perceptions may be frightening; interrupting the hallucinations by getting the patients to talk to you; developing a trusting relationship with patients; not touching patients without warning them beforehand; and protecting patients from harming themselves as a result of misperceptions by removing harmful objects.

Illusions

Illusions are a misperception or misinterpretation of an external stimulus. The patient actually perceives something in the environment but misinterprets what it is. Illusions are frequently the result of poisons, infections, drug overdose, alcoholism, or changes in the level of consciousness. Interventions include: removing the object that triggered the illusion; explaining what the object really is without verbally disagreeing with a patient's perception; letting the patient see or handle the object after calming down; allowing patients to have sense-related objects from home in their immediate environment when feasible (familiar pictures, pillows, or blankets); and minimizing unfamiliar objects in the patient's surroundings (provide night light to avoid shadows or remove pictures that are ambiguous). Take preventive measures by being aware of the patient's sensory level and then either reduce sensory overload or increase sensory stimuli. Patients who were overtly psychotic at the time of injury remitted the psychotic symptoms within a few days of the injury, although the secondary symptoms of psychosis remain.

TABLE 9–3 Neurotic Behavior Defined

Neurosis	Definition
Anxiety neurosis	Free-floating anxiety with acute episodes of *anxiety attacks* that may progress to *panic*. The individual experiences a sense of impending doom.
Phobic neurosis	Persistent fear of a specific place or thing that leads to avoidance. The individual gradually retreats from whatever is causing the anxiety (open spaces, crowds, or high places are some examples).
Obsessive-compulsive neurosis	Obsessions (persistent, distressing thoughts) and compulsions (persistent, uncontrollable urges to perform certain acts), both of which become time consuming and interfere with the individual's interpersonal relationships.
Hysterical neurosis	A loss or alteration in physical functioning that suggests physical disorder with no organic pathology but which is an expression of a psychological conflict.
Hypochondriasis or hypochondriacal neurosis	The predominant disturbance is an unrealistic fear or belief of having a serious disease despite medical assurance to the contrary. Preoccupation with such beliefs leads to impairment in social and/or occupational functioning.

- Assist patients in effective problem solving and give constructive feedback.
- Establish a daily routine for the patient that provides structure while decreasing anxiety.
- Focus on the current task or intervention under discussion and do not allow patients to digress.
- Assess patients for self-destructive behavior and take precautions as necessary.
- Evaluate outcomes.
- Link with community-based resources early to plan continuing support services.

Chemical (Drug/Alcohol) Dependency

Spinal cord injury is an overwhelming or catastrophic injury that affects the individual involved psychologically as well as physically. For many of these individuals, the loss of control, pain, dependence on others, depression, and anxiety lead to substance abuse. Recognized or not, these individuals are on a downward self-destructive spiral. They consistently deny that the valium they take for "spasm," the few beers they drink each day, or the marijuana they use regularly, is a problem. Yet, all of these substances prevent them from recognizing their fears and anxieties and learning to live with their disabilities.

All individuals develop ways to cope with problems because the desire to eliminate anxiety is universal. Chemically dependent individuals attempt to relieve anxiety through the use of a chemical substance without going through the usual problem-solving techniques. Consequently, these individuals seldom recognize what triggers their anxiety, nor do they learn how to eliminate its cause. The chemical substance used, be it drugs or alcohol, dulls the discomfort experienced when the individual is anxious. Anxiety is relieved temporarily but the problem still exists and the anxiety will return, causing the repetitive pattern of chemical abuse.

The causes of chemical dependency are not completely understood. Theories of etiology generally fall into three groups: psychological, biochemical, and genetic. It is generally agreed that no basic personality disorder is inherent in chemically dependent individuals. Yet such individuals usually have a low tolerance for frustration and tendencies to seek immediate gratification and depend on others for their sense of well-being.

Chemical dependence refers to an individual's physiological and/or psychological dependence on a chemical substance with resultant impairment of the individual's functioning at home, school, work, or other area of life. Physical dependence means that the body has adapted to the presence of the chemical substance so that it is required by the individual to maintain functioning. If the chemical substance is withheld, withdrawal symptoms occur. The development of physical dependence is followed by the development of tolerance: as the body accommodates to the chemical substance, it requires increasing doses to maintain its effect. Psychological dependence means that individuals feel they cannot get along without the use of the chemical substance.

The damaging consequences of chemical dependence are extensive. This disease not only effects the individual but also has a severe impact on family, friends, and the community at large. Divorce rates, absenteeism, suicide rates, and the incidence of physical illness are much higher in these individuals than in the general adult population. Excessive chemical use is frequently implicated in homicides and automobile accidents. Despite the fact that chemical dependence is recognized as a major health problem, physicians as well as nurses display a degree of resistance and/or reluctance to identify and intervene with patients as well as peers. In many rehabilitation settings the chemically dependent patients are only recognized when they become problematic—returning from a pass intoxicated and abusive; too sleepy or "hung over" from

PERSONAL VIEWPOINT: BACK FROM THE EDGE

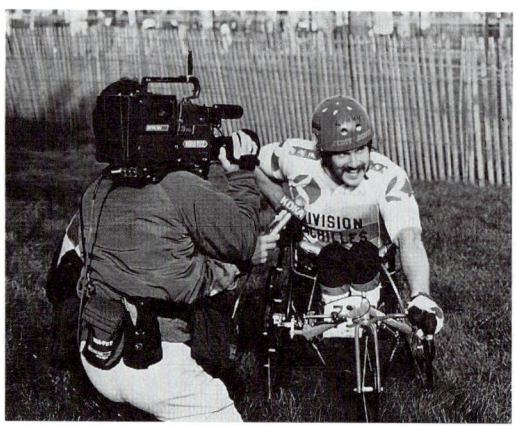

Kenny Carnes is a world-class athlete. He works at a skilled and demanding job 50 hours a week; he trains for his sport another 20 hours. He competes nationally and internationally. Carnes has won the Pittsburgh Marathon, shattering the course record by more than 10 minutes. Four days earlier he competed against nine of the top athletes in his field in a 52-mile road race in Washington, DC. Carnes has also placed second in the European Cup Super Marathon in Poland. Yet Kenny Carnes has only been racing for 18 months. He is paralyzed from the waist down. His sport is wheelchair racing.

He presents his story of adversity and self-destruction without regret and almost without emotion. He had a childhood that was derailed by pot, pills, and booze.

At 13, he started hanging out with a crowd of older boys who introduced him to dirt bike racing. One ride and he was hooked. He got a paper route and worked at a fast-food restaurant to make enough money to buy a bike. He knew early on that he could be the best.

Although Carnes had a stable home life, good schooling, plenty of discipline from loving parents, and church on Sundays, his older friends started giving him beer and marijuana when he was 13, and he quickly became an eager participant in the night moves of the neighborhood. He also became more and more adept on the racing circuit and gained the respect of a group older and more experienced than he. Soon he was sharing a pharmacopoeia of drugs and washing them down with beer and bourbon. Still, his behavior didn't interfere with his abilities on the racing circuit. He

became a nationally ranked racer and devoted all his spare time to his sport.

On a perfect spring day in Virginia, he started his last dirt bike race well in the back of the pack, but by midrace he was chasing second place. At the first jump, the number two racer lost control of his bike, and Carnes went over his handlebars trying to avoid the other driver. His own bike flew into the air and came down on top of him, breaking his back and paralyzing him from the waist down. At 18, Carnes' racing career was over. The hard part of his life had just begun.

By the time he was discharged from the hospital, he was chemically dependent on Valium. His girlfriend provided him with beer and marijuana on demand. The time he spent at the hospital in Virginia and at an upstate New York rehabilitation hospital passed in a blur.

In the following years, Carnes was frequently stopped for drunk driving. Most of the time, the charges were dropped. The police were reluctant to place an additional burden on a kid in a wheelchair.

There was some hope of a steady job and stability. During his tenure at the rehabilitation hospital, Carnes studied dental technology. For a year he apprenticed himself to a man who ran a dental lab on the second floor of his home. Each morning Carnes left his wheelchair at the bottom of a steep, narrow staircase and dragged himself to the lab, step by step. There he learned to mold and sculpt plaster, silver, and gold; a delicate and exacting pursuit that came naturally to him.

However, he started to deal drugs and sold LSD to an undercover narcotics agent. Carnes served a few months in prison, and then continued to abuse drugs and alcohol. He wrecked three vans and two cars in alcohol-related accidents. Less than a year after he left prison, he again sold drugs to an undercover narcotics agent. This time even the best legal representation failed to win him a reprieve, and he served 22 months in federal prison facilities.

When he was released, Carnes met a woman who would change his life. She was older than he and easily the most beautiful woman he had ever dated. Although she, too, was involved in drug use, they both resolved to turn their lives around. For the first time since his accident, Carnes felt fulfilled in a relationship—he was genuinely happy.

(Box continues)

PERSONAL VIEWPOINT (continued)

Their relationship ended tragically: On the way home after Thanksgiving with his parents, Carnes's van was struck by a drunk driver going more than 100 mph. He lost control of the van and struck a concrete retaining wall. Both his legs were broken. His girlfriend was killed instantly.

Once more, Carnes turned to substance abuse. After two DWI arrests, he lost his license for 10 days. Though it seems like a minor inconvenience when compared to the enormous setbacks in his past, this incident was a turning point. The fear of losing his license permanently, of being totally dependent on others to get around, led him to change his life. In August 1986, Carnes attended his first AA meeting. With the exception of a short relapse early in his recovery, he has been sober since then.

Shortly after the first AA meeting, Carnes became involved with the National Handicapped Sports club. Some club members challenged him to participate in a 10-kilometer road race, his first athletic challenge since his accident. He remembered what it felt like to be a competitor, and he found the desire and the determination to become a champion again.

Working out with members of National Handicapped Sports and the Achilles Track Club, organizations that promote sports and physical fitness for the disabled, Carnes finally came to terms with his disability. He admitted to himself that he was going to be in his wheelchair for the rest of his life. "Ever since my accident, I despised my disability. I didn't want to associate with other disabled people," he said. As he met other handicapped athletes, however, Carnes realized that his disability was comparatively minor. He saw the tremendous courage and determination of people much less fortunate and gifted than he and was transformed by their examples.

Carnes is recognized at each competition. The media attention he has received during his rapid rise in the ranks of wheelchair racing has made him a local celebrity. As he rolls around in the crowd before a race, runners approach him, shyly at first, congratulating him on a recent win or discussing strategies for upcoming races. He is relaxed and approachable until it is time to prepare for the race. He fully expects to win. As he explodes out of the starting line, the spirit soars—on wings and on wheels.

Candace Karu Carnes
Potomac, MD

chemical abuse to participate in therapies; or continually asking for valium, pain medication, or other drugs that alter the perceptions of the problems of living with a disability.

Due to the catastrophic losses of people with SCI, they are frequently characterized as being vulnerable to the abuse of drugs and alcohol. In fact, a review of the literature provides very little factual information about the prevalence of substance abuse in the SCI population. Burke (1973) noted a high incidence of alcohol and drug use among patients with SCI and suggested that such substances are used to relieve pain. Malec (1982) was interested in marijuana use before and after SCI and how the use of marijuana affected spasticity. A majority of the patients who used marijuana before injury continued this use after injury. The few formal treatment programs designed specifically for the disabled substance abuser have offered very little information on this population.

Frisbie and Tun (1984) studied the incidence of alcohol consumption before and after SCI. They found that the majority of patients in their study (67%) were habitual drinkers before SCI, and many of these individuals had consumed at least six drinks on the day of their injury. It was noted that several patients were using marijuana as well as alcohol. Their survey indicates that patients who consume alcohol after SCI usually developed the habit before injury. Kirnbakaran (1986) found similar results in a study of drug and alcohol misuse. The majority of patients (75%) acknowledged the use of alcohol before age 21 and before SCI. Conversely, the majority of drug users reportedly began using drugs after SCI. This study also indicates that both alcohol and drug misuse in these patients is far less than what has been reported in the general population of adults. In both of these studies, the disabling SCI was the motivating factor in the cessation or reduction of alcohol use. Further studies of the young adult population are needed to determine use or misuse of alcohol and/or drugs in this specific age group. Although the earlier studies were done by random sampling, the majority of the study population were white married men over 50 years of age who lived with their families.

Despite the lack of factual studies on the incidence of substance abuse, most health care professionals working with people with SCI are aware of many patients, particularly young adults, who deal with their overwhelming physical and emotional pain by abusing drugs, alcohol, or both substances. From the acute stage on, patients have access to a wide variety of addictive pain medication and muscle relaxants. Physicians as well as nurses find it easier to medicate a patient than to deal with the anger, anxiety, and frequently abusive behavior. Patients, staff, and family all avoid, and even deny, the problem. Patients readily collude with their care givers by focusing on the physical aspects of paralysis and denying any problem with drugs and alcohol.

There are two alternatives to managing patients with SCI who are prone to chemical abuse: prevention and treatment.

Prevention by necessity starts with the professional staff. The health care staff educated to treat disabilities must also receive basic training to recognize and intervene in behavior associated with substance abuse. Patients themselves must be made aware of the threat of chemical dependency if they cannot deal with the issues of disability. Pete Anderson* (Maddox 1987), a recovering alcoholic and an advocate for the disabled substance abuser, states: "If you look at the reasons why people with paraplegia or quadriplegia are admitted to hospitals, it's almost never for substance abuse. It's things like they have fallen out of their wheelchairs, they are malnourished, they have lost their personal care attendant or they have recurrent decubiti as a result of self-abuse." It is easier for the health care team to focus on the paralysis and resultant physical problems rather than the substance abuse.

Since disabled individuals are vulnerable to substance abuse, staff must:

- Avoid using drugs with high abuse potential.
- Avoid giving patients large supplies of abusive drugs to take home on pass.
- Consider tolerance and cross-tolerance of medications when dealing with the problems of insomnia, anxiety, pain, or muscle spasms.
- Avoid prolonged and indefinite use of valium.
- Educate family and/or significant other to the problems.

The paralyzed individual frequently needs someone's help to become or remain addicted to drugs or alcohol. That someone, called the *enabler*, or *co-dependent*, is usually found in the patient's immediate environment—a spouse, parent, significant other, doctor or nurse, an aide, or a well-meaning friend. Whether their activity is conscious or unconscious they harm the patient rather than help, and the patient remains chemically dependent. It is also not uncommon to hear knowledgeable health care professionals as well as family or friends state disabled individuals should be able to "enjoy" something in life—let them have their drugs or alcohol. In fact, they are giving up on the individuals' ability to be independent, responsible, and an effective member of the community. Treatment programs for disabled substance abusers are not yet common. The programs that do exist offer patients a good chance of recovery if they deal with the disability: grief, sexuality, independence, self-esteem, role within the family, as well as activities that enhance the individuals' ability to exist meaningfully in the community.

Treatment of chemical dependence disorders demands cross-consultation and collaboration with abuse specialists (Pires 1989). Conventional interventions that help disabled substance abusers include:

- Using disabled, recovering alcoholic/chemically dependent peer counselors
- Conducting therapeutic groups composed of both drug- and alcohol-dependent, disabled individuals
- Giving individuals responsibilities and holding them accountable for self-care, attendance at therapies and so forth
- Developing a therapeutic relationship
- Confronting substance abuse in a supportive manner, recognizing that the individuals may feel frightened and helpless
- Setting limits on behavior to help individuals regain control
- Recognizing and avoiding manipulative behaviors and/or staff splitting
- Being consistent in approach to individual care plans
- Ongoing education of individuals regarding disability as well as substance abuse. The educational process needs to be regularly reinforced to allow for anxiety and lack of readiness to learn intellectually as well as emotionally.
- Networking with support groups such as Alcoholics Anonymous and Narcanon to facilitate support for people after leaving the rehabilitation program
- Vocational counseling to assist in realistic goal setting and activities for reentry into the community
- Outpatient follow-up to provide support and to prevent problems from occurring as people adapt to home living
- Developing the plan of care with each person and setting mutually agreed, short- and long-term goals. Treatment goals need to focus on independent living in the community and must be individualized
- Providing suitable alternatives to substance abuse— swimming, painting, photography, wheelchair sports, travel, education, computers, gardening
- Educating the family or significant other regarding the disability and chemical dependency emphasizing their understanding the disease process and their role as co-dependent or enabler.

Ultimately the individuals must accept responsibility for themselves and the need for treatment that will allow them to become productive members of society.

*Executive Director of the Congress on Chemical Dependency and Disability, Gardena, CA. The goal of the Congress is to ensure that disabled individuals who also have alcohol and/or other chemical dependency problems receive accessible, high-quality treatment services.

REFERENCES

Aadalen, S. P., and Stroebel-Kahn, F. 1981. Coping with quadriplegia. *American Journal of Nursing.* 81 (8): 1471–1478. *Presents a description of coping with the physical and emotional trauma one of the authors experienced after becoming quadriplegic. Good discussion of adaptive mechanisms used by patient and family.*

Associated Press. 1989. *Holocaust survivors cope by suppressing their pasts. Washington Post Health* June 27.

Boyink, M. A., and Strawn, S. M. 1980. Spinal cord injury: Post acute phase. In *Comprehensive Rehabilitation Nursing.* Eds. N. Martin, N. B. Holt, and D. Hicks. New York: McGraw-Hill. *Overall assessment and planning, and related nursing care in later rehabilitation phase.*

Burke, D. D. 1973. Pain. *Paraplegia News* 10 : 297–313.

Buscaglia, L. 1975. *The Disabled and Their Parents.* Thorofare, NJ: Charles B. Slack. *In a very humanistic readable style, describes how disabled persons, their families, and even professionals can suffer more pain than is caused by the disability itself when competent, sound, reality-based guidance is not forthcoming. Chapter 13 deals with becoming disabled later in life. Highly recommended.*

Caplan, G. 1964. *Principles of Preventive Psychiatry.* New York: Basic Books.

Ernst, F. A. 1987. Contrasting perceptions of distress by research personnel and their spinal cord injured subjects. *Archives of Physical Medicine and Rehabilitation* 66 (1): 12–15. *This study replicates and extends the tendency among staff to overestimate depression anxiety and social discomfort while underestimating optimism. Also includes information for designing assessment tools and encourages application in personal clinical settings to measure levels of distress of patients and staff.*

Ferington, F. E. 1986. Personal control and coping effectiveness in spinal cord injured persons. *Research Nursing Health* 9 (3): 257–265. *Findings indicate that the significance of having control is an individualized matter and that detailed assessment may be necessary to obtain maximum benefit from participating in their own care.*

Frank, R. G., and Elliot, T. R. 1987. Life stress and psychologic adjustment following spinal cord injury. *Archives of Physical Medicine and Rehabilitation* 68 (6): 344–347. *Examines the impact of life events from contemporary perspectives. Patients who were experiencing higher levels of stress displayed more distress in adjustment to injury than those with lower levels of life stress, which was not mediated by the passage of time.*

Frank, R. G., et al. 1988. Age as a factor in response to spinal cord injury. *Archives of Physical Medicine and Rehabilitation* 67 (3): 128–131. *Examines further the role of age in response to catastrophic injury. Results reported that greater life stress correlates with more depressive symptomatology regardless of age.*

Freeman, D., and Trute, B. 1981. *Treating Families with Special Needs.* Alberta Association of Social Workers, Ottawa, Ontario, Canada (copublished by The Canadian Association of Social Workers).

Frisbie, J. H., and Tun, C. G. 1984. Drinking and spinal cord injury. *Journal of the American Paraplegia Society* 7 (4): 71–73.

Gunther, M. S. 1980. The threatened practitioner: work under stress. In *Comprehensive Rehabilitation Nursing.* Eds. N. Martin, N. B. Holt, and D. Hicks. New York: McGraw-Hill. *Skillfully analyzes the nursing service at work, explores factors that cause stress for the nurse, and focuses on management activities that help. Highly recommended.*

Hoff, L. 1989. *People in Crisis: Understanding and Helping* 3rd ed. Redwood City, CA: Addison-Wesley. *Straightforward approach using everyday language to teach people how to understand, identify, and help other people in crisis; includes information about helping self-destructive people and those whose health and self-image are threatened.*

Hohmann, G. W. 1975. Psychological aspects of treatment and rehabilitation of the spinal cord injured person. *Clinical Orthopedics and Related Research* 112 (Oct.): 81–88. *Discussion of "normal" reaction to the experienced loss, observations of people with preexisting psychopathology, and exploration of psychological aspects of pain, sexual adjustment, and the impact on the family. Gives insight into the process of adjustment. Highly recommended.*

Judd, F. K., and Burrows, G. D. 1986. Liaison psychiatry in a spinal injuries unit. *Paraplegia* 24 (1): 6–20. *Examines implications of mistakenly held beliefs about adaptation to injury in achieving both short- and long-term goals of rehabilitation.*

Judd, F. K., Burrows, G. D., and Brown, D. J. 1986. Depression following acute spinal cord injury. *Paraplegia* 24 (6): 358–363. *Describes successful treatment with antidepressant for those accurately diagnosed. Differentiates depressive illness from grief reaction with implications for rehabilitation.*

Kirnbakaran, V. R. 1986. Survey of alcohol and drug misuse in spinal cord injured veterans. *Journal of the Study of Alcohol* 47 (3): 223–227. *Study indicates that alcohol and drug abuse is far less than in the general population.*

Kozier, B., and Erb, G. 1991. *Fundamentals of Nursing.* 4th ed. Menlo Park, CA: Addison-Wesley. *Review of development of self-concept and self-esteem.*

Lawson, N. C. 1978. Significant events in the rehabilitation process: the spinal cord patient's point of view. *Archives of Physical Medicine and Rehabilitation* 59 (Dec.): 573–579. *Report of a research study using tape-recorded daily logs, hospital staff ratings, behavioral measure of verbal output, and an endocrine measure to determine significant events during hospitalization. Results suggest that prolonged depression is counterproductive to the rehabilitation process and that important people in the patient's life exert a most significant influence. Discusses programmatic implications.*

Leinart, B. K. 1979. Attitudes of nurses toward spinal cord injury patients. *Journal of Association or Rehabilitation Nurses* 4 (Jan./Feb.): 7–9. *A comparison of attitudes of nurses working in acute, intermediate, and rehabilitation areas; stresses the importance of professional attitudes as an integral force determining the degree of success in patient adjustment to disability.*

MacLean, S. 1981. Discharge planning for spinal cord injured patients. Unpublished material. University of British Columbia, Vancouver, BC. *Examines the rehabilitation process as it applies to three young quadriplegic patients.*

Maddox, S. 1987. *Spinal Network.* Boulder, CO: Sam Maddox, Publisher. *A true network and fine resource designed to connect persons* with spinal cord injuries to ideals, experiences, and resources in the spinal cord injury "community" to become aware of the variety of choices open to reach personal goals. Invaluable to injured individuals, families, and friends and also for health professionals for insight into the real world of disability. This resource is a must.

Malec, J. 1982. Cannabis effect on spasticity and spinal cord injury Archives of Physical Medicine and Rehabilitation 63: 116–118.

Morant, C. 1978. The role of a psychiatrist on an acute spinal cord injury unit. Unpublished material. Shaughnessy Hospital, Vancouver, BC. Focuses on the role of the psychiatrist in managing stress encountered by the interdisciplinary team.

Orbaan, I. 1986. Psychological adjustment problems in people with traumatic spinal cord lesions. Acta Neurochir (Wein) 79 (1): 58–61. Results from this study show that the level at which a lesion occurs has no effect on the adjustment process.

Ostrow, N. A. 1985. The psychiatric spinal cord injured patient. Spinal Cord Injury Nursing 2 (2): 18–19. Encourages introspective examination of our beliefs and actions and calls for liaison activities with those involved in counseling professions.

Pires, M. 1989. Substance abuse: The silent saboteur in rehabilitation. Nursing Clinics of North America 24 (1): 291–296. Calls for cross-consultation between rehabilitation and mental health specialists to help patients, families, and staff deal with this escalating problem.

Richmond, T. S., and Metcalf, J. A. 1986. Psychosocial responses to spinal cord injury. Journal of Neuroscience Nursing August, 18 (4): 183–187. Details the concepts of disturbances in self-esteem, powerlessness, functional grieving, and alteration in family process in the framework of nursing diagnoses.

Roglitz, C. 1978. Team approach in the acute phase of spinal cord injury. Journal of Neurosurgical Nursing 10 (3): 117–120. Focuses on the interaction between the nurse and the social worker to enhance staff communication, development, involvement, and understanding of others, which ultimately improves quality of individualized patient care.

Roy, C., Sr. 1976. Introduction to Nursing: An Adaptation Model. Englewood Cliffs, NJ: Prentice-Hall. Presents a model of nursing focusing on the nurse's role as a helper to patients in adapting to stress rather than a provider in meeting needs. In-depth exploration of self-concept, self-esteem, role function, the physical self and experiencing loss, and related problems in these and other areas.

Sadlick, M., and Penta, F. B. 1975. Changing nurse attitudes toward quadriplegics through use of television. Rehabilitation Literature 36 (9): 274–278. A technique for promoting more positive attitudes toward potential patient outcomes during rehabilitation.

Shontz, F. 1975. The Psychological Aspects of Physical Illness and Disability. New York: Macmillan. Superior background reading exploring cyclical adjustment to disability.

Steinglass, P. 1982. Coping with spinal cord injury: The family perspective. General Hospital Psychiatry 4: 259–264. Focuses on family responses and points out the need for staff to recognize coping mechanisms families use to cope with both acute and chronic phases of disability.

Szasz, G. 1980. A guide to the interpersonal skills of history-taking. Beta Release (Journal of the Canadian Diabetes Association) 5 (2): 2–8. A clear and concise practical overview, especially for the student professional, to enhance the skills of interviewing in clinical situations. Highly recommended.

Thomas, E. J. 1966. Problems of disability from the perspective of role theory. Journal of Health and Human Behavior 7 (1) Spring: 2–14. Examines with insight acquisition of new behaviors and roles.

Thompson, D. D., and Lott, J. D. 1980. Psychosocial redevelopment of the spinal cord injured person. Spinal Cord Injury Digest 2 (Winter): 6–9. Description of the psychosocial aspects of treatment, rehabilitation, and community environment and how these relate to reprocessing of Erikson's life span development stages.

Trieschmann, R. 1980. Spinal Cord Injures, Psychological, Social and Vocational Adjustment. New York: Demos Publications. Exclusively devoted to the psychosocial impact of SCI. Includes an exhaustive critique of the literature with a view to dispelling myths and stimulating research to develop future strategies.

Tucker, S. J. 1980. The psychology of spinal cord injury: patient-staff interaction. Rehabilitation Literature 41 (5–6): 114–121. Reviews and analyzes current knowledge about the psychology of spinal cord injury; focuses on the emotional reactions of the patient and the less-recognized but vitally important emotional reactions of the staff. The author is a psychotherapist and has a spinal cord injury herself. Extensive selective bibliography.

Vash, C. 1981. Disability as a transcendental experience: A personal perspective on learning to live with a disability. In Treatment of the Spinal Cord Injured—An Interdisciplinary Perspective. Eds. M. Eisenberg and J. Falconer. Springfield, IL: Charles C. Thomas Publisher.

Virginia Spinal Cord Injury System, University of Virginia Center and Virginia Department of Rehabilitation Services, Woodrow Wilson Rehabilitation Center, 1988. Virginia Spinal Cord Injury Care and Teaching Manual. 1980. Fisherville, VA: Author. Approach directed to patient and family regarding psychosocial and sexual issues.

Weller, D. J., and Miller, P. M. 1977a. Emotional reactions of patient, family, and staff in acute-care period of spinal cord injury: part I. Social Work Health Care 2 (Summer): 369–377. Describes and analyzes stages of adjustment in the acute postinjury period with treatment implications and their significance in later rehabilitation. Focuses on introductory material and patient responses.

———. 1977b. Emotional reactions of patient, family, and staff in acute-care period of spinal cord injury: part 2. Social Work Health Care 3 (Fall): 7–17. Considers emotional reactions of family members and staff with further implications for treatment.

Williams, J. M., and Kay, T. Eds. 1990. Head Injury, A Family Matter. Baltimore: Paul H. Brookes Publishing Co. Superb resource tackles tough issues from dealing with behavioral problems of individuals to divorce within families and presents models to deal with these consequences. Guidance applicable for those coping with spinal cord injuries.

Wool, R. N., et al. 1980. Task performance in spinal cord injury: effect of helplessness training. *Archives of Physical Medicine and Rehabilitation* 61 (July): 321–325. *Explores possibility of significantly influencing psychological recovery by using rehabilitation strategy aimed at providing success experiences.*

Wortman, C., and Silver, R. C. 1989. The myths of coping with loss. *Journal of Consulting and Clinical Psychology* 57 (3): 349–357. *Expectations of depression as inevitable following loss are examined. Mistaken assumptions held about loss fail to acknowledge variability in coping with loss and may lead professionals to respond in unhelpful ways to people for whom they care.*

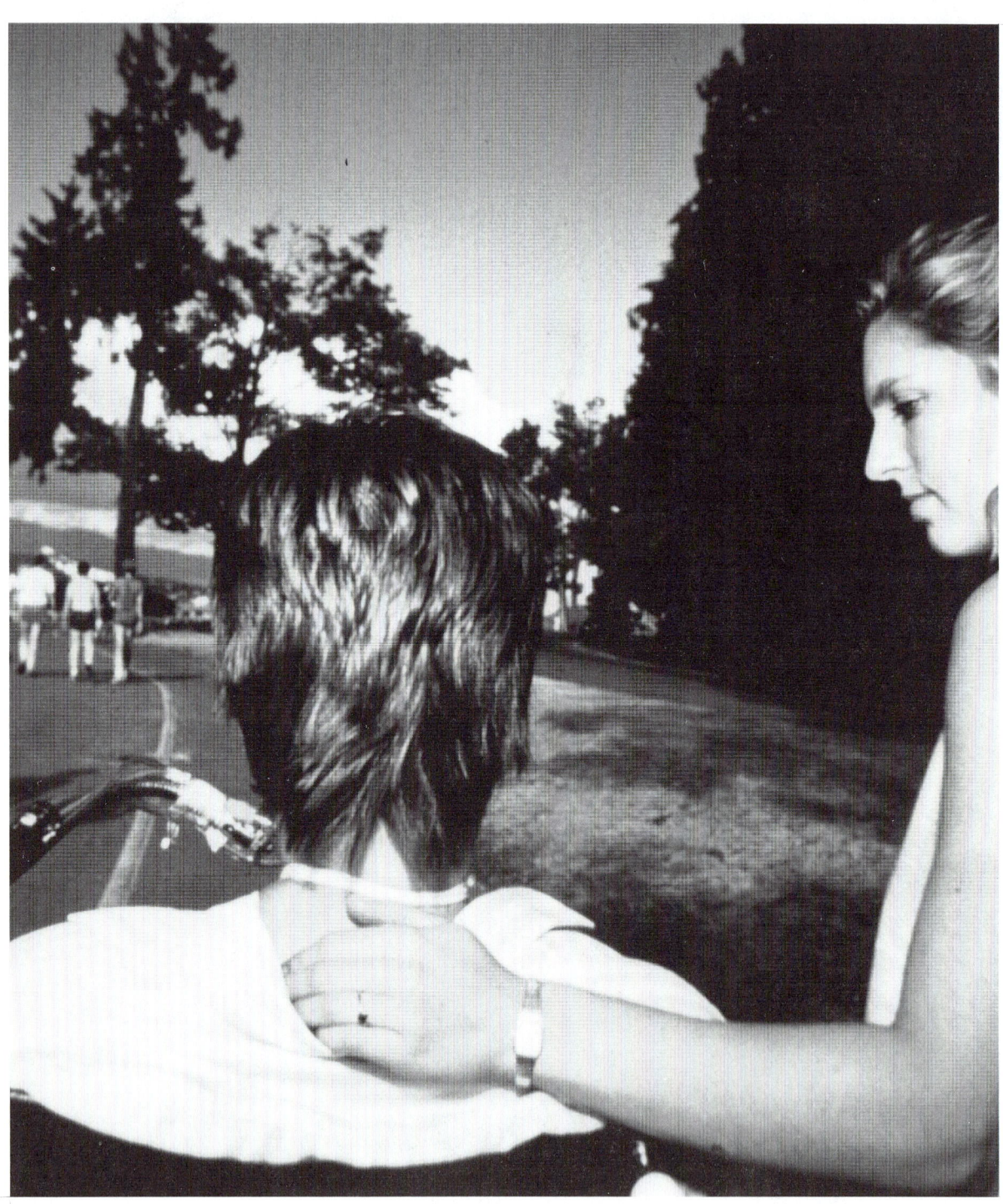

CHAPTER
— 10 —

Sexual Health Care*

George Szasz, M.D.

Chapter Outline

Sexual Health Objectives

- To understand the sexual consequences of SCI
- To understand current approaches to sexual health management
- To describe sexual health care methods for the nonspecialist care giver
- To develop communication skills to obtain and give sexual information
- To develop an awareness of personal attitudes, recognize personal limitations, and seek assistance when needed

*The help of Joan Stradiotti and Shirley Haliday, sexual health clinicians, is acknowledged.

A 52-year-old woman, married for 28 years and the mother of three sons, suffered an incomplete injury to the C_{6-7} segments in a car accident. Two months after her injury, and just after her husband left at the end of visiting hours, she turned to the nurse: "I think I want to talk to somebody about our sexual life. This was very important to my husband . . . to me too. You know . . . not that we are like kids, but we enjoy each other. I guess I can live without it, but it was so much a part of our life."

It is not surprising that this woman turned to her nurse for help, but what did she expect of the nurse? This is how the woman explained it: "I don't know. I didn't know who to talk to. I know that my husband is worried, but he's so shy. I suppose he could go to our family doctor, or the doctors here, but they're all so busy, and there's no privacy here. Actually I feel embarrassed about the whole thing. Talking about sex somehow doesn't fit in with all these sick people. . . . And here I am . . . middle aged, can't move my legs, can't even urinate without help. I guess I should worry about the legs and forget the sex part, and yet, I can't. I thought the nurse might have some answers. How do other women get over this? Is sex over? Or can I do something? Will I satisfy my husband? Will I feel anything? Will my husband ever look at me like he used to?"

This woman's questions are not unusual at all. In the last few years increasing numbers of patients, partners, and family members want intelligent exploration of their sexual dysfunctions and disabilities. Anticipating patients' requests for information, a number of spinal cord injury (SCI) units and rehabilitation centers have begun programs that consider patients' sexual needs. The role of the care givers in this has not been clear. For example, should care givers be involved in sexual care? If so, should this involvement be limited to informal and private discussions with the patient, or should it be a formally assigned task? In either case, should the interaction be reported at the team meetings? Should the patient's physicians be informed about the patient's concerns? Should care givers give advice? If so, what guiding principles should be followed? Who should set these? To whom should the care givers be accountable if something goes wrong, and who should give them feedback for excellence in the practice of sexual health care? What roles should be assumed by physicians, nurses, physical therapists, occupational therapists, psychologists, or social workers? Or should there be a separate "sexual health care service" staffed with specially trained personnel? If so, what would be expected of care givers, and how could they make the best use of such a service? The answers to these questions are now evolving. The purpose of this chapter is to help this evolution.

HEALTH CARE GOALS

Goals of health care for helping patients and families adjust to sexual consequences of SCI are:

- To provide a comprehensive service, including assessment and treatment of physical, social, and emotional components of patients' sexual functioning
- To make available early consultation services to all patients and families
- To offer continuous assessment, education, and therapeutic features to patients and families as they move through various stages of rehabilitation

SEXUAL CONSEQUENCES OF SPINAL CORD INJURY

Sexual Health and Sexual Losses

The meanings of *sexual health* and *sexual losses* vary greatly. For example, what is normal and healthy in sex, and how would one define a patient as sexually healthy? Put another way, at what point would health professionals want to be involved with a patient's sexual life to save that patient from sexual ill health, and at what point would health professionals say: "The treatment is finished; our tests show that you are now sexually healthy"? The consideration of this fundamental question has to be sidestepped in this chapter. Not enough is known about the biology of sexual behavior to declare that, for example, continuation of various sex practices is a condition of good health and therefore sexual health care is a must for every patient. Also, sexual losses mean different things to different people. For example, a surgeon was overheard to say: "If I had a spinal injury, the last thing I would worry about is sex." A nurse said: "I applied to work on this unit because they have a sex rehabilitation program here." A 24-year-old patient who suffered an incomplete lesion in the lower lumbar and sacral neurological levels said: "You know, it just kills me to think that I might never get it up, you know, hard like it used to be. I just don't feel like being complete. I feel sexless. There's a void . . . as if I wasn't a man anymore." A 42-year-old married man who suffered a complete injury to the T_{10-11} area commented: "We are just thankful to God that I survived. We have three healthy children. Sex was not that important to my wife, and now it's not important to me either." A staff member in an acute SCI unit was overheard to complain: "If he could get his mind off sex, he might do okay. Doesn't he understand that he has got to do his physical therapy?"

The surgeon who would not worry about sexual losses explained what he meant by saying, "As far as love is concerned, yes, at first, intercourse had a lot to do with it, but now our relationship doesn't stand or fall with it. If I were in this situation and had a choice, I would rather walk than get sexual feelings back. I can't see myself without my work." The nurse explained that to her, intimate physical acts were the way to express love and affection. She said, "I was married before. Sex problems were the cause of our deepest distress. Now I wish we could have gone for help." The young man said, "To me sex means pleasure. It's also a way to show how much I like my partner. I also wanted to have a child. It's the difference between being a boy and being a man." The older man said, "We used to enjoy intercourse. Stimulation with the hand? No! That's for kids. I don't think my wife would stand for that anyway! Best to forget it." The staff member who complained about a young man's preoccupation said: "Yes, of course, sex is important, but everything has its time and place. This is time for physical therapy, not for sex. Besides, this is a hospital, not a pleasure dome."

The variety of interpretations of what sex is about or what a sexual loss may represent makes it virtually impossible to organize a sexual health care service with the universality, urgency, and discipline of, for example, a bladder or bowel care program. An added complication is that although some patients are distressed enough to say that "life is not worthwhile" without access to the sexual options (whatever this may mean to the individual), most patients and their partners feel embarrassed about expressing sexual needs at any time, but particularly at the time of a physical crisis. The roots of these feelings are part of our cultural heritage, which still holds that sexual desirability and the right to sexual practices belong to the young, the healthy, the whole, and the beautiful. Even though these ideas have begun to change outside the walls of hospitals and long-term care institutions, the change within is slow. Some professionals unwittingly stifle patients' expressions of sexual problems because never having received training in this area, they are not sure how to assess or treat patients suffering from these problems. Many patients have a sense of foreboding about their sexual losses, but they have no words to specify their complaints, even if they have the courage to complain. This is why care givers may be approached with mumbled comments, like "I guess I will be a bachelor for life," or "Maybe my wife should get another man," or "I won't be attractive to him now."

Many patients will require a list to decide areas that might fall into the "sex" category. Staff members would also find the answers to specific questions valuable because these could reflect the patient's "sexual functioning status" before the injury at the time of admission to the hospital and at various occasions thereafter (Szasz 1987a).

A patient's sexual functioning status can be categorized in the following terms:

1. *Sexual response status* reflects the physiological ability of the patient to experience genital sensations, erection, ejaculation, vaginal lubrication, orgasm, pelvic thrusting, and other responses to stimulation.

2. *Sexual activity status* indicates the available motor functions that might be used, for example, for embracing, caressing, and intercourse.

3. *Sexual interest status* reveals the degree to which the patient wants to be involved in sex activities.

4. *Sexual behavior status* gives information about availability of partners and the skills in social interaction processes that may lead to sexual activities.

5. *Sex organ status* describes the anatomical integrity of the genitalia and the sexual problems caused by urinary drainage apparatus, genitourinary infections, or surgery.

6. *Fertility status* reveals evidence of the need or ability to procreate or the nature of contraception desired.

In the following pages these categories are discussed in more detail. Because these categories overlap, they will be grouped under three headings:

1. *Sexual response*
2. *Sexual practice* (including the interest, activity, and behavior status categories and the condition of the genitalia)
3. *Fertility* (including contraceptive issues)

The section on *sexual response* will be the largest, because the physical methods of its assessment will also be included.

Sexual Response

In conceptualizing the sexual physiological damage in SCI, it is useful to think of the sexual response as a complex reflex. Like other reflexes, this one requires certain stimuli to initiate reactions, nerve tracks to carry the stimuli to various centers, returning nerve tracks, and organs that react. One characteristic of the sexual response is that the reaction of the genitalia sets off further stimuli, which in turn escalate the intensity of the sexual response. Another characteristic of this response is that eventually the whole body becomes involved in the process so that apart from genital changes there may be changes in muscular tension, blood pressure and heart rate, and perhaps even the level of certain hormones circulating in the body. The stimuli may be "mental"—erotic materials, situations, or thoughts—or "touch"—applied to the genitalia or to other parts of the body. Rhythmic rubbing action applied to the genitalia is usually the most effective stimulating action in a person with intact neurological pathways. If carried on long enough, such stimulation may lead to a full sexual response. In men the genital aspects of this response include erection of the penis and orgasm. The male orgasm has two parts: an inner tension caused by the secretion of seminal fluid, and the pleasurable release of this tension in the ejaculation of the seminal fluid. In women these two parts of the orgasm are not well identified, but the orgasmic experience starts with a suffusion of warmth in the vaginal area, increase in the lubrication, and strong inner tension, and ends with pleasurable release.

Rhythmic rubbing of the breasts, neck, inner thighs, perineum, or perianal areas may also produce high sexual tension and may lead to orgasmic responses. It is not understood yet how the brain identifies a stimulus as sexual or nonsexual. For example, stimuli arising from washing the genitalia, examining the breast, dressing or undressing, combing hair, or body contact when lifting could be identified as sexual by the brain of the receiver, even though the giver or doer (the nurse or the physician) had no sexual intention at all. The nerve tracks in the brain and the neural reactions necessary to translate a situation or an action into a sexual response are also not well understood.

Spinal Cord Centers for Erection and Vaginal Lubrication

There seem to be two spinal cord centers for the neurological management of the penile erection and the vaginal lubrication process—the S_{2-4} and the T_{11-12}-L_1 regions. Stimuli from the genitalia are carried to the sacral center by the pudendal nerve and by autonomic sensory pathways that have not yet been clearly identified.

Mental stimuli are processed in the brain and are carried through as yet unidentified spinal cord tracks to the centers at the lower thoracic and high lumbar segments. The activities arising out of these two centers are controlled by higher centers in the brain, but the location of the brain centers is not clear. It is likely that the spinal cord centers to do with erection (and possibly with vaginal lubrication) receive continuous inhibitory signals from the brain so that erection may occur only when these signals diminish or stop. It is not clear whether additional excitatory stimuli are needed in the relevant spinal segments of neurologically intact persons.

In a complete injury of the spinal cord, the brain becomes disconnected from the spinal cord segments below the lesion. The erection centers located in those segments become liberated from the brain's controlling influence and thus erection becomes a reflex function.

Spinal Cord Centers for Ejaculation and Orgasm

The neurological site of the mental or sensory aspect of orgasmic experience is not known. The physical events associated with orgasm, including the internal vaginal changes in women and the process of ejaculation in men seem to be located in the T_{12}–L_{1-2} and the S_{2-4} segments. Although the erection and ejaculation functions seem to be mediated through similar areas of the spinal cord, each of these functions can occur in the absence of the other.

With regard to ejaculation, studies on animals suggest that the T_{12}–L_2 spinal cord segments are responsible for sperm transport along the vas deferens, contraction of the seminal vesicles, injection of semen into the prostate, initiation of prostatic fluid secretion, and closure of the internal bladder neck. The S_{2-4} spinal cord segments are thought to send both somatic and parasympathetic signals to release the external sphincter and to activate contractions of the urethra. These contractions, along with the pelvic muscle contractions mediated by somatic nerves, cause the forward ejaculation of the seminal fluid.

Although there is no comparable female response, the vaginal changes (swelling of the vaginal wall, expansion of the inner third of the vagina, tenting, or dipping of the uterus into the vagina) are probably brought about by neurological action at thoracolumbar and sacral cord levels.

The neurological sites mediating the orgasmic sensations are not known. The lateral spinothalamic tracts (which also carry heat, cold, and pain stimuli) are probably the main signal conductors between the genitalia and the thalamus region of the brain.

Sexual Response with Complete Injuries

When SCI is complete at any level, the brain becomes isolated from signals arising in the genitalia. While erection and vaginal lubrication may still occur in response to either touch or mental stimuli, there can be no orgasmic response arising from or detected in the genitalia. However, pleasure sensations or intense sexual experiences are possible either through mental stimulation or physical stimulation of neurologically intact areas (particularly breasts, neck, earlobes, face, back of the neck). Some men and women with complete injuries describe these experiences as very similar to what they have known in their preinjury experience as an orgasm. Others say that "if an orgasm is like being at the peak of a mountain, then my present sensations are like being on the flat top of a small hill." Intense sexual experiences may also occur in the context of fantasy or dreams.

Erection responses in men with complete SCI at various levels are predictable in theory, but the clinical realities are influenced by a number of factors. If the complete injury is anywhere above S_{2-4}, the erection-mediating centers in the sacral area will be abandoned by the brain, and the centers will freely respond, so that any physical touch of the genitalia will evoke an erection response. Maintenance of this erection is dependent on repeat stimulation of the reflex arc.

If the complete SCI is in the S_{2-4} segments, the touch-stimulation-based erection will not be possible. However, in such a case erection based on the activation of the centers in the lower thoracic and high lumbar areas is still possible. Now the stimulus must be of the mental kind. Signals coming from the brain may activate the thoracolumbar center and may cause the beginning of an erection. However, mental stimulation is more likely to lead to a penile swelling than to a full erection. The reason for the qualitative differences between the strength of touch related to mental erection is not clear. Seminal fluid leakage may also occur during mental erection. This is probably brought about by the neurological impulses arising from the lower thoracic segments.

A proper ejaculation (usually expected in the course of sexual practices or in the form of nocturnal emission) rarely occurs in men with complete injuries. In some men oral stimulation of the tip of the penis or very active stimulation of the penis may lead to ejaculation (but not orgasm).

Two forms of artificial stimulation can be of value in causing ejaculation of seminal fluid: (1) through vibratory stimulation of the tip of the penis, and (2) electrical stimulation of the nerves close to the prostate gland. Both methods were first popularized by Brindley (1981). Since then a number of investigators have applied these stimulations to men with various SCI levels.

Vibratory stimulation of the penis is applicable only to men with injury above T_{10}. The reason for this seems to be that the vibration stimuli must excite both the S_{2-4} and the $T_{12}–L_{1-2}$ segments (as well as the connection between these segments) for ejaculation to occur. The vibrator method is useful for about 65% of men with SCI above T_{10}. The electroejaculation method has been adapted from veterinary science. Electrical stimuli are applied with various types of probes, which stimulate the peripheral nerves lying in the proximity of the prostate gland. This method is useful for about 70% of the men with SCI. It is not clear why some men do not respond to this form of stimulation. With both methods the ejaculation may be antegrade or retrograde,

and may be mixed with urine, so that the ejaculate may have to be cleaned in laboratory procedures before using for artificial insemination of the partner. See further comments in this chapter's section on fertility. Men with SCI in or above T_4 may experience autonomic dysreflexia when exposed to stimulation by vibrator or by electroejaculation techniques. Acute blood pressure elevation may be followed by severe headaches that may last for minutes or hours. For this reason, men with high SCI are discouraged from using the vibrator without consulting their physicians. Antihypertensive medications may prevent the occurrence of ejaculation-related autonomic dysreflexia.

The following examples illustrate some concerns about losses in genital sensations, ability to have predictable erections, ejaculations, vaginal lubrication, or orgasm. Table 10–1 and Figures 10–1 to 10–3 explain the reasons for the patients' problems. (Some of the explanations are provided in italics.)

A 36-year-old man, married for eight years, suffered a complete C_{4-5} injury. While still in the intensive care unit, he asked the nurse for a mirror to see his penis while he was being catheterized. "How come I have an erection when I can't feel anything? Will that last?"

(Complete injury to the C_{4-5} cord levels stops incoming signals from the genitalia from reaching the brain. There

TABLE 10–1 Guidelines to Expected Sexual Dysfunctions Following Complete SCI

	$T_{10}–L_1$ Segments or Above	$L_2–S_1$ Segments	$S_2–S_4$ Segments
Genital Sensations	Lost: communication between genitalia and the brain is interrupted	Lost: vague internal feelings possible; some visceral connections to brain still present	Lost: communication between genitalia and the brain interrupted
Erection (Touch)	Still possible: sacral segments intact; genital-sacral reflex connection intact. Called somatic or touch reflex erection	Possible: sacral reflex connection intact	Not possible: sacral segment destroyed and genital-sacral reflex lost
Erection (Mental)	Not possible: fibers coming to $T_{10}–L_1$ segments, bringing necessary signals, are interrupted	May be possible: sympathetic pathways from brain open to bring necessary signals to $T_{10}–L_1$	May be possible: $T_{10}–L_1$ segments intact and still able to mediate signals from brain; called mental or psychogenic erection
Ejaculation/Orgasm	Not possible: necessary genital-brain-genital contact lost	Cannot occur: necessary genital-brain-genital contact lost. Seminal flow possible because sympathetic fibers coming to $T_{10}–L_1$ may bring necessary signals	Not possible: genital-brain-genital contact lost. In male, seminal flow may be possible because signals originating in brain and coming through sympathetic fibers to $T_{10}–L_1$ can reach genitalia. For reasons not understood these signals may diminish mental erection
Erotic Mental Feelings	May be experienced: pulse rate and blood pressure changes possible if mouth, neck, and other intact areas stimulated	May be experienced: pulse and blood pressure changes possible if intact areas of body stimulated	May be experienced: pulse rate and blood pressure changes possible if intact areas of body stimulated

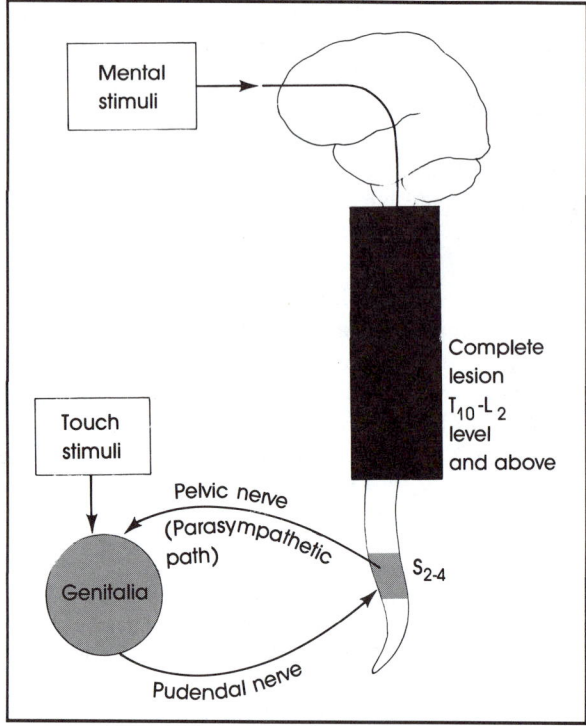

FIGURE 10–1 Complete injuries at T_{10}–L_2 or above allow touch erection/lubrication. Ejaculation and orgasm in men and orgasm in women is not possible from ordinary genital stimulation.

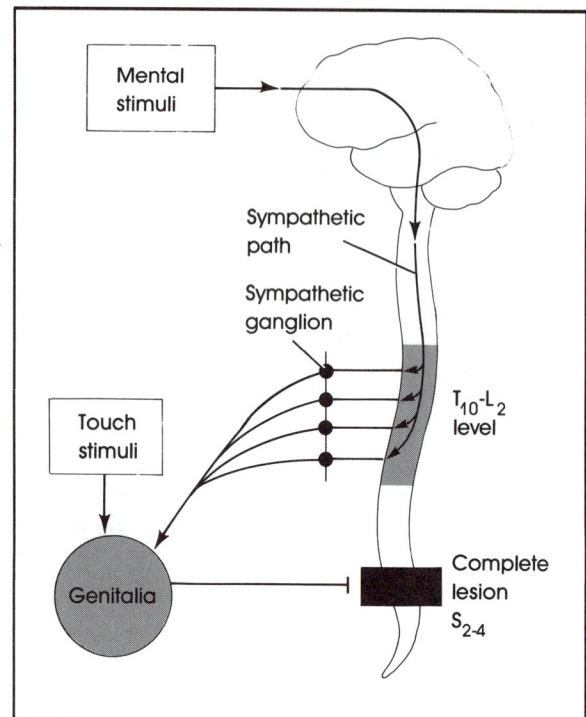

FIGURE 10–2 Complete injuries at S_{2-4} and below allow mental erection and seminal flow in men. Orgasm is not possible from genital stimulation.

will be no genital sensation or ejaculation and orgasm arising from genital stimulation. Brain control over erection has been released and touch will cause lasting erection.)

A 28-year-old man, unmarried but living with a female partner, was injured in the sacral area. He was already walking with crutches and braces when he said: "I can't understand it. I get a bit of swelling in my penis when I am in bed with her. Then I get a sticky fluid coming out of my penis—just a few drops—and then all the swelling is gone. It kills me! I feel like . . . I feel worthless. What's the use? I'm not even half a man."

(The sacral area was damaged, and potential for touch reflex erection is gone. Mental stimuli may get through the T_{10}–L_1 segments, causing some erection. The same fibers also carry signals for seminal flow. For reasons not yet understood, when flow occurs erection usually diminishes.)

A 42-year-old married woman with a T_{12} complete injury said: "Orgasm was very important to me. Any chance for it now?"

(Not from genital stimulation. Whenever the injury is complete, genital signals cannot get to the brain to generate neuromuscular tensions. However, she may become highly responsive to face, neck, and breast stimulation.)

Sexual Response with Incomplete Injuries

The effects of incomplete injuries on the sexual response depend on the damage to the specific pathways and cellular

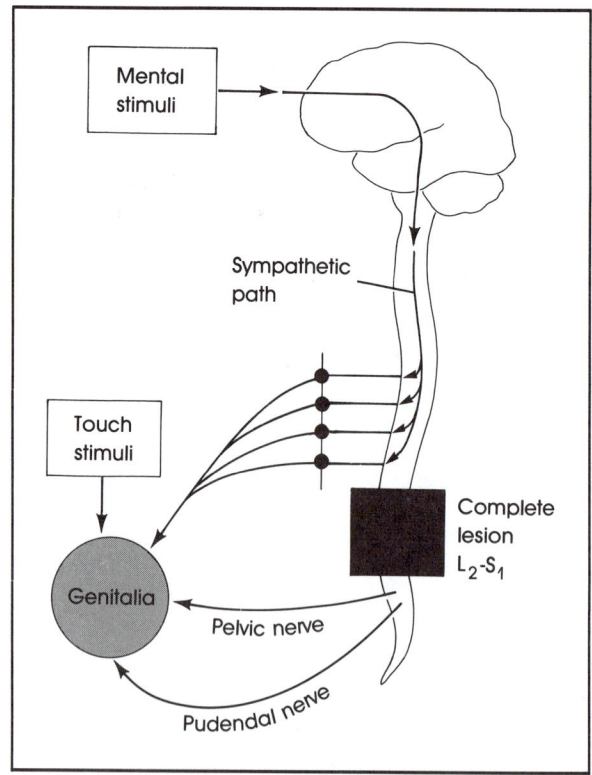

FIGURE 10–3 Complete injuries at L_2–S_1 result in a dissociated reaction. Both touch and mental erections asre possible in men, but these are not coordinated. Orgasm in men and women is not possible from genital stimulation.

structures. For example, in central cord lesions, the sexual response might not be disturbed. If a partial lesion involves the dorsolateral or ventrolateral sides of the cord, sensory or motor sparing may occur and some aspects of the response may be possible. If the lesion is a hemisection of the cord (Brown-Séquard's syndrome), some responses remain, but the eventual outcome is not predictable. Incomplete injuries are detailed in Chapter 4.

Some people falsely believe that the less complete an injury is, the more sexual functioning potential is retained. This is not usually so. Although complete damage still permits the functioning of certain necessary reflex arcs, it does so because the spinal cord segment is isolated from the brain. Partial damage may not only interfere with these arcs, but may permit the inhibiting influence of the brain to further interfere with reflex responses.

Diagnostic Tests

Two tests can determine if male or female orgasmic reactions might occur in response to genital stimulation.

1.   The *pain* or *heat/cold sensation test* is used to check out the sensory pathways between the genitalia and the brain. A pin or hot/cold stimuli are used to find out if the patient can feel pain or differentiate between various temperature levels in the genital region. These tests give information about the lateral spinothalamic tracts. The tracts are considered intact if a pinprick on the penis or on a woman's genital area is immediately perceived as sharp and painful (Figure 10–4), or if hot and cold stimuli are immediately and correctly identified.

2.   Another test requires the patient to *contract the anal opening on command*. This test provides information about the motor fibers going to the genitalia from the brain, along the fibers of the pyramidal tract systems. If the patient can correctly perceive pain, heat, or cold and is able to contract the anus voluntarily, the basic tracts are open for genital sensation and for male and female orgasmic reaction. If either one or both of these tests are negative, the patient will not be able to experience orgasm or ejaculation from ordinary genital stimulation because somewhere along these nerve tracts an injury has occurred, blocking signals from reaching the brain. Three reflexes are tested to clarify the situation with regard to reflex touch or mental erection:

- Squeezing the tip of the penis normally elicits the *bulbocavernosus reflex*. See Figure 10–5. This indicates that the sacral segments of the spinal cord are open, and reflex touch erection is likely to occur.

The significance of the bulbocavernosus for women is still not understood. The bulbocavernosus reflex can be tested in women by pressing the clitoris to elicit anal contraction.

- The examiner's finger is placed in the patient's anus to test for the *anal tone reflex*. See Figure 10–6. Contraction of the internal muscles over the

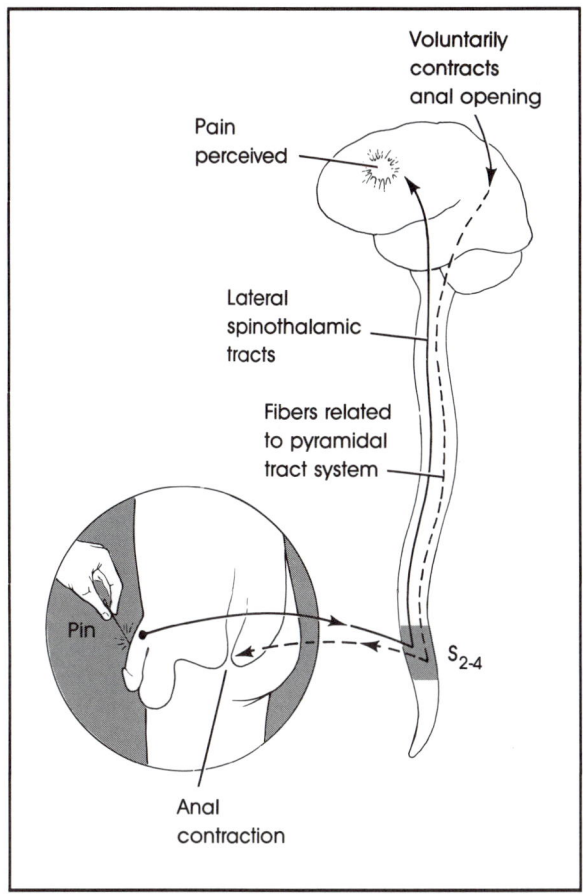

FIGURE 10–4   Testing the lateral spinothalamic tract and descending fibers of the pyramidal tract system. If both are open, genital sensation and orgasm are likely.

examiner's finger indicates that this reflex is still intact, which confirms that both the sacral and the lumbar segments of the cord are intact. When both the bulbocavernosus and the anal tone reflexes are present, the reflex touch erection is usually strong, because the level of the injury is higher up in the cord. When the bulbocavernosus and the anal tone reflexes are absent, touch reflex erections will be absent, too. However, mental reflex erections may occur if the cord injury is below the T_9 level.

Although the anal tone is tested in the same manner for women as for men, the significance of this reflex is not understood either.

- To find out if the injury is below or above the T_9 level, the examiner squeezes the testicles to elicit pain. See Figure 10–7. The sensory fibers of the testicle enter the spinal cord at the T_9 level. If the patient cannot feel any sensation when the testicles are squeezed, the lesion is above the T_9 level, and there is no possibility for mental erections, because the fibers necessary for this type of erection emerge at around T_{10-12}. However, if the patient experi-

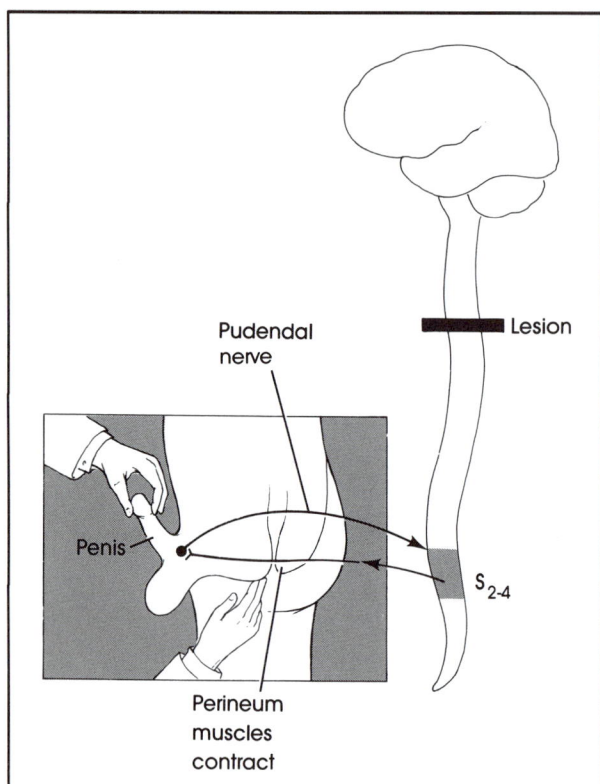

FIGURE 10–5 Testing the bulbocavernosus reflex in men. If present, sacral segment is open. Injury must be above sacral segments. In men touch erection is likely.

ences acute testicular discomfort, the injury is likely to be below T_{10-12}, and the chances are strong that mental erection may occur.

On rare occasions SCI occurs at L_2–S_1, so that the bulbocavernosus, anal tone, and testicular pain reflexes can be elicited, but there is no perception of pain in the genitalia, no anal tone, and no voluntary ability to contract the anus. In such a situation both mental and touch reflex erection may be expected, although of poor quality. Orgasm and ejaculation will still not be possible.

Dysfunctions Related to Time after Injury

When the reflexes begin to return after the initial period of spinal shock, some of the sexual responses may be exaggerated. For example, in a person with complete high quadriplegia, strong and lasting erections may occur in response to even the gentlest genital irritation. This response may last for days and must be differentiated from *priapism*, which is an erection due to clotting of the blood in the penis. If the erect penis becomes even more erect with touch or if erection subsides when touch is removed, the condition is not likely to be priapism.

Erection in response to mental stimulation may not appear for several months after the injury. It is not known why this time delay occurs.

Touch reflex erection is remarkably stable over the years. Men whose injury may have occurred 35 to 40 years ago still may experience this reflex. Mental reflex erection is subject to situational influences.

Other Factors Influencing the Sexual Response

An interesting feature of erections related to mental stimulation is that they may be accompanied by a flow of prostatic fluid. Often when this secretion appears, the erection weakens. The mental stimulation may be something seen, heard, imagined, or dreamed. Touching on the chest, neck, ears, or throat may also provide mental stimulation. Some women report orgasmic experiences during dreams or when strongly concentrating on erotic fantasy. Spinal cord injured men do not seem to have this facility. Erections resulting from mental stimulation may be subject to interference by concerns over ability to perform sexually, by preoccupations with other worries, by depression and anger, and by centrally acting sedatives or tranquilizers, including alcohol.

The somatic or touch reflex erection may be negatively influenced by some antispasticity medication. Both somatic

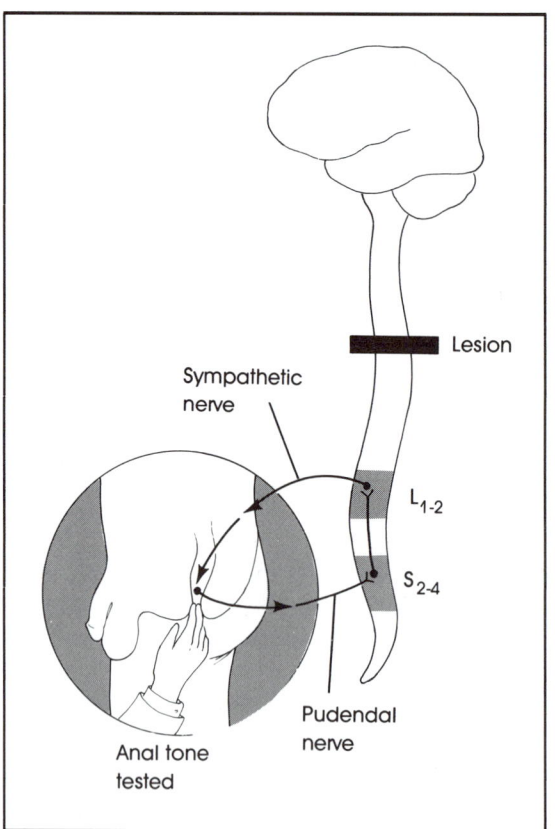

FIGURE 10–6 Testing the anal tone. If present, sacral and lower thoracic and high lumbar segments are open. Injury must be above L_1. In men touch erection is likely to be strong.

and mental reflex erections may be lost by an external sphincterotomy. Although no clear risk figures are available, reports suggest that less than 20% of the patients having the operation suffer this side effect.

Sexual Practices

Three categories of the sexual functioning status will be reviewed under this heading: sexual interest, sexual activities, and sexual behavior.

Interest

Sexual interest and disinterest are poorly understood even in the able-bodied person. *Interest* is often a combination of desire to experience certain sensations arising from caressing or genital play, the wish to be sexually useful to a partner, and the hope that one will be a desirable partner. Without regard to the extent of the injury, motivation to engage in various sex acts may be related to the need for intimacy, feelings of belonging, and pleasure; mutual search for orgasmic experiences; expression of love, affection, and passion; or a need for relief from anxiety and boredom.

A 24-year-old married woman suffered T_{12}–L_1 complete injury. One year after the injury she said: "You know, I'm really horny, and it's in my head. I never thought how much sex has to do with your head, but sitting in this wheelchair is like being isolated. I used to get a kick out of chasing my husband when he came out of the bathroom. Now I have to close my eyes and think back to the good old days."

Sexual *disinterest* can be caused by chronic pain, discomfort, malaise, and tiredness related to the complications of SCI. Sedatives, antispasticity medications, and psychotherapeutic drugs may temporarily depress interest level; and drab living quarters or the physical environment of hospitals or institutional settings may also diminish sexual interest.

Four weeks after his injury a 32-year-old unmarried man with an incomplete C_{6-7} injury said, "You know, sex just hasn't been on my mind at all. I'm not surprised, mind you . . . too much else on my mind. Also I haven't slept well for days. It worries me a bit. I used to be pretty active."

Still other negative factors include preoccupation and worry about finances, the job situation, and housing; relationship discord; depression and feelings of hopelessness; and sexual dysfunctions that either existed before the injury or were caused by the neurological damage.

On some occasions the partner's disinterest is more significant than the injured person's loss of zest.

A 57-year-old married man, injured at the C_{5-6} level at age 45 and now with complete quadriplegia, said: "Yes, I do get the occasional desire, but my wife just shut down. She says it doesn't bother her—why can't I just forget it, too?"

Sex activities may become a chore or a duty, or may turn into oppressing, distressful events.

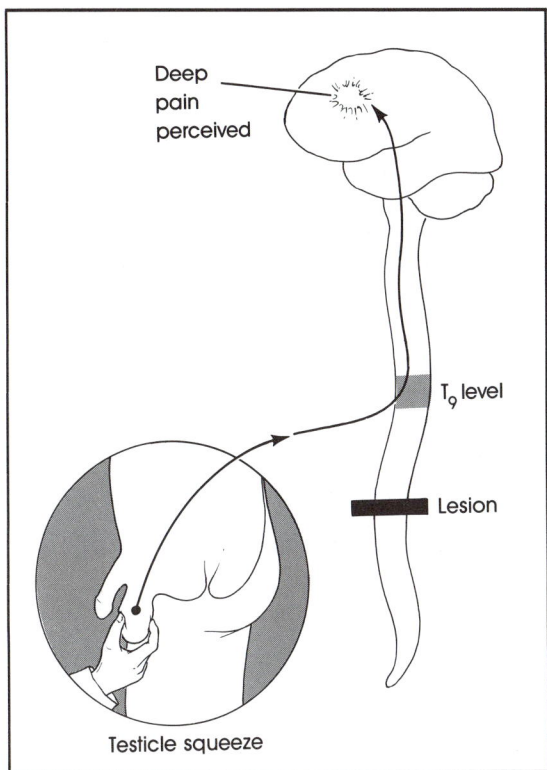

FIGURE 10–7   Testing for testicle-squeeze- induced pain. If present, injury must be below T_9. Mental erection is possible in men, sometimes with flow of seminal fluid.

One woman partner explained it this way: Before his injury he used to grab me while I was in the kitchen. I said "No! Don't do it!" But he knew I wanted it, so he carried on, and finally we just rushed into the bedroom. Now, I wheel him into the bedroom, help him transfer, take his pants off, and wash his penis after I take the condom catheter off. Then I get undressed, sit on top of him, and move till I get bored. I haven't had a climax since he was injured. Yes, I kind of want it, but this is just not my way!

Sexual Activities and Behavior

Sex acts may be classified as solitary (masturbation) and partner-related acts. The latter might be subdivided into caressing, kissing, genital fondling, oral sex activities, and vaginal and anal intercourse. Most of these activities may be carried out in a heterosexual or homosexual relationship. Homosexually oriented people with SCI may be concerned about rejection by heterosexual staff members, in addition to their concerns over other aspects of their disability.

Sexual behavior represents courting activities. The focus is on establishing or maintaining a relationship that includes sex activities. The behavior may vary in different cultures and within the cultural context individuals have their own customs. Presenting oneself as a desirable partner may require the ability to dance or drive a car; facility with words; or deeds, such as dressing, walking, and eating in socially approved ways. Strong social norms dictate what is right and wrong. Many people with SCI feel that they cannot compete with others under the existing rules; some feel totally unattractive and a burden on a partner.

People enjoying the company of friends with SCI may be concerned about points of etiquette. This concern is caused by a feeling of responsibility for the welfare of the person with SCI. The injured person is perceived as "ill," and people who are ill need looking after! Indeed, it is not unusual for a partner to approach a nurse and ask for information. "What is it like for a spinal injured person? How do they go to the bathroom? Do they need constant supervision? Is there sex for them?"

The sex partners of persons with SCI may also be concerned about fulfillment of their own needs:

> A 24-year-old woman partner of a 22-year-old man with a complete C_4 quadriplegia said, "What I really miss is his caresses. Sure I can sit on top of him, but his arms and hands are . . . just useless."

SCI causes several types of problems in the area of sexual activities and behavior.

1. Technical problems caused by the weakness or loss of function of arms, hands, and legs. Undressing, assuming desirable positions, holding, touching, stimulation with hands, and moving in rhythm with the partner may not be possible.

> A 42-year-old woman suffered a partial injury to the T_{4-5} level of her spinal cord. She had only vague sensations in response to hot/cold testing of her genitalia, and she was unable to contract her anal opening on demand. This indicated that it would be unlikely for her to experience orgasm from genital stimulation. This news did not concern her: What worried her most was the weakness in her legs. "I used to hold my lover close to me with my legs around his body. And I used to move. Now I am like a sack of potatoes. I won't be any use to him in sex."

2. Concerns over the appropriateness of acts other than intercourse. To many people the norm is having the erect penis inside the vagina. Manual or oral stimulation is often thought of as a preliminary act that leads to the "real thing." To some people anything other than intercourse is "perverse." Among nondisabled people, this focus on intercourse, rather than on enjoyment, is a major cause of erection dysfunction and loss of interest. Among people with SCI, this belief may inhibit any experimentation with sex acts other than intercourse.

> A 46-year-old man with complete injury in the sacral area complained: "We've been married for 24 years. The wife never wanted anything but intercourse. I told her I don't have erections. Why can't I rub you with the fingers? But she says that's not normal; she doesn't want to learn anything new like that; and besides, if I can't come, she doesn't want it either."

3. Worries about the possibility of being victimized.

> A 20-year-old man suffered a C_{6-7} complete injury. He revealed that in the past he had homosexual as well as heterosexual experiences. "My friends were sitting around the bed, and we talked about my strong erections. Michael said, You're lucky! You can get it from front and back and you wouldn't even know it! I don't like this idea of being used."

Others feel that they are already victims for rape. There are indeed reports of rape committed against women with SCI, but there are also stories about quadriplegic men whose reflex erections were capitalized on without consent by women.

4. Concerns about the genitalia and about bowel and bladder accidents. Both men and women tend to worry about offensive genital odors. Urinary cleanliness and menstrual hygiene care are discussed in Chapters 18 and 21. A recurrent concern among men is that their penises may have become smaller. They notice that when applying the condom drainage device, the shaft of the penis appears to be shorter than before. The reason for this is not clear. Perhaps the weakness of the pelvic floor is responsible for this change. In any case, when pressure is applied to the perineum, the penis becomes longer again.

Bladder and bowel accidents may occur more commonly when sex acts occur spontaneously. If there is time for planning, most people restrict their fluid intake and empty their bladder. Bowel accidents are more difficult to avoid, particularly if the routine calls for bowel care only every second or third day. Women may have more problems with this than men, presumably because the penis inside the vagina activates bowel reflexes. There will be further comments about these problems in the management section of this chapter.

People with SCI also report new possibilities.

> A 29-year-old married man, who had suffered a complete injury at C_{6-7} level six months before, said, "It was quite surprising! She never could come with me inside. I used my fingers. Now I can't move my hands so we said what the hell, there is that erect penis. So she sat on me and wow! She went over with a bang! It's better for her than before. I get a charge out of it, too."

Fertility and Contraception

Many people with SCI have urgent concerns about fertility and contraception. "If I can't be a father what else could we do?" "Is there some way to get sperms out of me?" "Can a person with a spinal injury adopt a child?" "My boyfriend has quadriplegia. Should we use a contraceptive?" "I used to be on the pill before my injury. Is this still all right to use?" "Will I fit in my wheelchair if I get pregnant?" "How can the baby come out of me if I cannot push?"

Women in their childbearing years are able to get pregnant despite their injuries, although it is not known whether they are as fertile as nondisabled women of comparable age.

The fertility of men with spinal injuries is very much subject to dysfunctions. The major issues are: *inability to ejaculate* with ordinary genital stimulation, and *the low percentage of motile spermatozoa* in the specimens recovered with vibratory stimulation of the penis or with electroejaculation techniques. (See Management.) However, even a small volume of seminal fluid, a very low sperm count, and a low percentage of motile spermatozoa show some capability for fertilization. Lack of erection ability or inability to experience penile sensations or orgasm is not a reliable indicator of fertility.

If infertility is proven in the man (Ver Voort 1987), adoption procedures or artificial insemination by donor are the currently available family planning methods.

If a couple's fertility is established, the question is who is going to assume responsibility for birth control. Experience has shown that in a stable couple relationship it is a shared responsibility, but usually the person who is most motivated and most able physically should be in charge of the birth control procedures. However, if the person is single or has casual relationships, it is important not to make assumptions about the partner's birth control measures. In such situations it is best for the disabled person to assume the responsibility for protection.

Methods of birth control can be viewed as "you-do-it" or "done-to-you" procedures. The you-do-it methods necessitate some motor and intellectual performance from the person. When these are lacking, the done-to-you methods are alternatives. Condoms and withdrawal are the you-do-it methods used by men. Both methods require a certain level of motor coordination for correct application. The you-do-it methods used by women include barrier creams and foams, the diaphragm, oral contraceptives, and natural family planning methods using mucous characteristics and/or rhythm methods. Appropriate insertion of anything into the vagina requires specific physical abilities. Few people think that oral contraceptives have complex requirements. Yet appropriate use of oral contraceptives includes a series of motor acts that may be beyond the abilities of some quadriplegic women. The done-to-you methods available to women include intrauterine devices, tubal ligation, and hysterectomy. Vasectomy is the only method currently available to men.

Virtually every birth control method is reputed to have some hazards. Some of these side effects are accentuated in the spinal injured because of the nature of the disability. For example, the thromboembolic hazard in the use of oral contraceptives containing estrogen may make this method inappropriate for a woman with SCI who spends a large part of the day in the wheelchair. Progesterone-based oral contraceptives may cause weight gain and contribute to depression. Intrauterine devices may be inadvisable when a woman cannot feel discomfort indicating possible uterine perforation or pelvic inflammatory disease, or when in-creased menstrual flow would be difficult to cope with. Tubal ligation has few if any contraindications specific to physically disabled people. Hysterectomy has the added attraction of reducing the hygienic problems associated with menstrual flow.

Pregnancy

In most women the preinjury menstrual pattern is reestablished within 6 months of the injury to the spinal cord. The timing of the return of the first menstrual period does not seem to be related to the level of the injury or the degree of its completeness. Fertility and miscarriage rates after SCI in sexually active women are similar to those in the general population (Ohry, Peleg, and Goldman 1988). A British survey by Robertson (1972) suggested that the incidence of stillbirth was significantly higher in women with SCI than in other women at that time. Another survey (Goller and Paeslack 1972) suggested that the rate of stillbirth, malformations, and disabilities were high in babies born to women whose pregnancies were conceived after the injury to the spinal cord. Current statistics are not available.

Pregnancy, labor, delivery, and postpartum experiences in the woman with SCI may be complicated by a number of problems (Nygaard, Bartscht, and Cole 1990). During the *pregnancy*, pressure sores, urinary tract infections, and anemia are common. Weight gain may interfere with the pregnant woman's usual methods of self-care, and she may require assistance with her transfers.

Labor may be painless for some women. Monitoring the state of the cervix after the 28th week of pregnancy will forewarn of the danger of unsuspected and unattended premature delivery. Increased vaginal discharge may also warn the pregnant woman and her attendants of impending labor. Other women, even with a complete injury, may recognize labor contractions as abdominal spasms, leg spasms, difficulty in breathing, and back pain (Wanner, Rageth, and Zach 1987). Autonomic dysreflexia (described in Chapter 16) is the major complication affecting the laboring woman with SCI above T_{4-6}. Bradycardia, flushing, sweating, tingling, nasal mucosal congestion, and headaches are among the early signs of dysreflexia. Characteristically, the hypertension, related to dysreflexia, occurs only during the contractions. In contrast, elevation of the blood pressure in preeclampsia of pregnancy is constant. Regional anesthesia such as epidural or spinal block is suggested for prevention and controlling autonomic dysreflexia during labor; however, the danger of long-lasting hypotension makes frequent monitoring of the woman mandatory. The symptoms and signs of autonomic dysreflexia stop with delivery.

During *delivery* perineal muscle spasticity of women with higher injuries may necessitate intervention with forceps.

PERSONAL VIEWPOINT: *Tamara Jean Marie Johnson*

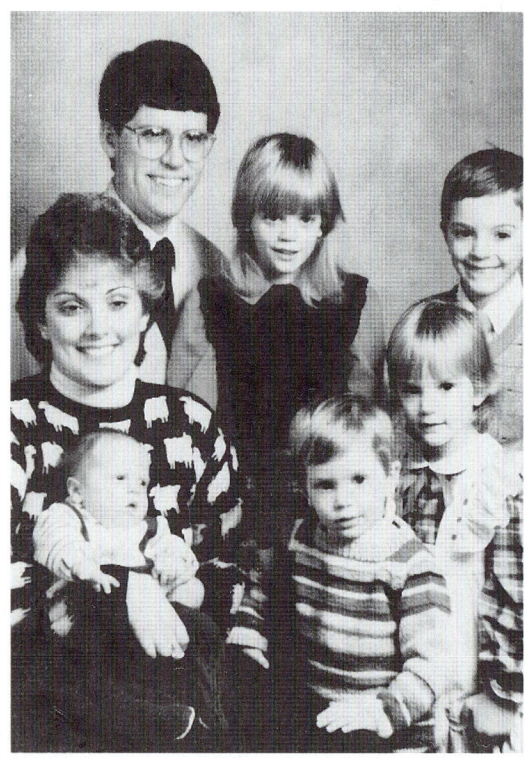

I live in Minneapolis with my husband, Todd, and our five children. When I was 14 years old, I was injured doing a back flip on the sand at a lake and have C_{5-6} quadriplegia.

I was very outgoing and looked forward to excitement and fun as a teenager. My life had centered around physical activity. Well, I think I am still active. After therapy, I continued in school and became class secretary, sports writer for our school newspaper, a compet-itor in wheelchair sports, and even princess during the St. Paul Winter Carnival. I enjoyed going to school dances in formals with nice young men. Shortly there-after I met my future husband, who was a senior nursing aide in the rehabilitation center where I was undergoing tendon transplants. We dated for 2 years before marriage. Todd is currently the Director of Human Resources at Courage Center, a nonprofit organization for physically disabled persons.

As a home executive, I do everything except mow the grass. The children, reading, craft projects, cook-ing, being outdoors, and being alone with Todd fill my time.

All our children were born vaginally without many complications, although three were premature. I was not declared high risk until the fifth pregnancy. Todd and I decided the physician needed a very good game plan to get me to my due date. He was thorough and addressed all of our concerns. The labor room staff was alerted regularly as to who I was and my progress. A chart with instructions for all the potential problems was reviewed weekly and updated. When you are in the minority, you must be assertive, even aggressive, for your own well-being.

I would like to see support groups for disabled women and resources for high-risk labor, delivery, and prema-turity. OB/GYN services need to be made aware of the needs of disabled women. Helpful experiences in-cluded staff taking time to get to know me as a person as well as a patient. They took a genuine personal interest in who I was and my future.

Tamara Jean Marie Johnson
Minneapolis, MN

Caesarean section is required only when other obstetrical indications are present.

Immediate *postpartum* complications are the same as those in women without spinal cord damage. The episiot-omy wound may become contaminated due to bowel or bladder incontinence. A mother may breast-feed her baby in bed or in her wheelchair. Emotional distress over physi-cal limitations in early baby care may be reduced by rehears-als and by a supporting family and additional attendant care if needed. The incidence of postpartum depression among women with SCI is not known.

Successful pregnancy outcome depends on teamwork. This includes prenatal education in preventive measures for the pregnant woman, her family, and her health care advi-sors. In prenatal management, give special attention to ongoing skin care, periodic checks for urinary tract infec-tions, maintenance of regular bowel function, treatment of anemia, and prevention of unsupervised deliveries. In labor special steps may be needed to ensure the early recognition and treatment of autonomic dysreflexia. In the postpartum period, the new mother may require assistance with her parenting skills (Ford and Duckworth 1987). Discussion of birth control plans should be done before the new mother leaves the hospital. The joy (but added weight) of holding a newborn baby while sitting in a wheelchair will necessitate diligent sacral skin care.

ONE-TO-ONE APPROACHES TO MANAGEMENT

Treatment can include *psychological* (verbal and guidance oriented), *pharmacological* (involving medications), *medical* (using medical technology), *physical* (using external devices, appliances), and *surgical* (using internal devices) approaches. A combination of these approaches may be used. Contact with the therapist may be short term, long term, regular or sporadic, open ended or time limited. Some of the treatment approaches may require involvement of the partner; sometimes a group format is used.

Psychological Approach

The goals of the psychological approach are to dispel myth, increase freedom of choice, and support the patient's right to feelings and to the expression of feelings. The methods may include *education* to increase biological and self-knowledge; *reassurance* about adequacy; *diminishing of hesitation* toward alternative sex activities; and *increasing acceptance* of viewing and touching one's own and the partner's body. These basic methods are often combined into more specific therapy formats. *Marital* and *communication therapies* are used to attend to interpersonal disagreements and to promote direct and intimate discussions between partners; *sex therapy* is applied to treat specific sex dysfunctions.

Sex therapy differs from other psychological treatment methods in two respects:

1. Its goals are essentially limited to the relief of the patient's sexual symptoms.
2. Its methods include prescribed sexual experiences.

These goals shift the couple's attention from intercourse and orgasm to giving and receiving pleasure. The couple learns that apprehensions about any sex act may cause erection, ejaculation, and orgasmic difficulties and may lead to sexual disinterest. An expectation of the therapy outcome is that as various nonintercourse sex acts are gradually accepted by the couple as pleasure-producing, those acts will be approached with less apprehension.

Sex therapy requires a degree of concentration on the sex problem and an exclusion of other problems for a limited period of time. For this reason, it is not often suitable to the life situation of people with acute or recent SCI. However, the components of the therapy, namely, education, reassurance, and sexual skills practice, can be used in various combinations and to appropriate levels of intensity just about any time after the injury. The prescribed sexual experiences represent the unique feature of this sexual care approach.

Using this approach in the case of the 46-year-old man with a complete injury in the sacral area who complained that his wife didn't "want to learn anything new," the patient and the partner would be educated about various pleasure-yielding physical activities. They would also be helped to become more comfortable with words expressing their sexual feelings and needs. All of this would help them acquire a wider appreciation of the range of so-called normal in sex practices. The wife would become more comfortable with viewing and touching his genitalia and would experience less disappointment with his lack of erection. She would gain more courage to guide her partner with language such as, "I like this. Now a little more pressure. Continue. Now higher," rather than, "That's no good. I don't know what I want. Try something else." The husband would worry less about intercourse being the one and only real sex act. Once relaxed, he might experience erection from mental stimuli and gain pleasure from stimulation of his face, neck, or lips.

Obviously, some people are more suitable for this type of an approach than others. To assess suitability, the person's main complaints have to be clarified first. For example, in the case considered here it would be important to establish whether the main problems are really lack of erection and worries over the wife's refusal to participate in sex acts other than intercourse. Other problems could be the man's disinterest in sex activities or his hidden fear of failure in an intercourse situation; his lack of genital sensation; or his worry over dribbling while being caressed. His wife may have lost sexual interest before the accident; she may or may not have been regularly orgasmic even with the penis inside her; and she may not now enjoy (or may never have enjoyed) the manner in which he stimulates her. On top of all this, hand or oral stimulation may be against her principles. The clarification of the man's problems involves a painstaking review of these possibilities. The therapist's approach is to ask questions in a nonthreatening way. For example, in trying to find out if the wife has been orgasmic before her husband's accident, the therapist might proceed as follows:

THERAPIST: Now I have to ask you a question about orgasms. Would this be all right with you? *(This is asking for permission.)*

WIFE: Okay.

THERAPIST: Well, I wonder if you have read that many women don't normally experience orgasms? *(This is preparation for acceptance in case she does not have orgasms.)*

WIFE: Yes.

THERAPIST: I wonder what your own experiences were? *(This is an open question, inviting more than a yes or no answer.)*

WIFE: Well, I had orgasms but always with intercourse. I don't know why. Maybe my mother told me never to touch myself.

The second step in the assessment is to review the couple's preinjury sexual interest level and sexual practices, including frequency, timing, location, and situations producing "turn on" or "turn off" of interest. Then postinjury sexual practices must be recounted and compared with preinjury experiences.

These two steps yield a rich store of data on the sexual functioning status of this couple, their sexual losses, the meaning of their loss, their beliefs about the right or wrong in various sex acts, their flexibility in this area, their interest in each other, and their willingness to evolve new activities. These are the resources or burdens that they bring to the therapy.

The third step would be a physical examination of the man. This would define the physiological limitations of his erection, ejaculation, and orgasmic process. Of particular interest in this specific example would be the testicle squeeze test (see Figure 10–7). If he felt acute deep pain in response to the squeeze, the chances for erections produced by mental stimulation would be very good. The physical exam would also review his ability to hold and caress his wife and move in bed and his urinary equipment requirements. The wife would be encouraged to participate in this examination to learn about his remaining potential.

In the fourth step of the assessment, the couple's sexual goals would be explored. A list would have to be developed of their desired acts, the desired frequency of these acts, and safeguards for privacy, birth control, and so on.

The fifth step would be a search for conditions that might contraindicate the use of the psychological sex therapy method. Contraindications include untreated depression, heavy use of tranquilizing medication, obvious evidence of marital strife, and lack of time to engage in the proposed program.

The sixth step would be a review of the other treatment approaches, in case they are applicable in the management of this couple's sexual difficulties in addition to, or instead of, the psychological methods.

Pharmacological Approach

Medications used to reduce anxiety, relax spasticity, or provide rest or pain-free periods may help indirectly, presumably because the person may feel more zestful. There are many medications, however, that, at certain dosage levels, interfere with interest and function. Drugs that may decrease interest and impair the sexual response include sedatives, analgesics, anticholinergic and anti-adrenergic drugs, muscle relaxants, estrogens, and the major tranquilizers.

The therapist must remember the sexual side effects of illness and of the medications used to treat the patient; must inquire systematically about changes in interest, erection, lubrication, and the orgasmic and ejaculation process; and may have to recommend alternate medications if untoward changes do occur.

Medical (Technological) Approach

Erection Enhancement with Intracavernous Injections

Erection may be enhanced using intracavernous injections. This therapy involves injection of vasodilating medication into the spongy erectile tissue of the penis. Papaverine either alone or in combination with phentolamine mesylate is a commonly used medication for this purpose. Recent experiences with prostaglandin E_1 suggest that this medication may become the preferred choice. Loading the syringe, plunging the needle into the side of the penis, and then injecting the medication into the spongy tissue of the penis is easily learned by men with lower injuries. The procedure may be difficult to carry out by men with injuries that affect hand and arm function. On occasion partners may wish to administer the injection. The physician usually administers test doses and determines the optimal amount of medication—the amount that produces an erection with onset in about 5 to 10 minutes and lasts for about 1 to 1 1/2 hours. A major problem with the intracavernous medication technique is that erections may last for several hours. Sustained erection beyond 6 hours may lead to permanent ischemic damage in the corpus cavernosum. Treatment of prolonged erection may include bedrest and avoidance of penile stimulation; if that is not successful then intracavernous injection of a sympathomimetic agent may be necessary to reduce the swelling. Occasionally blood may have to be aspirated from the penis. Men with SCI seem to be more susceptible to prolonged erection than other men whose erection problem is based on other etiology. It is not clear yet whether the sensitivity is related to nerve damage or to factors inherent in the relative youth of the SCI population receiving this treatment. A review of the ongoing use of the intracavernous injection among men with SCI suggests that the majority of the men and their partners are highly satisfied with the method, even though the man's genital sensation or ejaculatory capacity is unchanged. Reports of abuse of the injections (more than once a day) are rare.

The use of other medications for enhancement of erection is very limited. Testosterone (oral or intramuscular) may be indicated when the level of this hormone is consistently low. Yohimbine (a vasodilating drug usually taken by mouth) can cause intolerable dizziness, flushing, or headaches, without contributing to penile swelling. Other potions (often advertised in magazines) may have placebo effect, but are generally unhelpful.

Sperm Recovery: Vibratory Technique, Electroejaculation Procedure, and Pharmacological Stimulation

The effect of SCI on the ejaculation process has been outlined earlier in this chapter. Three useful techniques have emerged in the last few years for recovering spermatozoa in men with SCI: the vibratory technique, the electroejaculation procedure, and pharmacological stimulation.

The *vibratory technique* is applicable mostly to men with injuries above T_{10} (Szasz and Carpenter 1989). An electric vibrator capable of running at a speed of between 18 to 120 oscillations per second, with a 2 to 3 mm amplitude of back and forth motions, is applied to the glans penis. In response to this stimulation the reflex erection is temporarily lost (the physiological reason for this is unclear); rhythmic abdominal, hip, and leg spasms occur, culminating in ejaculation in about 65% of the men. The procedure usually takes 1 to 5 minutes. Urination may follow the ejaculation. The ejaculation may be retrograde (into the bladder) in men with sphincterotomy. Men with T_4 injury and above often experience severe headaches during ejaculation because of autonomic dysreflexia caused by this procedure. The dysreflexia may be partially controlled by premedication with an antihypertensive agent. Reflex erections return after a short time. Many men feel tired for varying lengths of time following this procedure.

The *electroejaculation procedure* involves electrical stimulation of the peripheral nerves responsible for the ejaculation process. Electrodes are applied to the posterior surface of the prostate gland. A 200 to 300 mAmp current at 15 to 20 volts is delivered at various frequencies. About 70% of men with SCI (regardless of the level or the degree of completeness) respond to this procedure. Anal spasms and leg and hip spasms are common during the electrical stimulation. The procedure is usually painful in people with incomplete injuries. These people usually require a brief anesthetic. The ejaculation may be antegrade (out through the penis) or retrograde, into the bladder. Results of sperm analysis of specimens obtained by vibrator or by electroejaculation seem to be similar. Usually there are a high number of well-formed spermatozoa, but only 10% to 25% of these are actively motile. The reasons for this are not understood. One thought is that the temperature control mechanism of the testicles is affected by the injury.

Pharmacological stimulation using intrathecal (spinal) injection of neostigmine and subcutaneous physostigmine have been tried by various investigators. Less than half of various groups of men with SCI responded with ejaculation. It is unclear how these medications stimulate ejaculation: one suggestion is that these medications depress skeletal muscle reflexes; another is that they stimulate the lumbar reflex centers directly. Both of these medications are reported to have serious side effects.

Several pregnancies have been reported by couples who have used the vibrator at home and inserted the ejaculate in the vagina. Attempts are now being made to develop an electroejaculation apparatus for home use by couples. In most instances, however, a more organized method is required. The urine in the bladder may have to be neutralized so that the destructive effect of the urine on semen is reduced. The recovered spermatozoa may have to be concentrated, the fast-moving spermatozoa may have to be separated from the slow movers, the prepared specimen may have to be inserted intracervically or into the uterus. The woman partner also has to be prepared in some instances, which may require hormone assays and ultrasound detection of ovulation checks. In some instances in vitro fertilization has been carried out with success. The impression is that about 30% to 50% of couples going through the various methods of artificial insemination by a man with SCI are successful.

Physical Approach

The goal of the physical approach is to give technical assistance to patient and partner in the physical aspects of sex activities. Promotion of independent movement, dressing and undressing, cleanliness, and secure bowel and bladder management are part of this approach. Occupational and physical therapists may wish to conceptualize a bedroom scene and apply principles of the daily living skills (DLS) training toward the requirements of sexual interaction.

Patients may need technical advice about preparation for, engaging in, and disengaging from sexual activities (Szasz 1987b).

Preparation

The spinal cord injured person may have to plan for and rehearse many of the activities that others take for granted. Preparations may include bladder and bowel check, disconnecting urinary and drainage devices, oral hygiene, moving to a bed or other suitable place, transfers, positioning, and undressing.

The skills for independent management of these activities are described in other chapters. Many people however, prefer a degree of continuity in sexual activities, and the partner may elect to help the quadriplegic person disrobe, help the partner into bed, or elect to conduct their activity in the wheelchair. (Szasz 1987b provides an illustrated reference.) New partners may first need guidance as to the complexities of wheelchair management, undressing, and catheter or hygiene routines. A recent partner may be surprised at the skills required and energy expenditure needed for activities that come easily to most people. Many couples find it useful to keep towels or perhaps a dish close by, in case of urinary or bowel accidents, or to clean off perspiration or genital fluids.

Bowel and Bladder Hygiene. Individuals may wish to plan ahead and reduce fluid intake in the 2 or 3 hours preceding sex activities. When fluid intake is restricted and the bladder emptied just before sex, urinary accidents are unlikely. Men using condom drainage may disconnect their apparatus. Some men prefer to use a fresh condom to catch small amounts of leakage during sexual play.

Spinal cord injured women with indwelling catheters may disconnect the catheter, fold it back, and tape the end to the lower abdomen or groin area. Men with indwelling catheters may first disconnect their catheters, then close off the end of the tube. After producing a reflex erection, they bend the free portion of the catheter back on the erect penis. Finally, they may apply a condom to cover the erect penis and the catheter. Lubricant on the condom may facilitate easier entry into the vagina.

Stomas. Some persons with high quadriplegia may have a tracheostomy, with or without a ventilator. They may need to learn the best positioning for easy breathing and the continuous action of the ventilator.

Ileostomies, colostomies, and urinary bags should not produce undue complications to sexual practices. Preparation may include emptying the bags and assuring that the adhesive holding the appliance binds well. Some people may wish to wear an apronlike garment to cover the bags.

Engaging in Sexual Activities

Manual Stimulation. Quadriplegic persons may wish to use the fingers, hands, arms, nose, lips, ears, and hair to rhythmically caress their partners. Some of the activities are best accomplished if the partner is positioned within reach of the disabled partner or the partner moves against, for example, the immobile hand. Other activities may be managed with the movements quadriplegic people learn to manipulate various objects. For example, the penis may be held between the heels of the quadriplegic person's hands, or an overhead sling may be adapted to permit rubbing of the vulva or clitoral area of the well-positioned female partner. Principles of tenodesis may be adapted to breast or genital stimulation. The back or side of the hand may prove to be softer than the fingers in caressing the face, breasts, or other desired areas. Aids and splints may be used in several ways. For example, caressing may be accomplished using a hand splint covered with sheepskin or other soft material.

Caressing the person with SCI may require considerable guidance. The injured person may need to indicate both the areas still sensitive to touch and those that might be hypersensitive or even painful to caressing. The other partner may need to prepare for longer periods of stimulation.

The method devised for caressing or the time spent on touching each other is not, perhaps, as important as knowing what the partner requires at that particular time. Directions to each other, therefore, may lead to exploration of a wide variety of high-quality experiences.

Oral-Genital Sex Acts. These acts may require body positioning by the able partner. Adequate hygienic preparation reduces concerns over the degree of cleanliness of urinary or bowel openings. When the act is applied to the quadriplegic person, urinary flow may occur in spite of normally adequate bladder management. Spasticity in the adductor muscles of the hips and thighs may temporarily trap the head of the partner. If stopping the activity for a few moments does not reduce the spasticity, gentle, steady pressure on, for example, the knee, may reduce the muscle tension. Sometimes medication may be required to prevent spasticity. However, some persons with higher injuries may enjoy the rhythmic contraction of the hip and leg muscles in response to active genital stimulation.

Gagging, choking, or not getting enough breath may be a problem for the quadriplegic person engaged in oral sex. Experimentation with these acts and becoming proficient in giving clear signals to the partner to move are the ways to manage these situations.

Intercourse. Sexual intercourse provides both emotional closeness and physical pleasure. Suitable positioning may require assistance by the partner or application of techniques of self-positioning in bed. The various methods of turning, moving down the bed, and the use of an overhead bar for bed mobility can be well applied here.

Sitting on top of the injured male may provide for the comfort, mobility, and stimulation required by the female partner. This position also provides for a face-to-face view that may offer additional stimulation.

Women with low SCI may prefer to lie on their backs, with their legs separated. Spasticity in women with higher injuries may make this position impractical. On occasion, pillow support under the knees helps to open the legs. Other women may wish to lie on their sides, with one or both knees pulled up. In the man-on-top position, the quadriplegic woman may have to pay attention to her freedom of breathing. She may have to tell her partner to avoid pressing on her chest. Leg spasticity may allow for holding the partner.

Intercourse in the wheelchair may be an alternative to lying down. The quadriplegic man would ease forward in the chair so that his partner is able to straddle him. Similarly, the injured woman can slip forward in the chair and the partner kneel between her legs.

The mechanics of intercourse require thrusting the penis in the vagina in a rhythmic manner. The quadriplegic man lying on his partner may contribute to this action by using his skills to roll from side to side. On his back, he may wish to use his overhead strap to produce a bouncing motion in rhythm with his partner's movements. Lubricating jelly applied to the penis may reduce chafing the vaginal opening and the vaginal wall.

Spasticity occurring during intercourse may add to the rhythmic movement, but in men with high injuries, severe leg spasms may make intercourse difficult. Gentle, steady pressure on the legs may release the spasms. Occasionally medication may be required to control extreme sensitivity to touch.

The soft penis of the injured male can be "stuffed" into the vagina. This technique is easier to accomplish with the man on top and the partner's legs drawn up. The partner moves her buttocks so that she can guide the well-lubricated soft penis into her vaginal opening. She can then contract her vaginal opening in a rhythmic manner and gently move her hips to expose herself to the desired stimulation.

Disengaging from Sexual Activities

The technical aspects of disengaging include bathing or washing the genitalia, getting dressed, and transferring back into the chair, and may take as much energy and organization as preparation for the activity.

For some people, the period after sex activity may be characterized by elated feelings and strong energy. Other people find they have become quite tired. Some couples find they can go only so far, and then have to rest or stop. Yet others might feel frustrated and angry that they cannot achieve their objectives.

The psychological aspect of disengaging is clearly important. This time period may be of value to debrief each other about the preparations, the positions, the preferred ways of stimulation, the nature of the responses, the newly discovered potentials, and the plans for next time. On a more specific level, the patient may need assistive devices.

Assistive Devices

Some couples may wish to enhance their sexual experiences through technical means. Vacuum-principle external penile prostheses, penile rings, dildos, and vibrators are external methods to assist with erection or sensation.

Vacuum-principle devices come in two forms. The Correctaid erection assistance device is an elongated cylinder made of a soft, transparent silicone rubber with walls thick enough to support the penis. The flaccid penis is placed into this device. Air is removed from the inside of the device through a tube built into the wall of the sheath. The gentle vacuum created in this way slowly draws the penis into the device. The penis looks erect inside the prosthesis. Intercourse is certainly possible. The device may be difficult to put on without help if the user's hands are not fully functional. Penile sensation (if spared) is greatly reduced inside the cylinder. The partner may need extra lubricant applied to the outside of the device to prevent vaginal discomfort. The Correctaid device requires penile length and girth measurements in accordance with the manufacturers' recommendations.

The Erectaid is different from the Correctaid in that the penis is not covered by a sheathing. A firm cylinder is placed over the flaccid penis. Air is removed from the cylinder by means of a small hand pump. The penis becomes engorged with blood and slowly becomes erect. At that point a thick rubber ring is placed at the base of the erect penis to retain the blood inside the penis, and the cylinder is removed.

Rings may capture blood in the penis and thereby produce and maintain erection. They come in several forms, some flexible, others more rigid. Any of them may be effective sometimes, if applied to a partially swollen penis. Placing the ring on the penis requires a degree of manual dexterity that may not be available to the spinal cord injured. The risks of using rings are poorly documented, but medical concerns include causing skin damage to the penis, damage to the erectile tissue inside the penis, and even bruising of the urinary passage in the penis.

Dildos are rubbery or hard casings that fit over the soft or semierect penis. The casings may be held on with suction devices, adhesives, or straps. The purpose in using dildos is to provide stimulation inside the vagina.

Some couples may enjoy using these implements; others may find them strange or repulsive. Common sense must rule. If the appliance is of value and acceptable to the couple, then it might have a place in the management of their sexual life.

Stimulation may be enhanced by battery-driven or electric *vibrators* used by either partner for several purposes. An able-bodied partner may enjoy the sensation of vibration on the body as well as on the genitalia. To provide this stimulation, the quadriplegic person may need to use a wrist-driven flexor-hinge splint to assure a good grasp on the vibrating appliance. The cord injured man or woman may enjoy the vibration sensation on the neurologically intact areas of the body. Application of the vibrator to the tip of the penis or the clitoral area may produce abdominal and leg spasms. These spasms may become rhythmic and in some instances be accompanied by internal feelings of tension even though the genitalia itself may be insensitive to touch. In persons with high injuries, the application of the vibrator to the genitalia may also cause extragenital responses, including elevation of pulse, respiratory rates, and blood pressure. Some quadriplegic persons may experience headaches in such situations. For this reason, the use of a vibrator on the genitalia of men or women with high injuries is discouraged. The application of the vibrator for sperm recovery purposes is described in the medical approaches section of this chapter. The vibrator may cause skin abrasions or burns on the skin.

Surgical Approach

The *surgical approach* to the management of sexual problems is limited to insertion of internal penile prostheses (Green and Sloan 1986). These devices are either firm or flexible rods or fluid-filled, cylinderlike structures inserted into the erectile tissues of the penis. Some devices need to be pumped up when erection is desired. The pump is located inside the scrotum and both the activating and the releasing process requires strong finger power. The quadriplegic person may need assistance from the partner. The device makes possible a reliable erection of the penis. While long-term outcome studies are not yet available, current

PERSONAL VIEWPOINT

At the age of 35, Gus sustained a spinal injury at T_9, resulting in complete paraplegia at that level. His wife, Kate, was 33 years old and their two children were 10 and 7 years old at the time of the injury.

Gus was referred to the sexual health care clinician when he expressed concern that his wife might leave him. The clinician described the service and reassured him that many men worry about their marriages. Gus said he feared that he could not get an erection and that his wife might become sexually frustrated.

Kate admitted that she had many anxieties, including sexual tension. She was embarrassed talking about sex but said that their sexual life had been very important to her.

In subsequent visits during the next two weeks, Gus revealed that he and his wife had, in their 12-year marriage, explored a variety of sexual activities including mutual oral and manual genital stimulation and intercourse in various positions. Physical touch was important to him even though he did not feel it. The findings also indicated that touch erections would be possible, but mental erections, ejaculation, and orgasm would likely be lost.

With Gus's permission, the clinician interpreted these physical findings to Kate in a separate interview. Kate said she enjoyed and needed physical touching and caressing, but preferred orgasms through intercourse. She admitted that she would like to initiate sexual play, but felt shy and therefore did not. Although their sexual play was varied, she said it was not unusual for them to talk to each other about their feelings and desires.

The clinician emphasized to both partners that the initial test results were not final and that the genital assessment would be repeated. It was suggested that they might wish to begin to explore various body sensations that might offer sensual feelings and to monitor changing feelings and responses to genital touching. A private room was made available to them for this intimate experimentation and testing of their remaining sexual abilities.

Kate said she had touched her husband's penis when they were cuddling together and observed a reflex erection. Although she was distressed that he could not feel her touch, the experience was comforting to both, and they were interested in attempting intercourse.

Physical examination with Kate present showed that Gus could trigger his bladder to empty, remove his condom, and clean his penis without assistance. Examination of his mobility for sexual activity showed that he could undress and transfer himself to bed, but he needed assistance with his shoes and socks. He could assume a supine or side-lying position and could easily move his arms and body to caress and stimulate his wife. A major problem area was their difficulty in talking openly about their sexual desires. Following another interview together, Kate was able to tell Gus that she would like to initiate some sexual play. He was pleased.

Before his first weekend pass home, Kate and Gus said they hoped to have intercourse. He was worried, however, that she would not be satisfied sexually, because he couldn't move his pelvis and be as physically active in intercourse as he had been in the past. Kate was worried that she might hurt his back if she sat on top of him, and both were uncertain about how they would sleep together for the first time.

After consulting with the orthopedic surgeon, the clinician was able to reassure them that Gus's back was stable and that Kate would cause him no harm. After the weekend, they said that although the experience was different for both, Kate was able to come to orgasm. Gus was pleased that he could satisfy her in this way, and he himself felt physically relaxed after their sexual play.

Soon after, Gus was discharged from the rehabilitation center. The clinician maintained contact with the couple to help them continue reestablishing their sexual relationship in the transition from hospital to home.

---

experiences suggest that the inflatable prosthesis is more applicable to the needs of people with SCI than are rigid devices. The major concern with both is that pressure sores may develop in the shaft or in the perineum.

A secondary benefit of the inflatable prosthesis is that it makes it easier to use the condom for urinary drainage. The prosthesis does not promote ejaculation and it does not restore sensation to the penis. It seems to be of greatest value to patients with incomplete injuries, many of whom have unreliable and incomplete reflex erections.

Choosing the Right Approach(es)

An educational or psychological approach is the most appropriate early choice. This approach includes the clarification of the problem and a positive stock taking of the personal and relationship resources still available. Ongoing educational and supportive discussions may then lead to realistic goal setting. Modified sex therapy combined with physical assistance may be applicable if the physical dysfunctions are minimal or if they are accepted. When the main concern is erection dysfunction and the couple's goals unalterably involve intercourse, various medical, medicinal, or surgical approaches may have to be considered. *Parenthood* issues may require one of the technical solutions to sperm recovery. However, even when medical, surgical, or technical methods are available for the management of a specific problem, the couple's total situation needs to be considered, including religious beliefs (Rucker, Szasz, and Carpenter 1988). For example, the intracavernous injection method may ensure an erect penis, but this may not meet the personal requirements of a partner. To some people, the somewhat mechanical aspect of an induced or enhanced erection may not be considered sexually attractive. The psychological approach, dispelling myth, increasing freedom of choice, supporting the person's right to feelings and their expression, may prepare the couple for the inclusion of newer approaches to their intimate lives.

Treatment approaches might be less direct or less definitive if a person without a partner asks for help than when an interested couple inquires about specific sexual issues. A marital rather than sexual approach may be indicated if not only the couple's "bedroom" but their "living room" is in turmoil.

The situation may be different when help is sought a few years after the acute rehabilitation phase. The person with SCI may have a new vocation; settled financial issues; or have a new partner. Often both partners know what help they need and ask for realistic assistance, such as, for example, enhancement of the erection. Sometimes the sexual issue is not a specific consequence of SCI; rather it is a symptom of intrapersonal or interpersonal difficulties. Although the symptoms of such problems may be sexual, the individual's emotional struggle may have to be assessed by counseling specialists.

Treatment Approaches with Children

Little is known about the sexual concerns of young children with SCI. Parents, however, might have grave concerns about the sexual future of the injured child. Some parents prefer to withhold information from children about the likely losses, particularly in terms of fatherhood. Other parents encourage an outgoing life-style for their injured children. Both groups hope for ultimate adaptation, but the first group believes there is a specific time in the growing person's life when sexual issues should be dealt with, while the second hopes that adaptation will come through daily experiences in school, sports, and friendships over a long period of time.

There is some evidence that exposing injured children to the tumults of daily experiences is better in the long run than saving them from uncertainties until they are more mature. Formal sexual assessment and management efforts are probably out of place for very young children. However, sexual assessment seems to be appropriate, with parental permission, for pubescent boys and girls. Preliminary discussions with parents are important because they need to know what the sexual counselor will present to the child. If the parents prefer to withhold sexual information, even after discussion with the counselor, then, at least under current social arrangements, this is their right.

The situation is different if a teenager has had preinjury sexual experiences that represent adult behavior. Although the parents' approval should still be sought, if it is not forthcoming, a second professional opinion should be requested. If it is in agreement, sexual assessment and management should be carried out when requested by the person. In the prescription of contraceptives, the same safeguards may be applied.

One dilemma is in the use of a prosthetic device for young persons. For example, in 1978 a 16-year-old boy suffered a L_1–S_4 injury. He had no erectile response to physical touch or to mental stimulation. He was sexually active before his injury and gravely concerned about his sexual life. There was no change in his situation 2 years later. A decision was made to proceed with an implant. In the short run, this worked well. However, presumably he will live another 40 to 50 years. New medical and technical advances that became available in the last few years may make the decision to proceed with the surgical approach look like a mistake.

Parents of youngsters with SCI may develop sexual problems of their own. The reasons for this are not clear, but there seem to be several factors. Adult couples who see sexual practices as "stolen pleasures" rather than as means of closeness often break off sex activities when they feel oppressed, guilty about, or preoccupied with, the gravity of their child's situation. One parent is often in the hospital for days at a time, and is almost forced to or inadvertently neglects other members of the family. This distancing may lead to a break in the couple's sexual routines and difficulty picking them up later. Couples often stop talking to each other because they are so sad and they do not wish to cause each other more distress. These circumstances may lead to sexual disinterest and erection or orgasmic problems. It is clearly the professional's role and responsibility to mention to parents that interpersonal conflicts, including sexual ones, are not unusual features in the life of the injured person's family.

INSTITUTIONAL APPROACHES TO MANAGEMENT

Although one-to-one approaches may be stated with some degree of rationality, institutional approaches are still fairly haphazard (Novak and Mitchell 1988). During the last 40 years there have been three administrative approaches to the sexual concerns of patients and partners.

1. To *deny* or repress sexual expressions. The philosophy behind this approach is partly that sex is an inappropriate area for professional exploration; that the patient's whole attention should be focused on return to work; and that it may be a further strain on the patient to learn about the sexual disabilities on top of other problems.

2. To *tolerate* expressions of sexual needs and even to offer some answers or suggestions when this appears to be appropriate or when one or two interested nurses or other health professionals are willing to get involved. This approach is usually haphazard and often undertaken with only token support from the medical staff. It is characterized by a well-meaning surge of interest in the plight of *some* patients; exclusion from consideration of the needs of the *young* and the *old*; dependence on a few interested staff members; and a wait-and-see attitude in most of the nursing staff and the medical staff. If an untoward incident occurs, such as a phone call from a wife who is upset that "someone talked sex with my husband," the staff member involved may be reprimanded and memos ("I don't wish to have my patient exposed to sexual counseling" or "there will be no sexual discussion in the intensive care unit") may fly!

3. To *organize a program* of sexual rehabilitation.

The Organized Approach

An organized program has to have clearly defined goals that are acceptable to the staff members. There must also be a clearly stated outline of the nature of the specific services required, the type of personnel who will be responsible for offering various aspects of this patient-partner care service, and their relationship to the other team members. The relationship has to be spelled out in terms of the referral methods and the role of staff members "before the specialist arrives," the methods of reporting back to staff members, and the inclusion of reports in the agenda of team meetings. A protocol must be drawn up to introduce the service to the patient and the family and to communicate with the staff of the next institution assuming the care of the patient. The plan must provide ongoing staff education and introductory education for new staff members; coordination with other programs; means of supervision, consultations, backup services, and in-service training programs; materials, supplies, and physical space for various required procedures. In ad-

dition there may be a need for a protocol to manage conflicting areas for the staff. For example, the staff may have to agree whether this type of service is appropriate for children, or whether to provide a private room for undisturbed experimentation by a couple.

A Model of the Organized Approach

The Sexual Health Service in Vancouver, BC, is one of the few models of the organized approach. British Columbia has a population of 3.5 million. Approximately 120 persons suffer SCI each year. More than 90% of these people are transported to an acute SCI unit within the first 48 hours of injury. After an average stay of 6 to 8 weeks in the acute setting, most of the patients are transferred to the G. F. Strong Centre, an active rehabilitation facility. The average stay in that institution is about 3 to 6 months. Some of the patients go home, where necessary alterations have been made to accommodate wheelchair living; others go to apartments specifically designed for people with SCI; and a small proportion, for example, those requiring respiratory assistance, go to specialized accommodation. In the long run, the patient's family physician looks after medical matters, with appropriate referrals to, for example, urological care. The patient may also reenter the rehabilitation center for further occupational or physical therapy.

The Sexual Health Service is an integral part of the acute ward, the active rehabilitation setting, and the long-term rehabilitation institution. Sexual health clinicians are specially trained and prepared for their role. Each clinician has a background in one of the health care professions. The specialized training focuses on sexual interviewing, assessment, and management of the sexual consequences of SCI and other severe disabilities. The clinicians also receive training in how to present in-service education to staff members and rehabilitation counselors. In addition, the clinicians may develop specialized skills in, for example, erection enhancement with pharmacological means, or fertility management. While the day-to-day operation of the Sexual Health Service is looked after by the sexual health clinicians, the medical staff members of the Sexual Health Service provide medical consultations and are involved in the erection enhancement and sperm recovery programs. The medical personnel are based in a sexual medicine unit. This unit is a teaching and research division of the Faculty of Medicine, University of British Columbia, in close relationship with psychiatric, urological, and gynecological departments.

Persons with SCI may enter the sexual health care system in several ways. In the acute setting, the nursing staff makes the referrals to the sexual health clinician. The patient is followed by the clinician to the active rehabilitation setting. Once discharged from the rehabilitation center, the patient may come back to the Sexual Health Service at any time, although notification of the patient's physician is required. Those patients in the rehabilitation setting who have not been through the acute SCI unit have to be referred by their rehabilitation physician; people living in the community may be referred by their family physicians. These patients are then admitted to the Sexual Health Service as outpatients. Consultations with the sexual medicine specialists are arranged internally by the sexual health clinicians. The financing of these services is derived from the British Columbia Medical Plan and Hospital Services, a tax-based "medicare" for all residents of Canada.

In the last 15 years, virtually all persons in British Columbia with SCI and their partners had some (even if minimal) contact with the Sexual Health Service. The service is also well known by rehabilitation counselors of the Canadian Paraplegic Association, who travel around the province and remind their clients that sexual health care is available to them if and when they need it.

The sexual health clinician's work involves several steps:

1. *Soon after admission.* The primary nurse tells the patient that there is a specialized care service and that the sexual health clinician will visit the ward later. The existence of the service is also brought to the attention of the partner and family.

2. *Introductory visit.* The first visit is often arranged by the primary care nurse, who is most informed about the patient's (or partner's) needs. At the first visit the clinician may only briefly outline the sexual rehabilitation process. When the patient expresses sexual concerns, the clinician might clarify these immediately, offer limited information, or prepare the patient for an assessment. Usually the clinician would acknowledge the patient's concern and make arrangements for a more thorough assessment at a later date.

3. *Assessment.* The timing for the major assessment is determined by the patient's readiness—the patient or the partner may ask to see the clinician (the clinicians are easily accessible); or the staff working with the patient notifies the clinician when the patient (or partner) brings up sexual or sex-related questions. The sexual health clinicians are part of the care team and participate in, for example, the weekly patient review meetings. Patient readiness for assessment is often decided at those meetings.

If a partner is available, first a private assessment is made of the partner's past experiences, present sexual tensions, and methods of resolution. The partner is then invited to participate in the patient's assessment, which includes a physical examination.

This assessment deals with each of the six categories of the patient's sexual functioning status (see the section on sexual consequences of spinal cord injury in this chapter). Specific alternatives are then explored and on occasion demonstrated. For example, the partner may want to see how to bring on a reflex erection, or both may want to know what position in intercourse may be most feasible. Some patients may want to know about sexual aids.

In the acute setting, a private room is made available to the couple for their unobserved use at their convenience. In the active rehabilitation phase the couple is encouraged to practice during home visits. A record of the assessment is summarized under the various headings of the sexual functioning status list. After review with the patient and partner, the summary is placed in the chart. No final diagnosis is made because the patient's physical and social circumstances may change in the future. Follow-up, therefore, becomes very important.

4. *Follow-up visits.* Follow-up visits are carried out to correct areas of confusion and misinformation, to monitor changes in the patient's sexual functioning pattern and marital and social relationships, and to encourage experimentation with alternative sex activities. The follow-up includes preparation for discharge and periodic progress visits thereafter.

Some patients do not wish to have follow-up visits. Other patients wish to delay experimentation and begin their probings in their home environment. Patients who have no partners may be encouraged to experiment by themselves.

5. *Long-term care.* The sexual health clinicians are available for consultations over the telephone and for repeat visits. A significant portion of the patients come back to the Sexual Health Service 4 to 5 years after discharge from the rehabilitation setting. By that time some of the unmarried persons have entered into significant relationships, and others have gone through divorce and now have a new partner. Some people have not been able to form relationships and feel that their future chances as a partner depend on their sexual integrity. Among men, the leading concerns are problems with erection and infertility. After reassessment of the situation, some of these men may be referred to the self-injection clinic (for intracavernous injections) or the sperm recovery project, for a review of and assistance with the fertility issues.

Outcome evaluations of this program are inadequate. In this service the objective of the patient care services is to provide treatment on the basis of assessment. This requires a highly individual approach to each patient and a range of goals that can be very broad, from reassurance and relief gained through accurate information, to a reorientation of the patient's perspectives about the acceptable range of sexual expression.

Immediate and retrospective reviews indicate that in nearly all instances the clinician's interaction with patients and partners leads to a clear definition of the patient's functioning in sex response, sexual activity capabilities, interest level, fertility status, and urinary-bowel hygiene relevant to sex activities. About two-thirds of the patients and partners are able to refocus their sexual expectations on goals consistent with their physical disabilities. This process may take several months or several years. It is not yet possible to assess the relative significance of a number of factors, such as the clinician's input, the behavior of the existing partner (or the appearance of a new partner), the success of vocational reorientation, or the financial status of the family.

One important observation is that the nature and severity of the injury are not the important determinant of the outcome of the sexual rehabilitation. Two factors that seem to help the patient refocus and work toward realistic sex-related goals are (1) active, varied, and satisfying sex relationships before the injury and (2) an interested and adventurous partner. If these factors are missing, or if one or both partners are consumed by anger related to the catastrophic injury, it is more difficult for the clinician to help the couple to achieve significant goals in the short-term treatment.

Personal Viewpoints in this chapter illustrate the complexities of the sexual rehabilitation process and the involvement of a partner.

PRACTICE METHODS FOR NONSPECIALIST HEALTH CARE PROFESSIONALS ————

Although a sexual rehabilitation program may have to be provided as a specialty service, it cannot function without the interested and knowledgeable support of other staff members. Patients do not approach nurses, therapists, psychologists, social workers, brace makers, and even housekeepers with their sex-related concerns. If there is a specialist backup, both patients and team members might feel more at ease discussing sex issues. One nurse said, "The conversation could always be closed by me telling the patient, 'Why don't you go see the sex counselor?' or 'I don't know the answer to this, but I'll ask the sex specialist.'" But even without a specialist around, patients want to explore their sexual situations. The nonspecialist might consider three basic approaches to patient inquiries: *detection* of concerns; *clarification* of the complaints, questions, or concerns; and *information* giving.

Detection of Concerns

A patient's sexual concerns may surface

- Directly in the form of well-formulated questions or statements
- Indirectly through various sex-related comments, innuendos, or behaviors; through noncompliance with the rehabilitation program; or through behaviors that interfere with the nurse's work
- In response to questions in nursing histories or other forms of inquiry by the nurse

The purpose of case finding is to legitimize the patient's sex-related inquiries. It is a way to say that "sex is spoken here," however haltingly. Care givers can explain their limited qualifications for sexual counseling, assist patients by clarifying the concern, offer information, or help patients to find out about better sources of information.

Direct Inquiries

Mrs. Smith, the 52-year-old woman (discussed at the opening of this chapter), married for 28 years and the mother of three sons, suffered an incomplete injury to the C_{6-7} segments of her spinal cord. Two months after her injury she turned to the nurse: "I think I want to talk to somebody about my sex life."

This is direct sexual inquiry. This kind of plea for help gives care givers an opportunity to acknowledge the appropriateness of this question, to state their own limitations in this area, and to invite further revelations from patients on a low anxiety level.

NURSE: Oh, I'm glad! You're feeling comfortable enough to talk about sex *(acknowledgment)*. I guess you know that I don't have special training in sexual counseling, but I would be glad to listen. Would I do? *(This indicates limitation and invites further information.)*

PATIENT: I'd like that, if you would listen.

NURSE: I might have to ask you a few questions too. *(This is asking for permission to explore when appropriate.)*

PATIENT: I could talk to you.

NURSE: Should we arrange a time then? Like around 2 o'clock, just after your treatment? *(This gives an official seal of approval to the discussion, lowering the anxiety level.)*

Others might approach the care giver with clear-cut questions: "I don't feel my penis. Does this mean that I can't have sex anymore?" or "How long will my reflex erection last?" or "Which position would we use while my brace is on?" or "Could you tell me about artificial insemination?" Again, the response to these inquiries should contain an acceptance of the question and a statement of the care giver's limitations in this area. Then it is up to the patient to continue the conversation. For example, if the care giver is unable to answer the patient's inquiry, a statement like this would be appropriate: "This is a very important question. I just don't know the answers. Would it be all right with you if I check out who could help you with this?" If the questions are within the care givers' sphere of knowledge, they may begin to clarify the patients' worries and offer appropriate information. These methods are discussed later.

Indirect Expressions

Examples of *indirect expressions* of sexual concerns include repetitive references to one's past sexual prowess; repeated compliments about the therapist's desirable physical attributes; jokes with sexual connotations; hypothetical questions like, "If you were my wife, would you want to go to bed with me?"; or statements like, "Maybe my husband should find another woman. I will be useless to him," or "I think I'll be a bachelor forever." Patients may make sexual propositions to care givers or may expose their bodies, ask for genital care more often than required, hold onto the nurse when it is not appropriate, or attempt to caress the care giver's face or body.

PATIENT: *(for the third time in half an hour)* Say, you still did not answer me. Would you come to bed with me?

NURSE: Jim, I am not upset with what you are saying, but I want you to know that I don't want to go to bed with you. Is this clear? *(This rejects the patient's behavior but not the patient.)*

PATIENT: Clear, Shmeer. How am I supposed to know what I can do?

NURSE: You're worried? *(This open question invites more information.)*

PATIENT: Worried?!

NURSE: Well, you know, some of the other men are worried that they can't get an erection, or that they can't meet women, and so on. What would concern you most? *(This is clarification mixed with reassurance that patient's worry is not unique.)*

Without making too much fuss, the nurse defused a bothersome situation and gave an opportunity to the patient to express his sexual concern directly. The nurse was now able to respond to the patient's concern and at the same time proceed with other tasks without having to dodge inappropriate requests.

Sometimes what the patient does or says is not an indirect expression of sexual concerns or desires, but behavior representing indirect complaints about the treatment program, or concerns over not making good progress in recovery. The task here is to find out what these expressions really mean. For this reason, other members of the team should know about the individual's experiences with the patient. Often other staff will report similar experiences; by comparing notes they may uncover a pattern of patient behavior that clarifies the problem and indicates the appropriate action.

Doug, a 28-year-old man, married six weeks, suffered a C_{6-7} injury. Two months after his injury he was being prepared for his first weekend home visit. Although usually a cooperative and well-motivated patient, he became abusive to the staff, yelled at his wife, and refused to participate in physical therapy. When the physical therapist suggested to him that the exercise would help him to transfer into his bed, he said: "You'd think I'm training for my second honeymoon."

Doug's nurse picked up on this and attempted to clarify.

NURSE: Is that the way you feel?

PATIENT: What way?

NURSE: Like you're going on your honeymoon?

PATIENT: Are you kidding?

NURSE: Well no, but I can imagine that you might feel some pressures. *(This is acceptance of feeling.)*

PATIENT: What the hell are you talking about?

NURSE: Well, we somehow haven't talked about you and Jane being in the same bed. *(This directs the interview toward the sexual area.)*

PATIENT: Maybe we didn't talk because it's none of your business.

NURSE: Perhaps not. Have you talked with Jane about this? *(This is further directing.)*

PATIENT: No. What's there to talk about?

NURSE: Well, this first visit home is kind of an experiment. *(This focuses the discussion.)*

PATIENT: So?

NURSE: It might be worthwhile to make a plan. What is it that you and Jane want to experience? *(This focuses with an open question.)*

PATIENT: There you are. Sex raises its ugly head.

NURSE: I did not say sex, or intercourse, or erection, or orgasm. Maybe the two of you want to try something, maybe not. What I am saying is that you and Jane may want to agree before the weekend what your plans are. She might just want to know how the two of you can be side by side. *(This gives options and responsibilities to the patient.)*

PATIENT: Yeah. Hm . . . Is this written down somewhere?

NURSE: Well, no; but when Jane comes in today, we could make a list together.

PATIENT: I wouldn't mind it.

This brief illustration shows how the nurse disarmed the patient's angry outburst, clarified the main concern, and helped the patient acknowledge his hurt and fear. The patient now could explore alternatives with dignity. The nurse accepted sexual issues as part of the person's daily life and used common sense and interviewing skills to handle the situation. The next three examples show some of the problems encountered when inquiries are ignored or misinterpreted:

Joe, a 39-year-old married man, suffered a C_{6-7} complete injury. An external sphincterotomy was proposed to assist him with his urinary flow. Although at first he seemed pleased with the suggestion, rather abruptly he started to berate the nurse who usually assisted with his catheterizations. Joe also said, "I'm going to sue that doctor if he doesn't do it right." These and similar outbursts were quite uncharacteristic of his previous behavior. Eventually, just a few days before the scheduled operation, his wife told the head nurse that the patient was "petrified with worry because he heard from other men that his erection will be lost after this surgery." When the nurse explained to him that "it would not likely happen," he was still unsatisfied but agreed to the surgery.

His erection failed to materialize for about 6 weeks after the operation. Although this was not unusual following this type of surgery, Joe was depressed, uncooperative, and refused to be treated by the urologist involved. Even after the episode was over, he remained withdrawn and angry. Looking back on this situation, the nurses agreed that the patient was labeled "an angry man" and no concerted attempt was made to investigate the sexual causes for his behavior, even though the nurses knew that many patients are concerned about this operation.

Russ, a 28-year-old unmarried man, suffered an incomplete C_{6-7} injury. While still in the intensive care unit he wanted to know about his chances to become a father. When someone suggested to Russ that the answer to this was way down the line, he became angry, asked to see a specialist to find out if the "sperms could be taken out of me and somehow frozen for later use." His request was ignored and his subsequent outbursts were explained at the team meeting as "loss of self-image" or a "struggle to reestablish his image."

Two weeks later his girlfriend arrived from out of town and revealed that she was ten weeks pregnant. She also told the nurse that just before the accident they were planning to have her then seven-week-old pregnancy aborted because of their interpersonal difficulties. Now their dilemma was whether she should go ahead with the abortion or have the baby; and if so, should they separate now or get married and see how things would go?

In the light of this story, the patient's extreme agitation to have his sperm checked was not unreasonable. He had to know whether the baby she carried was his last chance to become a father. In this instance, however, the staff acted in a judgmental way and did not clarify the concerns. The patient lost his trust in the staff members and robbed himself of the opportunity to express his concerns, to hear others' reactions, and to consider the various alternatives for resolving the difficult situation. Parental pressures also forestalled further discussions. The couple got married; she had the baby; two months after that they separated and later divorced.

Barbara, an 18-year-old woman (with an incomplete C_{6-7} injury), was engaged in a lighthearted conversation with a male physical therapist about fashions and clothing styles while doing her exercises. Discussion focused on the differences between "sexy" and "sensuous" clothing, and she turned to him for an opinion.

One would not immediately identify this conversation as a cry for help, yet Barbara recalled the incident several months after her discharge from the unit. She said, "I desperately wanted to know, am I attractive enough for a man to have interest in me sitting in a wheelchair, and do I still come across as a sensuous person in a wheelchair? But nobody heard my questions!"

Sexual Concerns and Patient Histories

Medical, nursing, social work, psychology, and physical or occupational therapy histories have room to gather information about sexual concerns during assessment.

NURSE: Now I have a question about sexual functioning. Many persons have some worries about this. Have you or your wife (husband) had any concerns in this area? *(This is a form of reassurance, "My questions are routine; you are not the only one who might have some problems.")*

PATIENT: I'm not so sure I know what you mean.

NURSE: Can I give you some examples of some common concerns? *(This is asking for permission.)*

PATIENT: Uh-huh.

NURSE: Well, many men (women) wonder if they will be able to satisfy their partners; others worry whether they will be able to get some satisfaction; and others worry whether they can still become fathers or mothers. *(This is clarification.)*

PATIENT: Yes, to all!

NURSE: You know, these are difficult areas for everybody, I am glad that you don't mind talking about them. We don't have a sex specialist on the ward, but we will get the best information to you over the next few weeks. *(This gives reassurance, states limitations, and asks permission to continue.)*

PATIENT: You mean everybody will know about my problems?

NURSE: These problems are just as important as your other difficulties. We will respect your privacy. The doctor and two or three of the nurses looking after you will have to know about these concerns so that you can get the best information. *(This is explanation, forewarning.)*

PATIENT: I guess that's okay.

NURSE: Would you like a pamphlet that mentions sex problems?

PATIENT: No, not now. I will wait till I can talk to you about this again.

NURSE: Okay. But be sure to bring up these questions again if you feel that your questions haven't been dealt with! *(This puts some responsibility on the patient.)*

The early introduction of the idea that "sex is spoken here" lowers the patient's anxiety that this area might be ignored. It also helps the staff members: the sexual concern will be part of the problem list now, and it will be a relatively easy task to approach the patient again some appropriate moment in the future with: "You may remember, when I took your history, you said that you were worried about some sexual issues. Would this be the right time to talk about it?"

Other ways of letting the patient know about sexual care services would be in a pamphlet describing the services offered in this treatment unit. Some patients prefer to read about sexual alternatives, rather than discuss them. For example, a 45-year-old wife of a doctor suffered a T_{12}–L_1 fracture with complete paraplegia. She thought sexual health care was a "wonderful idea," but she preferred to "read about it rather than talk." She studied the few pamphlets the nurse gave her but did not ask any questions. She, however, introduced other female patients to her reading material.

Another way of introducing this topic may come from interested staff members—for example, a social worker, physician, or psychologist—who take on the responsibility of describing how these concerns can be looked after on the unit.

Clarification of Concerns

Once a patient's complaint or concern is out in the open, it has to be clarified. To which of the six categories of "sexual concerns" listed earlier in this chapter does the patient's complaint belong? Is it a worry about erections and orgasms, loss of interest, loss of the partner's interest, new relationships, active participation in sex acts, or managing urinary or bowel control during a sex act? Is it a concern about becoming a father or mother, or about contraception? Clarification translates the patient's diffuse worries into manageable bits. It also reassures patients that their concerns are not unique. The following example shows how clarification helped the 52-year-old mother of three mentioned in the first part of this chapter.

NURSE: Here I am. We have at least 15 minutes now.

PATIENT: I hope I'm not holding you up. I don't even know where I should start! I've never known anybody with my type of injury before. Does it cause any sex problems?

NURSE: Well, you know, just the other day one of the other patients said exactly the same thing and asked the same question. (*This reassures the patient.*)

PATIENT: You mean other people ask about sex, too? That makes me feel better. I thought I might get reprimanded or something.

NURSE: More and more people want to get proper information now. But sex means so many things. How would you feel if I asked you a few questions to find out what areas concern you?

PATIENT: Well, I only thought about intercourse, but why don't you go ahead. I *am* glad you're here.

NURSE: You did mention intercourse. (*This lets the patient set the limits.*)

PATIENT: Yes, that's a worry. Could my husband lie on top of me without doing more damage to my spine?

NURSE: You mean when the fracture is healed?

PATIENT: Well, certainly not now! Or do people want this in the hospital? (*The patient is now set up to receive information.*)

NURSE: Most people want to be hugged and held. That can be done here, certainly. And when your fracture is healed, it would be perfectly safe. Your husband may have to place your legs so that he can position himself.

PATIENT: So you say that we could try intercourse later? I must tell him tonight! You know, I *know* he just did not dare to ask me!

NURSE: There might be other areas that you want to check out, too.

PATIENT: I'm sure, but this is the best news yet. Let's leave it at this; then later I can ask you more.

In this instance this is all that the patient wanted to handle. Now that she had developed a special trust in the nurse, she would later ask for more information.

Information Giving

Information giving is a form of "sexual first aid." It is most appropriate when the patient already has a specific concern about sex. Giving specific information is an organized approach to the patient's distress. Once the main complaint is isolated and the reason for the timing of the question is understood (for example, after a visit by family, a television program, diagnostic comments by a medical attendant, or comments by other patients), the nurse has a good opportunity to clarify misinformation and provide relevant new information. Equally important is how to close the brief discussion. This may consist of a promise for more information, a check with someone more expert in the situation, or a discussion with the partner.

The care giver will have to accept the patient's statements without cover-up or offering false hope; clarify specific complaints and misinformation; and if it appears to be in the best interest of the patient, arrange for a visit with someone more familiar with the issues.

Megan, a 49-year-old woman, suffered a low thoracic level, incomplete injury. She was divorced but had a partner who entered the picture after her injury. He visited her frequently, but she became depressed after the visits and then gradually lost interest in her bowel training and physical therapy. Although they had access to a private room for sex experimentation, Megan refused to go there after the first visit. Eventually she told him that he should find another partner. He opened up the possibility of a sex problem when he asked the nurse about "another position." In the process of clarification Megan eventually revealed to the nurse that she used to be proud of her ability to "move my seat and satisfy my partner." Unable to do her customary movements she felt useless as a sex partner and as a person. The nurse asked her permission to check with the physical therapist about alternate positions. The physical therapist devised a small band that helped keep the patient's ankles together and let her "clasp" him. By the time this was discussed and tried out, the patient's partner was able to convince her that he loved and enjoyed her *as she was.*

The following are a few techniques that may help the care giver in giving sexual first aid:

1. *Ask for permission.* Whenever a new sexual area is about to be discussed, a good approach is to ask: "Can I ask you a question about your relationship?" or "I would need to know if you have experienced an erection in the last few days. May I ask you about this?" If the patient says "No. I don't want to talk about it," the care giver can safely reply: "I'm glad I asked you first. I wouldn't want to invade your privacy." Although the care giver should stop this line of questioning, the reason for the patient's somewhat frightened reply may need to be investigated.

2. *Be specific.* Most patients find it easier to deal with well-stated questions than generalities. For example, "What sort of erection did you notice this morning?" is a question that can be answered with some specificity. "What was going on down below this morning?" is such an unclear way of asking that the answer might not be trustworthy.

3. *Avoid irrelevant questions.* A useful rule is to ask oneself: "Why did I ask this? Could I explain the reason for my question if the patient challenged me?" If the answer is "yes," the question was not irrelevant.

4. *Start with reassurance.* "Many women with spinal injury go through periods of loss of interest, but tell me . . . this loss of sexual interest that's concerning you now . . . have you ever experienced it before your injury?"

5. *Proceed from least sensitive to more sensitive areas.* "I wonder . . . in your conversations with your friends, have you heard about self-stimulation? Have you read about it? What sort of feelings have you had about it? Many young children stimulate themselves—what was your experience as a child? What has your experience been in the last few years?"

6. *Use language that is clear to the patient.* The language can be medical, slangy, or earthy, depending on the patient's needs and the care giver's comfort. Patients sometimes say "organism" meaning orgasm; "pee-nuts" instead of penis; "clidoris" instead of clitoris. In these instances correction may be embarrassing, but letting the patient know that "not that it makes any difference, but here we usually say *orgasm*" may be helpful.

Practicing to Provide Care

Care givers need to practice to fulfill a role in sexual health care. Even if they have a great deal of knowledge about the sexual consequences of SCI and the best of intentions, they may feel so awkward, vulnerable, and concerned about causing hurt to the patient that a sexual conversation is impossible. One way to acquire the necessary confidence is to practice various conversations. Alternating roles, care givers can rehearse various ways of detecting concerns, or giving sexual first aid. Audiotape or videotape equipment is useful because it is possible to review style, sound level, points of hesitation, methods of reassurance, clarity, and so on.

In some institutions the staff participate in desensitization programs, which include viewing explicit sexual films, discussing reactions to sex-related words, and describing sex acts. The value of these programs is not clear. Perhaps a more fundamental approach to acquiring a facility with sexual conversation is to reflect on the fact that health professionals are motivated in their work by their desire to help people. There is plenty of evidence that sex problems are distressing to most patients. Their desire to talk and enthusiasm about receiving information usually motivates health professionals to help. This motivation leads care givers to seek more knowledge, better communication skills, and sometimes, a position in an environment where the sexual consequences of the patient's disability are formally considered.

REFERENCES

Brindley, G. S. 1981. Electroejaculation: Its technique, neurological implications and usage. *Journal of Neurology, Neurosurgery and Psychiatry* 44: 9–18. *This is the first major statement about electroejaculation in men with SCI.*

Ford, J. R., and Duckworth, B. 1987. *Physical management for the Quadriplegic Patient.* 2d ed. Philadelphia: F. A. Davis.

Goller, H., and Paeslack, V. 1972. Pregnancy damage and birth complications in the children of paraplegic women. *Paraplegia* 10: 213–217.

Green, B. G., and Sloan, S. L. 1986. Penile prostheses in spinal cord injured patients: Combined psychosexual counselling and surgical regimen. *Paraplegia* 24 (3): 167–172. *Describes experiences with 40 spinal cord injured patients who have received penile prostheses as well as early sexual counseling.*

Novak, P. P., and Mitchell, M. M. 1988. Professional involvement in sexuality counseling for patients with spinal cord injuries. *American Journal of Occupational Therapy* 42 (2): 105–112. *A national survey indicates that although sexuality counseling in the total rehabilitation of the spinal cord injured patient is considered a priority, many of the professionals surveyed did not conduct sexuality counseling as part of their job.*

Nygaard, I., Bartscht, K. D., and Cole, S. 1990. Sexuality and reproduction in spinal cord injured women. *Obstetrical and Gynecological Survey* 45: 727–732.

Ohry, A., Peleg, D., and Goldman, J. 1988. Sexual function, pregnancy, and delivery in spinal cord injured women. *Gynecology and Obstetrics Investigation* 9: 281–283.

Robertson, D. N. S. 1972. Pregnancy and labor in the paraplegic. *Paraplegia* 10: 209–212.

Rucker, B., Szasz, G., and Carpenter, C. 1988. Legal, ethical and religious issues related to fertility enhancement of men with spinal cord injuries. *Canadian Journal of Rehabilitation* 1 (4): 225–231.

Szasz, G. 1987a. Sexual function in the spinal cord injured. In *Management of Spinal Cord Injuries*. Eds. R. F. Bloch and M. Basbaum. Baltimore: Williams and Wilkins, pp. 410–447. *Outlines the process of sexual assessment in persons with SCI.*

Szasz, G. 1987b. Sexual management. In *Physical Management for the Quadriplegic Patient*. Eds. J. R. Ford and B. Duckworth. Philadelphia: F. A. Davis, pp. 377–395. *Focus is on physical management of sexual problems in persons with SCI. (Illustrated.)*

Szasz, G., and Carpenter, C. 1989. Clinical observations on vibratory stimulation of the penis in men with spinal cord injury. *Archives of Sexual Behavior* 18 (6): 100–103. *Outlines step-by-step the physical and mental reactions during the vibration process that leads to ejaculation in some men with SCI.*

Ver Voort, S. M. 1987. Infertility in spinal cord injured male. *Urology* 29: 157–165. *Reviews the current understanding of sterility in men with SCI.*

Wanner, M. B., Rageth, M. D., and Zach, G. A. 1987. Pregnancy and autonomic hyperreflexia in patients with spinal cord lesions. *Paraplegia* 25: 482–490.

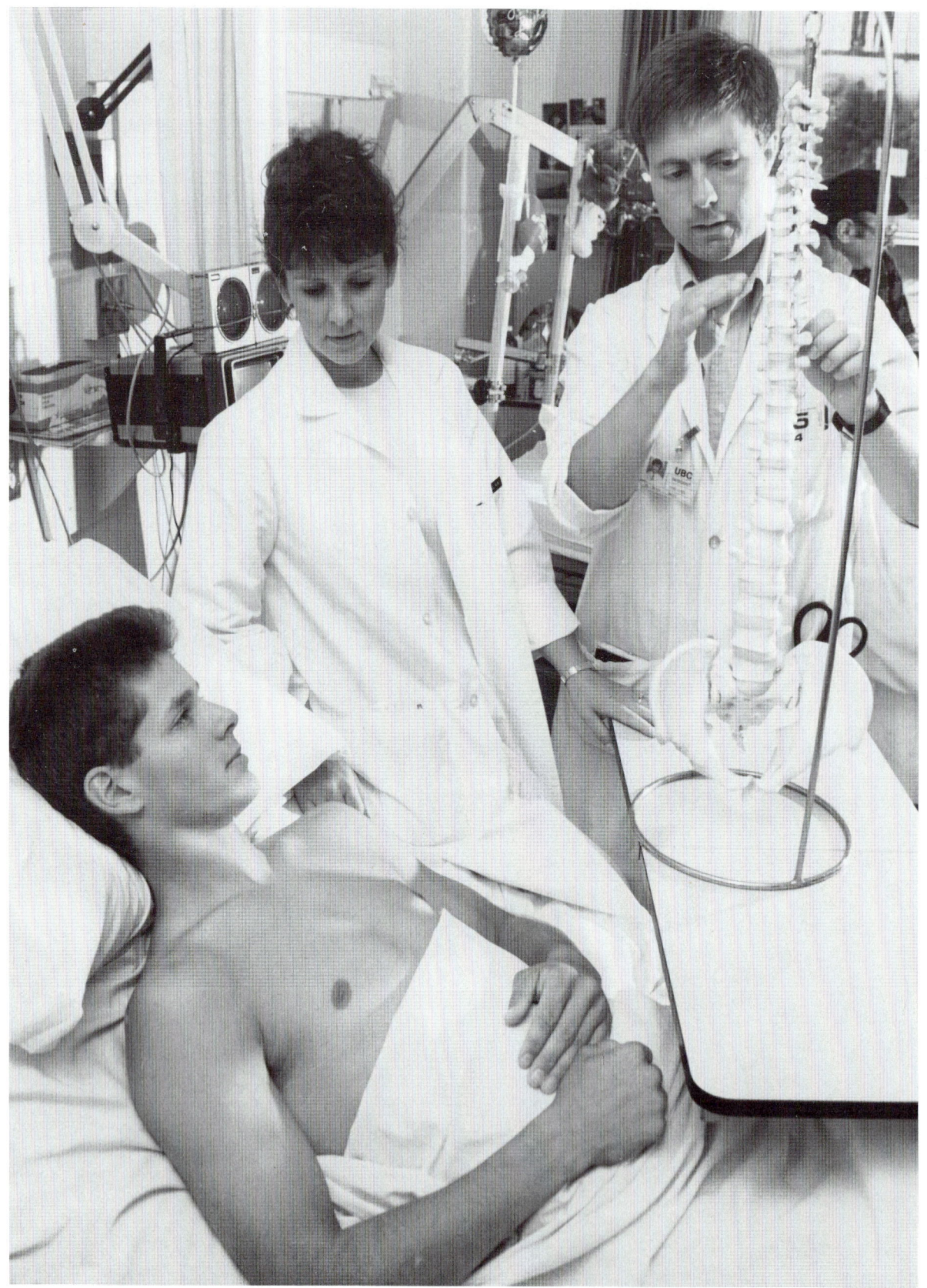

CHAPTER
— 11 —

Individual and Family Health Education[*]

Chapter Outline

HEALTH CARE GOALS
FACTORS TO CONSIDER WHEN PLANNING AND
CONDUCTING EDUCATION
  Self-Concept and Self-Esteem
  Age and Developmental Stage
  Educational Background and Life Experience
  Emotional Aspects
  Physical Health
  The Therapeutic Environment
A PROCESS FOR PATIENT AND FAMILY HEALTH
EDUCATION
  Assessment
  Goal Setting
  Implementation
  Evaluation
REFERENCES

Health Education Objectives

- To identify patient and family health education goals and develop an educational process
- To define learning and describe factors that affect learning
- To identify desirable qualities that enhance the role of the nurse as educator
- To assess learning needs, develop behavioral objectives, implement educational activities, and evaluate the teaching-learning process

.*This chapter was developed with the assistance of Jane Andrew, O.T.,
M.Ed., Patient and Family Health Education Coordinator; G. F.
Strong Rehabilitation Centre, Vancouver, British Columbia.

Significant benefits will accrue to patients, families, and staff from a planned, coordinated health education program. The following are among the very pertinent reasons for developing a planned patient education program:

- Planned patient education programs offer a means to obtain information that can better equip patients to make decisions and [act to] safeguard their well-being and . . . meet their own health care needs.
- Planned patient education programs help ensure that the patient receives correct, nonconflicting information from each staff person involved, that is, the patient experiences continuity and consistency of the educational component of care. [American Hospital Association 1979: 41–42]

The total adaptation of patients and families to a different life-style is the most significant goal of the rehabilitation program. Therefore, patients and families should be given maximum opportunity to explore new health habits, roles, responsibilities, and social functioning. This may require that time be made available from the more traditional rehabilitation program. Learning to cope with leisure time, particularly after discharge, is one such nontraditional area that must be included in the health education process.

In this chapter, patient and family health education is defined as *any information or knowledge, skills or techniques, and attitudes needed by an individual and family to understand and manage the effects of the disability and maintain optimal health.*

HEALTH CARE GOALS ————————

Successful health education of people with spinal cord injuries (SCI) and their families significantly contributes to the entire rehabilitation process.

We are witnessing a change in the attitude of the health professional and the consumer toward patient education. The consumer rights movement, the requirements of governmental and accrediting agencies, and today's emphasis on prevention of health problems attest to this change. With this change comes the challenge of providing accumulated knowledge with a fresh approach. [McCormick and Gilson-Parkevich 1979: preface]

The goals of patient and family health education are:

- To acquaint the patient and family with the extent of disability and the treatment approaches that are being used
- To effect attitudinal/behavioral changes in patients and families so that they will assume an active role in rehabilitation and in the maintenance of optimal

health, including management of the disability throughout life

Implicit in the goals of patient and family education is the principle that the patient and family have a right to be part of the process of determining rehabilitation goals. Health care workers must not allow their dedication and expertise to abridge this fundamental right. In order to make informed decisions about and commitments to their participation in the rehabilitation process, patients and families must be properly informed about the extent of residual disability, the services available in the rehabilitation process, and the functional and other outcomes that may depend on the rehabilitation process. The patient and family must then realize they are responsible for the consequences of their decisions and resultant actions.

In order to achieve the goal of patient and family participation in decision making, the "system" and the entire treatment team must not only permit it but also actively encourage it. In practice this means that the patient must be involved in determining the goals of the rehabilitation and life care plans. The patient, family, and staff must clearly state and mutually understand their expectations and responsibilities very soon after injury. The discussion should include the reasons for admission, services to be provided, effort required, estimated length of stay, and expected outcomes of the various stages of the rehabilitation process. If the participants' expectations and acceptance of responsibilities are not congruent or compatible, the educational process attempts to bring the patient and family to active participation. When there is agreement and involvement, the patient and family will find the ensuing process meaningful and relevant and will commit to it.

FACTORS TO CONSIDER WHEN PLANNING AND CONDUCTING EDUCATION ————————

Learning is a process that results in a behavioral change or the acquisition of a skill. To illustrate these definitions let us consider the education necessary to promote optimal urinary function. Activities to attain this goal may include the performance of intermittent catheterizations. Knowledge of the basic anatomy and function of the urinary system, the principles of emptying the bladder at specific regular intervals, and the rationale for using selected techniques will help the patient understand why catheterizations promote optimal urinary function. The information constitutes the knowledge base. The actual physical skill of catheterization is the technique used to meet the goal. It is usually easier to teach the patient and family appropriate knowledge and skills. However, the key question is whether the patient or the family will use the skills; this brings up questions of attitude. The attitudinal component of education is a complex issue involving interest and value judgments supporting the application of acquired knowledge and skills. The behavioral changes made as a consequence of learning help patients and families assume an active role in health care.

Learning is affected by many factors, both internal and external: the abilities of the patient and family and the therapeutic environment. Although health advancements and technology increase the physical pace of rehabilitation, psychosocial adaptation usually occurs at a slower rate. These barriers to learning point to the need for ongoing educational opportunities. Community resources, knowledgeable in disability-related health care issues, are increasing, but vary slowly.

Some internal factors that affect learning for patients and their families are self-concept and self-esteem, age, educational background and life experience, emotional status, and physical health.

Self-Concept and Self-Esteem

As people mature, self-concept evolves from that of a dependent personality to that of a self-directed adult with the need to be seen by others as self-directing.

> Adults have a need to be treated with respect, to make their own decisions, to be seen as unique human beings. They tend to avoid, resist and resent situations in which they feel they are treated like children—being told what to do and what not to do, being talked down to, embarrassed, punished, judged. Adults tend to resist learning under conditions that are incongruent with their self-concept as autonomous individuals. . . . Once an adult makes the discovery that he can take responsibility for learning, as he does for other facets of his life, he experiences a sense of release and exhilaration. [Knowles 1972: 40]

In the aftermath of SCI, a patient's and family's self-concept and self-esteem are particularly vulnerable. The sensitive professional will be aware of this fact and will take measures to promote feelings of self-worth and minimize feelings of helplessness. To enhance readiness to learn, try to strengthen the learner's self-image and promote self-confidence. Implementing the general interventions outlined in Chapters 9 and 10 will help provide psychological support, which in turn promotes learning. For example, the critical care nurse who has skillfully involved the patient and family in nursing care activities communicates recognition of their capabilities and of the importance of their involvement. This preparation develops interest and fosters positive attitudes toward personal health care in the future.

It is important to continue to involve the patient and family in planning, implementation, and evaluation of health education. This gives the patient an opportunity to see the relevance of learning the activity at hand and thus be more committed to it. If we accept the principle that the patient is the ultimate decision maker and is responsible for the consequences of decisions and actions, in other words is self-directing, we must give the patient as much opportunity for input and involvement as possible during learning (Shaw 1981).

Age and Developmental Stage

The patient's age and related developmental stage are important factors in the educational process. Throughout life, growth encompasses fulfillment of such new roles as mate, parent, community member or leader, son or daughter of aging parent, or pensioner.

It is important to understand how normal fulfillment of maturational roles must be integrated with health education. For example, a teenager may be exclusively concerned with appearance and attractiveness to the opposite sex. This concern reflects a normal learning need to establish sexual identity and begin the process of exploring what qualities are desirable in a future partner. To proceed with educational aspects of care before attending to personal appearance may be devastating and completely block learning. The adult who is dependent on assistance for a bowel procedure may have difficulty accepting help from a family member because it endangers the patient's perceived role as a spouse or independent son or daughter. The elderly are often worried about burdening their families. If returning home and remaining there is to become a reality, possible changes in roles must be assessed with great care and insight.

The physiological aspects of aging also affect learning. The possibility of diminished visual and auditory faculties, general physical deterioration, and slowed thought processes must be considered.

Educational Background and Life Experience

Knowledge of educational background and life experience give some idea about a person's interest in maintaining health and the ways in which a person learns. Generally, the higher the level of education, the greater the working vocabulary and exposure to learning. Depressed socioeconomic status or cultural difference can often hamper the person's understanding of the English language (Doak, Doak, and Root 1985).

Life experience can provide a helpful background conductive to learning; or it may be detrimental if a behavior has to be unlearned. For example, establishing controlled regularity with a neurogenic bowel dysfunction depends largely on dietary intake. The patient who practiced good dietary habits before injury will achieve regulation of bowel movements more easily than a patient whose dietary habits must be unlearned and then corrected. Generally, the older the person is, the greater the tendency to be rigid, which makes behavioral change more difficult.

Emotional Aspects

Sensitivity to the learner's present emotional feelings is a key factor affecting learning. Disinterest, increasing agitation, or openly expressed hostility signal underlying concerns that interfere with learning.

> Sensitivity to the patient's anger, fears, and problems is an essential element in a flexible educational program. If, for example, a patient suffers an emotional reverse due to frustration in physical therapy, no teaching is attempted until feelings of inadequacy or rage have been ameliorated. Or, if a patient seems singularly disinterested in the lesson of the moment, and the nurse perceives concern about a family problem, the lesson is explored. Efforts are then initiated to help with the resolution of the problem before further attempts at teaching are made. [Engstrand 1979: 17]

Psychosocial adaptation following SCI is a major factor to consider, particularly if denial is a problem with either the patient or the family. When hoping for a "miracle cure" negates all else, encourage the patient to focus on the disability as it is today, and emphasize how important it is to maintain optimal health in case any function should return. This approach usually resolves some of the patient's inner turmoil and helps the patient and family become more open to learning.

Physical Health

When people are ill, the amount of strength and energy they are able to devote to learning is limited. However, Stauffer (1980: 56) injects reality into the situation when she states that whether the patient is "feeling angry, sick, depressed, or just plain miserable, he must absorb an amount of information comparable to a difficult college course, and absorb it well enough to put into immediate daily use once he goes home."

The most stressful times in terms of physical illness for people with SCI are the initial recovery period after injury and when infections or setbacks are experienced during the rehabilitation program. During these times, however, health education can continue by developing interests and fostering positive attitudes about involvement in health care.

The Therapeutic Environment

One key concept in ensuring successful patient and family health education outcomes is that of helping an adult learn—that is, demonstrating observable attitudes and behaviors that communicate a sense of concern or interest, patience, and a desire to share knowledge, skills, expertise, and points of view acquired through formal training and experience. This emphasizes the role of the professional as *facilitator* and *resource person*, rather than an authority figure. The total concept of adult education in health care is that professionals have a responsibility to share information and expertise that is vital to maintaining health and to do so in a way that is meaningful for the patient and family—a partnership for managing the effects of disability.

The patient and family must feel at ease. A relationship that is open to communication and is respecting and constructive will best help the patient and family learn. A positive interpersonal relationship between the nurse and the learner is essential to the process. Primary nursing is also conducive to health education because it fosters a continuous nurse-patient and nurse-family relationship.

A PROCESS FOR PATIENT AND FAMILY HEALTH EDUCATION

Progressing through each phase of a problem-solving process—assessment, goal setting, implementation, and evaluation—provides a systematic method to ensure that the care provided is geared to the individual needs of the patient and family. This method is also applied when providing patient and family health education (Hanak 1991). Consider how the following basic questions illustrate this process.

1. What does the patient and family need or want to learn? What change in behavior is desired? Why is it important that the patient and family learn? (Assessment)

2. What will the patient and family be able to do and how well at the conclusion of the teaching/learning? (Goal setting or establishing behavioral objectives)

3. On what basis should the education be organized? How should the educational content or material be presented? What teaching aids will facilitate learning? (Implementation)

4. How will the educator, patient and family determine if learning occurred? (Evaluation)

The educator must draw on both professional and personal experiences to assess learning needs and determine educational content; to develop behavioral objectives, which can then be evaluated; to find creative ways of communicating, encouraging learner participation, and facilitating feedback; and to apply behavioral change theories.

Peer resource persons are increasingly used to encourage patient participation in rehabilitation. Role modeling can break down barriers to learning. Disabled persons also act as resource persons for health care professionals.

Assessment

Two major components constitute the broad assessment involved in patient and family health education: learning needs directly related to maintaining health and managing disability, and the psychosocial and other needs of the patient and the family. On an individual basis, consider factors that affect learning while identifying specific learning needs. Flexibility is an important concept in health education. Integrating awareness of such factors as the person's self-concept, self-esteem, and physical and emotional health enhances learning. For example, if the patient is emotionally upset or physically ill, deal with these issues before presenting an educational activity.

The scope and depth of the teaching-learning process involved with severe disability can be overwhelming for both the health professional and the patient and family. the complexity of this situation strongly emphasizes the need for a systematic, coordinated approach to learning on an interdisciplinary level to determine what information is needed; to ensure consistency of content; and to include appropriate team members in determining, implementing, and evaluating educational objectives.

Throughout this book specific educational needs are addressed. Several primary areas include neurogenic bladder and bowel dysfunction, care of the skin, and respiratory and cardiovascular system management, as well as various aspects of nutrition, physical activity, independent daily living skills, and psychological adjustment. Although professionals may be well aware of learning needs, the patient may not be as receptive for a variety of reasons. The initial exploration may appear to be limited in terms of what the patient wants to know, but developing awareness of what the patient needs to know is part of the educational process.

Timing is an important factor. Adults tend to view education as a process necessary to cope with a present problem (Knowles 1972; Bartlett 1985). If, for example, a patient is preparing for an initial outing, it is more meaningful to learn how to apply a condom and what to do if an "accident" should occur than it is to learn about medications and bladder infections. The latter information is more relevant when the patient is about to go back to work, because bladder infections may cause absenteeism from the job.

The task is to communicate clearly what behaviors are necessary to meet the desired objectives, to clarify the patient's wants and needs, and to present realistic alternatives (Shaw 1981). For example, when teaching essentials to prevent pressure sores, the nurse must explain reasons for skin breakdown and present preventive measures necessary to avoid pressure sores. If the patient has difficulty understanding the significance of this education, one reinforcement measure is to demonstrate how unpleasant the alternatives are. The personal cost of ineffective behaviors can sometimes be demonstrated to the learners by confronting them with the consequences of failure (Engstrand 1979). A pressure ulcer is deforming and its appearance grotesque. Yet visual examination of pressure sores and a discussion of how they developed can motivate patients to learn preventive behaviors.

Goal Setting

Throughout the rehabilitation process it is important to communicate what behaviors are required to meet the goals of planned patient and family health education. A model that clearly conveys the expectations of the health professional allows the patient and family to identify what they know now and what they need to know in the future to maintain optimal health and manage the disability. This kind of communication is facilitated by developing specific behavioral objectives.

For the purposes of this chapter, *behavioral objectives* are statements that express, in demonstratable terms, what is to be learned and, when appropriate, how well. Behavioral objectives include the use of action verbs, such as *states*, *demonstrates*, and *performs*, so that learning can be described precisely and, consequently, evaluated. Words such as *understand* or *appreciate* are too vague and should be avoided. Behavioral objectives specify criteria or standards of acceptable performance that relate directly to identified learning needs.

Table 11–1 is a checklist of the necessary educational objectives related to management of a bowel program. It can also be used to identify learning needs and as an evaluation tool. To initiate the teaching-learning process, discuss the objectives with the patient and family. To evaluate learn-

TABLE 11–1 Bowel Management Education Checklist

Name _____

INSTRUCTED (insert signature and date)		OBJECTIVES	EVALUATED (insert signature and date)	
Patient	Family Member		Patient	Family Member
		1. States how SCI affects bowel function		
		2. Explains 2 reasons for developing a bowel program		
		3. Explains 4 important factors in developing a bowel program		
		4. Performs or describes how to instruct others with bowel evacuation techniques		
		5. States how to evaluate effectiveness of bowel program		
		6. Describes medications related to bowel management including indications for use, precautions when administering, and side effects		
		7. Describes 4 potential problems and solutions		

ing, ask the patient to demonstrate or state the specific objectives. This form can be adapted to the entire teaching program and must be supported by a formalized body of information to provide consistency in teaching the content. If such a guideline is unaccompanied by supportive material, it means something different to everyone. For example, the third objective reads: *Explains four important factors in developing a bowel program.* In order to achieve and evaluate this behavioral objective, precise information about nutritional and fluid intake, physical activity, planning a consistent evacuation time, and developing a responsible attitude should be specifically documented. The seventh objective—*Describes four potential problems and solutions*—requires supportive information including measures to prevent, recognize, and relieve symptoms of constipation, diarrhea, hemorrhoids, and autonomic dysreflexia. If this information is not available, one staff member may consider only prevention as a potential problem, while another may focus only on relief of abnormal symptoms.

Inconsistency in educational activities causes confusion, discouragement, and incomplete education for the patient and family. As a result, the patient and family may not take their active role in managing the disability and main-

taining health, and the desired behavior change is less likely to occur.

Implementation

Having established behavioral objectives related to specific learning needs, it is important to review the documented content, specifically, what is to be taught. Implementing the teaching process requires decisions to be made about who will do the teaching and when, how, and where it will occur. Implementation involves organizing learning experiences in a systematic way, selecting resource materials, and supporting desirable changes in behavior.

Patient and family health education should be an integral and scheduled part of the total rehabilitation program, offered as routinely and consistently as any other health care service. Staff and patients should schedule educational activities during day hours, rather than relegating education to spontaneous sessions during evenings or on weekends when the patient is more likely to be tired, interested in visiting, or other leisure activities. Scheduled sessions may be planned on both an *individual* one-to-one and a *group* basis. For example, many aspects of patient and family health education require teaching on a one-to-one basis because of the intimate nature of the tasks involved; however, a nurse may establish group sessions to teach the basic essentials of bowel, bladder, or skin care, which are common to everyone.

Health education is usually done on a one-to-one basis and often on the spot—that is, during care or assistance with an activity. On-the-spot teaching can be effective for reinforcing learning and providing practical application of knowledge or a skill, but it is not always the most effective method for teaching and learning because it is not the prime purpose of the activity. Teaching a skill by repeated demonstrations can only be effective if the steps and procedures are consistent among the various staff from whom the patient is learning. Without documented procedures, points may be taught somewhat differently by different staff members. This difficulty is compounded by the lack of scheduled time for educational programs. Formalized programs provide consistency, are more efficient in terms of staff time, and therefore make the overall teaching program more effective.

Printed and audiovisual materials enhance the learning process but do not replace the educator or facilitator. When selecting or developing supplemental educational materials, keep in mind that

- The most effective materials are liberally illustrated and speak simply and directly to the problem without medical jargon. This material is comprehensible to people with limited reading ability and not offensive or insulting to those with more education.

- Aids should be accessible and easy to use. Videotape and slide-tape presentations are the most likely formats for audiovisual material although interactive computer programs are now available (VIVA! 1991).

- Audiovisual materials can be tied in to reference material from the patient library. Flexible library hours will accommodate families as well as patients.

- "Workbook" teaching manuals for the patient and family can be used continuously and extensively following discharge.

Although teaching aids may be planned and produced in-house, an increasing amount of material can be purchased, often at a low cost. Manuals are designed specifically for people with SCI and their families. For instance, PVA (Hammond, Umlauf, Matteson, and Perduta-Fulginiti 1989) offers a complete and inexpensive resource. A free service cataloging all SCI audiovisual materials is offered through Texas Institute for Rehabilitation and Research (1991). See the Resources at the end of this book.

Review the contents of these valuable resources to ensure their timing and relevance, and plan comprehensive educational activities.

It is important to give recognition and support when desirable changes in behavior occur. Behavior is sensitive to influence by consequences. When met with positive reinforcement, such as praise or encouragement, that behavior is most likely to be repeated in the future. If a behavior elicits a negative consequence, such as criticism or a disinterested response, that behavior is less likely to be repeated in the future. Health care professionals use this behavioral approach with varying degrees of intensity and awareness. For example, as a subtle way to reinforce positive peer influence, more and more rehabilitation facilities design group interaction with spinal cord injured individuals living in the community as role models.

Patients may need help with personal problems or concerns to be more open in learning experiences. In addition, those specifically trained in the behavioral sciences are a valuable resource to the nurse engaged in clinical application of behavioral change theories to help patients learn faster.

The combined expertise of health professionals and innovative educators seems most likely to improve teaching techniques and stimulate learning (Engstrand 1979; Smith 1987). See the Resources at the end of this book for specific educational materials.

Evaluation

"Basic to all processes of creativity is the ability to evaluate . . . to select, to reject, and to critically determine the value of what has been done" (McCormick and Gilson-Parkevich 1979: 153).

Evaluation is an ongoing shared process by which the nurse and the patient and family can determine whether learning has occurred. Evaluation is directly related to the behavioral objectives documented in the planning process. When learning is defined in terms of a behavioral change or a capability, it can be evaluated. Most often the shortcoming in health education is the lack of evaluation. Without criteria or standards supported by specific content, it is difficult to determine when and how adequately an activity has been learned.

There are many ways to evaluate learning. Some methods include open discussions, direct questioning and observation, return demonstrations, and comparison of pretest and posttest results. Written tools should be simply designed and easily tabulated; checklists or rating scales are good formats. The checklist in Table 11–1 is an example of a simple evaluation tool.

The following points should be kept in mind when selecting methods to evaluate learning (University of British Columbia 1977: 67):

- Exactly what is it that you want to find out? Whether the learners "know" something? Whether they "can do" something? How they "feel" about something? [Evaluating attitudes is far more difficulty than evaluating knowledge and skills.] Be sure to specify that "something" as clearly as possible.

- What does common sense tell you would be the best way to find out? Have the learners answer questions—written or oral? Have them carry out a procedure? Have them solve a problem of some kind? Have them teach another patient? Have them role play back to the nurse?

- How much time is available? How much help do you have (or do you need)? Interviews and skills demonstrations require a low learner-instructor ratio.

- How important is the element you are considering evaluating? Something the learners *must* know or be able to do, or just something that would be "nice"?

Evaluation should occur throughout the educational process to measure the extent to which learning has occurred. Patient and family health education is increasingly gaining recognition as an integral process that most significantly influences the ultimate outcome of rehabilitation. Therefore, evaluation data may not only indicate necessary changes in teaching techniques and learner participation, but they may redirect the entire rehabilitation process.

REFERENCES

American Hospital Association. 1979. *Implementing Patient Education in the Hospital.* Chicago: Author. *Includes definitions and reasons for and guidelines to development of education in health care.*

Bartlett, E. E. 1985. Forum: Patient Education Introduction: Eight Principles from Patient Education Research. *Preventive Medicine* 14: 667–669.

Doak, C., Doak, L., and Root, J. 1985. *Teaching Patients with Low Literary Skills.* Philadelphia: J. B. Lippincott. *Filled with practical approaches to assist health care professionals improve the chances that poor readers will understand their health care instruction.*

Engstrand, J. L. 1979. A nursing challenge; effective patient education. *Journal of Association of Rehabilitation Nurses* 4 (5): 15–18. *Presents a relevant overview of the educational process in rehabilitation; offers valuable guidelines for nurses involved with spinal cord injured patients and focuses on preventable complications of disability, in this case pressure sores.*

Hammond, M.C., Umlauf, R. L., Matteson, B. and Perduta-Fulginiti (Eds.). 1989. *Yes, You Can! A Guide to Self-Care for Persons with Spinal Cord Injury.* Washington, DC: Paralyzed Veterans of America (PVA). *A most welcome resource, this 374-page manual (available in three-ring or bound format) is packed with easy-to-retrieve information on everything from physical needs to resources needed in the community. Valuable glossary of terms and abbreviations. Practical approach is highlighted by wallet card to cut out and fold for management of autonomic dysreflexia. Great chapters on recreation, driver's training, attendant care, and home modifications. Highly recommended for preparation for discharge from formal rehabilitation and thereafter.*

Hanak, M. (Ed.). 1991. *Educational Guide for SCI Nurses: A Manual for Teaching Patients, Families and Caregivers.* Jackson Heights, NY: American Association of SCI Nurses (AASCIN). *A wonderful resource for effective and comprehensive teaching. Each need, such as respiratory management or sexual function, is presented with objectives, content outline, suggested questions, and return demonstrations to aid in* evaluation. *Excellent preparation for community living. Section on community resources includes education, employment, and recreation issues. The flexible design permits development of individualized programs.*

Knowles, M. S. 1972. *The Modern Practice of Adult Education.* New York: Association Press. *Classic text on principles and methods involved in adult learning.*

McCormick, R. D., and Gilson-Parkevich, T. 1979. *Patient and Family Education: Tools, Techniques, and Theory.* New York: John Wiley and Sons. *Practical guidelines for designing, presenting, and evaluating educational activities in a pediatric setting.*

Shaw, L. 1981. The patient as an adult learner. *Association of Operating Room Nurses Journal* 33 (2): 233–239. *Uses a problem-centered approach to adult learning; focuses on preparing the nurse to teach and on assessing the patient's readiness to learn in a hospital environment.*

Smith, C. E. (Ed.). 1987. *Patient Education: Nurses in Partnership with Other Health Care Professionals.* New York: Grune and Stratton. *With a detailed theoretical and research base, provides advanced information on comprehensive rationale, legal aspects, and results of studies on patient education. Health promotion included throughout.*

Stauffer, S. 1980. A master-plan for teaching the patient with spinal cord injury. *Registered Nurse* (July): 56–60. *A brief overview of major educational areas.*

Texas Institute for Rehabilitation and Research (TIRR). 1991. *Educational Resources on SCI.* Houston, TX: Author. *The project, supported by American Spinal Injury Association (ASIA) and an Education and Training Foundation of the Paralyzed Veterans of America (PVA/ETF) grant, focuses on identifying all audiovisual educational materials that are available in the specialty of spinal cord injury and on developing a comprehensive data base to serve as a central information resource and retrieval center.*

University of British Columbia, Department of Adult Education. 1977. *Program Planning Guide for Health Professionals.* Vancouver, BC: Author. *Presents principles of planning continuing education.*

VIVA! 1991. *Spinal Injury Series*. Dallas, TX: Health Enhancement Learning Program, Inc. *VIVA! is a computer-based patient education system that provides self-care information to people with SCI. The system can be completely controlled by voice commands or a keyboard. Supplements education by staff and promotes independent learning at the patient's own pace. Reimbursement for hospital use is possible. Introductory unit includes information on the spine, bladder and bowel programs, dysreflexia, skin, and respiratory and sexuality issues. In English and Spanish. Offers patient manuals, on-site training, off-site training, and extended phone support.*

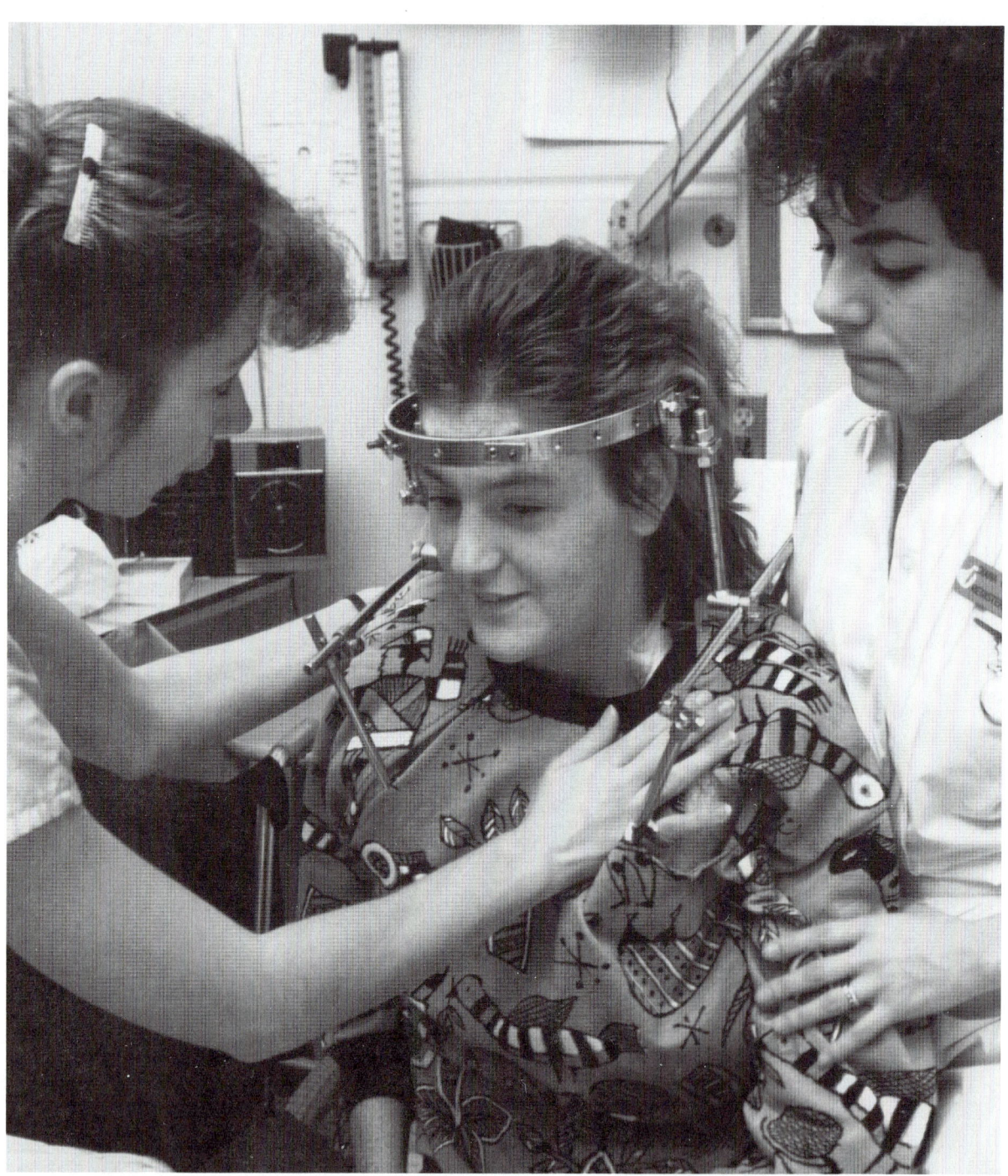

CHAPTER
— 12 —

Developing a Therapeutic Milieu on a Spinal Cord Injury Unit*

Audrey Nelson, R.N., M.N., Ph.D.

Chapter Outline

*A version of this material appeared in *SCI Nursing Journal*, 1990: Vol. 7, pp. 44–64.

Health Care Objectives

• To describe the process of reintegrating newly injured SCI patients

• To identify and explain the four phases of reintegration
• To describe helpful and unhelpful staff interventions in each phase of reintegration

THE PROCESS OF REINTEGRATION

Optimal rehabilitation is a creative and individualized process of reintegration that prepares a person to cope with physical limitations, architectural barriers, and societal prejudices while simultaneously feeling intact and valued.

There are four phases of reintegration: buffering, transcending, toughening, and launching. *Buffering* is the nurturing and protective process of lessening, absorbing, or protecting the newly injured patient with SCI against the shock of multiple ramifications of the injury and the indignities of being a patient. The transcending phase helps people with SCI recognize and rise above culturally imposed limitations and negative beliefs about people with disabilities. The *toughening up* process focuses on compensating for physical limitations, gaining independence, and maintaining social interactions without "using" the disability. Finally, the *launching* phase exposes the disabled individual to the real world, explores the range of options for living in the community, promotes autonomy and decision making, and enables the person to leave the rehabilitation program.

Phases of the reintegration process are not always clearcut. The need for buffering may resurface at intervals throughout hospitalization. For example, when the person develops complications, or during emotional crises and other traumatic events, staff need to offer support. Rehabilitation staff must learn when to protect and buffer the patient and when to be tough and unwavering. Patients progress through the buffering, transcending, toughening, and launching phases at different times. Furthermore, each team member may be in a different phase of the reintegration process. For example, a patient may be in the toughening up phase with the therapists and nurses, while the vocational counselor is just beginning a relationship with the patient and is in the process of buffering the patient.

Reintegration is thus a complex and difficult process for both patients and staff. Many of the effective strategies used by experienced rehabilitation staff are not apparent to new staff and the families of patients. Much of what experienced staff do to enhance a therapeutic milieu is intuitive and difficult to articulate to newer staff members—in fact, it may be misunderstood. When new staff are oriented, they may not see the informal interactions that promote positive rehabilitation outcomes. Timing is the critical determinant in whether a staff member is

buffering or promoting dependency when interceding and helping a patient. Frequently, newer staff perceive toughening up behaviors as mean, hostile, uncaring, and unprofessional. Furthermore, it is difficult, if not impossible, for staff to help patients transcend negative stereotypes if they themselves harbor negative attitudes about people with disabilities.

BUFFERING

Newly injured patients with SCI can easily become overwhelmed with the number of changes, limitations, and personal affronts facing them (Hohmann 1975; Lewis 1983). In addition to dealing with the injury itself, the patient must find the physical and emotional resources to cope with the day-to-day stressors caused by extended hospitalization and a strenuous rehabilitation program. The patient loses a sense of control over life, privacy, modesty, possessions, familiar daily routine, sleep, sexual relationships, and leisure activities.

Buffering is the nurturing and protective process of helping people gather physical and emotional strength to build a reserve of psychic and physical energy for the strenuous rehabilitation program that lies ahead. Buffering helps ease the transition into the unique environment of the rehabilitation unit. Time is needed to adjust to the new environment as well as to orient the person effectively to the rehabilitation program. People with SCI who are effectively buffered are able to establish a trusting, comfortable relationship with the staff. They feel confident in the proposed treatment and in the "right place."

When to Buffer

The most important time to buffer a patient with SCI is when the person is first admitted to the rehabilitation unit. Buffering gives the person time to adjust to the new surroundings and develop a rapport with staff and other patients, and mobilize coping resources and physical stamina for participation in the rehabilitation program.

Second, it is appropriate to buffer patients during a crisis situation, when resources are quickly depleted. Family crisis can occur, distracting the person from the rehabilitation program. Setbacks within the rehabilitation program can evoke feelings of despair and frustration and need to be buffered—for instance, physical complications such as pressure areas or equipment failure, such as electric wheelchair malfunctions. The physical environment and ward routines may contribute to the depletion of coping resources. For example, excessive dependency on staff for basic needs can be a chronic source of frustration. Sleep deprivation, isolation, poor staff-patient communication, depression, and lack of staff-patient rapport can significantly contribute to inability to cope. Furthermore, people on extended bedrest need more buffering than people who are more mobile.

Third, buffering is appropriate when the person is experiencing something for the first time. Persons need to be buffered before and after the first public wheelchair outing, the first weekend pass, and the first day in therapy. Other milestone firsts that cause anxiety include the first independent wheelchair transfer, first accidental bowel movement, first time falling out of the wheelchair, and seeing a friend for the first time after the injury. Last, buffering is crucial as the person approaches discharge from the rehabilitation unit.

Process of Buffering

Establishing Rapport

Staff-patient rapport is initiated with the welcome to the unit on admission. The welcome is most effective when the majority of the multidisciplinary team members participate by briefly stopping by the person's room, introducing themselves, discussing their role in the rehabilitation program, and acting genuinely concerned. These visits should take place within the first 24 hours of admission, delayed only when the person is medically unstable. Also, it is helpful to have other patients welcome the new arrival.

Continuity in personnel facilitates the rapport-building stage. Assigning the same therapists and nurses for the entire hospitalization allows the staff and person to get to know each other. This continuity becomes especially important in the later stages of reintegration.

The person's family/significant others also play a critical role in establishing rapport. Because the patient cannot move freely and is often confined to bed in the early stage of rehabilitation, the family can provide the person with information about the unit. They wander around the halls and report back, orienting the person to the new surroundings. Family members also try to get the rehabilitation staff "invested" in working with their relative by being charming, for instance, or demanding.

Interactions between injured persons and staff are nontraditional in that the relationships are built on friendship rather than professional distance. These friendships are meaningful to those who are far removed from their ordinary circle of family, friends, and acquaintances. People are much more critical of staff who are underinvolved rather than overinvolved. Most staff believe that personal attention facilitates motivation and enthusiasm to participate in rehabilitation (Brodsky and Platt 1978).

Recognizing and Attending to Needs

The second phase of buffering requires that the staff and individual mutually recognize and tend to critical needs—physical, social, emotional, and material. Persons follow through with self-care more readily and cope better with the stress of illness and disability when they feel their needs are being understood. Individuals consistently identified staff competency as a prerequisite for adequate caring and buffering strategies.

Individuals on bedrest feel isolated. There is too much time for reflecting on their injuries and losses. Knowing how difficult it is to cope with bedrest, more mobile other patients can make frequent visits. They visit, tell what is happening on the ward, see if they need anything, offer to get them a soda or candy bar, buy them shampoo, play cards, and so on. Individuals who are more personable and well liked are visited more frequently than those who are crotchety, depressed, or angry. Attractive people with a good sense of humor receive many visits, especially if they show sincere appreciation towards the visitor. Lastly, visits to individuals on isolation precautions for infectious conditions are strictly curtailed. Patients fear isolation precautions and avoid these rooms whenever possible.

Information about unaccustomed bodily sensations and the physical effects of injury are especially important. Individuals are usually most interested in specific information about *their own particular injuries* and find information about SCI offered in classes and teaching booklets less valuable.

Building Up

The third phase is building the injured person up physically and emotionally. Rehabilitation philosophy mandates that individuals do as much for themselves as possible; yet, there are appropriate times in rehabilitation to "do for" the patient. Buffering may also include acts to preserve physical and emotional energy. For example, a person with a C_5 quadriplegia who is learning to use a fork may reach a point of frustration where therapeutic efforts no longer apply. Experienced rehabilitation staff will stop the person before this point and finish the feeding. This assures that the patient will try again at the next meal, rather than giving up. There is a fine line between averting a crisis and fostering dependency.

Hooking the Person into the Program

The fourth and final phase of buffering involves "hooking" the person into the program. This "sales job" assures that the person has been indoctrinated into the unit's philosophy and will fully participate in the program. The rehabilitation staff, environment, and program are made as enticing as possible. Patients believe that with hard work and motivation they will accomplish multiple goals.

One of the ways other patients and staff make the unit appealing is to emulate home as much as possible. An intimate environment is created by bringing in family-style food. The food is shared equally between patients and staff. There is a ritual of food gift-giving in which both staff and patients participate. Reasons for giving food include: giving disabled people some control over the food they eat, promoting nurturing, expressing gratitude, promoting staff solidarity, and celebrating.

Informal support systems emerge as patients and families share and learn from each other. There is a sense of belonging and being part of the intimate group of patients and staff on the unit. This rapport is the earliest form of acceptance postinjury and gives patients courage in other relationships. It brings with it many of the obligations and responsibilities of dealing with family members for example, support, respect, and intimacy. The staff talk to patients about themselves and others on the unit. There is a lot of joking and teasing among staff and patients. This sharing results in the unit having loose patient-confidentiality boundaries. Staff admit that patients know everything that is going on within the unit. Staff must learn how much information to share with patients. Loose patient confidentiality on the unit makes patients invested in the unit, personalizes patients (secrets are not kept from them), and makes patients look beyond themselves and their injuries and feel empathy towards others. Interestingly, patients do not mind that staff talk about patients (even if it is about them). Patients also admit that the close feeling of family between staff and patients serves to make them feel obligated to do their best and work harder.

Staff legitimize and facilitate the patient community on the unit. This informal community becomes active in the evening. Functions of the patient community include (1) enculturating persons with new injuries to the unit and to live with a SCI, (2) encouraging mutual support, (3) assuring adequate patient education—for example, staff tell patients to "ask around" before making up their minds whether to do intermittent catheterizations, indwelling catheterization, or suprapubic catheterization, and (4) allowing patients to ask other patients questions they would not ask staff—perhaps sexuality-related issues are most common.

Buffering versus Fostering Dependency

One crucial difference between buffering and fostering dependency is in the timing. Buffering occurs when a patient has inadequate coping resources to manage a situation—either because the situation is new, or because the patient's resources have been depleted. However, when a person is capable of coping, this level of nurturing fosters dependency and robs the person of self-esteem.

Buffering involves a minimum reduction in autonomy and saves the person from failure or total frustration. In the early stages of recovery, there is no way to avoid some level of dependency. It should not, however, be continued simply because staff routines are geared to a certain level of illness. Every person's range of competency should be reviewed and incorporated into the rehabilitation program (Keith 1968). Buffering is, however, a temporary strategy for preserving physical and emotional resources. A person cannot be permanently shielded from society.

TRANSCENDING

The general public holds many negative attitudes toward persons with disabilities (Dunn 1982; Nelson 1987). Unchecked, these attitudes can severely restrict and limit the potential of people with SCI. For example, disabled people are viewed as less socially skilled, more dependent, more politically conservative, and more personally "good." Furthermore, a disabled person is also assumed to be fragile and easily hurt, both emotionally and physically (Dunn 1982). Transcending is the process of rising above these culturally imposed limitations and negative beliefs about people with disabilities (Vash 1981).

Because many negative attitudes and stereotypes create barriers for people with SCI in the community, the situation could be framed as more of a social than a physical problem (Stubbins 1984). Unfortunately, the problem is rarely viewed in this way, and often individuals with SCI feel that these societal reactions are brought on by their own social ineptness. *Transcending* is the process of helping persons with SCI recognize and rise above these culturally imposed limitations and negative beliefs about people with disabilities (Vash 1981).

Conditions

Disabled people face new challenges and barriers that will require transcending throughout their lives. While in the hospital, patients are first confronted with negative stereotypes when interacting with newer staff and family members who are not fully socialized in working with disabled people. Effective rehabilitation staff have learned to see many life options for people with SCI. Accepting the stereotypes of how a person in a wheelchair should act severely limits life options and choices related to vocation, social relationships, intimacy, and recreation. Each person should be viewed as unique, with the treatment program flexible enough to accommodate their individualized strengths, weaknesses, and life ambitions.

Research has shown, however, that rehabilitation staff are just as biased and have just as many negative stereotypes about people with disabilities as the general public (Bell

1962). This is gradually improving as disabled people increasingly join the mainstream. Staff with negative attitudes toward the disabled are likely to feel helpless and hopeless when interacting with people with SCI and easily transmit these feelings to both the patients and families (Adler 1972). These staff people vacillate between feeling pity and intense rage. They tend to ignore the competencies the person may have to complete tasks independently. Their efforts are geared toward making themselves, as care givers, feel better and needed, and they get angry when these efforts are not appreciated by patients.

People farther along in the rehabilitation process are most adept at helping newly injured people transcend. Therefore, the rehabilitation environment should promote this. Having experienced many of the social and physical barriers in the community, peer counselors—people who have completed rehabilitation—are in a better position to help the more recently injured place these experiences into perspective and develop strategies to combat them.

The unit philosophy can facilitate or impede the process of transcending. Rehabilitation staff who take a more optimistic approach are in a better position to help the newly injured transcend (Phillips et al. 1987). A rehabilitation program that focuses on control, challenge, and commitment (Pollack 1987) fosters hardiness and ability to withstand societal prejudices and physical barriers present in the community.

A staff-patient relationship that focuses on sharing things about one's self is critical. Maintaining professional distance in rehabilitation gives the message, *I am the professional, I am a step above the patient.* Staff-patient interactions based on partnership, rather than the typical professional distance, are essential to validating that the person is a fully functioning, valued human being.

Flexible treatment programs that manage each individual with SCI as unique restore a sense of self. Zealousness to create optimal SCI units often results in an overemphasis on structure and organization that interfere with staff's ability to see each person as an individual.

Process of Transcending

The process of helping newly injured patients and their families transcend negative stereotypes is accomplished by staff and peer counselors. Transcending must occur throughout life: new situations and different social barriers will emerge long after the initial rehabilitation program. However, this process must begin during the initial rehabilitation program so that goals and life plans are not limited by preconceived notions about what is proper for people with disabilities. Transcending is facilitated less by formal educational offerings than by observations of how people are managed on the rehabilitation unit. Staff attitudes and beliefs are readily transmitted to both the patients and their families. The following strategies help people transcend:

using "ideology pushers" to socialize individuals, evaluating how ward routines and the environment might depersonalize individuals, socializing staff to reject the negative stereotypes about persons with disabilities, and making dependency invisible.

Using Individuals as Ideology Pushers

Successful SCI units promote a positive unit ideology that supports the attainment of many preinjury life choices, goals, and dreams, An indoctrination process is essential. Certain people can serve to perpetuate the unit milieu by acting as "ideology pushers." An *ideology pusher* is a person who, by virtue of being consistently present while others move in and out of the ward, coupled with strong commitment to a particular philosophy of care, socializes new people to the therapeutic values and beliefs of the ward (Strauss et al. 1964)—helping them to look for options where they see barriers.

Evaluating Depersonalization Effects

Another important factor in facilitating the transcending process is to assure that the unit environment and program treat people like adult human beings. Depersonalization impedes the transcending process. Malfunctioning equipment, insufficient quality or quantity of supplies, bureaucratic procedural delays, lack of privacy, and inflexible unit routines all serve to detract from a person's feeling valued.

Another way to depersonalize people with SCI is by unnecessary exposure of genitals. It is not uncommon for people with SCI to sleep nude as a convenience for staff. A small towel or fig leaf is draped over the genital area. Individuals are also exposed unnecessarily because staff forget to close curtains or pull the door shut when providing care. Intrusive, intimate procedures such as bowel care are particularly embarrassing for people. If these depersonalizing aspects of the environment are not kept in check, they diminish the individual's ability to respond emotionally, essentially destroying the capacity to experience shame and disgust.

Socializing Staff to Reject Negative Stereotypes about People with Disabilities

Inexperienced staff can feel anxious because they do not know how to act or respond to persons with SCI. they may feel that it is inappropriate to show direct sympathetic concern, and yet if they ignore the level of injury, they are likely to make impossible demands. As a result, it is not uncommon for staff to speak guardedly with everyday expressions suddenly taboo, such as "taking a walk" (Goffman 1963). A staff nurse describes the subtle effects of communication in patient interactions.

> I talk to these guys [patients] like they were a friend of mine. I tease them. Sometimes I say, "Hey, walk down with me to the Xerox machine." They don't get upset

about it. Some of them can roll a lot faster than I can walk or even run. You've got to get past the point where you are afraid you are going to hurt them or you might extend the injury. And the other thing we do is we don't call them patients. I call them guys—I say, "Yes, my three guys are up today."

Making Dependency Invisible

Dependency is the aspect of SCI that people find most difficult. Experienced SCI nurses can make dependency invisible. Subtle efforts to distract by talking, sharing things about themselves, joking, touching, and hugging while efficiently completing necessary procedures serve to make much of the dependency invisible. On the other hand, new or unskilled staff become so task oriented that they magnify dependency. When dependency is magnified people respond with embarrassment, hostility, detachment, or apathy.

TOUGHENING UP

Experienced rehabilitation staff and peer counselors believe that newly spinal cord injured persons should not be pampered, but rather toughened up if they are to make it in the real world. They feel that if things are made too easy, the family care givers will not be able to cope after discharge and the injured person's relationships with others will suffer, destroying the support system essential to community adjustment.

The toughening-up process focuses on compensating for physical limitations, gaining independence, and maintaining social interactions without using the disability. People who use their disabilities con others into helping with things they could do but are not inclined to do (Dunn 1975).

Conditions for Toughening

Staff Considerations

The key to effectively toughening newly injured people lies in experienced, well-trained staff. Inexperienced staff are usually unable to push patients or toughen patients up. Not yet fully socialized to the unit philosophy and still harboring some of society's negative stereotypes about disabled people, newer staff tend to want to help rather than push. Often, they are confused by the mission of the toughening-up process and may actually view these actions as cruel, heartless, and unprofessional.

Those staff end up doing things for patients to make themselves feel better without regard to the patients' futures. When the ratio of inexperienced to experienced staff increases, the burden of toughening up falls on fewer people.

Continuity of staff assignments is essential. Staff-patient conflicts are likely to arise when nurses and therapists assigned to a particular person give consistent treatment. A

person who does not really know a nurse is less likely to respond positively to toughening-up strategies. Even though the experienced staff person possesses excellent toughening-up skills, without an established base of trust and rapport during the buffering phase, the person is likely to respond in an angry and defensive manner.

Optimally, the rehabilitation program is designed to maximize contact between newly injured people and peer counselors. The latter are extremely effective in providing critical feedback to newly injured people on both behavior and attitude. Other persons with SCI are best able to point out more adaptive responses because they have been through the same kind of experience. Peer counselors won't let the newly injured feel sorry for themselves or complain.

People who fully participate in all program activities and work hard are most likely to elicit more attention and positive regard from staff. The relationship between self-care and rehabilitation outcomes was explored by Malec and Neimeyer (1983). Based on follow-up an average of 7 months postdischarge, the best predictor of posthospitalization self-care behavior seems to be the level of self-care behavior displayed during the rehabilitation hospitalization. The results emphasize the importance of pushing people to complete self-care during rehabilitation.

In order to stress self-care during hospitalization, ward routines need to be reconsidered. Sometimes routine tasks of daily living such as awakening, dressing, washing, grooming, and eating are often pressed to completion without involving the injured person so that the person paradoxically can be made ready for therapy (Gubrium and Buckholdt 1982). When staff take over for the person in an effort to save time, realistic life problems cannot be exploited as learning opportunities.

Taboo against Depression, Anger, and Complaining

The social environment of an optimal rehabilitation unit fosters a taboo against depression, anger, and general complaining behavior. People with SCI claim staff consistently overestimate the extent of depression experienced during rehabilitation (Klas 1970; Lawson 1976). Their premise is that hospital routines—such as intermittent catheterizations and turning patients every 2 hours—lead to sleep deprivation that causes irritability and feelings of isolation.

The benefits of making depression taboo on a rehabilitation unit have only recently been recognized. Much of the coping literature in the 1970s was influenced by Kubler-Ross's (1975) work on death and dying. Importance was placed on patients' progressing through phases of grief so as to foster adaptation to the injury (Kerr and Thompson 1972; Roberts 1972; Stewart and Rossier 1978). The pervasiveness of this stage theory in both the thinking and practice of rehabilitation professionals resulted in what Wright (1960) called the "requirement for mourning." However, no data have substantiated the necessity or value of grieving over the losses incurred from SCI. Staff feel they have seen many people do very well with SCI. People with SCI indicate that the more staff permit the newly injured to get depressed, the more staff validate the dismal nature of their condition and reveal their own negative attitudes about people with disabilities. Furthermore, depressed patients do not socialize, therefore their contacts with peers and staff are limited and less helpful. A unit taboo against depression sends out a strong message to people with SCI that staff value them and have confidence in their ability to contribute to society.

Process for Toughening

The toughening-up process begins when the person is able to get out of bed and independently move about the unit. Toughening starts slowly with subtle teasing and coaxing and gradually moves to overt taunting. Toughening strategies vary based on the extent of disability and how long the person has been injured. More recently injured people toughened less than others. Also the more extensive the injury the less tough staff are. Self-starters get toughened less.

Peer counselors are most skilled at toughening up the newly injured. Critical feedback on behavior is provided to minimize conflict between the newly injured and family members or the staff. Criticism is usually buffered through the use of humor. Sometimes people are singled out for teasing as a way to get behavior in line. Open confrontation is also used when it is warranted, for instance, when a person is abusive to staff or family.

Staff use several strategies to toughen a newly injured person. Using humor, teasing, and avoiding depression, anger, and complaining behaviors have already been discussed. Additional strategies for toughening include hard work, competition, praise, demonstrations, criticism, threats, refusal to assist, and exposure to both peer counselors and the outside world.

Hard Work

Most patients spend about 4 to 6 hours per day working in active rehabilitation. Working includes such activities as physical, occupational, and correctional therapy; recreational outings, learning and/or completing daily living skills (DLS), talking with staff, and participating in ward activities. During the toughening-up process, staff expectations of performance become higher. Persons are expected to complete DLS to the degree their functional limitations permit. Therapy workouts become longer, more strenuous and complex.

A certain level of *competition* is fostered. Patients, particularly those new to the ward, look for other people at the same level of injury to compare with themselves. They note how long the other people have been injured, what kind of

return they experienced, their functional level, and attitude. It is common to hear, "If that guy can handle it, I can, too." These comparisons serve to encourage patients, or even shame them, into working harder. For example, an individual with a C_5 level injury who complains that feeding oneself is too time consuming and messy may find that staff have intentionally seated this person across from another person with C_5 or higher level injury who can use a fork without difficulty. Therapists might foster competition by announcing, "Hey, look at Bob doing those push ups—can you do that many?" In the course of doing therapy, nurses and therapists continually make use of such comparisons to motivate.

Another means of motivating the patient to work harder is through the use of *praise*, compliments or other forms of positive reinforcement. The nurse might say, "Try it again, hang in there," or, "That's the way." Positive feedback that was most appreciated focused on invisible progress, such as fluidity of movement, degree of effort, quality of movement, attitude, affect, energy level, tolerance, and endurance. Staff deliberately set small goals that can be accomplished in short time frames so that patients experience success.

Criticism

Society tends to withhold negative feedback from disabled people, which distorts reality and fosters dependency. Staff who attempt to be as honest as possible are most helpful—even though it may create temporary discomfort. In the long run, it is better for a person to be criticized in the context of the helping environment of the rehabilitation unit than to learn these skills in the outside world where social encounters may result in excessively traumatic feedback. The person is likely to respond to a traumatic social event by avoiding further social encounters or reverting to using the disability to manipulate social encounters. As one staff member stated, "Rehabilitation gives people the opportunity to learn to deal with people, and if you learn you get your way by crying or acting out, then you'll do it more often. On the other hand, if you get your way by being a nice guy and being friendly and happy, you'll get along better here and in the real world." Negative feedback is immediately given to the person even for small favors such as asking a friend to get a glass of water. People who continue to use their disability are teased by other patients who may mimic their feigned helplessness. Peer counselors and staff tell stories about patients who managed to alienate family and friends with this kind of behavior. Open confrontation is the most helpful response when a patient is caught using the disability.

Furthermore, for the most part, complaining is not tolerated. A quadriplegic person can complain to a paraplegic person but probably not to another quadriplegic person. A paraplegic person can complain to someone with an incom-

KNOWING HOW HARD TO PUSH

Knowing when and how hard to push a patient is a critical challenge. Newer staff tend to provide more assistance to patients than what is needed. As one person stated, "What we really need is more time and less help from staff." An experienced rehabilitation nurse and a patient describe this art of gauging when to assist a patient and when to stand back and wait.

It is hard for nurses to know when to push and when not to push. But I guess I have to say that staff need to learn to push more. The majority of people that are newly injured will always allow staff to do a lot of things for them. They have it in their head, "Oh, no, I am crippled now, I can't do this" which has got to be erased. There is no room for unnecessary dependency. When staff do something for the patients they are capable of doing for themselves, they are fostering that dependency. They are turning them into cripples. New staff are notorious for doing that.

But on the other hand, you have to know when to back off. You have to be tough, but there is a point that you reach when it is no longer helpful. You don't want to reach that point of frustration. You have to know when it is time to say, "Well, that was a very good try, here, let me help you" and you do it—like opening a package of crackers or carton of milk. Once you have reached that level of frustration it doesn't serve any

purpose to continue. Each individual reaches that point at a different time, and that is what makes it very hard to gauge. Every person is unique, and some are more fragile than others.

To be really successful, both staff and patients need to know how far to push; they need to push as far as they can but to stop before the person has gotten too frustrated to benefit from the experience. Staff have to communicate among themselves about how successful this person was the day before so that they don't get conned into doing it for the patient the next day. But then again, the other patients have to have that information, too, if they are going to help out. It is easy to con and easy to be conned on this floor. You've got to have solid information to be able to function and to help the person as much as you can help him.

There is a big difference, though, between getting tough with the patient and getting angry. Inexperienced staff do not always see the difference. When they watch an experienced staff member get tough with a patient, they interpret that it is acceptable to get angry, talk back, or freely ventilate their own feelings to the patient. Patients are able to discern the staff member's underlying motivation: whether it is to help the patient become more independent, as in the case of toughening up, or that the nurse is frustrated, angry, or too busy.

plete injury while the person with incomplete injury cannot complain to anybody. It is important that patients understand during this toughening-up phase that they do not have unique rights, they will not be treated differently, and regardless of their injuries, they are responsible for their behavior.

Threats

Positive feedback is designed to motivate by encouragement, but threats are designed to encourage by setting limits on or guidelines for behavior (Gubrium and Buckholdt 1982). A nurse might say, "If you don't watch your fluids, you'll end up with a Foley catheter."

Staff have various resources at their disposal for backing up threats. Staff control whether they will assist a patient, how much attention a patient receives, and recommendations related to weekend passes and discharge. Staff indirectly threaten by withholding attention and favorable regard when a patient does not work hard or acts out. Of course patients differ in their susceptibility to be influenced by threats. Some people remain uninfluenced by staff threats,

whereas others are quite susceptible. Regardless of how effective they are in shaping behavior, they are used by nurses and therapists regularly to help motivate and toughen patients.

Refusing to Assist

During the toughening-up process, staff openly confront any person (staff or family member) who tries to take too much initiative in helping. New staff, friends, and family members of a newly injured person are warned not to participate in direct care when the person is capable. Responses to these warnings vary. A few people were impressed positively when they noticed the busy staff patiently waited for patients. However, many people did not fully appreciate or understand the reason for the patient to struggle and wanted to offer assistance. In those instances, staff would explain, "We are letting him try on his own," or "It is important she learns how much she can do for herself." The dangers of overindulgence and pity were cited. People who were not convinced this was the best approach refrained from assisting the patient further when in direct view of staff, but protected the patient from the effects of toughening wherever possible.

It was not always clear as to the degree of autonomy expected from patients or how much the staff should help patients do things they could do for themselves (Brodsky and Platt 1978). Anger was directed toward those patients who were always asking for things and appearing to be more helpless and needful than other patients.

Interactions with Other SCI Individuals

Experienced staff were instrumental in promoting positive and timely interactions between injured persons. Staff linked patients through a formal process called *networking*. Loose patient confidentiality facilitated therapeutic patient interactions, assuring that patients had adequate information to intervene effectively. Specifically, the staff would share pertinent patient information with more experienced people with SCI in hopes that they would "talk with the new guy" and "handle the problem."

Room assignments were another way staff exposed more experienced people with SCI to new rehabilitation patients. Careful consideration of each patient's roommates allowed staff to shape patients' behavior indirectly, provide role models, and promote socialization to the ward. For example, patients who complained and gave many reasons why they could not participate in various aspects of the rehabilitation might find their rooms changed. The new roommate, not by accident, would be a much more independent person at the same level of injury. In completing day-to-day activities and DLS, the person who had been injured longer would effectively communicate expectations for behavior, while acting as a role model.

LAUNCHING ——————————

Ultimately, patients are toughened in preparation for discharge and the process of launching. It is easy for patients to grow dependent on staff. The rehabilitation unit represents both safety and comfort when compared with the outside world. The toughening-up process serves to remind patients that they eventually need to leave the hospital to reap the full benefits of freedom and autonomy.

Expected Outcomes of Launching

As persons become exposed to the real world, it is expected that they will adopt a more realistic appraisal of the injury when faced with day-to-day realities of life. Hope continues to play an important role, but the practical aspects of daily living are reinforced. Patients begin to look toward the future and make decisions about how to alter their life-styles to accommodate injury. They actively solve logistical problems related to securing accessible housing and transporta-

tion. In some cases, care givers need to be identified and trained. Careful consideration is given to vocational plans, strategies to promote family and social relationships and plans for leisure activities.

Vulnerability is defined as the susceptibility to destruction and defeat (Henry 1973). Society fosters vulnerability by playing on fears of economic insecurity, fears of outsiders, and so on. The function of vulnerability is to promote dependency and exaggerate the image of those who could harm us or protect us. One of the goals of launching is for individuals to say, "I may be stronger than I think" as opposed to "I am afraid" (Henry 1973).

Conditions

Staff Who Communicate in a Timely and Effective Manner

As patients begin to take more responsibility for their treatment and rehabilitation outcomes, it is imperative that staff keep the person informed and included in all aspects of decision making. Rehabilitation programs often create formal communication links through patient care conferences or team rounds. These formal communication strategies often fall short of their intended goals because the person feels too intimidated and outnumbered to participate fully. Informal one-to-one communication or small informal groups are preferred. Individuals and their families frequently cite a lack of one-to-one discussions with the physician—especially the first and last few weeks of the rehabilitation stay.

Timeliness of information is also critical. In one rehabilitation program, individuals were provided an opportunity to take part in goal setting through participation in "intake conferences," attended by multidisciplinary team members, the individual and family. Each individual had three conferences during rehabilitation: initial, intermediate, and final. Actually, however, goals were identified in separate, earlier meetings of the social worker, psychologist, nurse, physician, therapists, and other team members, with the conference serving as a vehicle for team communication.

Lack of privacy detracts from effective communication. Due to convenience of staff, frequently intimate conversations are held in full view of other patients and staff, such as in the patient's room. This is especially problematic during rounds, a daily walking team meeting where each person's progress is discussed. Rounds also can be dehumanizing if the team members discuss individuals as if they were not in the same room. Persons are expected to ask questions and contribute to the discussion during rounds, but most are too intimidated by both the crowds and lack of privacy.

Program that Fosters Autonomy

Staff cannot rehabilitate people who do not choose to participate fully in the process. Learning reintegration skills occurs as individuals increase their role in planning and making decisions for themselves. Yet hospital routines generally limit capacities for increased self-directed behavior. Many people find these routines comforting and quickly acquiesce to the all-pervasive authority exercised over them. This iatrogenic dependency detracts from successful reintegration and serves to delay the launching process. On the other hand, gradually increasing the level of participation and decision making fosters autonomy and better prepares people for discharge. Successful rehabilitation staff are able to gauge readiness for participation and allocate decision-making freedom. Ideally, the rehabilitation process indicates a steady increase in the persons' capacities to plan, decide, and control their own behavior.

Promoting Goal Setting

Patients enter the SCI rehabilitation program with varying levels of life experience in goal setting and goal attainment. However, even people who are most adept at goal-setting strategies find their limited knowledge of SCI impedes their ability to set realistic and appropriate goals. For this reason, staff involvement in the early stages of rehabilitation is intensive. Later, staff involvement in setting goals tends to decrease as patients become more knowledgeable about SCI and are subsequently encouraged to take more initiative in setting individualized goals.

Goal setting in SCI rehabilitation serves two major purposes. First, goals provide markers for determining progress. These markers provide the stimulus for ongoing positive feedback to individuals and in a sense motivate them to continue to work hard. Second, the process of goal setting gives individuals critical cues about the extent of the disability as well as what can be expected from staff, the rehabilitation program, and life (Gubrium and Buckholdt 1982).

Providing Markers for Measuring Success

As individuals move through the rehabilitation program, more attention is paid to progress and goal attainment. Staff give individuals cues as to the progress they see. For example, a nurse might say, "Well, I think you ought to start going to the dining room for your meals," or, "Have you thought about going out on pass for the weekend?" Staff provide patients with cues to keep them on course and provide markers for noting when progress has been made.

Gubrium and Buckholdt (1982) described three ways to view progress in rehabilitation. First, the linear model characterizes progress in a steplike fashion with small increments occurring with each day of therapy. Second, progress can also be viewed in stages. Little or no change occurs for a period of time and then at some critical point the person leaps to a new stage of recovery. The third model is more spontaneous: individuals go from little or no progress to a remarkable gain, perhaps approaching recovery almost overnight. Each model allows for regression.

Typically in SCI rehabilitation, staff view progress in a linear fashion. They are able to see many nuances of progress that are invisible to individuals—improved balance, less effort and concentration necessary to complete a task, increased confidence, smoother movements, and so on. Individuals, on the other hand, tend to view progress as more stagelike, focusing only on such goal attainment as the ability to transfer independently, without noting the gradual increase in balance and muscle strength.

Individuals gauge progress in terms of being dependent or independent in completing a task, as in the statement, "I couldn't do this and now I can." From their perspective, the following milestones indicate progress: getting up in the chair for the first time, independent transfers, doing bowel care and catheterizations by oneself, eating by oneself, dressing oneself, going on recreation trip for the first time, first pass overnight, and setting a discharge date. Individuals also gauge progress through cues they get from other patients or the staff.

Staff have a more complex system of gauging progress. For example, muscle strength is graded on a scale from 1 to 5. (See Table 4–6.) Staff also evaluate the level of assistance a person might require, such as dependent, partial assist, stand-by assist, and independent. In addition, staff monitor the quality of movement, self-confidence, speed, amount of effort expended to complete a task, the ability to solve problems, and the number of assistive devices used (less is better). Staff also place a heavy emphasis on attitude. For example, a good sign is when a person stops being egocentric and becomes concerned about family and others.

Unit Environment That Is Linked to the Real World

The SCI unit environment is the testing ground for newly injured people to practice creative ways to adjust to the environment. However, many rehabilitation units fall short of reintegrating people with SCI into the community because staff are not familiar with what it is like to be in a wheelchair and are not informed about what is required to live successfully in the community. The rehabilitation program is not systematically linked with the real world in a way that enables people to learn how to apply what is learned in the hospital to the home setting.

For example, the unit environment is carefully designed for wheelchair accessibility. Unfortunately, the real world is not arranged quite so conveniently. As one patient described,

> Everything in the hospital is exceptionally convenient—level floors, accessible facilities for shower and bowel care. The real bummer is when you leave here and you get outside. Your social life goes to an absolute zero because most people have steps to their homes. So even though you may have a large circle of friends and associates, you are rarely in anyone's home other than your own because nobody has ramps—nor would you expect them

to build the ramps just to have you over. In a sense, the hospital sets you up. It is easy here because everything is so accessible.

The narrow doors at home, the steps you look at with no way to get up; a ramp so steep you really have to push hard and strain to get up—you may fall out of your chair a few times at inopportune moments. But in this rehabilitation unit, the new guys don't face falling out of their chairs or straining to get somewhere. The real world is full of curbs and stairs. It's two different worlds, and you've got to get the new patients to start seeing that.

Process of Launching

Introducing Rehabilitation Patients to the Real World

There is a wide gap between being able to survive successfully on a SCI unit and being able to survive at home. Staff cannot simply assume patients will be able to transfer the knowledge and skills gained in the unit environment to their home environment; it is not an easy task. Furthermore, patients need to experience life outside the unit before they can fully appreciate and apply what they have learned in rehabilitation. Launching exposes patients gradually to obstacles and limitations they have not considered while in the hospital. Recreational trips, followed by weekend passes, provide patients with short glimpses of what life will be like after discharge from the hospital. The patient begins to experience the full range of deprivation and limitations imposed by SCI. Comforting during this stage is inappropriate and encourages continued depression. Using kind firmness, staff demand that patients participate to facilitate more positive outcomes. The goal is to help them attempt things they can easily accomplish. Seemingly insurmountable problems are broken down into small workable pieces (Lazarus 1971).

It is fairly common for patients to deal with their fears through avoidance. They may be reluctant to go on a recreational outing where they will encounter strangers who will stare at them. They may not ask for weekend passes fearing family responses. Fear of returning to the community can be so great that many patients sabotage their rehabilitation programs to delay discharge. Peer counselors often are more aware of this avoidance tactic than staff, who frequently misinterpret avoidance as disinterest or a lack of commitment. Persons injured previously frequently tease those with newer injuries into participating in these activities by openly confronting the persons' worst fears.

Occasionally, patients obstruct their rehabilitation progress. A neutral, matter-of-fact response toward this is better than agreeing or arguing.

Exploring the Range of Options for Living in the Community

Staff are frequently unaware of strategies to help with the transition from hospital to home. Experienced SCI nurses learn to ask critical questions to assess the unique living environment to which the individual will be returning. Peer counselors can provide valuable information and an empathetic ear to those with newer injuries. Efforts to link inpatient and outpatient services are essential to provide feedback on how to adjust the overall rehabilitation program to enhance the launching process.

The quality of launching preparations varies. Persons who are either under- or overdemanding are apt to be shortchanged in the amount of attention and individual instruction they receive from the staff. The amount of progress a person makes significantly impacts on the launching process.

Guidance in how to handle difficult situations can minimize future trauma. Peer counselors can joke and tell stories of their most embarrassing experiences—an accidental bowel movement or falling out of the wheelchair. These discussions prepare those with newer injuries for worst-case scenarios. Staff offer encouragement and reward creative problem solving. Those with older injuries are asked to show others how to do things in different ways.

Promoting Autonomy and Decision Making

Patients on a rehabilitation ward recognize early in the hospital stay that specific behaviors influence health outcomes. Staff coach patients on how they can help themselves achieve their goals. Guidelines for expected behavior are clearly delineated.

Initially, however, some people do not recognize the link between their participation in rehabilitation and future health outcomes. It is as though they passively wait for improvements in health status to derive from some source other than themselves. Slowly, they begin to recognize that their own efforts directly influence rehabilitation outcomes (Gubrium and Buckholdt, 1982).

Enabling Persons to Leave the Rehabilitation Program

As discharge plans emerge, persons experience a sense of excitement as well as impending doom. They have many fears about their injuries. They worry about how their friends and family will respond to them, whether they will lose their jobs, and whether they will be attractive to the opposite sex.

Eventually, they progress to the point where they can safely manage their own care. This means either the patient can independently complete DLS or can competently direct the actions of the care giver. Patients become afraid although this is masked with increased joking, teasing, laughter, and practical jokes. Launching is a stressful period for both staff and patients. It is inevitable that patients will encounter difficulties and make mistakes. Furthermore, since rehabilitation is not really over at the time of discharge, staff are left with the feeling of unfinished business.

The process of launching is usually initiated by the staff. Discharge is considered appropriate when most of the goals have been met and staff determine that the patients can safely take care of themselves.

Networking is a way for staff to link patients from the same hometown or those with similar interests to facilitate adjustment to injury. Both inpatients and outpatients are networked. The function of networking is to enculturate the individual to living with SCI.

People view the SCI unit as a safe place to which to return, if needed. Intermittent phone contact between former patients and staff is not uncommon several years after discharge. The unit has wedding invitations, vacation postcards, funeral announcements, and birth announcements posted on the bulletin boards attesting to the familylike ties the staff maintains.

Patients describe the comfort the unit provides in terms of backup support, information, and friendships. As one person stated, "It is nice to know that you have support and friends here at the rehabilitation center and that this support system is always going to be here. You always have someone in your corner."

Degrees of Launching

Launching can be described in terms of readiness—appropriate, delayed, or premature. Appropriate launching occurs when the individual, family, and staff are in agreement about the timing of the discharge. Delayed launches are typically the result of one or more individuals who sabotage discharge plans. For example, a family member will decide the injured person cannot move in at the last minute, a person will refuse to participate in discharge planning, or a staff member will plead with the team for more time to achieve certain goals. At times, launching is initiated by individuals—for instance, when the person begins to question the benefit of continued hospitalization. Even though the staff feel discharge may be premature, if the person is persistent, launching efforts are initiated. Also some people may be prematurely launched by the staff if they refuse to participate in the rehabilitation program. Even after a person has been launched, it is assumed that the reintegration process continues.

Furthermore, staff differentiate between rehabilitation successes and failures. Failures are often viewed as rehabilitation stalemates—a success that hasn't yet happened.

RECOMMENDATIONS FOR PRACTICE AND RESEARCH

Key elements in developing a therapeutic milieu on an SCI unit have emerged from patients' attitudes, beliefs, and behavior on SCI units.

The problems people with SCI face after discharge from a rehabilitation center are mostly social problems, rather than problems of individual adaptation to injury. Most SCI units are designed to focus on individual patients, ignoring the reality of the society to which they will return. Hospitals are designed to achieve the goals of delaying death, defeating illness and complication from injuries, and seeking health in patients (Taylor 1970), but in SCI rehabilitation this view is shortsighted. Conceptualization of disability as a functional incapacity (Haber 1973) negates society's response to the disabled people in the community. SCI units that are not clearly linked to the real world will fail in attempts to reintegrate persons into the community.

A second major implication focuses on the critical role others with SCI play in the rehabilitation of those with new injuries. People more experienced with SCI have a wealth of information to share with patients and staff. Patients want reciprocal relationships, which are more satisfying than relationships in which one consistently receives more than one gives (Cogswell 1968). Facilitating personal relationships among individuals optimizes opportunities to teach as well as to learn; to share their lifetime of joys, experiences, frustrations, sorrows, and skills for survival (Cogswell 1967; Leviton 1970). Even the most difficult individual will frequently respond well when asked to help another person with SCI on the ward.

It is not true that only the best or most successful people are suited to offer assistance to more recently injured people. In fact nearly everyone with SCI can offer valuable information, emotional support, physical assistance, experience, or diversional activities. Successful SCI units capitalize on this wealth of expertise and facilitate these interactions.

Importance of Nontraditional Staff-Patient Relationships

Staff are usually instructed to beware of becoming emotionally involved with patients. Nurses, for instance, are taught to maintain a certain professional demeanor and distance. It is considered unprofessional for nurses to talk to patients about themselves or other patients. In fact, however, nontraditional staff-patient relationships are instrumental in helping patients with SCI reintegrate into the community.

A staff-patient relationship that focuses on intimacy and sharing things about oneself helps patients transcend the negative stereotypes about persons with disabilities. Comfortable staff-patient partnerships model how relationships can develop when disability is not the crucial factor.

Because staff attitudes and beliefs are readily transmitted to both the patient and family, staff new to SCI rehabilitation need to replace negative stereotypes about persons with disabilities with more constructive ideas. Orientation needs to go beyond the teaching of bowel care and bladder training to include attitude assessment and coaching to promote comfort in interactions to make dependency invisible. Most important, newer staff need to discard the blinders that limit life options for disabled people. Staff should facilitate each patient's pursuit of preinjury goals, ambitions, and dreams to the fullest extent possible.

There is a widely held belief that negative feelings and depression are highly contagious and should be avoided at all costs. Staff support this notion. To get on with the business of rehabilitation, the taboo against depression and anger is necessary to ensure the patient has the physical and psychic energy to participate in rehabilitation. Patients who are depressed or hostile during rehabilitation rarely benefit from the hospitalization and are likely to fail at the reintegration process.

Informal support systems emerge as patients and families share and learn from each other. There is a sense of belonging and being part of the intimate group of patients and staff on the unit. This comradery is the earliest form of postinjury acceptance and gives patients courage in other relationships. It brings with it many of the obligations and responsibilities of dealing with family members—helping, support, respect, and intimacy.

Many people with SCI think too much emphasis is placed on improving care versus finding cure. Myths and stories of miraculous cures and medical miracles pervade many discussions. Patients who can walk are viewed with a mixture of awe, excitement, and envy. People with quadri-

RESEARCH NOTE

The process of reintegration provides direction for future research in the fields of nursing, rehabilitation, and medical anthropology.

Although more recent studies have challenged the belief that depression and grief are phases of adaptation essential to the adjustment of people with SCI (Kleinman and Good 1985; Katz, Gordon, Iversen, and Myers 1978; Trieschmann 1988; Dinardo 1971; Kalb 1971; Lawson 1976), most rehabilitation staff still endorse this idea. Further research is needed in this area, related to the long-term effects of depression or lack of depression during rehabilitation on the postrehabilitation functioning of people with SCI.

Exploring patients' perspectives of the period immediately after the initial rehabilitation hospitalization is needed to clarify aspects of the launching process. The first 6 months postinjury are considered to be critical for patients, and yet very little is known about what happens in the patients' homes after discharge. Patients allude to a process of "going crazy" that eventually is replaced with established routines. More information could help staff anticipate problems and provide guidance to the newly injured.

Furthermore, teaching is at the core of the rehabilitation process, and yet rehabilitation staff have little information about timing and specific strategies for effective teaching. Multiple cognitive, psychosocial, and attitudinal education is provided, using both structured and unstructured methods. However, staff are unsure which methods work and which are ineffective. What is the nature of the experience of relearning self-care after SCI? What factors determine a patient's readiness to relearn self-care? What do patients perceive as obstacles or facilitators of the relearning process? Because rehabilitation and patient education are so closely aligned, further study in this area is imperative.

Information that would significantly contribute to the literature on SCI involves staff-patient boundaries. Given that effective staff-patient relationships are nontraditional, what boundaries should staff observe? Staff state they know how far they can go, and yet these boundaries remain unclear and create staff dissension. Intimate relationships, dating, and marital relationships are a source of concern for many SCI staff and need to be explored further.

The size of the unit and mix of patients on the unit were identified by many patients as a significant feature of the success of this program. These critical issues, as well as those of staffing levels and the effects of staff turnover on the quality of the rehabilitation program, would be of immense value. Organizational factors that facilitate or impede the reintegration process also need to be explored further.

This process of reintegration was derived from patients' perspectives on a SCI unit. Although this model has multiple implications for clinical practice and administration, its applicability to other SCI units needs more exploration as well.

plegia wish they had the use of their hands, paraplegic people wish they had bowel and bladder function, and people with incomplete injuries wish they had more strength and balance. Hope plays an important role in the lives of everyone with SCI, regardless of how long they have been injured.

REFERENCES

Adler, G. 1972. Helplessness in the helpers. *British Journal of Medical Psychology* 45: 315–326.

Bell, A. 1962. Attitudes of selected rehabilitation workers and other hospital employees toward the physically disabled. *Psychological Reports* 10: 183–186.

Brodsky, C., and Platt, R. 1978. *The Rehabilitation Environment*. Lexington, MA: Lexington Books.

Cogswell, B. 1967. Rehabilitation of the paraplegic: Processes of socialization. *Sociological Inquiry* 37: 11–26.

Cogswell, B. 1968. Self-socialization: Readjustment of paraplegics in the community. *Journal of Rehabilitation*: 11–13.

Dinardo, Q. 1971. *Psychological adjustment to spinal cord injury*. Unpublished doctoral dissertation, University of Houston.

Dunn, M. 1975. Psychological intervention in a spinal cord injury center: An introduction. *Rehabilitation Psychology* 22 (4): 165–178.

Dunn, M. 1982. *Social Relationships and Interpersonal Skills: A Guide for People with Sensory and Physical Limitations*. Virginia: Institute for Information Studies.

Goffman, E. 1963. *Stigma: Notes on the Management of Spoiled Identity*. New York: Simon & Shuster.

Gubrium, J., and Buckholdt, D. 1982. *Describing Care: Image and Practice in Rehabilitation*. Cambridge: Oelgeschlager, Gunn & Hain, Publishers.

Haber, L. 1973. Disabling effects of chronic disease and impairment. II. Functional capacity limitations. *Journal of Chronic Diseases* 26: 127–152.

Henry, J. 1973. *On Sham, Vulnerability, and Other Forms of Self-destruction*. New York: Vintage Books.

Hohmann, G. 1975. Psychological aspects of treatment and rehabilitation of the spinal cord injured person. *Clinical Orthopaedics and Related Research* 112: 81–88.

Kalb, M. 1971. *An examination of the relationship between hospital ward behaviors and post-discharge behaviors in spinal cord injury patients*. Unpublished doctoral dissertation, University of Houston.

Katz, V., Gordon, R., Iversen, D., and Myers, S. 1978. Past history and degree of depression in paraplegic individuals. *Paraplegia* 16: 8–14.

Keith, R. 1968. The need for new model in rehabilitation. *Journal of Chronic Disability* 21: 281–286.

Kerr, W., and Thompson, M. 1972. Acceptance of disability of sudden onset paraplegia. *Paraplegia* 10: 94–102.

Klas, L. 1970. *A study of the relationship between depression and factors in the rehabilitation process of the hospitalized spinal cord injured patient*. Unpublished doctoral dissertation. University of Utah.

Kleinman, A., and Good, B. (Eds.). 1985. *Culture and Depression: Studies in Anthropology and Cross-Cultural Psychiatry of Affect and Disorder*. Berkeley, CA: University of California Press.

Kubler-Ross, E. 1975. *Death, the Final Stage of Growth*. Englewood Cliffs, NJ: Prentice-Hall.

Lawson, N. 1976. *Depression after spinal cord injury: A multimeasure longitudinal study*. Unpublished doctoral dissertation, University of Houston.

Lazarus, A. 1971. *Behavior Therapy and Beyond*. New York: McGraw-Hill.

Leviton, G. 1970. Professional-client relations in a rehabilitation hospital setting. In *Rehabilitation of Psychology*. Washington: American Psychological Association, pp. 215–247. Ed. W. S. Neff.

Lewis, K. 1983. Grief in chronic illness and disability. *Journal of Rehabilitation* (Aug./Sept.),: 8–11.

Malec, J., and Neimeyer, R. 1983. Psychologic prediction of duration of inpatient spinal cord injury rehabilitation and performance of self-care. *Archives of Physical Medicine and Rehabilitation* 64: 359–363.

Nelson, A. 1987. Normalization: The key to integrating the spinal cord injured patient into the community. *SCI Nursing* 4 (1): 3–6.

Phillips, L., Ozer, M., Axelson, P., and Chizeck, H. 1987. *Spinal Cord Injury: A Guide for Patient and Family*. New York: Raven Press.

Pollack, S. 1987. Adaptation to chronic illness: Analysis of nursing research. *Nursing Clinics of North America* 22 (3): 631–643.

Roberts, A. 1972. Spinal cord injury: some psychological considerations. *Minnesota Medicine* 55: 1115–1117.

Stewart, T., and Rossier, A. 1978. Psychological considerations in the adjustment to spinal cord injury. *Rehabilitation Literature* 39 (3): 75–80.

Strauss, A., Schatzman, L., Bucher, R., Ehrlich, D., and Sabshin, M. 1964. *Psychiatric Ideologies and Institutions*. London: The Free Press of Glencoe.

Stubbins, J. 1984. Rehabilitation services as ideology. *Rehabilitation Psychology* 29 (4): 197–210.

Taylor, C. 1970. *In Horizontal Orbit: Hospitals and Cult of Efficiency*. New York: Holt, Rinehart and Winston.

Trieschmann, R. 1988. *Spinal Cord Injuries: Psychological, Social and Vocational Adjustment*. New York: Demos Publications.

Vash, C. 1981. Disability as transcendental experience: A personal perspective on learning to live with a disability. In *Treatment of the Spinal Cord Injured—An Interdisciplinary Perspective*. Eds. M. Eisenberg and J. Falconer. Springfield, IL: Charles C. Thomas Publisher.

Wright, B. 1960. *Physical Disability: A Psychological Approach*. New York: Harper & Row.

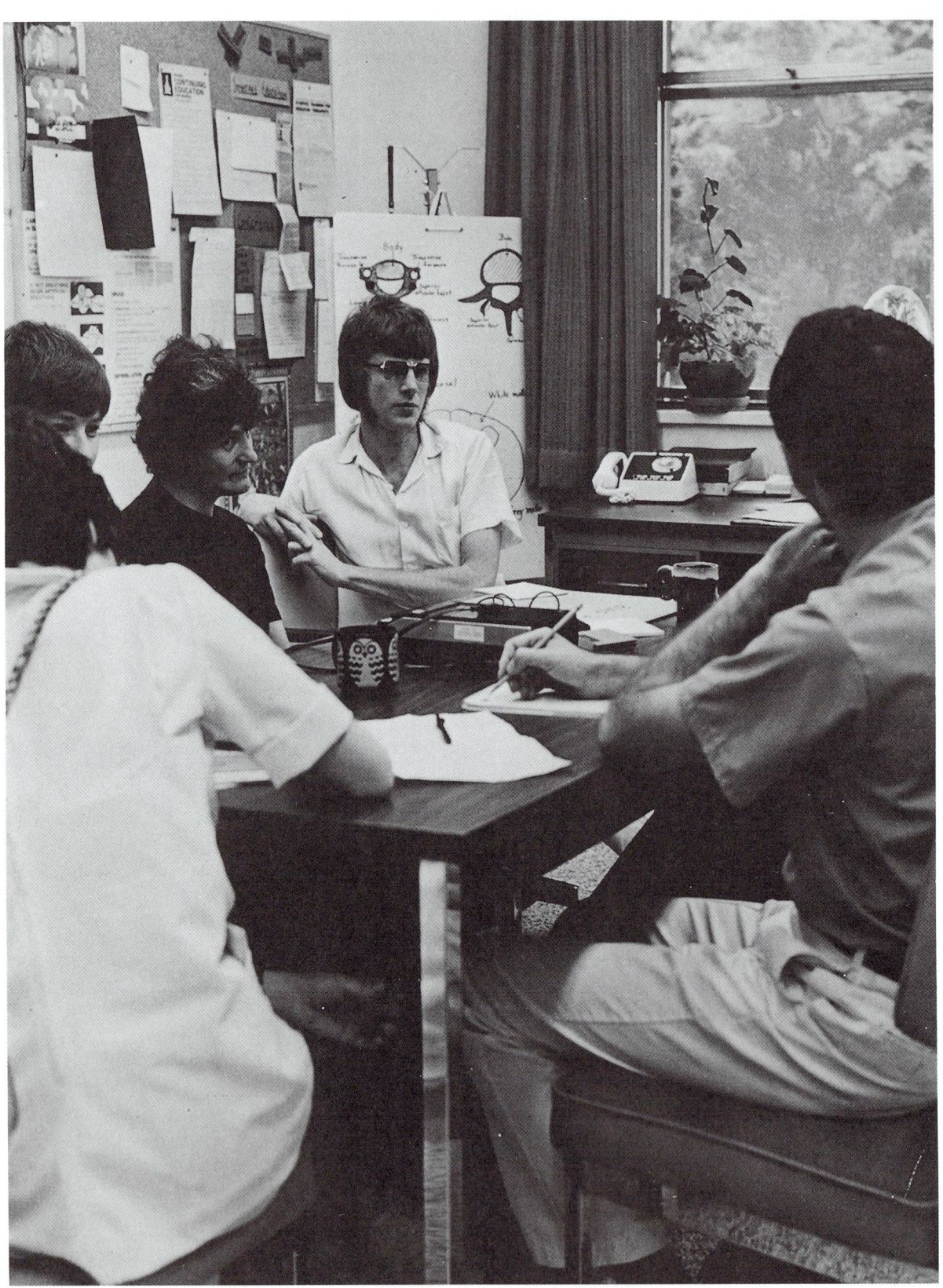

CHAPTER
– 13 –

A Practical Guide to Team Functioning in Spinal Cord Injury Rehabilitation*

Michael Dunn, Ph.D., Noreen Sommer, R.N., M.S.N., and Hank Gambina, M.S., L.M.F.C.C.

Chapter Outline

Objectives

- To describe the challenges of working as a member of a SCI team
- To identify the strengths of the team in SCI rehabilitation both for patient care and individual staff satisfaction
- To suggest concrete ways that team members can strengthen and maintain team functioning

*The help of Irene Saperstein, L.C.S.W., Louis Moffett, Ph.D., and Antonette Zeis, Ph.D., is acknowledged.

REHABILITATION GOALS

The concept that rehabilitation goals are best supported by well-functioning teams has been endorsed by many rehabilitation groups (Melvin 1989) and by organizations that set standards of care for rehabilitation (Joint Commission on Accreditation of Healthcare Organizations, Commission on the Accreditation of Rehabilitation Facilities, Department of Veterans Affairs). Many articles praise the virtues of team functioning, but research demonstrating its usefulness (see Halstead 1976; and Trieschmann 1988 for reviews); manuals showing how to develop a team; or clinical guides to increasing its effectiveness (Wise, Rubin, and Beckard 1974; Ducanis and Golin 1979; Smith, Moore, and Gilso 1983) have not been as available. For an excellent review of the literature on team functioning and a scholarly explication of its components see Browne and Bishop (1980) and Katz, Halstead, and Wierenga (1975). SCI rehabilitation, by virtue of the complexity of the disability, the variety of disciplines involved, and the relatively long-term interaction of staff with patients, makes a persuasive argument for the necessity of a team approach.

This chapter examines how staff and patients of an SCI injury rehabilitation center operate as a team, the difficulties involved in being a team member, and the advantages of the team both for patient care and for individual growth and job satisfaction. The remainder of the chapter then discusses specific ways in which individual members of the team can facilitate team functioning and enhance their own performance and satisfaction as team members.

TEAM CHALLENGES

Teamwork is difficult. Team functioning evolves and develops in sequential phases, described by Tuckman (1965) as forming, storming, norming, and performing. In the *forming* phase, individuals enter the team relationship, take on significance for each other, and begin to define themselves as a team. They set expectations of behavior for themselves, each other, and the team as a whole. The goal is to develop a sense of unity in order to meet their individual and team goals effectively.

In this process of developing a team, there may be a *storming* phase to determine distribution of power, or control, and to set alliances. This unsettling stage is important because it further defines roles and relationships, and specifies goals more clearly. The *norming* phase usually follows. Roles and functions are further defined and individuals are either reintegrated into functioning roles or become discouraged and leave the team. *Performing* is the ongoing business of the team, the outcome of the above process. Naturally, all these processes continue throughout the

team's existence. When the manner in which the team functions is threatened, the process begins anew.

Rehabilitation takes place in a complex web of organizational and professional issues, economic constrains, inadequate staffing patterns, maladaptive communication, personal issues, games patients and staff play, and other difficult situations all of which contribute to the challenge of mastering the role of team member.

Organizational and Professional Issues

Rehabilitation professionals work in a complex power structure. In addition to hospital administration that of necessity views rehabilitation from a primarily economic perspective, the director of rehabilitation is seldom the director of the professional service. It is often a vague system with multiple bosses and multiple responsibilities. Administrators have varied knowledge of and interest in SCI rehabilitation and therefore are often unable to provide consultation and support based on knowledge of the specialty.

Professional issues make team functioning more problematic, because one's profession may not emphasize a rehabilitation model of treatment or interdisciplinary team functioning.

Professional leaders are sometimes threatened by the individual staff member's identification with the SCI rehabilitation team rather than with the profession. Even with enlightened professional leaders each individual is required to balance professional autonomy and expertise with team goals. These are not easy choices, and each team member may struggle with divided loyalties or professional constraints at one time or another.

Who is responsible for *what* and *who* does *what* to or with *whom* can be misunderstood by patients and other staff. Roles and responsibilities may be ambiguous and vary according to the institutional or professional structure. Often, treatment guidelines for professional staff show that interventions overlap because of a commitment to shared responsibility.

Professionals receive training in their specialty, but few receive any formal training or supervised experience in how to integrate their specialty with those of others or how to function as part of a team. Professional schools teach how crucial and significant their profession is and how much it can do rather than how much it depends on other professions to accomplish its goals.

Economic and Staffing Constraints

In this age of increasing costs and decreasing resources, the cost of team functioning is a consideration. Very few studies have examined the cost/benefit ratio of the team approach (but see Ham, Regan, and Roberts [1981] for such an analysis of a small team), so it is easy to argue that economic factors discourage a team approach.

Where fee-for-service is a way of life, some rehabilitation facilities have a difficult time billing for team meetings, staff intervention, and training, partly because of the as-yet-unproven efficacy of team intervention. Some facilities, however, add a fixed amount to everyone's bill for reimbursement of team activities.

Formal team meetings are difficult to schedule and are expensive in staff time and effort. Thus, even when reimbursement is not an issue, time for communication and team functioning is at a premium. In some teams, meetings can only be held early in the mornings so as not to interfere with therapy times, but this in turn may prevent nurses from attending the meetings. The staff may believe that the meetings are important, but restlessness occurs if topics are discussed that the whole team does not believe are relevant or if the total meeting is too long.

Staffing constraints exist in every organization. There seldom seems to be enough people to work in a facility or never the correct distribution of specialists. There is frequently more work to be done than staff can do. Therefore, lack of success and satisfaction may be blamed on an insufficient number of trained staff.

Communication Patterns

Communication is difficult. It is a skill that requires vigilance because patterns change, and people change, which influences the manner in which the team communicates. Some research (Rintala et al. 1986) has examined the communication patterns in one team meeting about patients in a rehabilitation setting and found that there was a large discrepancy between what the team members considered to be ideal team communication patterns and what actually occurred. For example, "The physical content area was overemphasized (65%) and the psychosocial area was underemphasized (14%) when compared with the perceived needs of the patients" (Rintala et al. 1986: 118). To avoid or reduce these discrepancies, team members are encouraged to implement the methods of improving team communication described in this chapter.

Personal Issues

The personal needs and conflicts of the individuals who work on an SCI unit have an impact on team functioning and patient care. Important issues for the patient and team include why one wants to work in a rehabilitation setting, what the work of a SCI center is considered to be, and what is a rehabilitation setting. Who does what to whom is important, but so is the *Why*.

Staff entering a SCI center may have had limited, if any, contact with disability. In the education and socialization of new staff, it is important to consider the concept of personal threat (Gunther 1981) and how it affects one's interaction with other staff and patients. If one is fearful about SCI happening to oneself, then one's treatment of the person with SCI may be too optimistic, too patronizing, or too solicitous.

Gunther (1981) also discusses the difficulties for the team when individual staff members try to resolve personal developmental issues such as adolescent rebellion or parenting through their interaction with other staff and patients. For example, a therapist might conspire with a patient to break the rules because he or she may have authority problems; or a nurse may be overly manipulated by a patient who acts like father, son, or spouse.

Team members who have problems with authority may challenge leadership or lead in an authoritarian manner when status is more important than outcome.

Team functioning is interfered with by people with low self-esteem who try to be the best of everything, the expert, the star or the person who has to have a special relationship with the patient. This type of individual seeks praise by placing personal gain before team effort. A well-coordinated team strikes a balance among members with various expertise.

Issues concerning sexuality may also be unresolved and interfere with the ability to understand and intervene appropriately with patients' sexual concerns. See Chapter 10. Hohmann (1975: 12) suggests a number of caveats in this regard, for example:

- Avoid forcing your morality and convictions on the patient.
- Do not assume that once the topic is discussed that you can leave it alone.
- Do not make sex an all or none sort of experience.

Attitudinal Issues

It is important for all people who work in the field of SCI to be aware of the impact of their own attitudes about disability on their job performance and ability to function as team members. Being aware that in the general population, ambivalence and conflict about disability often lead to people with SCI being overpraised and undercriticized (Dunn 1982) helps the team members realize the importance of learning to give honest feedback for the patient's benefit as well as their own.

Studies have shown that rehabilitation staff have widely varying, but generally negative, attitudes about disability. Singleton, Cole, and Long (1979) found that those professionals who have the most contact with patients had the most negative attitudes.

In addition, many rehabilitation staff cannot predict well the emotional concerns of people with SCI. Bodenhamer, Achterberg-Lawlis, Kevorkian, Belanus, and Cofer (1983) have shown that staff predicted more depression and less anxiety and optimism than the patients reported. Trieschmann (1988) has reviewed the literature on depression and

SCI and concluded that staff tend to overpredict depression in SCI. See Chapters 9 and 12.

Difficult Rehabilitation Situations

Table 13–1 shows situations that were rated difficult to manage at an inpatient SCI center and an outpatient SCI facility. At the outpatient facility, the items that were difficult to manage were mainly issues about sexuality. Even though these situations did not happen to many of the staff persons, they were especially uncomfortable about these incidents. At the inpatient facility, however, the unique situations that were the most difficult to manage were excessive complaints, patients showing dislike of the staff or who did not try to get better, and family members asking when the patient is going to walk out of the hospital. It can be seen that the first three situations happened quite frequently and were highly rated in terms of difficulty. It appears from this study that the inpatient staff at the time had more trouble with anger and patients who did not cooperate, whereas at the other facility, the difficulties concerned sexual issues. Few professionals are trained to deal with situations like these.

Within the context of difficult staff/patient interactions, games refer to indirect, passive ways of interacting with other, more powerful individuals in such a way as to accomplish one's goals or gain an advantage. Patients in a rehabilitation setting characteristically feel a lack of control and consequently may attempt to regain that control or obtain an emotional response from the staff through problem behavior. For instance, they may try to play the staff against each other: a patient may tell the nurse that the therapist said something was okay, and then tell the therapist the nurse said it was okay. They may also do this to staff on different shifts. Effective team functioning depends on individual staff members' learning how to deal with these games so that the team is not split. Sometimes helping may mean saying *no* to a patient's request in the context of a consistent team approach.

TABLE 13–1 Situations that Staff Encounter in a Rehabilitation Setting Rated as Difficult to Handle, Awkward, or Embarrassing

	Items Most Difficult to Manage	Discomfort*	Frequency of Occurrence**
Both Inpatient and Outpatient SCI Facilities	Being put down by another staff member in front of a patient	3.73	39%
	Doctor comes in during treatment, ignores staff member and patient, and begins procedure	3.60	55%
	Patient who is vulgar, abusive, and offensive	3.42	79%
	Taking care of a patient who is uncooperative	3.39	85%
	Doctor tells patient something with which other staff do not agree	3.31	64%
Inpatient	Patient who complains excessively	3.25	76%
	Taking care of a patient you know doesn't like you	3.22	60%
	Patients who don't try to get better	3.19	61%
	Family says, "When is he going to walk out of here?"	3.09	42%
Outpatient	During a transfer, patient repeatedly kisses you on the neck	3.35	2%
	Patient makes a sexual advance during a treatment	3.31	33%
	Paraplegic person makes fun of a quadriplegic person	3.24	6%
	Patient asks, "What do you and your partner do sexually?"	3.20	12%

*The mean discomfort on a 1 to 5 scale with 1 being low and 5 being high.
**The percentage of staff to whom that situation had occurred. From Dunn (1983a).

TEAM STRENGTHS

Organization, Power, and Influence

Teamwork provides a stable structure and therefore a consistent response to patients. Even though staff sometimes complain about too many meetings, the patient benefits from opportunities for staff to discuss issues, plan interventions and strategies, include patients in the treatment plan, and give feedback in a formal manner.

Team members who work toward common goals form highly cohesive groups. Intense relationships facilitate group consensus rather than individual decision making. Reaching consensus is a powerful experience and reinforces the notion that there is power in numbers as well as the belief that the team is unique from every other team. Affirmation by other team members can be a great reward for a job well done.

The team can also exert power and influence on patients. This influence adds to the power of numbers at meetings with patients and affects patient compliance. Because of the team's diversity, there often is at least one team member who gets along well with a particular patient and can assume an advocacy role.

The team also has an influence over external forces. When the team speaks as one voice, there is more credibility than when one team member speaks. The team is also more willing to take risks than the individual because the responsibilty is diffused. However, be careful to avoid so-called *group think* when no one individual takes responsibility.

Mutual Support

Complexity and conflicting opinions help individuals learn to work with diversity and to know the norms of the team. Shared discussions and consensus promote mutual support and prevent burnout. Open discussion promotes the understanding that there are no right answers. Mutual support also involves sharing explanations of another's behavior and offering reinterpretations of what might otherwise be interpreted as inappropriate behavior.

Multiple Leaders

Another advantage of the team approach in rehabilitation is the opportunity for different team members to take the lead in various situations. Fordyce (1971) discusses the essential elements of a rehabilitation team leader—abilities to facilitate group and interpersonal communication, to yield authority effectively, to supervise, and to possess a wide range of rehabilitation knowledge. He acknowledges as do other researchers that these qualities may not exist in the same individual at all times. One of the strengths of the team is its ability to adjust to changing leaders in the face of changing demands, and the well-functioning team has different leaders for different tasks.

STRENGTHENING AND MAINTAINING THE TEAM

Supporting Others

It is important to make a conscious effort to diffuse competition and splitting among members of the team. Avoid rewarding tattletales and do not allow scapegoating. For example, when a patient is late for a therapy appointment, the team does not tolerate or agree with staff who say, "Nursing didn't get the patient up on time." The well-functioning team looks at the situation, discusses the problem of scheduling, and talks in a team manner. For example, "Let's go back and look at the schedule again to see if *we* can find the problem." It is unproductive and destructive to team functioning to scapegoat other team members. It is better not to allow complex patient-care situations to be opportunities to compete with or blame each other.

In place of competition the well-functioning team looks for opportunities to find a team member doing something worthy of praise or applause. Try to applaud one another for doing a good job with a particular patient or project. Support and celebrate in a public forum the individual professional accomplishments of team members, such as presentation of a paper, development of a new form or procedure, election to office in a professional society, or publication of an article.

Find opportunities to celebrate team functioning, which requires attention to the function and process of the team. For example, say, "I think we did a good job with this patient. It was difficult and we worked well together. I think it's great that this patient's been rehabilitated without dividing us." Another example is, "We're doing a good job giving a consistent message and I think this patient is going to do well as a result." Using *we* instead of *I* or *you* messages supports the team process.

Assisting other staff to disown a problem is a supportive team function. People in the helping professions often have an overdeveloped sense of responsibility and often feel that negative events or outcomes are somehow their fault. The team can help individuals realize that the patients' problems are not theirs. Team members can contribute to the resolution of the problem and are responsible for what they do individually, but the problem or problems do not belong to them. Team members can be helped to avoid feeling guilty when they cannot make patients realize their full potential. The avoidance of guilt does not involve giving up, but it does mean sharing a team strategy and the belief that the solution to the problem does not rest with any one team member.

It is helpful for a team member to adopt a model of coping rather than a model of mastery. Trying to project a perfect model of professional and/or personal competence discourages other team members from taking risks, asking for help, or giving feedback. It also takes a toll on the apparently perfect person. Discussing and demonstrating how one copes with one's own difficulties helps develop these skills in others.

In the effort to give team support to one another, it is better to avoid *shoulds* or *musts*. Believing in a "just world" causes believers to feel worse than they need to feel when they make a mistake because they believe they have broken the rule as well as causing difficulty for another person. Additionally, they do not feel as good as they might when they do well because they feel that they only did what they *should* have done.

It is helpful to acknowledge that there are many equally effective answers to any problem. There are many different ways to reach the same goals and there is no reason to insist on having the only right answer. Each team member has an area of expertise and can assist the others along the way.

Support Group Activity

A variety of group activities occur in one form or another at most rehabilitation centers, and with some attention and effort by the team members these activities can support and reinforce team functioning as well as accomplish specific goals.

The patient planning meeting is a group activity that involves members of the team sharing responsibility for planning with patients. When planning is viewed as a team function with the patient as a member or partner of the team, a format can be developed that enhances team functioning and benefits both the patient and the team (Bonifay 1989). Each team member has an important part to play and is accountable for a specific area of the plan. However, it is most helpful to the patient and team members if there is a free flow of information and the patient and team members are free to ask questions. The team develops norms and rules such as speaking directly to the patient, selecting the meeting leader, inviting the patient to sit at the head of the table, and preparing the patient in advance for the meeting. In addition to the stated goal of the meeting—to plan—these meetings represent a regular opportunity for team members to work together, assign responsibility, understand roles, prevent splitting, build group spirit, and plan interventions. The team can seek feedback from patients and family members as well as each other on ways to improve the meeting.

In some facilities, team meetings occur for the stated purpose of group support and discussion. A problem-solving approach may be taken as well as providing an opportunity to share feelings. These meetings may take the form of the facilitator asking what the staff wish to discuss. Usually individual patients are brought up for discussion and in the context of specific discussion, general principles are derived and applied to other situations. Asking other staff how they handle the situation facilitates sharing feelings as well as arriving at different approaches. Other techniques, such as advice giving and role playing, also have been used with success. A recent evaluation of such meetings (Dunn 1989) reveals that the staff felt that the meetings were practical, concrete, and entertaining; they had learned that many staff shared the same feelings about specific problems; they wanted the meetings to continue at the same frequency and duration; and they had learned new techniques for dealing with patients and other staff.

Gans (1987) describes another approach in which the patient is interviewed by a psychiatrist in the presence of the treatment team. He feels that this procedure facilitates staff-patient interaction by modeling interviewing skills and showing the staff how their own behavior may influence the patients.

Planning social events can be viewed as opportunities for social interaction and good practice for the team in solving problems, distributing tasks, and making decisions without the added pressure of patient-care problems and outcomes.

The effort made to socialize new team members is an investment in future team functioning. Some of this socialization is truly social in the usual sense of the word, for example, making sure that someone accompanies the new employee to the cafeteria for lunch, showing them which table the SCI staff usually occupies in the lunch room, and introducing all students, interns, and new employees to the staff.

The new staff member needs to be socialized and oriented to the professional culture of the SCI unit as well. Assigning a mentor to new staff and providing adequate opportunities to observe all team members, to see what their work includes and how they interact with staff and patients, assist with this process. In addition to sharing information about professional roles and functions, experienced staff usually model a style that reflects comfort with disability, a skill seldom included in basic professional education. Encouraging the staff to seek assistance from the team when they do something for the first time can result in the new staff members' feeling the benefit of team support very early in their SCI experience.

Taking the opportunity to educate the team together is a way to support the team. Not only are information and skills imparted, but people get to know each other as individuals as opposed to disciplines. An example of a specific class is a one-day workshop on sexuality and SCI (Lloyd and Dunn 1981). It includes a didactic lecture on the physical, social, communication, and cultural aspects of sex and SCI as well as discussion of sexual counseling techniques. In addition, there is behavior rehearsal on potentially difficult sexual encounters the staff may have with patients (Dunn 1983b).

Other types of team experiences are group education on the psychosocial consequences of SCI team functioning and behavior rehearsal of typical patient interactions, difficult patient encounters, and problematic team issues (Dunn 1983a). These experiences offer opportunities to learn new skills, practice old ones, decrease anxiety about applying these skills with people with disabilities, become more comfortable with other disciplines, learn that others share the same difficulties and feelings, and, most important, feel closer to one another. Table 13–2 gives guidelines for behavior-rehearsal exercises.

Three different kinds of situations are used, common patient interactions, difficult patient interactions, and team

TABLE 13–2 Suggested Guidelines for Staff-Training Groups on Managing Rehabilitation Situations

I. Introduction
   A. Rationale: The opportunity to rehearse and get feedback increases comfort level and skill.
   B. Staff are asked to rehearse situations that SCI staff have found difficult to manage or discomforting
   C. Reassurances to participants:
      1. It is difficult to be the staff person because of the element of surprise.
      2. There are no absolute wrong or right answers.
      3. One's professional reputation is not on the line.
      4. You're not doing psychotherapy; choose many short interactions, rather than one in depth.
      5. Have some fun.

II. Demonstration
   A. Ask a participant to suggest a situation for leaders to do.
   B. Model a discussion about how to select roles and how to practice a situation.
   C. Model handling a situation and the feedback process.

III. Break into random groups
   A. Try to put different disciplines in each group.
   B. Each group will designate one "patient," one "staff member," and one or two "observers" to give feedback.
   C. The "patient" selects a situation from an envelope (in order to make the situation a surprise for the "staff member") and acts it out as suggested.
   D. The "staff member" will respond and interact for a short time; the "staff member" will determine the length of the rehearsal.
   E. The "observer" will give constructive feedback (See Table 13–4 for helpful suggestions on constructive criticism).
   F. Then roles will change; a new situation will be chosen so that each person will have an opportunity to be "patient," "staff member," and "observer."
   G. The process can continue until all the situations are used.

and team-family interactions. These are shown in Table 13–3. Some situations involve specific statements while others describe a troublesome incident.

Sharing the responsibilities for the development of a patient and family education curriculum as well as the classroom teaching for the education classes can be an affirming activity for the team. It provides an additional opportunity for the individual members of the team to share their individual professional expertise with patients and families and each other. The team decisions about what needs to be learned is an additional opportunity for building team consensus.

Preparing patient and family manuals, SCI center brochures, preparing team lectures, articles, book chapters, and doing team research are examples of group projects. Not every discipline will be or can be part of every group project, which protects team members' time as well as gives opportunities for different configurations of team members to work together. These projects serve the same team building functions as do the other group activities.

Environmental Influences

The environment in which the team works is an important aspect of team functioning. Seemingly minor changes in the workplace can have an impact on communication, job satisfaction, motivation, and patient interaction. One study, for example, found that feedback to staff was ineffective in increasing patient time in therapy (Kennedy, Fisher, and Petersen 1988). An environmental change, however, such as banning smoking in the Day Room, increased group participation in therapy.

A good example of how the environment can influence team functioning is provided by the process of destruction, construction, and reconstruction with which one team had to deal for 2 years as its unit was expanded from 30 SCI beds to 60. As a result of noise, dust, schedule disruptions, uncertainty, dark patient rooms (necessitated by reconstruction), and so forth, team morale went down while turnover and anger increased to a new high. Under conditions of such environmental stress, it may be helpful to emphasize team functioning. Change, even change for the better, is a stressor that should be acknowledged and faced by the team.

Team functioning can be improved when the space for team meetings is large enough to accommodate a circle so that all team members are seated in an egalitarian fashion. This promotes group discussion, eye contact, and cohesiveness. The physical format of a meeting can initiate change, just as can an explicit decision by the team (Halstead et al. 1986).

If the spatial configuration of the SCI unit does not allow team members to be near each other, communication and understanding suffer. For example, some large rehabilitation facilities have therapy departments on separate floors from the patient care areas, and opportunities for commu-

TABLE 13–3 Role-Play Situations Used in Teaching Team Functioning

Kind of Interaction		Kind of Interaction	
Common Patient Interactions	Patient says, "I'm old. I'd rather be dead than injured."	Difficult Patient Interactions	Patient always says, "I can't do that," but does it elsewhere, for example, transfer.
	Patient seems to forget constantly, and when reminded, refuses, for example, to go to therapy.		Patient who doesn't try to get better and says, "I'm just going to wait until I can walk out of here."
	A paraplegic person makes fun of a person with quadriplegia by saying, "You call that a handshake, you wimp?"		Patient says, "Let's do it."
	Patient tries to intimidate staff member by saying, "I'm going to my congressman because you're not doing your job."		Patient is vulgar, abusive, and offensive.
	A quadriplegic person gets a patient who can walk to do things for him that he could do for himself.		Even though patient attempted a transfer before he was trained and fell on the floor, he says, "Why didn't you help me? It's your fault!"
	Patient says, "I just feel like giving up."	Team and Team-Family Interactions	Another staff member disagrees with you about a treatment in front of a patient.
	Patient makes a sexual advance during a treatment.		Mother says to patient, "Have faith in God and you'll walk again."
	An angry patient almost runs into a staff member with his wheelchair.		Doctor comes in during treatment, ignores staff member and patient, and begins procedures.
	Patient expresses a lot of pain and feels helpless about being able to do anything about it.		Doctor tells patient something with which you do not agree.
Difficult Patient Interactions	Patient asks, "What do you and your partner do sexually?"		Spouse says, "Will he walk out of here?"
	Patient says, "Not you again!" to a staff member whom patient does not like.		Family of one patient tells another patient, "You'll get as much recovery as our son did."
	During a transfer, patient repeatedly kisses staff member on the neck.		Patient with a hangover doesn't go to therapy and staff member says, "Let him skip therapy. What else does the poor guy have?"
	Patient refuses to use a splint even though it prevents damage to himself.		Doctor interrupts your procedures to talk with the patient about another treatment.
	Patient asks staff member for a date and staff member doesn't want to go with him.		Being put down by another staff member in front of a patient by saying, "We don't have any trouble transferring when I'm working with you, do we?"
	Patient complains excessively.		

nication between nurses and therapists thus require an effort. Some teams report that they work as well as they do because they are all crammed together into a small space. Proximity can facilitate awareness of the similar problems that other disciplines have with patients and can provide the opportunity for observation of problem solving skills.

When external circumstances are not under one's control, they can be used as a way of promoting group unity. When there is no one entity to blame, such as in a nursing shortage, the team can grow closer by discussing the problem and brainstorming how the team can compensate for

it. Of course, it is helpful to assume an attitude that problems can be a growth experience.

Interpersonal Skills

Well-functioning team members need to be able to assess adequately the system in which they function. System problems are often interpersonal problems, and the ability to assess the system is necessary in order to understand and facilitate group functioning. Contact is the cornerstone— being available when needed, being open to other disciplines on the team, listening, and contributing to conversations. Feeling comfortable in expressing one's feelings and looking forward to the consequences helps other team members do the same.

Assessing the system is also important because at times the team becomes the patient. Sometimes problems that the team has with a particular patient or staff member are more usefully considered in terms of the *team's* problem rather than an individual's problem. Effective team members recognize this and contribute to understanding the situation. Monitoring and assessing the team functions in formal ways such as quality assurance/peer review not only include looking at what one's colleagues are doing in relation to patients, but also in relation to each other.

In addition to this kind of assessment, a formal, standardized instrument can occasionally be useful. The team also benefits by stopping for a moment in the course of everyday work to examine what it is doing. Assessment results offer a good opportunity for the team to discuss its functioning. The Ward Atmosphere Scale (WAS) (Moos 1974, 1987) used mainly in psychiatric settings, offers a beneficial way of examining rehabilitation wards (Sutkin 1980). It can be an informative and useful tool to examine how the atmosphere of the ward is perceived and what aspects of team functioning could be changed or reinforced. It consists of 100 items relating to the manner in which the milieu is perceived by the respondents (patients and/or staff) on 10 different scales, Involvement (I), Support (S), Spontaneity (SP), Autonomy (A), Practical Orientation (PO), Personal Problem Orientation (PPO), Anger and Aggression (AA), Order and Organization (O), Program Clarity (PC), and Staff Control (SC).

Romano (1980) discusses other ways of evaluating staff problems. Less important than the measure, however, is the idea that each team member be sensitized to the necessity for monitoring team process and discussing that process with other team members.

Every team member should attempt to understand the problems that can weaken the team and to work on maintaining the team system. Concentrating on the task is necessary but often not sufficient for team functioning or patient change.

New team members often do not realize that their presence alone is insufficient to guarantee acceptance by the team. It is necessary that they demonstrate to the team that they can be a part of the solution and a useful, productive team member. Established team members also have to produce in order to solidify and legitimize their positions. They also contribute by joining the team socially after work, attending ward parties, and being visible members of the system. They enter into the team's social structure by participating.

One of the most important interpersonal skills is reinforcing others with praise, knowing when and how to give and receive it. The team functions much better and the members feel better about themselves if praise for accomplishments, both individual and collective, are freely given and honestly accepted.

Principles for giving praise are:

1. Try to praise accomplishments as soon as possible.
2. Always praise effort.
3. Praise closer and closer approximations to the goal.
4. Praise both publicly and privately.
5. Praise individual as well as group accomplishments.

Accepting praise involves:

1. Thank the praiser for being aware and expressing praise in public and private.
2. Do not belittle the efforts being praised.
3. Share the praise with other team members if appropriate.

In the context of good team functioning, sometimes the best approach to maladaptive behavior is simply to ignore it. Walking quietly out of the room, looking away from a person, or changing the subject can be very effective in limiting the behavior without raising the level of conflict.

Talk in a "team" manner:

"I guess we have different approaches to pain management. Let's see if we can work out a team approach."

"We all may have difficulties with this patient."

"We did a great job with that person."

Personal Stress Reduction

An important aspect of professional behavior is caring for oneself. The strength one has to care for the team comes from taking care of and supporting oneself. It is difficult to support team members when one loses sight of one's own needs. For example, a team member who has too heavy a personal or work schedule may need to set limits and choose not to take part in a team project, so that the next team endeavor can be undertaken with renewed vigor.

It is important to seek honest feedback from team members regarding one's performance as a team member. It is also important to receive this feedback nondefensively, and to listen closely to others' perception. In seeking feedback, ask team members to be specific and check their communication to assure that it is clear. Table 13–4 provides principles of constructive feedback.

Taking a day off occasionally is usually difficult for people who have a highly developed sense of responsibility. A day's respite, however, tends to rejuvenate and reenergize an individual to be a more functional team member. Taking enjoyable time while at work may accomplish the same purpose. For example, attend an interesting conference or in-service workshop, become involved in an enjoyable project, or work with an enjoyable patient. Scheduling difficult patients at the beginning of the day and successful patients at the end of the day helps one leave work with a better attitude.

TABLE 13–4 Characteristics of Constructive Feedback
Adapted from Bergquist and Phillips (1975)

1. Descriptive, not evaluative
2. Specific, not general
3. Focuses on behavior, not the person
4. Not meant to make one feel better
5. Directed at behavior the receiver can do something about
6. Solicited, not imposed
7. Well timed
8. Sharing information, not giving advice
9. Involves the amount of information the receiver can use
10. Concerns what is said and done, or how, not why
11. Checked to ensure clear communication
12. Checked to determine degree of agreement from others
13. Followed by attention to the consequences of feedback
14. A step toward authenticity

Realize the value of taking small steps and be comfortable at times with approximations to the goal. Being pleased with a patient's ability to assist with transfers makes it easier to move to the next step of independent transfers. This successive approximation leads to more satisfaction and serves to solidify and strengthen team spirit as well as enhancing the outcome of many team endeavors.

The team can help each team member set realistic goals. It is easier to determine what is realistic and to prioritize when the process is shared with others. It is also important to recognize which battles to fight and where to focus one's energy.

In any system or bureaucracy there is bound to be inefficiency. Things seldom work the way they should, and one should not focus on these inefficiencies at the expense of making progress toward one's goals. Resolving inefficiency is less important than striking a balance and prioritizing intervention strategies.

Furthermore, people in helping professions often expect more of themselves than they expect from others, which produces stress and leads to disappointment and low self-esteem. This type of perfectionism leads to an array of personal and team problems. It is more helpful as a professional to accept certain personal limitations. Try not to make the same mistakes repeatedly, and instead view problems as an opportunity to rethink how to handle the situation. Although this approach does not lead to perfection, it leaves team members better off personally and professionally than when they started.

A sense of humor among team members and patients relieves tension and anxiety and puts things in perspective. Individuals who learn to enjoy one another tend to have a

better working relationship, and fostering humor in a rehabilitation setting is crucial to team functioning.

Interdisciplinary Coordination Strategies

Strategies that encourage team functioning serve to acquaint each member of the team with the roles, knowledge, and skills of the other members, as well as provide an opportunity to practice team skills in specific situations.

It is helpful to teach one's skills to other team members whether they be psychosocial, nursing, or physical or occupational therapy skills. This gives strength to the team as a whole without lessening one's individual expertise. Role diversification or blurring serves to unite the team and leads to a more coordinated team functioning if done in a purposeful and sharing way. Sharing information and skills also serves to expand individual roles and helps provide consistency of treatment (Mullins 1989).

All team members at one time or another can participate in choosing which patients room together. This decision belongs to all team members, not solely to nursing staff. Different disciplines know the patients' levels of psychosocial functioning, daily living skills (DLS) status, and motivation, and can use their knowledge to maximize the therapeutic value of appropriate roommate selection.

All team members may wish to facilitate a patient network. For example, sending an experienced person with SCI to visit a newly injured person can be useful for both patients. Valuable peer modeling takes place and, most important, this strategy helps to integrate the patients into the team. See Chapter 12 for a further explanation of this important concept.

The emphasis in a rehabilitation center is on concrete services rather than theoretical or abstract goals. A philosophy of rehabilitation is required; however, specific services bring the philosophy and goals to fruition. For example, DLS and attendant care training, facilitating the search for affordable and accessible housing, and training in social skills are all practical, concrete interventions. Concentrating on the outcome rather than personality variables facilitates team functioning.

If team members from different disciplines meet together with patients, team functioning is strengthened and patients benefit. Team members learn what others do and thus broaden their intervention strategies. Patients profit both from the individual expertise and from the interaction and role modeling of the team members.

CONCLUSION

The multiple systems that are affected by SCI and the various disciplines needed to treat people require a team approach. This chapter has presented some of the strengths and weaknesses of interdisciplinary team functioning in terms of both patient care as well as the job performance and satisfaction of team members. More important, it has suggested how team functioning can be developed, improved, and maintained. Working as a member of an SCI team is not an easy task and requires that the whole team attempt to maintain it. In that attempt the true satisfaction and worth of the team emerges.

REFERENCES

Bergquist, W., and Phillips, S. 1975. *A Handbook for Faculty Development*. The Council for the Advancement of Small Colleges in association with the College Center of the Finger Lakes.

Bodenhamer, E., Achterberg-Lawlis, J., Kevorkian, G., Belanus, A., and Cofer, J. 1983. Staff and patient perceptions of the psychosocial concerns of spinal cord injured persons. *American Journal of Physical Medicine* 62 (4): 182–193.

Bonifay, R. 1989. Methods, measurements and results of using the philosophy of patient participation as a total care plan. *SCI Psychosocial Process* 2 (1): 6–11.

Browne, J., and Bishop, D. 1980. Team functioning: A professional versus lay perspective. In *Behavioral Problems and the Disabled*. Ed. D. S. Bishop. Baltimore: Williams and Wilkins.

Ducanis, A., and Golin, A. 1979. *The Interdisciplinary Health Care Team*. Germantown, MD: Aspen Systems Corp.

Dunn, M. 1982. *Social Relationships and Interpersonal Skills: A Guide for People with Sensory and Physical Limitations*. Falls Church, VA: Institute for Information Studies.

Dunn, M. 1983a. The Rehabilitation Situations Inventory: An instrument to assess discomfort in rehabilitation staff. Paper presented at the American Congress of Rehabilitation Medicine, Los Angeles, CA.

Dunn, M. 1983b. Sexual questions and comments on a spinal cord injury center. *Sexuality and Disability* 6 (3): 126–134.

Dunn, M. 1989. Staff groups. From a workshop entitled *Therapeutic groups: Theory and practice*, presented at the third annual meeting of American Association of SCI Psychologists and Social Workers, Las Vegas.

Fordyce, W. 1971. Psychology, social work, and medicine. *Archives of Physical Medicine and Rehabilitation* 52: 9.

Gans, J. 1987. Facilitating staff/patient interaction. In *Rehabilitation Psychology Desk Reference*. Ed. B. Caplan. Rockville, MD: Aspen.

Gunther, M. 1981. The threatened practitioner: work under stress. In *Comprehensive Rehabilitation Nursing*. Eds. N. Martin, N. Holt, and D. Hicks. New York: McGraw-Hill.

Halstead, L. 1976. Team care in chronic illness: A critical review of the literature of the past 25 years. *Archives of Physical Medicine and Rehabilitation* 57: 507–511.

Halstead, L., Rintala, D., Kanellos, M., Griffin, B., Higgins, L., Rheinecker, S., Whiteside, W., and Healy, J. 1986. The innovative rehabilitation team: An experiment in team building. *Archives of Physical Medicine and Rehabilitation* 67: 357–361.

Ham, R., Regan, J., and Roberts, V. 1987. Evaluation of introducing the team approach to the care of the amputee: the Dulwich study. *Prosthetics and Orthotics International* 11: 25–30.

Hohmann, G. 1975. Reactions of the individual with a disability complicated by a sexual problem. *Archives of Physical Medicine and Rehabilitation* 56: 8–13.

Katz, S., Halstead, L., and Wierenga, M. 1975. A medical perspective of team care. In *Long Term Care: A Handbook for Researchers, Planners, and Providers*. Ed. S. Sherwood. New York: Spectrum.

Kennedy, P., Fisher, K., and Petersen, E. 1988. Ecological evaluation of a rehabilitative environment for spinal cord injured people: Behavioural mapping and feedback. *British Journal of Clinical Psychology* 27: 239–246.

Lloyd, E., and Dunn, M. 1981. Staff sexuality education in spinal cord injury. Paper presented at American Congress of Rehabilitation Medicine, San Diego, CA.

Melvin, J. 1989. Status report on interdisciplinary medical rehabilitation. *Archives of Physical Medicine and Rehabilitation* 70: 273–276.

Moos, R. 1974. *Evaluating Treatment Environments: A Social Ecological Approach*. New York: Wiley.

Moos, R. 1987. *The Social Climates Scales: A Users Guide*. Palo Alto, CA: Consulting Psychologists Press.

Mullins, L. 1989. Hate revisited: Power, envy, and greed in the rehabilitation setting. *Archives of Physical Medicine and Rehabilitation* 70: 740–744.

Rintala, D., Hanover, D., Alexander, J., Sanson-Fisher, R., Willems, E., and Halstead, L. 1986. Team care: An analysis of verbal behavior during patient rounds in a rehabilitation hospital. *Archives of Physical Medicine and Rehabilitation* 67: 118–122.

Romano, M. 1980. Staff problems in rehabilitation. In *Behavioral Problems and the Disabled*. Ed. D. Bishop. Baltimore: Williams and Wilkins.

Smith, R., Moore, C., and Gilson, L. 1983. Development of interdisciplinary team effectiveness. Presented at the 60th annual session of the American Congress of Rehabilitation Medicine.

Sutkin, L. 1980. Spinal cord injured patients' perceptions of ward atmosphere following assertiveness training of nursing staff. In *Communication in a Health Care Setting*. Eds. M. Eisenberg, J. Falconer, and L. Sutkin. Springfield: Charles Thomas.

Trieschmann, R. 1988. *Spinal Cord Injuries: Psychological, Social and Vocational Rehabilitation*. 2d ed. New York: Demos.

Tuckman, B. 1965. Developmental sequences in small groups. *Psychological Bulletin* 53.

Wise, H., Rubin, I., and Beckard, R. 1974. Making health teams work. *American Journal of the Disabled Child* 127: 537–542.

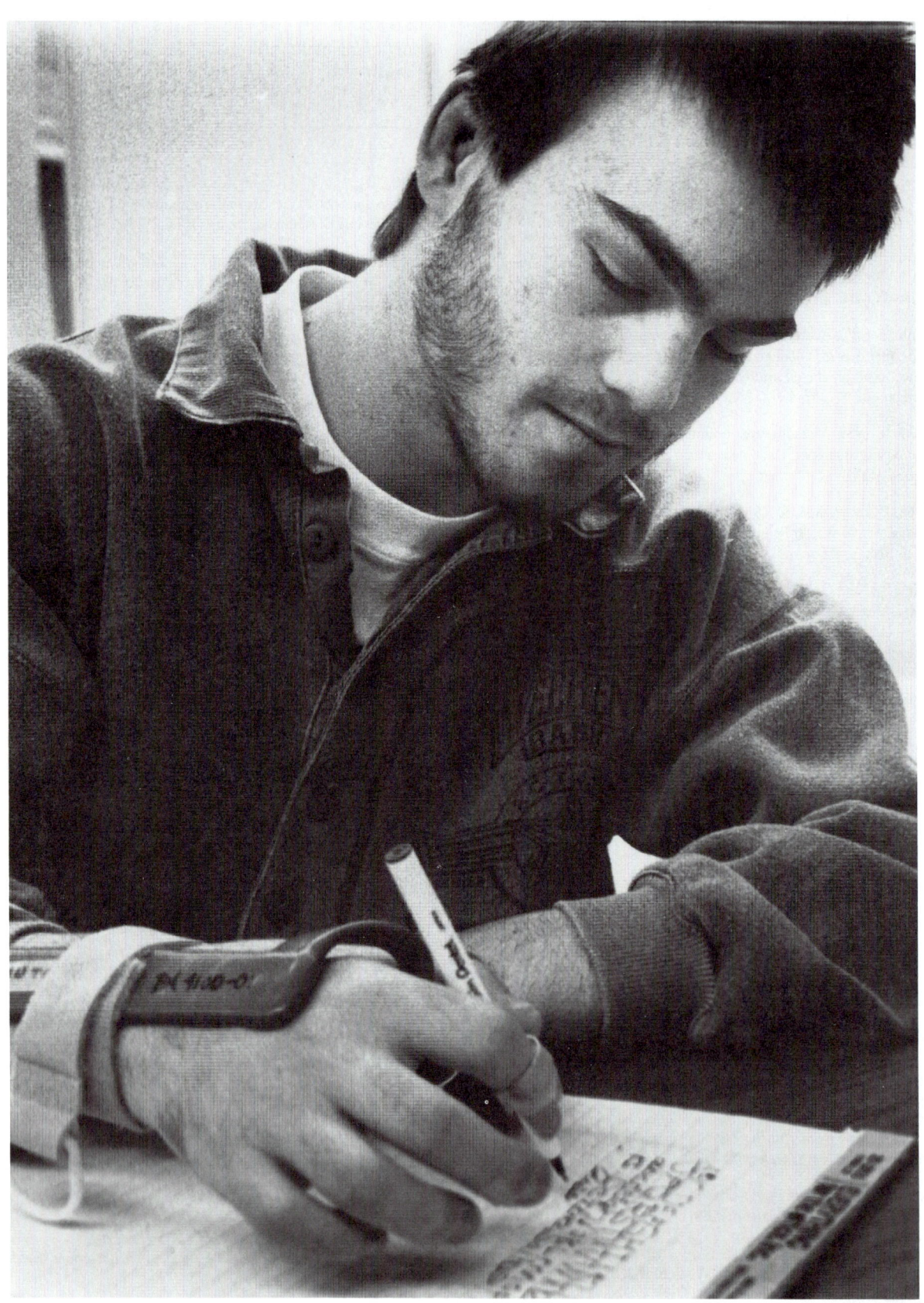

CHAPTER
— 14 —

Case Management Services

Tim Gust, Ph.D.

Chapter Outline

Health Care Objectives

- Identify the variety of case management roles currently in the insurance and health delivery settings
- Identify the common functions of case managers
- Determine meaningful overlap coordination between case managers on behalf of the SCI client
- Identify the benefits for the SCI client of effective case management

NEED FOR CASE MANAGEMENT

As society becomes ever more complex, the various health and rehabilitation services become less understandable even though sometimes more available. Specialists sometimes have defined their roles and functions so narrowly as to preclude the ability to communicate or coordinate with each other.

Concurrently, society emphasizes the desirability and even necessity for consumer involvement and patient choice in health and rehabilitative services. If the complexity of health delivery specialization precludes effective communication between and among the professional disciplines, how can the consumer be expected to make informal choices?

These problems point to the need for a new generalist in the health and rehabilitation field, *the case manager.*

But even more pressure for effective management of patients has come from the insurance industry and the government. The payers of rehabilitation are concerned with the ever-rising costs of care and with obtaining a fair return for their rehabilitation investment. This investment is substantial for the individual SCI patient—just one decubitus, for example, may cost in excess of $60,000.00 to repair!

Case management involves various methods of monitoring, managing, and facilitating health care; processes that have been practiced for many years by physicians, nurses, social workers, physical therapists, and state rehabilitation counselors. The first formal case management demonstration was funded by the U.S. Department of Health, Education, and Welfare in 1971 (Merrill 1985). Merrill defines case management as a process of organizing services and resources to respond to an individual's health care problem.

Case managers have been viewed as patient advocates who can both save employees money and guide them through the bewildering medical care system. Hembree (1985) gives examples of effective case management in which savings of more than $100,000 per case were attained.

More specific to physical medicine and rehabilitation, Dixon (1988; 1989) has described the issues and process of case management with the traumatically brain injured population. A catastrophic injury with long-term sequelae, brain injury rehabilitation with its resultant complex case management needs is similar to the rehabilitation case management process in spinal cord injury (SCI).

Case management exists today in rehabilitation because of cost containment. In fact, the insurance industry often calls case managers "cost-containment consultants," whose objective is to save money. Accelerating health care costs, increasing numbers of survivors, and entitlements of Workers' Compensation are some of the main factors precipitat-ing the need to contain costs by managing them more efficiently and effectively.

Case management ensures that people with SCI progress along a continuum of healing and physical restoration to eventual restoration of self-esteem, dignity, and personal identity as capable people.

Figure 14–1 clarifies the somewhat complex case management situation. Significant overlap exists within the case management process in rehabilitation. The description and discussion that follow use the major headings in Figure 14–1.

THE REHABILITATION PROCESS

Figure 14–1 describes the involvement of people with SCI and their families in the rehabilitation process from pre-injury life-style, through trauma and rehabilitative services, and eventual postinjury life-style. No time line is given in the figure, but experience suggests that 6 months, at the very least, to 3 years or more may be required for people with SCI to develop a satisfactory postinjury life-style. For some individuals the process may stop at the physical restoration, functional performance, or personal identity restoration phases with the individual unable to progress beyond these stages.

HEALTH AND REHABILITATION FACILITIES

Responding to the needs of people with SCI thrust into the process, hospitals and rehabilitation facilities provide an ever-widening range of services. Figure 14–1 lists some of the key medical and vocational personnel who have traditionally provided direct health services plus case management. Many rehabilitation personnel function in case management roles at various stages of the rehabilitation process. The most notable examples of rehabilitation clinical practitioners providing case management are the trauma nurse, the physiatrist, the social worker, and vocational rehabilitation specialist.

The Professional Disciplines

Nurses
Nurses have historically coordinated and managed services for people with SCI. They have a unique role and function during trauma and intensive care as they assist trauma physicians in communicating with significant family mem-

The Rehabilitation Process	Preinjury → Trauma→ Medical → Physical → Functional → Personal Identity→ Postinjury Life-style Stabilization Restoration Performance Restoration Life-style
Health and Rehabilitation Facilities	• Trauma nurse coordinator (see ch. 6) • Trauma/SCI physician specialists • Rehabilitation team case managers Patient & Family • Physiatrist • Vocational rehabilitation specialists (see ch. 33) • Independent rehabilitation specialists Internal Case Managers • Rehabilitation corporate case managers
Insurance Industry Payers	• Reinsurance case managers External Case Managers • Insurance company case managers • Independent case managers
Federal and State Government	• V.A. medical, rehabilitation, and vocational specialists • State rehabilitation counselors Internal Case Managers

FIGURE 14–1 Professionals involved in case management during the rehabilitation process.

bers and in educating other trauma and ICU staff relative to the unique needs and management of SCI.

In contrast to the trauma physician who often cannot take significant time with the family, and the social worker who may not be aware of the unique health and rehabilitative management needs of patients, the nurse can bridge the situation, spending consistent time with family members, explaining SCI in general and unique problems and progress of patients in particular. Especially in critical care settings the RN case managers contribute significantly to the progress of people with SCI by educating families concerning continuing treatment options.

Social Workers

Social workers often facilitate the management of patients by planning the discharge from the hospital. Review of options, insurance benefits, federal and state entitlements, and other financial factors deal with significant concerns of patients and families at the time of SCI trauma.

Effective financial management is required to determine appropriate and available rehabilitation facilities for people with SCI. Admissions reviewers at each rehabilitation facility carefully screen prospective patients for financial acceptability. The social worker facilitates patient management by knowing the financial requirements of the prospective facilities as well as the financial capabilities of each family.

Although the main reasons for social worker involvement are often finances and discharge planning, the social worker also helps patients and families come to terms with SCI. This helps families and patients gain perspective and develop the social relationships they will need to reintegrate the person with SCI into the community.

Physiatrists

Physical medicine and rehabilitation is the medical specialty most notably identified with providing comprehensive medical services to people with SCI. Although other specialists in orthopedics, neurology, and urology are often

THE PHYSIATRIST: THE PROTOTYPICAL PHYSICIAN CASE MANAGER

WHAT IS PHYSICIAN CASE MANAGEMENT?

Physician case management has been an integral part of good patient care for years. Because physicians have the greatest power to prescribe, coordinate, and control expensive health services, it is logical that they balance this authority with accountability for adequate resource use.

THE PHYSICIAN CASE MANAGER CONCEPTUAL FRAMEWORK

Physicians have five basic categories of clinical functions: as

1. Healer
2. Expert
3. Coordinator
4. Rationer
5. Educator

Figure A situates these roles on two axes: a vertical axis that has at one end a patient service orientation and at the opposite end a health care system orientation; and a horizontal axis that has a clinical orientation at one end and a managerial orientation at the other.

THE PHYSIATRIST AS TRADITIONAL CASE MANAGER

In the 50 years that physiatry (physical medicine and rehabilitation) has been in existence as a recognized medical specialty, it has gained distinction by its clinical focus not only on the purely medical, but also on the functional, psychosocial, educational, financial, vocational, recreational, biomedical, and community aspects of care.

Following completion of medical school and internship, the physiatrist undergoes 3 years of residency training during which emphasis is placed on the development of high levels of skill in the direction of a rehabilitation team as well as the ability to negotiate with community, private insurance, and governmental agencies.

By virtue of the expense and complexity of caring for catastrophically injured people with SCI, physiatrists have long been sensitized to cost-benefit analyses and externally originated review. For example, distinguishing between needs and wants with respect to expensive items of adaptive equipment is routinely done by the

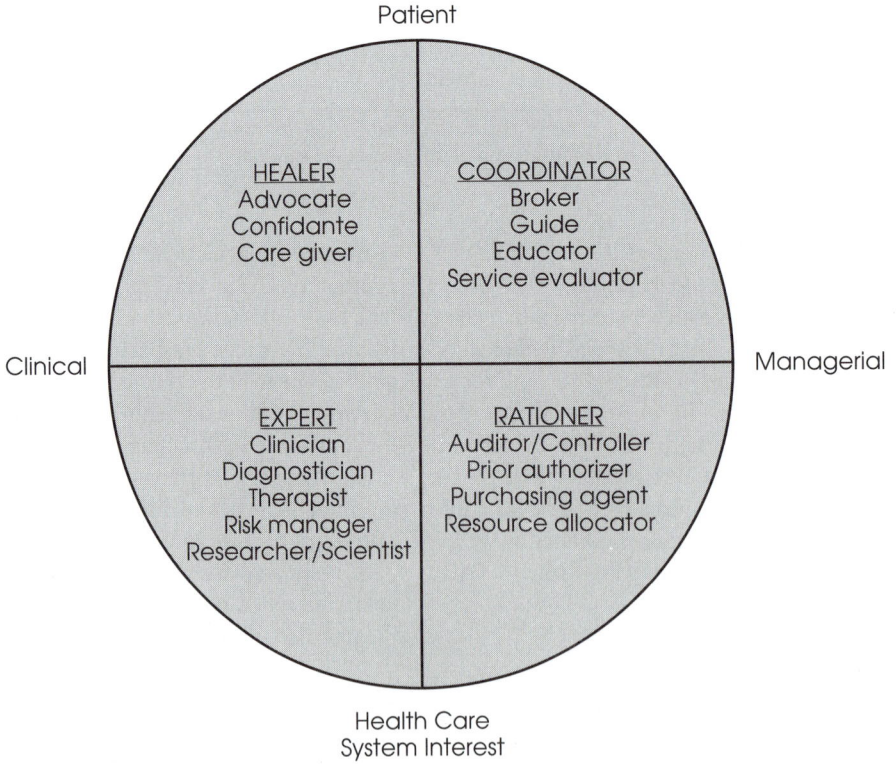

FIGURE A   (Adapted from Hurley 1986.)

(Box continues)

THE PHYSIATRIST: THE PROTOTYPICAL PHYSICIAN CASE MANAGER   (continued)

psychiatrist in order to limit unnecessary expense and to foster optimal adaptation to disability.

More recently, the development of programmatic and model systems approaches to SCI rehabilitation has resulted in an increased emphasis on improved efficiency of care in conjunction with measurement of outcomes and cost effectiveness.

Outcomes need to be considered on an acute, as well as a long-term, basis, and not only in terms of costs, but also in terms of improved health and quality of life. The option that is cheapest now may not be the most cost effective in the long run.

Physiatric assessment, planning, coordination, and monitoring frequently become a lifelong process. Currently, primary care physicians in the community rarely have enough exposure and experience with spinal cord injured individuals to develop the base of knowledge, skill, and attitudes that provide for the highest quality of care for this relatively small population with very specialized needs.

PHYSIATRIC CASE MANAGEMENT OBJECTIVES

The objective of the physiatrist in SCI rehabilitation is to restore physically challenged individuals to the highest possible levels of health, independence, productivity, and self-esteem. The primary roles of the physiatrist include care giver, coordinator, educator, advocate, reviewer, and counselor, from the time of acute injury and continuing potentially on a lifelong basis.

The physiatrist's practice style includes direct treatment and education to minimize complications that increase morbidity and resource consumption, with the expectation that as time goes on patients will become educated, skilled, and empowered to take over many of these skills and ultimately function as their own case managers, using appropriate consultants as needed. This is consistent with the overall rehabilitation goals of helping individuals with SCI become active and informed managers of their own cases rather than passive consumers of medical services.

THE PHYSIATRIC CASE MANAGER'S RESPONSIBILITIES

Roles of physiatrists may vary according to the setting in which they function and the inclinations. See Figure B. A physiatrist may have a predominantly clinical and patient orientation, a primarily managerial or system orientation, or a balance of all.

For example, as a HEALER, the physiatrist serves as:

- Advocate (for the patient's need to receive further therapeutic services in the face of cost containment and rationing systems)
- Agent (certifies for the Department of Motor Vehicles that a patient can drive using appropriate adaptive equipment)
- Confidante (responds to a patient with marital difficulties who confides family problems and requests help in reestablishing intimacy with a spouse)
- Care giver (supports a newly injured teenager who grieves over the inability to walk and run)

As an EXPERT, the physiatrist functions as:

- Clinician (elicits a medical history and examines the patient, then advises a home health agency on an appropriate care plan)
- Diagnostician (evaluates progressive weakness of a person with quadriplegia regarding possibilities, such as syringomyelia or progressive peripheral denervation)
- Therapist (provides treatment for spasticity)
- Risk manager (advises a female patient with paraplegia regarding the additional risks of thromboembolism while using oral contraceptives)
- Researcher/scientist (oversees treatment of a patient with computerized functional electrical stimulation and collects clinical information as part of a cooperative multiinstitutional study)

As a COORDINATOR, the physiatrist serves as:

- Broker (identifies and refers suitable candidates for sponsorship by the state department of vocational rehabilitation and subsequently certifies work capacities for the employer)
- Guide/escort (helps a pregnant quadriplegic woman prepare for her labor and delivery by talking to her obstetrician and anesthesiologist about the recognition and treatment of autonomic dysreflexia)
- Educator (provides information about the crucial role of health maintenance procedures to minimize complications on a lifelong basis)
- Service evaluator (meets on a regular basis with the health care team to review response to treatment and to update the program)

As a RATIONER, the physiatrist functions as:

(Box continues)

THE PHYSIATRIST: THE PROTOTYPICAL PHYSICIAN CASE MANAGER *(continued)*

- Auditor/controller (maintains contact with external review organizations to determine whether treatment is in compliance with policy benefits)
- Prior authorizer (completes on behalf of a review organization the necessary forms authorizing substance abuse treatment for a paraplegic person who has become addicted to Valium)
- Purchasing agent (decides about the type of equipment to be purchased for a home exercise program and recommends a vendor who has a good track record on maintenance)

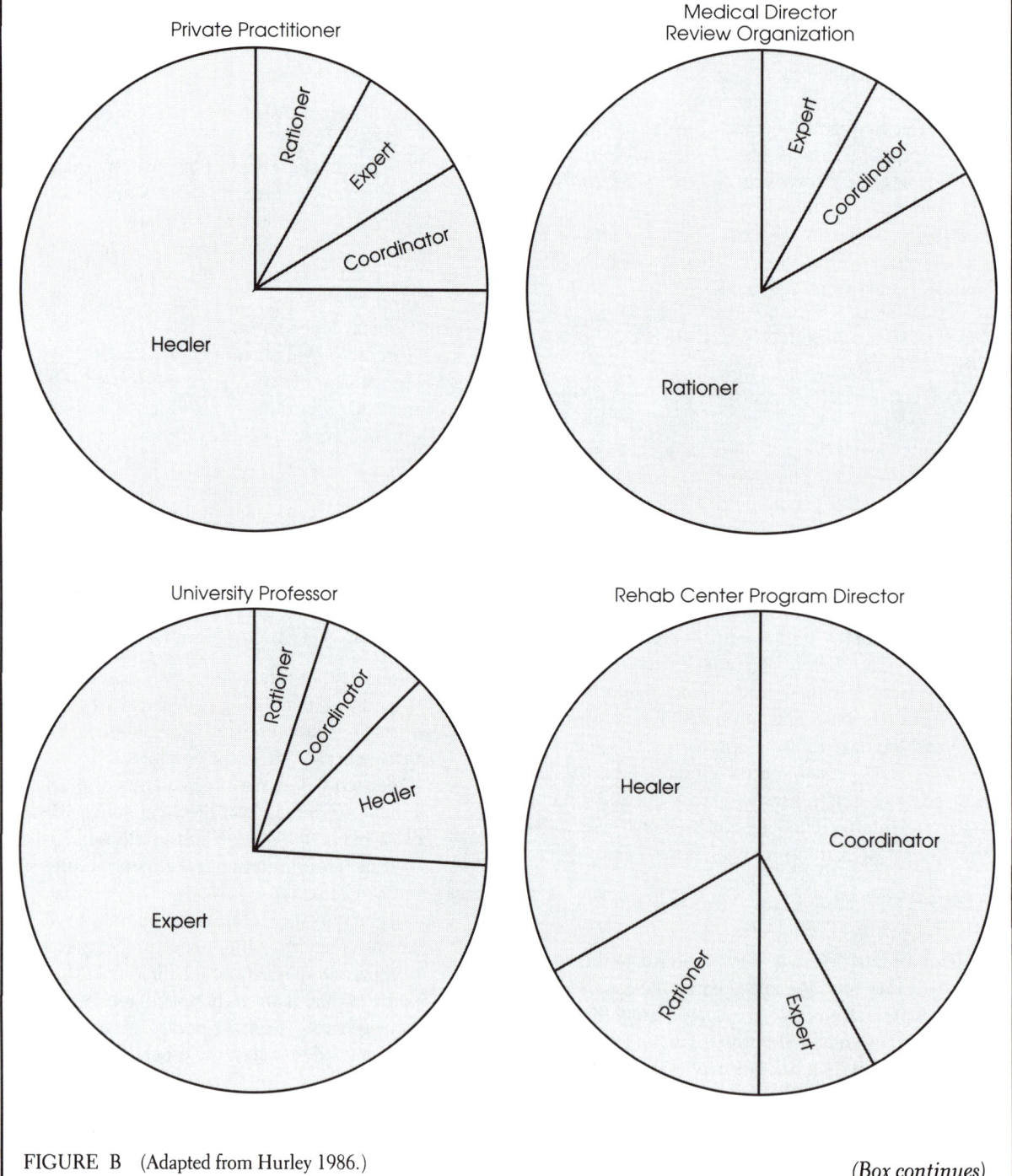

FIGURE B   (Adapted from Hurley 1986.)

(Box continues)

THE PHYSIATRIST: THE PROTOTYPICAL PHYSICIAN CASE MANAGER   (continued)

- Resource allocator (decides for patients with a per diem and total cap on health care benefits which combination of services would be the best use of the available resources)

DETERMINANTS OF THE SUCCESS OF PHYSIATRIC CASE MANAGEMENT

- Case management occurs in the context of the physician-patient encounter in a supportive and informed environment.
- The physiatrist has long-term relationships with medical and other health care providers, and those community, governmental, business, educational, vocational, and transportation resources that have the highest level of expertise in meeting the needs of individuals with SCI. This facilitates acquisition, negotiation, and monitoring of appropriateness of services.
- The physiatrist's care is reviewed by quality assurance and utilization review committees of each hospital's medical staff under the supervision of the hospital board and licensing agencies.
- The physiatrist has not only the authority, but also the ultimate legal accountability, for the design and implementation of treatment and for possible detrimental results of cost-containment mechanisms. This liability is significant when errors in decisions regarding the authorization of health care services may lead to increased disability or death.

ARRANGING FOR ENHANCED EFFECTIVENESS OF THE PHYSIATRIST AS CASE MANAGER

- The physiatrist who subspecializes in SCI rehabilitation could become the primary care physician case manager for these persons on a lifelong basis.
- The physiatrist must be paid a fair fee for case management services based on time consumed, administrative costs, and case complexity.
- The physiatrist's management skills should be cultivated and fostered by feedback, peer review mechanisms, resource consumption data, and budgetary performance data.
- The physiatrist's approach to planning, coordinating, and providing care should include specific mechanisms for input not only by the interdisciplinary health care team, but also by patient and family, insurance and employer representatives, nonphysician care coordinators, and community agencies whose input can assure that the patient receives necessary services in an effective, efficient, logical, ethical, and cost-effective manner.

Julie G. Madorsky, M.D.
Medical Director, Spinal Cord Injury Program
Casa Colina Hospital for Rehabilitative Medicine
Pomona, CA

involved, the physiatrist is the key physician with a holistic, comprehensive view of the patient.

The case management role most often carried out by the physiatrist is that of medical or clinical management of the patient during acute medical rehabilitation. Injury to the spinal column and cord must be carefully managed, as well as respiratory and nutritional problems, contractures, and skin breakdown. Yet the physiatrist must oversee an entire program of personal as well as physical restoration.

Vocational Rehabilitation Specialists

Master's degree in rehabilitation from an accredited university program constitutes the basic qualification of the vocational rehabilitation specialist (VRS). Although special emphasis in training is placed on knowledge of the world of work and the worker, the VRS also is concerned with the entire disability process from medical to community reentry. The VRS may also specialize in the evaluation of the

vocational potential of the patient and the social or psychological aspects of disability for people with SCI and the subsequent quality of their lives.

The VRS must work closely with the physiatrist as well as other rehabilitation team members to coordinate and develop a plan of services that will appropriately enhance the injured individual's long-term vocational potential.

Recently rehabilitation facility team case managers and rehabilitation corporate case managers have become full-time case managers. This internal case management permits better monitoring and management of the service delivery of its own clinicians, improved cost containment, and increased consumer satisfaction with care.

Full-Time Case Managers

As rehabilitation facilities have become more specialized and sophisticated, rehabilitation case managers have become involved as managers of rehabilitation teams. In addition, some rehabilitation organizations have developed a continuum of facilities or corporate structure in order to respond to the evolving needs of the patient from trauma to community reentry. These corporations have established a rehabilitation "corporate case manager."

Both of these case managers are usually recruited from the ranks of clinical rehabilitation specialists, especially vocational specialists, social workers, nurses, and to a lesser extent, speech pathologists and physical and occupational therapists.

Within a rehabilitation facility, case management is increasingly a step up the management career ladder. This is in contrast to the department head or discipline director who usually becomes specialized in the management of only one discipline group such as physical therapy or speech language pathology.

Rehabilitation Team Case Managers

The primary role of the team case manager (TCM) is the effective coordination and leadership of the team of rehabilitation professionals such that services are delivered to people with SCI in the most efficient manner possible. The effective TCM works to obtain consensus among team members and emphasizes the positive functional performance of the person with SCI as the ultimate goal.

Objectives/Goals. The TCM must not only seek the highest level possible of independent functioning for the SCI patient, but also minimize the time and personnel effort devoted to the outcome. A second objective of the TCM is to keep the referral source informed and pleased with both the process and result of the rehabilitation process of each patient. The external case manager (ECM) and the TCM (or internal case manager) work very closely together to identify and enhance individual goals for the person with SCI.

Yet a third and equally important objective is the maintenance of a healthy and productive rehabilitation team with minimal burnout and turnover and maximal creativity in rehabilitation service delivery.

This TCM then functions in relationship to the following constituents: (1) rehabilitation facility management, (2) the person with SCI and family, (3) the rehabilitation team, and (4) the referral source and/or payer.

Functions. The functions of the TCM include, but are not limited to, the following:

1. Participate in the review and decision process of accepting referrals of people with SCI
2. Help team members develop a consensus regarding the outcome goals for patients
3. Lead and direct the rehabilitation team in developing individualized rehabilitation plans
4. Maintain communication with physicians and payer referral sources regarding and during the entire rehabilitation process
5. Maintain communication with clients and families regarding and during the entire rehabilitation process

6. Maintain highest quality and quantity of rehabilitation service delivery while taking into account the financial resources available from the payer for each client

Rehabilitation Corporate Case Managers

Because some rehabilitation hospitals and facilities have diversified ways of providing a continuum of services, a corporate structure has evolved to encompass the various rehabilitation facilities and programs involved. In this corporate system, there may be a corporate case manager (CCM).

The primary role of the CCM is the effective coordination of team case managers (TCM) to provide consistent service delivery across all facilities within the corporation. The CCM also maintains effective relationships with referral sources that enhance overall service delivery and maximize referrals.

Objectives/Goals. The overall goal of the CCM is identical to the TCM's—the highest level possible of independent functioning for the person with SCI. Objectives include: (1) maximizing profit levels of the corporation, (2) balancing the patient's length of stay with the patient's need and resources, (3) recruitment, training, and maintenance of an effective contingent of TCMs, and (4) maintenance of a regular communication link with referral sources to resolve clinical delivery issues not resolved by the TCM.

Functions. The CCM functions include, but are not limited to, the following:

1. Maintain and review information systems relative to referrals and referral sources
2. Maintain and review information systems relative to patient status from admission through service delivery, discharge, and follow-up
3. Communicate regularly with referral sources regarding all aspects of service delivery to patients they have referred
4. Recruit, employ, train, and maintain TCMs such that a consistency of service delivery across all facilities is maintained
5. Communicate regularly with facility and program directors relative to program evaluation, external accreditation agencies, and program function
6. Provide clinical and case management consultation as needed to TCMs in the facilities

THE INSURANCE INDUSTRY: THIRD-PARTY PAYERS

As Workers' Compensation, major medical, and disability insurance have become more available in our society, the insurance industry has sought to reduce liability through various cost-containment measures.

The external case manager (external to the rehabilitation or health service facility) has emerged as a potent force in the area of disability management and eventual cost containment.

Case managers are now found in the reinsurance and insurance industry as well as in large and small case management companies and the independent practitioners who accept referrals from the insurance industry.

Many case managers are registered nurses, but a more substantial number are members of the vocational rehabilitation profession, possessing master's or doctoral degrees.

External Case Managers (ECM)

The external case manager (ECM) provides case management services from outside the rehabilitation service facility. This external position can make possible an unbiased impression of the patient's needs and the treatment provided by the rehabilitation service.

The ECM can provide quality control of the rehabilitation services provided to patients. This occurs as the ECM consults with payers, families, physiatrists, and entire rehabilitation teams. The ECM approaches the rehabilitation of people with SCI from the perspective of the complete picture, from trauma to vocational placement and community reentry.

ECMs may be employees of insurance companies, employees of large or small case management firms, or self-employed rehabilitation practitioners. Most ECMs have a medical rehabilitation background gained through education or experience, with the largest disciplines represented by registered nurses (RNs) and vocational rehabilitation specialists.

Disability case management (Matkin and Wallace 1985) is a term that appropriately encompasses the complete spectrum of medical case management and vocational case management. Registered nurses may manage the cases of people with SCI through the entire rehabilitation process. However, vocational rehabilitation specialists coordinate the vocational phase of the process. As Matkin and Wallace (1985) indicate, it is important that medical and vocational issues be perceived concurrently rather than sequentially in order to provide the best benefits to patients.

Reinsurance Case Managers

As shown in Figure 14–1, specialists in rehabilitation may work for large insurance companies that insure the smaller insurance companies from whom individuals or businesses purchase policies. These reinsurers employ rehabilitation specialists to monitor the claims arising within insurance companies issuing policies to individuals or businesses. When a catastrophic injury is identified by the reinsurer, a reinsurance case manager will monitor the case, sometimes by suggesting that a case management firm be consulted on a continuing basis, and in other instances by working directly with the claim representative. Having a knowledge of rehabilitation facilities nationwide is helpful to reinsurance specialists who provide case management consultation from a broad national perspective.

The goal, as with all insurance case management, is the containment of costs in the short term and the reduction of liability in the long term, along with identifying the most appropriate rehabilitation services for the claimant.

Insurance Company Case Managers

Some major insurance companies employ their own case managers (primarily rehabilitation nurses) who work closely with claim representatives to meet the goals of reducing liability for the insurance company while identifying and monitoring the most cost-effective rehabilitation services for the claimant.

These case managers perform services similar to their counterparts who work for large case management firms or who work independently. The main difference is their source of referrals and the entire marketing and referral process. As an employee of the insurance company, the rehabilitation case manager has a single identified source of referrals, the claim representatives. Marketing is primarily a process of providing education to claim representatives and others within the insurance company to assure that referrals are made in an appropriate and timely manner. The case manager identifies and coordinates the services required for people with SCI from initial point of contact through community reentry.

Independent Case Managers

Independent case managers (ICM) are not direct employees of the insurance industry. They include members of large and small case management firms and independent practitioners. Also, some insurance companies have developed wholly owned companies to provide case management services. Although employees of the subsidiaries can be considered in this category, there may be a more direct relationship between the insurance companies and the subsidiary case management firms than if the firms were completely independent.

The roles and functions of independent case managers are the same as those of direct employees of the insurance industry, except for the increased effort required to develop and maintain a case management firm.

The "dual bottom line," a balanced emphasis on both financial management and clinical management considerations of the rehabilitation business, must be given ade-

THE ROLE OF REGISTERED NURSE IN SCI INSURANCE CASE MANAGEMENT

WHAT IS NURSE CASE MANAGEMENT?

In 1988, an American Nursing Association (ANA) Task Force published the first standards for case management for inclusion in the Association of Rehabilitation Nurses (ARN) Performance Criteria for Medical Case Management.

ANA/ARN defines case management as "a process in which proactive, individualized, and cost-effective health care services are identified, coordinated, implemented, and evaluated on an ongoing basis for individuals who have sustained an injury/illness."

The ANA/ARN categorizes case managers based on place of employment:

- Internal Case Manager (ICM)
  - Insurance based (ICM-IB)
  - Facility based (ICM-FB)
- External Case Manager (ECM)

However, the same goals, professional accountability of individual practitioners, qualifications, and quality assurance standards apply regardless of the place of employment. ICM-IB confront unique challenges and opportunities in maintaining these high professional standards because of their unique employment setting. Like their colleagues in facilities and in external, independent case management firms, they are accountable both to professional and business standards. Yet, lack of peer contact and support presents unique challenges in adhering to professional standards. Nevertheless, the duty of their employers to manage high-cost cases over long periods of time provides a unique opportunity to redefine case management continuity of care.

The typical injured/ill person cared for by an ICM-IB lives in a rural area with a primary treating physician who is not a SCI specialist. The ICM-IB often collaborates with the hospital and physician to transfer the person to a SCI expert for first-year inpatient treatment. Subsequently, out-of-town discharge planning and home care is then coordinated through an ICM network. The ICM conducts postdischarge home visits, identifies unforeseen problems, and arranges for re-evaluation based on individual needs. If the employing insurer's benefits provide for lifetime care or have unlimited ceilings, the ICM-IB can follow a particular person for life.

Whether insurance benefits are for life, the insurer's incentive is to manage lifetime care costs because for many, the major lifetime cost is attendant care. The ICM-IB coordinates hometown resources for outpatient treatment with the expert resources of the rehabilitation facility to address the inpatient and lifetime outpatient continuum of care.

The ICM-IB can assess individual progress and regression over time and analyze the normal aging process for each individual. Long-term continuity of care is a factor that few other types of case managers have.

The ICM-IB communicates with as many as 20 disciplines, initiating ideas, carrying messages from one to the other, and obtaining clarification. Both verbal and written communication are coordinated, not only among the health care team, but also between the health care team and the financial decision-making member of the team, the claim representative. Two factors differentiate the communication of the ICM-IB: preestablished co-worker trust with the claim representative, whose timely financial decision making is essential to outcomes, and health care synthesis of both the hometown and out-of-town treatment teams' recommendations into a cohesive plan of action.

Other nurse case managers must earn claim representative trust and may or may not be able to research hometown care alternatives.

COORDINATION OF APPROPRIATE HEALTH CARE ALTERNATIVES

Like their counterparts, ICM-IB must identify the appropriate health care alternative before coordinating the services through personal experience and through a network of colleagues who conduct on-site visits. However, the position of the ICM-IB also involves coordination long after discharge from the rehabilitation facility. All case managers coordinate the timing of hometown services with dates of discharge, but the ICM-IB also implements additional service needs long after initial home care has been established

Timing is essential: services must not be provided too early, before they are needed, or too late, after problems have been exacerbated and coping skills have been altered.

Coordination of appropriate health care alternatives at the correct time for the individual's specific needs over a time continuum is the essence of both quality of life and cost management.

Stephanie Johnson, R.N., C.I.R.S., Manager
Rehabilitation and Disability Management
The Aetna Casualty & Surety Company
Hartford, CT

quate consideration. The independent consultant or the employee of the independent case management firm must attend equally to these two aspects of the bottom line or the business will eventually suffer.

FEDERAL AND STATE GOVERNMENTS

Other sources have detailed the case management function of federal and state government health and rehabilitation agencies. See especially Casell and Mulkey 1985. Comcare, in the Australian system, is presented as an innovative international model of preventive case management in Chapter 1.

The most representative example of rehabilitation case management within the government are those individuals in the Department of Veterans Affairs (VA) and rehabilitation counselors in the divisions of vocational rehabilitation within each state and territory of the United States.

Department of Veterans Affairs (VA)

VA services are typically available for veterans and eligible family members. Medical, rehabilitative, and vocational services along an entire spectrum are usually coordinated by VA counselors whose function is similar to internal case managers within nongovernmental rehabilitation facilities.

The VA's network of inpatient hospitals and outpatient facilities provides comprehensive medical and vocational rehabilitation services to veterans who are victims of SCI. Also, because these facilities have a teaching function, there is a rotation of physicians and other rehabilitation specialists through the Physical Medicine and Rehabilitation Unit.

In the outpatient setting, VA counseling psychologists often provide the case management function for veterans. In concert with vocational rehabilitation specialists, they work toward community reintegration and vocational placement of veterans with SCI.

State Vocational Rehabilitation

Authorized in 1920 to provide rehabilitation services to disabled nonveterans, this federal-state partnership has as its goal the identification, retraining, and vocational placement of individuals disabled by SCI and many other physical and mental impairments.

State rehabilitation agencies provide comprehensive rehabilitation services to individuals traumatized by accident or disease who show potential for recovery and eventual return to the community. Through careful coordination of benefits, state rehabilitation counselors seek to use all other insurance or other entitlements before authorizing state monies for payment of rehabilitation services to people with SCI. *Division of Vocational Rehabilitation* is the most typical name for this state agency. In some states it is called Bureau of Vocational Rehabilitation (BVR) or Office of Vocational Rehabilitation (OVR).

The first case management of impaired and disabled people began with this cadre of men and women in the states and territories of the United States. Their cumulative knowledge and experience, supplemented by university educational and training programs, formed the basis of the present professional organization to which case managers now belong.

GENERAL GOALS AND OBJECTIVES AND THE PROCESS OF CASE MANAGEMENT

The goal of all types of rehabilitation case management for people with SCI is their satisfactory rehabilitation. However, the definition of "satisfactory rehabilitation" depends on who is paying the cost of the rehabilitative services.

An individual injured on the job and eligible for Workers' Compensation benefits may be perceived as "satisfactorily rehabilitated" only if or when returned to work.

In contrast, an individual injured in a family outing who is covered by group health insurance may only receive trauma and acute medical care for medical stabilization and may have no rehabilitation benefits. For rehabilitation services, these people may have to resort to some combination of governmental funding such as MediCare or Medicaid.

For a complete overview of the process of case management, refer to the excellent resources presented by Cassell and Mulkey (1985), and Roessler and Rubin (1982), which deal with case management and insurance rehabilitation in depth.

A brief outline of the case management process within the scope of disability case management as described by Matkin and Wallace (1985) suggests that (1) medical care costs and resultant disability costs, (2) selection of the client for rehabilitation, (3) initial evaluation and assessment of the case, and (4) planning and developing rehabilitation goals must be taken into account.

In contrast, Cassell and Mulkey (1985) address the business aspects of health and rehabilitation as they describe three models or strategies of case management: the process model, the marketing model, and the accounting model. They also describe in detail effective management control, decision making, time management, and specifics of caseload management such as case recording and documentation. These functions must be carried out in a manner acceptable to several different groups.

Variations in process are common, but experience suggests the following basics:

1. Identification and acceptance of referrals
2. Initial interview and evaluation of patient, family, and significant others
3. Assessment of medical problems and prognosis for level of disablement
4. Prediction of functional outcomes of rehabilitation and community reentry status regarding home and work
5. Monitoring of the physical restoration phase and development of clear vocational goals
6. Monitoring of the vocational development phase and development of community-living goals
7. Monitoring of the community reentry process and estimation of needs and costs of lifetime follow-up, including physical and emotional needs and any other case management

Some of the functions include but are not limited to:

1. Case finding, marketing, and education of referral sources
2. Information gathering, including initial interviews with patients, families, significant others, and obtaining all available medical records
3. Organizing, coordinating, and developing initial plans based on available data
4. Negotiating with key people including family members, medical service providers, and payers concerning the rehabilitation plan
5. Identifying rehabilitation service providers and facilities relevant to the needs of the specific person with SCI being referred
6. Referral coordination and plan development with the rehabilitation provider or facility chosen by the patient and family
7. Coordination and monitoring of the rehabilitation plan and patient progress with the internal case manager and rehabilitation team
8. Continuing relationship with the referral source and/or payer to assure adequate cost containment
9. Projection of disability level and overall functional capacity of the person with SCI at the completion of active rehabilitation in order to help the payer identify lifetime liability and necessary services
10. Identification of resources within the community to provide needed rehabilitative services for people with SCI at various levels of restoration

STRESS, PRESSURE, AND THE CASE MANAGER

All occupations exert pressure on individual workers. The job of case manager, however, has special stressors that

should be understood by individuals. The most outstanding pressure is the requirement to satisfy so many constituents or customers, who include the person with SCI; the family and significant others; the referral source; the payer; the medical staffs of the trauma center, specialized medical center, and rehabilitation facility; and the staff of the relevant vocational rehabilitation facilities.

Another important consideration is that the person with SCI, for whom all these services are being managed, did not choose to be a consumer and is often not compliant or easily satisfied. Distraught family members likewise do not readily respond to a case manager who is initially an outsider to the medical trauma team.

Finally, the rehabilitation case manager, as a member of one of the rehabilitation/health disciplines, maintains a responsibility to the ethics of the profession. The responsibility to balance cost containment with the needs of the person with SCI, the pressure exerted by the family, and the marketing of rehabilitation services are a few aspects of the ethical pressure felt by the case manager.

Kreider (1987) suggests some of the qualifications and skills important for the successful case manager: a background in Workers' Compensation and insurance, good communication skills, and assertiveness in dealing with claim representatives on the one hand, and the rehabilitation team on the other. Case managers must be mature professionally as well as personally in order to be competent advocates for people with SCI while containing costs for the payer. See also Chapter 8 for legal implications during the early postinjury period. Professional organizations for case managers are listed in the resources at the end of this book.

FUTURE PERSPECTIVES

The present status of disability or rehabilitation case management is so dynamic as to make its description as a field or profession extremely difficult. The National Association of Rehabilitation Professionals in the Private Sector (NARPPS) to which a significant number of case managers belong, has a current membership of approximately 3550 across the nation. Mr. Richard La Fon, executive director of NARPPS, estimates that there may be from 16,000 to 20,000 individuals providing disability case management in the United States today (La Fon 1989).

Approximately 5% of case managers are employees of insurance companies, 20% are employed by large case management firms, and 25% by small case management firms; the remaining 50% operate as independent practitioners either as sole proprietors or in small partnerships. La Fon (1989) estimates that approximately 65% of the NARPPS membership has a vocational rehabilitation background and 35% has a nursing background. The latter membership category is growing faster than the former.

In addition to developing sections for medical, vocational, forensics, and other specialists, NARPPS is currently developing medical case management standards for eventual national application. NARPPS has also recommended to the Commission on Certification of Insurance Rehabilitation Specialists (CIRS) that their name be changed to Certified Case Manager. Finally, NARPPS is suggesting its own name be changed to the International Case Management Association (La Fon 1989).

The Head Injury–Special Interest Group of the American Congress of Rehabilitation Medicine is also continuing its work to develop standards of practice for rehabilitation case managers in the specialty area of traumatic brain injury, which have implications for SCI.

Kreider (1987) projects that over the next 10 years, case management will become a specialized field and be crucial to the survival and growth of rehabilitation programs.

This field of specialization will continue to evolve into a fully developed profession. Furthermore, there will likely be conflicts among the factions representing the public versus private sectors, employees of insurance companies versus independent companies and practitioners, and those people who maintain a specialty in medical case management versus those maintaining a specialty in vocational case management.

All practitioners of disability case management, regardless of professional discipline or employment setting, must have a professional degree as well as firsthand clinical experience with the disabled clients they represent. In addition, courses and/or seminars in understanding the payer sources of health care and rehabilitation are essential. It is hoped that graduate curriculums and continuing education programs will meet the needs of this emerging profession.

REFERENCES

Cassell, J., and Mulkey, S. 1985. *Rehabilitation Caseload Management: Concepts and Practice.* Austin, TX: Pro-Ed.

Dixon, T. P. 1989. Systems of care for the head injured. In *Physical Medicine and Rehabilitation* (State of the Art Reviews 3 [1]). L. J. Horn and D. N. Cope. Eds.

Dixon, T. P., Goll, S., and Stanton, K. S. 1988. Case management issues and practices in head injury rehabilitation. *Rehabilitation Counseling Bulletin,* 31: 324–344.

Hembree, W. E. 1985. Getting involved: Employees as case managers. *Business and Health* (July/August): 11–14.

Hurley, R. E. 1986. Toward a behavioral model of the physician as case manager. *Social Science Medicine* 23: 75–82.

Kreider, J. 1987. Editorial: The new case manager. (National Association of Rehabilitation Facilities) *Rehabilitation Insurance Report* 3 (5).

La Fon, R. 1989. Personal Communication with the Executive Director of the National Association of Rehabilitation Professionals in the Private Sector (NARPPS).

Matkin, R., and Wallace, C. 1985. *Insurance Rehabilitation.* Austin, TX: Pro-Ed. Inc.

Merrill, J. C. 1985. Defining case management. *Business and Health* (July/August): 5–9.

Roessler, R., and Rubin, S. 1985. *Case Management and Rehabilitation Counseling.* Baltimore, MD: University Park Press.

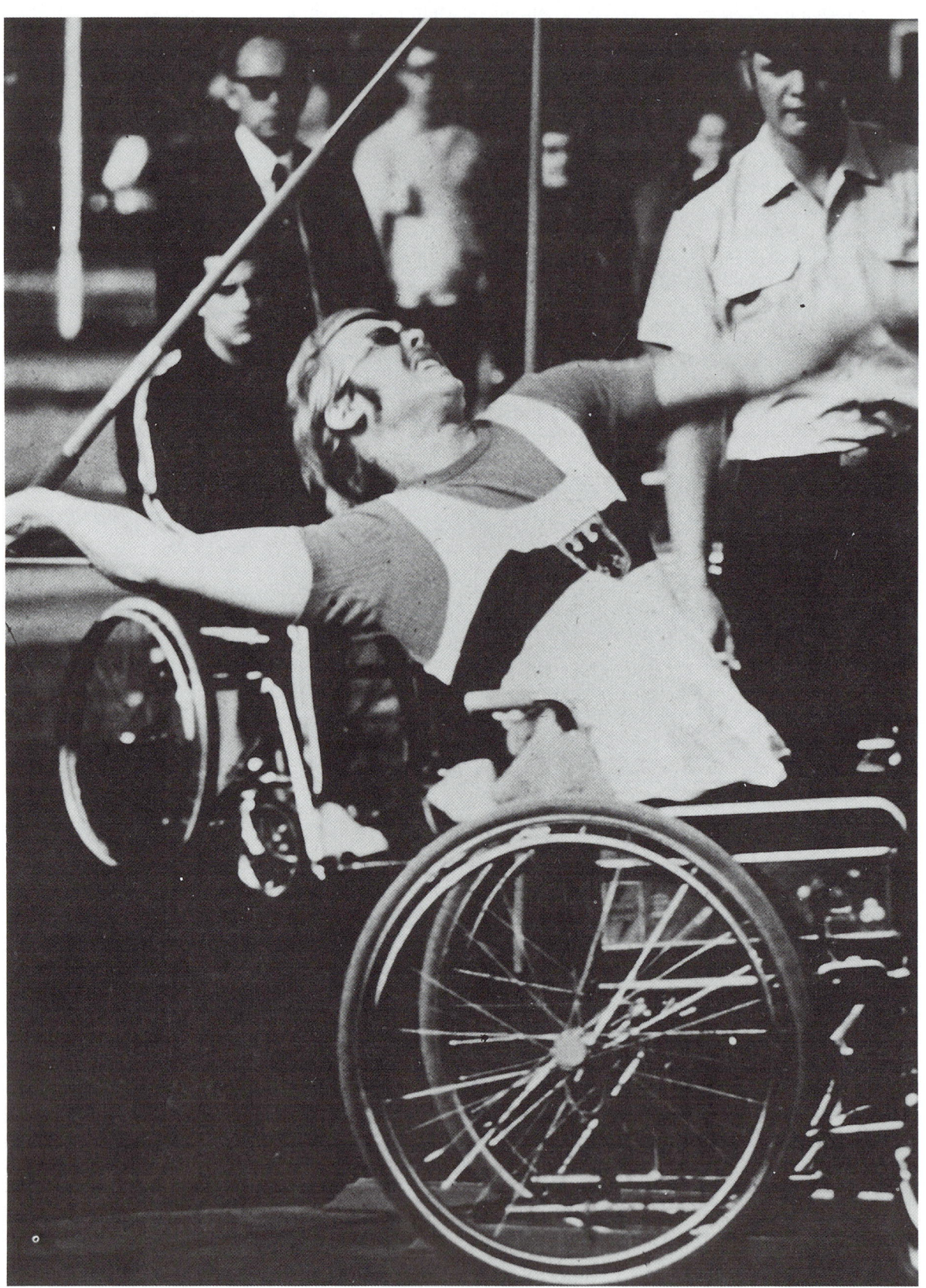

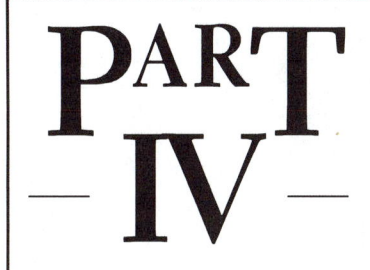

PART IV

MAINTAINING OPTIMAL PHYSIOLOGICAL FUNCTIONS

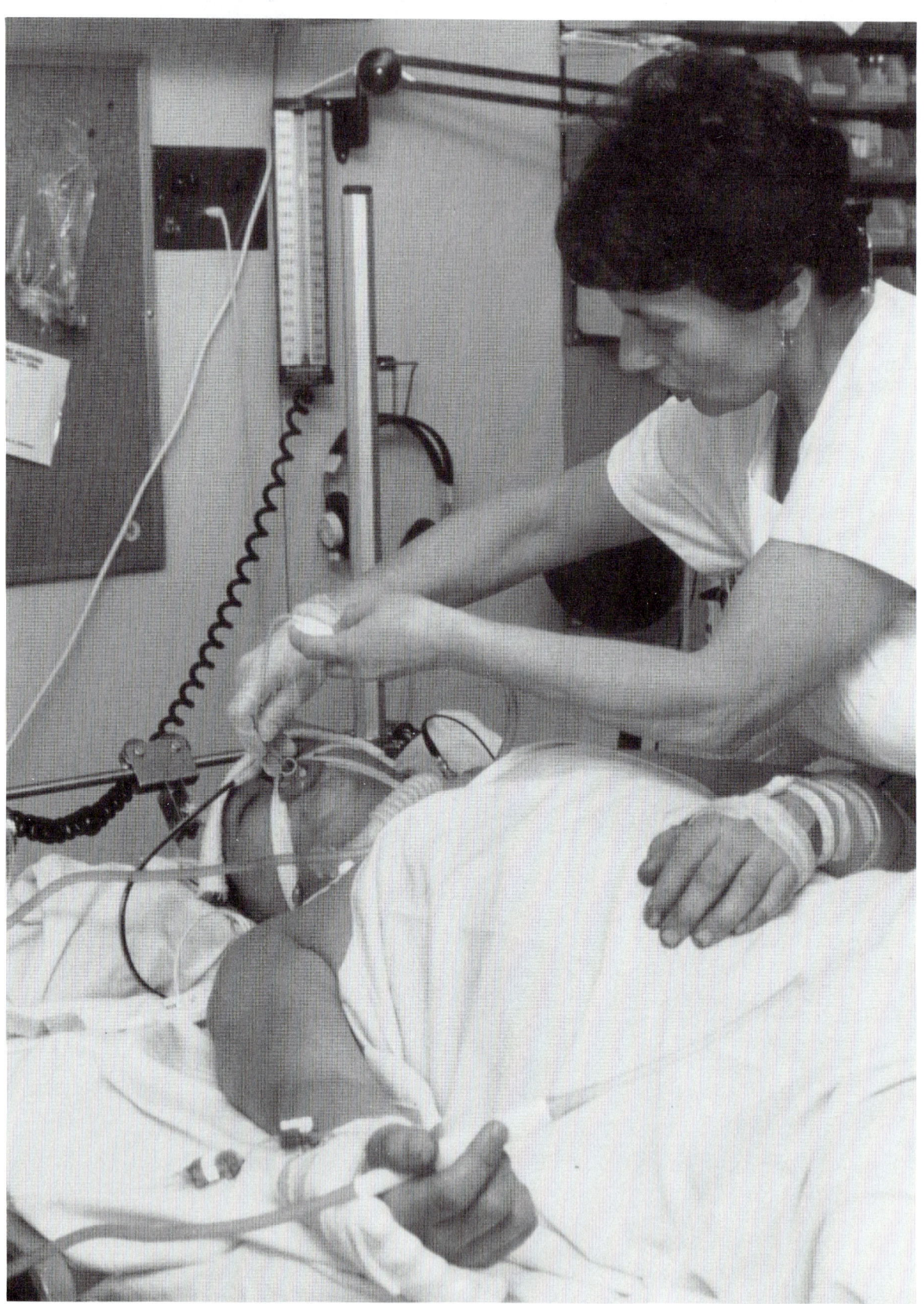

CHAPTER
— 15 —

Promoting Optimal Respiratory Function[*]

Chapter Outline

[*] This chapter was developed with the assistance of William Donovan, M.D., and Fina Canave Jimenez, R.N., M. Ed.

Chapter Outline

Health Care Objectives

- To explain how respiration is impaired by SCI, correlating anticipated dysfunctions with the level of cord injury sustained
- To describe assessment techniques and diagnostic procedures and measures that promote ventilation, pulmonary gas exchange, and gas transport
- To describe respiratory support systems and options, indications for use, and related care
- To enhance patient comfort, confidence, knowledge, and sense of being in control
- To educate individuals and families regarding lifelong pulmonary health care, including ventilator dependency

Respiratory insufficiency is a most serious threat to many patients with spinal cord injury (SCI). Those with quadriplegia and high paraplegia must be considered to have some degree of respiratory compromise that may lead to life-threatening complications. The degree of insufficiency depends on many factors, including the extent of neurological impairment to the respiratory muscles, associated trauma and general response to trauma, and the patient's preexisting condition and age.

Care of patients with SCI demands a well-defined and coordinated team approach guided by a pulmonary medical specialist to ensure successful outcomes (Whiteneck et al. 1989: 7–112). Because pulmonary compromise is a leading cause of death, interdisciplinary care requires a *consistent* approach to routine assessment, prophylactic treatment, expert evaluation, and education of new staff members as well as patients and families (Clough, Lindenhaur, Hayes, and Zekary 1986).

Roles and responsibilities of physicians, nurses, and physical and respiratory therapists must be clearly outlined and organized. Detailed communication is essential among team members because of overlapping responsibilities, especially when complex, round-the-clock care must be provided. Inadequate or untimely interventions result in serious complications, extended stays in critical care areas, and delayed rehabilitation—costly in both human and economic terms.

THE RESPIRATORY SYSTEM

Respiration is a three-part process involving ventilation, pulmonary gas exchange, and transport of gases. Respiration occurs when the respiratory muscles—the diaphragm, intercostal muscles, and to a lesser extent the accessory and abdominal muscles—move air to and from the lungs, permitting *alveolar-capillary diffusion*, the exchange of oxygen and carbon dioxide gases between the alveoli of the lung tissue and pulmonary capillaries.

Oxygen and carbon dioxide are transported in the blood to and from body cells, enabling *cellular respiration*, the metabolic process of oxygen use and carbon dioxide excretion. Transport of these gases depends on adequate cardiac output, red blood cell count, and hemoglobin. Most of the oxygen is carried in the hemoglobin of the red blood cells. Most of the CO_2 is carried in the return circulation as biocarbonate (HCO_3) inside the red blood cells. CO_2 is a key factor in the acid-base balance of the body.

Ventilation, the basic act of breathing, requires an adequate partial pressure of oxygen (PaO_2), an intact respiratory drive or means of delivering the gas mixture to the alveoli, clear airway passages, and normal compliance (elasticity) of the lungs. Breathing also depends on stable musculature and skeletal structures of the thorax and abdomen.

The lungs are suspended in the flexible thoracic cage, which is bound by the sternum in front, the spinal column in back, the rib cage encircling, and the diaphragm below. See Figure 15–1. Each lung has a covering of visceral pleura, which is closely related to the parietal pleura lining the thoracic cavity. The lung has no muscle tissue itself and does not actively contract but responds directly to the muscular expansion and contraction of the thorax. *Inspiration* requires effort because it expands the thorax in three directions (anteroposterior, lateral, and vertical). This expansion creates a negative (subatmospheric) pressure in the lung, pulling air into the alveoli. Normal *expiration*, a much more passive phase, occurs because the chest muscles relax and the thorax and the lungs recoil, returning the thoracic cage to its resting position.

The Respiratory Muscles

The *diaphragm* is a strong sheet of muscle separating the thoracic and abdominal cavities. See Figure 15–2. It is convex above and concave below. The diaphragm is attached to the lower border of the rib cage and inserts into a common central tendon. As the muscle fibers contract, the diaphragm flattens, lowering the upper dome shape to pull downward and enlarge the thoracic cage. It also pushes abdominal viscera downward. Diaphragmatic action is the dominant force involved in normal, quiet breathing. Normally the diaphragm accomplishes 40% of inspiration while the external intercostal and accessory muscles are responsible for the remaining 60% (Wetzel 1985).

The *intercostal muscles* are a large number of small muscles located between each pair of ribs (Figure 15–3). Contraction of the *external intercostal muscles* elevates the rib cage, leading to expansion of the chest wall. These muscles may be responsible for 30% to 35% of effective ventilation (Cheshire and Flack 1978–1979).

The *accessory muscles* of breathing are the *sternocleido-mastoid* and *scalene muscles* located in the neck and upper chest. The accessory muscles help elevate the upper rib cage during inspiration (Figure 15–4).

The major muscles of expiration are the *abdominal muscles* (Figure 15–5), aided by the *internal intercostal muscles*. The muscles of the anterior abdominal wall decrease the size of the thoracic cage by pulling downward and inward

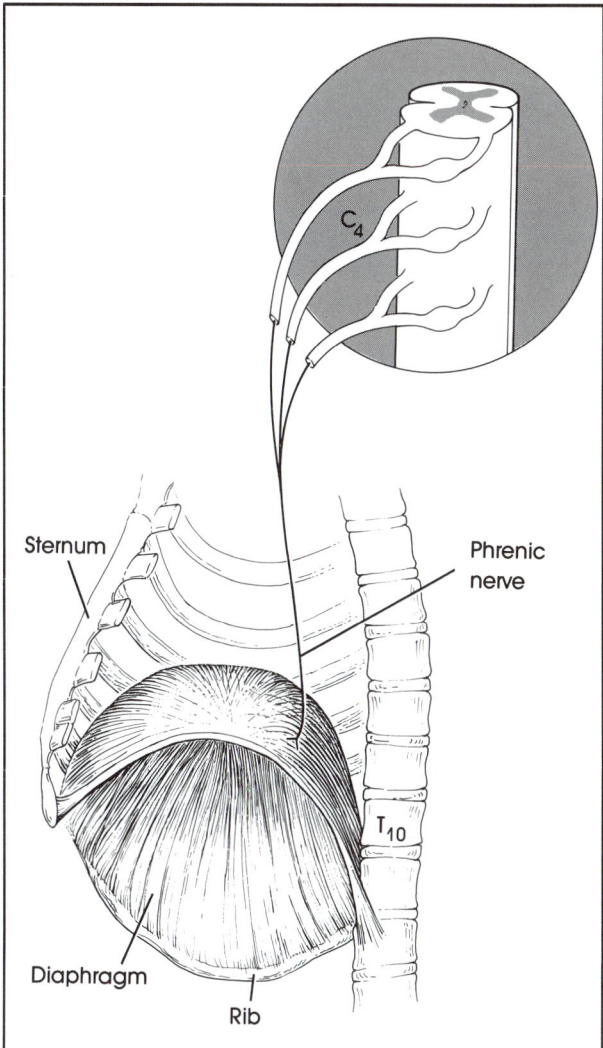

FIGURE 15–2   The diaphragm, the most powerful muscle for breathing, receives innervation from the C_4 cord segment with lesser contributions from C_3 and C_5 cord segments.

on the rib cage and forcing the abdominal viscera upward against the diaphragm. These muscles provide resistance to a working diaphragm and thus help return the thoracic cage to its resting position.

Neurological Control of Breathing

Neurological control of breathing requires adequate neural drive from the respiratory center in the medulla and intact neural pathways. It involves complex interactions between the central and peripheral nervous systems and the respiratory muscles. The central nervous system provides both *voluntary control (cortical)* and *involuntary control (autonomic)* to regulate respiration. An example of voluntary control is the breath control used in singing. Autonomic control regulates breathing during sleep. Normal respiration

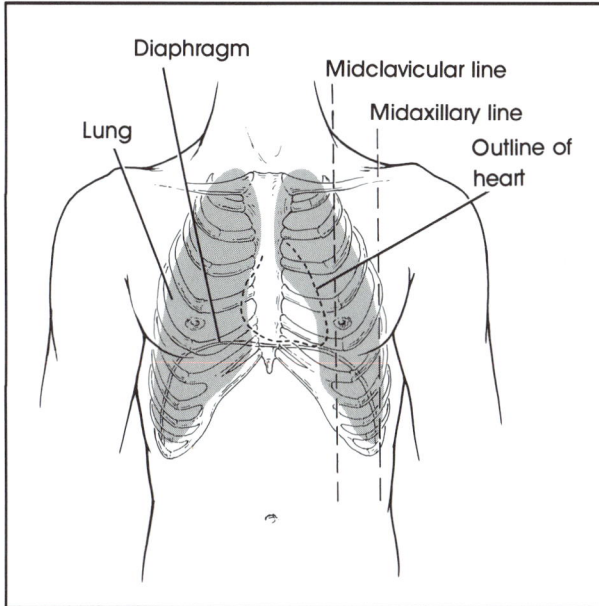

FIGURE 15–1   External chest landmarks in relation to underlying respiratory structures.

in the adult occurs at a regular, rhythmic rate of 14 to 20 breaths per minute, inspiration being shorter than expiration.

The diaphragm is innervated by the phrenic nerve arising primarily from the fourth cervical cord segment but receiving small contributions from the third and fifth cord segments. The intercostal muscles are innervated by the intercostal nerves from T_{1-12}. The sternocleidomastoid muscle is innervated by the cranial nerve XI and the scalene muscles by the cervical cord (C_{2-7}). The abdominal muscles are innervated by the lower thoracic cord (T_{6-12}).

Intimately tied to the neural drive regulating respiration are feedback mechanisms made possible by chemoreceptors, mainly sensitive to CO_2 levels in the blood. For various reasons, SCI adversely affects cardiac output, altering gaseous exchange and thus affecting respiratory function. See Chapter 16 for a detailed discussion.

CONSEQUENCES OF SPINAL CORD INJURY

Impaired Pulmonary Function

Depending on the level of cord injury, paralyzed patients may have difficulty preserving neural drive to the breathing muscles and maintaining a clear airway on their own. Varying degrees of failure of the muscles of respiration to ventilate may result from SCI.

Impairment of ventilation is reflected by a high arterial partial pressure of carbon dixoide ($PaCO_2$), that is, difficulty exhaling the end products of respiration, resulting in retention of CO_2. Impairment of gas exchange is reflected by low arterial PaO_2.

Spinal cord injury at or above C_4 causes diaphragmatic paralysis and loss of spontaneous respiration (*complete apnea*), requiring permanent ventilator support. Injuries near this level may result in weakened diaphragmatic movement. One side may function and not the other. Lesions occurring below the cervical plexus (C_{1-4}) may allow partial or full diaphragmatic function, but respiratory function will be subnormal due to involvement of the remaining muscles of breathing.

When diaphragmatic control is preserved but autonomic function is impaired from damage to the reticulospinal system (C_{1-3}), patients with quadriplegia are predisposed to *sleep-induced apnea (Ondine's curse* or *central alveolar hypotension)* during the first 3 to 5 months postinjury (Zeluff et al. 1977). (In ancient folklore, Ondine placed a curse on her unfaithful husband such that he would stop breathing when he next fell asleep.) The patient may be able to breathe normally when awake but "forgets" to breathe during sleep. Lethargy and headaches may occur in the morning. If severe, hypoxemia can build to fatal levels.

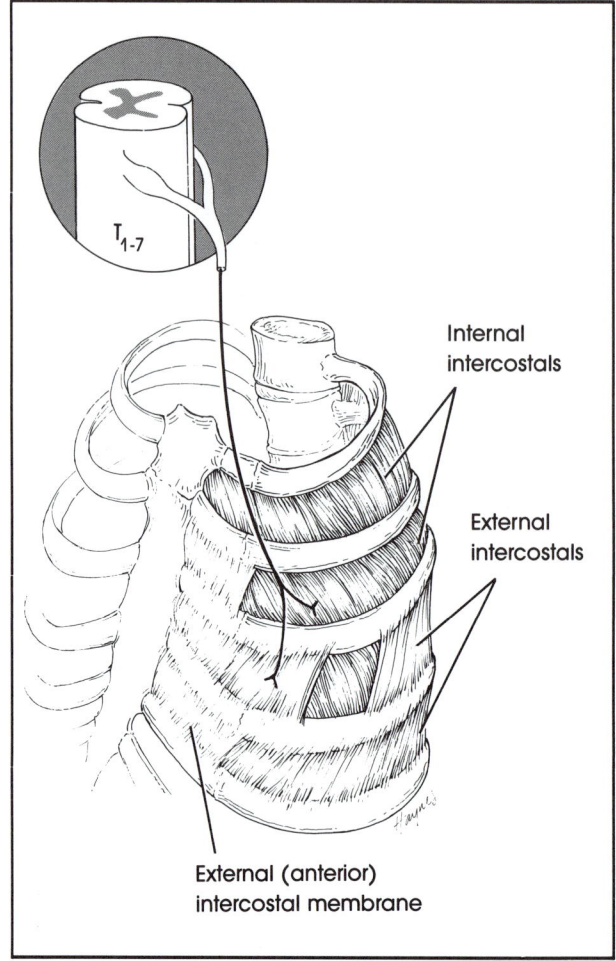

FIGURE 15–3 The intercostal muscles aid in chest expansion and are innervated by the T_{1-7} cord segments.

Following high thoracic or cervical cord injury, lack of chest and abdominal movement and difficulty raising secretions increase risk of atelectasis, decrease exchange, and permit alveolar collapse. This contributes to chronic alveolar hypoventilation resulting in hypoxemia, in which retained secretions (as with atelectasis) obstruct alveoli with mucus and prevent ventilation.

Injury to the lower thoracic cord at or above T_{6-12} causes impairment of the intercostal and abdominal muscles, which limits the ability to cough and exhale forcefully. Table 15–1 summarizes anticipated respiratory dysfunction following SCI.

Other Factors Associated with Respiratory Compromise

Associated trauma includes *chest trauma*, most commonly fractured ribs occurring with thoracic spine fractures; *trau-*

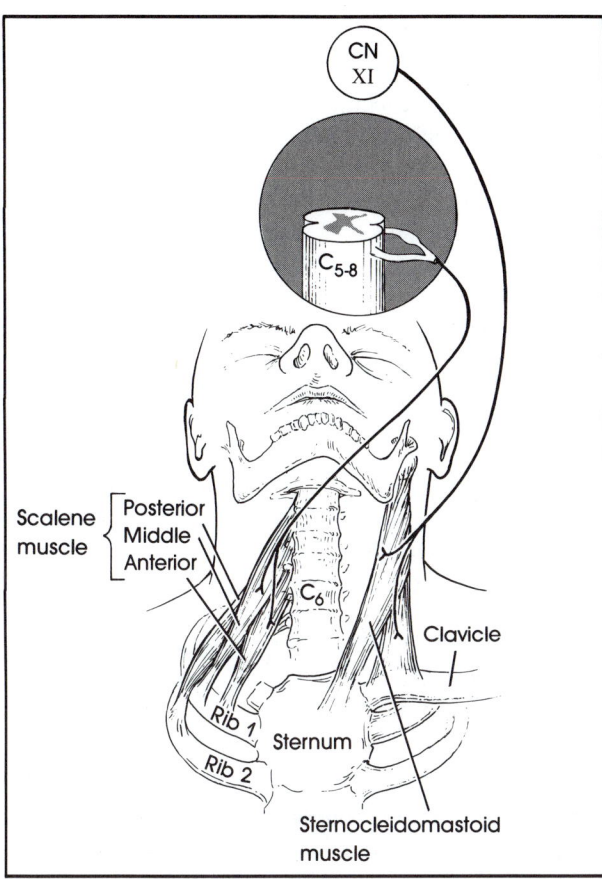

FIGURE 15–4 The accessory muscles are most often preserved following a cord injury, and therefore they become overworked. They elevate the upper rib cage during inspiration and are innervated by the cranial nerve XI (spinal accessory) and C_{2-7} cord segments.

matic brain injury, with accompanying depressed neural drive; *neurogenic (spinal) and hypovolemic shock* that diminishes the oxygen-carrying capacity of the circulating blood; and *aspiration*, suspected with unconscious patients and water-related accidents, that causes a severe inflammatory reaction. Any associated trauma compounds risks of respiratory insufficiency.

Preexisting pulmonary and related risk factors include preexisting pulmonary disease or infections, thoracic surgery, smoking history, cough or sputum, dyspnea, shortness of breath on exertion, low activity tolerance, obesity, allergies, asthma, and anemia. During the prehospital and transport period, systemic fluid overload with resultant fluid overload of the lungs is not uncommon.

Age is an important factor. Older patients often have problems that resemble those of heavy smokers and people with chronic obstructive pulmonary disease. Reduced compliance with some chest wall rigidity and less lung elasticity occurs. Cleansing mechanisms of the respiratory tract are also less efficient (Spence and Mason 1979).

ASSESSMENT OF RESPIRATORY FUNCTION

All care givers need to know how to perform an adequate assessment of respiratory function because difficulties can develop rapidly at any time—soon after injury, during rehabilitation, and for persons with quadriplegia, throughout life. Only by comparing assessment parameters on a continuing basis can deterioration or improvement of function be detected. Be familiar with the patient's history and physical assessment as noted on the medical record and from communication with other team members. Knowledge of the patient's general response to the management plan and the specific response during the preceding 24-hour period is necessary.

The initial assessment establishes baseline data for future comparison, identifies which respiratory muscles are dysfunctional, and provides information about actual compromises and potential problems that may occur.

Physical Assessment

Observation of the Airway

Check for airway obstruction, commonly associated with injuries to the cervical spine and loss of consciousness.

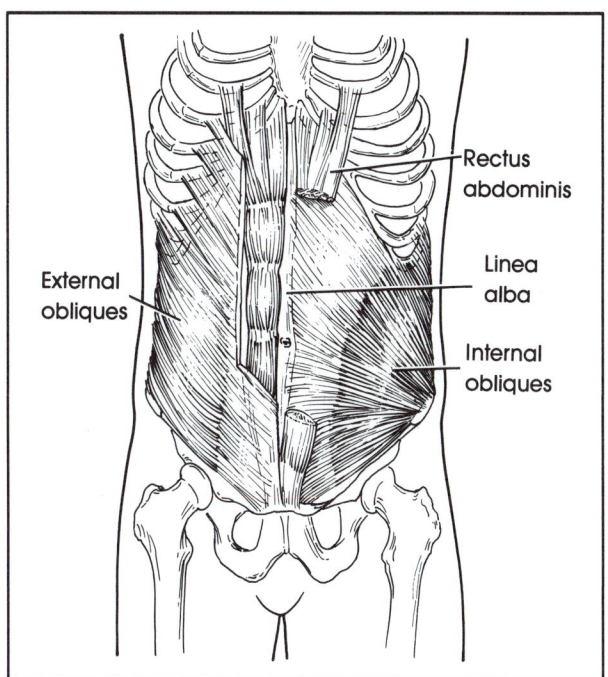

FIGURE 15–5 The abdominal muscles, innervated by the T_{6-12} cord segments, must be intact to produce a forceful cough. Ineffective coughing is a major cause of respiratory insufficiency for persons with SCI.

Aspiration of vomitus, especially during the first 48 hours, is a potentially fatal complication for the patient with decreased coughing ability (Burke and Murray 1975). Severe nasal congestion is also common and troublesome for people with quadriplegia. This may be due in part to the interruption of the cervical sympathetic fibers supplying the face and nose (Carter 1979). Eventually, swallowing difficulties and choking on retained secretions or food may become problematic for those with high quadriplegia. Become familiar with individual signs and symptoms.

Characteristic signs of ineffective airway clearance include:

- Restlessness and agitation
- Poor chest expansion
- Abnormal or diminished breath sounds on auscultation; audible rattling, gurgling respiratory sounds
- Pale or dusky color of facial skin, cyanosis of oral mucous membranes
- Alterations in pulse rate from baseline bradycardia

For patients with artificial airways, also note:

- Visible secretions at tracheostomy tube orifice
- Changes in respiratory status: abrupt rise on pressure gauge on ventilator

- Resistance in passing suction catheter (mucus plug)
- Inspection for ventilation

Chest assessment requires knowledge of external chest landmarks in relation to underlying respiratory structures. Review Figure 15–1. Assess thoracic shape and size, respiratory rate and rhythm, chest expansion, and abdominal movement. Procedure 15–1 summarizes chest assessment techniques.

Thoracic shape and size is normally symmetrical and smaller in the anteroposterior dimension than the lateral dimension. Look for unusual shaping or bony protuberance, which will necessitate modifying procedures for turning, positioning, and fitting to allow for adequate chest expansion.

Respiratory rate and rhythm may not be immediately affected postinjury, but may change dramatically due to fatigue or the exertion required to talk or eat. Note an increased rate of shallow respirations, an early sign of respiratory insufficiency.

Chest and abdominal movement may be abnormal. *Paradoxical respiration (abdominal breathing)* is a familiar condition in quadriplegia. The intercostal muscles do not move, and the diaphragm is the sole remaining muscle of

TABLE 15–1   Neurological Control of Breathing and Anticipated Dysfunctions Following Spinal Cord Injury

| Muscles of Breathing | | Segmental Nerves | Cough Function | Vital Capacity (VC) | |
Inspiration	Expiration			Acute	Long Term
Accessory Muscles		CN XI, C_1, C_2	Absent (nonfunctional)	5–10% of normal (500–600 ml)	Ventilator-dependent for life
Diaphragm		C_3, C_4, C_5, C_6	Absent (nonfunctional)	20% of normal (1250 ml)	Most ventilator-free (especially C_4 and C_5) (some part-time) 50% of normal
External Intercostals	Internal Intercostals	C_7, C_8, T_1		30–50% of normal	60–70% of normal
		T_2, T_3, T_4	Weak		
	Abdominals	T_5, T_6, T_7, T_8, T_9, T_{10}	Fair	75–100% of normal	Nearly normal
		T_{11}, T_{12}, L_1 to S_5	Strong	Normal	Normal

Procedure 15–1 Chest Assessment

Purpose

To determine the patient's respiratory status, especially to detect retained secretions and to evaluate the effectiveness of the therapy. The techniques of inspection, palpation, percussion, and auscultation are included.

Action	Rationale
1. Place the patient supine and remove clothing or bed covers below the waist.	To observe all the muscles used in breathing, especially the diaphragm, a good view of the chest *and* abdomen is necessary.
2. Inspect chest for abnormal shape or asymmetry.*	
3. Count respiratory rate.	An increased rate of shallow respirations is an early sign of respiratory insufficiency.
4. Observe pattern of respiratory rhythm.	Be alert for periods of sleep-induced apnea in quadriplegic patients.
5. Observe chest expansion and abdominal movement. Describe chest expansion as normal, increased, or decreased. (Further assessment requires spirometry.)*	Signs of abnormal or increased work of breathing include: • Exaggerated use of accessory muscles in the neck and shoulders • Paradoxical or abdominal breathing • Inability to breathe deeply • Inability to cough
6. Palpate the chest with fingers on each side of the rib cage, thumbs pointing toward the sternum. Observe movement of your hands as the patient breathes.*	As the patient breathes, thumbs should move apart equally. A symmetry of chest expansion exists if they do not. A condition such as fractured ribs may caused asymmetry of chest expansion. Tactile fremitis or vibratory tremors may also be felt on palpation of the chest wall.
7. Percuss the chest systematically by tapping the chest from the apices to the bases of the lungs. Compare from side to side and at each level. Also percuss diaphragmatic excursion on the posterior chest.*	Abnormal dullness on percussion is indicative of retained secretions.
8. Use a stethoscope to auscultate all lobes of the lungs. Proceed systematically as for percussion.*	Retained secretions cause: • Bronchial sounds • Diminished breath sounds • Increased or decreased fremitus • Adventitious sounds (rales and rhonchi)
9. If possible, place patient prone and repeat techniques.	The prone position can aggravate breathing by limiting impaired chest expansion and abdominal movement.
10. Observe the posterior chest for spinal curvatures.	Spinal curvatures impair chest expansion and may have predisposed the patient to initial injury.
11. Observe amount and nature of secretions.	
12. Check VC and compare with baseline data.	A reduced vital capacity indicates deterioration in pulmonary function.
13. Interpret serial comparison of arterial blood gas analysis.	Early deterioration in respiratory function is detected by a decrease in PaO_2 and/or an increase in $PaCO_2$ values.
14. Collaborate with physician to determine significance of chest X-ray findings.	Chest X rays are of limited value in early detection of retained secretions because microatelectasis, which causes small airway closure, cannot easily be seen.

*The halo-thoracic brace limits the use of these techniques.

breathing. The paralyzed muscles of the thoracic cage are passively drawn inward with inspiration (as the diaphragm descends) and expand with expiration (as the diaphragm ascends) (Tyson et al. 1978). This reversal of normal ventilatory movements is easily recognized (Metcalf 1986). In the unconscious patient paradoxical breathing is the most important diagnostic sign of cervical injury.

Note that quadriplegic patients tend to overwork the accessory muscles. These patients may be observed attempting to heave deeply, with excessive neck and shoulder movements, to compensate for the loss of chest movement.

Chest Assessment

Use the techniques of palpation, percussion, and auscultation to assess vibrations transmitted throughout the respiratory system (Holloway 1988). See Procedure 15–1.

In *palpation*, the hands are placed on the patient's chest to determine whether chest expansion is symmetrical. The initial assessment is usually limited to the anterior chest because the patient is supine due to necessary immobilization.

Percussion involves tapping the chest to assess the position, size, and density of underlying structures. When percussed, normal lung tissue has a resonant sound. Diminished vibrations occur when structures are more solid. This dullness may be heard normally, as over the heart and liver, or abnormally when large amounts of retained secretions clog lung tissues.

Check breath sounds of ventilator-dependent persons at periodic intervals to assess air movement and secretion accumulation. With time, patience, and practice, a trained ear can accurately auscultate breath sounds during mechanical ventilation, noticing any subtle signs of respiratory insufficiency.

Auscultation of the chest using a stethoscope is used to determine breath sounds, voice sounds, and adventitious or abnormal sounds.

Breath sounds are described as *vesicular*—soft, quiet sounds heard over much of the lung as air passes into the alveoli (particularly on inspiration); *bronchial*—loud, tubular sounds heard over the major bronchi and trachea (mainly on expiration); and *bronchovesicular*—a combination of the two. Bronchovesicular sounds occur when the bronchi come close to the lung surface, which is mainly at the apices and between the scapulae posteriorly. Diminished or absent sounds indicate abnormality. Location is also important. Bronchial sounds should not occur where vesicular sounds should be, and so on.

Voice sounds are transmitted through the respiratory system and can be detected as vibrations on the chest wall. These vibrations are termed *fremitus*. An increase in fremitus, as occurs with consolidation of a lung, or decrease or absence of fremitus, as occurs with obstruction of a bronchus, indicates abnormality.

Listening for *adventitious sounds* superimposed on breath sounds is probably the technique used most frequently by nurses. As with assessment of vital signs, it is not the isolated assessment, but the comparison of data to indicate deterioration or improvement, that is most helpful. For example, it is important to listen to the patient's chest before and after a session of chest physical-therapy to determine the effectiveness of the treatment. The chest should be auscultated in a systematic fashion similar to that used in percussion.

Describing adventitious sounds can be confusing, as a wide variety of terms are used in the literature. For clarification it is better to describe the characteristics of abnormal sounds rather than simply to label them. The most common descriptions are of rales and rhonchi. *Rales* are continuous, moist, crackling, or bubbling sounds that are more evident on inspiration as air passes through alveoli that are partially collapsed or filled with fluid. *Rhonchi* are discontinuous, drier sounds—sometimes described as musical, whistling, or wheezing sounds—that are more evident on expiration as air passes through a tracheobronchial tree that has been narrowed, by lung secretion, for example. Occasionally, a pleural rub or grating sound of breathing may be heard.

Assessment of Coughing Ability

Patients with quadriplegia and high paraplegia have difficulty producing an effective cough. Assessment in patients with high paraplegia is more difficult because they may appear to be breathing normally. Close observation, however, may show that they cannot easily take deep breaths and cough effectively, or that their respirations are primarily diaphragmatic (abdominal).

Evaluate cough force, using a classification system such as that of Rinehart and Nawoczenski (1987):

- *Functional*: Able to raise secretions by a normal, forceful cough without assistance
- *Weak functional*: Able to clear secretions from the airway but unable to expel the secretions without assistance
- *Nonfunctional*: Unable to inhale or exhale with any functional force and cannot move secretions out of the airways or expel secretions without major assistance

Typically, attempted weak functional and nonfunctional coughs sound very quiet, are nonproductive, and occur in rapid succession. Movement in the throat is not accompanied by chest expansion. The person is in obvious distress, with a flushed face and frightened appearance and needs assistance to cough.

Coughing primarily requires strong abdominal muscle contractions to build up the high pressures that force air out of the lungs. This cleansing mechanism is essential for removing foreign particles or mucus from the bronchial tree.

Observe for the following signs that secretions are being retained:

- Moist, unproductive cough
- Increased rate of shallow breathing

- Dyspnea
- Repeated ineffective attempts to cough
- Abnormal bronchial sounds, diminished breath sounds, increased or decreased fremitus, adventitious sounds.

Extrathoracic Signs and Symptoms of Distress

Observe for:

- Sternal indrawing
- Trachea tug
- Nasal flaring
- Facial tension
- Shortness of breath

Also note cardiovascular signs related to respiration (see Chapter 16):

- Compensatory tachycardia
- Poor color ranging from peripheral cyanosis involving the extremities to central cyanosis (detected by a bluish tinge of the lips, tongue, and mucosa of the mouth)
- Subtle changes in level of consciousness such as restlessness, irritability, or confusion (progressing to coma if unarrested)

Never underestimate the negative effects of severe pain, anxiety, or agitation on respiratory function. Listen to the patient. If the patient claims difficulty in breathing, immediately assess the total respiratory situation, including the chest and related systems and, if in use, the artificial airway and mechanical ventilator. If the patient is still not comfortable, it is best to check the arterial blood gases or use noninvasive pulmonary gas measurement techniques.

Diagnostic Procedures

Pulmonary Function Tests

Assessment of pulmonary volumes, capacities, and pressures, especially procedures that can be done at the bedside, is useful in prevention, recognition, and treatment of pulmonary complications in patients with SCI. Evaluate on the basis of consecutive readings, rather than an isolated reading, to determine the trend.

The amount of air in the lungs can be divided into four pulmonary (lung) volumes: tidal (TV), inspiratory reserve (IRV), expiratory reserve (ERV), and residual (RV) volumes. Two or more pulmonary volumes combine to form the pulmonary (lung) capacities: total, inspiratory, vital, and functional residual capacities. Table 15–2 defines these terms and gives both normal values and values for persons with SCI. As research and management techniques improve, abnormal values once considered acceptable will likely not remain so.

Vital capacity (VC) is the most important value for patients with SCI. VC indicates the ability to take a deep breath and to cough effectively. It can be measured quickly and easily at the bedside with a spirometer. With appropriate exercises, the VC will improve (Brown, Scharf, and Melia 1988). See Figures 15–6 and 15–7. Without using bronchial hygiene techniques, the VC may worsen, possibly necessitating mechanical ventilation for an interim period.

> Patients with spinal cord injury at C_5 and below have a forced vital capacity (FVC) that may be expected to be about 30% of predicted normal in the acute stage. Patients with injury at C_4 usually have smaller FVC. A significant increase of the FVC can be expected within five weeks of injury with an approximate doubling at three months. Patients in whom the FVC decreases to less than 25% of predicted normal are likely to develop respiratory failure requiring ventilator support. [Ledsome and Sharp, 1981: 44]

Cheshire and Flack (1978–1979: 163) explain:

> It is in the context of the ability of the patient to handle a respiratory infection that the vital capacity becomes of critical importance. In the patient with respiratory infection, the greater the vital capacity, the greater the ability to move secretions from the alveoli to the airways, hence minimizing the chances of consolidation and the complications of inadequate gas exchange in the alveoli. The majority of quadriplegic patients are unable to bring secretions to the mouth, but with an adequate vital capacity they are able to bring secretions to the airways, and with assisted coughing, can bring secretions from the airways to the mouth.

Arterial Blood Gas Analysis

Adequate or insufficient gaseous exchange in the lungs is reflected by arterial blood gas analysis. Again, serial evaluations are essential.

Analysis includes PaO_2, $PaCO_2$, and a measurement of the acid-base balance (HCO_3 or base excess). See Table 15–3 for normal values and values following SCI. Desired values depend on the time interval after injury and indicate the presence or absence of the following conditions:

- Hypoxemia (systemic), insufficient oxygen in the blood
- Hypercarbia, a buildup of CO_2 in the blood, often associated with inadequate chest movement and hence inadequate ventilation
- Respiratory acidosis, indicated by the acid-base balance, caused by hypoventilation
- Metabolic alkalosis, measured by a rise in pH and HCO_3, while $PaCO_2$ remains within normal limits. Metabolic acids are lost through vomiting and nasogastric tube drainage.

Pulmonary Gas Analysis

Noninvasive techniques to measure pulmonary function are convenient alternatives to drawing blood. Values correlate closely to blood gas analysis; thus, trends can be predicted by comparing initial pulmonary function readings to arterial blood gas findings.

Oxygen saturation (SaO2) is usually measured by small, battery-operated monitors with receptors secured on extremities, such as the ear lobes, fingers, or toes—hence the term *ear* or *pulse oximetry* (Schroeder 1987). See Table 15–2.

End tidal volume of carbon dioxide (ETCO2) is measured in a sample of expired air. Receptors are placed in the expired air flow from an established endotrachial or tracheostomy tube. An acceptable range of ETCO2 is 38 to 45 mg, close to the acceptable values of arterial CO_2 measurements. See Table 15–3.

Chest X ray

Serial chest X rays are also valuable for assessing pulmonary status and in evaluating treatment of such complications as pneumonia. The initial chest X ray, taken on admission, establishes baseline data and detects associated trauma and preexisting pulmonary complications.

PREVENTIVE AND RESTORATIVE MANAGEMENT

Because impairment of ventilation with SCI is an *extrinsic* dysfunction, as opposed to an intrinsic disease process within the lungs, substitutions may be made for the respiratory muscles and the lungs will still function. This principle provides a base for treatment modalities.

A bronchial hygiene maintenance program promotes ventilation and humidification of the airways, prevents retention of secretions, builds muscular strength and endurance, and prevents pulmonary complications. To be effective, the manual and mechanical techniques selected must

TABLE 15–2 Lung Volumes and Capacities for Persons with Quadriplegia

Lung Volumes and Capacities	Definition	Normal Value* (±20% may be acceptable)	Stable Person with Uncomplicated Quadriplegia under Basal Conditions**
Lung volumes:			
Tidal Volume (TV)	Amount of air inspired and expired in normal quiet breathing	500 ml	350 ml
Inspiratory Reserve Volume (IRV)	Amount of air forcefully inspired in addition to the TV	3000 ml	Slightly subnormal
Expiratory Reserve Volume (ERV)	Amount of air forcefully exhaled below the TV	1100 ml	May be permanently decreased to virtually zero
Residual Volume (RV)	Amount of air left in the lungs after exhalation of TV and ERV	1200 ml	10% to 100% higher than normal
Lung capacities:			
Total Lung Capacity (TLC)	Total of all the volumes (TV + IRV + ERV + RV) (maximum volume to which lungs can expand)	5800 ml (avg)	Overall decrease
Inspiratory Capacity (IC)	TV + IRV	3500 ml	Decrease
Vital Capacity (VC)	TV + IRV + ERV (the single, most important test to assess coughing ability)	4600 ml (approx)	Initially 1150–1600 ml (25% to 35% of normal), improving to 2500–3000 ml***
Functional Residual Capacity (FRC)	ERV + RV: Amount of air left in the lungs after normal expiration	2300 ml	Within normal limits

*For young adult male (Kozier and Erb 1991). Normal values for females are about 20% to 25% less. Values may vary depending on age, build, physical condition, and position.

**Acceptable values may vary by more than 20%. Based on Cheshire and Coats (1966), Carter (1979), McMichan et al. (1980), and Ledsome and Sharpe (1981). It should be noted that as research and management techniques improve, abnormal values once considered acceptable will likely not remain so.

***If VC falls below 1 liter (25% of normal), ventilator support is indicated.

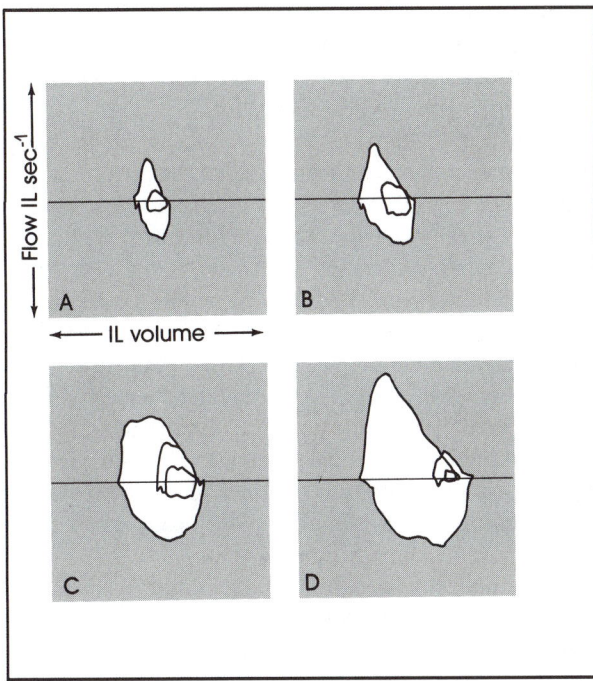

FIGURE 15–6 Changes in forced vital capacity (FVC) at intervals following SCI in five patients with injury at C₄ and in eleven patients with injury at C₅. Vertical bars indicate the standard error of mean. The asterisks indicate that the values are significantly different from the values measured at one week after injury. (From J. R. Ledsome and J. Sharpe, unpublished material.)

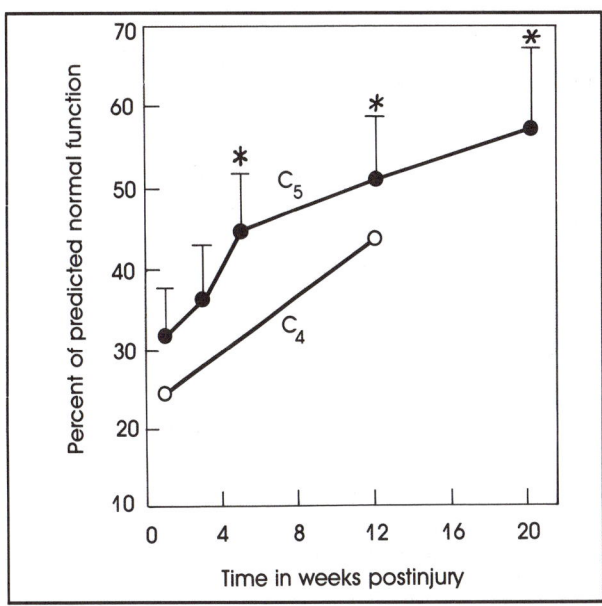

FIGURE 15–7 Changes in the maximum expiratory flow volume curves in one patient with complete C₅ quadriplegia at intervals following SCI. (A) On admission 24 hours after injury. (B) One week after injury. (C) Three weeks after injury. (D) Six months after injury. Note the significant increase in function as time progresses. (From J. R. Ledsome and J. Sharpe 1981.)

be practiced diligently to mobilize retained secretions from the lower airways to the upper airways where they can be suctioned or coughed up. Early mobilization, made possible by advanced medicosurgical techniques, has dramatically reduced problems associated with bedrest and stasis of secretions.

Maintaining an Open Airway

The first priority of respiratory care is to ensure a clear airway. Nasopharyngeal and oral suction of patients with quadriplegia and high paraplegia is intended only to remove secretions from the trachea and mainstem bronchi. In neurologically normal patients suctioning would also trigger a cough, but patients with quadriplegia and high paraplegia are unable to cough. They must rely on physical techniques

TABLE 15–3 Blood and Pulmonary Gas Analysis

Blood Gas Analysis		Normal Values	Recommended Postinjury Values
PaO₂		80–100 mmHg	At or above 80 mmHg
PaCO₂	More accurate reflection of alveolar ventilation in quadriplegia	36–44 mmHg (± 4 mmHg)	45–50 mmHg
pH		7.36 to 7.44	Should be normal
HCO₃		23–28 mEq/l	Should be normal
Base excess		+ 2.5 to –2.5 mEq/l	Should be normal
Pulmonary Gas Analysis			
SaO₂		85–90%	Close to normal
ETCO₂		38–45 mg	Close to normal

to move secretions from the alveoli to the mainstem bronchi. Placement of an oral airway, side positioning (which may involve emergency logrolling the patient), bag ventilation, intubation, and ventilatory support may be needed. Life-saving techniques must be adapted to reduce the risk of further neurological damage to the spinal cord. Chapter 5 describes these emergency procedures, and Chapter 6 outlines critical care, including nasogastric decompression to prevent aspiration of vomitus.

Patients with quadriplegia may tend to *gag or choke on food particles* as they gradually resume a full diet. If fed in the supine position or particularly if the head is in an extended position to realign the spine, a patient is even more likely to choke. During mealtimes, staff must provide adequate supervision and communication systems so that patients can get help if needed. Assisted coughing technique and/or oral suctioning, or the Heimlich maneuver (Texas Institute for Rehabilitation and Research 1986), will clear the airway. Have a portable suction machine handy in a communal dining setting and in therapy areas as well as at the bedside. Precautions with mechanically ventilated patients to minimize risks of aspiration must be taken (Irwin and Openbrier 1985). See also Chapter 17 concerning swallowing difficulties with high SCI.

Nasal congestion is common and troublesome, perhaps related to sympathetic nervous system interruption (Carter 1979). Turning the patient from side to side is most helpful. Adrenergic medications, for example, pseudoephedrine, are sometimes helpful. Nosedrops do little to alleviate the difficulty in the long term.

Regular Turning and Positioning

Regular turning and proper positioning play an important role in preventing secretion stasis in dependent areas of the lung and greatly speed the rehabilitation process. Judicious turning affects the other physiological systems. For instance, it improves circulation, although cardiopulmonary arrest is sometimes linked with sudden and profound position changes immediately after injury. See Chapter 16.

Even a minor adjustment to the patient's position promotes comfort and prevents *accumulation of secretions*. Hoffman (1977) monitored PaO$_2$ and PaCO$_2$ continuously in a patient on a ventilator and found remarkable improvement in arterial blood gas values within 15 minutes after a position change. Turn the patient every 2 hours or more frequently if desired. A patient may experience respiratory deterioration in a certain position; if so, avoid that position.

To *prevent cramping or restricting diaphragmatic movement*, position the patient in correct body alignment when recumbent and support good body posture when sitting.

Supine and *side-lying positions* are necessary for newly injured patients to immobilize the spine and prevent further neurological damage. *The prone position* aids drainage of

secretions and allows full percussion of the posterior chest. However, the position may be difficult to tolerate or contraindicated for the newly injured patient with chest trauma or for a patient on mechanical ventilation.

If the patient's abdominal muscles are paralyzed, breathing will be easier in the recumbent position than in the sitting position. Sitting upright creates a greater demand on the diaphragm because the downward pull of gravity on the abdominal contents causes the diaphragm to rest in a lower position than normal. Therefore, the resting length of the muscles is at a disadvantage. Abdominal binders/corsets offer support that minimize the effects of gravity. Apply so as not to extend over the rib cage, which would limit chest expansion

Good posture, when *sitting*, is important. Support of the trunk and spine in as normal alignment as possible is necessary to make breathing as effortless and effective as possible. If posture is poor, the chest will expand less, further compromising respiratory function.

Straps, individualized wheelchair fittings, orthotic devices, and occasionally the surgical insertion of rods for growing children, are some long-term measures used to achieve a desired position in the wheelchair.

Manual Bronchial Hygiene Techniques

Bronchial hygiene techniques, which include breathing exercises, assisted coughing (sometimes called the "quad" cough), and vibration and percussion (used with postural drainage), are manual techniques to move secretions centrally and clear the chest. When chest assessment identifies symptoms of retained secretions, treat promptly and vigorously, generally every 2 to 4 hours. Most seriously ill patients will not tolerate more than 15 minutes per session. Take into account the patient's tolerance and general condition to avoid fatigue. When the patient has a cold or congested chest, perform manual chest techniques more aggressively. Exhausting the patient defeats the purpose. See Procedure 15–2 for a helpful planning guide to minimize fatigue.

Breathing exercises build respiratory muscle strength and promote adequate ventilation. See Procedure 15–3. These exercises improve air entry to all parts of the lung by encouraging slow, relaxed, and deliberate deep breathing, concentrating on the diaphragm. Gradual progression to more difficult resistive exercises follows, according to principles of muscle exercise training used in athletic programs. See the Mechanical Bronchial Hygiene Techniques section in this chapter.

Assisted or diaphragmatic coughing (Procedure 15–4) helps move secretions centrally toward the trachea and mouth, and clears the airway of secretions or trapped food particles. All quadriplegic and many high paraplegic patients may use this technique throughout life (Brownlee and Williams 1987).

Procedure 15–2   Planning Chest Clearing Technique Sessions

Purpose

To improve effectiveness of chest clearing technique sessions and to conserve patient energy.

Action	Rationale
1. Coordinate interdisciplinary team members to plan treatments that coincide with regular turning times.	To promote rest and sleep periods for the patient.
2. Capitalize on peak periods when medications such as analgesics or bronchiodilators will be most effective.	To promote patient comfort and maximize action of medications.
3. Avoid mealtimes or oral feedings by 30 minutes.	To prevent aspiration.
4. Maintain adequate systemic hydration; avoid overhydration.	Adequate hydration liquefies secretions sufficiently for expectoration; overhydration leads to fluid accumulation in the lungs.
5. Carefully explain each session to patient (and family when necessary).	To maximize patient cooperation. Vigorous chest therapy can be initially frightening to both patients and families.
6. Check to see that the airway is clear before proceeding.	
7. Perform bronchial hygiene techniques. Preoxygenation with a higher percentage of oxygen before oral or tracheal suctioning may be used with all chest clearing techniques.	To move secretions centrally from alveoli to mainstem bronchi and trachea.
8. *Suction* as necessary immediately following sessions.	*Suctioning* is intended to remove secretions only. In neurologically normal patients it also acts to trigger a cough. But patients with quadriplegia and high paraplegia are unable to cough. They must rely on bronchial hygiene techniques.

Assisted coughing is best described as application of even and firm pressure on the diaphragm just below the rib cage as the patient exhales or attempts to cough. Hand placement is critical in order to prevent injury. Timing is also important. Communicate with the patient to establish some way—a nod or a blink, for instance—to signal when inspiration is complete.

Vibration and percussion (or clapping) are usually used in conjunction with *postural drainage* to dislodge and then remove mucus centrally to be expelled or removed. See Procedures 15–5 and 15–6. These techniques are used, for example, when the patient is on initial bedrest or has had a relapse caused by infection. A hand-sized mechanical vibrator can be used to enhance the effects of these techniques.

Reduce manual treatments as the chest clears, indicated by:
• Unlabored respiration
• Clear lungs on auscultation with air entry to all lobes
• Vital capacity and arterial blood and pulmonary gases within normal limits for the patient

Procedure 15–3   Breathing Exercises

Purpose

To ensure air entry to all parts of the lung by encouraging slow, relaxed, and deliberate deep breathing. This procedure can be used with incentive spirometry, which helps motivate the patient when VC can be measured to monitor progress.

Action	Rationale
1. Instruct patient to take deep breath in through nose and exhale through mouth (rate: 6 to 10 breaths per minute).	
2. Place hands on diaphragm to help patient focus attention (even though patient may not be able to feel your hand).	
3. If cervical traction is in place, provide prism glasses.	Restriction of head movements limits field of vision.

Procedure 15–4   Assisted Coughing

Purpose

To help the patient expectorate secretions when partial or complete paralysis of the abdominal muscles and inability to take deep breath reduce effective coughing and to prevent accumulation of secretions extending down the bronchial tree.

Action

1. Instruct patient to breathe in deeply and "double cough," that is, cough twice in succession without inspiration between.

2. Place forearm over upper abdomen and diaphragm. Place other hand over chest wall. Move hand around until most effective spot is found.

3. Maintain an even and firm pressure directed inward and upward and a "bounce" pressure as patient attempts to cough. Timing is crucial. Apply pressure *only* after inspiration is complete.

4. If patient is in chair, from behind place clasped hands over diaphragm and assist with a sharp pull inward and upward on cough or after inspiration. Paraplegic patients may fold arms over upper abdomen to assist own efforts, but quadriplegic patients need strong support.

Rationale

This adds more expulsion force for a more efficient cough.

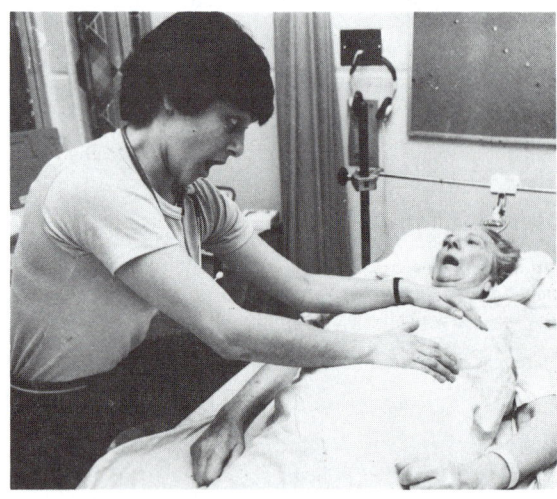

Strength requires weight of assistant's body but not sufficient to cause the patient pain.

Mechanical Bronchial Hygiene Techniques

If the patient's condition deteriorates despite chest physical therapy, consider mechanical techniques to enhance ventilation.

Incentive Spirometry

Incentive spirometry is based on the fundamental principles of neuromuscular exercise and behavioral psychology (Cheshire and Flack 1978–1979). The objective is to provide a practical means to increase the patient's VC and thus increase coughing ability to combat intercurrent respiratory infection. Neuromuscular exercise is based on repetitive and increasingly difficult movements, in this case to strengthen the diaphragm and other muscles of breathing. Gradually, the patient is able to take deeper breaths and exhale more forcefully. Operant conditioning techniques use positive reinforcement to encourage desirable behavior. When the patient's efforts to breathe deeply are acknowledged by positive consequences, such as praise from a nurse or other patients, this behavior is

more likely to be repeated again in the future. Thus the nurse's enthusiasm is a key influence on the success or failure of this technique.

The Spirocare Incentive Breathing Exerciser (distributed by Marion Laboratories, Kansas City, MO) is a device that provides positive feedback through its system of brightly colored lights and digital display to encourage the patient to perform sustained maximum inspiratory movements. The system is goal oriented. The desired volume range is selected and displayed on one panel. The measurements of the patient's efforts are displayed on the adjacent panel so that results can be compared directly.

Ventilatory Muscle Training

Ventilatory muscle training (VMT) can be safely instituted in the acute stage following SCI to improve ventilatory muscle strength and endurance (Hornstein and Ledsome 1986). VMT involves breathing through a T-shaped device with graded resistance placed on the inspiratory phase. Expiration is left unimpeded. Patients report decreased shortness of breath while talking or eating and increased

Procedure 15–5   Vibration and Percussion (Clapping)

Purpose

To dislodge and mobilize secretions in the bronchial tree. Secretions can then be expectorated or suctioned out. Used in conjunction with postural drainage.

Action	Rationale
1. Auscultate the patient's chest before each treatment.	To establish baseline data for comparison at end of treatment. This technique may be modified to find tremor in presence of rib fractures.
2. Place whole hands in contact with affected area of the chest wall. To vibrate chest, apply vigorous, rhythmical, intermittent pressure during expiration.	

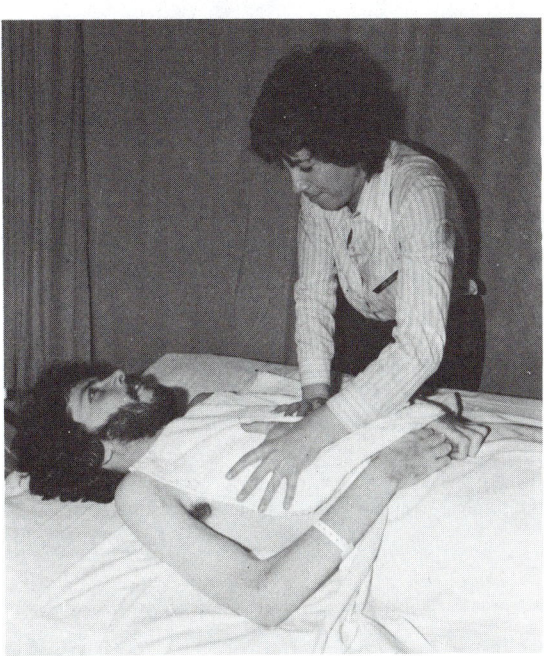 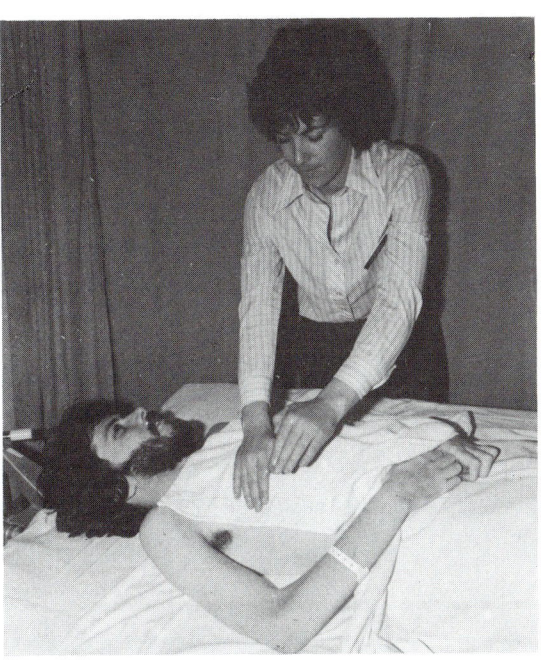

Action	Rationale
3. Place relaxed, cupped hands over affected area of chest and perform rhythmical percussion. This is called clapping.	This technique is contraindicated in the presence of rib fractures, pneumothorax, or acute cardiac disease, for example.
4. Work from more dependent to less dependent areas of the lung.	
5. If necessary, assist the patient to expectorate (as in Procedure 15–4) or suction out the secretions.	You may wish to hand ventilate the intubated patient on a mechanical ventilator; coordinate your efforts with the co-worker suctioning.
6. Auscultate the patient's chest after treatment.	This will determine the treatment's effectiveness.

voice projection. Control of saliva and less chance of choking on food may also be benefits that accrue when used on a long-term maintenance program

Graded weights placed on the upper abdominal area are another means of providing resistance during inspiration to strengthen the diaphragm. Inspirometers are used in conjunction with the weights to give feedback to the patient and evaluate effectiveness of the treatment. Belman (1988) describes all training methods in detail.

Intermittent Positive Pressure Breathing

Intermittent positive pressure breathing (IPPB) aerates and humidifies underventilated areas of the lungs of patients with quadriplegia, who are unable to sigh or deep breathe regularly. This alveolar distension may actually stretch the lungs and thorax and improve movement and distribution of gases.

At the first signs of chest congestion, aerosol medications such as bronchodilators and mucolytic agents may be ad-

Procedure 15–6   Postural Drainage (Trendelenburg Position)

Purpose

To promote gravity-assisted drainage of secretions. This position enhances effectiveness of vibration and percussion techniques. Unless contraindicated by associated injury, such as head injury, it is desirable to proceed with postural drainage with all spinal injured patients (within limitations of orthopedic alignment, tolerance, and type of immobilization bed in use).

Action	Rationale
1. Tip or tilt entire bed to lower head of bed approximately 18 inches.	This is possible on immobilization beds (Stoke-Eggerton tilting bed, the Wedge Stryker turning frame, and the ICU stretcher bed). Regular beds require placement of solid blocks under the foot.

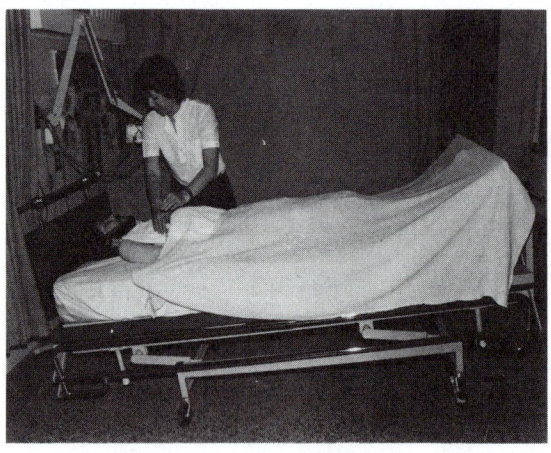

2. Place patient alternately in side-lying, supine, and prone positions.

3. To treat complications in specific lung segments, collaborate with physical therapist to choose approriate position.

When a patient is not allowed to sit up, the most difficult area to drain is the apices of the lungs. Sometimes tilt table therapy is possible.

---

ministered to enhance the effects of this deep-breathing technique. A typical treatment may consist of 2 ml of normal saline, 2 ml Mucomyst, 2 ml 1/4% Neosynephrine, and 0.3 ml Albuterol. Humidification is increased when sterile water is added to the nebulizer. The IPPB ventilators are used with a mouthpiece or tracheostomy adapter to enlarge airways and moisten and thin secretions.

Treatments are usually ordered every 4 to 6 hours. Each treatment must be followed with manual techniques sufficient to clear the chest of mobilized secretions. Suctioning may be necessary. As the chest clears, gradually discontinue treatments.

Ultrasonic Nebulization

The ultrasonic (electronic) nebulizer produces a fine non-heated mist from distilled water. It is used in conjunction with manual methods to clear the chest; to loosen thick, tenacious bronchial secretions further; to stimulate a cough reflex if possible; and to combat consolidation and atelectasis in the alveoli.

The mist created by the nebulizer is delivered to the patient by an oxygen flow system. Treatment sessions must not exceed 10 minutes and *must* be followed immediately by clapping, vibrating, and assisted coughing with postural drainage to clear the chest; otherwise, a dangerous excess of fluid remains in the lungs. Treatments are contraindicated if the patient has fluid retention, pulmonary edema, or bronchospasm resulting from inhalation of the mist. Medications are not compatible with this system; ultrasound may degrade the drug, and calculation of the dosage inhaled is unreliable.

Oxygen Therapy

Supplemental oxygen may be administered when signs of respiratory deterioration appear. Because paralyzed patients breathe through both nose and mouth in an effort to compensate for limited chest expansion, oxygen is generally delivered via face mask and *must* be humidified to prevent drying of mucosa and secretions. A regular mask is used to deliver an oxygen concentration of 40% to 60%; a mask with an attached rebreathing bag yields a higher concentration; and a Venturi mask, designed with increased exhalation ports to prevent rebreathing CO_2, delivers lower concentrations of 24% to 40%.

An Artificial Airway

An artificial airway may be needed at the scene of the accident or on admission to the emergency room. However, because secretions tend to accumulate gradually and respiratory parameters that indicate impending respiratory failure are acquired over time, elective intubation is more common. Anticipated dysfunction and length of time the patient is expected to be intubated influence the type of airway selected.

Psychological preparation for elective intubation can help relieve the fear and anxiety associated with the discomfort, total dependency, and inability to talk. Reassurance that this is a temporary measure offers some relief, but it is more important to establish a system of making the patient's needs known. As this problem is most severe when the patient is on a mechanical ventilator, it will be discussed in that section.

Endotracheal Intubation

Endotracheal intubation is useful for emergency or for short-term intubation. Endotracheal tubes extend from the nose or mouth to the trachea, at least 3 cm above the carina. The nasotracheal route is preferred for cervical injuries as less manipulation of the head and neck is required during insertion.

It is dangerous to wait too long before placing the endotrachial tube. If the VC is 1.0 liter to 1.5 liter or less, secretions are copious, fever is present, or fatigue is impending, intubate to minimize the risk of hypoxia, pneumonia, and other complications.

Tracheostomy

A *tracheostomy* is selected for long-term management (longer than one week). It is useful for the quadriplegic patient or the paraplegic patient with preexisting lung conditions or severe chest injury. This airway is essential for the quadriplegic patient requiring permanent mechanical ventilation and is used when a patient is intolerant of an endotracheal tube.

It is also dangerous to wait too long to perform a tracheostomy. If the conditions leading to intubation do not reverse within a few days, they will usually not reverse in 2 weeks. Tracheostomy may not only be life saving but can prevent the complications of prolonged intubation such as subglottic stenosis, intubation granulomas, and tracheomalacia. Also the weaning process may proceed gradually without a 1- or 2-week delay.

Tracheostomy tubes are inserted during an operative procedure. The surgeon makes a horizontal incision between the second and third tracheal rings just large enough to admit the tracheostomy tube. A tracheostomy is ideally an elective procedure but may be undertaken as an extreme emergency measure. Advantages include ease of removal of secretions, reduction of anatomical dead space to reduce the work of breathing, less chance of tube displacement, and increased patient comfort. Complications include that of the procedure itself, hemorrhage, tracheal trauma, and airway obstruction.

As a safety precaution, whenever a tracheostomy tube is in place, always keep a tube of the same size at the patient's bedside. A sterile tracheostomy dressing tray, with retractors or tracheal dilator forceps, should also be close at hand to facilitate emergency tube replacement.

There are two main types of tracheostomy tubes:

1. The *disposable Portex-plastic cuffed tube.* Most patients requiring a tracheostomy will also require initial mechanical ventilation. Portex-plastic cuffed tubes are recommended because they provide a good seal for the respirator. The inflated cuff occludes the space between the tracheostomy tube and the trachea to prevent air from escaping. The wide-bore tube with a soft cuff (high residual volume) is recommended to facilitate suctioning, minimize pressure on the trachea, and prevent tracheal necrosis. The cuff must be deflated periodically to relieve all pressure on the wall of the trachea. The patient can also speak when the cuff is deflated.

2. The *reusable metal tube (uncuffed)* is for long-term or permanent situations. See the Permanent Respiratory Support section in this chapter.

Mechanical Ventilation

Patients with very high cord injuries suffering instant diaphragmatic paralysis will require immediate resuscitation and lifelong ventilatory support. Occasionally patients with severe chest trauma may also need immediate artificial respiration. However, mechanical ventilation, like intubation, is usually an elective measure to manage respiratory deterioration. Deterioration is mainly caused by extreme fatigue as the work of breathing is increased or by neurological edema expanding to impair the muscles of breathing further. Particularly watch for ineffective rapid shallow breathing; increasingly noisy respirations; and approaching periods of apnea (or near apnea) leading to eventual signs of severe distress. When the patient will clearly not be able to maintain adequate respiratory function if the present course continues, mechanical ventilation is indicated. Capitalize on the observation time to prepare the patient and family psychologically for mechanical ventilation. It is important to minimize apprehension so the patient does not fight the machine and increase breathing difficulties.

Caring for spinal cord injured patients requiring mechanical ventilation demands detailed expertise, as for any critically ill, mechanically ventilated patient. However, paralyzed patients experience extrinsic lung dysfunctions (related to the muscles of breathing) as opposed to the majority of ventilated patients who suffer an intrinsic disease process of the lungs. Therefore management approaches differ. The following sections describe kinds of mechanical ventilators and summarize indications for their use and the potential physiological problems encountered with spinal cord injured patients.

Kinds of Mechanical Ventilators

The most commonly used ventilators are pressure-controlled or volume-controlled machines.

1. *The positive pressure-cycled ventilator*, such as the Bird Mark 7 or the Bennett PRII, ends the inspiratory phase when a preset pressure has been reached. If the airway is clear, the predetermined pressure will deliver the desired volume of gas. If the airway is obstructed or restricted in any way, however, the predetermined pressure will be attained earlier and only part of the volume of gas will be delivered.
2. *The volume-cycled machine* ends the inspiratory phase when a predetermined amount of gas has been delivered. Certain safety mechanisms abort the inspiratory phase if extreme pressures are reached while the ventilator is attempting to deliver the preset volume of gas. Volume-cycled machines include the Bennett MA–1 and MA–2, Ohio 560, Emerson, and Ergstrom ventilators.

For several reasons, the volume-cycled ventilator is more desirable for patients with SCI. Poor lung compliance and secretion retention problems make it difficult for the quadriplegic person to maintain a clear airway. Because airway closure causes the preset pressure of a pressure-cycled ventilator to be attained before the desired volume of gas is actually delivered, it is difficult to estimate from the preset pressure the actual volume of gas the patient is receiving. The pressure-cycled machine also increases intrathoracic pressure and thus can aggravate the already impaired venous circulation to the heart.

Each kind of respirator has a variety of modes to ensure inspiration:

- The *assist/control mode* assists patients to take a breath if they trigger the machine or delivers a breath if they fail to do so. This mode is desirable for patients with weak chest musculature or weak neural drive resulting in irregular respirations and is suitable for initial mechanical ventilation for most patients with SCI.
- *Assisted ventilation* is used when patients can initiate a respiration by triggering the ventilator to deliver the preset volume or pressure. This mode is used for patients with SCI when they are recovering from initial fatigue or neurological edema involving diaphragmatic function. At this stage, weaning should be considered.

- *Controlled ventilation* delivers a preset volume or pressure at the desired rate regardless of patient effort or lack of effort. This mode is needed by apneic patients, most notably ventilator-dependent quadriplegic patients with high cord injuries.
- It is also possible to change either the timing or pressure settings that influence the expiratory phase. The most frequently used expiratory maneuver for patients prone to secretion retention leading to alveolar collapse because of small airway closure is *Positive End Expiratory Pressure* (PEEP). PEEP is based on the fundamental principle of airway expansion on inspiration and airway collapse on expiration. PEEP maintains a positive pressure of 1 to 15 cm H_2O at the end of each expiration. To demonstrate this, take a deep breath, exhale part of it, and breathe in again. The pressure in the lungs is not allowed to return to normal atmospheric pressure and you have increased the resting volume of the lungs or the functional residual capacity (FRC). The application of PEEP causes alveoli to stay open longer maintaining oxygenation of pulmonary capillary blood. By combating small airway closure, it is possible to maintain or increase FRC and lung compliance and help prevent hypoxia and increased work of breathing. However, if the PEEP exceeds 20 cm of H_2O, a pneumothorax may develop. See the Pneumothorax section in this chapter.

Potential Physiological Problems Associated with Mechanical Ventilation

Major potential risks for patients with SCI who require prolonged mechanical ventilation include gastrointestinal problems, malnutrition, and retention of secretions with subsequent pulmonary infection and a pneumothorax. The long-term use of artificial airways also aggravates many of these potential problems in addition to necrosis associated with pressure on desensitized skin caused by the tracheostomy tube.

Paralytic ileus usually exists as a result of SCI perhaps only for a few days, but sluggish function of the gastrointestinal tract often persists. In addition to ileus, *air swallowing* can cause severe gastric dilation, which in turn hampers respirations. Severe emotional and physical trauma and major surgery increase the risk of *gastric ulceration* and *hemorrhage*. Nasogastric decompression and other management plans to control these complications are discussed in Chapter 17.

Maintaining optimal nutritional support is critical because patients with SCI frequently have a marginal nutritional status related to catabolic conditions from trauma, including surgery. Limited respiratory reserve is compounded by *malnutrition*, if present. Malnutrition affects respiratory muscle function by reducing muscle mass and strength; limited endurance and increased fatigue result. *Overfeeding*, especially carbohydrates, exacerbates respiratory distress in patients with marginal pulmonary reserve because of increased oxygen consumption and increased CO_2 production. (Respirations tend to become rapid and ineffective.) Complications of *underfeeding* result in catabolism of lean body tissue, including the respiratory muscles. A decreased immunocompetence from malnutrition increases the risk of pneumonia, and the loss of cardiopulmonary reserve complicates the weaning process. Chapter 17 describes malnutrition and calculation of supplements for critically ill SCI patients in detail.

Retention of secretions and subsequent *infections* are a constant threat for the patient with extrinsic lung dysfunctions. Constant and correct airway humidification and adequate systemic hydration will liquefy secretions for ease of removal. Continuation of a bronchial hygiene program is mandatory to minimize risks while on mechanical ventilation.

Meticulous sterile technique while suctioning the trachea is probably the single most important factor to prevent infection (in the acute stage). It is best to avoid excessive suctioning by choosing the most effective times to clear mobilized secretions—usually right after turning and promptly following bronchial hygiene techniques. Rigid cleaning schedules for equipment must also be followed. Tracheostomy site care is required every 4 to 8 hours. Consult with the physician about changing the tracheostomy tube weekly.

To minimize the risk of *tracheal necrosis*, Portex-plastic tubes with high residual volume soft cuffs are recommended for use with mechanical ventilation. As previously mentioned, this kind of airway ensures minimal pressure on the trachea at the cuff site. Tubing should be supported so that the tube itself is not malaligned and does not cause undue pressure on the trachea. Secure all tubing before and after turns.

A rare but serious complication that may develop even after extubation is a *tracheoesophageal fistula*. This necrotic complication is more likely to develop if a large nasogastric tube has also been used. Observe for oral or tube feeding in tracheal aspirate. During the early stages this is more commonly caused by difficulty in swallowing while the tracheostomy tube is in place. If tracheal aspirate is not found to contain food until 4 to 6 weeks after tracheostomy, it is more likely that a fistula has formed. The patient may complain of a severe burning sensation during and after meals; this is caused by food contamination of the fistula. Diagnosis is confirmed by X ray or endoscopy, and surgical repair is usually necessary.

Communicating during Mechanical Ventilation

Communication is a major concern for patients requiring mechanical ventilation. The longer the patient is mechan-

ically ventilated, the more complex the situation becomes as the need for communication becomes greater and greater. It is difficult to provide really helpful information and to ease the obstacles that are blocking communication. The nurse who is able to care effectively for a patient in this situation possesses wonderful skills much to be admired and is a valuable resource person. Such a nurse treats the patient with respect, appreciating what respiratory failure and SCI prognosis imply to the individual; manages the respirator and related equipment comfortably; minimizes the stressful effects of an intensive care setting; and establishes a basic communication system. The following measures help handle difficult situations when the patient becomes severely agitated:

- Consider the patient's preinjury personality to anticipate responses during illness. Often the social worker can obtain this information from family members.
- Consider internal sources of anxiety. The person dependent on a respirator is in constant fear of disconnection from the machine or possible mechanical failure that could lead to suffocation and death. Hypoxia may cause secondary confusion, and the physical and emotional trauma surrounding the sudden onset of paralysis will contribute to a severe anxiety state.
- Consider and try to eliminate environmental factors contributing to stress. Adverse effects are described as sensory deprivation or overload and sleep deprivation. Organize care to allow for much-needed sleep. It is generally valuable to create as "homey" an atmosphere as possible with colored linens, window drapes, and even posters on the ceiling. Chapter 6 offers further suggestions.

When delivering care, it is important to establish a trusting rapport to make the patient feel secure. If this is achieved, communication becomes much easier. Simple measures, such as protecting the patient's modesty or avoiding conversations "over" patients that do not include them are of utmost importance. *Gentle* moving of patients will convey messages of caring and concern. Patients may see the ventilator as a projection of themselves. Address the patient before making any ventilator adjustments. It is also helpful for nurses to introduce themselves, discuss the activities planned during the shift, and explain each procedure carefully. Much verbal support is needed.

Devices.   To facilitate communication a fenestrated, low-pressure, cuffed tracheostomy tube may be introduced for patients who swallow normally (see Figure 15–8). This device has a removable inner cannula that exposes an opening on the upper surface of the outer cannula, which allows the patient to talk during expiration. Unfortunately, suctioning may be difficult with this device. During insertion, the suction catheter tends to

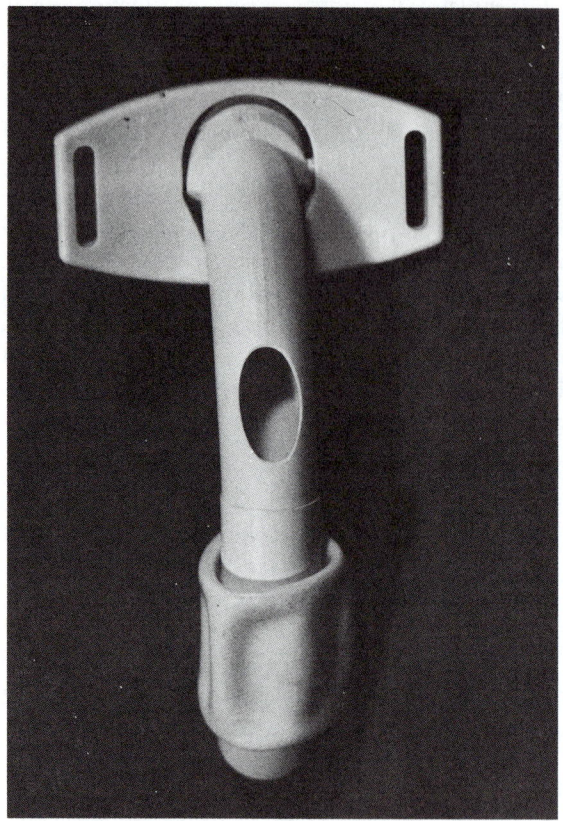

FIGURE 15–8   The Shiley fenestrated tracheostomy tube. (Distributed by Shiley Sales Corp., Irvine, CA 92714.)

catch on the window opening of the outer cannula. Reinsertion of the inner cannula at this point may push secretions back down into the lung. To accommodate the inner cannula, it is necessary to use a small catheter (French size 12), which is not large enough to remove tenacious or copious amounts of secretions. Also, if the patient has difficulty swallowing, food may be aspirated through the fenestration.

An innovative technique, still in the experimental stages, is the use of an *electrolarynx**. This is an artificial, electrically stimulated larynx that enables the patient to communicate quickly and effectively. Successful use depends on the patient's overall articulation ability and availability of a good placement site.

Eventually, patients with high cervical cord injuries, who will remain ventilator-dependent, will be able to talk. A portable ventilator system is compatible with the metal, uncuffed tracheostomy tube (size 6 or less) and, on expiration, allows for vocalization around the tube.

Nonverbal communication systems.   Most often some type of nonverbal system is needed to establish effective

*For more information on this largely experimental device, contact the Department of Speech Pathology, Northwestern Memorial Hospital (Wesley Pavilion), Chicago, IL.

communication. The most suitable approaches for patients without use of their upper limbs are scanning and encoding techniques.

In the *scanning technique*, a person presents various symbols or words to the patient, who remains passive until the correct item is chosen. Simple examples are:

- Yes/no guessing or questioning. Present the patient with choices, one at a time, or pose questions in such a way that only a "yes" or "no" answer is needed. This may require a system, such as one blink for "yes" and two blinks for "no." The questions include requests for information about pain, nausea, air hunger, or the need for suctioning. As sensation is diminished elsewhere, increasing awareness of discomfort over the head, neck, and shoulders is common, particularly headache or itchiness on the face. Include these questions and others about preferences and preexisting conditions.
- Scanning of a poster board. A poster board, or a set of cards on a ring, can contain a list of questions, commands, pictures, or symbols individualized to patient needs. The nurse can point to the choices individually and ask the patient to respond using the "yes" or "no" blink system.

Encoding techniques are techniques where the message items to be communicated are indicated by multiple signals from the patient. A simple example of this technique uses a vocabulary matrix like the one illustrated in Figure 15–9A. The patient specifies the word(s) of the message by indicating the two appropriate numbers; one in the horizontal column and the corresponding number in the vertical column. For example, if the desired word was *juice*, the patient would indicate number 5 from the horizontal line A and number 2 from the vertical line 0. The numbers can be indicated by using the blink method. An example of a more complex system is shown in Figure 15–9B. This requires a direct selector pointing to individual words and letters (note the letters are set up like a typewriter keyboard to prepare the patient for future skills that will require the use of a mouth stick). The patient again uses a blink system for indicating desired words.

The scanning techniques are simple to operate and require little effort on the part of the patient. Unfortunately such communication is slow. The encoding techniques provide a faster means of communication and an access to a larger vocabulary. They require, however, greater physical control and higher cognitive abilities than the scanning technique. For the spinal cord patient who requires a nonvocal communication aid for a short period only, a simple scanning device is suggested. Whatever system is used, *initiate* and *encourage* its use for the patient to become comfortable with it. For longer periods more sophisticated electronic environmental aids must be investigated by the interdisciplinary team.

LINE "A" FIRST	A 1	A 2	A 3	A 4	A 5	A 6	A 7	A 8
O 1	WHO	LEG	FOOT	PAIN	WATER	DOCTOR	P.T.	S.P.
O 2	WHAT	ARM	HAND	SCRATCH	JUICE	NURSE	O.T.	S.W.
O 3	WHEN	BACK	NECK	SUCTION	FOOD	BED		
O 4	WHERE	HEAD	EYES	TURN	HOT	WHEEL CHAIR		
O 5	WHY	NOSE	MOUTH	WASH	TISSUES	LIGHT	I	YOU
O 6	HOW	BOWEL	BLADDER	TIME	COLD	FAN	YES	NO

A

SUCTION	SCRATCH	FOOD	WATER	PAIN	YES	NO				
TIME	HOT	COLD	JUICE	TURN	I	YOU				
WASH	1	2	3	4	5	6	7	8	9	0
BED	Q	W	E	R	T	Y	U	I	O	P
LIGHT	A	S	D	F	G	H	J	K	L	;
FAN	Z	X	C	V	B	N	M	,	.	?
TISSUES	BOWEL	BLADDER	LEG	ARM	WHO	WHAT				
DOCTOR	EYES	HEAD	BACK	NECK	WHY	WHEN				
NURSE	P.T.	O.T.	S.P.	S.W.	WHERE	HOW				

B

FIGURE 15–9 (A) A vocabulary matrix as shown here is a simple example of an encoding system. (B) This matrix can become more complex with the addition of numbers and letters. Actual charts measure approximately 9 × 12 inches.

Liaison activities. To combat feelings of isolation and loneliness, provide a liaison between the patient and other team members or the family and visitors. For example, staying at the bedside to support the physician or visitor in their initial attempts to communicate can ease the situation and make the visit more meaningful. Also, patients frequently have questions about their treatments, such as "When can I eat?" or "How long will I be on this machine?" Try to clarify some of these concerns before the physician's visit, perhaps by talking to previously intubated patients for more ideas.

When verbal communication is not possible, the patient becomes increasingly aware of nonverbal communication. Facial expression, for example, can quickly communicate cheerfulness, anxiety, or frustration. In addition, touching patients, especially where their sensation is still intact, will enhance communication of feelings and concerns.

Discontinuing Mechanical Ventilation

Most patients with SCI require a gradual withdrawal or weaning process from ventilator support. Generally, the longer the time on the respirator, the weaker the muscles will be from progressive atrophy (Wicks 1989) and the longer the process. Withdrawal from ventilator support is *gradual* to increase the tolerance and strength of the respiratory muscles.

The Process of Gradual Withdrawal

Two methods for removing patients from mechanical ventilators are gradually increasing time periods off the ventilator and intermittent mandatory ventilation (IMV) while the patient is still maintained on the ventilator. Diaphragm strength is best developed by a program that alternates work or exercise periods off the ventilator with periods of complete rest on the ventilator. IMV encourages patients to breathe spontaneously while a controlled number of breaths per minute are delivered from the ventilator at preselected times. However, this method is not suitable for patients with muscle paralysis because it forces patients to work continuously to meet their oxygen requirements (Wicks 1989).

Benotti and Bistrian (1989) also suggest applying the muscle-training principles commonly used in regular athletic programs to strengthen the respiratory muscles. Because the respiratory muscles are also skeletal muscles, it is theoretically possible to design training in terms of measuring workload, duration of exercise and rest periods, number of repetitions, and rate of progression similar to training other muscles. See Chapter 24 for further explanation of exercise principles. This scientific approach is probably a more efficient weaning process.

Readiness to Begin the Process

As the patient's general condition stabilizes, neurological edema and spinal shock subside, and the diaphragm becomes stronger, the need for mechanical ventilation diminishes. The patient can gradually assume the entire workload of breathing spontaneously as lung function is restored, respiratory muscle strength and endurance improve, nutrition is adequate, and a desire or motivation to breathe independently develops. Specific signs of readiness include (Norton and Neureuter 1988):

- Maintaining normal arterial blood gas values (on room air)
- Maintaining clear airways
- A VC of at least 1.2 to 1.5
- Afebrile condition
- Chest X ray clear
- Related nutritional and metabolic stability
- A positive attitude (calm, rested, comfortable, motivated)

Adequate nutrition and metabolic stability are essential before undertaking an attempt to wean a person from a mechanical ventilator. Malnutrition is manifested by loss of muscle mass, including changes in the contractive properties of the muscles of breathing, and decreased energy, endurance, and respiratory reserves. Metabolic acidosis can cause an increase in the respiratory rate; metabolic alkalosis reduces oxygen delivery and predisposes patients to dysrhythmias and compensatory CO_2 retention.

During the weaning process, be careful to provide nutritional supplements, properly adjust amounts and types of feedings, and to replenish glycogen promptly during periods of rest. Proper management of bladder and bowel programs, especially to avoid abdominal distension, also eases the work of breathing. Ensure a stable blood pressure and pulse by caring for conditions such as postural hypotension or edema as well. Pain control and providing opportunities for diversional activities, followed by rest and sleep, are essential elements of a successful weaning process.

Adequate psychological preparation and interdisciplinary support reduce anxiety and fear of being unable to breathe and encourage patients to try. Depression invariably creates barriers to motivation. Most important is the patient's trust in the care giver who manages the periods off the ventilator. The care giver's skill, patience, and reassurance calm and relax the person, thereby promoting independent breathing.

Planning and timing are essential elements. The best time to initiate the process is when the patient is most rested. For example, after completing morning care, allow a rest period and then take advantage of peak periods of pain medication. Before beginning, the airway must be clear and the patient positioned properly—at first in the supine position for patients with quadriplegia or high paraplegia for most efficient diaphragm function. When the working diaphragm is supported by abdominal resistance, the VC will be greatest. Later when the patient is in a wheelchair, an abdominal binder can stabilize the abdomen and ease breathing.

Begin time periods off the ventilator for 15 minutes twice a day. Increase the periods depending on how the patient tolerates the process. Monitor progress before, during, and after initial periods by serial evaluation of VC, periodic arterial blood gas analysis, and noninvasive pulmonary gas measurement techniques (especially SaO_2 and $ETCO_2$ levels). Procedure 15–7 suggests a plan to integrate these measures.

Discontinuing the Artificial Airway

The quadriplegic patient, in particular, can rarely tolerate the removal of a tracheostomy tube in one step; thus a gradual process is necessary. Start discontinuing the artificial airway when the patient can maintain spontaneous respiration, maintain acceptable blood gas values on room air, and manage secretions effectively. An intact gag and swallow reflex should also be present.

Usually the larger Portex tube is replaced by a metal trachesotomy tube. Every few days change the tube to a smaller size to reduce the stoma size. Before starting to close the airway for short periods, the tube size should be 6 or less.

To facilitate gradual accommodation to closing the artificial airway, use a small plug to occlude the tracheostomy tube and allow intermittent periods of natural breathing and communication. The airway must be clear before inserting the plug into the tracheostomy tube. The patient may only tolerate this a few minutes each hour at first, but gradually increase the time until the tracheostomy is continuously plugged for 72 hours. Observe carefully throughout this 3-day period. Inability to tolerate the plugged tracheostomy tube when the patient has no difficulty with it unplugged suggests upper airway obstruction—for example, intubation granulomas, tracheal stenosis. Final extubation is per-

Procedure 15–7   Increasing Time Periods Off the Ventilator

Purpose

To withdraw the patient gradually from dependence on the mechanical ventilator by slowly increasing the time periods off the ventilator and, thereby, increasing the strength of the respiration muscles. Respiratory insufficiency must also be prevented.

Action	Rationale
1. Plan to initiate periods off ventilator when patient is most rested and comfortable.	To maximize patient tolerance to procedure.
2. Stay with patient, offer reassurance, and give constant feedback on progress.	To maximize patient cooperation and minimize fear. Psychological support is a key factor to ensure success.
3. Assess current respiratory status (both before and after the weaning period). Perform chest assessment and ensure that the airway is clear. Obtain arterial blood gases for baseline data, then use noninvasive pulmonary gas measurement techniques. Check the VC.	To prevent respiratory insufficiency, weaning criteria must be met.
4. Detach the ventilator source and attach a **T**-piece to the airway from a humidified oxygen source.	This is usually set 10% higher than the FIO_2 on the ventilator to compensate for less accurate control of inspired air.
5. Ask the patient to watch you breathe and to breathe with you.	This, in itself, will help to regulate breathing and minimize feelings of panic. Panic can lead to hypoxia and respiratory arrest.
6. Observe diaphragmatic movement and look for movement of accessory muscles in neck, shoulders, and abdominal muscles.	The objective of gradual removal of patients from mechanical ventilation is to activate these muscles.
7. Monitor pulse and respiratory rate every 5 minutes.	Respiratory distress is indicated by: • Tachycardia or an increase in the heart rate greater than 20 beats per minute from baseline • Tachypnea or an increase of respiratory rate greater than 30 breaths per minute
8. Continually observe general tolerance to procedure.	Be alert for additional signs and symptoms indicating respiratory distress: • Excessive apprehension • Extreme fatigue • Excessive sweating above the level of injury
9. If the patient is not too distressed, arterial blood gases may be drawn before returning to the ventilator to monitor patient's progress or monitor constantly O_2 saturation and/or End Tidal CO_2. Recheck VC (preferred method). Clarify with physician what fluctations are acceptable for individual patients and adjust timing accordingly.	Poor tolerance and therefore general indications to reduce time spent off the ventilator include: • A fall of PaO_2 to below 60 mmHg • A rise in $PaCO_2$ of more than 10 mmHg • A decrease in pH to below 7.25 (Adams 1979) Oxygen saturation indicated by oximetry should not fall below 60 mmHg.
10. Plan weaning periods to start "on the hour."	For ease in scheduling subsequent time periods off the ventilator.
11. Increase time spent off the ventilator gradually from 15 minutes twice a day, to 15 minutes each hour to a whole hour, then 2 hours, and so on as tolerated.	
12. Progress to full days off the ventilator and resume use only at night, then discontinue mechanical ventilation.	As quadriplegic patients are prone to sleep-induced apnea, careful evaluation should be made for *several nights* before mechanical ventilation is discontinued.

formed if the patient is breathing easily, vital signs are stable, and the VC and arterial blood gases are maintained at an acceptable level.

The Kistner tracheal button is another method. Remove the tracheostomy tube and replace with the Kistner button, which allows minimal inspiration of air while it occludes the stoma on expiration so the patient can talk. Most of the air is warmed and humidified as it is inspired through the nose and mouth. If a constant open airway is needed, a fenestrated tube will make communication possible. Techniques for extubation are described in Procedure 15–8. Hoarseness and sore throat can occur on extubation. No treatment is usually necessary. However, if this persists, indirect laryngoscopy should be performed to rule out vocal cord paralysis. The patient should be monitored for excessive fatigue, ease of respirations, maintenance of adequate VC, and stable vital signs. Should distress occur, reintubation may be necessary.

SPECIFIC MANAGEMENT OF PULMONARY COMPLICATIONS

Spinal cord injured patients are at risk of several serious respiratory problems. Risk factors include SCI above T_{10}, associated chest trauma, preexisting respiratory disease, older age, and smoking history. The importance of preventive and restorative measures, discussed in the previous sections, cannot be overstated. Always practice preventive measures to control risk factors. However, when any of these conditions develops, certain additional management approaches are necessary. The following sections describe respiratory complications and their consequences. The symptoms and specific treatment are also discussed. Table 15–4 gives optimal outcome criteria for evaluating the effectiveness of management approaches.

Procedure 15–8   Removal of Tracheostomy Tube

Purpose

To remove the tracheostomy tube without causing respiratory distress and to minimize patient discomfort.

Equipment

- Suction apparatus
- Scissors
- Sterile glove
- Light gauze dressing (sterile)
- Micropore tape

Action

1. Explain procedure to the patient. Point out that the procedure is not painful but may stimulate coughing.

2. Have suction equipment close at hand.

3. Auscultate the patient's chest and clear airway, if necessary, before proceeding.

4. Snip the tie tapes.

5. Don sterile gloves.

6. Use a circular motion to quickly, but gently, remove the tube.

7. Cover the tracheostomy site with a light gauze dressing and micropore tape.

8. Change the dressing every 8 hours or when soiled. Wipe area with saline or sterile water and dry.

9. Assess respiratory status.

Rationale

To promote patient cooperation. Apprehension and panic aggravate breathing difficulties.

The curvature of the metal tracheostomy tube necessitates the movements described. Slight hyperextension of the neck also eases removal.

To avoid skin breakdown, do not use waterproof tape which will completely occlude the area and trap secretions.

Mucus can wet the dressing from the inside. Watch for food and liquids contaminating the dressing on the outside. Allow tracheostomy site to dry and heal naturally. Avoid repeated cleansings and harsh solutions.

TABLE 15–4 Optimal Outcome Criteria for Respiratory Complications

Respiratory complications	Hypoxia	Atelectasis and pneumonia	Pulmonary edema	Pulmonary emboli	Pneumothorax
Alert and oriented; no restlessness	X	X	X	X	X
Normal, unlabored respirations, 12–20 breaths per minute	X	X	X	X (No chest or referred pain)	X (No chest or referred pain)
Blood pressure and pulse within normal limits for patient	X (No internal bleeding)	X	X	X (No signs of internal bleeding)	X
Normal body temperature		X	X	X	X
Good color, free from cyanosis	X	X			X
Lungs clear on auscultation; normal air entry throughout lungs	X	X	X	X (Chest clear; free from pleural friction or signs of consolidation)	X (Trachea midline; symmetrical chest expansion; no evidence of subcutaneous emphysema)
Unproductive cough; sputum		X (Sputum free from infective organisms)	X (No evidence of excess sputum production)		
Arterial blood and pulmonary gas analysis within acceptable range	X	X	X	X	X
VC and pulmonary function values within normal limits for patient	X	X	X	X	X
Chest X ray clear without evidence of consolidation		X	X	X	X (No signs of lung collapse or mediastinal shift)
Lung scan normal or without signs of further deterioration				X	
ECG within normal limits (Free from signs of right-sided heart strain)	X		X	X	
No evidence of thrombophlebitis				X	

Hypoxia

Hypoxia is a diminished availability of oxygen to the body cells and can be caused by internal or external environmental factors. With SCI the fundamental causes of hypoxia are usually related to *impaired neural impulses to breathing muscles* which decrease ventilation; atelectasis ensues. The other major cause of hypoxia is *hemorrhagic or neurogenic shock*, which leads to low cardiac output and decreasing volumes of circulating blood to transport bases.

Increased rapid, shallow breathing; noisy respirations, dyspnea, pale color; tachycardia; and restlessness or irritability are early symptoms of hypoxia. Extrathoracic signs and symptoms will develop eventually if hypoxia is severe.

Management

- Give oxygen supplement as ordered by physician. If high concentrations of oxygen by mask are ineffective, intubation and mechanical ventilation need to be considered.
- Confirm cause with physician and initiate treatment as ordered for underlying condition.

Expected Outcomes

Evaluate effectiveness of treatment according to level of outcome criteria reached:

- Normal, unlabored respirations at a rate of 12 to 20 breaths per minute
- Blood pressure and pulse within normal limits for patient
- Alert and oriented
- Good color, free from cyanosis
- Arterial blood gases within acceptable range of PaO_2 80 to 100 mmHg and $PaCO_2$ 35 to 45 mmHg

Atelectasis and Pneumonia

Atelectasis is a partial or complete collapse of the lung. Alveoli and blood vessels may be involved, leading to diminished blood flow and decreased gaseous exchange to the affected area. *Microatelectasis* or early small airway closure is scattered and not detectable on chest X ray. This subtle problem is a danger to any postoperative or immobilized patient.

Pneumonia results in inflamed, edematous alveoli, blocked with fluid. The lungs become saturated, heavy, and solid, thereby inhibiting gaseous exchange and creating an environment prone to inevitable *infection*. Bacteria, viruses, or aspirate of foreign material are prime causes of infection and inflammation.

Due to immobilization, poor chest expansion, and inability to cough effectively, patients with SCI are predisposed to *hypostatic pneumonia*. Gravity pulls the mucus to the dependent side of the bronchioles. The upper surfaces of the bronchioles then tend to dry out and crack, providing sites for infection, while the lower surfaces allow mucus to pool and become more easily obstructed.

These two conditions, related to secretion retention, are discussed together, as the goals and interventions are similar.

Observe for signs and symptoms of retained secretions, the earliest of which is a *moist cough*. Note the amount and nature of any sputum. Perform a routine chest assessment,

and be alert for dullness on percussion, tactile fremitus, and presence of rales and rhonchi. Examine diagnostic findings for abnormal arterial blood gases, a lowered PaO_2 and/or elevated $PaCO_2$, decreased VC, and signs of consolidation on chest X ray.

Management

Specific management focuses on removing secretions, providing adequate lung examination, and preventing or controlling infection.

- Maintain systemic hydration and bronchial hygiene program.
- Promote lung expansion. High pressures, gradually increased to 40 cm H_2O, may be indicated.
- Give oxygen supplement as ordered. The physician may increase the FIO_2 or flow rate. If mechanical ventilation is in use, the physician may increase the sigh mechanism in frequency and/or volume to ensure adequate deep inflation of the lungs. PEEP may be applied to keep small airways open longer.
- Liquefy secretions for ease of removal. Ensure adequate humidification of all supplemental oxygen. The ultrasonic nebulizer may also be used followed by techniques to mobilize and remove liquefied secretions.
- Remove severe, massive mucus plugs during bronchoscopy (a procedure offering direct visualization and access to the larger airways).
- Observe carefully for signs and symptoms of infection. Monitor temperature rectally every 4 hours (or more frequently if elevated over 40°C [104°F]) and observe sputum for increased amounts or purulence. Take daily specimens for culture and sensitivity. Prevent or control infection by using meticulous suctioning techniques and take measures to avoid any other systemic infections, such as a bladder infection, that will decrease the patient's general resistance.
- Administer therapeutic courses of antibiotic drugs as ordered. Report culture and sensitivity results before beginning antibiotic courses to prevent development of resistance. Because there is a high risk of this complication in long-term care, use prophylactic drugs cautiously.

Expected Outcomes

- Unlabored respirations at a rate of 12 to 20 breaths per minute
- Normal body temperature
- Unproductive cough or sputum, free from infective organisms
- Lungs clear on auscultation
- Chest X ray clear without evidence of consolidation
- PaO_2 80 to 100 mmHg and $PaCO_2$ 35 to 45 mmHg
- Vital capacity within normal limits for patient

Pulmonary Edema

Pulmonary edema causes the lungs to swell and become heavier with fluid, which increases the work of breathing and makes gaseous exchange more difficult. Although pooling of blood in the pulmonary system is most often associated with failure of the left side of the heart, in spinal cord injured patients, particularly those with quadriplegia, this can be due to fluid overload. Too much fluid may have been infused in the mistaken effort to treat neurogenic shock in the same manner as hypovolemic shock. See Chapter 6. A buildup in pulmonary capillary pressure ultimately causes rapid transudation of fluid into the alveoli and interstitial spaces of the lung.

Observe for signs of dyspnea, cough, and hypoxia. Note any amounts of pink, frothy sputum or chest congestion such as rales, which indicates fluid-filled alveoli.

Management

Management of pulmonary edema centers on decreasing venous return to the heart to assist movement of fluid out of the alveoli into the venous circulation, and maintaining adequate ventilation and perfusion.

- Minimize physical and emotional stress to decrease work of the heart and take measures to alleviate shock and avoid pulmonary complications.
- Prevent a positive fluid balance in the body. Maintain a detailed intake and output record. Be sure to include amount and type of fluids administered during transport.
- Take measures to decrease venous return to the heart and help move fluid from alveoli into the systemic circulation. Elevate the head of the bed if possible. Administer intravenously rapidly acting diuretics and cardiotonics as ordered by the physician. Measures such as application of rotating tourniquets to decrease circulating blood volume are contraindicated due to the decreased blood pressure associated with paralysis. Observe for unstable autonomic nervous system control causing sudden onset of shock or respiratory distress.
- Cautiously administer small doses of IV morphine as ordered to decrease respiratory rate, alleviate pain, and control apprehension. Stay with patient.
- Insert Foley catheter for accurate output record. (Intermittent catheterizations are not practical when hourly output should be monitored.)
- Give supplemental oxygen as ordered. Use of IPPB may be contraindicated because the positive pressure created in the chest tends to slow venous return to the heart. Also, if the patient is mechanically ventilated, cautious therapeutic use of PEEP may be desirable to minimize collapse of, or help reopen, alveoli.

Expected Outcomes

Evaluate effectiveness of treatment according to level of outcome criteria reached:

- Unlabored respirations at a rate of 12 to 20 breaths per minute
- Blood pressure and pulse within normal limits for patient
- Lungs clear on auscultation
- Pulmonary function tests and arterial blood gas values within normal limits for patient
- No evidence of excess sputum production
- No evidence of fluid imbalance

Pulmonary Emboli

Occlusion of a pulmonary vessel by an undissolved mass circulating in the bloodstream is known as *pulmonary embolism*. This condition is a major complication during the acute stage. The great majority of pulmonary emboli arise from deep vein thrombosis (DVT) in the legs or pelvic veins (Casas et al. 1977-1978). See Chapter 16. The danger from pulmonary emboli varies greatly depending on the location and extent of resultant lung ischemia. Small emboli may subside undetected, while a massive embolus may cause respiratory arrest.

Patients with SCI are subject to a number of factors that place any patient at risk: prolonged bedrest, recent surgery, hip or extremity fractures, possible deterioration of nutritional status, obesity, advancing age, preexisting heart disease or lung complications, and, of course, thrombophlebitis with subsequent DVT. During the most critical period, that is, for approximately 3 to 5 weeks after injury, spinal shock compromises the situation even further when flaccid paralysis virtually eliminates muscle tone.

Early detection is the best defense against pulmonary embolism. Be constantly alert to subtle or nonspecific changes in the patient's clinical condition, especially during the first 6 weeks after injury, when incidence is greatest. For example, a low-grade fever without evidence of infection may be the only indication that the patient is in potential danger.

To manage pulmonary emboli, inhibit formation of thrombi by preventing venous stasis, avoiding trauma to or pressure on venous walls, and minimizing effects of hypercoagulability of the blood.

Management

- Take measures to promote venous return to the heart and to protect venous walls from undue pressure or trauma. Avoiding dehydration will help maintain normal blood viscosity and clotting time. Detect thrombophlebitis promptly to enable initiation of early treatment. Chapter 16 fully describes how to care for these conditions including DVT.

- Observe for sudden onset of hypoxia, rapid respirations, or dyspnea. The patient may complain of difficulty "catching my breath." Tachycardia and pyrexia are usually present, and the patient is apprehensive. Chest pain may be absent, decreased, or referred due to sensory loss. On chest auscultation, a pleural friction rub or signs of atelectasis or consolidation may be evident. Symptoms may vary from mild to severe.

- Recognize the possibility of fat emboli in those patients with long bone fractures when petechiae are seen, particularly on the chest and neck.

- Stay to calm patient and provide psychological support.

- Provide complete bedrest. Return the patient to bed if up. To help ease breathing, elevate the head of the bed if possible or change patient to side-lying position and remove restrictive braces or clothing. Be sure to communicate the plan to other team members because occupational therapy and physical therapy activities will need to be modified or stopped.

- Give supplemental oxygen as ordered.

- Initiate emergency measures to combat shock or institute cardiopulmonary resuscitation if indicated. Massive emboli that often occur bilaterally are a major cause of death in the early stages. Many times there is no evidence of preexisting DVT. Some patients have a feeling of impending doom and complain of difficulty in breathing or light-headedness before a sudden arrest situation occurs.

- Prepare patient for a battery of tests to confirm diagnosis and assess extent of lung involvement. A diagnostic workup should include complete blood work; arterial blood gases, which may show a drop in PaO_2; chest X ray, which may show evidence of infarctions; and an ECG, which may reveal right-sided heart strain. Nonspecific results are frequently valuable to rule out other conditions. *Lung scanning* has proven more specific for pulmonary embolism than other tests. A radioactive substance (administered intravenously) travels with the blood to outline flow to the lung tissue. Where blood flow is decreased or absent due to ischemic changes (caused by pulmonary emboli or other lung disorders), uptake of the radioisotope will not be possible. A photograph of the results is taken. Areas of normal perfusion will be dark; ischemic areas will be light. Repeat all these tests for serial evaluation.

- Administer anticoagulant therapy as prescribed to prevent further embolization discussed in conjunction with the management of DVT in Chapter 16.

Expected Outcomes

Evaluate effectiveness of treatment by level of expected outcome criteria reached:

- Effortless respiration at a rate of 12 to 20 breaths per minute
- Stable vital signs and normal body temperature
- Chest clear on auscultation, free from pleural friction or signs of consolidation
- Blood work, arterial blood gases within normal limits for patient
- ECG within normal limits (free from signs of right-sided heart strain)
- Chest X ray clear
- Lung scan normal or without signs of further deterioration
- No blood in sputum, nasogastric aspirate, urine, or stool and patient free from other signs of internal bleeding
- No evidence of thrombophlebitis

Pneumothorax

A *pneumothorax* is defined as air in the pleural cavity, that is, air between the parietal pleura of the lungs and the visceral pleura of the chest wall. An *open pneumothorax* occurs with a perforation of the parietal pleura and chest wall providing a continuous opening to the outside air. A *closed or spontaneous pneumothorax* occurs with a rupture of the visceral pleura or underlying lung tissue. When the lung collapses the pleural tear closes. A *tension pneumothorax* is very dangerous because a valvelike tear allows air to pass in but not out. Risks may vary depending on size; a small, spontaneous pneumothorax may respond to oxygen therapy and bedrest while the air is slowly reabsorbed, but larger ones will create a medical emergency. Patients with SCI are most subject to the development of a closed pneumothorax as a complication of mechanical ventilation. There are several risk factors: copious secretions leading to complications such as airway obstruction, bronchitis, or pneumonia; and invasive procedures done in the chest region such as thoracentesis or cardiopulmonary resuscitation (CPR).

A patient fighting the respirator can raise intrathoracic pressures to dangerously high levels, as will application of high pressures of PEEP. One of the principal cautions regarding the use of PEEP is that of ensuring the adequacy of venous return. By elevating the intrapulmonic pressure, and to some extent the intrathoracic pressure, the venous return may decrease (because quadriplegic patients lack sympathetic tone and are unable to raise the venous pressure by vessel constriction to overcome the elevated intrathoracic pressure). As stroke volume decreases, the heart rate increases. Be alert for the development of tachycardia (not ordinarily a feature of quadriplegia) and for further respiratory embarrassment, which could lead to the development of a *pneumothorax* —a not uncommon occurrence when the PEEP exceeds 20 cm of H_2O.

A patient with fractured ribs may also develop a pneumothorax. Discussion in this section focuses on spontaneous pneumothorax developing as a major complication of mechanical ventilation.

Management of a pneumothorax involves evacuating air from the pleural cavity, reexpanding the lung, and preventing infection.

Management

- Recognize onset of pneumothorax immediately. A sudden onset of persistent, stabbing chest pain is the usual symptom. The spinal injured patient may not be able to feel this due to sensory loss or may not be able to communicate discomfort when on the ventilator. The first sign may well come from the ventilator itself when a *sudden increased and sustained pressure is required to ventilate the patient* (peak inspiratory pressure) (Fuchs 1979). Look for signs of hypoxia (tachycardia, tachypnea) and increased dyspnea progressing to distress. Sometimes subcutaneous emphysema on the chest and neck is apparent. The affected side of the chest may be enlarged and fixed (without movement with respiration). On auscultation, breath sounds will be diminished or absent. Look for signs of mediastinal shift (such as a tracheal tug) toward the unaffected side. A chest X ray may show signs of lung collapse and mediastinal shift.
- Notify the physician. Immediately hand ventilate the patient to help prevent high pressures of air from entering the pleural cavity and causing progression to a tension pneumothorax. If possible, elevate the head of the bed.
- Assist physician with chest tube placement and establishment of continuous chest tube drainage.
- Monitor serial chest X rays daily to evaluate improvement or deterioration.
- Administer analgesics, bronchodilators, and antibiotics or steroid preparations (to avoid secondary infection) as ordered by the physician.

Expected Outcomes

Evaluate effectiveness of treatment according to level of expected outcome criteria:

- Alert and oriented
- No chest or referred pain
- Normal respirations at a rate of 12 to 20 breaths per minute
- Symmetrical chest size and expansion
- Normal air entry throughout lungs
- No evidence of subcutaneous emphysema
- Trachea midline
- Blood pressure, pulse, and temperature within normal limits for patient; normal color

- Chest X ray clear without signs of lung collapse or mediastinal shift

LIFETIME RESPIRATORY HEALTH

Long-Term Implications

When assessing people with quadriplegia or high paraplegia who have been paralyzed for some time keep in mind changes in respiratory function that are considered acceptable in light of permanent disability and adjust baseline data as follows:

- Thoracic size and shape. A decreased anterior/posterior diameter caused by intercostal atrophy or contractures may lead to a rigid rib cage (Thomas 1977: 251). As VMT is practiced more, chest *stiffness* will probably decrease. Posture changes (tendency to slump over in the wheelchair) need careful attention because poor posture severely limits respiratory function.
- Chest movement. Anticipate permanent paradoxical breathing. The respiratory rate and rhythm should remain normal at a rate of 12 to 20 breaths per minute.
- Pulmonary function tests. Generally speaking, the overall total lung capacity decreases. A TV of 500 ml and a minimal VC of 1500 ml is considered acceptable under normal conditions, but a VC of 2000 ml is needed to handle a respiratory infection. The ERV, which measures ability to cough, is virtually absent. Review Table 15–1.
- Arterial blood gas analysis. A PaO_2 greater than 80 mmHg and a $PaCO_2$ less than 45 mmHg is considered acceptable. Acid-base balance should be within normal limits.

Patients with injury higher than the T8 level will frequently require assisted coughing and may find postural drainage and clapping necessary to keep the chest clear. However, secretions should be free from infection at all times.

Based on assessment, continue with preventive measures or refer to appropriate resources such as family physician or physical therapist. Remain alert for recurrent respiratory tract infections, keeping in mind that there may be underlying causes such as limited activities, depression, or poor nutrition.

Health Education

Injured persons and families need to know how the level of injury affects breathing or coughing and how to prevent and treat upper respiratory tract infection. Bronchial hygiene programs for quadriplegic and high paraplegic persons focus on hazardous complications associated with retained secretions, primarily pneumonia. Individuals should learn preventive measures to protect themselves from predisposing environmental factors.

Perhaps the single most dangerous factor hampering respiratory health is *smoking*, but despite its obvious evils, many individuals are unable to give it up. Gadgetry has even been developed to enable quadriplegic people to smoke independently! At least such devices promote safety by avoiding burns to the skin or surrounding environment. After prolonged stays in critical care areas where smoking is obviously not possible, some patients are able to quit outright. However, especially outside the hospital setting, the persons themselves must resolve to change.

Avoiding people with a cold or flu, dressing appropriately for the weather to avoid extreme changes in body temperature, and eating a well-balanced diet keep up general resistance and minimize risk of infection. Annual flu shots are recommended.

Should chest congestion or a cold occur, patients and families should understand the importance of a high fluid intake (2500 to 3000 ml) per day unless contraindicated), deep breathing exercises, assisted coughing, postural drainage and clapping, and use of a humidifier. Appropriate team members, such as the community health nurse, should assess the home setting to ensure that these measures are feasible. Individuals should take their temperature and call the family physician at the first sign of congestion.

Some people require a permanent tracheostomy. This and other techniques of caring for the ventilator-dependent quadriplegic person are discussed in the next section of this chapter.

For a review of general information on assessment and implementation of education programs for patients and families, see Chapter 11.

PERMANENT RESPIRATORY SUPPORT SYSTEMS*

Many options are available for people who require permanent respiratory support (Chapter 29). Portable, wheelchair-adaptable ventilators make mobility and independence possible. Other devices allow some people freedom from the ventilator for part of the day. Still others can breathe by using an internal phrenic nerve pacemaker to stimulate the diaphragm. Today even persons with high-level injury to the spinal cord are still able to achieve optimal health, an independent life-style, and adapt to losses of functional ability. Care givers are now challenged to meet the needs of tech-

nology-dependent individuals outside critical care settings (Kirby 1989); International Ventilator Users Network 1991).

Portable Ventilator Systems

To many people with high quadriplegia, the portable ventilator represents independence. This life-support system designed for permanent use is technically sophisticated yet practical: it is simple to use, dependable, economical, and, most important, mobile. Portable ventilator systems provide more choices in respiratory care for persons with high quadriplegia and ultimately improve quality of life (Fuhrer et al. 1987).

The primary respiratory goal for people with high quadriplegia is to establish and maintain *reliable* respiratory support systems that will provide adequate ventilation and lung tissue perfusion. For this to occur, the various components of the support systems must interact efficiently and the disabled person and care givers must collaborate to ensure special considerations are met.

The four basic portable components of a permanent ventilator support system are

- Artificial airway and its components
- Portable suction unit
- Portable mechanical ventilator
- Manual ventilating (resuscitation) bag

Backup systems for all components must be kept readily available. Electrically operated equipment requires planning for power failures. Make arrangements with the community fire department, hospital, paramedics, and local utility companies before discharge.

Special Considerations When Planning and Assessing Ongoing Care for Ventilator-Dependent Persons

The health care team must plan early for the purchase of appropriate specialized equipment so that it is available when the person needs it; otherwise, progress may be significantly hampered. This involves financial considerations (Indihar and Wacker 1986) and psychosocial preparation of the individual and family for using the equipment. Chapter 29 addresses and integrates these vital concerns.

The person is ready for the transition to portable ventilation when these criteria are met:

- Stabilization of vertebral column injury, autonomic nervous system impairment, and general medical condition.

*This section was contributed by Fina Canave Jiminez, R.N., M. Ed.

- Clear lungs, with no evidence of pulmonary infection or disease
- Toleration of room air at FIO_2 of 21% without additional oxygen. Occasionally higher FIO_2 may be necessary.
- Acceptable pulmonary function tests and blood gases determined by the person's baseline.
- Toleration of tracheostomy tube, preferably uncuffed.
- Good sitting tolerance to maintain portable equipment.

Acceptance of new equipment depends on minimizing fear and anxiety. Prepare thoroughly: familiarize persons with the new ventilator equipment and the sensations to expect, and reassure them constantly. Also essential are assigning the same care givers consistently and involving the individuals and families themselves. Listen to the person's questions.

Arrange meetings with other ventilator-dependent persons who have adjusted to portable breathing equipment or on-site visits to long-term and home care settings. Use success stories of ventilator-dependent persons living in the community to encourage positive attitudes. See Chapter 29 for more suggestions about helping persons adjust to lifelong ventilator dependency.

Accommodation to a portable system should be gradual for the sake of physical and psychological well-being. Initial periods on portable equipment may progress from 15-minute intervals to a few hours, then gradually to permanent use. Throughout this process monitor blood oxygen tension levels by arterial samples or ear or pulse oximetry. As always, serial comparison with baseline data obtained while the person was on a larger ventilator best indicate the level of tolerance to the portable one.

Select the peak flow or inspiratory time, volume, and rate controls as ordered by the attending physician. A typical setting might be a respiration rate of 10 to 12 breaths per minute and TV of 800 ml or 15 ml/kg with a cuffed tube or 100 ml with an uncuffed tube to compensate for air escaping around the tracheostomy tube and to prevent microatelectasis. Control settings may be altered slightly for patient comfort.

The *transition* from constant observation in a critical care setting to independence on a portable ventilator requires close monitoring balanced by opportunities to gain freedom and confidence. Ongoing assessment increasingly relies on individual response rather than on sophisticated diagnostic analysis.

Permanent disability changes respiratory function, necessitating adjustment of acceptable baseline data. For instance, persons on long-term mechanical ventilation with an uncuffed tracheostomy tube may not have normal $PaCO_2$ levels. One person on a ventilator with an uncuffed Jackson tracheostomy tube has had a $PaCO_2$ of 15 to 18 with a pH consistently between 7.40 and 7.45 for 15 years without ill effects. In general, the $PaCO_2$ level is irrelevant as long as the pH is in a good range (Peterson 1989).

Ongoing assessment for ventilator-dependent persons evaluates whether ventilation is adequate. Note characteristics of ineffective breathing pattern (dyspnea, shortness of breath, abnormal blood gases, cyanosis, change in rate and quality of ventilatory pattern, altered chest excursion) and impaired gas exchange (confusion, somnolence, restlessness, irritability, hypercapnea, hypoxia, alteration in baseline pulse rate or bradycardia. Monitor VC, SaO_2 (Figure 15–10) and $ETCO_2$ levels (noninvasive), and presence and degree of fatigability, noting trends and how they relate to the ventilator setting and its functioning.

Inspection for hydration of airway is a constant concern and observation of the adequacy of humidification includes:

- Respiratory secretion characteristics including color, odor, amount, and consistency. Thick, sticky, or absent secretions on suctioning probably indicate inadequate humidification
- Thick mucus plugs
- Breath sound abnormalities

A chain of events can occur in the lower airways when humidification of inspired air through the upper airway is inadequate (Allen 1966; Benson et al. 1969):

1. Impairment of ciliary activity
2. Impairment of mucus movement
3. Inflammatory change and necrosis of ciliated pulmonary epithelium
4. Retention of viscid, tenacious secretions with secondary encrustations
5. Bacterial infiltration of mucosa
6. Atelectasis
7. Pneumonia

Consider *environmental factors* such as room heating and air conditioning systems, and climatic or weather changes.

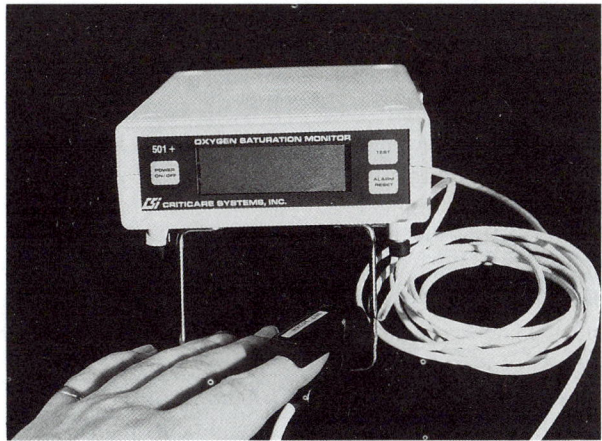

FIGURE 15–10 The noninvasive oxygen saturation monitor is useful for serial evaluation and spot checks.

The cooler and drier the inspired air, the greater the humidity deficit and the more water and heat the body must supply. Carefully monitor body temperature and obtain a culture and sensitivity of the tracheal aspirate if infection is suspected.

Continuing assessment and *care* of persons on portable ventilators focuses on promoting optimal respiratory function and recognizing respiratory insufficiency. Assess the person carefully when changing machines or switching from wall to battery power. If the person complains of not receiving enough air, consider problems in addition to those previously mentioned, including a ventilator that performs properly on wall power but inadequately on battery power. The person may feel that not enough air is being forced into the lungs or that the respiratory rate is too slow. In this situation, substitute another ventilator and have a maintenance service investigate the mechanical problem.

The Artificial Airway (Permanent Tracheostomy)

To sustain an artificial airway, the *reusable metal tube (uncuffed)* is more suitable for long-term or permanent use. Uncuffed tubes provide a vital means for access to a controlled airway. Additionally they protect the lower airway and ease maintaining tracheobronchial hygiene. They ease removal of secretions and decrease the effort involved in breathing by reducing physiological dead space.

The stabilized ventilator-dependent person can "talk around" this uncuffed tube as air escapes through the mouth and nose on expiration. Uncuffed tubes permit the person to talk while on mechanical ventilation. Air is expired directly around the uncuffed tracheostomy tube, over the vocal cords, and out through the mouth and nose. With practice, a person can time speech with the cycling of the ventilator. It is also possible to eat freely.

Double cannula stainless steel and hard plastic tracheostomy tubes are widely used for long-term airway maintenance with mechanical ventilation because they are easy to insert and clean and are durable. Metal tubes such as the Jackson tracheostomy tube tend to cause less local tissue reaction, less mucus production, and may be left in place longer than the plastic types (Peterson 1989; Giovanni, Keeney, and Plummer 1986). Also, the lining of the trachea and the skin at the tracheostomy site do not adhere to such tubes, reducing the risk of necrosis. Because they last longer, metal tubes are less costly than disposable plastic tubes. The hard, rigid, plastic tubes may cause pressure necrosis and discomfort.

Metal tubes are available in narrow diameter and short lengths to provide the smallest functional artificial airway possible. Correct size is important. For adults, Jackson-type sizes 5, 6, and 7 are most frequently used. The higher the number, the larger the external diameter. Metal tubes have

two parts: the outer cannula and a removable inner cannula, with an obturator with blunted end for insertion. An appropriate-size adapter connects to the air tubing of the ventilator (Figure 15–11). For normal use, the inner cannula remains locked in place inside the outer cannula. The proximal part of the tracheostomy tube is the flange to which ties are secured to fasten it to the neck of the patient. Once the outer cannula is secured with tie tapes, the inner cannula can be removed as needed for cleaning without changing the tracheostomy tube. Use normal saline or hydrogen peroxide to remove crusting and return and lock the inner cannula into place again. A weekly change is usually sufficient, unless secretions increase.

Other tracheostomy tubes for long-term mechanical ventilation include the fenestrated tracheostomy tube that has an opening or a "window" into the posterior wall of the outer cannula. It directs air through the upper respiratory tract, making speech possible.

The tube selected depends on the needs of the individual: the person's anatomic airway contours, physiological requirements, minimal or absence of tissue reaction or trauma, economy, and comfort.

When a tracheostomy is well established, the dangerous possibility of it closing over when the tube is removed is almost nonexistent. Review Procedure 15–9. Always take safety precautions when washing or bathing: prevent soap, water, or shampoo from entering the tracheostomy

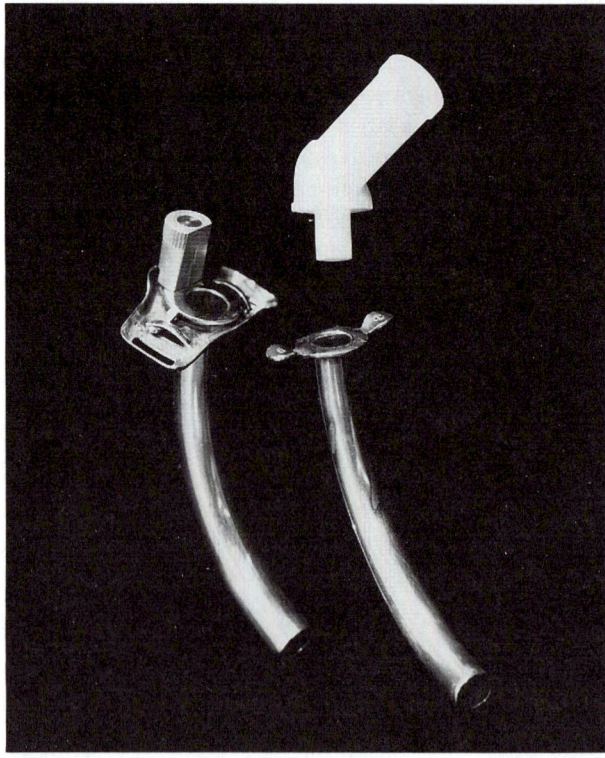

FIGURE 15–11 Metal tracheostomy tube: Outer cannula, inner cannula and adapter. (Obturator for insertion not shown)

Procedure 15–9   Changing Tracheostomy Tube

Purpose

To change the tracheostomy tube either for cleaning or to reduce size of stoma.

Equipment

- Metal tracheostomy tube set including an obturator, inner and outer cannula, and tie tapes
- Rigid plastic adapter for connection between the tracheostomy tube and the respiratory fitting
- Oxygen source
- Sterile gloves and masks

- Scissors
- Tracheal dilators (Trousseau)
- Spare Portex-tube within easy reach
- Sterile dressing tray; tracheostomy dressing
- Hand resuscitation bag
- Suction equipment and catheter

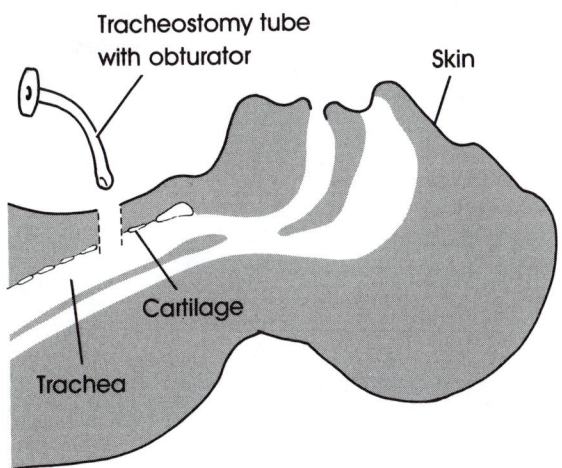

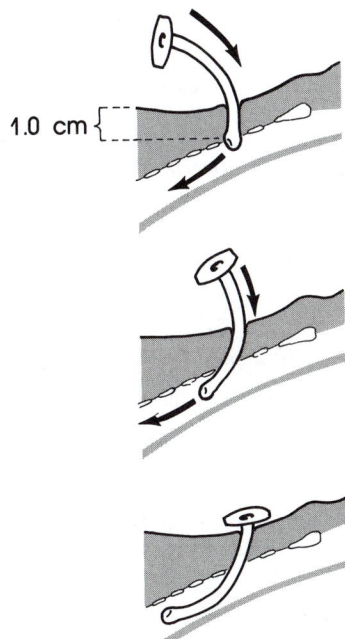

Action

1. Explain procedure to the patient. Point out that the procedure is not painful but may stimulate coughing.

2. Check suction equipment for working order. Connect catheter (correct size for tracheostomy tube) to suction tubing. Leave suction turned on.

3. Have hand resuscitation bag with tracheostomy adapters and an oxygen source at hand.

4. Have a set of tracheal dilator forceps on hand.

5. Open dressing tray and tracheostomy set and prepare sterile field.

6. Rinse tracheostomy adapters with sterile water and place at edge of sterile field.

7. Place sterile lubricant on sterile field.

Rationale

This helps relieve fear and gain the cooperation of the patient. If the patient is apprehensive or panics during the procedure, breathing difficulty will be aggravated.

In an emergency, equipment must be immediately available.

Emergency equipment is useless unless connecting adapters fit correctly.

Should the tube become accidentally dislodged, these special forceps will open the stoma and allow air entry.

Adapters are often soaked in antiseptic solutions.

(Procedure continues)

Procedure 15–9   Changing Tracheostomy Tube (continued)

Action	Rationale
8. Don sterile gloves and check to see that the inner cannula fits easily into the outer cannula. Also check to see that the tracheostomy adapter attaches securely to the inner cannula.	Technically the sterilized components of metal tracheostomy sets are interchangeable, but with use this is not always so.
9. Place the obturator inside the outer cannula and apply a small amount of sterile lubricant to the tip of the obturator. The tracheostomy dressing may be placed around the tube at this time.	
10. Suction patient to clear airway if needed and preventilate with a couple of "sigh" breaths before disconnecting the ventilator.	This increases patient tolerance to procedure.
11. Snip the tie tapes and deflate the cuff before removal. Use your dominant hand for maneuvering the metal tracheostomy tube.	
12. Using one hand (nondominant hand), quickly but gently remove the Portex-tube; with the other hand insert the metal tracheostomy tube. Advance the tip of the obturator approximately 1.0 cm (about 3/8 to 1/2 inch) to allow entry into the trachea; continue advancement using a continuous circular motion.	Attention must be directed toward the curvature of the metal tracheostomy tube, which necessitates the movements described. Slight hyperextension of the neck also eases insertion.
13. Immediately remove the obturator; insert the inner cannula (which has the adapter already attached); and connect the respirator tubing.	
14. Allow the patient several respirations, then proceed to suction through the new tracheostomy tube.	This ensures the patency of the new artificial airway.
15. Auscultate the chest and observe for chest wall expansion.	This is necessary to check for adequate air entry.
16. Secure tube with the tapes. Knot tapes rather than tying in a bow.	This prevents accidental extubation.
17. Place a piece of elastic over the respirator tubing at the tracheostomy connection site and anchor to each side of the outer cannula.	This prevents accidental dislodging of respirator tubing.
18. Assess respiratory status.	

by placing a protective shield over the tracheostomy tube. When showering, direct water spray at chest level or lower.

Use lightweight, swivel-type connectors that can pivot freely, and lightweight ventilator tubings to prevent pulling on the tube. Move persons smoothly to avoid excessive tugging on the tracheostomy tube.

Maintaining Airway Patency

Ineffective airway clearance exists when an individual is unable to clear secretions or obstructions from the respiratory tract to maintain airway patency (McLane 1987). Maintaining adequate fluid intake and an adequate bronchial hygiene program to mobilize secretions is necessary throughout life to reduce risks. Maintaining a bronchial hygiene program is easier for younger persons with healthy lungs than for those with a history of smoking,

allergies, repeated respiratory infections or preexisting lung disease.

Suctioning is the key to maintaining airway patency (an open airway). This procedure removes secretions from the trachea and mainstem bronchi when normal mechanisms for coughing to clear secretions are impaired. Suctioning is most effective following bronchial hygiene techniques. Persons well established on a portable ventilator may be able to inform the care giver of the need for suctioning. Signs of ineffective airway clearance are described in the Physical Assessment section of this chapter.

Frequency of suctioning varies considerably from one individual to another. Suctioning is rarely necessary on an hourly basis unless pulmonary complications are evident, and it should never be done routinely. There must be evidence of tracheal secretions. Unnecessary suctioning may irritate the mucosa and stimulate secretion production. Therefore, take care to perform suctioning gently to avoid any tracheal trauma. Performed correctly, it is an atraumatic procedure. Mid rotation and gradual withdrawal of the suction catheter, with application of intermittent suction, minimizes mucosal damage and aspirates secretions more effectively.

When suctioning a person, especially one with high quadriplegia, be alert for an abnormal vasovagal response that may cause severe bradycardia or possibly cardiac arrest (Mathias 1976). See Chapter 6. Use gentle technique and prevent hypoxia to minimize this risk. Stop suctioning immediately if the person looks or feels faint (syncope). Check pulse and reestablish ventilation. Let the person rest and then resume the procedure. Always weigh airway patency against the potential risk of suctioning.

Suctioning poses other potential hazards to both the care giver and the person. Take every precaution when there is risk of Acquired Immune Deficiency Syndrome (AIDS), including wearing gloves, protective goggles, and a mask or mouth shield when performing manual ventilation. Many authorities recommend considering everyone's blood, body fluids, and secretions hazardous (Mapp 1988).

Unless an emergency makes it impossible, use good *handwashing* technique before starting any suction procedure. Sterile technique is required during the acute phase, but *clean* technique is generally used for suctioning in long-term care and home settings. Clean technique is practical and convenient, reducing costs for supplies by more than 80% compared to sterile technique. It is not associated with increased infection in the home setting (Walsh and Kirkpatrick 1988). Clean aseptic tracheostomy care techniques are as safe in terms of level of infection as are sterile techniques (Harris and Hyman 1984). Variations of methods may be equally effective.

Choose the right size suction catheter. It should be large enough so that secretions do not block it, yet small enough to enter the airway. A rule of thumb is that the suction catheter should not occupy more than one half of the inside diameter of the tube being suctioned (Shapiro, Harrison, Kazmarek, and Cane 1985; Harper 1981). Select a soft, smooth, pliable catheter that is firm enough not to collapse when suction is applied. It should have a molded open end and side holes to prevent mucosal trauma and be long enough (20 to 22 inches) to pass the tip of the tube easily (Shapiro et al. 1985). Many disposable catheters are too stiff unless warmed—which is inconvenient. Rubber catheters, especially the cheaper variety, tend to become brittle with repeated sterilization.

Suction catheters should have minimal friction resistance passing through the tracheostomy tube. Catheters made of siliconlike material decrease friction; water does not adhere to them so they do not require lubrication. Suctioning should never exceed 15 seconds at negative pressure of 80 to 120 mmHg. When the suction catheter is placed on the airway and vacuum is applied, room air (21% oxygen)

enters around the catheter. Bagging with enriched oxygen at this stage is not necessary.

Prolonged suctioning removes air from the tracheobronchial tree. It may be necessary to give manual ventilation or reconnect the person to the ventilator for at least five breaths before repeating the suctioning process. Observe the person's facial gestures and check for cues.

Do not forget to suction the stoma around the tracheostomy tube for any visible secretions and do not reinsert the catheter into the trachea. Visible secretions can also be removed with lint-free tissue wipes. Lint irritates the airway.

Ventilatory support must be reestablished immediately after suctioning. Reconnect the person to the ventilator. Cover the end of suction-connecting tubing with gauze sponge, plastic bag, or other protective covering between suctioning events.

During suctioning, observe for significant changes in nature of secretions (blood-tinged or tenacious secretions). Slight bleeding indicates overly vigorous suctioning technique and the application of high suctioning pressures. Thick sticky secretions on suctioning may indicate inadequate humidification or may be a complication of systemic dehydration or pulmonary infection. This may require instillation of 3 to 5 ml of normal saline into the tracheostomy tube at the beginning of the suctioning procedure followed by giving a few breaths with the ventilator or a manual resuscitator bag. How much saline to instill depends on how often the person needs suctioning and the tenacity of secretions. As much as 10 ml may be needed to loosen and remove thick mucus or plugs (Mapp 1988). Use of a unit-dose squeeze vial of normal saline is recommended, because it is efficient and poses less risk of bacterial contamination than a stock or multidose vial. When instilling with a syringe, use without a needle.

Reusable catheters are good for home care. Rinse any parts that have been in contact with mucus. To clean, thoroughly rinse with cold tap water; boil for 5 minutes. Soak the catheter in a mixture of equal parts of water and hydrogen peroxide to loosen secretions. As an alternative when rushed or traveling, soak the catheter in a basin of vinegar solution (one part vinegar to two parts water) and rinse. Place in a dry towel for storage. Order two sets of inner parts (bottles and tubing) for flexibility and convenience when cleaning. A foot-operated (nonbattery) suction apparatus, although outdated, is a useful backup system. A 60 cc large syringe or manual suction traps (Deelee Sputum traps with filters for care givers' protection) are also useful in emergencies or when traveling.

Insert suction catheter 6 to 10 inches in adults in order to ensure adequate depth. If the catheter is not passed beyond the end of the artificial airway, secretions can accumulate at the end of the tracheostomy tube and cause complete airway obstruction (Beland and Passos 1981).

The proximal end must have an opening that neutralizes the vacuum in the catheter without turning off the suction apparatus, allowing the vacuum apparatus to remain on without subatmospheric pressure being transmitted to the catheter. When suction is desired, the proximal hole is occluded with the thumb and the vacuum transmitted to the catheter. The proximal hole must be larger than the internal diameter of the catheter so than when unoccluded there will be less resistance to room air entering the proximal hole than tracheal air through the distal tip. This ensures that tracheal suctioning will occur only when the proximal hole is occluded.

Providing Adequate Humidification

The upper airway cleanses, heats, and humidifies inspired air and thus maintains hydration of the mucous blanket, part of the pulmonary defense mechanism that cleans the lungs through its ciliary activity and appropriate mucus production (Wanner 1979). Mucus viscosity is primarily dependent on its water content.

Maintain 100% humidity and warmth (35°C to 37°C) of inspired air to prevent tenacious to dried, retained secretions. If an artificial airway is used, these secretions collect on the ends or sides of the tracheostomy tube and within the airway itself, but with appropriate humidification and warmth of inspired air, this crusting and obstruction is rare, and results in less frequent changing of tracheostomy tubes. Persons with high quadriplegia need humidifiers to warm and humidify inspired air. See the section on humidifiers in the Mechanical Ventilation section of this chapter. Also, *maintain adequate systemic hydration orally* (2 to 3 liters per day) to prevent the production of thick and tenacious mucus.

Minimizing Airway Contamination

Respiratory equipment, artificial airways, and interruption of normal defense mechanisms in the respiratory tract caused by SCI increase the risk of infection. Understanding distinctions among the concepts of contamination, colonization, and infection, as described by Shapiro and associates (1985), is helpful.

When bacteria are present where they do not normally exist, the area is said to be *contaminated*. Regardless of how well an artificial airway is maintained, airway contamination is inevitable. Respiratory equipment such as the ventilator circuitry are also subject to bacterial contamination. *Colonization* occurs when an organism is present without evidence of infection. Cultures of sputum obtained from persons with artificial airways usually will be positive; thus colonization is to be expected (Comhaire and Larry 1981). Preventing bacterial colonization may be a worthwhile area for investigation, but it is impossible. *Infection* is the presence of inflammation secondary to a microorganism. Do not confuse contamination or colonization with infection of the airway. Despite the strictest airway maintenance

procedures, the risk of lower airway infection is always present. Infection must be clinically diagnosed (fever, increase in the white blood cell count, positive laboratory data, change in color, amount, and consistency of secretion, presence of abnormal breath sounds, chest X-ray evidence of pulmonary infiltrates) and treated with appropriate antibiotic therapy; contamination and colonization must be evaluated but are not treated.

Care meticulously for the permanent tracheostomy site, a primary site of bacterial colonization. Whenever the tube is changed closely observe for redness, swelling, bleeding, purulent drainage, and the condition of the surrounding skin. Care for the skin at the tracheostomy site daily or as necessary with hydrogen peroxide—do not use powder or lotion. Tracheostomy ties are also usually changed when caring for the stoma. The person must know the early signs of infection of the trache site and respiratory tract and learn and establish a preventive maintenance program before hospital discharge.

Always properly clean and disinfect respiratory equipment. Care givers must use aseptic techniques when handling and setting up respiratory equipment. Use single-person ventilator circuits; schedule regular changes of suction and ventilator tubings and filters; carefully drain condensation out of tubing so it does not stagnate.

Securing the Airway and Breathing System

Maintaining a secure connection between the person's tracheostomy tube and breathing system is critically important, a major factor in planning for potential independence and safety at home. Accidental disconnection is a universal concern, but few antidisconnection mechanisms exist.

Disconnection is most likely between the tracheal tube connector and the adapter, humidifier connections, and exhalation valve connections, as well as misthreaded cascade jar assembly. Sometimes care givers establish connections in the breathing system too gently or loosely. Also, spasms, high pressure in the breathing circuit, various movements of the breathing system or the patient, water in the circuit, and the weight or tension of the tubing can apply enough force to disconnect the equipment inadvertently. Reusing disposable parts and repeated disassembly or sterilization can also contribute to disconnections by diminishing the strength of assembled connections or by compromising the integrity of other parts of the breathing circuit (Janowski 1984).

Several types of antidisconnection devices and methods are available including straps, hooks, adapter knobs, springs, locking connectors, and even rubber bands that secure the tracheostomy and loop over the connector (Carter 1987). A tracheostomy adapter lock system has been developed recently. The Pearson Lock—a one-piece, hardplastic adapter—has a spring-loaded pin on the outer cannula of the metal tracheostomy tube that securely locks the adapter into place. The graspable lock allows easy access to the airway for suctioning or emergency purposes. See Figure 15–12.

Take the following safety precautions against accidental disconnection of the patient's airway and breathing system (Janowski 1984):

- Be constantly aware of the possibility of disconnection.
- Always respond immediately to the patient, then to the machine, every time the alarm sounds.
- Secure tracheostomy tube with knot tapes rather than tying in a bow.
- Arrange and support ventilator tubing so that tubing does not pull on the tracheostomy tube.
- Secure all tubing before and after turns.
- Check that alignment of the patient's head and neck is in neutral position.
- Check the entire breathing system and airway thoroughly when a disconnection is suspected.
- Twist, rather than push, components together to make connections more reliable.
- Prevent high-pressure buildup in the breathing circuit. Keep tubing drained of condensation and maintain adequate airway.
- Regularly retrain and review the skills of care givers in the use of equipment.

No matter how sophisticated the technology, the best insurance against accidental disconnection is the responsi-

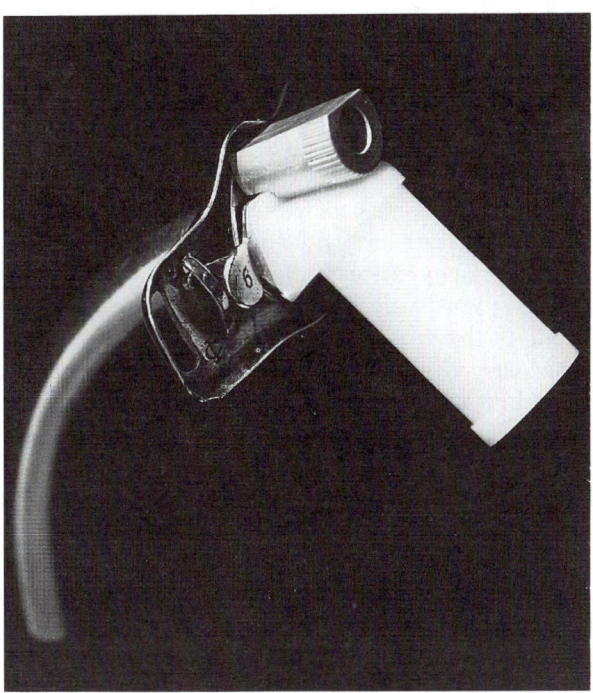

FIGURE 15–12 The silver Pearson Lock (Pearson Centre, Vancouver, BC, Canada) fits above the white adapter.

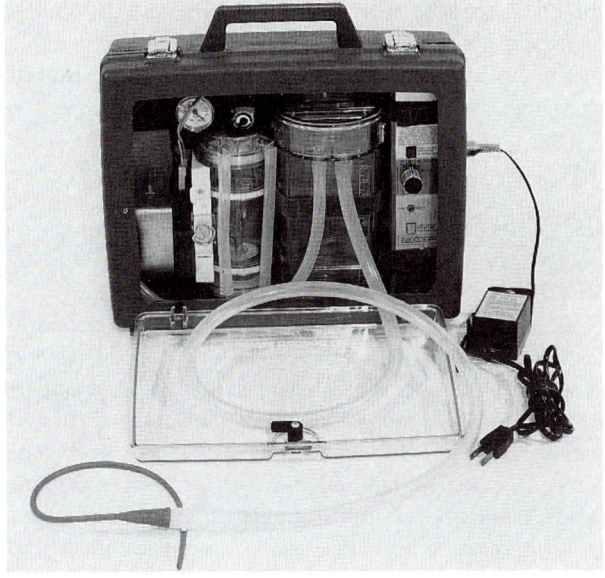

FIGURE 15–13 The Laerdal Suction Unit.

ble care that experienced care givers provide ventilator-dependent persons (Janowski 1984).

The Portable Suction Unit

Portable suction units run on internal and external battery power as well as standard or car-lighter outlets. An example is the versatile Laerdal Suction Unit,* an emergency aspirator used in rescue vehicles (Figure 15–13). Be familiar with the power source, operating time, principles of operation, and maintenance procedures.

The Laerdal unit is a high-vacuum, free air-flow system well suited for tracheal suction. It has four components: a power pack and control panel containing internal batteries and power selection switch; a piston-driven motor pump unit that creates a vacuum in the attached cylinder; a vacuum bottle that collects aspirated material; and suction tubing to which a T connector and catheter can be attached. This equipment is mounted in a small briefcase-size carrier.

Operating time depends on battery capacity, load during practical use, and voltage. Realistic operating times for continuous suction on fully charged internal batteries are 60 to 80 minutes at half-power (6V) and 35 to 40 minutes at full strength (12 V). Full power supplies a powerful suction of 600 mmHg and an airflow of 30 liters per minute. Full to half strength is generally sufficient power to aspirate normal respiratory secretions.

The batteries in portable suction units can accept a continuous charge without overcharging from a wall outlet, the most convenient source among available charging options. Recharging may take 14 to 16 hours. Equipment

*Laerdal Medical Corporation, 136 Marbeldale Road, Tuckahoe, NY 10707.

should be checked every 30 days. Be sure to establish and follow an appropriate charging routine. Newer portable suction units can operate on AC current and have reduced charging time and built-in pressure gauges.

The Portable Ventilator and Breathing Circuit

Ventilator Characteristics and Features

Users and care givers must know the characteristics and features of the ventilator and circuit in use; be aware that accepting a portable ventilator is a gradual process; understand respiratory management principles; and prevent and manage common problems associated with long-term ventilator support. Be familiar with the mode of operation, power requirements, the operating time, indicators and controls, the mobility of the user, the ease of positioning the ventilator, and the maintenance of the equipment.

The portable ventilator operates on room air and is designed for use with a pneumobelt, a mouthpiece, or, for high spinal cord injured persons, a tracheostomy. Most portable ventilators weight 26 to 30 lb allowing easy transport. Volume ventilators are widely used.

A portable ventilator pushes air into the lungs as a piston pump moves back and forth inside a cylinder. The speed and rate of movement of the piston are controlled by an electronic motor. When the piston moves forward, it pushes air from the cylinder into the lungs via the circuit. When the piston pulls back, it fills the cylinder with room air for the next breath. Exhalation is thus natural. The piston does not pull air from the lungs: the elastic lung tissues naturally recoil.

The LP6, a microprocessor-controlled volume ventilator, operates on a brushless motor-driven piston, a time-cycled device with variable volume and rate control (Figure 15–14).* The unit's power source is either a 110-volt AC current (wall outlet) or a 12-volt DC auto battery (external) for wheelchair, automobile, or air travel. A limited internal battery is used primarily as a backup system for short periods such as during transfer of a patient from one power source to another. The unit should be plugged into a wall outlet unless the person is moving around in the wheelchair.

The LP6 unit automatically selects the power source, choosing first the AC current, for an indefinite operating time, then the external battery for as long as 24 hours (when

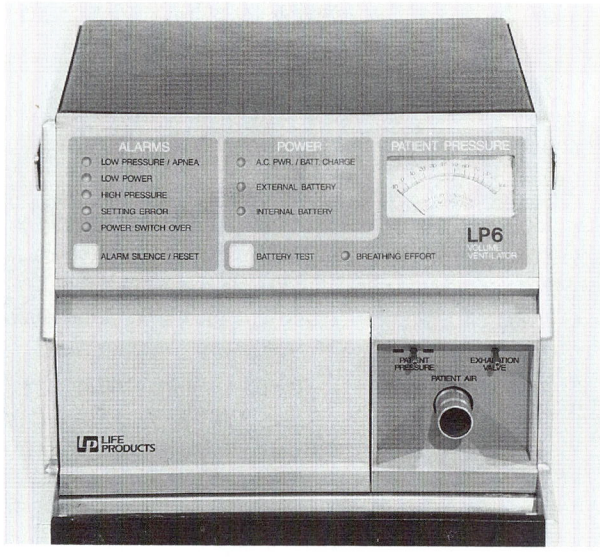

FIGURE 15–14   The LP6 volume ventilator.

fully charged), and finally the internal battery for as long as one hour. Actually, realistic estimates of reliability are 12 to 16 hours for the external battery and 45 minutes for the internal battery, after which times older units may switch back and forth between power sources, creating alarm and risk of ventilator failure. Therefore, be sure the external battery is sufficiently recharged to last as long as desired.

The LP6 automatically recharges whenever the unit is connected to a wall outlet (whether or not the unit is operating). Charging time is about 1.5 times the operating time, thus, 8 to 10 hours operating time requires that the unit be plugged in 12 to 15 hours. Other units without this powerful feature may not allow the person as much time up as desired; a standard heavy-duty battery charger is then usually needed. Some portable ventilators have to be set to the "charge" position to recharge the battery effectively. Other ventilators automatically charge in any mode position, for example, the Lifecare PLV–100. Whatever the system, it is essential to understand, adopt, and follow a recharging policy.

The LP6 has simplified indicators and controls covered by a magnetic door to prevent accidental change of settings. The front control panel may face either forward or upward. The rate control is adjustable from 1 breath-per-minute increments to 20 breaths-per-minute, and 2 breaths-per-minute increments to 38 breaths-per-minute, and the volume control is adjustable from 100 to 2200 ml. The LP6 emphasizes delivery of a preset volume of air, adjusting pressure from -10 to +100 cm H_2O. There are also audible and visual alarms for high or low pressure and power failure. Lights indicate the power source in use. Supplemental oxygen may be added into the circuit or ventilator intake.

Cleaning and maintenance are as important for ventilators as for artificial airways. Hospital procedures are more

*Examples of volume ventilators include the LP6 (Aequitron Medical Inc., 14800 28th Ave. North Minneapolis, MN 55447); Bear 33 (Bear Medical Systems Inc., 2085 Rustin Ave., Riverside, CA 92507); Companion 2800 Portable Volume Ventilator (Puritan Bennett Corporation, 4865 Sterling Dr., Boulder CO 80301, Life Care PLV–100, 5606 Central Ave., Boulder, CO 80301); and the Thompson MiniLung previously referred to as the Bantam Respirator (also of Puritan Bennett Corporation). Because the LP6 is particularly suited for persons with SCI, it is used as a model to describe portable mechanical ventilation.

rigid than at-home procedures and include sterilization because of the risk of infection from cross-contamination. Dust the ventilator with a damp cloth and change the bacterial filter every 2 to 4 weeks. Vendors can provide monthly preventive maintenance and check functioning of home respiratory equipment. O'Donahue and colleagues (1986) recommend checks of TV, rate, pressure, and alarm functions, calibrating them if necessary; check of filters; and regular review of overall function and maintenance per manufacturer's specifications. Also evaluate personal adjustment to the machine and ability to troubleshoot the ventilatory support system.

Ventilator Alarms

Ventilator alarms are necessary for safety. However, many portable ventilators are not equipped with reliable alarm systems. There are two basic categories of built-in ventilator alarms: high pressure and low pressure alarms to signal disconnections, leaks, or blockages in the circuit, and electrical outage alarms. Because of concerns that a power outage or ventilator failure may invalidate all built-in alarms simultaneously, an independent, battery-operated, external (not part of the ventilator) low pressure alarm such as the Ventronics low pressure alarm is recommended (Carter 1987). Every care giver must know how to respond to ventilator alarms. Plan emergency procedures and be able to use a manual resuscitation bag.

Humidifiers

A portable *humidifier* with a passive condenser is located in the air hose assembly in the LP6. Active humidification with the addition of any standard in-line humidifier is also possible. the two kinds of humidifiers commonly used for long-term mechanical ventilation are the *water reservoir*, such as a cascade humidifier (Figure 15–15A), and the *hygroscopic condenser*, such as the "artificial nose" (Figure 15–15B). The latter is not as effective as the former for extended use but can be used for short periods of time or transport. Moisture generated during expiration can be used during the next inspiratory phase. Some individuals may not need external humidification for brief periods. (O'Donahue et al. 1986)

Not all water reservoir models monitor temperature or have alarms to signal high gas temperature or low water level. Failure to monitor temperature may cause thermal injury to a person's airway. Place a temperature probe in the breathing circuit as close to the individual as possible.* Keep the water level in the jar at the recommended level as marked on the reservoir. Distilled water is preferred. Do not allow the water level to fall below the refill line because that would decrease effective humidification. Always place the humidifier below the level of the person to prevent backflow of water to the lungs.

The Breathing Circuit

A *breathing circuit*, the connection between the person's breathing tube and ventilator, pushes air from the ventilator to the user. Inspired air from the ventilator goes through a humidification system to avoid drying of the airway secretions. The components include a 7-inch flex hose attached to the tracheostomy tube adapter, an exhalation valve or manifold, and ventilator hoses or tubings with attachments

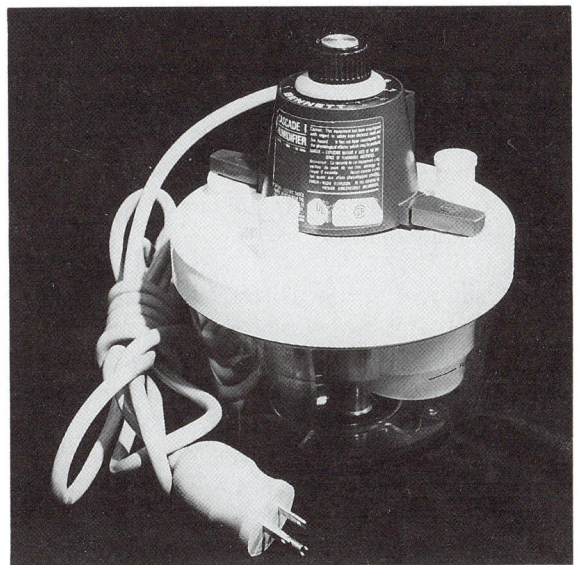

A

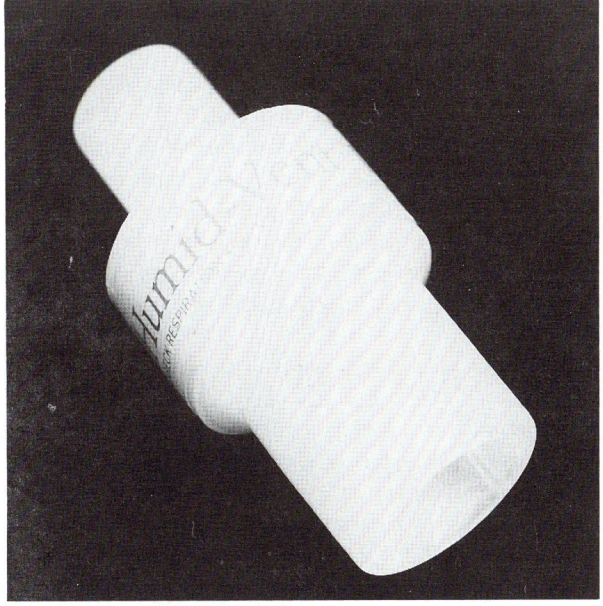

B

FIGURE 15–15 A cascade humidifier (**A**) and an "artificial nose" (**B**).

---

*Disposable and permanent probes are available from Intec Medical, Inc., 2220 East 40 Hwy., Blue Springs, MO 64015.

to the humidifier. A secure fit between connections in the circuit prevents leaks and disconnection.

Before connecting the person to the ventilator, complete the recommended routine safety check (LP6 Ventilator Users' Manual 1988).

1. *Check the prescribed settings on the control panel.*
2. *Check alarm signals* (both audible and visual) by turning ventilator to an operating mode and pushing the alarm silence/reset button.
3. *Check high pressure alarm by blocking circuit.* Confirm that the alarm signals when pressure gauge exceeds high pressure limit.
4. *Check low pressure alarm by disconnecting circuit.* Confirm that alarm signals when pressure meter indicates that pressure has not achieved low pressure setting for two consecutive breaths.
5. Before connecting the person, *check volume* being delivered at the user end of the circuit on ventilator volume control with a respirometer.

If the ventilator does not function correctly, contact a dealer or alternate. A backup ventilator is needed immediately whenever the ventilator in use malfunctions or fails. Have an emergency procedure for times when a backup system is not available.

Ventilator circuits may be *disposable* or *reusable*. Due to lower cost, the latter are often preferred for long-term care. Two or three circuits are generally recommended for home care. Frequency of circuit changes and cleaning techniques vary but clean rather than sterile technique is usually recommended. For home use, this equipment should be washed in warm water and dishwashing detergent to remove all foreign matter, followed by soaking in a vinegar solution (one part vinegar to two parts water) then rinsed and completely air dried. Clean tubing should be kept in plastic bags in a clean, dry area. Circuit changes in long-term or home-care settings may be necessary only two or three times a week (O'Donahue et al. 1986). A study of ICU patients demonstrated that persons receiving circuit changes at 24 hours had a higher rate of infection than those at 48 hours (Craven et al. 1986). These data also indicate that less frequent tube changes are more cost effective and beneficial.

The Manual Ventilating Bag

The *manual ventilating or resuscitation bag* is a vital accessory for ventilator-dependent individuals and must be available at all times. Various models incorporating different types of valves are available today. Choose a ventilating bag made of pliable material if it is easy to compress; continued use is less tiresome. Dismantle the apparatus and check that the valve is inserted correctly to allow a free intake of air. Squeeze the bag and check for leaks. For individual use, keep the 6-inch flex tubing with appropri-

ate-size tracheostomy adapter attached to the bag, and store the unit in a plastic drawstring bag on the wheelchair or at the bedside.

To perform manual ventilation or "bagging," first squeeze the resuscitation bag to check integrity of the valve. Connect the bag directly to the tracheostomy via an appropriate-size adapter. Inflate the person's lungs by squeezing the bag with both hands. Administer 12 to 15 breaths-per-minute or ventilate at the appropriate rate for the person.

Wash the manual resuscitator bag after each use with soap and water until all foreign material is removed and then soak in a solution of three parts water to one part vinegar for 15 minutes (Brown 1985).

Other Respiratory Support Devices and Techniques

Phrenic Nerve Pacers

A phrenic nerve pacer (diaphragm pacing) can provide needed ventilatory support for some high quadriplegic persons in the home or community. It generates breathing through electrical stimulation of the phrenic nerve causing the diaphragm to contract. Electrodes are surgically implanted around the phrenic nerve either in the thorax or neck.

First implanted by Judson and Glenn in 1966, phrenic nerve pacemakers are infrequently used (Lake 1988). Successful candidates must have an intact phrenic nerve, that is, the lower motor neurons must be preserved so the reflex arc is able to react to the electric charge of the pacemaker. The spinal cord must also be free from trauma at the C_4 segmental level. Because this cord level corresponds with the more frequently injured C_{3-5} vertebrae, the possibility of phrenic pacing is relatively rare for people with SCI. However, if injury is sustained at the C_{1-2} vertebrae and the C_4 segmental level is intact, a pacemaker can be used. After spinal shock passes, prognosis can be determined by fluoroscopic examination, to visualize diaphragmatic excursion, and transcutaneous nerve conduction studies to determine phrenic nerve response to electrical stimulation.

The phrenic nerve pacemaker is an external, battery-operated, transmitter-antenna unit that activates internal implants. It has three major components: an electrode cuff, implanted in the neck or thorax circumventing the phrenic nerve near its origin; a receiver unit, secured internally in a subcutaneous pouch just below the rib cage; and an external transmitter-antenna unit (D'Agostino and Welch 1979).

When the phrenic nerve is stimulated, the diaphragm descends, pulling air into the lungs. To activate the phrenic nerve, a current flows from the transmitter to the antenna, then to the internal receiver to the electrode cuff, which stimulates the diaphragm to move. A person with quadriplegia may need as long as 3 months to build tolerance to full pacing.

Lee, Mathews, and Yarkony (1989) describe several pacing schedules: for instance, bilateral diaphragm pacing for 8 hours during the day and unilateral pacing alternating every 8 hours at night. They report that any of several maintenance pacing schedules can be adopted as long as adequate ventilatory support is maintained. Detailed instructions for gradually establishing a pacing schedule during the postoperative period are presented in the original works of D'Agostino and Welch (1979) and more recently Carter (1987).

The usual goals of care apply: maintain adequate ventilation, identify and manage potential problems, promote psychological acceptance, and provide comprehensive education. Knowing how the pacer works is of course helpful in maximizing the effectiveness of the device.

Once the patient is stable, continuing care focuses on recognition of complications of phrenic nerve pacing, including temporary or permanent damage to the phrenic nerve from injury or lack of blood supply, fatigue of the diaphragm from excessive stimulation, implant site and respiratory infections, and equipment failure. The latter may be due to damage to any of the phrenic nerve stimulator's parts or battery failure (Carter 1987; Callahan and Taylor 1985). For the high quadriplegic person on a phrenic nerve pacer, Carter (1987) recommends having a backup ventilator when problems or complications occur.

The Pneumobelt

The pneumobelt is a corsetlike device applied around the abdominal area that assists ventilation during expiration rather than inspiration. It has three components: corset, inflatable bladder, and lightweight tubing connected to a portable positive pressure ventilator (pump). See Figure 15–16. The pump cyclically inflates the inner bladder within the corset, compressing the abdominal wall and causing the diaphragm to rise. This results in active expiration. Conversely, when the bladder is deflated, the diaphragm and abdominal contents fall, producing passive inspirations.

Miller, Thomas, and Wilmot (1988) describe the following protocol for pneumobelt training for people with high quadriplegia:

1. Select individuals based on motivation, medical stability, and absence of marked abdominal wall obesity or spasticity.
2. Fit the pneumobelt while the person is supine, with the corset's horizontal upper border approximately two finger breadths below the costophrenic junction and the curved lower border fitted tighter than the upper part.
3. Position the person for optimal ventilation in a semi-reclining or sitting position in a wheelchair (between 65° and 85° angle).
4. Use a portable positive-pressure ventilator, such as the PLV–100, with the pneumobelt. Average settings are 12 to

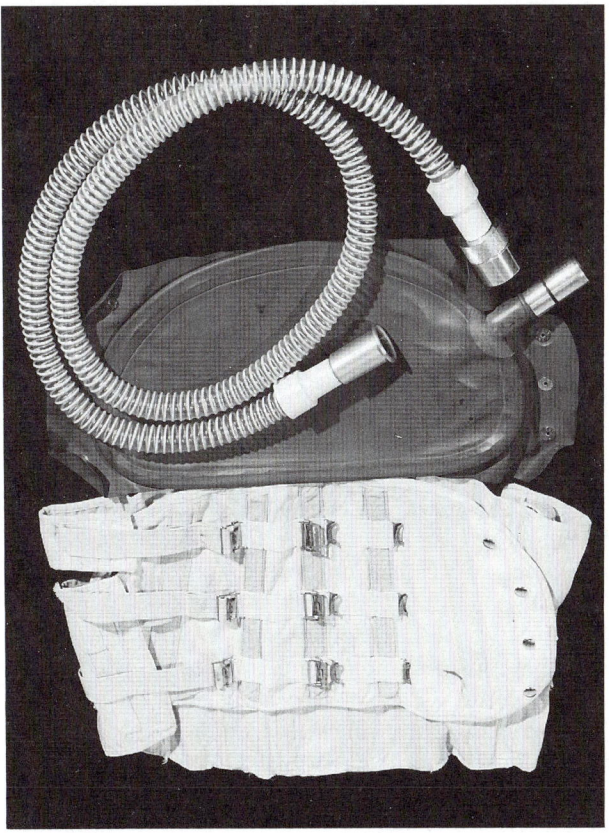

FIGURE 15–16 The pneumobelt (corset) and tubing for connection to a portable positive pressure ventilator.

14 breaths-per-minute with routine pressure attaining +58 to +60 cm H_2O pressure. If the person has a tracheostomy, it must be plugged.
5. Begin with 20- to 30-minute trial periods, adjusting to 2 to 16 hours of continuous use. Tolerance varies greatly and is measured by exhaled volumes and serial pulmonary and/or blood gas analysis.

Other measures include minimizing problems and discomforts by, for instance, teaching to avoid eating large meals to prevent abdominal distension from stomach gas; checking skin daily for signs of breakdown such as abrasions associated with incorrect corset application; and dressing the individual carefully so that clothing does not catch on the corset buckle.

Monitor and encourage the person's adaptation to using the pneumobelt. Evaluate the effectiveness of the pneumobelt frequently, based on:

- No evidence of respiratory insufficiency
- Satisfactory blood gases for person's baseline
- Adequate range of exhaled volumes
- Increased self-esteem and quality of life indicated by increased mobility and activity, improved speech, esthetics, safety, and health

- Individual and family know how to use the pneumobelt effectively and can direct other care givers about the device

Techniques to Relearn Breathing for Short Periods

A most important feature of care of persons with ventilator-dependent quadriplegia is to help them relearn breathing. A degree of safety and psychological comfort is gained if a person can learn to breathe independently for short periods. It may not be possible for some, but people with respiratory quadriplegia consistently emphasize that everyone must try.

Relearning breathing takes place several months after injury due to neck immobilization and spinal shock. It involves strengthening the remaining accessory muscles of breathing, primarily the scalene muscles of the neck. Glossopharyngeal breathing (frog breathing), perfected for people with polio, is not as useful for people with spinal cord injuries that cause respiratory paralysis, probably because they have lost sensation and proprioception which polio victims retain. Occupational and physical therapists can teach exercises that enhance neck control and head balance; mouthstick activities are also helpful. A progressive weaning program gradually increases the FVC and begins with intervals as short as 30 seconds for some people. Independent breathing periods should never be so long that the person tires or panics. Follow the principles outlined in the section on gradual withdrawal from mechanical ventilation in this chapter, keeping in mind that the goal may only be to breathe independently for a few minutes. It is important to practice independent breathing daily if muscle strength is to be maintained.

Complications Related to Respiratory Support Systems

Complications of long-term or permanent tracheostomy mechanical ventilation include accidental extubation or disconnection; partial or complete obstruction of the tube with secretions; mucosal damage resulting in tracheal stenosis; and tracheoesophageal fistula and infection. Complications can occur despite the best preventive management.

Accidental Dislodgement of the Tracheostomy Tube

Care givers should be thoroughly prepared for the unexpected dislodgement of the tracheostomy tube. Be familiar with Procedure 15–9, which explains how to change the tube under normal conditions. Additional emergency procedures include:

- Use the spare tracheostomy tube set with ties, hemostat, and scissors that should be within easy reach. If another tube is not available, however, reinsert the old tube. Direct it back and downward rather like inserting a nozzle into a gas tank. If the tube is difficult to insert, pass the obturator through the stoma or spread the stoma with a hemostat to reopen the tract. After reinserting and securing the tube, remove the obturator and suction to clear the airway if needed. Reconnect to ventilator. In the rare instance that the tracheostomy tube cannot be reinserted, ventilate by mask-to-mouth or mouth-to-mouth breathing and cover the stoma.
- Promptly reestablish artificial airway and ventilation.
- Identify the cause of the accidental extubation and take every possible step to prevent recurrence.
- Be sure emergency equipment—spare tracheostomy tube set with ties, hemostat, and scissors—is easily accessible for another emergency.

Airway Obstruction

Partial or complete occlusion of the artificial airway may be caused by thick secretions or plugs within the lumen of the airway. Accumulated secretions can easily obstruct an airway especially when tubes without inner cannulas are used (Hardy 1973). Other causes are misplaced and incorrectly sized tracheostomy tubes: for example, a cannula that is too long can impinge on the carina or tracheal wall.

Airway obstruction is indicated by the sudden rise in airway pressure reading on volume ventilators, decreased tidal volume, or signs of hypoxia. A further problem for individuals with artificial airways is inadequate humidification of the mucosa and mucous blanket of the tracheobronchial tree. When water and heat are not supplied by the nose to inspired air, water is extracted from the mucous lining in the lower airway, which can lead to the inspissation of the mucus secreted in the lower airway (Beland and Passos 1981).

When the artificial airway is occluded, take the following steps to relieve the obstruction:

1. Liquefy secretions by instilling 5 to 10 ml normal saline into the tracheostomy tube followed by a few breaths with the ventilator or a manual resuscitator bag to disperse saline. Suction to remove the thick secretion or plug.
2. Relieve the impingement of the tube bevel on the carina or tracheal wall by simple manipulation of the tracheostomy tube.
3. If steps 1 and 2 are ineffective, remove tracheostomy tube and replace. Ventilation must be established. Reconnect to ventilator.
4. Identify the cause(s) of the obstruction and redouble efforts to prevent recurrence.
5. Check that respiratory status returns to acceptable normal level for patient.

Tracheoesophageal Fistula

A tracheoesophageal fistula may also be an early or late complication and can occur both after and during long-term ventilation. It results from necrosis of the posterior wall of the trachea when the tracheostomy tube is improperly positioned. Tube-fed persons are at greater risk due to the pressure of the nasogastric tube on the esophagus.

Signs and symptoms may be nonspecific. Observe for oral or tube feeding contents in tracheal aspirate or a severe burning sensation during or after meals; this is caused by food contamination of the fistula. Confirm diagnosis by X ray or endoscopy. Surgical intervention is usually necessary.

Lower Airway Infections

In addition to vigilant hydration and preventive care, be constantly on the alert for signs and symptoms of pulmonary infection. Control infection with meticulous suctioning technique and take measures to avoid other systemic infections that will further lower the person's general resistance. Ensure adequate hydration and humidification and administer antibiotic therapy as ordered. Check that respiratory status returns to normal for the person, that respiratory secretions are free from specific infective organisms, body temperature is normal, and a chest X ray is clear without evidence of consolidation. Make sure the person, family, and care givers know how to maintain good pulmonary hygiene and are doing so.

Stomal Infections

Infection in the stomal site is diagnosed clinically by redness, inflammation, fever, change in character of stomal discharge to purulent and foul odor. The type of infective organism is indicated by a culture. When a stomal infection occurs, ensure adequate hydration and humidification and build the person's general resistance to infection. Review and carefully implement preventive measures, and be sure the person, family, and care givers understand and practice proper maintenance of the stoma site.

Tracheal Stenosis and Granuloma Formation

Scarring of the trachea—*tracheal stenosis* and *granuloma formation*—is caused by the healing process at a stricture site of the airway and may occur from 1 week to 2 years after tracheostomy. Incidence among persons with cuffed tracheal tubes ranges from 1% to 65%. It occurs less frequently with uncuffed tubes and is then usually located where the distal end of the tube irritates the tracheal wall. Other causes are tracheal infection and movement, and weight or tension on the tracheostomy tube due to irritation to the tracheal mucosa (Shapiro et al. 1985). Signs of a stricture such as difficulty suctioning when no thick secretions or plugs are present, airway obstruction, and dyspnea may indicate tracheal stenosis. A tracheal obstruction less than 50% seldom results in clinical symptoms (Andrews 1971). As always, minimize trachea irritation by suctioning gently, avoiding tugs on the ventilator tubing connections, and other pre-

ventive measures. Surgical intervention may be required but healing and repair can present a complex series of events (Hsu et al. 1987).

Ventilator Complications

When a ventilator alarm sounds, the first priority is to maintain the person's respiratory status and assure adequate ventilation. Table 15–5 summarizes user-related and ventilator-related problems and their characteristic signs (Shapiro et al. 1985). Respond immediately. Never violate this basic rule: treat persons, not machines! Emergency procedures include:

- If the person is in respiratory distress and the problem cannot be corrected immediately, ventilate with a manual resuscitation bag or any way possible.
- Check for disconnections or poor connections.
- Check that air flows freely through the corrugated tubing attached to the tracheostomy tube. If not, replace tube.
- Check the cascade gasket and make sure the lid is secure.
- Check the exhalation valve and diaphragm for a free flow of air. The valve may not be positioned correctly or the diaphragm may be wet. Dry the diaphragm and reset it.
- If the problem is still not resolved and the indicators are set at the desired readings, change the entire assembly.

Respiratory Deterioration

Respiratory deterioration is mainly caused by tracheobronchial obstruction or ventilator malfunction. Benvenuti (1979) explains:

> If ventilation is inadequate (as determined by patient response, comfort, and excursion of the chest), check the patient for mucus plugs or for increased secretions and the need for suctioning before considering the equipment as the source of the problem. Thus, it is important to know the patient well—his frequency of suctioning, the character of his secretions, and his normal breath sounds.

First assess and care for the *person* as previously described, and then the equipment. Always look for any signs warning of an emerging problem. Identify and minimize such general problems as poor cardiovascular status, abdominal distension, pain, agitation, or inability to sleep, which may interfere with respiratory function. Observe the nature and rate of respirations, particularly watching for ineffective, rapid, shallow breathing; increasingly noisy respirations; and approaching periods of apnea (or near apnea) leading to eventual signs of severe distress. Recognize the onset of such pulmonary complications as hypoxia, atelectasis, pneumonia, and pulmonary edema.

TABLE 15–5   Common User- and Equipment-Related Problems with Mechanical Ventilation

User-Related Problems	Defining Characteristics	Equipment-Related Problems	Defining Characteristics (Indicators)
Hyperventilation (person ventilated too fast or with too much air)	• Increased respiratory rate • Low $PaCO_2$ • Dyspnea • Lightheadedness	Holes or tears in circuit tubing leading to leaks in the system	• Audible air leak coming from ventilator circuit • Ventilator gauge or dial does not register prescribed amount of volume • Low pressure alarm sounding
Hypoventilation (person ventilated with too little air)	• Dyspnea • Increased $PaCO_2$ • Decreased oxygen saturation and PaO_2 • Tachycardia • Lethargy and drowsiness • Anxiety and restlessness • Audible air leak	Blockage from kinks or water in tubing	• High pressure alarm sounding • Gurgling sound
		Disconnect between ventilator and patient	• Ventilator gauge or dial registering that no volume is being delivered • Low pressure alarm sounding
Increased airway pressure	• Audible respiratory secretions • Airway pressure alarm sounding • Abnormal breath sounds	Ventilator failure	• Ventilator gauge or dial registers no volume delivered • Low pressure alarm sounding • Ventilator not cycling
Thick secretions, mucus plugs	• Secretion thick, difficult to suction • Resistance in passing suction catheter • Low oral fluid intake and ventilator humidification	Incorrect ventilator settings	• Ventilator gauges and controls register different readings from prescribed rates • Alarms may sound
Infection	• Changes in sputum—color, amount, and consistency • Fever • Positive laboratory data	Humidifier (cascade): decreased water supply, overfilling of reservoir, incorrect temperature, leaks	• Dry, hot gas when cascade humidifier becomes dry • Rain-out in tubing occluding gas flow • Pulmonary burns
Tracheal injury	• Blood-tinged mucus		
Pneumothorax (barotrauma)	• Dyspnea • Diminished breath sounds • Weak, rapid pulse • Sudden increase in airway pressure or decrease in TV readings		
Dislodged tracheostomy tube	• Apnea • Bradycardia • Color changes • Anxiety and restlessness		

Adapted from Grassback 1986; Blodgett 1987; and Winters 1988.

REFERENCES

Adams, N. R. 1979. The nurse's role in systematic weaning from a ventilator. *Nursing* 9 (8): 35–41. *A comprehensive, well-illustrated guide describing weaning with a T-piece or with intermittent mandatory ventilation (IMV) and weaning from a tracheostomy. Includes criteria for beginning the process, related nursing care, and a sample weaning flow sheet.*

Aequitron Medical. 1988. *LP6 Ventilator Users' Manual*. Minneapolis, MN: Author.

Allen, D. 1966. Application of the ultrasonic nebulizer in infants and children. In *Proceedings of the First Conference on Clinical Application of Ultrasonic Nebulization*. Chicago, IL.

Andrews, M. J., et al. 1971. Incidence and pathogenesis of tracheal injury following cuffed tracheostomy with assisted ventilation:

Analysis of a 2-year prospective study. *Annals of Surgery* 173 (249).

Beland, I., and Passos, J. 1981. *Clinical Nursing: Pathophysiological and Psychosocial Approaches*. New York: MacMillan, pp. 371, 382.

Belman, M. 1988. Ventilator muscle training. In *Current Respiratory Care*. Eds. R. Kazmarek and J. Stoller. Philadelphia: B. C. Decker, pp. 223–226.

Benotti, P. D., and Bistrian, B. B. 1989. Metabolic and nutritional aspects of weaning from mechanical ventilation. *Critical Care Medicine* 17 (2): 181–185. *An in-depth look at the relationship between nutrition and metabolism and respiratory function with guidelines for management based on principles common to muscle exercise training.*

Benson, D., et al. 1969. Systematic and pulmonary changes with inhaled humid atmospheres. *Anesthesiology* 30: 199.

Benvenuti, C. 1979. Independence for the quadriplegic: the Bantam respirator. *American Journal of Nursing* 79 (5): 918–920.

Blodgett, D. 1987. *Manual of Respiratory Care Procedures*. 2nd ed. Philadelphia: J. B. Lippincott, p. 218.

Brown, B. 1985. Infection control guidelines for home respiratory therapy. *Dimensions in Health Service* 62 (8): 28–39.

Brown, R., Scharf, S., and Melia, S. 1988. Spinal Cord Injury. In *Current Respiratory Care*. Eds. R. Kazmarek and J. Stoller. Philadelphia: B. C. Decker, pp. 316–320.

Brownlee, S., and Williams, S. 1987. Physiotherapy in the respiratory care of patients with high spinal injury. *Physiotherapy* 73 (3): 148–152.

Burke, D., and Murray, D. 1975. *Handbook of Spinal Cord Medicine*. London and Basingstoke: MacMillan Press. *Brief focus on acute respiratory and metabolic management of the quadriplegic patient.*

Callahan, M. J., and Taylor, W. 1985. Respiratory complications. In *Nursing Spinal Cord Injuries*. Ed. N. M. Woll. Totowa, NJ: Rowman & Allanheld.

Carter, E. R. 1987. Respiratory aspects of spinal cord injury. *Paraplegia* 25: 262–262.

Carter, E. R. 1979. Medical management of pulmonary complications of spinal cord injury. *Advances in Neurology* 22: 261–269. *Presents major principles of respiratory insufficiency; summarizes problems common to the typical, the older, and the high-level quadriplegic patient; and focuses on several unique problem such as pleural effusion and cardiac arrest.*

Casas, R., et al. 1977–1978. Prophylaxis of venous thrombosis and pulmonary embolism in patients with acute traumatic spinal cord lesions. *International Journal of Paraplegia* 15: 209–214. *A review of incidence and prevalence of deep vein thrombosis, its complications, and the prophylactic use of calcium heparin (a European perspective).*

Cheshire, D. J. E., and Coates, D. A. 1966. Respiratory and metabolic management in acute tetraplegia. *International Journal of Paraplegia* 4: 1–23. *Detailed correlations between the respiratory and metabolic aspects of acute management. Describes concepts and principles of maintaining adequate alveolar ventilation while promoting optimal nutrition and fluid and electrolyte balance.*

Cheshire, D. J. E., and Flack, W. J. 1978–1979. The use of operant conditioning techniques in the respiratory rehabilitation of the tetraplegic. *International Journal of Paraplegia* 16: 162–174. *Based on the principles of neuromuscular exercise and behaviorist psychology, incentive spirometry is described as a way to improve respiratory function. Respiratory rehabilitation is designed to help the quadriplegic patient clear secretions and combat respiratory infection. Interprets conflicts in existing literature about mechanisms of breathing after SCI. Highly recommended.*

Clough, P., Lindenhaur, D., Hayes, J., and Zekarny, B. 1986. Guidelines for routine respiratory care of patients with spinal cord injury. *Physical Therapy* 66 (9): 1395–1402. *A practical guideline for physicians, nurses, and physical and respiratory therapists. Outlines tasks for each group with special emphasis on overlapping roles and the need for interdisciplinary education.*

Comhaire, A., and Larry, A. 1981. Contamination rate of sterilized ventilators in an ICU. *Critical Care Medicine* 9: 546–548.

Craven, D. E., et al. 1986. Risk factors in pneumonia and fatality in patients receiving mechanical ventilation. *American Review of Respiratory Disease*: 130.

D'Agostino, J., and Welch, P. 1979. The phrenic pacemaker. *Nursing* 9 (5): 41–50.

Fuchs, P. L. 1979. Understanding continuous mechanical ventilation. *Nursing* 9 (12): 26–33. *Concise overview of continuous mechanical ventilation with clinically relevant suggestions for recognizing and solving common problems.*

Fuhrer, M., Carter, R., Donovan, W., Rossi, C., and Wilkerson, M. 1987. Postdischarge outcome for ventilator-dependent quadriplegia. *Archives of Physical Medicine and Rehabilitation* 68 (June): 353–356.

Grassback, I. 1986. Troubleshooting ventilator and patient related problems. *Critical Care Nurse* 6 (4): 58–70.

Hardy, K. L. 1973. Tracheostomy: Indication, techniques and tubes. *American Journal of Surgery* 126: 300.

Harper, R. 1981. *A Guide to Respiratory Care: Physiology and Clinical Applications*. Philadelphia: J. B. Lippincott, p. 261.

Harris, R., and Hyman, R. 1984. Clean versus sterile tracheostomy care and level of pulmonary infection. *Nursing Research* 33 (2): 80–85.

Hoffman, J. 1977. Arterial blood gas analysis as a basic criterion for the management of the neurosurgical patient. *Journal of Neurosurgical Nursing* 9 (1): 29–33. *Integrates pulmonary assessment and intervention techniques for patients with head and spinal cord injuries; includes chart of blood gas analysis for a patient with quadriplegia during the first 14 days after injury. Illustrates anticipated decreased pulmonary function before recovery.*

Holloway, N. 1988. *Nursing the Critically Ill Adult*. 3d ed. Menlo Park, CA: Addison-Wesley.

Hornstein, S., and Ledsome, J. 1986. Ventilatory muscle training in acute quadriplegia. *Physiotherapy Canada* 38 (4): 145–149. *Discusses methods, timing, selection of patients, and measurements indicating positive results of VMT. Very encouraging.*

Hsu, S., et al. 1987. Glottic and trachial stenosis in SCI patients. *Paraplegia* 25 (2): 136–148.

Indihar, F., and Walker, N. 1986. Experience with a prolonged respiratory care unit—revisited. *Chest* Oct. (4): 617–620.

International Ventilator Users Network (IVUN). 1991. *Gazette.* International Network Institute, 4502 Maryland Ave., St. Louis, MO. *Provides excellent resource with written materials for individuals and care givers.*

Irwin, M., and Openbrier, D. 1985. Feeding ventilated patients safely. *American Journal of Nursing* May: 544–546.

Janowski, M. J. 1984. Accidental disconnections from breathing systems. *American Journal of Nursing:* 241–244.

Kirby, N. 1989. The individual with high quadriplegia. *Nursing Clinics of North America* 24 (1): 179–191. *Focuses on respiratory support, aided communication, and technology-assisted environmental control.*

Kozier, B., and Erb, G. 1991. *Fundamentals of Nursing Concepts and Procedures.* 4th ed. Menlo Park, CA: Addison-Wesley.

Ledsome, J. R., and Sharpe, J. 1981. Pulmonary function in acute cervical cord injury. *American Review of Respiratory Disease* 124 (1): 41–44. *Research has implications to improve management of pulmonary function.*

Lee, M., Mathews, P., and Yarkony, G. 1989. Rehabilitation of quadriplegic patients with phrenic nerve pacers. *Archives of Physical Medicine and Rehabilitation* 70 (July): 549–552.

Loke, J. 1988. Diaphragm Pacing. In *Current Respiratory Care.* Eds. R. Kazmarek and J. Stoller. Philadelphia: B. C. Decker.

McLane, A. (Ed.). 1987. Classification of nursing diagnosis. *Proceedings of the Seventh Conference.* St. Louis: C. V. Mosby.

McMichan, J. D., et al. 1980. Pulmonary dysfunction following traumatic quadriplegia. *Journal of the American Medical Association* 243 (6): 528–531. *A current study of pulmonary complications in 22 quadriplegic patients. Concludes that vigorous pulmonary therapy is associated with increased survival, fewer pulmonary complications, and less need for mechanical ventilation. Documentation of serial pulmonary function tests demonstrating marked decrease in respiratory function immediately after injury with significant improvement over time.*

Mapp, C. 1988. Trach Care. *Nursing* July: 36–40.

Mathias, C. 1976. Bradycardia and cardiac arrest during tracheal suction—Mechanisms in tetraplegic patients. *European Journal of Intensive Care Medicine* 2: 147–156.

Metcalf, R. 1986. Acute management phase of persons with spinal cord injury: A nursing diagnosis perspective. *Nursing Clinics of North America* 21 (4): 589–598. *Includes concise, informative sections on ineffective secretion clearance, airway maintenance, and breathing pattern.*

Miller, H. J., Thomas, E., and Wilmot, C. 1988. Pneumobelt use among high quadriplegic population. *Archives of Physical Medicine and Rehabilitation* 69: 369–372.

Norton, L. C., and Neureuter, A. 1988. Weaning the long-term ventilator-dependent patient: Common problems and management. *Critical Care Nurse* 9 (1): 42–52. *Comprehensive assessment and management of the many related problems such as malposition and bowel problems that must be addressed for successful outcomes. Excel-lent tables include forms for preweaning assessment, problem identification, and nursing management strategies.*

O'Donahue, W., Giovanni, R., Keeney, T., and Plummer, A. 1986. Long-term mechanical ventilation. Guidelines for management in the home and at alternate community sites. *Chest* 90 (1). Special Supplement.

Peterson, P. 1989. Pulmonary physiology and medical management. In *The Management of High Quadriplegia.* Eds. G. Whiteneck et al. New York: Demos Publications.

Rinehart, M. E., and Nawoczenski, D. A. 1987. Respiratory care. In *Spinal Cord Injury—Concepts, Management and Approaches.* Eds. L. E. Buchanan and D. A. Nawoczenski. Baltimore, MD: Williams and Wilkins, pp. 61–80. *A physical therapy perspective of respiratory care clearly outlining concepts and management techniques.*

Schroeder, C. H. 1987. Pulse oximetry: A nursing care plan. *Critical Care Nurse* 8 (8): 50–67. *An in-depth look at the background, principles, indications, limitations, and advantages of oximetry. Prepared for CE enrollees with a multiple-choice examination following.*

Shapiro, B., Harrison, R., Kazmarek, R., and Cane, R. 1985. *Clinical Application of Respiratory Care.* 3d ed. Chicago: Yearbook Medical Publishing.

Spence, A., and Mason, E. 1979. *Human Anatomy and Physiology.* Menlo Park, CA: Addison-Wesley. *Presents foundations in anatomy and physiology, which include the effects of aging.*

Texas Institute for Rehabilitation and Research (TIRR). 1986. *Management of Choking Victim in a Wheelchair.* Houston, TX: Author. *Videotape program teaches how to identify a person in distress and dislodge foreign particles through the Heimlich maneuver. Intended for rehabilitation professionals, students, and personal care attendants.*

Thomas, E. L. 1977. Nursing care of the patient with spinal cord injury. In *The Total Care of Spinal Cord Injuries.* Eds. D. S. Pierce and V. H. Nickel. Boston: Little, Brown, pp. 249–297. *Focus on long-term assessment and optimal maintenance management of respiratory function.*

Tyson, George W., et al. 1978. *Acute Care of the Head and Spinal Cord Injured Patient in the Emergency Department.* Charlottesville, Va: Department of Neurosurgery, University of Virginia. *Includes recognition of impending or manifest respiratory insufficiency in emergency care. Concise overview of emergency care, including neurological assessment and preparation of the patient for transport. Highly recommended.*

Walsh, J., and Kirkpatrick, P. 1988. Home discharge of the ventilator-assisted patient. In *Current Respiratory Care.* Eds. R. Kazmarek and J. K. Stoller. Philadelphia: B. C. Decker, p. 248.

Wanner, A. 1979. Clinical aspects of mucociliary transport. *American Review of Respiratory Disease* 116: 73–125.

Wetzel, J. 1985. Respiratory evaluation and treatment. In *Spinal Cord Injury.* Ed. H. A. Adkins. New York: Churchill Livingstone, pp. 75–98. *A well-researched and illustrated physical therapy perspective giving an abundance of specific predictions and values correlated with the level of cord injury sustained.*

Whiteneck, G., et al. 1989. *The Management of High Quadriplegia.* New York: Demos Publications.

Wicks, A. 1989. Ventilator Weaning. In *The Management of High Quad-riplegia*. Eds. G. Whiteneck et al. New York: Demos, pp. 141–149.

Winters, C. 1988. Monitoring ventilator patients for complications. *Nursing* (June): 38–41.

Zeluff, G. W., et al. 1977. Ondine's curse. *Heart Lung* 6 (6): 1057–1063. *Discussion of pathophysiology and differential diagnosis of apnea or near apnea on the high cervical cord injured patient; includes descriptions of phrenic nerve testing and surgical considerations to resolve the problem.*

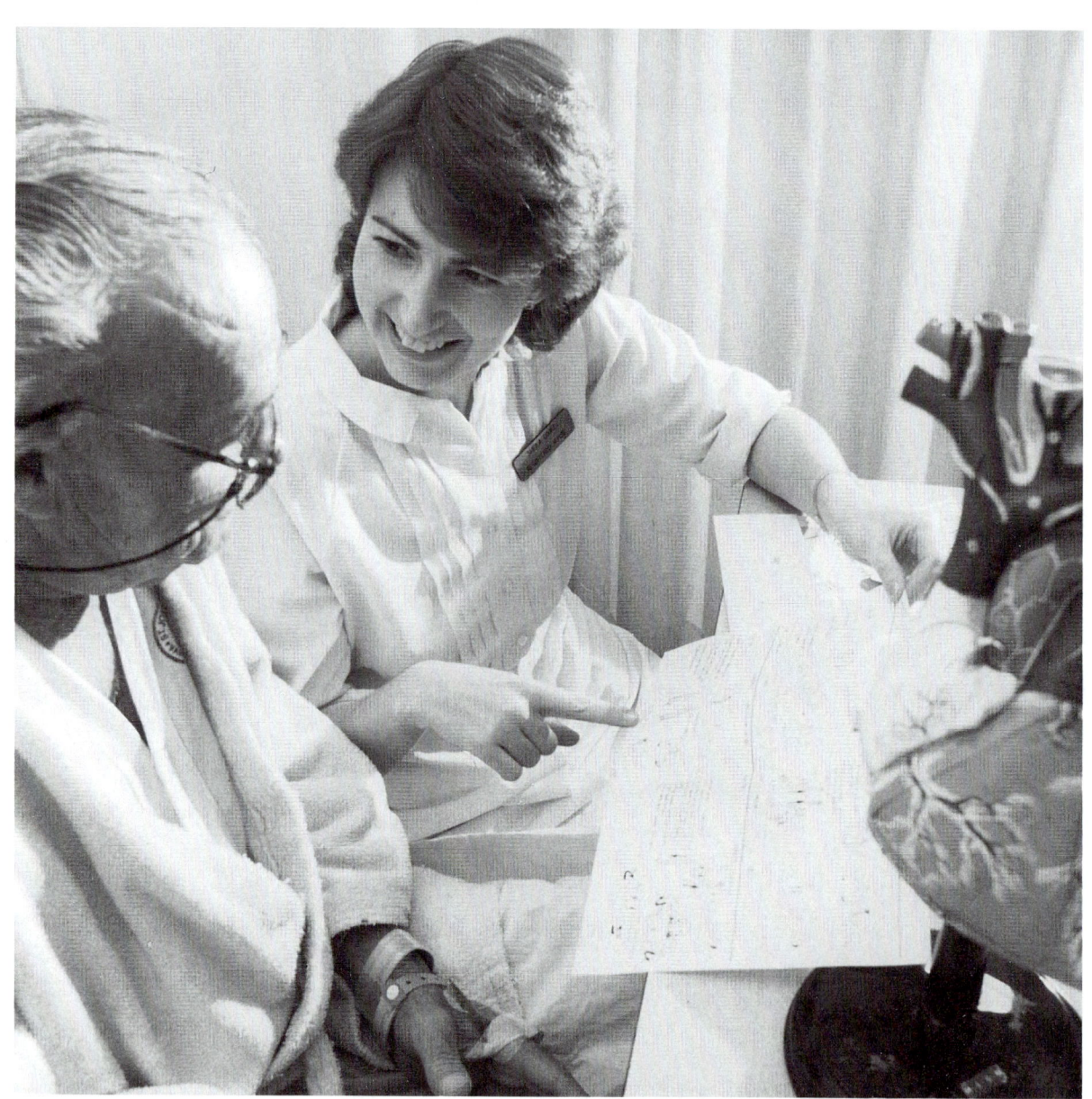

CHAPTER
— 16 —

Regulating Cardiovascular Function and Body Temperature

Chapter Outline

Health Care Objectives

- To explain how neural control of heart rate, systemic vascular resistance, and body temperature control are impaired by SCI

- To describe patients who develop circulatory and temperature regulation problems and to identify risk factors and methods of assessment and management
- To focus on preventive care and health education
- To describe long-term implications associated with cardiovascular function and regulation of body temperature

The cardiovascular system is the transport system that perfuses and nourishes all body organs and tissues and removes nonessential elements from body cells to maintain a desirable environment within the body. The autonomic nervous system influences the heart and blood vessels and provides regulatory control of the heart rate and blood pressure. Closely related is the regulation of body temperature, similarly dependent on autonomic control of blood vessels (vasoconstriction and vasodilation) and sweat glands.

The stability of the internal environment is threatened when intricate communications between the autonomic and central nervous systems are disconnected as a result of SCI. The higher the level of cord injury, the more complicated the effects become, as greater body area is involved. Both the short-term consequences, which tend to be extreme, and the gradual adaptation to long-term effects are hampered further by the hazards of immobility. Health education and planning are integral aspects of care for life.

The goals for health care are:

- To stabilize heart rate and blood pressure
- To prevent or control stimuli from triggering an exaggerated autonomic nervous system response that could be life threatening
- To minimize negative effects of a passive vasodilation of the systemic vascular system below the level of cord injury
- To promote fitness for life

IMPAIRED CARDIOVASCULAR FUNCTION AS A RESULT OF SPINAL CORD INJURY

The Cardiovascular System

Cardiac Output

Cardiac output is defined as the total volume of blood pumped by the heart per minute—approximately 5 liters per minute (at rest). Cardiac output is computed by multiplying the *heart rate* by the *stroke volume* or amount of blood ejected into the systemic circulation with each ventricular contraction (*afterload*). The cardiac output is determined by the amount of blood returned to the heart (*preload*) and the heart rate. In addition to the heart's effectiveness as a pump and the rate at which it pumps, circulation depends on the blood volume and viscosity of circulating blood.

Blood Pressure and Pulse

Blood pressure is a complex mechanism reflecting functional integration of the neurological and cardiovascular systems, and its measurement is a basic indicator of adequate tissue perfusion. Blood pressure is directly related to *cardiac output* (heart rate and *systemic vascular resistance*). Similarly, the *pulse* reflects adequacy of circulation in general and can also be used to assess specific blood flow to the periphery.

Neurological Control of Circulation

Heart Rate

The heart derives innervation from both the sympathetic and the parasympathetic divisions of the autonomic nervous system. Powerful sympathetic stimulation increases the heart rate and strengthens cardiac contractions, a vital response involved with the body's stress response, "fright or flight" mechanism. In a normal resting state there is little sympathetic influence on the heart. The major determinant of the heart rate at rest is the parasympathetic tone. Parasympathetic fibers reach the heart via the *vagus* nerve.

Systemic Vascular Resistance

Systemic vascular resistance is determined by the length and radius of the blood vessels and to a lesser extent blood viscosity. The vascular network responds to local tissue needs and to the central and autonomic nervous systems.

Local control of blood flow is very important and functions independently to a great extent. Local blood vessel activity is based primarily on oxygen need and levels of carbon dioxide accumulation in the tissues themselves. Decreased oxygen levels in the tissues draw blood flow; increased levels of carbon dioxide shunt blood away from the affected area. The heart is also capable, to a certain extent, of adjusting pump action according to the preload volume.

Central control of blood flow and vessel resistance is accomplished by the combined actions of the vasomotor center in the brain stem and the sympathetic division of the autonomic nervous system. (Numerous other intricate factors are involved including the actions of higher brain centers on the vasomotor center and sensitive feedback mechanisms located throughout the body.)

The *vasomotor center* is located in the reticular formation of the pons and medulla and is greatly influenced by the hypothalamus and other higher brain centers. With SCI, vasomotor tone is impaired mainly due to interference with neural, rather than humoral, control of vasoconstrictor fibers.

The *sympathetic vasoconstrictor system* is responsible for maintaining vasomotor tone. It is capable of rapidly shunting blood from the peripheral circulation to more vital organs when preparing the body for stress defense. Vasoconstrictor fibers are distributed, with rare exception, to all the blood vessels of the body, but most abundantly to the arterial vessels. The supply is especially rich in the kidney, spleen, and skin of the limbs. Vasoconstriction can be accomplished by direct *neural stimulation* of the blood vessels. Secretion of epinephrine and norepinephrine from the adrenal medulla is described as *humoral stimulation* and also causes vasoconstriction. Neural stimulation provides rapid action, while humoral control produces long-lasting chemical effects throughout the body. The sympathetic nervous system also carries vasodilator fibers for innervation of specific secretory sites, but these are of less significance in circulatory control. The blood vessels do not receive parasympathetic innervation.

Sympathetic stimulation alters the radius of blood vessels, thus directly changing the resistance of these vessels and regulating blood flow through the tissues (Guyton 1976). Changing the rate of flow in these numerous and widespread blood vessels ultimately alters the total amount of circulating blood, which plays a major role in cardiovascular stability.

Cardiovascular Dysfunctions after Injury

Injury to the spinal cord has the greatest effect on the function of the sympathetic nervous system, which arises from the thoracolumbar portion of the spinal cord.

- The *level of cord injury* has a profound effect. Upper thoracic and cervical cord injuries result in severe disruption of sympathetic control to the heart and vascular network. Loss of sympathetic control is aggravated by the unopposed parasympathetic influence (preserved from the undamaged cranial outflow of the autonomic nervous system).

- Injury to the spinal cord at the T_6 segmental level or above will interfere with the sympathetic nervous functions of preparing the body for stress and maintaining vasomotor tone. Injury below the T_6 level allows at least partial sympathetic function to continue. With lower lumbar or sacral cord injuries, the sympathetic nervous system remains intact but loss of reflex activity below the level of injury impairs vasomotor control to the lower limbs.

- High paraplegic and quadriplegic patients are in the most danger of cardiovascular disturbance as evidenced by *hypotension and bradycardia*. The fall in the blood pressure and heart rate, with parallel decrease in cardiac output, is explained by the loss of vasoconstrictor tone and lack of sympathetic tone to the heart (Guha and Tator 1988). When circulation is slowed blood tends to pool in the abdomen and lower limbs.

- The *time factor*. The number of days or weeks postinjury changes the profile of reflex activity from that of complete loss (spinal shock), through a recovery phase, to that of exaggerated responses. See Chapter 6. With the passing of spinal shock, segmental sympathetic reflex activity provides some degree of compensatory function. Although a lower blood pressure and pulse rate may persist, cardiovascular function will eventually stabilize.

- The *age factor*. Older patients have diminished cardiac reserve and cannot withstand the increased demands placed on the heart as well as younger people can. The heart becomes a less effective pump as valves thicken and become more rigid, which causes incomplete filling and emptying of the heart with each contraction. Similar loss of arterial elasticity diminishes blood flow mainly to the extremities and the brain. The aging process, then, makes patients more susceptible to congestive heart failure, hypertension, and ischemic heart diseases. This places the older paralyzed person in double jeopardy of developing cardiac insufficiency.

- *Associated trauma*. Blood loss from trauma associated with SCI is not uncommon. The importance of distinguishing hypotension due to hemmorhagic versus spinal shock is addressed in Chapter 6.

- *Preexisting cardiovascular disease and related risks*. It is important to note any preexisting cardiovascular disease. The patient may be well aware of a previous cardiac condition or may only describe subtle changes, such as fatigue on exertion or swelling of extremities, indicating circulatory problems. Complaints of dyspnea, palpitations, and especially chest pain should be investigated thoroughly. Pain can also be associated with vascular occlusion problems, as with intermittent claudication in the lower limbs.

Preexisting cardiac disease is not prevalent with SCI because the majority of patients are young, athletic, and have slow resting heart rates reflecting preinjury fitness. When bradycardia as a result of cervical injury is superimposed, this can become a problem. The risks associated with poor nutrition, obesity, and/or substance abuse must also be taken into account.

DISTURBANCES OF THERMOREGULATION AFTER SPINAL CORD INJURY

General Factors Influencing Body Temperature

The *heat regulation center* or "thermostat" of the body is located in the hypothalamus at the base of the brain. Input is received from thermosensitive receptors in the skin, the abdominal viscera and spinal cord (to a lesser extent), and central thermoreceptors in the hypothalamus itself that respond to actual changes in the temperature of the circulating blood. Thermoregulatory activity is further influenced by conditions resulting in fever and by environmental temperature changes. The following descriptions of heat production and heat loss are based on the works of Guyton (1976) and Castle and Watkins (1979). Explanations of abnormal control of these mechanisms associated with cord injury are based on the works of Guttman (1973) and Johnson (1971).

Production of heat in the body is actually the amount of energy released when food is metabolized. The rate at which this process occurs is called the metabolic rate and is usually measured under basal conditions. Factors that mainly affect the basal metabolic rate, and therefore directly alter body temperature, are exercise or activity, actions of the sympathetic nervous system, and production of the thyroid hormone. The actual temperature of the circulating blood is also able to accelerate or decrease metabolism.

Again, as in control of circulation, the sympathetic nervous system is most powerful in maintaining immediate physiological control of body temperature. People also adjust clothing and indoor temperatures to protect themselves from changes in the environmental temperature. Fluctuating levels of thyroid hormone production respond, but only gradually. For example, prolonged exposure to the cold, such as in the beginning of winter, will stimulate production of the thyroid hormone to increase the basal metabolic rate, but the response takes several weeks.

Neurological Control of Body Temperature

Thermogenesis, or conservation of body heat when the circulating blood becomes abnormally cool, relies on the anterior hypothalamus to raise body temperature by stimulating mechanisms to vasoconstrict peripheral blood vessels and increase metabolism and muscular activity, including shivering.

Sympathetic vasoconstriction of the blood vessels of the skin diminishes blood flow to the periphery, thus decreasing the amount of heat loss to the atmosphere. Heat is thereby conserved by circulation of the warmed blood within the internal structures.

Sympathetic stimulation to increase body metabolism produces additional heat. Release of epinephrine into the tissues immediately increases the need for oxygen; this requires acceleration of cell metabolism and thus increases heat production.

Increased muscular activity also produces additional body heat. This may be voluntary, as with vigorous exercise, or an autonomic response to increase muscle tone. Progression to the reflex action of shivering, characterized by rapid muscle relaxation and contraction, is a most powerful mechanism and can almost double heat production in the body. Piloerection, or goose bumps, also occurs as small muscle contractions erect hair follicles. (This is of benefit to lower mammals with thick fur as a means of trapping air to increase thermal insulation.)

Thermolysis, or reduction of body heat, is stimulated when circulating blood becomes abnormally warm and relies on the posterior hypothalamus to stimulate mechanisms to lower body temperature. The thermoregulatory mechanisms act primarily to dilate skin blood vessels.

Disturbances of Temperature Regulation after Injury: Poikilothermia and Hypothermia

Injury to the spinal cord above the thoracolumbar outflow of the sympathetic nervous system disconnects thalamic thermoregulatory mechanisms, mainly:

- Absence of vasoconstriction and loss of the ability to shiver to conserve body heat
- Loss of thermoregulatory *sweating* to dissipate heat

The inability to maintain a steady internal temperature and thereby assume the temperature of the environment is a condition known as *poikilothermia*. Acute and chronic loss of vasomotor tone and passive vasodilation below the level of cord injury tend to cause continual loss of body heat resulting in *hypothermia*. This response is severe in the early stages. The loss of ability to sweat to cool the body also exists. The degree of dysfunction is directly proportional to the body area experiencing loss of thermoregulatory mechanisms. Persons with quadriplegia, in particular, cannot maintain a desirable body temperature if they are not protected from changes in the environmental temperature.

Body temperature also tends to decrease with age. A temperature of 95°F (35°C) is not uncommon; therefore, a temperature of 99.5°F (37.5°C) can be a significant fever in some elderly patients (Kozier and Erb 1991). Adaptation to changes in the environment is slower due to sluggish action of thermoregulatory mechanisms. For example, older patients find it difficult to keep warm and cannot tolerate as much increased activity at high temperatures.

ASSESSMENT OF CARDIOVASCULAR STATUS AND BODY TEMPERATURE

Physical Assessment

The physical examination reveals the patient's current cardiovascular status and includes cardiac assessment, vascular assessment, and assessment of other related body systems. Observation of body temperature is also described in this section. Preinjury cardiovascular health and risk factors must be taken into account.

Cardiac Assessment

Purely cardiac problems are not particularly common in patients with SCI and are not emphasized here. The techniques of *inspection, palpation,* and *auscultation* are used to obtain precise information about the heart. See Procedure 16–1.

Vascular Assessment

Impairment of vasomotor control as a result of SCI may cause short- or long-term changes in the systemic vascular system. Techniques involved in vascular assessment are *inspection and palpation of the extremities, and measurement of the blood pressure and pulse.* See Procedures 16–2 and 16–3.

Assessment of Related Body Systems

Inadequate circulation can be reflected by altered function of other body systems, and examination of pulmonary and renal function and the central nervous system, in particular, should be included in general assessment of the cardiovascular system. Respiratory function is affected by cardiac function; left-sided heart failure, for example, causes blood to pool in the pulmonary system, which leads to pulmonary edema. Renal and cardiac functions are also interdependent. Urine output will decrease to conserve blood volume when compensating for an abnormally low blood pressure. Observation of the level of consciousness is most important as increased restlessness, irritability, or subtle behavioral changes may well be the first signs from the central nervous system of poor oxygenation from inadequate blood flow.

Assessment of Body Temperature

Methods used to determine body temperature include palpating the skin and, of course, measuring by thermometer. For techniques used see Procedure 16–4. Because of extreme lability, determine body temperature regularly. A daily basis is recommended for an 8- to 12-week period. Early detection of a fever (often low grade) is frequently the one and only sign of occult infection—a deep vein thrombosis, for example. Closely observe the high paraplegic and quadriplegic patient for disturbance of temperature regulation, especially for hypothermia during the phase of spinal shock. Guarding against extremes in hot or cold weather remains problematic throughout life.

Diagnostic Findings

Hemodynamic Monitoring

Hemodynamic Monitoring, through direct placement of catheters in the atria (for obtaining central venous pressure) or pulmonary or systemic arteries, measures cardiovascular pressures and allows arterial or venous blood samples to be obtained without repeated vascular punctures. The advantage of hemodynamic monitoring must be carefully weighed against the increased possibility of complications including infection; thrombosis, and possibly emboli formation; perforation of the vessels of the lungs or heart; dysrhythmias (specifically preventricular contractions) or a myocardial infarction. General range of motion exercises—with careful support of the limb and continuous assessment of circulation to the distal portion of the limb—are mandatory.

Electrocardiogram

The *electrocardiogram (ECG)* is a most valuable and frequently used diagnostic test to aid in the identification and treatment of cardiac dysrhythmias. Meticulous skin care and changing of lead sites are essential to prevent skin breakdown when leads are placed on an area of the chest that is without sensation.

Chest X Ray

A *chest X ray* must be included on admission to provide information about heart size, signs of enlargement, calcification of cardiac structures, and alterations in blood flow in relation to the pulmonary circulation.

Procedure 16–1 Inspection, Palpation, and Auscultation of the Heart

Purpose

To assess the current cardiac status. (Holloway 1988)

Action

1. Inspect and palpate the chest wall. Locate the heart and determine size by describing cardiac borders in relation to external landmarks of ribs, intercostal spaces, and imaginary reference lines, e.g., midclavicular or midsternal lines. Palpate the *point of maximal impulse* (PMI)

2. Auscultate heart sounds and describe in terms of intensity, frequency, quality, and duration.

3. Auscultate heart sounds in a systematic fashion from the aortic area, to the pulmonic area, to the tricuspid area, and finally to the mitral or apical area.

Rationale

The *precordium* is the chest area overlying the heart. Note any lifts, heaves, or abnormal pulsations or vibrations of the precordial area.

Auscultation techniques allow assessment of heart sounds created by blood flow inside the heart during each cardiac cycle. Heart sounds are low and may be hard to hear, making auscultation difficult. The first sound corresponds to the beginning of ventricular systole (*lubb* sound) and the second sound corresponds to the end (*dupp* sound). Normally a longer pause (the *lubb-dupp pause*) occurs after the second sound. This relationship remains throughout the normal cardiac cycle, and these two sounds may be heard throughout the precordial area.

To assess specific valve action, it is best to auscultate in a systematic fashion. Murmurs are heard when blood flow within the heart becomes turbulent. These usually result from obstruction, valvular defects, or abnormal vascular communication between compartments of the heart. Abnormal sounds may reveal specific problems, such as valvular insufficiency or stenotic changes.

Procedure 16–2 Inspection and Palpation of the Extremities

Purpose

To assess vascular status, especially to detect impairment or obstruction of venous blood flow.

Action

1. Inspect and palpate both upper and lower extremities. Check and compare extremity pulses.

2. Watch carefully for developing edema in the hands and arms of quadriplegic patients, as well as in the feet and ankles of all paralyzed patients. Always compare limbs bilaterally. Watch for dependent edema when the patient is mobilized.

3. Constantly examine the skin for local lesions.

4. Examine the involved extremity *distal* to the lesion for increased warmth, redness, and swelling.

Rationale

Good circulation to the extremities ensures that the skin is warm and dry, pink (if the patient is Caucasian), and free from any swelling. The skin will reflect inadequate circulation by abnormal pallor, a mottled appearance, or a cyanotic tinge. Coolness of extremities and presence of edema also indicate poor circulation.

Vasomotor inactivity associated with paralysis causes blood to pool in the extremities. Gravitational forces, especially when a sitting position is assumed, further complicate the situation by overcoming the abnormally low pressure of venous blood returning to the heart.

Initially, lacerations, hematomas, bruises, or even burns may be sustained at the time of injury. During the course of rehabilitation, pressure areas or accidental trauma may occur. Observe these surface areas closely, because stasis of circulation slows the healing process, and the underlying venous structures may be damaged.

These signs indicate an obstruction to venous return. The greatest potential danger is the development of a deep vein thrombosis, predisposing the patient to pulmonary embolism. For more detailed information on general skin assessment and care, see Chapter 21.

Procedure 16–3   Measurement of Blood Pressure and Pulse

Purpose

To assess systemic circulation, which reflects the general cardiovascular status. The pulse is also measured to assess systemic circulation. More specifically, it is used to evaluate blood flow to selected body parts (e.g., the pedal pulse [*dorsalis pedis*] is included in assessing circulation to a lower limb).

Action	Rationale
1. Obtain the blood pressure.	The blood pressure indicates the pressure at which blood is forced through the arteries; the systolic pressure is produced when the ventricles contract and the diastolic when the ventricles are at rest. The normal blood pressure range for an adult is generally 110 to 140 mmHg systolic and 60 to 80 mmHg diastolic.
2. Observe for *hypotension* immediately after injury (80 to 90 systolic is common for patients in spinal shock).	Systolic pressures less than 100 mmHg are considered hypotensive. Due to spinal shock, and sometimes hypovolemic shock caused by multiple injuries, all patients may experience an initial fall in blood pressure. High paraplegic and quadriplegic patients will eventually develop a constant low blood pressure. Experience has shown that quadriplegic patients have a blood pressure of about 100/60 mmHg when resting and an even lower pressure when sitting up.
3. Observe for episodes of *hypertension* when spinal shock subsides.	A pressure of greater than 160 mmHg systolic or 100 mmHg diastolic is described as hypertensive. Episodes of hypertension, reaching extremely dangerous levels, can be associated with the autonomic crisis called autonomic dysreflexia.
4. Take the pulse and describe in terms of rhythm and volume.	The pulse rate is generally between 60 and 100 beats per minute in the adult and of a regular rhythm and normal force.
5. Observe for *bradycardia* immediately after injury.	Bradycardia describes a pulse rate less than 60 beats per minute and tachycardia a pulse rate greater than 100 beats per minute. Bradycardia after injury is due to spinal shock. Tachycardia at this time is a symptom of internal or external bleeding associated with the initial trauma.
6. Keep Atrophine 0.4 or 0.6 mg on hand for a heart rate less than 40 beats per minute.	

Blood Gas Analysis

Arterial blood gas analysis detects insufficient gaseous exchange and is regularly monitored, especially with patients experiencing actual or potential pulmonary compromise. Also useful are serial comparisons of oxygen saturation and end tidal carbon dioxide measures. Chapter 15 reviews blood and pulmonary analysis.

Blood Work Analysis

Blood work analysis to examine serum enzyme levels may be useful to detect ischemic heart problems. Certain enzymes are released from damaged tissues, and the enzyme levels peak between 24 and 72 hours after a myocardial contusion or infarction. Spinal cord injury itself is not associated with increases in serum enzyme levels unless there is significant damage to skeletal muscles. Assessment is incomplete without consideration of general blood work results.

PREVENTIVE AND RESTORATIVE MANAGEMENT

Maintaining Adequate Circulation

To control and/or minimize the effects of *hypotension and bradycardia*, care focuses on preserving adequate heart rate, maintaining desirable blood volume and composition, and promoting blood flow in the systemic vascular system. Measures discussed in this general section are largely preventive. As seen with respiratory function, *early mobilization* has greatly reduced complications, and *vigorous physical therapy to unaffected limbs* has done much to enhance cardiopulmonary reserve.

Procedure 16–4   Assessing Body Temperature

Purpose

To determine the measures required to help the patient maintain a desirable body temperature, a vital diagnostic sign.

Action	Rationale
1. Palpate the skin surface of the body with the back of the hand, rather than the fingertips.	The back of the hand is more sensitive to temperature changes.
2. Note areas of warmth or coolness and also moisture content.	The body surface may be the same throughout; or cooler in areas of poor circulation; or warmer in localized areas, indicating a problem such as soft tissue pressure or thrombophlebitis. The skin may be dry (as in spinal shock) or moist and clammy (as in hemorrhagic shock).
3. Obtain an oral temperature.	The normal range of an oral temperature is 36° to 37°C (96.8° to 99.6°F).
4. Obtain a rectal temperature. Gently insert a *well-lubricated* thermometer and *hold* in place.	A rectal temperature is considered most accurate in measuring core body temperature and will measure 0.4°C (0.7°F) more than an oral measurement. Rectal temperatures are recommended for patients in shock or coma, restless or uncooperative patients, or patients receiving oxygen or mouth-breathing (most quadriplegic patients mouth-breathe). Extra care must be taken to avoid rectal trauma when the patient is without rectal sensation and is subject to sudden position change from involuntary leg spasms.
5. Be alert for *hypothermia* early after injury, and in the postoperative and elderly patient.	Most patients with SCI suffer from subnormal temperatures due to spinal shock, hypovolemic shock, exposure to the elements at an accident scene, and the air-conditioned surroundings of emergency rooms.

Preserving Cardiac Function

1. *Prevent hypoxia.* A diminished flow of oxygen in the systemic circulation may progress to myocardial hypoxia in the heart. The most common causes of simple systemic hypoxia in patients with SCI are:

- Paralysis of the muscles of breathing leading to respiratory compromise
- Neurogenic (spinal) and/or hemorrhagic shock, which lowers cardiac output

It is important, then, to determine the cause of hypoxia and initiate early treatment. To review identification of patients at risk and treatment of pulmonary complications resulting in hypoxia, see specific management in Chapter 15.

2. *Minimize workload of the heart.* Physical and psychological insult, which both occur readily with paralysis, easily increase the workload and oxygen consumption of the heart. In reaction to stress, the heart receives increased amounts of epinephrine and becomes more irritable; this may cause electrical instability and dysrhythmias. This less effective circulation, in turn, decreases oxygenation of vital organs including the heart itself.

To avoid excess cardiac stimulation, promote adequate rest and psychological comfort to reduce stress. See Chapter 9.

General measures to protect the patient from the invasive atmosphere of a critical care unit have been described in Chapter 6. As the rehabilitation process progresses, monitor the patient closely for signs of fatigue associated with increases in physical activity. Carefully observe people with a history of poor tolerance for exercise before injury, such as the obese or the elderly. Therapy programs can be modified if necessary.

Another important measure is to ensure regular evacuation of the neurogenic bowel to avoid any added strain on the heart. Maintaining bowel function is discussed in Chapter 19.

3. *Maintain desirable blood volume and composition.* Prevent or promptly treat fluid and electrolyte imbalances. Adequate nutrition and hydration, are described in Chapter 17. A decrease in the volume of circulating blood may result from hypovolemic or neurogenic shock. Still commonly encountered is initial volume overload, in a mistaken effort to combat neurogenic shock. Especially with the older person, congestive heart failure and pulmonary edema may be problematic.

4. *Initiate and maintain pharmacological control of blood pressure as ordered.* Hypotension due to neurogenic shock

can be treated by medications such as dopamine hydrochloride (Intropin), a sympathomimetic amine. This powerful drug increases cardiac output directly by stimulating the heart muscle and indirectly by stimulating the release of norepinephrine. Dopamine hydrochloride must be carefully titrated, using an infusion pump, to maintain the target blood pressure. Onset of the effect is rapid, within 5 minutes, and duration of action is about 10 minutes. Be alert for adverse reactions of dysrhythmias and watch insertion site for signs of infiltration, which will cause necrotic changes.

Promoting Blood Flow in Paralyzed Limbs

1. *Assist venous return to the heart.* As all patients with SCI suffer from some loss of strength and ability to move in addition to initial total immobilization, an appropriate activity level must be provided immediately to prevent circulatory complications. Early mobilization with postural changes and wheelchair activity greatly decreases the hazards of immobilization caused by venous stasis.

Encourage as much activity as possible within limits of orthopedic stability. Active or passive range of motion exercises are essential for patients on bedrest. A physical therapy program based on the level of injury and patient tolerance should be initiated soon after admission.

Introduce mobilization from bedrest to wheelchair activities gradually by a *graded* activity program to avoid circulatory collapse. This is evidenced by the frequently encountered and closely related problems of *gravitational* or dependent *edema* and *postural* (orthostatic) *hypotension*. Ways to prevent or forestall these complications, which are particularly severe with quadriplegia, are described in the section on specific management in this chapter.

Elevate paralyzed limbs while in bed or in the wheelchair. The following measures may need to be maintained continuously during bedrest if the problem is severe. Otherwise they may be used during rest periods or at night only.

- Elevate and support limbs with pillows and select arm and foot boards for immobilization beds.
- Elevate foot of bed 10 to 15 degrees only (to avoid inguinal congestion), unless contraindicated when countertraction is required for cervical injuries.

The following technique may be used while the patient is in the wheelchair rather than returning the patient to bed.

- Tip the chair backward and elevate legs to rest or recline on bed or couch. See Figure 16–1. Elevated leg rests for special problems may be required.
- Practice tipping chair every 2 to 3 hours while up. After meals, in between therapy, or when watching television may be convenient times.

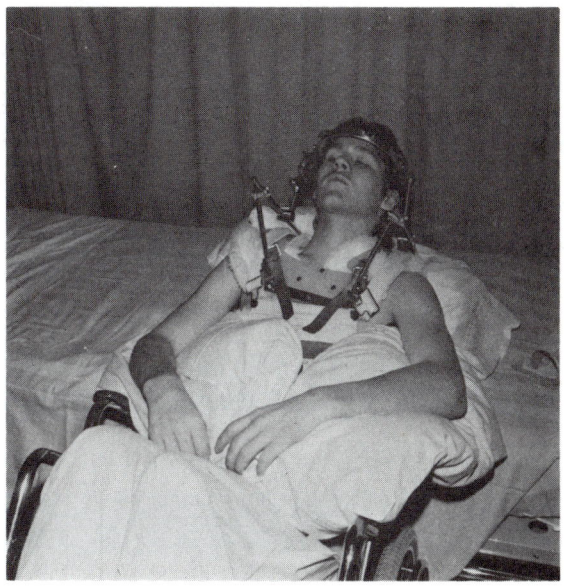

FIGURE 16–1 A convenient rest position.

Provide compression forces to muscle bellies and joints. Antiembolitic (elasticized) stockings and ace or tensor bandages are used to exert a supplemental force on the veins. These measures are specifically indicated with edema, postural hypotension, or thrombophlebitis. Correct application and care are essential to avoid blocking circulation.

Antiembolitic stockings are generally preferred for convenience and ease of application. A variety of sizes and strengths of stockings are available on the commercial market. Some come in small, medium, and large sizes. Others must be individually measured to fit the foot, calves, and thighs. To ensure a correct fit, obtain measurements following a rest period, when edema has subsided. See Procedure 16–5.

Tensor bandages are not as convenient and tend to slip when a patient sits up in the wheelchair.

Tensor bandages are required when the patient has an arterial line, when there are associated leg injuries or open areas on the skin, or when elasticized stockings are not large enough to fit. To promote circulatory return, use spiral turns, wrapping upward from the foot; wrap the entire leg, as far up the thigh as possible; and use circular turns only to anchor and terminate bandaging (using circular turns on the entire leg would impede rather than promote circulatory return). To avoid abrasions to skin without sensation, secure the tensor with one-inch adhesive tape rather than metal clips.

Whatever method is used, success depends on a good fit and correct application. Be sure to apply *before* the patient is mobilized. Continuous monitoring of circulation to the toes and heels is necessary and stockings or bandages must be removed every 4 to 8 hours for inspection and care of the skin. Be alert to the dangers of arterial occlusion from the tourniquetlike action of the elastic bandages causing com-

Procedure 16–5   Obtaining Leg Measurements

Purpose

To compile serial data to detect early swelling that may indicate onset of thrombophlebitis, which may lead to pulmonary embolism. Strict accuracy must be obtained for measurements to be of any value.

Action	Rationale
1. Measure ankle, calf, and thigh circumferences on admission.	To provide baseline data.
2. Obtain measurements at the widest point of the ankle, calf, and thigh.	To provide continuity, some settings prefer calf and thigh measurements to be obtained at a mandatory distance from the kneecap—for instance, 6 or 8 inches (20 cm).
3. Mark the leg with a black felt pen to indicate area to be measured. Apply the tape so that it is centered on the line before measuring.	To facilitate accuracy of serial measurements.
4. Obtain serial measurements in the morning before any activity.	If the patient is up before measuring, gravitational edema may give a false reading.
5. As a preventive measure, repeat measurements on a weekly basis.	To detect swelling early that may be indicative of thrombophlebitis.
6. Repeat measurements daily if swelling is present.	To monitor swelling and response to treatment.
7. Record measurements.	Measurements can be conveniently recorded on a flow sheet as shown below.

Leg Measurements

	Left	Right
Thigh	_____inches/cm	_____inches/cm
Calf	_____inches/cm	_____inches/cm
Ankle	_____inches/cm	_____inches/cm

Action	Rationale
8. Compare measurements of one leg with the other and with baseline data. Look for any discrepancies.	Swelling of one leg may be an early sign of thrombophlebitis. Findings of 1.5 cm increase in size (as compared with baseline or admission measurements) or a 1.5 cm discrepancy (when compared with the unaffected leg) is considered significant for males; a 1.2 cm measurement is considered significant for females.

partment syndrome and/or ischemic necrosis (Kirshblum and Zafonte 1989).

2. *Avoid local trauma to blood vessels.* Regular turning to relieve pressure and positioning the patient correctly to reduce pressure on body prominences help ensure adequate circulation to the skin. Positioning, support, and protection of the extremities, including the arms of quadriplegic patients, are important whether the patient is on bedrest or sitting up in a wheelchair. (Chapter 20 describes specific positioning methods on various immobilization beds.)

Generally, measures to prevent, recognize, and treat skin breakdown will in turn prevent undue pressure on internal vein structures. Avoid venous punctures in the legs at all costs. Be sure to alert lab technicians to avoid this hazard when obtaining blood specimens. An IV site in the leg should be selected only under extraordinary circumstances. Also, attend promptly minor cuts, blisters, or skin abrasions on the legs and feet. Due to paralysis, the healing process is slow and extra care is needed to prevent infection.

Maintaining Desirable Body Temperature

To maintain desirable body temperature, care focuses on protecting the patient from the environment. *Hypothermia* in the immediate postinjury period is common. Measures to help conserve and dissipate body heat are needed.

Helping Conserve Body Heat

1. Prevent undesirable cooling of the body. Maintain a desirable environmental temperature of 21°C (70°F) whenever possible. The quadriplegic patient (without blankets) in a constant environmental temperature of 21°C (70°F) will stabilize at a body temperature of 35°C (94° to 95°F) (Cheshire and Coates 1966). This slight degree of hypothermia may be beneficial during the initial postinjury period when hypoxia is most likely to occur. The lowered body temperature decreases the basal metabolic rate, thereby reducing oxygen requirements and reducing the work of breathing. Although there may be immediate therapeutic advantages to this spontaneous cooling, the patient is generally kept covered until complications are ruled out. Later, if patients are going to be outside for activities, or even for a short period during transport, provide warm clothing or covering to protect them from the climate. Carefully observe inactive, poorly nourished, or elderly patients who have difficulty keeping warm at the best of times.

2. Take measures to warm the patient. A blood-warming system may be needed. A hot beverage, a warm bath, or an extra cover, for example, may make the patient comfortable. Keep the patient dry at all times to prevent rapid heat loss. Never use hot water bottles and electric heating devices that may burn desensitized skin.

The postoperative patient with SCI can readily develop hypothermia. Immediate placement of warmed blankets on the patient in the recovery room usually prevents further problems.

3. Care for the quadriplegic patient with excessive diaphoresis of the upper body. Sometimes periods of *profuse* sweating above the level of injury are thought to be a mechanism triggered to compensate for loss of thermoregulatory sweating below the level of injury. This is most uncomfortable and distressing although the condition tends to stabilize eventually. The patient must be kept dry to *prevent chilling*. Changes of bed linen or clothing may be necessary every few hours. "Drenching" of bed linen is not uncommon. Flannel sheets or towels used to wrap the patient's torso are most absorbent. Dehydration may occur.

When the problem is prolonged or interferes with daily activities, oral anticholinergic drug therapy can be used to suppress the overactive sweat glands. However, anticholinergic side effects may also produce undesirable reactions, such as urinary retention.

Periods of excessive sweating may be induced by reflex action of the sympathetic nervous system. Underlying conditions, such as increased bladder pressure from infection or straining with a constipated stool, may cause reflex sweating. Unlike the desired diaphoresis associated with temperature control, the cause of these diaphoretic episodes must be identified and treated.

Helping Dissipate Body Heat

1. Prevent undesirable warming of the body. Avoid the outdoors if temperatures are extremely high, especially if high humidity is a factor, or remove extra clothing during exercise or therapy periods to allow heat loss. The patient's oral temperature may well average 38°C (100° to 101°F) at this time (Thomas 1977).

A fan can be used to cool a warm patient (constant air flow aids heat loss by convection). Adjust air conditioning if possible. Another idea, often used by wheelchair athletes, is to carry a water spray bottle. The water vapor sprayed on the skin acts like perspiration to promote heat loss through evaporation.

2. Recognize, investigate, and treat fever promptly. An elevated temperature is a particularly valuable diagnostic sign, as sensory loss frequently renders the patient unable to localize or describe pain associated with infection or other underlying disease processes.

- Detect onset of fever. Frequently the patient will feel chilled, complain of general malaise, fatigue, headache, and loss of appetite, and the skin will be warm and dry to the touch. Monitor temperature rectally every 2 to 4 hours, or more frequently, to reveal fever pattern. Observe pulse and respirations. Hyperventilation may occur as oxygen requirements increase approximately 18% with each 1°C rise in body temperature.

- A constant fever pattern, of sudden onset, is usually associated with infection. Urinary or respiratory tract infections are common culprits in patients with SCI. Immediately check for concentrated, foul-smelling, or sedimented urine. Perform a chest inspection and note any signs of congestion. Check for a moist, productive cough that may indicate early secretion retention. A persistent low-grade fever can be associated with thrombophlebitis. Check the lower extremities for any signs.

- An intermittent fever pattern, in which the temperature is elevated for periods and then returns to normal during a 24-hour time span, may indicate an allergic drug reaction, gram-negative bacteremia, or septicemia. This can be very difficult to diagnose. Check the patient's drug profile. Note any penicillins or barbiturates in particular that may cause an allergic reaction. Often a blood culture, obtained when the temperature is next elevated, will be ordered.

- Alert the physician to an elevated temperature. Before specifically treating the source of the suspected infection, obtain urine, sputum, throat, and wound specimens for culture and sensitivity to indicate specific antibiotic therapy. As paralyzed patients are prone to a number of infections over a long-term period, cautious use of antibiotics in the early stages is important to avoid building up a drug resistance.

- Administer antipyretic drugs as ordered to act directly on the vasomotor temperature control center and take measures to promote heat loss from the body surface. Fanning and tepid sponging are usually sufficient to maintain the body temperature around 37.8°C (100°F). Alcohol sponges have a tendency to dry the skin. The use of ice packs or an electric cooling blanket introduces the added risk of "burning" the patient's insensitive skin and is rarely necessary. Should the patient begin to shiver above the level of the injury, stop the cooling measures in use. The shivering mechanism actually generates heat. The patient may even need to be warmed temporarily to alleviate shivering.

- Replace fluid loss and maintain adequate nutrition. Increase fluid intake to 3000 ml daily unless contraindicated by other conditions. As the basal metabolic rate increases with fever, there is a dramatic increase in the amount of calories needed. Nourishing liquids, such as milk shakes or eggnogs, are usually most acceptable to the anorexic patient. Soup or broth is good, too. Intravenous therapy for fluid and electrolyte replacement may also be necessary.

SPECIFIC MANAGEMENT OF CARDIOVASCULAR COMPLICATIONS

Cardiac Dysrhythmias

Patients with severe *cervical* cord injury are especially prone to irregularities of heart contractions, cardiac dysrhythmias. Disruption to the autonomic nervous system decreases sympathetic stimulation to the heart and allows parasympathetic influence to predominate. Autonomic imbalance exists. Abnormalities, namely bradydysrhythmias, supraventricular dysrhythmias, and primary cardiac arrest must be anticipated to peak during the initial postinjury period and taper off over the next 6 weeks (Lehmann, Lane, Piepmeier, and Batsford 1987). Preexisting cardiovascular status and related risk factors will increase the severity of cardiac dysrhythmias.

Severe instability of the cardiovascular system is prolonged for patients with high quadriplegia. A most dangerous phenomenon may occur. Stimulation, such as rapid changes of body position when turning or tracheal suctioning, is believed to trigger an *abnormal vasovagal response*. Massive activation of the parasympathetic system, made possible by the intact cranial outflow portion, is unchecked by the usual sympathetic antagonism; therefore stimulation to the heart is strong enough not only to slow, but also to stop, the heartbeat.

To care for patients with cardiac dysrhythmias,

- Minimize risk conditions to stabilize heart rate and blood pressure.
- Preserve adequate cardiac output by maintaining optimum heart rate and sufficient systemic perfusion.
- Diagnose and initiate treatment early to prevent progression of symptoms causing fatal complications.

Management

1. Provide general measures, as discussed previously in this chapter, to

- Prevent systemic hypoxia and therefore myocardial hypoxia
- Minimize workload of the heart to decrease oxygen requirements
- Maintain desirable blood volume and systemic composition
- Promote vascular circulation to avoid complications of dependent edema and postural hypotension

2. Maintain normal fluid and electrolyte balances. Surprisingly severe fluid and metabolic imbalances can and usually do accompany SCI. It is postulated that increased mineralocorticoid activity leads to sodium retention and potassium depletion (Burke and Murray 1975). A positive sodium balance causing overhydration adds to circulatory overload. More important is the severe loss of potassium. *Hypokalemia* delays restoration of smooth muscle function, particularly in the cardiac muscle; irregularities can thus develop. The body's buffer systems are severely taxed by pulmonary and renal involvement, which further aggravate the situation. Administer fluid and electrolyte replacement therapy as ordered and monitor.

3. Measure hourly intake and output. Since the interpretation of vital signs can be confusing and not reflect the seriousness of the clinical situation, end organ perfusion (kidneys) is considered a critical indicator. A *minimum output of 30 cc per hour* indicates adequate cardiovascular function (McCagg 1986).

4. Alleviate pain and promote physical and emotional rest to minimize stress response activated with the sympathetic system. This minimizes stimulating effects of increased catecholamines circulating in the blood, characterized by premature contractions.

5. *Avoid vagal stimulation leading to uncontrolled brady-cardia or cardiac arrest in quadriplegic patients.* Suction patients cautiously, especially those with an artificial airway. Even manipulation of the endotracheal tube can elicit this undesirable response. To minimize risk:

- Preoxygenate the patient on 100% oxygen before and after suctioning to minimize the risk of hypoxia-induced dysrhythmias. Observe a time limit of 10 to 15 seconds when applying suction to avoid blocking patient's air supply.
- Bagging with a *manual resuscitator* for several breaths to increase the heart rate before suctioning has also proven effective. When the vasovagal stimulus does reduce the heart rate, the abnormal response is minimized.
- Keep Atropine on hand to reverse uncontrolled bradycardia.
- Avoid turning patients quickly. Although poorly understood, cardiac arrest has occurred following a sudden change of position. Turning may create an undesirable stimulus. Without time to develop a local homeostasis, the passively dilated venous network may simply be unable to shunt blood adequately to accommodate the position change. For this reason, early use of turning frames for those with cord injury at or above T_6 can cause problems.

6. Constantly observe patients with preexisting heart disease or those at risk of developing cardiac involvement. Some factors to be alert for are advanced age, severe emotional strain, severe pulmonary or renal involvement, a history of smoking, and diabetes. There should be frequent consultations between physicians and other care givers concerning continuous ECG monitoring, need for pain relief, and need for oxygen for high-risk individuals. Confirm preexisting diagnosis and initiate treatment measures to alleviate effects of primary disease.

7. Observe for deterioration in current cardiac function associated with dysrhythmias. Are dysrhythmias to compensate for decreased heart rate or is there another reason? Look for signs of decreased *cardiac output*, mainly reflected by depressed level of consciousness, failing cardiac signs, and poor renal function as follows:

- Note subtle changes in the level of consciousness, such as dizziness or slow mentation, which can indicate hypoxia.
- Note falling blood pressure and pulse rate and rhythm irregularities. Compare apical pulse with peripheral pulses to detect any pulse deficit.
- Be alert for decreased urinary output (less than 30 cc/hour is cause for alarm).
- Be alert for signs of heart failure. Increased central venous pressure, jugular vein distension, venous engorgement of abdominal vessels, liver tenderness, anorexia, nausea and vomiting, and general-

ized dependent edema suggest right-sided heart failure, which causes backup of blood in the systemic circulation. Left-sided heart failure causes backup of blood in the lungs and creates pulmonary signs such as dyspnea, rales, and wheezing; cyanosis; pulmonary edema; and hyperventilation leading to respiratory alkalosis. Finally, more generalized symptoms, such as severe apprehension with accompanying chest pain, poor color, and clammy skin with diaphoresis, may well indicate a myocardial infarction.

8. Detect dysrhythmias by continuous monitoring. The ability to identify a normal sinus rhythm, detect abnormalities, and initiate appropriate interventions is important. Obtain an electrocardiogram rhythm strip and attach to chart on a regular basis and when abnormal rhythm occurs. Note and record time of onset, duration, and frequency of dysrhythmia. Collaborate with the physician to determine acceptable parameters for the heart rate and number and pattern of premature ventricular beats allowed. If the patient is hemodynamically stable, intervention may not be warranted. If dysrhythmias worsen, however, cardiac output can fall to dangerous levels. A sudden onset of bradycardia is dangerous, whereas a gradual onset is a compensatory method to improve stroke volume and maintain cardiac output that is commonly seen with quadriplegia.

9. Administer cardiac suppressants and stimulants, diuretics, and oxygen therapy as ordered. Also administer analgesics as ordered. Assess pain and anxiety levels frequently. (Often small intravenous doses of analgesics every 2 hours are most effective.)

10. Detect abnormal laboratory findings (primarily blood hematology, chemistry, electrolytes, and urine and serum osmolality) and respond appropriately. Monitor arterial blood gas analysis.

Expected Outcomes

Evaluate effectiveness of treatment by level of outcome criteria reached:

- Pulse 60 to 100 beats per minute of regular rate and rhythm, no pulse deficit, peripheral pulses of equal rhythm and volume bilaterally
- Blood pressure within normal limits for patient (100/60 mmHg is acceptable for a recumbent quadriplegic person)
- ECG in regular sinus rhythm without evidence of premature beats (or within acceptable rate and pattern as decided by physician)
- Heart action able to maintain adequate central and systemic perfusion as evidenced by alert and oriented mental state, absence of elevated venous systemic or pulmonary pressure, no chest pain (angina), and urinary output within normal limits, usually 2 to 3 liters per day (30 ml/hour minimum)

Dependent Edema

Edema is the swelling of body tissues from excessive fluid accumulating in the interstitial spaces. The source of edematous fluid is the blood plasma (Kozier and Erb 1991). During circulation the blood plasma enters the capillary from the arterioles and filters into the interstitial space. Fluid, electrolytes, and nutrients are delivered and waste products are removed in this space between the capillaries and the tissue cells. Normally, approximately 90% of the fluid reenters the capillary at the venule end and is reabsorbed into the systemic circulation. The remaining 10% is reabsorbed by the lymphatic system.

Several factors may interfere with this fluid exchange at the capillary level to result in edema. The most common cause, however, is an increase in venous pressure at the reabsorption end of the capillary. When reabsorption is not possible, fluid is trapped in the interstitial spaces and nourishment and removal of waste products at the cellular level is decreased. This is also true of patients with SCI. Due to disturbed vasomotor control and decreased tone in paralyzed limbs, circulatory return to the heart is poor, which increases venous pressure. Sluggish venous return is overcome by gravitational forces and *dependent* or *orthostatic edema* occurs. Dependent edema is characterized by bilateral, pitting edema in dependent body parts that is relieved by position changes. Spinal shock aggravates this complication.

To care for persons with dependent edema,

- Promote venous return to the heart to assist movement of edematous fluid back into the systemic circulation
- Prevent complications.

Management

1. Encourage as much activity as possible within limits of orthopedic stability while on bedrest and in the wheelchair. Avoid extended periods of time without a position change or incorrect positioning of limbs that will block circulation. Protect the patient from skin breakdown or other local trauma to blood vessels. Take measures to relieve episodes of postural hypotension.

2. Inspect extremities carefully for evidence of any swelling, especially during early mobilization, as most problems occur at this time. Check lower extremities every few minutes during initial tilt-table mobilization and again on return to bed following early wheelchair activity. *Edema can also occur in dependent areas while the patient is in bed.* Check the sacral area, the hands and arms of quadriplegic patients, and the lower extremities, especially if countertraction is being used (when the bed is tilted with the head raised and foot lowered). Be sure to support upper and lower extremities securely on arm boards, foot boards, or pillows. When the patient is in the wheelchair, paralyzed limbs

must always be supported. Elevated wheelchair leg rests are available. Techniques used to position patients on a variety of immobilization beds are described in Chapter 20. Positioning the patient in a wheelchair is discussed further in Chapter 22.

3. Consult physician if edema does not subside with overnight bedrest or if unilateral or sudden edema occurs. Although dependent edema is most common, other complications, such as cardiac failure or thrombophlebitis, must be ruled out. An X ray of the involved extremities may be needed to determine undetected or pathological fractures or *heterotopic ossification* (Chapter 20).

4. Apply elasticized stockings or tensor bandages, which aid venous circulation as described in the Preventive and Restorative Management section of this chapter.

5. Perform range of motion exercises according to an individualized program. Collaborate with the physician and physical therapist to plan passive exercise programs. Forced movement of edematous joints may cause additional trauma.

Expected Outcomes

Evaluate effectiveness of treatment according to level of outcome reached:

- No evidence of sacral or extremity swelling; if minimal dependent edema is present, it should be relieved with rest or position change
- Skin extremities warm to touch without evidence of breakdown
- Full range of motion possible in all extremities without evidence of contractures or pain
- Blood pressure and pulse within normal limits for patient without evidence of severe and prolonged hypotension
- Urine output balanced with fluid intake without evidence of fluid retention
- Hematocrit, hemoglobin, and red blood cell count of blood plasma within normal range

Postural Hypotension

Postural or *orthostatic hypotension* is a dramatic fall in the blood pressure when the upright position is assumed. The pathology involved is similar to that causing gravitational edema in people with SCI, that is, disturbed vasomotor control decreasing the blood supply returning to the heart. Again, injuries sustained at or above T_{4-6} interfere with sympathetic stimulation to the abdominal viscera and lower extremities. Blood tends to pool in these structures, and the sluggish circulation is overcome by gravitational forces when the patient attempts to sit up in bed or transfers to the wheelchair. Blood literally rushes to the patient's feet, and the body is unable to make the necessary blood pressure adjustments to preserve circulation to the head, neck, and chest areas. The higher the level of injury, the greater the effects become. Prolonged bedrest is an aggravating factor with any patient, but quadriplegic patients have the most difficulty.

General adaptation to this problem does occur, usually within a year after injury. The critical time is during early mobilization from bed to the wheelchair. This process must be undertaken very *gradually* but *must commence as soon as possible to stimulate adjustment* (Mathias and Frankel 1986: 334).

To care for persons with postural hypotension,

- Forestall blood from accumulating in the abdomen and lower extremities when the upright position is assumed
- Prevent complications, such as blackouts or fainting spells, until compensatory function develops

Management

1. Assist the patient to adjust to position changes. Activity is permitted within the limits of orthopedic stability but the mobilization process must be undertaken gradually according to the patient's tolerance. Thomas (1977) recommends progressions in elevating the head of the bed for increasing periods of time before the patient sits at 90 degrees. When the patient can tolerate one-half hour at 30 degrees, increase elevations in stages until 80 to 90 degrees can be tolerated for one hour. Although a reclining back chair may be needed initially, sitting in a wheelchair can then be attempted. A tilt table can be used in a similar fashion. The physical therapist usually supervises the use of this equipment, but it is a good idea to know how to lower the table should a hypotensive episode occur. Monitor the patient's blood pressure before and after each significant position change and compare with baseline data. The systolic pressure should not drop below 80 mmHg.

Other measures used to prevent hypotensive episodes are the application of long-leg antiembolitic elastic stockings, tensor bandaging of the legs, and abdominal binders. The classic many-tailed scultetus binder may be used, but the straight cotton or elastic abdominal binders are more convenient, especially for repeated use. See Figure 16–2. Do not allow any abdominal binder to extend over the rib cage, making chest expansion more difficult. It should reach from the gluteal fold to the waist. Be sure to apply all supports before getting the patient up.

For extreme or prolonged bouts of postural hypotension, medication such as ephedrine may be given 20 to 30 minutes before mobilization.

2. Carefully observe the quadriplegic patient during early mobilization for signs and symptoms of *hypotension*. Often the patient can alert you to its onset. Due to cerebral anoxia weakness, dizziness, pale color, and blurred vision deteriorating to blackouts, or fainting may occur.

3. Promote venous return to increase the blood pressure should a hypotensive episode occur. Immediately lower the

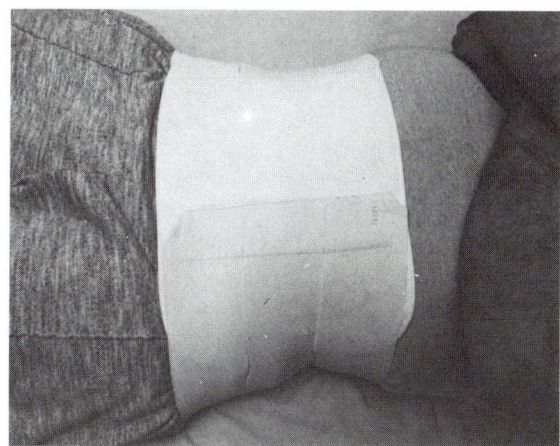

FIGURE 16–2   An elastic abdominal binder with Velcro closures; note correct position to allow for free expansion of rib cage for ease with breathing.

tilt table or head of bed. If the patient is up, quickly tilt the wheelchair backward and lower the chair back (Figure 16–3). Instruct the patient to breathe deeply and assist expiration by placing a hand on the diaphragm. This movement may elicit a vasoconstriction reflex in the chest. Within a few minutes the blackout will usually disappear, and the wheelchair can be slowly returned to its normal position. If these measures are not successful, return the patient to bed, elevate the foot of the bed, and notify the physician.

4. If an episode should occur when the patient is alone, the patient can bend forward to relieve symptoms. To avoid injury from falling out of the wheelchair, secure a safety strap around the lower chest of quadriplegic patients. Provide close supervision and restrict off-ward activities during the early stages.

5. Prepare patient and family to alleviate anxiety should problems occur. Often the patient can alert you verbally of a blackout coming on. Tell the family to notify a staff member and teach them how to alleviate the problem.

Expected Outcomes

Evaluate effectiveness of treatment according to level of outcome reached:

- Alert and oriented
- Blood pressure maintained within normal limits for patient, usually 90/60 mmHg for the stabilized quadriplegic person
- Pulse within normal limits for patient
- Physical strength within normal limits for level of injury sustained
- Patient able to state signs and symptoms of possible onset of hypotensive episodes to alert others

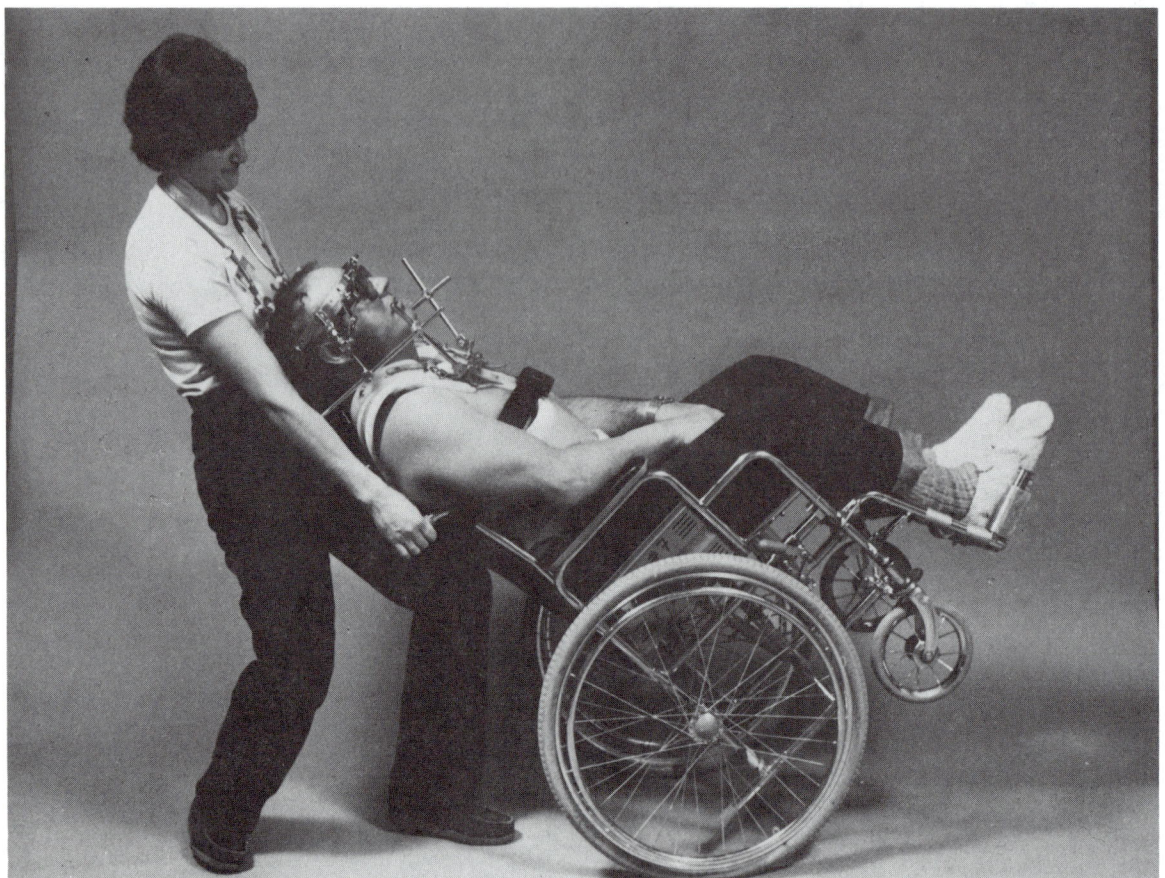

FIGURE 16–3 Promptly tilting the wheelchair back to a reclining position usually prevents or alleviates a fainting spell.

Autonomic Dysreflexia

All interdisciplinary staff must be familiar with the syndrome of *autonomic dysreflexia* or *hyperreflexia*. Autonomic dysreflexia is mainly characterized by a sudden, severe headache secondary to an uncontrolled elevation of blood pressure. If untreated, the *hypertension* may progress to fatal complications, such as cerebral hemorrhage or an acute myocardial infarction.

Most quadriplegic people experience autonomic dysreflexia at some time after the spinal shock period has subsided. Although this autonomic response is most frequent and unpredictable during the first year or so after injury, it occurs throughout life.

Autonomic dysreflexia is caused by a variety of stimuli, creating an exaggerated response of the sympathetic nervous system (comprising the thoracolumbar outflow of the autonomic nervous system) due to lack of control from higher centers. This condition occurs mainly when the level of injury is at the T_{4-6} segmental levels or higher (see Figure 16–4). When injury is sustained below this level, enough of the sympathetic nervous system is usually preserved to avoid this abnormal functional response.

The condition of autonomic dysreflexia is precipitated by specific stimuli from localized areas below the level of injury, mostly from the abdominopelvic region (Taylor 1974). The most frequent source of stimuli is an overdistended bladder. Rectal stimulation, bowel impaction, urinary infection, calculi, or instrumentation (particularly when associated with internal bleeding to some degree) are also common offenders. Later in the rehabilitation process, pressure sores, operative incisions, or perhaps an ingrown toenail, may also cause problems. Even pregnancy, but most especially labor, can elicit this undesirable response (Wanner, Rageth and Zach 1987). The mechanisms involved in this unique condition are (Figure 16–5):

1. Local stimuli (for example, from a distended bladder) enter the spinal cord and ascend to the level of cord injury where communication to the brain is interrupted. An enormous sympathetic reflex response is activated.

2. The result: blood vessel spasticity in the abdominal and pelvic organs and vasculature of the skin. This spasticity causes vasoconstriction to an area so rich in blood supply that the body's blood pressure rises quickly.

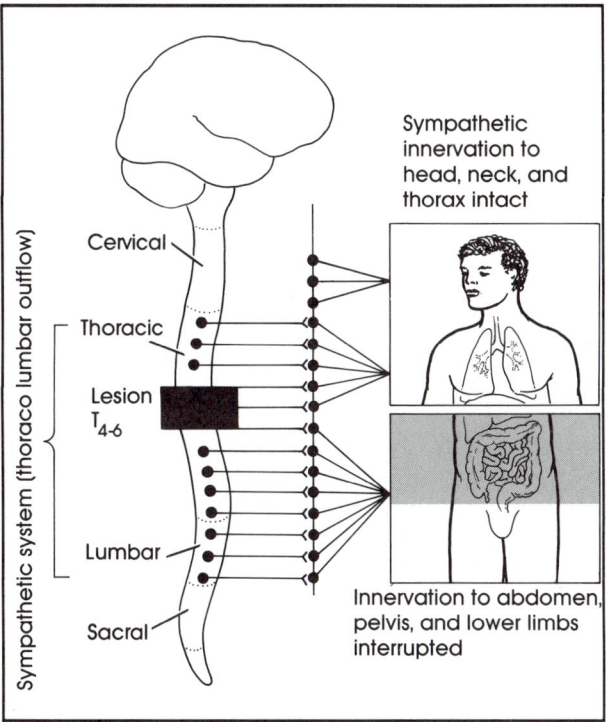

FIGURE 16–4 Significant interruption of the sympathetic nervous system is evident with an injury at the T_{4-6} cord segments or above.

3. Messages indicating this sudden hypertension travel by *systemic routes* other than the spinal cord (communication from distended receptors in the aortic arch and carotid sinuses) to the vasomotor center in the brain. To compensate, the parasympathetic division of the autonomic nervous system lowers the blood pressure by slowing the heart rate and attempting to dilate all blood vessels. Some impulses may be effective, as normal parasympathetic (cranial) outflow is preserved, but other impulses are blocked by the cord injury, thus preventing communication with the lower thoracic and sacral autonomic outflow.

4. *The result:*
Overactive sympathetic vasodilation above the level of injury causing the sudden onset of:

- Headache (due to elevated blood pressure) of a pounding, severe nature
- Elevated blood pressure. (Compare with baseline data. Blood pressure of 140/90 may be considered high for some; others may experience obvious extremes of blood pressure of 300/160.)
- Profuse sweating, flushed face, blotchiness of skin above the level of injury, and goose bumps
- Nasal stuffiness or obstruction
- Apprehension, very frightened
- Bradycardia (from unbalanced parasympathetic influence)

To care for patients with autonomic dysreflexia,

- Recognize immediately the onset of this condition and initiate measures to lower the blood pressure
- Remove or control stimuli and prevent dangerous or fatal complications such as cerebral hemorrhage
- Prevent recurring episodes

Management

1. Minimize risks of abnormal autonomic responses from local stimuli, and especially provide optimal bladder and bowel care (see Chapters 18 and 19):

- During the intermittent catheterization program, ensure a desirable balance between intake and output. Monitor IV fluids carefully to prevent over-hydration or warn patients against drinking several glasses of fluid at one time. Urinary output for each catheterization (including the preceding manual expression measurement) should not exceed 600 ml.
- When the patient has an indwelling catheter, promote unobstructed, gravity-assisted drainage at all times.
- Take measures to prevent urinary infection, reflux, and calculi formation that could serve as a focus for abnormal stimuli.
- Observe the postoperative patient closely. Following any invasive diagnostic procedures or surgery involving the urinary tract, hemorrhage or clots may block a catheter and cause overdistension of the bladder.
- Provide regular and reliable bowel program. Keep stool soft. Avoid incomplete emptying and constipation.

2. Closely observe the patient with quadriplegia or high paraplegia. The patient may experience an isolated incident of autonomic dysreflexia or develop autonomic dysreflexia signs following certain procedures. Be aware of those factors associated with earlier episodes to prevent recurrence.

3. Be alert for signs and symptoms, indicating the onset of autonomic dysreflexia.

4. If up in the wheelchair, return the patient to bed and elevate the head of the bed or hold the patient in the sitting position to lower the blood pressure. Postural hypotension is induced in the sitting position. Avoid placing the patient in a chair as it is more difficult to check the possible source of stimuli. During a crisis situation, care will require two or three staff members simultaneously to monitor the blood pressure every few minutes and check for a possible cause.

5. Remove the causative stimuli if possible.

- Check the bladder for overdistension, the most frequent cause. If the patient is on an intermittent catheterization program, catheterize immediately regardless of how recently the last procedure was performed. If there is an indwelling catheter, look

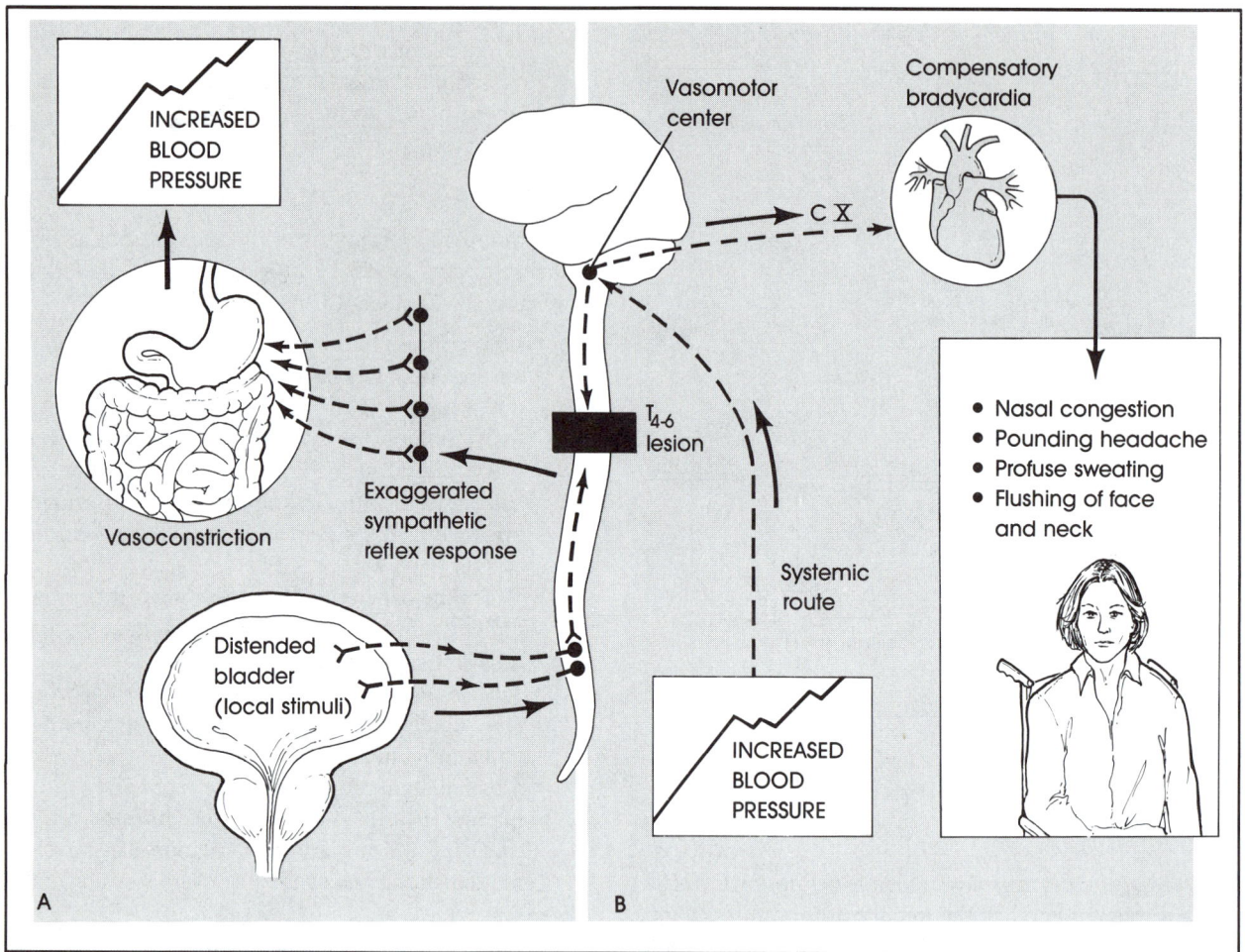

FIGURE 16–5   (**A**) Local stimuli enter the spinal cord; upgoing communication is blocked by injury at T$_{4-6}$ segmental levels (or above); an exaggerated sympathetic reflex response is activated. (**B**) Communication via systemic routes activates the parasympathetic nervous system, but inhibitive downgoing messages are blocked by the T$_{4-6}$ lesion; parasympathetic response in the cranial outflow overcompensates, causing a number of symptoms experienced above the level of injury.

for kinks in the tubing, plugged connections, or a full leg bag—anything that may obstruct the urinary flow (Taylor 1974). Immediately irrigate or change the Foley catheter if obstruction persists using anesthetic gel as lubricant.

- Check the lower bowel for stool. Bowel problems often cause onset of autonomic dysreflexia during routine evacuation measures. Gently and gradually try to remove stool manually. If symptoms persist, *stop* procedure. Resume cautiously if symptoms subside. This may require instillation of an anesthetic gel 10 minutes before resuming.

6.   Consult the physician promptly if first aid treatments are not successful. Although the techniques mentioned are usually effective, miscellaneous problems need to be identified and treated. For example, if profuse bleeding and clotting occur following a urological procedure, the patient

will probably have to return to the operating room for surgical intervention.

7.   If the blood pressure does not return to normal, administer antihypertensive drugs as ordered. During a crisis situation, intravenous medication is required. To counteract massive sympathetic outflow immediately, intravenous ganglionic blocking agents such as Himethaphan (Arfonad) should be used; nitroprusside sodium (Nipride, Nitropress) and diazoxide (Hyperstat IV) also act rapidly and have a direct vasodilatory effect (McGuire and Kumar 1986). Comarr (1977) recommends hydralazine hydrochloride (Apresoline) (20 mg per ml) cautiously given 0.5 ml at a time. Should extreme hypotension occur, an antidote to the ganglionic blocking agents, such as metaraminol bitartrate (Aramine), should be kept on hand. A rebound hypotension is common, so drugs must be administered cautiously and effects must be monitored carefully. If the hydralazine

hydrochloride fails to lower the blood pressure, a low spinal anesthetic may be given to calm local reflex activity in the abdomen or the lower extremities. This is a rare occurrence. These medications should be located in a prominent place for convenience. Some centers use the emergency cart. A lumbar puncture tray to administer the spinal anesthetic should also be easily accessible.

Once the entire episode has passed, an elevated blood pressure and other symptoms may persist, requiring less potent, oral, antihypertensive medication. The dosage may be titrated as indicated by the blood pressure.

8. Monitor the patient's blood pressure and pulse every 4 hours for 24 hours following a crisis. The autonomic nervous system tends to remain unstable when the body's reaction has been severe.

9. Provide psychological support. The exaggerated sympathetic response is accompanied by an increased circulation of catecholamines, which increase anxiety. The patient may feel apprehensive and agitated and find it difficult to rest. Explain the body's reaction and make the patient comfortable to promote sleep.

10. Reconsider the causes of autonomic dysreflexia for each patient, and initiate management to prevent further episodes if possible. For example, if rectal stimulation during bowel procedures precipitates an attack, insert a local anesthetic, such as Nupercaine ointment 1% 10 minutes before evacuation.

Should a patient experience headache, a rise in blood pressure, and diaphoresis every time voiding is imminent (these may be described as "autonomic signs"), a course of medication may be tried to quiet the hyperactivity of bladder contractions and relax tight sphincters to help emptying.

11. Provide patient and family education. At an appropriate time, the patient must be adequately prepared to cope with this emergency situation outside the hospital setting. A medic alert system accompanied with a wallet-size instruction card is highly recommended (Hammond, Umlauf, Matteson, and Perduta-Fulginiti 1989). See Figure 16–6.

Expected Outcomes

Evaluate effectiveness of treatment according to level of outcome criteria reached:

- Blood pressure within normal limits for patient (usually 90/60 mmHg for a quadriplegic person in the sitting position)
- Pulse rate within normal limits for patient without evidence of bradycardia
- Patient comfortable without signs of hypertension (no headache, signs of increased intercranial pressure, or signs of heart failure indicating hemorrhage)
- Nasal passages clear

TO WHOM IT MAY CONCERN:

I have suffered a spinal cord injury at the level of T_6 or above; therefore, I am subject to a syndrome known as Autonomic Dysreflexia. The symptoms are caused by an overwhelming discharge of the sympathetic nervous system. If not treated promptly, it can lead to a CVA or death.

Possible Causes:

Irritation of the bladder (overdistension, infection, stones, plugged catheter), distension of the bowel, menstrual cramps, pressure sores, ingrown toenails, pregnancy.

Signs and Symptoms: (May have only 1 or 2 of these):

Hypertension, severe headache, flushing or blotching of skin, gooseflesh, nasal congestion, slow pulse, feeling of great anxiety, sweating.

Treatment:

1. Help me sit up
2. Find and correct the cause:
   a. If using indwelling catheter, check system for kinked tubing or clogged catheter. Irrigate catheter with no more than 30 cc solution. If unrelieved, remove catheter and catheterize.
   b. If not using indwelling catheter, catheterize immediately.
   c. If no relief, apply nupercainal ointment to rectum and gently remove any feces present.
   d. Check skin for irritation.
3. Employ emergency medical treatment if symptoms continue.
   Some suggested treatments include:
   1. Amyl Nitrite ampules by inhalation or
   2. Nitroglycerin tablets SL 0.15 mg–0.3 mg or
   3. Apresoline 10–20 mg IM or IV or
   4. Hyperstat 300mg IV or
   5. Regitine 5 mg IM or IV

(Courtesy of National Rehabilitation Hospital. Washington, DC, © 1989. Reprinted with permission.)

FIGURE 16–6 A wallet instruction card for autonomic dysreflexia.

- Skin warm, dry, pink (if the patient is Caucasian), and without blotchiness or excessive sweating above the level of injury
- Patient calm or able to sleep
- Patient able to state signs and symptoms and causes of onset of autonomic crisis to alert staff member
- Individual and family actively involved in management with a preventive focus and problem solving; prepared to take appropriate actions when living in the community

Thromboembolitic Disease (Deep Vein Thrombosis)

Deep vein thrombosis (DVT) is the development of a blood clot in the venous structures. It is particularly common in the abdominopelvic region and lower extremities. Sometimes *thrombophlebitis,* or inflammation of a venous pathway, can be identified before the clot or *thrombus* matures.

A clot—consisting of intact and ruptured platelets that adhere to the blood vessel wall—protrudes slightly. The platelets cause the precipitation of fibrin and other blood elements, which then form the mature thrombus. Once formed, a thrombus can grow in size as more platelets and blood elements stick to it. A thrombus can partially or completely occlude a blood vessel or break free from the blood vessel wall and travel in the bloodstream, at which point it becomes an *embolus.* The embolus is most dangerous when it enters the pulmonary circulation and obstructs blood flow to lung tissue. *Thromboembolitic disease* (TED) refers to this process.

Stasis of venous circulation, changes or trauma to the vein wall, and hypercoagulability of the blood—all consequences of SCI—can precipitate formation of thrombi. Therefore, all patients with SCI are susceptible. Additional risks include: advanced age, poor nutritional status, obesity, smoking, preexisting heart disease, lung complications, associated hip or long bone fractures, and recent (especially abdominal) surgery.

During the first 3 months postinjury, 15% to 100% of patients may develop DVT. Occurrence varies with the diagnostic tests used. Unfortunately, there is no consensus on how to prevent DVT (McCagg 1986). For instance, no well-defined, adequately controlled studies of prophylactic anticoagulation methods have been reported to date (Lammertse 1989).

Some specialized SCI centers rely on passive motion exercises (rigorously and consistently performed) and early mobilization. They may also use antiembolitic elastic stockings and pneumatic compression stockings. They avoid even low doses of anticoagulants, which may further reduce oxygen supply to the damaged spinal cord. Furthermore, after spinal surgery, anticoagulants increase the risk of occult bleeding or hemorrhage at the operative site and in other body systems (VanPheteghem and Belanger 1990).

Presently, however, widespread use of low-dose anticoagulation is practiced because the risk of thromboembolism is believed to be high compared to the risks of prophylaxis. Pulmonary emboli are the most common, and can be fatal.

Once a thromboembolitic complication does occur, a full anticoagulation regimen is generally begun. If bleeding complications cannot be controlled, or if risks are too high, an inferior vena cava filter should be considered (Lammertse 1989).

The clinical picture is complicated by the fact that the person with SCI cannot feel the classic sign of pain in the affected part. *Fever,* frequently low grade and occurring at night, when no other source can be found, may be the earliest, and possibly the only, clinical sign of an otherwise occult thromboembolitic process (Weingarden, Weingarden, and Belen 1988).

The increased use of the RotoRest Treatment Table is also suggested as beneficial in reducing the incidence of DVT because the patient is in perpetual motion, changing position up to 200 times per 24 hours (Becker, Gonzalez, and Gentili 1987; Green, Green, and Klose 1980). More research concerning this kinetic measure to reduce cardiopulmonary and other complications of immobilization would be welcomed.

Functional electrical stimulation (FES), addressed in general in Chapter 24, applied to the calf muscles to increase circulation may also have a role to play in the future.

To care for patients with thromboembolitic disease,

- Promote venous return and inhibit formation of thrombi
- Detect thrombophlebitis early, and prevent or control DVT
- Prevent pulmonary emboli

Management

1. Discourage clot formation by promoting venous return to the heart, increasing the rate of blood flow in the peripheral vascular system, and preventing blood pooling in the extremities:

   - Encourage as much activity as possible within limits of orthopedic stability. If the patient is on bedrest, active and passive range of motion exercises are essential. Be sure to include a full range of passive exercises to the lower limbs during morning and evening care. *Also perform ankle-pumping exercises, about five times on each foot after every turn.* A physical therapy program designed according to level of injury and patient tolerance should be initiated soon after admission. Early mobilization with postural changes and wheelchair activity greatly decreases the risk factors.

- Apply elastic stockings or tensor bandages correctly to exert a compression force on the veins.
- Position limbs carefully to avoid gravitational edema.
- Encourage smokers to quit. Nicotine in cigarettes is believed to constrict the veins, thus slowing blood flow.

Protect venous walls from trauma or pressure as follows:

- Turn and correctly position the patient every 2 hours. Generally, measures taken to prevent skin breakdown will prevent undue pressure on internal vein structures. Take care to prevent pressure on the susceptible popliteal space behind the knee, a point at which lower limb circulation can be easily obstructed, especially in the supine position. *Never put pillows under the knees or use a knee gatch when a patient is sitting in bed.* Elevate the entire foot of the bed on blocks if necessary. When a patient is in the side-lying position, be sure to place a pillow between the legs. Without a pillow, the legs pressing against each other will compress the veins.
- Avoid venous punctures in the legs at all costs. Be sure to alert lab technicians when obtaining blood specimens to avoid this hazard.
- Promptly attend to minor cuts, blisters, or skin abrasions on the legs and feet. The healing process is slowed due to already compromised circulation, and extra care is needed to prevent infection and subsequent blood vessel irritation.

Minimize effects of hypercoagulability and promote normal clotting as follows:

- Prevent or alleviate dehydration, thus avoiding an increase in blood viscosity.
- Question women of childbearing age who may be taking birth control pills. Research shows this pseudopregnancy state, accompanied by a slight increase in blood coagulability, may also be a predisposing factor in increasing the tendency for clot formation. The physician will likely order discontinuance of birth control pills, at least temporarily.
- Administer *prophylactic* anticoagulant therapy as prescribed by physician. The desired effects of preventing thrombosis must be carefully weighed against complications of uncontrolled bleeding.

2. Monitor the high-risk patient closely for thrombophlebitis, especially during the 3 to 5 weeks immediately after injury when the incidence of thrombus formation is greatest.

Patients with high, complete quadriplegia and those with multiple trauma and/or with persistent infection are particularly at risk, as are obese and elderly patients.

3. Monitor body temperature regularly for at least 6 weeks after injury. A low-grade fever, unaccompanied by apparent infection, often indicates thrombus formation. The time it takes to get a quick temperature before the daily activities start is always well spent; it can provide valuable baseline data for detecting a host of problems. Low grade fever pattern associated with TED generally spikes at night during the first 3 months postinjury (Weingarden, Weingarden, and Belen 1988).

4. Observe lower extremities of all patients daily. During morning care is a convenient time. Thrombophlebitis is often discovered by astute nurses and therapists during routine activities. Expose the legs from the groin to the feet. Compare legs bilaterally. Look for any combination of the following signs or symptoms:

- Skin warm to the touch in a localized area. An increased temperature in the affected leg often occurs several days before other signs. If the patient has had a heavy blanket on, expose the legs for 10 minutes to assume room temperature. To increase sensitivity to temperature variation, place your hands in cold water for a few minutes before examination and then use the backs of your hands. Compare various parts of each leg at the same time to detect any variations.
- Asymmetric enlargement in comparison of thighs, calves, or ankles. Obtain leg measurements immediately on admission and compare daily if swelling is suspected. See Procedure 16–5 for further information on technique.
- Swelling and/or redness following the course of a vein. Inspect the calves and popliteal areas closely.
- Possible increase in spasticity of affected limb.
- Low-grade fever without other apparent cause. Remember that due to sensory loss the classic Homan's sign or induction of pain on movement will not be present.
- A thrombolitic complication should also be suspected when investigating occult sources of syncope (fainting), pleural effusion, pulmonary infiltrate and hypoxia (Lammertse 1989: 137).

5. If thrombophlebitis is suspected, maintain bedrest and minimize limb movement until the diagnosis is confirmed and further activity orders are obtained.

6. Prepare the patient for diagnostic tests. Clinical evaluation is unreliable 50% of the time. To detect thrombi the two most widely used noninvasive screening procedures are Doppler ultrasound and venous occlusion plethysmography. The two highly accurate diagnostic procedures—125I-labeled fibrinogin uptake scanning and venography—may be used to confirm the diagnosis but are invasive and present the drawback of dislodgment of any thrombus formation (Chu et al. 1985). If thrombi are present, a lung scan will detect any embolization to pulmonary vessels. Coagulation studies are also included.

7. Administer anticoagulant therapy as ordered by physician. Low-dose heparin (such as 5000 to 7500 IU every

12 hours) is the drug of choice for prophylaxis for several reasons: rapid action, lack of interaction with other drugs, relative ease of neutralization, and low incidence of side effects (Watson 1974). Administration would be contraindicated for patients with brain injuries or with gastric, genitourinary, or other signs of internal bleeding. Heparin is most effectively absorbed intravenously and is generally given via a heparin lock by slow infusion over a 5-minute period. Observe the site for signs of infection or infiltration.

8. Adjust anticoagulant medication and dosage as ordered. To protect patient against excessive anticoagulation, clotting and prothrombin times and/or platelet counts are frequently monitored (usually 30 minutes before the next dose of medication is due) to adjust dosages accordingly. Maintaining the prothrombin times at 1.3 to 1.5 the control value will prevent recurrence and minimize the risk of bleeding complications—an important consideration for patients in active rehabilitation (Lammertse 1989; Weingarden, Weingarden, and Belen 1988; McCagg 1986).

Observe closely for any signs of frank bleeding in sputum, nasogastric returns, urine, or stool. Obtain periodic specimens for occult blood. Minimize intramuscular injections, as bleeding from injection site may persist. The patient is usually anticoagulated until the clinical picture has stabilized and gradual mobilization is resumed. To prevent a state of hypercoagulation, the dosage of heparin is reduced *gradually* as oral anticoagulants are initiated over a 5- to 7-day period. Sometimes aspirin is used for its antiplatelet property in preventing thrombus formation. Oral anticoagulants especially tend to be incompatible with many drugs. Check with the hospital pharmacist about interaction with other medications the patient is receiving.

9. If not already done, apply elastic stockings or tensor bandages to exert a compression force on the veins. *Never* use heat treatments on insensitive skin to promote circulation.

10. Carefully elevate the affected limb to promote circulation. Specific activity will be ordered by the physician. Prolonged immobilization may aggravate venous stasis, but some form of inactivity is warranted to minimize the chances of dislodging clots.

A conservative approach includes bedrest for 5 to 10 days with the foot of the bed elevated 10 to 15 degrees (with the hip and knee extended). Range of motion exercises are restricted to the upper extremities.

A more liberal approach includes bedrest for a few days only; legs elevated when up in the wheelchair; and maintenance of a full physical therapy program without exercises to the affected limb.

11. Take measures to avoid postural hypotension and autonomic dysreflexia. Sudden changes in blood pressure could dislodge thrombi.

12. Be constantly alert for signs of embolization to the pulmonary circulation, characterized by sudden onset of hypoxia; rapid, shallow respirations or dyspnea; and severe apprehension. Chest pain may be absent, decreased, or referred due to sensory impairment. Symptoms may vary from mild to severe, depending on the extent of lung involvement. For assessment and interventions, see Chapter 15.

Expected Outcomes

Evaluate effectiveness of treatment by level of outcome criteria reached:

- Lower extremities free from signs of swelling, redness, or localized warmth along the course of a vein
- Leg circumference measurements symmetrical and within normal limits as compared with baseline admission data
- No evidence of increased spasticity
- Body temperature normal
- Anticoagulation studies (clotting and prothrombin times and platelet counts) within acceptable limits for patient
- No signs of blood in sputum, nasogastric aspirate, urine, or stool, and patient free from other signs of internal bleeding
- Ultrasonic recordings and venogram normal without signs of thrombus formation
- Effortless respirations at 12 to 20 breaths per minute without signs of hypoxia or chest discomfort

HEALTH EDUCATION ————

Persons with SCI need to know how their level of injury affects their circulation and body temperature. They must learn measures to promote circulation and avoid hazardous complications associated with blood pooling in the extremities, primarily dependent edema, postural hypotension, and thrombophlebitis. The ever-present danger of autonomic dysreflexia and environmental factors predisposing the person to extreme changes in body temperature should also be included. The program is directed toward the quadriplegic and high paraplegic person, but circulatory difficulties can also be a problem for the person with a lower motor neuron or flaccid paralysis from a lumbosacral injury.

Keeping active, elevating legs periodically during the day on a chair, and taking general measures to relieve pressure on skin and body prominences are general preventive measures. Swelling in the feet, lower legs, and hands of quadriplegic people tends to be a long-term problem. If swelling is not controlled by general measures or does not disappear with overnight rest, a physician should be notified.

Once mobility is established, postural hypotension is not generally a long-term problem, but it may cause dizziness or blackouts in the early stages when individuals are out on day or weekend passes. Include instructions on how to prevent fainting. If the problem occurs when getting out of bed, instruct them to prop the patient on pillows for 15 to 20 minutes beforehand.

Prepare selected individuals for an autonomic dysreflexia crisis, emphasizing prevention and early recognition. Teach how to check bladder and bowel; instruct them to go immediately to the nearest emergency facility if symptoms do not subside. Recommend that quadriplegic persons carry some type of medical alert information.

Teach how to prevent overheating by avoiding direct sunlight in hot weather; staying indoors during extreme heat and humidity; being alert for symptoms of heat stroke (light-headedness, headache, fainting, nausea, and vomiting); and drinking 8 to 10 glasses of fluid per day. Emphasize that body temperature should never be over 37.8°C (100°F). Teach about effective cooling measures: sponging, water spray, fanning, and air conditioning.

Alert people to avoid chilling in cold weather by wearing extra protective clothing. This is an important consideration for people involved in winter sports. Stress never to use hot water bottles or electric heating devices because loss of sensory warning systems makes it difficult to prevent burns to the skin, which are difficult to heal.

For general information on education programs and workbooks for patients and families, see Chapter 11.

LONG-TERM IMPLICATIONS

Physical Consequences

When assessing a quadriplegic or high paraplegic person who has been paralyzed for some time, keep in mind changes in cardiovascular function and control of body temperature that are considered acceptable in light of permanent disability. Adjust baseline data as follows:

1. A chronic, passive degree of vasodilation below the level of injury. However, within a year or so, local reflex activity will resume to provide some compensatory function in vasoconstriction.
2. An average blood pressure of 100/60 mmHg for an uncomplicated stabilized quadriplegic person. A slightly lower pressure of 90/60 mmHg is common in the sitting position.
3. A lowered pulse rate of 60 beats per minute.

The quadriplegic person may always require elastic stockings and occasionally an abdominal binder to control gravitational edema. If edema does not subside overnight, is of sudden onset, or occurs only on one side, further investigation is needed. Prolonged postural hypotension is also abnormal.

Signs of autonomic dysreflexia can usually be avoided as the person becomes more familiar with bladder and bowel management. However, severe, sudden episodes can occur spontaneously at any time after injury. Autonomic dysreflexia is a constant complication to anticipate. Take several precautions and collaborate with a physician if a woman becomes pregnant. See Chapter 10.

Based on your assessment, help the person continue with preventive measures or refer to a family physician or follow-up rehabilitation center if a problem is suspected. Be alert for skin breakdown in all patients with poor circulation. Sometimes underlying problems, such as cardiac failure or inability to provide self-care, will arise.

Fitness for Life

Cardiovascular disease is now the leading cause of death for persons with SCI (Le and Price 1982), the same as for the general population.

Advancements in medical and surgical techniques and more potent and effective drugs to control such other complications as upper urinary tract infections, have brought about this change. A growing interest in aging with a disability and in fitness and related nutrition will help minimize risks associated with coronary artery disease. See Chapter 33.

Fitness and sport, for recreation *and* for health, are as important for people with disabilities as for everyone else. The trend toward early integration of fitness and sport into formal rehabilitation programs is believed to enhance therapeutic goals and promote active participation for life. See Chapter 24. Athletically active people with SCI appear to have less need for medical care and require less rehospitalizations than do their nonactive counterparts (Stotts 1986). Metabolic studies comparing athletic people with SCI to those who are not athletic suggest that desirable high-density lipoprotein cholesterol is lower with inactivity, presumably increasing the risk of coronary heart disease (Brenes, Dearwater, Shapera, LaPorte, and Collins 1986).

Similarly, a focus on health education to prepare persons for managing the effects of disability is advocated as a key to healthy living. Preparation to deal with long-term, related implications, such as obesity associated with an inactive life in a wheelchair, for example, frequently requires a behavioral change. Nutritional counseling, promoting foods rich in fiber and low in cholesterol and calories, needs to be linked with psychosocial support to bring about the desired outcome.

More research into the related risks and combating the consequences of a sedentary life-style for persons with disabilities is needed. Another priority is to provide better access to resources to maintain health, functional abilities, and vocational and recreational pursuits (Brown et al. 1987; Curtis 1986). Finding meaningful ways to integrate injured persons into the mainstream of life is the strongest motivator to keeping fit, eating right, and staying healthy.

REFERENCES

Becker, D. M., Gonzalez, M., and Gentili, A. 1987. Prevention of deep vein thrombosis in patients with acute spinal cord injuries: Use of rotating treatment tables. *Neurosurgery* 20 (5): 675–677. *Results suggest but do not prove that rotating treatment tables prevent proximal deep vein thrombosis.*

Brenes, G., Dearwater, S., Shapera, R., LaPorte, R., and Collins, E. 1986. High density lipoprotein cholesterol concentrations in physically active and sedentary SCI patients. *Archives of Physical Medicine and Rehabilitation* 67 (7): 445–450.

Brown, M., et al. 1987. Unhandicapping the disabled: What is possible? *Archives of Physical Medicine and Rehabilitation* 68 (4): 206–209.

Burke, D., and Murray, D. 1975. *Handbook of Spinal Cord Medicine.* London and Basingstoke: Macmillan Press, Chapters 4 and 6. *Brief overview of temperature control and venous drainage complications.*

Castle, M., and Watkins, J. 1979. Fever: Understanding a sinister sign. *Nursing* 9 (2): 27–33. *A review of normal body temperature control, fever patterns, pyretic agents, and related nursing care.*

Cheshire, D., and Coates, D. 1966. Respiratory and metabolic management in acute tetraplegia. *International Journal of Paraplegia* 4: 1–23. *Includes literature review and summarizes causes of hypothermia following SCI; explores possible clinical advantages of permitting spontaneous cooling (p. 8).*

Chu, D. A., et al. 1985. Deep vein thrombosis: Diagnosis in spinal cord injured patients. *Archives of Physical Medicine and Rehabilitation* 66 (6): 365–368.

Comarr, A. 1977. Autonomic dysreflexia. In *The Total Care of Spinal Cord Injuries.* Eds. D. Pierce and V. Nickel. Boston: Little, Brown, pp. 181–185. *Summarizes etiology and characteristics and focuses on medical management of crisis situations; includes preventive aspects and patient and family education.*

Curtis, K. A. 1986. Health, vocational and functional status in spinal cord injured athletes and non-athletes. *Archives of Physical Medicine and Rehabilitation* 67 (12): 862–865.

Green, B., Green, K., and Klose, K. 1980. Kinetic nursing for acute spinal cord injury patients. *Paraplegia* 18 (3): 181–186.

Guha, A., and Tator, C. 1988. Acute cardiovascular effects of experimental SCI. *Journal of Trauma* 28 (4): 481–490.

Guttman, L. 1973. *Spinal Cord Injuries Comprehensive Management and Research.* Oxford: Blackwell Scientific Publications. *Classic text on all aspects of spinal cord injury.*

Guyton, A. 1976. *Textbook of Medical Physiology.* 5th ed. Philadelphia: W. B. Saunders. *Detailed presentation of local (neural) control of blood flow to tissues and body temperature regulation.*

Hammond, M., Umlauf, R., Matteson, B., Perduta-Fulginiti, F. 1989. *Yes, You Can! A Guide to Self-Care for Persons with Spinal Cord Injury.* Washington, DC: Paralyzed Veterans of America (PVA).

Holloway, N. 1988. *Nursing the Critically Ill Adult.* 3d ed. Menlo Park, CA: Addison-Wesley.

Johnson, R. 1971. Temperature regulation in paraplegia. *International Journal of Paraplegia* 9: 137–143. *Technical descriptions of heat production, heat loss, and the local effect of ambient temperature following SCI.*

Kirshblum, S., and Zafonte, R. 1989. Dangers of elastic bandage immobilization of the spinal cord injury patient. *Abstracts Digest, Annual Meeting, American Spinal Injury Association,* Las Vegas, p. 34.

Kozier, B., and Erb, G. 1991. *Fundamentals of Nursing: Concepts and Procedures.* 4th ed. Menlo Park, CA: Addison-Wesley, pp. 376–380. *Review of tensor bandaging procedures and application of binders.*

Lammertse, D. 1989. Medical management of high quadriplegia. In *The Management of High Quadriplegia.* Eds. G. Whiteneck et al. New York: Demos Publications.

Le, C. T., and Price, M. 1982. Survival from chronic disability. *Journal of Chronic Disabilities* 35: 487.

Lehmann, K., Lane, J., Piepmeier, J., and Batsford, W. 1987. Cardiovascular abnormalities accompanying acute spinal cord injury in humans: Incidence, time course and severity. *Journal of the American College of Cardiology* 10 (1): 46–52.

Mathias, C. J., and Frankel, H. L. 1988. Chapter 16. In *Spinal Cord Injury Medical Engineering.* Eds. D. Ghista and H. L. Frankel. Springfield, IL: Charles C. Thomas Publisher, pp. 323–345. *Addresses cardiovascular disorders and their management in both acute and chronic disability. This text had its origins in NATO Advanced Study Institute and is an excellent reference for interdisciplinary study.*

McCagg, C. 1986. Postoperative management and acute rehabilitation of patients with spinal cord injuries. *Orthopedic Clinics of North America* 17 (1): 171–182. *Emphasis on all aspects of rehabilitation, beginning at the moment of injury. Review article of up-to-date trends and controversies.*

McGuire, T. J., and Kumar, V. N. 1986. Autonomic dysreflexia in the spinal cord injured. What every physician should know about this medical emergency. *Postgraduate Medicine* 80 (2): 81–84, 89. *Review indicates aggressive drug therapy if removal of stimulus is not effective.*

Stotts, K. M. 1986. Health maintenance: Paraplegic athletes and non-athletes. *Archives of Physical Medicine and Rehabilitation* 67 (2): 109–114.

Taylor, A. 1974. Autonomic dysreflexia in spinal cord injury. *Nursing Clinics of North America* 9 (4): 717–725.

Thomas, E. 1977. Nursing care of the patient with spinal cord injury. In *The Total Care of Spinal Cord Injuries.* Eds. D. Pierce and V. Nickel. Boston: Little, Brown, pp. 249–297. *Implications for nursing management in long-term care to maintain optimal body temperatures.*

VanPheteghem, K., and Belanger, L. 1990. Acute Spinal Cord Injury Unit, University Hospital, Shaughnessy Site, Vancouver, BC. Personal communication.

Wanner, M. B., Rageth, C. J., and Zach, G. A. 1987. Pregnancy and autonomic dysreflexia in patients with spinal cord lesions. *Paraplegia* 25 (6): 482–490. *Discusses the increased likelihood of earlier onset of labor pains, the perception of labor pains, general management, and epidural and general anesthesia.*

Watson, N. 1974. Anticoagulant therapy in the treatment of venous thrombosis and pulmonary embolism in acute spinal injury. *International Journal of Paraplegia* 12: 197–201. *Detailed article favoring selected use of anticoagulants.*

Weingarden, S. I., Weingarden, D. S. and Belen, J. 1988. Fever and thromboembolic disease in acute spinal cord injury. *Paraplegia* 26 (1): 35–42. *A 3-year retrospective study of the occult thromboembolic disease process.*

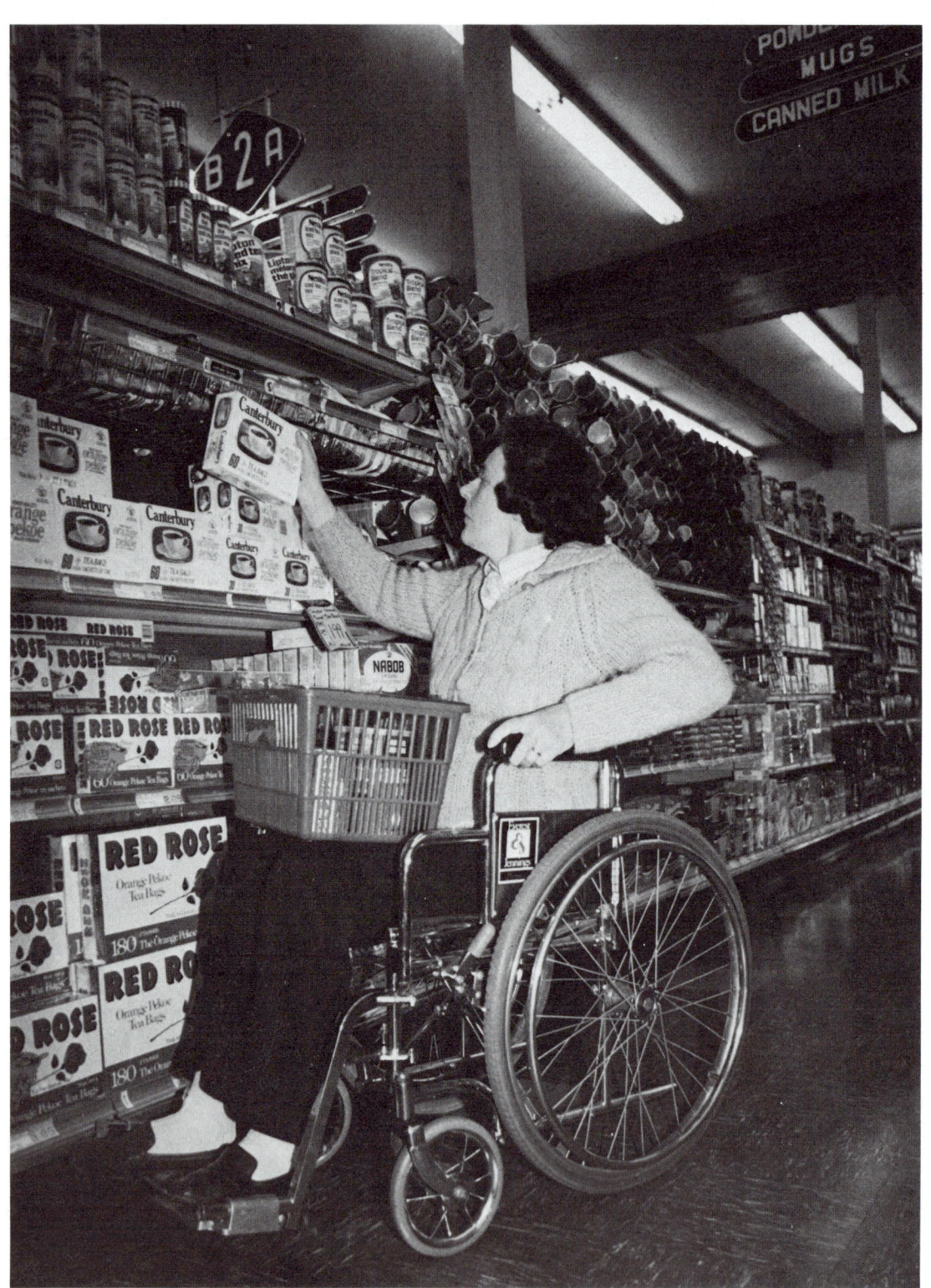

CHAPTER
— 17 —

Maintaining
Optimal Nutrition*

Chapter Outline

Health Care Objectives

- To identify and implement goals of optimal nutritional management
- To describe neural control of the gastrointestinal system and changes in function and nutritional requirements following SCI
- To assess patients' ability to feed themselves and provide appropriate adaptive aids and assistance
- To focus on preventive care and health education

*This chapter was developed with the assistance of Rosemary Cox, R.D.

Nutrition contributes directly to physical and mental health as well as to resistance to infection and disease. Although maintaining optimal nutrition favorably influences the outcomes of the rehabilitation process, it nevertheless presents some unique problems for patients with spinal cord injury (SCI).

Strength and muscle mass begin to decrease rapidly, and dramatic weight loss is not uncommon during the initial postinjury period. Recovery from massive trauma, in the face of permanent disability, frequently results in malnutrition that continues.

Being knowledgeable about nutrition is not enough. Disabled persons must eventually overcome barriers (both physical and sometimes financial) encountered in shopping for groceries, preparing meals, and perhaps even eating independently.

The goals of such nutritional management are:

- To prevent morbidity from nutritional complications
- To prevent or minimize occurrence of malnutrition by accurately providing nutrients for energy and to build, repair, and maintain body systems
- To help individuals reach and maintain, but not exceed, ideal body weight
- To help regulate bladder and bowel programs
- To promote physical and emotional strength, energy level, and ability to participate in daily activities
- To help persons with disabilities develop a continuing plan for food selection, shopping, meal preparation, and assistance with diet and eating as required.

CHANGES IN NUTRITIONAL STATUS FOLLOWING SPINAL CORD INJURY

The Gastrointestinal System and Changes in Neural Control

The gastrointestinal system, or alimentary canal, is a long tubular structure extending from the mouth to the anus and is composed largely of varying layers of smooth muscle. The digestive process is largely controlled by the autonomic nervous system, with the exception of such voluntary acts as chewing, swallowing, and controlling defecation. Generally, with the exception of the distal colon and rectum, innervation to the digestive apparatus is affected only temporarily by SCI.

The gastrointestinal system readies food for absorption and metabolism and eliminates the largest volume of waste products from the body. Digestion requires a number of motor, secretory, and sensory functions. Although the di-

gestive tract receives innervation from both the parasympathetic and sympathetic divisions of the autonomic nervous system, the parasympathetic division is by far the more significant. The sympathetic nervous system contributes antagonistic control to balance activities of motion and secretion, but it is generally less significant in daily functions. For a review of the general characteristics of the autonomic nervous system, see Chapter 4. In general, unchecked parasympathetic activity results in enhanced glandular secretion (that is, pancreatic and gastric) and relaxed junctional sphincters, such as the pylorus and ileocecal valve. Autonomic nervous system imbalance and release of the external anal sphincter from central control are responsible for the majority of the gastrointestinal complications of SCI.

Motor Functions

Motor functions are necessary to propel food through the digestive tract. Parasympathetic stimulation, which is transmitted almost entirely by the vagus nerve from the cranial outflow, maintains tonic contractions (tone) and produces stronger rhythmic contractions when ingestion of food distends the gut. These propulsive movements are referred to as *peristalsis*. With the exception of the immediate postinjury period when reflex activity is suppressed by spinal shock, motor functions of the gastrointestinal tract largely remain within normal limits following SCI.

Secretory Functions

Secretory functions are associated with the chemical digestion of food. The parasympathetic nervous system stimulates production of saliva and other gastric juices to aid in this function. Patients with quadriplegia or high paraplegia may experience *hyperchlorhydria*, a highly acidic condition that occurs most frequently with cervical cord injuries, because the vagus nerve (parasympathetic) is preserved and the thoracolumbar innervation (sympathetic) is interrupted. Stimulation of the vagus nerve causes the secretion of a strong acidic gastric juice, while sympathetic stimulation causes the secretion of a weak, alkaline mucoid juice. When quadriplegia causes interference with sympathetic stimulation, neutralization is diminished and hyperacidity can occur (Pollock and Finkelman 1954).

Sensory Functions

Sensory functions are closely associated with regulation of dietary intake. Some local element of preserved sensation is believed to occur, since the sensations of hunger and satisfaction remain unchanged following SCI. The most significant factor is diminished or lost sensory warning mechanisms in the abdominal area. Although referred pain sometimes ascends to the upper body, this loss of pain can disguise or make acute abdominal distress difficult to recognize. Diagnosis relies heavily on radiographic and laboratory findings.

Metabolic and Nutritional Responses

Metabolic and nutritional responses after SCI indicate that calorie requirements decrease from the moment of injury and remain low throughout life. People with SCI appear to have a reduction in their energy needs proportional to the amount of muscle that has been denervated (Kolpeck et al. 1989; Cox, Weiss, Posuniak, Worthington, Prioleau, and Heffley 1985). The combination of disuse and denervation atrophy significantly correlates with the level of injury, and not the duration of time since injury (Shizgal, Roza, LeDuc, Drouin, Vollemure, and Yaffe 1986). For example, daily energy expenditures and basal metabolic rates measured in persons with high quadriplegia reflected activity levels concomitant with their profound motor deficits; persons with low quadriplegia varied a great deal depending on their abilities, personalities, interests, and motivation; while those with paraplegia were within the normal range when compared to an average population of healthy men (Mollinger et al. 1985). These baseline data suggest that energy needs must be calculated specifically for the SCI population, rather than in comparison to standards for able-bodied people (Lee, Agarwal, Corcoran, Thoden and DelGuercio 1985). Without dietary control, weight gain becomes a problem beginning about one year following the injury.

ASSESSMENT OF NUTRITIONAL STATUS

Nutritional assessment begins with a review of the patient's history for factors that change nutrient needs or interfere with nutrient intake, absorption, and/or digestion. The physical assessment reveals the patient's current nutritional status rather than identifying risk factors. Unfortunately, there is not one specific test for nutritional assessment. Careful interpretation by an experienced clinician of multiple assessment parameters, with consideration given to the nonnutritional factors that may affect these parameters, is critical to an accurate assessment.

Nutritional History

To determine the patient's knowledge, interest, and previous eating habits, discuss a typical breakfast, lunch, dinner, and snacks. During this discussion note special diets, food allergies, likes and dislikes, fluid intake, and any sociocultural factors that may influence the diet. For example, certain ethnic groups prefer diets excessively high in carbohydrates and fats or low in fruits and vegetables; certain foods may be prohibited for religious reasons; and lack of money often restricts food selection.

Also ask about tendencies toward indigestion, diarrhea, or constipation that influence dietary intake. Weight control frequently emerges as a significant problem when adapting to physical disability, therefore, inquire about preinjury weight variation. People with significant weight variation are at additional risk.

Physical Assessment

General Appearance and Vitality
A well-nourished person appears alert and responsive, has healthy looking hair and skin, and is not overweight or underweight. Some early signs of poor nutritional status include easy fatigability, listlessness, inattentive or even irritable behavior, and anorexia. Emaciation, pallor, muscle wasting, and edema can also occur. The mucous membranes of the eyes may look dry or "glassy," and conjunctiva may be too pale or too red. The skin may be dry, or there may be evidence of skin breakdown or lesions.

Anthropometric Data
Height, current weight, usual weight, and ideal body weight are the most useful and easily assessed anthropometric data. Less frequently, muscle mass and body fat are measured. Clinical measurements of mid-upper arm circumferences (as an indicator of muscle mass) and triceps skin fold measurements obtained with special calipers are of limited value as indicators of body fat tissue and are difficult to interpret. A margin of error exists because of variations in the quality of calipers, inconsistent techniques, and failure to account for individual variations in muscle mass associated with disuse atrophy for those with quadriplegia.

Bioelectric Impedence in Body Composition Analysis
Bioelectric impedence in body composition analysis is an accurate method to measure total body water, lean body mass, and body fat.* An impedance measurement consists of two components: resistance and reactance. Body fat has low amounts of fluid and conducting electrolytes, making it a high-resistance electrical pathway. Lean tissues, however, have high amounts of water and conducting electolytes, making them a low-resistance electrical pathway. This analysis can thus help in modifying and personalizing nutritional needs and planning of exercise programs.

The Gastrointestinal System
Initial assessment of the gastrointestinal system should determine whether the gut is functional and should rule out complications, thus determining how nutritional needs will be met. Swallowing problems are not uncommon for patients with cervical cord injury, particularly when the neck

*Manufactured by RJL BODY COMPOSITION ANALYZER INSTRUMENTS, 9930 Whittier, Detroit, MI 48224.

must be slightly hyperextended to promote healing of the fractured spine. See Chapter 20.

The patient with a tracheostomy may also have swallowing problems. The nearness of the artificial airway to the esophagus interferes with movement of the larynx and relaxation of the upper esophageal sphincter, necessary to allow food to pass (Logemann 1983).

Feelings of nausea, diaphoresis, and general discomfort frequently signal problems with bowel and bladder elimination. Maintaining regular and reliable programs are essential to promoting a good appetite. Depression and emotional factors, too, must always be assessed in relation to anorexia.

Use Procedures 17–1 and 17–2 to assess chewing and swallowing ability and gastrointestinal function.

Functional Ability

Patients with quadriplegia experience varying degrees of difficulty feeding themselves because of paralysis/weakness of the upper extremities. Collaborate with occupational therapists to complete a detailed assessment of upper extremity muscle function and provide individualized aids to assist with feeding. In addition to the care and application of these devices, also be aware of psychological stresses to patients using them. Patients easily become frustrated when relearning basic eating skills. Eating is a very social activity and mealtime can sometimes trigger stressful reactions. Refusing to eat or overeating can signal a deeper existing depression.

Laboratory Findings

Certain laboratory findings reveal abnormalities suggestive of nutritional deficiencies. However, nonnutritional factors frequently make accurate interpretation difficult. Routine urine and blood analysis may reveal: protein, glucose, and acetone in the urine; low hemoglobin and hematocrit; reduced serum albumin, prealbumin, transferrin, retinol binding protein, and total protein; abnormal cholesterol levels; and abnormally low serum electrolyte concentrations. Other miscellaneous blood and urine tests may be

---

Procedure 17–1   Assessing Chewing and Swallowing Ability

Purpose

To identify problems associated with malnutrition and to promote safety by preventing choking and aspiration.

Action	Rationale
1. First examine the mouth.	Dental caries, absent teeth, and gum disease may be painful and hamper chewing ability. Young people may have impacted wisdom teeth. Periodontal problems with reddened, swollen, or spongy gums that bleed easily are most common in patients over 40. A major problem in the elderly is ill-fitting dentures due to shrinking gums.
2. Check for any swallowing difficulties.	Although not associated with SCI per se, a patient with a very high cervical cord injury may experience ascending edema, affecting the lower brain stem and subduing the swallowing reflex.
3. To check for gag reflex, brush the eyelash lightly with a piece of soft tissue.	Usually if the blink reflex is present so is an intact gag reflex.
4. Observe the tracheal aspirate for evidence of oral or tube feedings. Routinely add blue food coloring to all tube feeds in the critical care setting. Note if swallowing becomes painful (burning sensation) on a continuing care basis.	To distinguish oral and pulmonary secretions from aspirated tube feedings. A positive result will confirm the connection between the trachea and the esophagus. It may also suggest a rare but more serious complication, tracheoesophageal fistula. Differentiating the two requires radiology or endoscopy, but a fistula takes 2 to 4 weeks to develop, so a positive dye test before then probably indicates swallowing dysfunction (Holloway 1988). Although this problem usually disappears after the airway is removed, the patient requiring prolonged use may have difficulty meeting nutritional requirements.
5. Closely observe ability to swallow in patients who have just had a halo-thoracic brace applied or who are in cervical traction.	Maintaining the neck in the desired degree of hyperextension may cause swallowing difficulties. However, with very slight adjustment of the bars by the physician this problem can usually be solved. Traction-related problems can be more difficult to solve. Relying on liquid/soft diets is probably the best temporary solution. See Procedure 20–3.

Procedure 17–2   Assessing the Function of the Lower Gastrointestinal Tract

Purpose

To determine function of the lower gastrointestinal system, primarily to determine route(s) of nutritional intake possible. Perform an abdominal assessment, observe the consistency and frequency of stool, and look for systemic signs and symptoms of gastric upset.

Action	Rationale
1. Check the abdomen.	Normal bowel sounds are intermittent and vary in intensity but indicate a functional/usable gastrointestinal system. Be alert for absent, occasional, or weak sounds immediately following injury, indicating that the tract is still sluggish and absorption would be impaired. Flatus, stooling, and decreasing amounts of nasogastric returns are better indicators of returning gastrointestinal function.
• First, listen for bowel sounds by auscultating the abdomen in all four quadrants. • Next percuss and palpate the abdomen. • Note flatus, stooling.	The techniques of percussion and palpation should follow auscultation as manual pressure applied to the abdomen may change peristaltic activity. (Abdominal assessment is discussed further in Chapter 19.) The abdomen should be soft and flat without evidence of distension, swelling, or rigidity related to paralytic ileus.
2. Recognize physical discomfort.	When large portions of the body trunk are without sensation, appreciation of localized pain is not possible.
• In addition to the obvious signs of nausea and vomiting, be alert for generalized tension, malaise, anorexia, *shoulder tip pain* (the most common referred pain); and, in quadriplegic patients, headache, perspiring, or chills.	These signs and symptoms are indicative of abdominal abnormality.
• Above all, be alert for an increased pulse rate or an elevated systemic temperature and/or white blood count without other apparent cause.	This may signal acute abdominal distress or peritonitis, which may cause death if unrecognized or unchecked.
3. Examine bowel elimination patterns in detail.	Lack of control and bouts of constipation or diarrhea greatly affect the patient's nutritional status (see Chapter 19).

indicated to measure the end products of metabolism, namely, urinary urea nitrogen and creatinine excretion, to indicate the catabolism of protein.

Following SCI, anemia and hypoproteinemia are common manifestations. Also, a high elimination rate of serum albumin, an indicator of visceral protein status, is not uncommon. The creatinine-height index, which is determined by lean body mass or muscle and expressed as a percentage of normal, is a constant value regardless of dietary intake. Severe depletion is a significant complication, especially among patients with quadriplegia.

The following factors are positive indicators of nutritional risk (Peiffer, Blust, and Leyson 1981: 503–504):

- Body weight—more than 10% below the recommended ideal body weight
- Serum albumin—less than 3.0 g/dl
- Caloric intake—less than calculated maintenance or anabolic requirement
- Protein intake—less than calculated maintenance or anabolic requirement
- Hemoglobin—less than 12 g/dl

- Hematocrit—less than 37%
- Creatinine-height index—less than 60% of standard
- Persistently negative nitrogen balance

PREVENTIVE AND RESTORATIVE MANAGEMENT

Physical fatigue and psychological adjustment can directly affect a patient's appetite, and relearning feeding skills practiced since early childhood or being fed is almost unbearable for many patients. Dietitians, nurses, occupational therapists, physicians, and pharmacists must work closely together with counseling professionals to prevent malnutrition.

Interventions include:

1. Provide appropriate fluid intake. Routine intravenous solutions provide little nutrition. For example, a liter of 5% dextrose in water contains only 170 calories. Take steps to

prevent malnutrition as described in this chapter. Vitamin supplements are needed very early and fluids by mouth should be given as ordered as soon as active bowel sounds return. Fluid intake should be correlated with the selected bladder management program. See Chapter 18.

2. Encourage oral intake of food when the patient is able. Following the critical period, a high-protein diet with sufficient calories is needed to improve nutritional status. A high-protein diet may be defined by either grams of protein intake per kilogram of body weight *or* nonprotein calorie to nitrogen ratio. If the day's protein intake is beyond 22% to 25% of the total caloric intake, the protein will be used for energy and not for the desired building and restorative purposes. Measures to encourage eating include:

- Small, frequent feedings of preferred foods with as pleasant an atmosphere as possible.
- Calm, friendly assistance with feeding. Be patient, but firm, and do not rush. The quadriplegic patient will often develop hiccoughs if forced to eat too quickly.
- Social interaction. Bringing the patient to the dining table, or even in a bed to a communal dining area, encourages socialization and promotes the feeling of health rather than sickness and isolation.
- Often families can be most helpful with this aspect of care.

3. Take measures to prevent aspiration:

- If the patient is in cervical traction or must maintain the recumbent position on bedrest, use the *side-lying* position and tilt the entire bed up 20 degrees. Most specialized immobilization beds have a tilt control.
- If the patient is on a turning frame, position *prone*, not only for safety reasons but also to promote independence as it is easier for patients to feed themselves in this position. See Figure 17–1.

4. Ensure an adequate airway. Use manual techniques to clear the chest at least one half-hour before mealtimes. This allows the patient sufficient time to expectorate secretions and rest. To prevent aspiration, avoid chest physical therapy for 30 minutes following oral intake. Also, if the patient is being mechanically ventilated, be sure to inflate the cuff on the tracheostomy tube before feeding. Be sure suction equipment is readily available for high-risk patients. Test the equipment before each meal, particularly when mobile suction units are used in communal dining settings. Choking can be a particular problem, especially during the early stages, because of decreased coughing ability. Performing an assisted coughing maneuver (see Procedure 15–4) will usually dislodge food particles in the throat, but suctioning may be necessary to clear the airway. A soft diet is easier to tolerate should choking be a recurring problem. Groher (1984) stresses the preventive importance of prefeeding management techniques.

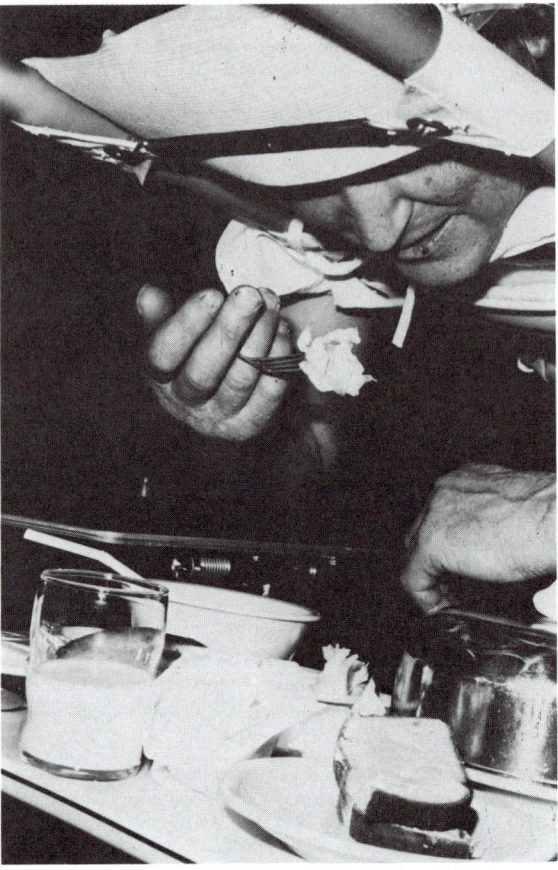

FIGURE 17–1 A quadriplegic man eating in the prone position on a Stryker frame.

5. Encourage good nutritional habits, including three regular meals and a well-balanced diet. An adequate diet includes recommended amounts of all major food groups: milk and milk products; meat and alternates; breads and cereals; and fruits and vegetables. The body requires proteins, carbohydrates, fats, vitamins, minerals, and water. Table 17–1 outlines nutrients, major food groups, sources, functions, and any changes in requirements of each following injury—typically a high-protein, moderate-calorie diet, high in fiber and fluids. Also initiate and maintain regular bowel habits to avoid constipation and diarrhea. For specific bowel management, including high-fiber intake and sources, see Chapter 19.

6. Encourage as much activity as orthopedic stability allows. Maintain range of motion and other specific exercises of unaffected limbs to promote digestion, aid in elimination, and minimize protein breakdown, thus ensuring that weight is gained as lean muscle rather than adipose tissue.

7. Provide patient and family education. Nutritional counseling should develop or reinforce good eating habits. Although the dietitian is mainly responsible for this teaching program, others have many opportunities to help put

TABLE 17–1 Nutritional Needs of the Spinal Cord Injured Patient

Nutrient	Food Groups; Best Food Sources	Function	Requirements Following Spinal Cord Injury
Protein	MILK and MILK PRODUCTS MEAT and ALTERNATES, e.g., meat, fish, poultry, eggs, milk, and cheese. Lower quality: soybeans, nuts, breads, cereals, dried beans and peas, and other legumes.	1. To build, repair, and maintain muscle, nerve, connective, and epithelial tissue. Protein accounts for tough fibrous nature of hair, nails, ligaments, and muscular structures. 2. To constitute essential components of enzymes, hormones, antibodies, and other blood proteins. These affect internal environment, stability, and metabolism.	1. Increased supply is needed to: • Repair severe bone and ligamentous injuries • Heal associated wounds • Minimize negative nitrogen balance and rate of loss of lean body mass (including that from respiratory and cardiac muscles) which is difficult to restore • Prevent skin breakdown • Fight infections such as those of the respiratory and urinary systems
Carbohydrates (Fiber)	BREADS and CEREALS FRUITS and VEGETABLES, e.g., whole grain breads and cereals, fresh fruit, raw vegetables, rice, pasta, and potatoes.	1. To supply readily available energy. 2. To provide roughage needed to regulate elimination of solid wastes. Fiber is a complex carbohydrate not broken down by mechanical or chemical digestion. Fiber absorbs many times its weight in water to soften stools and eliminates toxins and waste products more rapidly.	1. Adequate supply is needed to provide energy for basic functions in response to illness, e.g., increased respiratory effort of quadriplegic patients during acute phase. Respiratory muscle glycogen (stored carbohydrate replacement) is necessary during weaning from mechanical ventilation. 2. Increased fiber in the diet is generally needed to promote bowel control. Fiber must be increased gradually to avoid cramping and discomfort. Adequate/increased fluid intake must accompany increased fiber intake.
Fats	MEAT and ALTERNATES MILK and DAIRY PRODUCTS, e.g., whole or 2% milk, cheese, meat, fish, poultry, nuts, oils, butter, and margarine.	1. To provide a concentrated form of reserve energy, which is stored in adipose tissue and has high calorie value. 2. To protect and insulate body. 3. To promote normal growth and development.	1. Normal supply is required. 2. Reduced supply is required for overweight patients. In addition to the general health hazards of obesity, mobility problems and susceptibility to skin breakdown increase.
Vitamins A	ALL FOOD GROUPS dark green or yellow-orange fruits and vegetables, e.g., carrots, squash, apricots, and spinach; milk and dairy products; and liver.	1. To play dynamic role in metabolism. Absence of vitamins results in malnutrition and specific deficiency diseases. 2. To promote normal energy growth and development and resistance to infection.	1. Supplements almost always required in early stages. 2. Vitamin C in high doses is given to provide acidic environment in bladder to reduce infection.
B Complex	whole grain cereals and breads, organ meats, and eggs		
C	citrus fruits, juices, tomatoes, strawberries, broccoli, and canteloupe		

(Table continues)

TABLE 17–1 Nutritional Needs of the Spinal Cord Injured Patient (continued)

Nutrient	Food Groups; Best Food Sources	Function	Requirements Following Spinal Cord Injury
Vitamin			
D	fortified milk and margarine		
E	vegetable oils, wheat germ, whole grain breads and cereals, and margarine		
K	green and yellow vegetables		
Minerals	ALL FOOD GROUPS	1. To control many chemical mechanisms in the body such as fluid balance, blood volume, and acid-base balance.	1. Specific deficits measured by blood chemistry in early stages and replaced accordingly.
Calcium	milk, cheese, and yogurt		
Phosphorus			2. Calcium and phosphorus deficits occur with paralysis and immobility.
Iron	liver, red meats, whole grain breads and cereals, and green leafy vegetables	2. To provide rigidity to bones and teeth.	
Potassium	fruits and vegetables	3. To regulate excitability of muscular and nervous systems.	
Sodium	salt and high-protein foods		
Water	MILK and MILK PRODUCTS FRUITS and VEGETABLES, e.g., beverages, soups, milk, and juices	1. To provide a medium for all body fluids (secretions and excretions). In fact, the body requirements for water exceed food.	1. Measures to correct dehydration or fluid overload must be initiated according to fluid profile.
			2. Water requirements generally increase especially when fiber intake is increased. Bladder and bowel programs largely depend on regulated intake of 2000 to 3000 ml daily.
		2. To aid digestion and elimination.	
		3. To regulate body temperature.	
		4. To make possible all body functions.	

recommendations into practice. Education involves self-care skills and encouragement of independence with eating, which is discussed at the end of this chapter.

SPECIFIC MANAGEMENT OF POTENTIAL NUTRITIONAL COMPLICATIONS

Paralytic Ileus

Paralytic ileus is the absence of normal peristalsis in the small bowel, which allows fluid and gas to accumulate. It is common with all levels of injury to the spinal cord. Its exact cause is unknown, but it is probably related to temporary autonomic nervous system interruption. Onset and severity differ although patients with complete quadriplegia are likely to suffer the most. Many times ileus lasts only for a few days, but a sluggish gut may persist for some time.

Management of paralytic ileus involves preventing aspiration of emesis and providing adequate hydration and nutrition.

Management

1. Give nothing by mouth from the moment of injury until the physician has ruled out all paralytic ileus 48 to 72 hours later.

2. Observe all patients with SCI for the onset of paralytic ileus throughout the 72-hour postinjury period. Loss of bowel sounds may occur immediately following injury or

may be delayed up to 48 hours. Carefully check the patient with quadriplegia for delayed onset. Unrecognized ileus can cause sudden death in the quadriplegic patient during the first 48 hours when decreased coughing ability leads to aspiration of stomach contents, which results in respiratory arrest (Burke and Murray 1975).

3. Auscultate the abdomen to detect presence or absence of *bowel (peristaltic) sounds*. Place the diaphragm of the stethoscope lightly against the abdominal wall and listen to all four quadrants. Normally, peristaltic bowel sounds are heard as gurgling sounds (at least five sounds per minute). Bowel sounds may be described as present, fleeting (occasional), faint, or absent. Bowel sounds are absent during ileus.

4. Be alert for developing abdominal distension. Measure abdominal girth at level of umbilicus every 8 hours. Progressive abdominal distension may contribute to respiratory difficulties by restricting the movement of the diaphragm and, if untreated, may lead to nausea and vomiting. When ordered, insert a nasogastric tube to decompress the stomach and reduce the risk of vomiting. To minimize gastric irritation, select an air-vented tube and attach to gravity drainage or low intermittent suction. Observe nature of aspirate, and record volume.

5. Check lower bowel for presence of stool. Any stool should be gently removed manually with a well-lubricated, gloved finger. Do not give enemas as fluid will only accumulate and aggravate the situation. A well-lubricated rectal tube in place for 30 minutes at a time, to avoid pressure on desensitized bowel lining, may help relieve flatus.

6. Maintain nothing by mouth and administer intravenous replacement therapy. If untreated, dehydration and electrolyte imbalance are dangers as large volumes of fluid are trapped in the gut and unavailable to the general circulation.

7. Monitor intake and output, including gastric returns, and vital signs as ordered or more frequently according to nursing judgment.

8. Monitor blood hematology and chemistry daily.

9. Detect passing of paralytic ileus by reduced nasogastric returns, return of bowel sounds, and passing of flatus or stool.

10. Be alert for prolonged paralytic ileus, again especially in patients with complete quadriplegia. If ileus persists for longer than 48 to 72 hours hyperalimentation should be considered to supply adequate nutrition. Depending on preexisting nutritional status and expected resolution of ileus, hyperalimentation may be considered earlier. Be alert for any signs of symptoms of gastric ulceration and bleeding.

Expected Outcomes

Evaluate effectiveness of treatment according to level of outcome reached:

- Gastric aspiration of less than 50 ml in 24 hours
- Active bowel sounds with passing of flatus or stool
- Abdomen flat without evidence of distension
- Blood hematology and chemistry within normal limits without evidence of bleeding or electrolyte imbalances
- Adequate urine output without signs of dehydration

Gastric Ulceration and Bleeding

Neurogenic gastroduodenal ulceration and bleeding is a severe complication of SCI but may pass unrecognized because the paralyzed person cannot feel the classic symptom of severe or burning abdominal pain. The literature suggests that early detection and management could avoid a number of fatalities (Kewalramani 1979). The terms *stress ulceration* and *acute peptic ulceration* are used to describe gastrointestinal hemorrhage that occurs following SCI or other physical trauma. Patients with severe cervical cord injury, often with respiratory insufficiency and/or multiple injuries, and those who have undergone early operative procedures are most likely to develop gastric ulceration. The incidence of acute ulceration is probably close to 5% (Burke and Murray 1975; Kewalramani 1979).

Insult to the autonomic nervous system may cause local circulatory disturbances in the gastric mucosa, which are of paramount importance in initiating the process of ulceration and hemorrhage. Abnormal vasodilation or vasoconstriction may cause ischemic changes, which become a focus for ulceration. Excessive production of acidic gastric juices may further erode existing necrotic areas, particularly in quadriplegic patients, in whom parasympathetic irritation is unchecked because of damage to the sympathetic system.

Whatever the mechanism, increased acid secretions tend to accumulate and combine to form increased risk of stress ulceration.

Preexisting gastrointestinal problems, severe psychological reaction to injury, steroid therapy, and/or parasympathomimetic (cholinergic) drugs further predispose the patient to gastric ulceration.

Steroid therapy to minimize postinjury edema within the spinal cord has largely been abandoned because the increased risk of gastric bleeding outweighs the questionable benefits. On the other hand, newer, nonirritating nasogastric and nasoduodenal tubes have reduced the risk of gastric irritation/erosion.

To care for people with gastric ulceration, detect early and understand the significance of slightly abnormal clinical findings, control hemorrhage, and promote the healing of gastric mucosa.

Management

1. Take preventive measures to minimize risk. For example, prevent or recognize and treat systemic *hypoxia* early (see Chapter 15). Take precautions to decrease local gastric

irritation when a nasogastric tube is in place; always use an air-vented tube attached to gravity drainage or low intermittent suction.

2. To combat hyperacidity, administer antacid regimens or H₂ blockers as ordered. Davidoff (1987: 84) recommends a sump nasogastric tube with constant low suction to monitor gastric acidity (and decompress the abdomen). Measure gastric pH hourly and titrate with antacids to maintain a level above 4.5.

3. Be alert for evidence of bleeding in the gastrointestinal tract: an unexplained drop in blood pressure (systolic pressure 85 mmHg or below); an acute drop in hematocrit or hemoglobin (less than 10 gm %); nausea and vomiting; frank hematemesis; abdominal distension; nasogastric returns that look like coffee grounds, are blood tinged, or show frank fresh blood; and stools that are loose and tarry (melena) or show occult blood on laboratory examination. The onset of acute gastrointestinal hemorrhage usually occurs within 7 to 14 days after injury. It may present as a slow perforation, which is difficult to diagnose because lack of sensation eliminates the classic signs of abdominal pain, tenderness, and muscle guarding. *Shoulder tip pain*, which is referred pain, is a classic sign but not always present.

4. Differentiate between gastric bleeding and the relatively common problem of paralytic ileus, Wilmot and Walsh (1973) emphasize:

- *Hemorrhagic shock* is not evident in paralytic ileus unless the ileus has been untreated and the patient has been allowed to progress to a much more serious state of acute gastric dilation.
- *Shoulder tip pain* is never present in paralytic ileus; if it is present, immediately think of perforation.
- *Vomiting* is not present in paralytic ileus (unless it is untreated) but is present in early perforation.

5. Prepare the patient for diagnostic tests. An abdominal flat plate will reveal air in the peritoneum caused by gastric dilation. The patient may be too sick to undergo an upper GI series with a contrast media or a gastroscopy. The physician may wish to use peritoneal lavage to rule out peritonitis. Washings should be free from blood, gastric contents, or infection.

6. Institute the following measures as ordered to control gastric bleeding:

- Insert nasogastric tube and attach to low-pressure, intermittent suction.
- Give continuous iced saline lavage.
- Administer antacids.
- Administer blood transfusions and IV replacement therapy.

Surgical intervention may be indicated in rare or unusual cases.

7. Discontinue corticosteriod therapy as ordered, to avoid the associated side effect of gastric irritation.

8. Control pain with analgesics and/or muscle relaxants as ordered.

9. Monitor vital signs and intake and output to assess tissue perfusion.

10. Monitor patient's response to treatment by obtaining daily specimens for blood hematology and chemistry and stool specimens for occult blood. Daily measurements of abdominal girth may also be needed to check amount of distension.

11. As rehabilitation progresses, along with appropriate antacid therapy, alleviate discomfort by temporarily limiting known gastric irritants such as black and red pepper, chili powder, regular and decaffeinated coffee, cocoa, and other sources of caffeine and alcohol. Traditional bland diets are no longer advised; it is best simply to avoid foods that bother a particular individual (Pemberton, Moxness, German, Nelson, and Gastineau 1988). Patients may also benefit from small, frequent meals during the acute stage of gastric ulceration.

Expected Outcomes

Evaluate effectiveness of treatment according to level of outcome criteria reached:

- Regular pulse at rate of 60 to 100 beats per minute
- Blood pressure within normal limits for patient (90/60 mmHg is considered acceptable for the patient with quadriplegia)
- Urinary output approximately 60 ml per hour
- Blood hematology and chemistry within normal limits for patient
- Nasogastric returns free from occult or frank blood with a pH above 3
- Stools free from occult or frank blood
- Patient comfortable without feelings of nausea, referred pain, or abdominal distension

Malnutrition during Critical Period

Despite immediate life-threatening problems that often appear to overshadow nutritional needs, maintaining optimal nutritional support is vital to cardiopulmonary and hemodynamic life-saving measures during the critically ill period following SCI. The major potential complication, *malnutrition*, can develop rapidly (Schlichtig and Ayres 1988). The nutritional risk factors of major trauma and stress, plus the effects of paralysis, are compounded by the growth and maturation needs of a predominately young population and require an extensive nutritional plan (Vizuete 1989) and aggressive nutritional support (Kaufman, Rowlands, Stein, Kopaniky and Gildenberg 1985).

Especially during the first 2 weeks following injury, SIC has a negative effect on nutritional status (Laven et al. 1989). Limited research indicates that spinal cord injured patients represent a unique population that does not seem to exhibit the hypermetabolic response frequently observed in other critically ill patients.

Nutritional Responses Following Spinal Cord Injury

The body stores three primary fuel sources—carbohydrates, fats, and proteins (*endogenous* stores). *Catabolism* is the process by which these stores are broken down and converted into usable energy and requirements for maintenance. Following an immediate decrease in the metabolic rate due to severe injury, metabolism increases rapidly to levels above normal.

Energy requirements are initially met by catabolism of stored carbohydrates in the form of *glycogen*. However, in the acute period, carbohydrate stores are rapidly depleted following injury.

Certain glucose-dependent cells include those of the brain and spinal cord, red blood cells, kidney tissue and fibroblasts at the edge of wound healing. To meet energy requirements in this stressed state, the body is then forced to make glucose by the breakdown of protein found in lean muscle mass. *Gluconeogenesis* is the synthesis of glucose from noncarbohydrate sources and one of the primary responses to traumatic injury/stress (Kinney, Jeejeebhoy, Hill, and Owen 1988). Obligatory protein breakdown to meet energy requirements (as opposed to its usual function of building and repairing tissue) releases amino acids from skeletal muscle tissue protein (and also viscera) to provide substrates for conversion into glucose. Nitrogen, a waste product of protein metabolism, is excreted in the urine. Gluconeogenesis plus a concomitant decrease in new protein available for normal synthesis for the total body occurs and a *negative nitrogen balance* ensues. Nitrogen balance is a function of nitrogen intake minus nitrogen excretion. A negative nitrogen balance indicates a catabolic state. Protein losses from catabolism can be measured by laboratory analysis of nitrogen excreted in the urine. By comparing it to the nitrogen in exogenous intake, the degree of negative nitrogen balance is estimated. Each gram of negative nitrogen balance indicates an approximate loss of 30 g lean body tissue (Lugerner and Cox 1988), that is, a negative 12 g N_2 balance = loss of 360 g (0.8 lb) lean body tissue. The loss of greater than 20 g per 24 hours is frequently seen in the early stages following SCI. A negative nitrogen balance can continue with SCI beyond the postinjury phase. A portion of obligatory protein catabolism is thought to be associated with disuse and denervation atrophy that accompanies paralysis.

Malnutrition is evidenced by:

- Accelerated loss of weight, muscle mass, strength, and function
- Decreased immunocompetence and resistance to infection
- Dehydration and electrolyte imbalances
- Dramatic respiratory responses causing impairment of pulmonary function, most notably, inability to wean from mechanical ventilation (Chapter 15)
- Poor wound healing
- Increased risk of skin breakdown, recurrent bladder infections, and bowel irregularities
- Generalized weakness and fatigue that prolongs convalescence and delays rehabilitation

Nutritional Requirements

The basal energy expenditure equation developed by Harris and Benedict in 1919 is the most widely used method for calculating energy requirements. To this, various percentages are added for major stress, trauma, infection, and medication, perhaps increasing calculated energy needs by 20 to 50%.

However, literature available regarding energy metabolism (caloric expenditure) of acute and stable spinal cord injured patients indicates that they have reduced caloric needs in proportion to their level of injury and degree of muscle denervation (Cox et al. 1985; Laven et al. 1989; Kolpeck et al. 1989). Cox and associates observed a requirement of 22.7 kcal/kg/day in 15 quadriplegic patients compared to 27.9 kcal/kg/day in 5 paraplegic patients. Most critically ill patients require caloric intakes in the range of 30 to 40 calories per kg per day. Kolpeck and associates concluded that quadriplegic patients should receive only 80% of their predicted caloric needs (as calculated with the Harris-Benedict equation), which was consistent with other studies to date.

Normal persons require 0.8 grams of protein/kg to maintain protein equilibrium, but critically ill patients with SCI may require from 1.5 to 3.0 g protein per kg, depending on the clinical status, calorie balance, other nutritional parameters, and the degree of negative nitrogen balance.

Nutritional Support

The goal of nutritional support is to maintain caloric balance while providing sufficient protein to minimize the negative nitrogen balance. Provide the calories for energy and nitrogen substrates (protein) the patient actually needs. Approximately 60% of the total daily calories should be from carbohydrates, 15% to 20% protein, and 20% to 30% fat (a concentration found in many enteral products). Up to 60% of total caloric requirements as glucose is effective in reducing nitrogen excretion; beyond that level, glucose is converted into fat yielding more CO_2 than O_2.

During critical illness it is important to determine energy needs as accurately as possible. Critically ill patients frequently have altered fuel metabolic mechanisms and, as such, frequently cannot compensate for excessive quantities of any nutritional substrates—more is not necessarily better. Take into account that SCI patients have less than predicted needs and avoid *overfeeding*.

Overfeeding frequently produces various iatrogenic side effects. An excessive *dextrose* load causes:

- Hyperglycemia that, if significant, will require exogenous insulin for control.
- Increased CO_2 production. Too much CO_2 increases the patient's respiratory effort in an attempt to reduce these abnormal levels, which in turn may lead to respiratory failure (hypercapnia) in critically ill patients with marginal pulmonary reserves.
- Fatty liver.
- Elevated SGOT, SPGT, and serum alkaline phosphatase.

An excessive protein load causes:

- Azotemia
- Increased minute ventilation
- Dehydration

An excessive fat load causes:

- Hypertriglyceridemia
- Increased intravenous fat may cause decreased O_2 diffusion, especially if pulmonary function is impaired as with quadriplegia, because pulmonary vasoconstriction is produced.

Preventive and restorative management.

1. *Immediately consult a registered dietician or nutritional support team as soon as possible (within 24 hours) postinjury to complete a nutritional assessment, determine calorie and protein requirements, and set time frame (within 48 to 72 hours) for initiation of nutritional support (oral, enteral, or parenteral).*

2. Carefully monitor patients at risk of developing malnutrition; patients with quadriplegia who have impaired (marginal) pulmonary function; patients with multiple (especially abdominal) trauma; those requiring surgical intervention; and patients with an elevated temperature. The underweight patient (or one who abused drugs or alcohol before injury) with preexisting depletion is at greater risk also.

3. Assess the function of the gastrointestinal tract. Depending on the functional status of the gut, the routes for nutritional support are chosen. Table 17-2 summarizes information relating to nutritional support. Listen for bowel sounds. If bowel sounds cannot be detected, the gastrointestinal tract is considered to be nonfunctional. Fleeting or faint sounds may indicate that the tract is still sluggish and that absorption would be impaired—required amounts of fluids to deliver the desired calories and protein would be poorly tolerated.

4. Administer *total parenteral nutrition* (TPN) as ordered, which should be implemented by the third postinjury day, after the patient has had an opportunity to stabilize. A highly skilled team must implement and monitor TPN. Be especially alert for hyperglycemia as the TPN rate is increased. Check urine glucose every 6 hours with chemsticks and monitor blood glucose regularly.

5. When the gut is functional, begin enteral nutrition (oral, nasogastric, nasoduodenal, or jejunostomy feedings) as ordered. Gastrostomy feedings are less common in the critical care area but have a place in the long-term management of persons with high quadriplegia with dysphagia.

Transitional feeding, introducing enteral feedings before TPN is discontinued, or encouraging oral intake before tube feedings are discontinued, may be a long process. Generally patients should be consistently taking greater than 50% of their nutrition orally or by tube feedings before TPN is discontinued.

Advanced techniques, tubes, and formulas have made tube feedings safer, nutritionally complete and adequate, and more comfortable for the patient. New feeding tubes are smaller, softer, and more pliable, and these improvements reduce the risks of aspiration, tube irritation to the throat and gastric mucosa, and pressure necrosis of the esophageal and tracheal wall. Insertion can be difficult if the patient is uncooperative or if cervical traction or a halo is in place. It is *easier and safer to place the SCI patient in a side-lying position* during insertion.

6. When the patient has a neurogenic bowel, problems with absorption and diarrhea may be more pronounced. Enteral feeding problems (mechanical, gastrointestinal, or metabolic) must be approached aggressively. The following techniques to establish feeds, promote absorption, avoid constipation, and control diarrhea may be helpful (Kohn and Keithly 1987):

- Begin lactose-free, isotonic (1.0 cal/cc) formulas at full strength, typically at an infusion rate of 50 cc/hr. If gastric residuals aspirated are less than 150 cc over an 8-hour period (indicating gastrointestinal tolerance), feedings can be advanced in 25 cc increments every 8 to 12 hours until nutritional goals are met. Nausea may indicate delayed gastric emptying. If gastric residuals are consistently greater than 150 cc, metaclopromide 5–10 mg may be given two to three times daily.
- Administer feedings at room temperature to avoid cramping.
- Give continuous feedings at a consistent rate versus a rapid, intermittent, or bolus rate.
- Use fiber-containing formulas as an effective means of controlling diarrhea; bulking agents may also be given two or three times per day.
- Administer antidiarrheal agents as ordered.
- Evaluate medication profile for drugs that are associated with gastrointestinal side effects, especially antibiotics or steroids. Oral preparations are particular culprits.
- For profuse diarrhea, culture stools for *clostridium difficile,* an infection associated with toxins that

TABLE 17–2 Enteral and Total Parenteral Nutritional (TPN) Support: Key Points

Choice of feeding route depends on the patient's general condition and on the functional ability of the gastrointestinal system. Formula choice is determined by caloric and protein needs, volume constraints (fluid restrictions), macronutrient composition, and metabolism.

	Enteral Nutrition	Total Parenteral Nutrition (TPN)
Definition	Enteral nutrition refers to the administration of nutrients via the gastrointestinal tract when the gut is functional, but oral intake is inadequate or not possible. • Oral or tube feedings via nasogastric, nasoduodenal, gastric or jejunal routes • Preserves gut function; decreases incidence of metabolic and infectious complications; cost effective	Total parenteral nutrition (TPN) refers to the administration of nutrients via the intravascular route, when nutritional needs cannot be met through the enteral route (because the gut is nonfunctional). • Preserves and/or replenishes lean muscle tissue • Administration of protein with adequate nonprotein calories to meet energy requirements so that protein will be used to build and repair tissues (normal function) and not be wasted to meet energy requirements (as evidenced by negative nitrogen balance)

Formula Components	• Amino acids (proteins)
	• Carbohydrates
	• Fats
	• Vitamins, minerals, and trace elements
		• Amino acids
		• Nonprotein calories (carbohydrate and fat)
		• Additives (electrolytes, vitamins)
		• Vitamin K 10 mg IM is given each week unless contraindicated while patient is receiving anticoagulant therapy (common for the spinal cord injured patient with the risk of deep vein thrombosis)
		• IV fat emulsion to boost caloric intake and provide essential fatty acids
		  • Administration of 500 cc of 10% lipids over 24 hours two to three times per week to prevent fatty acid deficiency
		  • May be infused simultaneously with amino acid/dextrose solution via a central or peripheral line

Types of Formulas	• Polymeric (contain higher molecular weight forms of protein, carbohydrate, and fat; used in patients with completely functional GI tract; some contain dietary fiber)
	• Peptide-based or elemental (consist of predigested and easily absorbed forms of nitrogen; greater amounts of carbohydrate and smaller amounts of fat; hyperosmolar and not suitable for oral use; used for patients whose digestion and absorption is impaired as with a sluggish neurogenic bowel)
	• Modular (supply one single nutrient; used to modify the nitrogen, carbohydrate, and lipid content of polymeric or elemental formulas)
		• Central TPN infusion (high dextrose concentration)
		  • Standard solutions generally contain 4.25% or 5.00% amino acids, 25% dextrose final concentration for use with IV fat emulsions
		  • A continuous mixed fuel system (carbohydrates given with 10% or 20% IV fat emulsion) preferable for critically ill patients;
		  • 1 bottle (500 cc) of 10% IV fat emulsion two to three times per week for more stable patients
		  • IV fat emulsions piggybacked into central line if peripheral access is limited
		• Peripheral or central infusion (low dextrose concentration)
		  • Standard solutions generally 4.25% amino acids, 10% dextrose final concentration
		  • Requires continuous infusion of 20% fat emulsion at a rate dependent on patient's caloric need to assure amino acids are used for protein synthesis
		  • Primary calorie source: lipid (low concentration of dextrose limits carbohydrates as a calorie source)
		  • Often given piggyback to prevent phlebitis in the peripheral veins
		• Mixed fuel central
		  • Standard solutions generally contain 5% amino acids and 25% dextrose final concentration
		  • For use with continuous IV fat emulsion given at a variable/rate depending on caloric need and other factors for optimal calorie/nitrogen ratio if administered with one to three liters of amino acids/dextrose solution per day

(Table continues)

TABLE 17–2 Enteral and Total Parenteral Nutritional (TPN) Support: Key Points (continued)

	Enteral Nutrition	Total Parenteral Nutrition (TPN)

Formula Selection	• Takes into consideration
	  • Diagnosis of associated trauma or preexisting disease
	  • Caloric and protein needs
	  • Biochemical indicies
	  • Volume considerations
	  • Presence of malabsorption or maldigestion
	  • Tolerance of current feeding
		• Similar selection process

Method of Administration	• Nasogastric
	  • Accepts higher osmotic loads and volume without cramping, diarrhea, or fluid and electrolyte shifts
	  • Tubes are easily placed
	  • Bolus feedings are more physiological and stimulate digestion by gastric distension
	  • For patients with SCI the risk of aspiration is significant due to esophageal compromise combined with impaired muscles of breathing from paralysis; inability to raise the head of the bed 30° because of cervical traction or thoracolumbar bracing
	
	• Nasoduodenal
	  • Preferred for patients with delayed gastric emptying, or those at risk of aspiration
	  • Small-bore tubes are more comfortable for the patient
	  • Placement of tubes more difficult and accidental dislodgement may occur
	  • Small bowel poorly tolerates rapid infusion or sudden rate changes; may cause fluid and electrolyte shifts resulting in cramping, distension, and diarrhea
	
	• Gastrostomy
	  • For patients with long-term tube feedings, gastric tubes are less unsightly; offer less frequent reflex of feedings; wide-bore tube allows for administration of blenderized table food as well as medications
	  • May be indicated in long-term management for selected persons with high quadriplegia who have major paralysis of swallowing muscles
	  • Disadvantages include skin excoriation and leakage of contents intraperitoneally (most serious without sensation intact); tube displacement and outlet instruction; potential for fistula formation; and the constant danger of aspiration for the person with ventilator-dependent quadriplegia
	
	• Jejunostomy
	  • May be either feeding or needle catheter
	  • May be useful in postoperative management if the small bowel is functional; minimize risk of aspiration; and avoid use of TPN
	  • Must be administered continuously to minimize diarrhea, which is common until the small bowel adapts
		• Depends on the anticipated duration of therapy and the nutritional requirements of the patient which in turn dictates the formula to be used
		
		• High dextrose concentration TPN (centrally infused)
		  • Central venous cannulation, ideally the superior vena cava, allows for rapid absorption of hypertonic solutions with less chance of phlebitis and thrombosis
		
		• Low dextrose concentrations (less than 10% final concentration) for peripheral infusion
		  • Reserved for patients who are going to be without oral intake for a shorter time or for those adjusting to enteral diets
		  • Also good for patients being weaned from mechanical ventilation (reduced carbohydrate) or for patients with glucose intolerance
		
		• Requires good peripheral access
		• IV site change necessary every 48 hours to prevent phlebitis in peripheral veins
		• IV fat emulsion (intralipids) given as a calorie and fatty acid source
		• Piggybacked into TPN solution on separate infusion pumps

(Table continues)

TABLE 17–2   Enteral and Total Parenteral Nutritional (TPN) Support: Key Points (continued)

	Enteral Nutrition	Total Parenteral Nutrition (TPN)

Complications	• Mechanical complications
	  • Pharyngeal irritation, esophageal/mucosal erosion, otitis media
	  • Tube blockages from thick formulas or crushed medications and tube dislodgements
	  • Aspiration related to changes in gastric motility and altered gag reflex aggravated by malposition
	  • Coughing or nausea and vomiting from tube displacement
	  • Management of complications determined by assessment of tube size (use as small a bore tube as possible), patency, and placement; dilution of feeds; ensuring a position as upright as possible; avoidance of bronchial hygiene techniques immediately after feeding; and regular replacement and hygiene of tubes
	
	• Gastrointestinal complications
	  • Cramping, distension, flatulence, and diarrhea that may be related to rate, volume, concentration, and type of formula; bacterial contamination; concurrent drug therapy; fecal impaction; and absorption problems associated with malnutrition/hypoalbuminemia or compromised pancreatic function
	  • Management strategies: Hygienic preparation of lactose-free, lower-fat formulas given gradually at increasing rates to increase tolerance; alterations in rate, volumes, and concentrations of formulas as needed; evaluation of drugs for offending agent; administration of antiflatulents; establishment of a reliable bowel program adding bulk and fiber-containing formulas to combat low residue feedings; reconsidering an elemental diet or TPN if necessary
	  • Nausea, vomiting, and high gastric residuals (related to inadequate or delayed emptying from a partial ileus) that may plague spinal cord injured patients
	  • Management strategies: holding of feeds and a resumption at a slower rate with lower fat or diluted formulas; adminsitration of antiemetics, metaclopromide
	
	• Metabolic complications of underfeeding or overfeeding:
	  • Hyperglycemia (stress, diabetes), or hyponatremia (inadequate intake of sodium in relation to water intake)
	  • Management strategies: regular monitoring to detect abnormalities that can be accumulative; correcting hydration problems; adjusting formulas and giving supplements (Vitamin K) as needed
		• Metabolic complications much more pronounced and of a more rapid onset than with enteral feedings
		  • Judicious assessment of the protein-caloric needs of spinal cord injured patients in light of the unique needs of that population the key. Significant decrease in the estimated caloric requirements in relation to the level of injury due to disuse and denervated muscle atrophy factor (present from the moment of injury)
		  • Common results of overfeeding: further compromise of impaired respiratory function and hyperglycemia
		  • Underfeeding with not enough protein to support growth and maturational needs in this predominantly young patient population also a problem
		  • Complex electrolyte imbalances, insulin requirements, anemia, and congestive heart failure
		  • Management: astute and continuous assessment/monitoring to avoid problems; adjustment of infusion rates; alter protein-calorie ratio; correct deficiencies and/or reduce or increase specific electrolytes and formula contents and additives; and/or modify volume
		
		• Catheter-related complications
		  • Sepsis of catheter if cultures of all other sources of infection remain negative and fever persists; (significantly reduced by strict protocols for insertion and care)
		  • Pneumothorax, air embolism, and laceration to the vein itself due to insertion of the catheter
		  • Mechanical problems with central venous catheters: kinking, cracking, and thrombosis; possible need for catheter replacement and site change

Based on Lugerner and Cox 1988. Adapted with permission of the publisher.

produce a colitis caused by intestinal flora changes from antibiotics.

- Check for possible bacterial contamination of the formula. Although formulas are prepared commercially under sterile conditions, contamination may occur when transferred to delivery systems or when hanging at room temperature for long periods of time. Furthermore, patients receiving antacids or cimetadine are at greater risk because the protective functions of gastric acids are neutralized or, with jejunal feedings, bypassed.
- Examine rectum for *fecal impaction* when patients have liquid stools oozing around the blockage. Manual extraction of stool, if possible, and an enema to ensure a clean bowel are essential before a regulated bowel program can be initiated.

8. Occasionally, tube feeding is necessary for a severely depressed person who is unwilling or unable to eat. Feelings of hopelessness, despair, and not wishing to live with the imposed disability are often expressed. Arranging visits with a person with a similar SCI may help both the patient and the care givers gain perspective.

Serious depression needs psychiatric treatment and some people nevertheless will not wish to live. Ethical dilemmas regarding forced feeding cannot be sorted out until patients have an opportunity to look objectively at all their options. Ethical concerns surface more often when SCI is severe. See Chapter 29.

Expected Outcomes

- Trend of less negative, followed by consecutive positive, nitrogen balance studies to signal that catabolism has been slowed, ceased, or replaced by a stable anabolic rehabilitation phase.
- Conditions requiring enteral or parenteral nutrition improved and then alleviated
- Able to take an adequate diet orally

Continuing Malnutrition

Continuing malnutrition throughout the rehabilitation period is a common occurrence, involving as much as 66% to 70% of the general rehabilitation population (Newmark, Sublett, Black, and Geller 1981; Arego and Koch 1986).

Possible explanations for protein–calorie malnutrition, which lowers resistance to infection and is implicated in cardiopulmonary insufficiency that totally hampers rehabilitation efforts, include:

- Chronic, inadequate nutritional support/intake
- Recent acute catabolic processes
- Depression affecting eating habits
- Chewing or swallowing difficulties
- Difficulty feeding oneself, embarrassment and/or rushed, unrelaxed assistance

- Indigestion related to air swallowing, delayed emptying and impaired or irregular bowel control, perhaps associated with misuse of laxatives
- Recurrent infections
- Protein loss from decubiti
- Concurrent drug therapy for various reasons associated with gastrointestinal side effects. Antibiotics, especially tetracycline and sulpha drugs, and potassium preparations are common offenders. Also medications causing drowsiness, such as Valium for spasticity, play havoc with mealtimes.
- Dependency on substance or alcohol abuse (see Chapter 9)

Metabolic problems of persons with SCI cited by Arego and Koch (1986) stressed hypoalbuminemia and associated loss of immune function, subnormal levels of Vitamin K, and altered levels of urinary calcium and other electrolytes.

Although often unrecognized, continuing malnutrition is not uncommon for patients with SCI and requires and responds to dietary treatment and diverse interdiscliplinary interventions.

Expected outcomes include:

- Adequate nutritional support/intake
- Blood chemistry and hematology within normal limits for patient
- Improved wound healing, improved skin tolerance, fewer recurrent bladder infections, and more reliable bowel control
- Higher energy levels and physical stamina so that patient can enter into rehabilitation activities

Weight Management

Weight control is singled out as a specific (and a most visible) problem, because great fluctuations in body weight are apt to occur during the first year after injury. A poor appetite may persist for weeks postinjury. However, as mobility and strength return, undesirable weight gain is just as likely to occur. Spinal cord injured individuals have lower caloric requirements and dietary intake needs to be adjusted to altered activity levels. Overeating can also be linked to depression and changes of perceived body image. A wide discrepancy between a minimum and maximum weight that the individual can remember may be an *early* indication that weight control is a problem.

Maintain acceptable weight for body height and build (as determined for each individual, not just from charts!) by providing a well-balanced diet that includes a variety of foods from each of the four main food groups, and by encouraging maintenance of recommended dietary intake.

Management

1. A complete nutritional consultation is necessary to identify potential problems with eating habits and determine the patient's current status. Consult with the dietitian

and the patient to determine ideal body weight and develop realistic goals. Recommended weights for the stabilized person with SCI are slightly less than those recommended for the general population. The East Orange Veteran's Administration Center has established that for the patient with a paraplegic injury, the recommended weight is 10 to 15 lb (4.5 to 6.8 kg) below the Metropolitan Life Insurance ideal body weight for a given height and frame size (Peiffer, Blust, and Leyson 1981: 501). For the patient with a quadriplegic injury, the recommended weight is 15 to 20 lb (6.8 to 9.0 kg) below that in the Metropolitan Life Insurance table. Although the dietitian is primarily responsible for nutritional counseling, nurses and others have a major responsibility in observing dietary intake and identifying any physical or emotional problems that may need referral to other team members. Involvement of the patient, and often the family, is essential.

2. Care for the underweight patient. A poor appetite may be associated with physical or emotional stress. When major physical problems are ruled out, simple fatigue and low energy levels will naturally suppress the appetite. There is a delicate balance between conserving strength and energy and promoting independence. For example, patients may be fed breakfast and dinner but attempt lunch on their own. Encourage as much participation as possible and praise the patient when successful. Encourage friends or relatives to assist with meals. Often they can bring in appetizing snacks. Also offer high-protein, high-calorie drinks between meals.

Be constantly aware that the underweight, malnourished patient is much more susceptible to pressure and other factors that cause skin breakdown. Frequent turning, correct positioning, and meticulous attention to general cleanliness habits are required. Specialized beds or equipment may be used to minimize risk and prevent skin problems.

Emotional stress may contribute to anorexia. Be sensitive to patients who are embarrassed when they cannot feed themselves; are easily frustrated when trying to achieve feeding skills; and express feelings of hopelessness and depression or act out. Care givers should collaborate with counseling professionals to develop an approach to these deep-rooted problems. Sometimes patients are better left to their own devices; others prefer the peer support and positive social interaction of communal dining. Occasionally a patient may withdraw and completely refuse to eat. Not eating and feeling their "bodies are dead" are signs of severe depression, rather than a normal reaction to an abnormal situation, and a psychiatrist should be consulted. The patient may need antidepressant medication in conjunction with other therapy.

3. Care for the patient who overeats. Some patients feel eating is the only pleasure left in life and tend to consume large meals, frequent high-calorie snacks, and too many soft drinks. When activity is decreased this combination leads to rapid weight gain that is difficult to reverse. Be sure patients are aware of the high-calorie foods in their diet. The hospitalized patient's eating habits can be curtailed to a certain extent, but when the patient goes home, self-motivation is the key. Ongoing counseling may be needed to promote feelings of self-worth. Obesity in patients confined to wheelchairs makes transfers more difficult, hampers ability to shift weight to avoid skin breakdown, and generally makes such things as dressing or attendant care far more tiring and complicated.

Expected Outcomes

Evaluate progress toward weight control by levels of outcome reached:

- Body weight acceptable for height and body build
- Normal muscle mass and body fat distribution
- Caloric intake regulated to amount of energy expended
- Adequate nutrients from all four basic food groups included in daily intake

DAILY LIVING SKILLS (DLS)

Persons with Paraplegia

The person with paraplegia has little problem eating independently. During the initial stages, when the recumbent position must be maintained, it is much easier and safer to eat in the prone position on a turning frame or in the side-lying position on a regular bed.

When a person is ready to return home, thought must be given to redesign of the kitchen for wheelchair accessibility, especially if the patient is a homemaker. Many rehabilitation centers, under the direction of an occupational therapist, have preparation classes for home-living skills and offer advice on design following home assessment. Problems such as reaching over sinks, counters, stoves, and shelves must be considered. Managing to grocery shop is another important area of education. See Figure 17–2.

Persons with Quadriplegia

For the person with quadriplegia the simple task of eating may be very complex. Close collaboration with the occupational therapist is needed to help the individual achieve as much independence with eating as possible. The therapist will complete a detailed assessment of muscle power in the upper extremities to determine the patient's ability to use arms and hands. Appropriate aids and/or splints may then be selected or designed and fabricated for individual use. Nurses should be familiar with the care and application of these individualized aids and must be aware of the exact amount of assistance each patient requires.

Developing self-care skills is a very creative process, and much depends on each patient's interest, motivation, and cooperation, as well as physical capabilities. It is also a changing process. The amount of assistance required during the beginning stages of rehabilitation is not necessarily the degree of assistance that will be required throughout the person's life. With ongoing therapy and practice, existing muscles do strengthen, and coordination can improve.

There are increasing numbers and varieties of self-care aids currently available. Particularly sophisticated are the bioengineering aids being developed to help individual patients eat independently. The ability to feed oneself depends on three basic movements: movement of the fingers, including ability to stabilize a utensil; ability to flex (drop) and extend the wrist; and ability to move the arm sufficiently to bring food to the mouth. Adaptive aids capitalize on existing abilities to support these basic movements.

Patients who can move their fingers may interlace utensils between their fingers and manage with minimal assistance to set up a tray, reach a straw, cut meat, and so on. Others may need padded utensils, which are easier to maneuver. See Figure 17–3. (This can be accomplished by wrapping IV tubing around a fork even when the patient is in the intensive care unit!) If the finger function is very weak the universal Palmer cuff may be used. See Figure 17–4. Utensils are inserted into a pocket on the cuff. A splint may be added to help stabilize a weak wrist and enable the patient to take advantage of any arm movement. See Figure 17–5. Dynamic splints may be used to convert wrist power for a pincher grasp. See Figure 17–6. When arm movement is impaired, sling supports can be added to help the patient overcome gravity and allow sideways movement to bring food to the mouth. Such support systems may take the form of an overhead suspension system or of bilateral swivel arm supports attached to the sides of the wheelchair. Patients who sustain injury at the C_{1-4} level must rely on others to feed them.

The quadriplegic person will also require assistance with kitchen design for wheelchair living. More adaptations will be needed to contend with upper extremity weakness, which makes opening containers, cutting food, and handling household items more difficult.

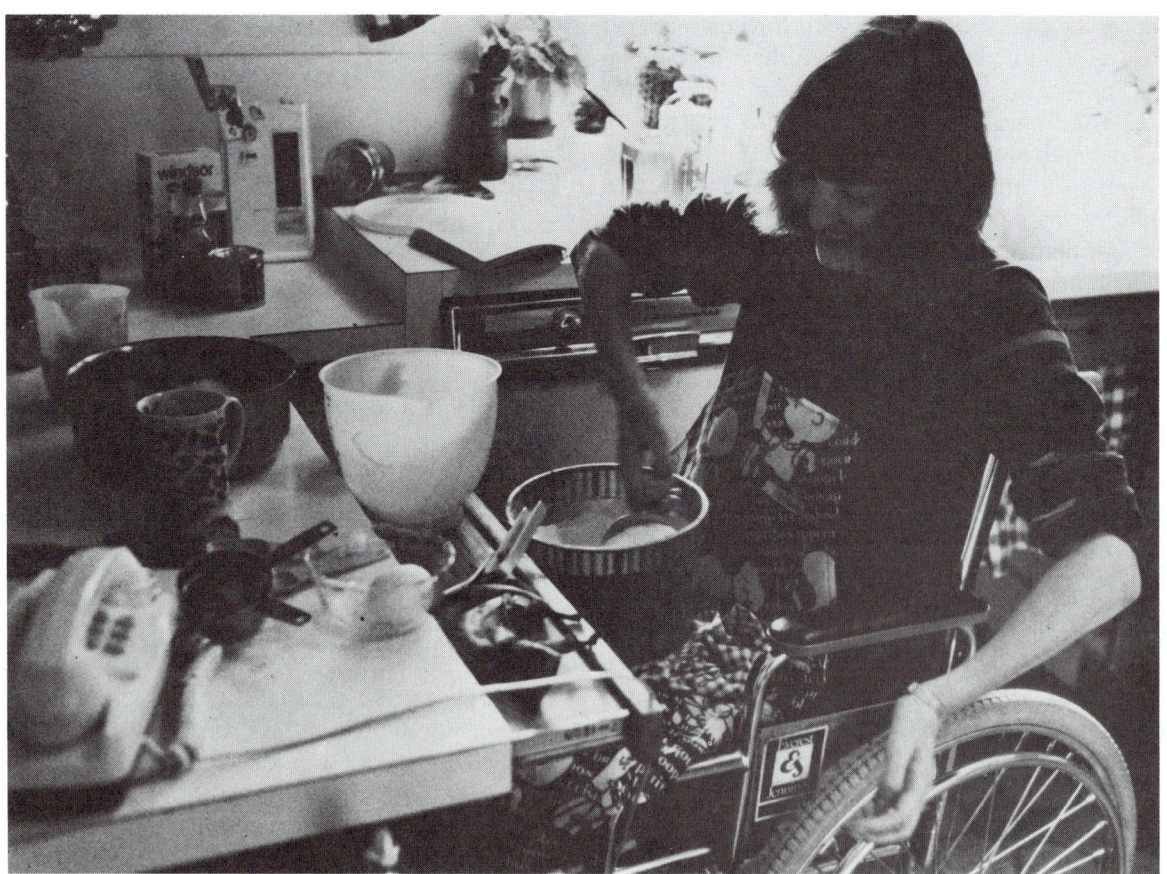

FIGURE 17–2 A quadriplegic woman cooks independently.

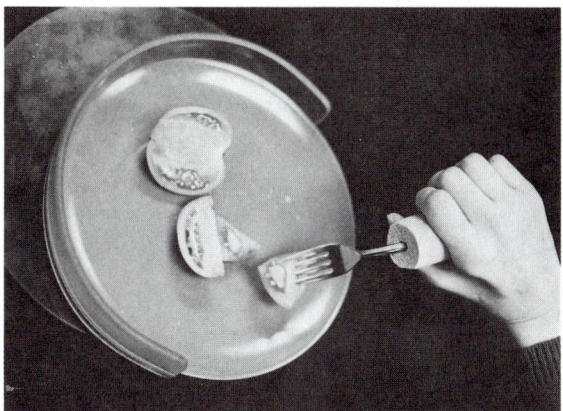

FIGURE 17–3   A quadriplegic woman using a padded handle on a fork. The nonskid plate mat and plate guard shown here are also commonly used aids.

NUTRITIONAL EDUCATION

1.   What types and amounts of food should be included in a daily menu?
2.   What does protein do for the body? What foods are high in protein? Why is it important to eat more protein if a pressure sore occurs?
3.   What about calories? Why is it important not to be overweight? or underweight?
4.   What amount of fluid is recommended? How are bladder and kidney stones prevented? Do dairy products cause kidney stones?
5.   How much fiber is necessary to help regulate a bowel program? What are good sources and why are extra fluids needed?

These basic questions must be answered for management of nutrition throughout life following SCI (Craig Hospital 1984; Germany and Plak 1982). See Chapter 11 for general guidelines regarding patient and family education. Patients and families must know the importance of *moderate* calorie intake, high protein, high fiber, and lots of fluids. Also encourage enjoyment of a variety of foods.

Although many young people seem to crave junk food, be creative. Try to think of interesting ways to incorporate nutritious foods into the diet (Galbreaith 1976). For example, get together with nutritionists and occupational, physical, and recreational therapists to introduce baking—with horse bran if necessary, salad days, ways to promote sex appeal of a healthy body, anything! Outings to introduce ethnic foods, new tastes, and follow-up education may help.

Perhaps colleagues who help people with diabetes change their eating patterns have applicable ideas, and community

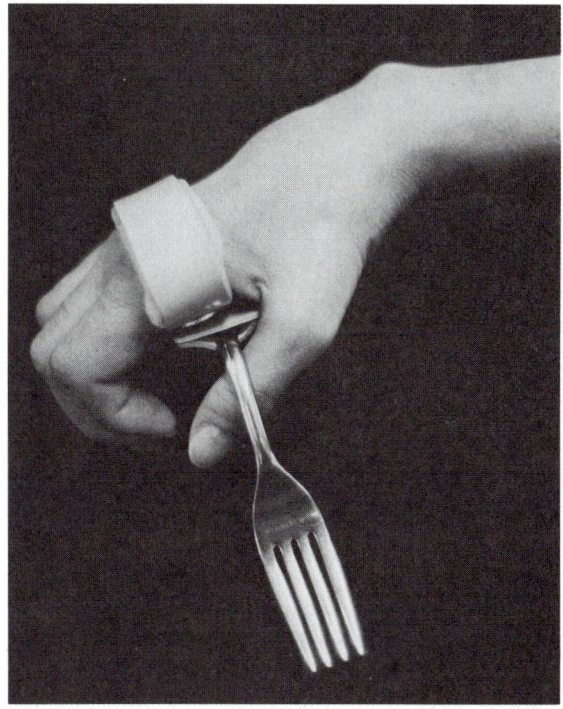

A

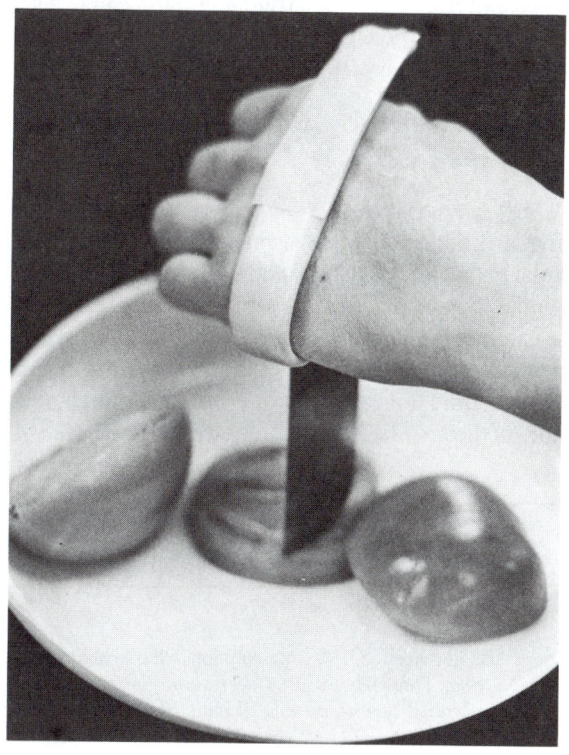

B

FIGURE 17–4   (A) A fork is inserted into the universal Palmer cuff. (B) Using a special knife attached to a cuffed device, a patient cuts food with a rocking motion.

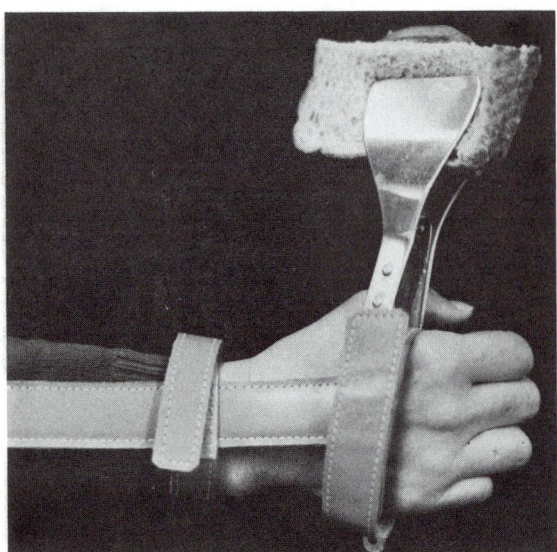

FIGURE 17–5   A splint may be added to stabilize the wrist, pictured here with a sandwich holder.

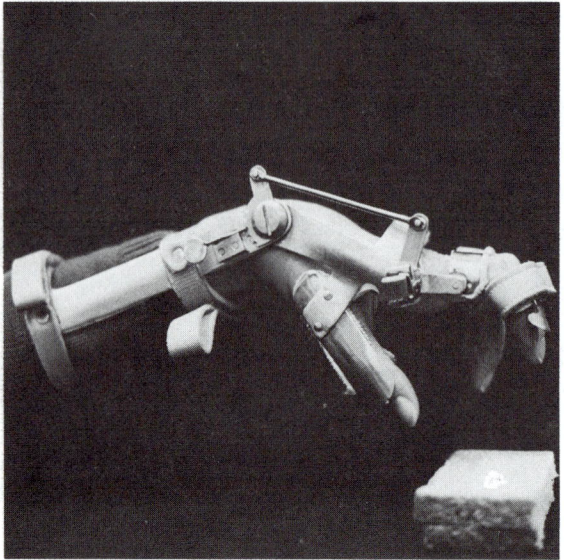

FIGURE 17–6   A dynamic splint converts movement of the wrist in a pincher grasp, enabling this person to pick up a sandwich.

groups such as Weight Watchers have useful techniques for encouraging good eating habits.

Most important, do not act as though eating is one of the only pleasures left in life. Good nutrition and energy to interact with life help individuals with SCI embrace opportunities.

LONG-TERM IMPLICATIONS

Long-term nutritional management for disabled people is similar to that for the general population. Good nutrition is essential to good health. The same nutrients are required; the caloric need simply decreases with less activity and denervation atrophy. People with SCI require constant adequate fluid intake to promote urinary function and plenty of dietary fiber to regulate bowel elimination.

Be alert for a variety of problems. For example, homemaking tasks may become too burdensome for one reason or another. consultation and referral may be necessary to initiate appropriate interventions: perhaps an occupational therapist to update skills, some actual assistance in the home, or encouragement to attend a community weight loss program.

Through the normal course of aging, and during periods of illness or rehospitalization, nutritional requirements change and eating patterns may need modification. Obesity is a widely identified problem for people with SCI and nothing but comprehensive services addressing all aspects of disability will help to alleviate the underlying causes (Marshall 1986). As with the nondisabled population, fitness and healthy eating decrease the risks of heart disease.

REFERENCES

Arego, D. E., and Koch, S. 1986. Malnutrition in the rehabilitation setting. *Nutrition Today* July/August. *Cites malnutrition as a common, often unrecognized, occurrence in the rehabilitation patient. Discusses assessment and treatment to deal with the range of psychosocial to frank mechanical problems contributing to this state.*

Burke, D., and Murray, D. 1975. *Handbook of Spinal Cord Medicine.* London and Basingstoke: Macmillan. *Introductory overview of gastrointestinal complications; includes paralytic ileus, acute gastric dilation, acute peptic ulceration, bowel obstruction, and acute abdomen.*

Cox, S., Weiss, S., Posuniak, E., Worthington, P., Prioleau, M., and Heffley, G. 1985. Energy expenditure after spinal cord injury: An evaluation of stable rehabilitating patients. *The Journal of Trauma* 25 (5) 419–423. *Study reveals patients have a reduction in their energy needs proportional to the amount of muscle denervated. Patients tend to become obese on uncontrolled diets.*

Craig Hospital. 1984. *Spinal Cord Injury Handbook.* Englewood, CO: Author. *Provides sophisticated guide to patient education, including nutrition.*

Davidoff, R. A. (Ed.). 1987. *Congenital Disorders and Trauma.* Vol. 4. *Infections and Cancer.* Vol. 5. *Handbook of the Spinal Cord.* New York: Marcel Dekker. *Very readable series offering a broad and com-*

prehensible survey of current knowledge about the spinal cord, both from a clinical and research viewpoint.

Galbreaith, P. 1986. *Tiptoeing Through the Kitchen*. Fort Worth, TX: Sunshine Publishing. *Healthy recipes with focus on quickness and simplicity of preparation and clean up.*

Germany, Y., and Ptak, K. 1982. *Nutrition for Spinal Cord Injuries*. Birmingham: University of Alabama. (Available through the Department of Dietetics, University of Alabama Hospitals/UAB, 619 South 19th Street, Birmingham, AL 35233). *Invaluable patient education booklet stressing the partnership and necessity of fluids and fiber for lifelong management.*

Groher, M. E. 1984. *Dysphagia: Diagnosis and Management*. Boston: Butterworth's. *Examines the pathophysiology of evaluation and management of swallowing disorders. Chapter 6 explores prefeeding management, training, and the use of adaptive equipment for people with high quadriplegia.*

Holloway, N. 1988. *Nursing the Critically Ill Adult*. 3d ed. Menlo Park, CA: Addison-Wesley.

Kaufman, H., Rowlands, B., Stein, D., Kopaniky, D., and Gildenberg, P. 1985. General metabolism in patients with acute paraplegia and quadriplegia. *Neurosurgery* 16 (3): 309–313. *Study of 14 patients during the initial 10 to 14 day postinjury period, with follow-up nutritional assessments that showed marked nutritional deterioration; suggests aggressive nutritional support on a routine basis.*

Kewalramani, L. 1979. Neurogenic gastroduodenal ulceration and bleeding associated with spinal cord injuries. *Journal of Trauma* 19 (4): 259–269. *A review of 24 patients: signs and symptoms, management, and updated exploration of etiological factors.*

Kinney, J. M., Jeejeebhoy, K. N., Hill, G., and Owen, O. E. 1988. *Nutrition and Metabolism in Patient Care*. Philadelphia: W. B. Saunders.

Kohn, C. L., and Keithly, J. K. 1987. Techniques for evaluating and managing diarrhea in the tube fed patient. A review of the literature. In *Nutrition in Clinical Practice*, pp. 250–257. American Society for Parenteral and Enteral Nutrition.

Kolpek, J., Ott, G., Record, K., Rapp, R., Dempsey, R., Tibbs, P., and Young, B. 1989. Comparison of urinary urea nitrogen excretion and measured energy expenditure in spinal cord injury and nonsteroid-treated severe head trauma patients. *Journal of Parenteral and Enteral Nutrition* 13 (3): 277–280. *Study suggests that a different mechanism promotes the increased nitrogen excretion observed in these two populations.*

Laven, G., Huang, C., DeVivo, M., Stover, S., Kuhlemeier, K., and Fine, P. 1989. Nutritional status during the acute stage of spinal cord injury. *Archives of Physical Medicine and Rehabilitation* 70 (Apr.): 277–282. *Study designed to help clinicians establish guidelines for meeting nutritional requirements of patients during initial hospitalization.*

Lee, B., Agarwal, N., Corcoran, L., Thoden, W., and DelGuercio, L. 1985. Assessment of nutritional and metabolic status of paraplegics. *Journal of Rehabilitation Research and Development* 22 (3): 11–17.

Logemann, J. 1983. *Evaluation and Treatment of Swallowing Disorders*. San Diego: College Hill Press.

Lugerner, S., and Cox, R. 1988. *Washington Hospital Center Nutritional Support Manual*. 2d ed. Washington DC: Washington Hospital Center. *Extremely helpful pocket-size manual prepared by a nurse and dietitian. Packed with theoretical and practical information for bedside use.*

Marshall, D. 1986. Nutrition care: An evolving service. *Caring* 8 (5): 30–31. *Focus on potential role of dietitian and wellness in home care.*

Mollinger, L., Spurr, G., Ghatit, A., Barboriak, J., Rooney, C., Davidoff, D., and Bonguard, R. 1985. Daily energy expenditures and basal metabolic rates of patients with spinal cord injury. *Archives of Physical Medicine and Rehabilitation* 66 (July): 420–425. *Study measuring basal metabolic rate and daily energy expenditure revealed that high quadriplegic persons expend significantly less energy than other groups. Data provide a basis for establishing guidelines for average needs of spinal cord injured patients.*

Newmark, S., Sublett, D., Black, J., and Geller, R. 1981. Nutritional assessment in a rehabilitation unit. *Archives of Physical Medicine and Rehabilitation* 62: 279–282. *Interdisciplinary assessment perspective.*

Peiffer, S., Blust, P., and Leyson, J. 1981. Nutritional assessment of the spinal cord injured patient. *Journal of American Dietetic Association* 78 (5): 501–505. *Study of nutritional status of 18 patients with SCI, which showed that these patients are nutritionally at risk.*

Pemberton, C., Moxness, K., German, M., Nelson, J., and Gastineau, C. 1988. *Mayo Clinic Diet Manual*. 6th ed. Philadelphia: B. C. Decker. *A handbook of dietary practices, intended as a reference tool for dietitians and medical and nursing staff. Contains detailed material on dietary fiber and gastric irritants.*

Pollock, L., and Finkelman, I. 1954. The digestive apparatus in injuries to the spinal cord and cauda equina. *Surgical Clinics in North America* 34: 259–268. *Examines the normal and altered motor, sensory, and secretory functions of the digestive tract.*

Schlichtig, R., and Ayres, S. 1988. *Nutritional Support of the Critically Ill*. Chicago: Year Book Medical Publishers.

Shizgal, H., Roza, A., LeDuc, B., Drouin, G., Villemure, J., and Yaffe, C. 1986. Body Composition in Quadriplegic Patients. *Journal of Parenteral and Enteral Nutrition* 10 (4): 364–368. *Examines a variety of factors that may contribute to malnutrition in the early stages and explains the importance of correction of the malnourished state.*

Vizuete, S. F. 1989. Nutritional management in acute spinal injury. In *The Management of High Quadriplegia* Eds. G. Whiteneck, et al. New York, New York: Demos Publications, pp. 77–93. *Detailed overview of nutritional assessment and management from the initial postinjury period throughout rehabilitation for persons with high quadriplegia. Strongly advocates establishment of protocols to manage complex needs. Excellent resource for entire interdisciplinary team.*

Walters, K., and Silver, J. R. 1986. Gastrointestinal bleeding in patients with acute spinal injuries. *International Rehabilitative Medicine* 8 (1): 44–47. *Reviews incidence and presentation of symptoms. Large study over 11-year period documented mean occurrence was 22.5 days postinjury.*

Wilmot, C., and Walsh, J. 1973. Abdominal emergencies in acute spinal cord injuries. *Proceedings from Veterans Administration Spinal Cord Injury Conference* 19 (Oct.): 202–205. *Includes incidence, causes, and types of abdominal trauma and signs and symptoms emphasizing how diagnosis, not treatment, is the greater problem.*

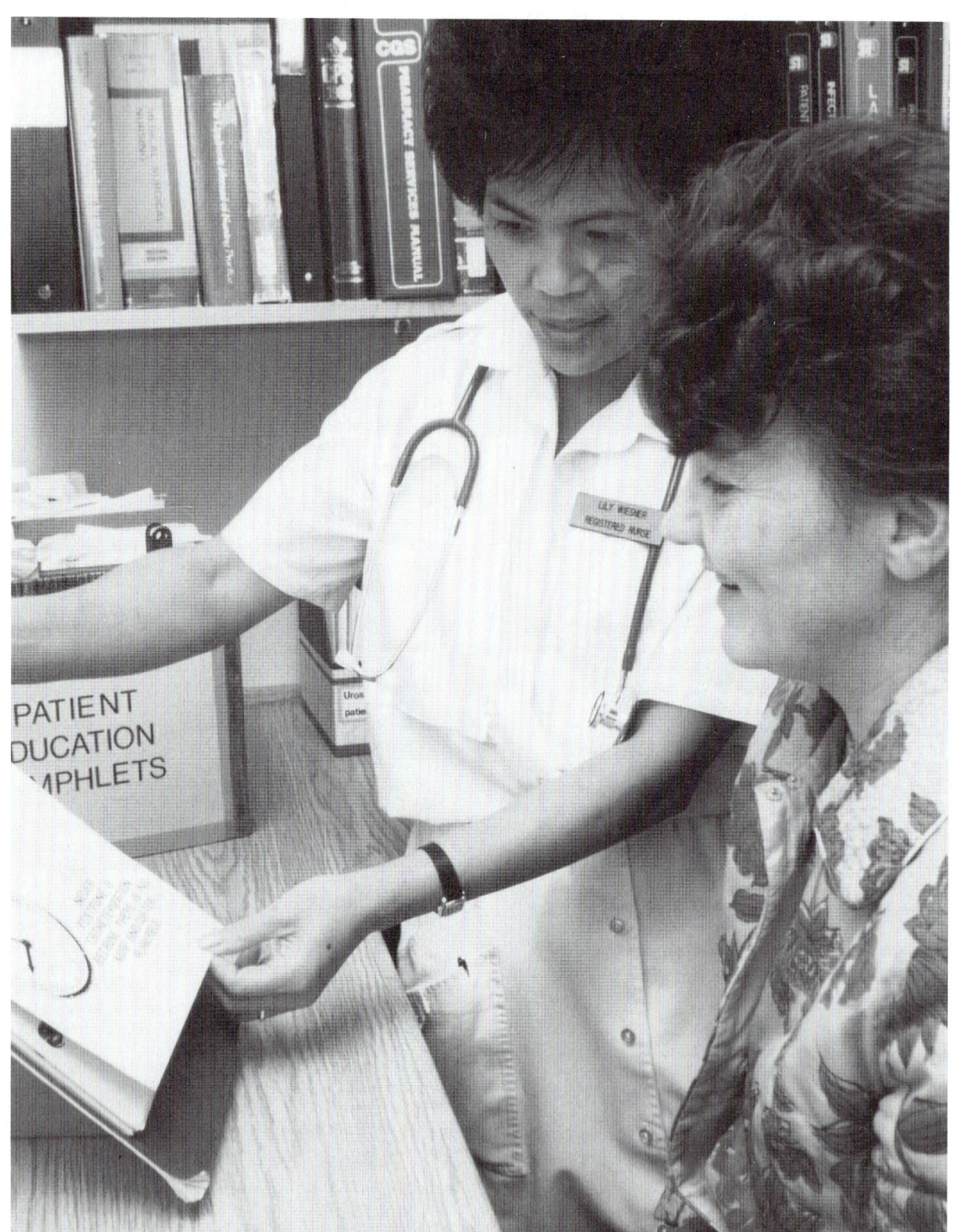

CHAPTER
— 18 —

Maintaining Urinary Function

Chapter Outline

Health Care Objectives

- To identify health care goals of urinary care correlating dysfunctions with the level of SCI sustained
- To describe assessment and diagnostic tests for urinary dysfunctions
- To describe methods of bladder management suited to the individual
- To focus on preventive management and health education
- To describe long-term implications and the vital follow-up care

Patients with spinal cord injuries (SCI) experience both neurogenic *bladder* and neurogenic *sphincter* dysfunctions that affect urinary storage and emptying capabilities. Loss of voluntary control of voiding, alterations in bladder capacity and in the power of the bladder to contract, changes in the degree of resistance of the urinary sphincters controlling urinary outflow, and lack of coordination of these functions result. Consequences of injury may impose partial or complete losses of either a temporary or permanent nature. Over time, complications frequently result in actual physical changes, such as overstretching or scarring of structures within the urinary tract, leading to further impairment of function well beyond the effects of the initial injury.

Loss of control can be embarrassing, disrupt daily activities, and sometimes lead to complete social isolation. Moreover, until recently, severe renal problems were the major cause of death in patients with SCI. This threat, although no longer as great, is still present. Hence the management of the urinary tract is of the utmost importance in a comprehensive care program for life. The success of the plan ultimately depends on acceptability to each individual but is greatly influenced by skilled, professional care.

The goals of health care are:

- To ensure adequate bladder filling and as complete emptying as possible to avoid stasis of urine and preserve a *low pressure* system
- To prevent bladder overdistension which would create an undesirable *high pressure* system
- To preserve the function of the upper urinary tract
- To prevent or control infection and other complications
- To achieve a reliable and socially acceptable urinary management program that individuals can manage independently or can teach others to perform
- To educate individuals and families in essential components of long-term urinary tract management

IMPAIRED URINARY FUNCTION AS A RESULT OF SPINAL CORD INJURY

The Urinary System

The urinary tract, or system, consists of the kidneys, ureters, bladder, and urethra.

Each of the two *kidneys* is located in the retroperitoneal area on either side of the midline, at the point where the last rib joins the spine.

The kidneys filter waste products from the blood and maintain essential body substances at a constant level. They excrete and conserve nutrients according to body need, regulate volume and composition of body fluids by excreting water, maintain acid-base balance, detoxify and excrete waste products, and influence blood pressure by controlling blood volume (which largely depends on the sodium content) and vascular space (which is affected by hormonal production).

After formation in the kidneys, *urine* passes into the collection system through the *ureters*, in which peristaltic contractions propel the urine into the bladder. The point at which the ureters join the bladder is called the *ureterovesical junction*, a muscular, one-way, valvelike structure. Although not a true valve, the ureters normally penetrate the bladder at an oblique angle in such a way that the contracting bladder pinches off the ureters to prevent backflow or *reflux* of urine.

The *bladder* is a highly elastic muscular reservoir that collects, stores, and expels urine. Its wall is composed mainly of interlaced, smooth muscle layers collectively known as the *detrusor urinae*. Although this muscle functions automatically, it is controlled by the brain as voluntary control of continence develops. The triangular floor of the bladder or *trigone* admits the ureter and urethral openings.

The *urethra* leads from the bladder neck to the outside of the body. The urethra is much longer in males than in females.

Urethral sphincters are muscular structures also involved in the voiding process. The *internal sphincter* is the first valve in the bladder outflow tract at the base of the bladder. It is not a distinct anatomical structure but an elastic mechanism formed by bladder muscle fibers that pass around the origin of the urethra at the bladder neck. These structures close the bladder neck in the resting state, maintaining continence. The *external sphincter* is a well-defined ring of strong, striated skeletal muscle surrounding the urethra as it passes through the pelvic floor (or diaphragm). This structure provides voluntary control of voiding. In the male it lies around and below the prostate gland. In the female, it surrounds the middle of the urethra. The striated muscles of the pelvic floor also have a valvular action in voluntary control.

An important factor in normal bladder emptying is the coordinated ability of these muscles and sphincters to relax when the bladder contracts. Also important for normal voiding are freedom from obstruction and the ability to contract and increase outflow resistance in response to changes in intraabdominal pressure such as coughing, sneezing, or straining.

Neural Control of Voiding

Neural supply to the bladder musculature has both a voluntary and an involuntary component. Voluntary control is achieved by the brain communicating with the sacral portion of the spinal cord, which contains the *reflex voiding center*. The reflex voiding center is located in the S_{2-4} cord segments: *reflex arcs* are composed of *sensory neurons* communicating from the bladder to the cord and *lower motor neurons* that transmit stimulation from the cord to the bladder in response.

Three areas of the nervous system supply nervous stimulation to the bladder: the T_{11}–L_2 segments provide sympathetic stimulation (via the hypogastric plexus); S_{2-4} segments provide parasympathetic stimulation and a final pathway for voluntary motor control (via the pelvic nerves); and finally micturition centers in the pons and hypothalamus provide ultimate cerebral control. The *sympathetic nervous system* plays an important role in allowing bladder filling: to contain urine, sympathetic innervation simultaneously relaxes the bladder while stimulating the opposite effect of tonic contraction (closure) of the internal bladder neck sphincter. Thus, a combination of the parasympathetic, sympathetic, and central nervous systems controls the micturition cycle. See Figure 18–1.

Micturition can be described as a sequence of events involving sensory input when the bladder fills with urine, activation of the spinal reflex voiding center, stimulation and provision of cerebral control, and progression and termination of actual voiding. In the adult, a sensation of filling first occurs when the bladder contains 175 to 250 ml. An urge to void occurs when the bladder contains 350 to 400 ml of urine. If voiding is appropriate, a coordinated voluntary and parasympathetic response induces sphincter relaxation and bladder contraction for voiding.

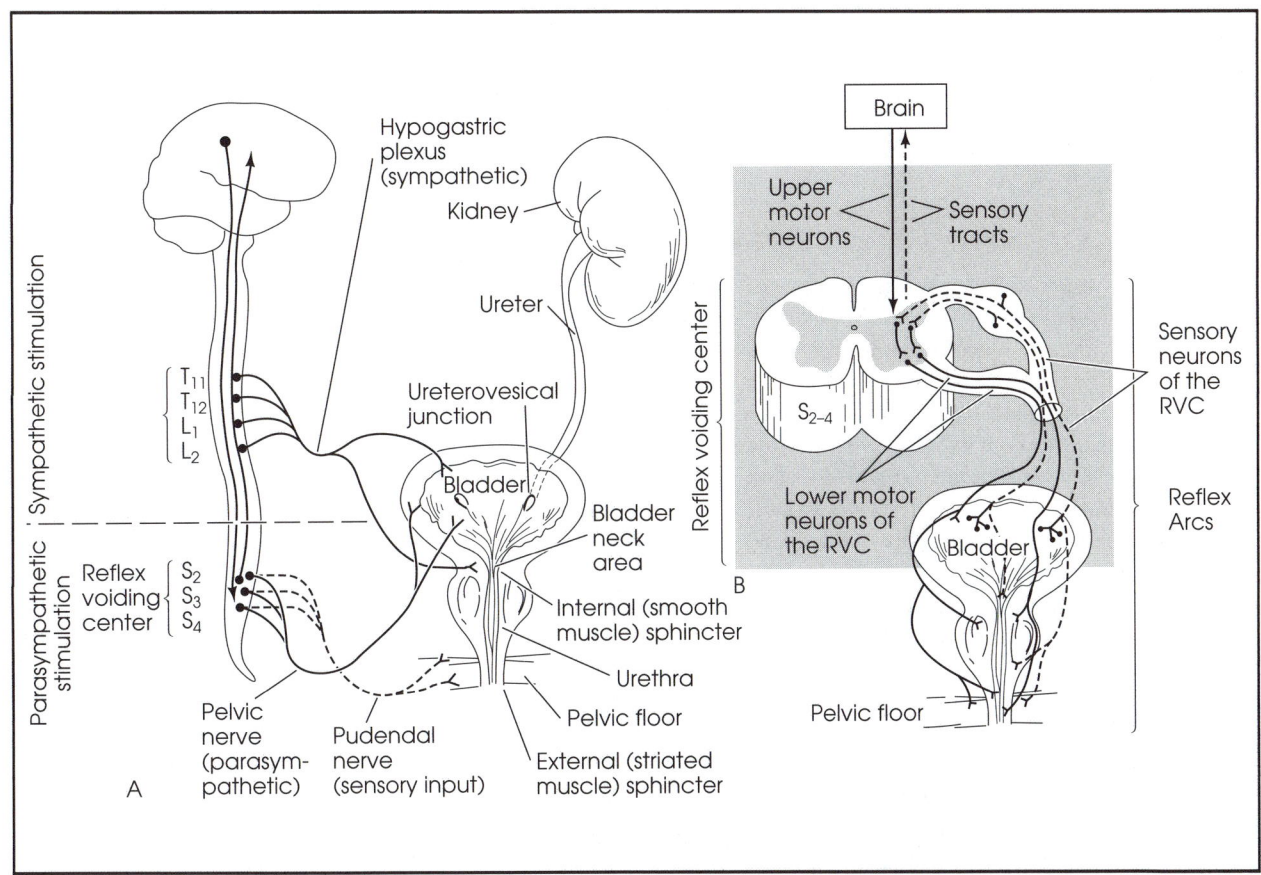

FIGURE 18–1 Neural control of the urinary system. (A) Innervation from the thoracolumbar sacral cord segments to the urinary tract is shown. (B) The reflex arc is shown in relation to the reflex voiding center.

When bladder fullness occurs in infants, transmissions to the sacral segment of the spinal cord cause the detrusor muscle to contract reflexly, resulting in spontaneous, involuntary urination. As the child develops, the brain assumes control over the reflex voiding center located in this sacral segment of the spinal cord. In the adult, cerebral inhibition suppresses the reflex, and individuals void only when the time and place are suitable.

In summary, normal bladder function is a cyclical, coordinated balance between retention (resistance) and expulsion (power) forces. The normal bladder has sensation indicating filling and the need for micturition. Residual urine (the amount left in the bladder) is normally nil and there is the ability to interrupt or initiate the stream of urine.

Dysfunctions after Injury

The kidney is not directly affected by SCI because the nervous connections do not appear to play an important role in kidney function. Production of urine is essentially unchanged. The bladder and sphincters, however, are composed of muscular tissues under autonomic and central nervous system control, and any disruption directly affects bladder sensation and function.

Interruption of communication pathways between the bladder and the reflex voiding center or between the reflex voiding center and higher cerebral centers will cause bladder and urinary outlet sphincter dysfunctions. The location of actual injury has a profound affect on the type and degree of neurogenic dysfunction.

Classification of the Neurogenic Bladder

Hyperreflexic (upper motor neuron) bladder profile. A *hyperreflexic* or so-called *upper motor neuron* paralysis of the bladder results when the level of cord injury occurs above the reflex voiding center in the sacral cord (supraspinal). Injury results in both motor and sensory dysfunction. Disconnection within the cord above the reflex voiding center causes loss of the sensation to void and loss of voluntary, coordinated control over the reflex voiding center (even though the sensory input and motor output reflex arcs remain intact). A hyperreflexic, *upper motor neuron*, or *spastic*, *automatic* bladder results. See Figure 18–2. During the spinal shock phase a spastic bladder will not be evident due to temporary loss of all reflex activity below the level of injury.

Patients with hyperreflexic bladders are unaware of the normal sensation of fullness and are unable to control voiding. When enough urine fills the bladder, stimulating the stretch receptors in the detrusor muscle, the simple reflex arcs contract independently, causing uncontrolled, spontaneous bladder contraction. A common additional problem is spasm of bladder sphincters, which prevents

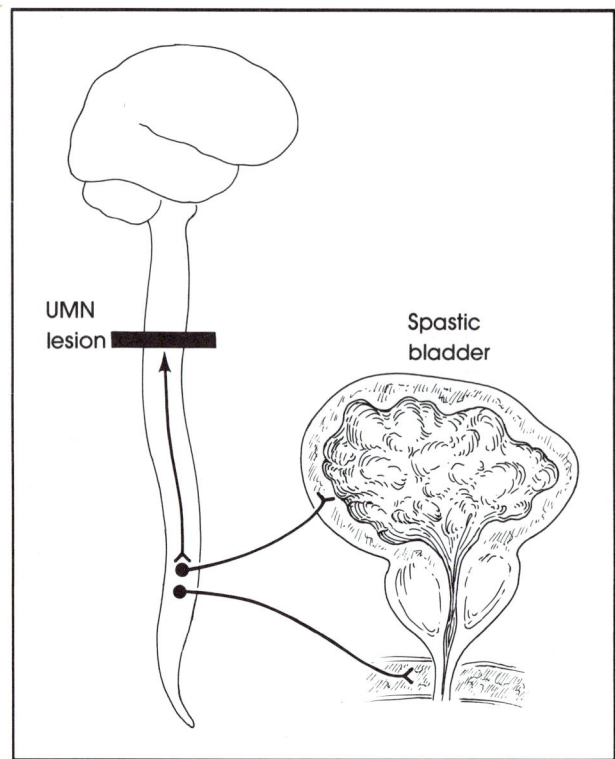

FIGURE 18–2 Dysfunction associated with upper motor neuron damage causes the bladder to become spastic (an automatic bladder).

expulsion of urine and causes overdistension of the bladder. The automatic bladder is inefficient in terms of emptying.

Areflexic (lower motor neuron) bladder profile. An *areflexic* or so-called *lower motor neuron* paralysis of the bladder results when injury to the sacral portion of the cord destroys the reflex voiding center itself. Interruption of sensory input and motor output reflex arcs at this level destroys communication with the intact sensory and motor tracts above the level of cord injury.

Reflex activity and bladder tone are diminished, which results in an *areflexic*, lower motor neuron, or *flaccid*, *autonomous bladder*. See Figure 18–3. The patient is unaware of the normal sensation of bladder fullness and is unable to initiate voiding. The bladder continues to fill with urine, but the patient is unable to void. Again, overdistension results. Preserved internal sphincter innervation (derived from the thoracolumbar level) is frequently displayed.

Mixed (upper motor/lower motor neuron) bladder profile. Incomplete injuries leave some neurons intact, preserving elements of motor or sensory functioning below the level of injury. For this reason, patients may be aware of bladder fullness yet have no voluntary control or only limited control over voiding. In this situation a *sensory* bladder exists. Some patients with incomplete injuries, for example,

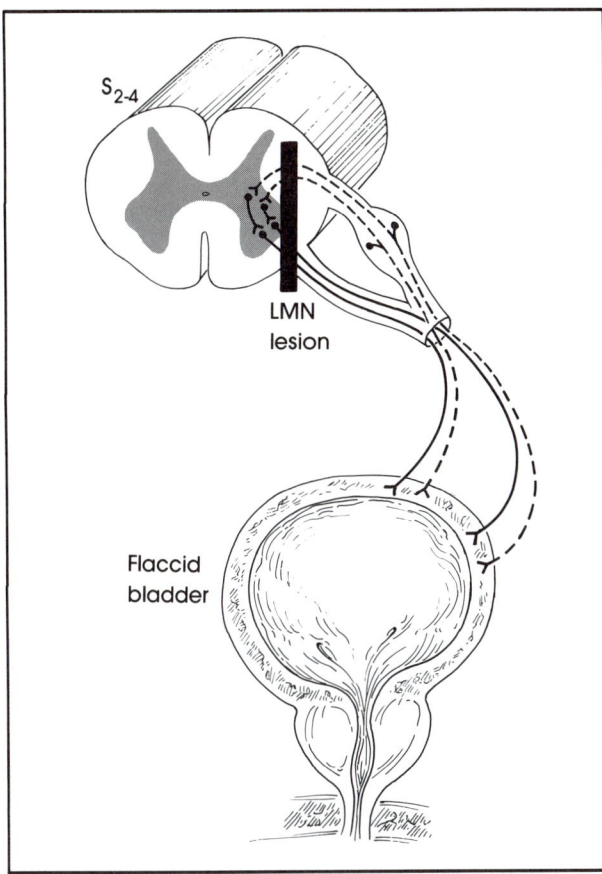

FIGURE 18–3 Dysfunction associated with lower motor neuron damage causes the bladder to become flaccid (an autonomous bladder).

those with Brown-Séquard syndrome, or central cord injury, eventually regain some degree of bladder control, which is hyperreflexic in nature and never perfect.

Injuries occurring at the conus–cauda equina junctions are more complicated, resulting in a *mixed*, or *spastic/flaccid*, *bladder*. A combination of spastic involvement of the external sphincter and flaccid involvement of the bladder, or the reverse, is possible. For example, preserved reflex activity in the pudendal nerve but not in the pelvic nerve may cause strong contractions of the external sphincter, preventing weaker detrusor muscle contractions from emptying the bladder.

A simplified classification of a neurogenic bladder due to SCI is outlined in Table 18–1.

Sphincter Classification

In addition to classifying the type of neurogenic bladder found after SCI, it is important to classify the type of sphincteric injury, because this influences treatment and prognosis greatly. One can classify the functioning of the internal and external sphincters as either spastic, normal, or flaccid in varying degrees.

Other Factors Associated with Urinary Dysfunctions

Associated Trauma

Associated abdominal trauma, bruising, or rupturing visceral organs or even the bladder itself often occur with fractures of the thoracic spine, high-velocity accidents, and sometimes seat belt injuries. Any patient with multiple injuries experiencing signs of neurogenic and/or hemorrhagic shock has decreased urinary output which must be carefully monitored. Any blood detected in the urine requires immediate investigation.

Preexisting Urinary Complications and Risk Factors

It is important to note any preexisting urinary infections or complications, including frequency, urgency, dysuria (painful or difficult voiding), burning sensation on voiding, and retention or incontinence. Also include a medication history.

Common causes of urinary problems are related to outflow obstructions, calculi formation, infections, or systemic problems affecting urinary production and output. For example, an enlarged prostate gland is a common cause of urinary obstruction in males. The female is more prone to bladder infections due to a much shorter urethra. Genitourinary and gynecological problems are common in the elderly and are sometimes complicated by diabetes, hypertension, or anemia.

Inadequate renal function can be reflected by altered function of other body systems, notably the cardiovascular and central nervous systems. Due to spinal shock, and sometimes to hypovolemic shock caused by multiple injuries, all patients experience an initial fall in blood pressure. Should severe hypotension decrease renal perfusion and cause acute tubular insufficiency, acute renal failure may result. If unchecked, uremia can cause drowsiness, confusion, altered thought processes, and irritability that may progress to twitching and convulsions.

ASSESSMENT OF URINARY SYSTEM FUNCTION

Physical Assessment

The physical assessment provides information pertinent to bladder function and potential for retraining. The neuro-

TABLE 18–1   Classifications of Neurogenic Bladder Dysfunction Following Spinal Cord Injury*

Upper Motor Neuron Dysfunction (Automatic, spastic, reflex bladder dysfunction)	Lower Motor Neuron Dysfunction (Autonomous, flaccid dysfunction)	Mixed Dysfunction
Level of injury occurs above the reflex voiding center in the sacral cord**	Level of injury damages the sacral portion of the cord involving the reflex voiding center.	Cord injury damages a portion of the reflex voiding center.
Generally associated with fractures of the T_{12} vertebra (T_{11} cord segment) and above	Generally associated with fractures to the lumbar and sacral spine (T_{12} cord segment and below).	Generally associated with fractures of the lumbar spine causing conus–cauda equina junction injuries.
Communication pathways between the brain and reflex voiding center are interrupted; communication pathways between the reflex voiding center and bladder are preserved (reflex activity is maintained after the passing of spinal shock).	Communication pathways between the reflex voiding center and the bladder are interrupted (loss of reflex activity); hence communication pathways to the brain are interrupted.	A combination of upper motor neuron/lower motor neuron dysfunction exists; for example, an upper motor neuron paralysis of bladder sphincters and a lower motor neuron bladder paralysis may exist concurrently.
The person is unaware of the sensation to void and may experience uncontrolled spontaneous voiding when enough urine fills the bladder to stimulate a reflex (spasmodic) contraction of the detrusor muscle.	The person is unaware of the sensation to void and does not experience spontaneous voiding; when urine fills the bladder, the bladder becomes overdistended, because there is no reflex activity to stimulate emptying.	The person may be unaware of the sensation to void and may or may not experience spontaneous voiding. A sensory bladder may exist; able to feel but unable to control voiding.

*Bladder dysfunctions are not clearly evident until spinal shock passes. An incomplete injury to the spinal cord results in varying degrees of preserved motor and/or sensory function below the level of injury sustained. For example, the person may be aware of the sensation to void but has limited or no control of micturition.

**The reflex voiding center is anatomically aligned with the T_{12} vertebra. Due to the expanding nature of SCI, anticipated voiding dysfunctions do not consistently correlate with the vertebral level of injury.

logical picture changes dramatically as spinal shock passes; thus, ongoing assessment cannot be stressed too strongly. Examination includes assessment of the abdomen, measurement of urinary output, inspection of the perineal and genital area, of urinary output and observation of sensation, voiding patterns, and other practical aspects of bladder management.

Assessment of the Abdomen

Inspection.   Inspect the abdomen visually for asymmetry, localized swelling, inflammation, or lacerations or bruises. Closely observe patients with fractures of the thoracic spine, because such fractures are usually caused by high-velocity accidents, which are commonly associated with abdominal injuries. Also note any scars that may indicate previous trauma or surgery.

Auscultation.   Auscultation is of limited value in assessment of urinary system function unless severe internal trauma or venous malformations are suspected. Bruits, swishing, or blowing sounds are abnormal.

Palpation.   Normally the abdomen is soft when palpated. When empty, the bladder lies behind the pubic bone; when full, it can be palpated in the lower abdomen. If distended, the bladder can expand to the umbilical region.

In a patient without sensation, gentle palpation may cause referred pain if the area is traumatized internally. Assessment by palpation is often restricted for fear of causing further damage when the patient is without sensory warning mechanisms.

Percussion.   Percuss the suprapubic area. If dullness rather than tympany occurs, the bladder is probably distended.

Measurement and Observation of Urinary Output

Perhaps the best indication of renal function and bladder status is the volume and nature of urinary output.

Measurement of urinary output.   Accurate and detailed measurement of intake in relation to output is of utmost importance during the first 48 to 72 hours after injury. A healthy adult's average hourly output of urine is 60 ml; less than 30 ml is dangerous when acute tubular necrosis may occur due to hypotension.

Measurement of urine volumes.   When intermittent catheterizations are first begun before voiding occurs, the total amount of urine obtained from a single catheterization is called a *bladder volume.* As spontaneous voiding, incontinence, or voiding induced with manual techniques occurs, the amount of urine obtained by catheterization after the bladder has been emptied by other means is called a *residual urine volume*. To obtain a true residual volume, catheterization must take place immediately after voiding. Portable renal ultrasound may also be used to measure residual urine volume, a noninvasive method that reduces unnecessary catheterizations (Cardenas, Kelly, Krieger, and Chapman 1988). Normal residual urine volume in a person without neurogenic bladder dysfunction is 0 ml.

Observation of urine. Note the color, odor, and concentration of urine. It is possible to detect hematuria, sediment, or mucous plugs on visual inspection. Simple dipstick tests can show the pH and protein content of urine. Specific gravity is measured with an hydrometer. Laboratory analysis is discussed in the section on Diagnostic Tests.

Inspection of the perineum and genital area. Inspect the perineal and genital areas for evidence of trauma—bruising, swelling, bleeding, and, particularly, urethral bleeding or discharge—that may indicate internal problems. Also note any evidence of infection. Remember that infection in any paralyzed part of the body is more difficult to heal, and vigorous treatment for minor irritations is necessary to prevent complications.

If the patient is male, examine the penis and scrotal folds carefully for skin ulceration and general cleanliness. Retract the foreskin in uncircumcised males to expose the glans penis.

If the patient is female, examine for evidence of vaginal infection or menstruation. Often the menstrual cycle is delayed by injury. Obtain the dates of the last menstrual period and a gynecological history.

When the female is in the supine position, it is safe to bend her knees gently, place her ankles together, and separate her legs (supporting the outer portion of the legs on pillows) to complete the examination.

Observation of Control, Sensation, Reflex Activity, and Voiding Patterns

Note any *voluntary control* of voiding. Since innervation to the anal sphincter is at the same level in the spinal cord as innervation of the voiding center, contraction of the anal sphincter on command suggests some voluntary control over initiating or stopping the urinary stream. Be sure to note any awareness the patient has of bladder fullness or spontaneous voiding. The quadriplegic person, for example, may perspire more when the bladder is full. Positioning often affects the patient's awareness of bladder fullness and ability to void. In particular the supine position inhibits voiding; the sitting position is used as soon as it is practical.

Saddle sensation (referring to the portion of anatomy in contact with a saddle when riding a horse) "is checked for intactness by means of light touch and pinprick of the penile skin, scrotal skin, and portions of the adjacent thighs and buttocks. If there is any sensation present, the lesion is

incomplete, and the sensory afferents (neurons) are relaying impulses to the brain" (Felder 1979: 98). This may be significant enough to establish some bladder control or at least a sensation of bladder fullness and awareness of the need to void. Sensation related to the passage of a catheter or sensitivity to cleaning of the perineal area or to bladder irrigations, if present, is also significant.

Reflex activity is noted as spinal shock passes. The *bulbocavernosus reflex* (see Figure 10–5) "is elicited by squeezing the glans penis or clitoris or by pulling gently on an indwelling catheter for a few seconds while a lubricated finger is in the rectum. In a positive test, as it is normally, the rectal sphincter can be felt to contract" (Johnson 1980: 300). Although the bulbocavernosus reflex is not the same as the voiding reflex, innervation is at the same level in the spinal cord. A positive reflex suggests the voiding reflex is intact. This test may be hyperactive in the hyperreflexive (spastic) bladder and is absent in the areflexic (flaccid) bladder.

Observe the *voiding pattern*. Compile a 24-hour record of output, accurately recording both volume and frequency. If the patient is incontinent, urine amounts can be approximated. A patient may be incontinent and continually leak urine or may suddenly pass large amounts of urine. Incontinence may be associated with stress, such as straining or coughing. Measure the amount voided (or estimate the amount of urine lost through incontinence) and the immediate postvoid residual urine to obtain an idea of the patient's bladder capacity. Table 18–2 highlights these observations.

Assessment of Practical Aspects Related to Bladder Management

Assessment of functional abilities. As mobilization begins, the patient's balance, coordination, and tolerance to the upright position must be considered. Although persons with uncomplicated paraplegia have the physical potential to become independent with bladder care, the initial use of thoracolumbar braces makes manual techniques to induce voiding and self-catheterizations more difficult. Quadriplegic patients require a detailed interdisciplinary assessment of hand and arm function and adaptive aids (Dailey and Michael 1977; Donovan 1977).

Assessment of potential for cooperation. The key to success in a bladder retraining program is related to patient motivation, reliability, learning ability, responsibility, and receptiveness. General difficulty adjusting to disability or cognitive impairment might impede the goals of the program.

Surely one of the most disruptive problems facing a person with SCI is the loss or alteration of bladder control. Maintaining bladder elimination is a major nursing responsibility requiring a special combination of knowledge, skill, and patience. "The knowledge, the conviction of its

TABLE 18–2 Bladder Assessment

Assessment Skill	Signs and Symptoms	Implications
Sensory testing of the saddle area	Absent sensation	Predictive of accompanying loss of sensation to the bladder; no sensation of bladder fullness; no control over voiding suggestive of lower motor neuron dysfunction
	Present (or limited) sensation	Predictive of accompanying bladder sensation; partial to full awareness of bladder fullness perhaps significant enough ultimately to establish voiding pattern
Testing of the bulbocavernosus reflex	Positive (or hyperactive)	Predictive of an intact reflex voiding center; suggestive of an upper motor neuron neurogenic bladder dysfunction
	Negative	Reflex absent during spinal shock. Ultimately predictive of damage to the reflex voiding center; suggestive of a lower motor neuron neurogenic bladder dysfunction
Observing voiding pattern over a 24-hour period	Incontinence with continual leakage of urine, sudden passing of large amounts of urine, or fluctuating output patterns	Indicative of an unregulated drinking pattern; inadequate timing of intermittent catheterizations or use of other techniques to induce voiding; urinary tract infection; incontinence with complications such as detrusor-sphincter dyssynergia; mobilization of dependent edema related to change of position from sitting to lying; variations in blood pressure due to orthostatic hypotension
Measuring residual urine	Unacceptable residual volume greater than 20% of bladder capacity	Unbalanced bladder; overdistension with susceptibility to reflux of urine and bladder infections

importance, the interest and the support of the nurse are essential factors for a successful program. Nursing intervention in this area needs to be *individualized, ingenious* and *rigorous* (emphasis added)" (Stryker 1977: 94). The techniques involved may be distasteful to some patients or impractical for others. Continued assessment must encompass the patient's capabilities and personal preferences. The nurse has a valuable contribution to make in helping the patient and family accept the preferred methods of urological care.

Another important factor is the support of knowledgeable staff and family members who will be involved in helping the patient to implement the program, particularly if the patient will be physically dependent for bladder care.

Diagnostic Tests

Diagnostic findings produce sophisticated data on bladder function and generally include the standard procedures discussed below.

Urine Examinations

Urine is a most important body fluid. The body must excrete urine to maintain its delicate balance of water and electrolytes and get rid of waste products. Frequently performed laboratory tests are urinalysis and urine culture and sensitivity. The following information is based on the work of French (1980).

Urinalysis. A routine urinalysis usually includes a description of appearance, pH value, specific gravity, and protein and sugar content. Microscopic examination of the sediment and screening for various other abnormal constituents are also included if requested. Since constituents of urine deteriorate rapidly on standing, a specimen not analyzed within the hour should be refrigerated. This is a most important nursing responsibility.

Normal urine is clear and may range from pale yellow to dark amber depending on the concentration. Diet, fluid intake, and certain drugs can cause changes in the appearance. Urine may be clouded by crystals, casts, blood cells or pus, amorphous material, or bacteria. Urine pH values from 4.5 to 7.5 or 8 are normal; however, normal urine is usually slightly acidic. Respiratory or metabolic acidosis causes the urine to be acidic (pH below 6). An alkalosis or infection may cause the urine to become alkalotic (pH above 6). Control of urinary pH may be desirable to prevent infection and calculi formation.

The specific gravity (SG) of urine ranges from 1.010 to 1.025. The SG is an indicator of urinary concentration. It depends on kidney function to concentrate or dilute urine and on the patient's status of hydration and periods of diuresis.

The SG can be measured approximately at the bedside by use of a hydrometer that works on the theory of displacement. Laboratory analysis measurements are more accurate, and a count of cells is included. An IVP using contrast media will produce false elevations of the SG for 24 hours or more following the procedure.

Urine culture and sensitivity. Bacteruria is a constant threat to patients with SCI. Urine is cultured when an infection is suspected. Observe urine carefully for alkaline pH, sediment, odor, or cloudiness that can indicate infection. Also monitor the systemic temperature.

A most important nursing responsibility is the collection and care of the specimen. During specimen collection, extreme caution must be taken to avoid contamination by penile or vaginal secretions, cleansing fluid preventing bacterial growth in the specimen, and improper handling of the specimen before laboratory analysis. Be sure to refrigerate the specimen immediately or ensure prompt delivery to the laboratory. The less expensive, more convenient dip slide technique is gaining popularity.

Catheterized specimens are the most common in patients with SCI. Early morning specimens are recommended for the most accurate analysis because urine is most concentrated at this time. Never take a specimen from a collection bag. Inform the lab if a patient is taking antibiotic or suppressant drugs.

BUN and Creatinine Levels

Urine is 95% water with electrolytes, bacterial toxins, certain pigments, hormones, and nitrogenous waste broken down from the metabolism of protein. The most plentiful waste products are *urea* and, to a lesser extent, *creatinine*. Urea nitrogen and creatinine both circulate in the blood but are largely excreted in the urine. The amounts excreted are proportional to the rate of production and the glomerular filtration rate. The following information is based on the work of Stark (1980).

Blood urea nitrogen (BUN) is normally 11 to 23 mg/100 ml. When urea is not being excreted adequately, the BUN level will rise. This is a helpful indicator when assessing renal function. However, several other factors unrelated to kidney function can cause an increase or decrease in BUN values:

- Protein metabolism is not constant and can be affected by poor nutritional status, excessive protein intake, infection, trauma, surgery, hepatic dysfunction, or certain medications such as corticosteroids or tetracyclines.
- The urea excretion rate can be altered by dehydration, vomiting, diarrhea, infection, surgery, and hypovolemia, all of which alter blood volume and reduce the glomerular filtration rate.

The BUN is therefore examined with the creatinine level to give a more exact reflection of kidney function.

Creatinine blood levels are normally 0.6 to 1.2 mg/100 ml. Creatinine is an end product of muscle metabolism. Since the muscle mass of the body seldom changes rapidly, creatinine levels are generally constant unless kidney failure has begun.

Carefully observe the BUN/creatinine ratio. This is normally 20:1. When the BUN rises, but the creatinine remains normal, look for any physiological reason that can cause decreased blood flow to the kidney, which will reduce the glomerular filtration rate or increase protein catabolism. Be alert for low fluid intake, chronic hypotension, and urinary infection as causes of volume depletion and low perfusion of the kidneys. Also consider depleted nutritional status, fever, bleeding from stress ulcer, and corticosteroid therapy as possible causes of increased protein catabolism. Reaction to trauma or surgery may cause BUN levels to vary. When the BUN and creatinine both rise, suspect kidney disease with nephron damage.

For lifelong surveillance other tests are more helpful. By the time creatinine levels change, kidney damage could be quite advanced. Creatinine production, being related to muscle mass and altered by atrophy associated with paralysis, appears to be lower than that of the able-bodied population; error in interpretation is thus possible (Mohler, Ellison and Flanigan 1986). BUN levels vary with fluid intake and output and also tend to be low in spinal cord injured persons educated to drink more fluids than average.

Intravenous Pyelogram

The intravenous pyelogram (IVP) is considered a diagnostic cornerstone because it gives overall information about the urinary system. An IVP is a series of X rays in which the "absence, presence, location, size, and configuration of each kidney as well as of the filling of renal calyces, pelves, and outlines of ureters can be determined. Some idea of the lower urinary tract is also obtained" (Winter and Morel 1977: 65–66). An IVP will provide baseline data for future comparisons and rule out any gross abnormalities of the urinary system.

Preparation for the patient should include a determination of any history of allergy to contrast medium or iodine and an explanation of the procedure, its purpose, and the reason for physical preparation. Preparation usually includes omission of food and fluids from midnight on the night before the procedure to improve concentration of the opaque contrast medium in the urinary system and produce a clearer X ray, and bowel evacuation because the kidneys lie retroperitoneally and fecal material or gas may cause shadows on the film. Physicians unfamiliar with SCI care may routinely order vigorous laxatives. Such cathartics are contraindicated for people with a neurogenic bowel because they increase incontinence and are unpredictable in action. Nausea, vomiting, fainting, and even blackouts or signs of autonomic dysreflexia can occur. Scheduling the test on a day of routine evacuation or when using a rectal suppository is usually satisfactory.

A plain X-ray film of the kidneys, ureters, and bladder is taken first. A radiopaque contrast medium intravenously outlines anatomical structures. During this time the patient must be observed for any allergic reactions. Serial X rays are taken over a 20-minute period. The last film of the series is usually a postvoid film. Empty the bladder by the current bladder program in use. The table must be padded with one-inch foam rubber or a soft sheet to protect the bony prominences. Anticipate increases in output following test because the contrast medium is a diuretic.

Cystoscopy

A cystoscopy is an examination with a lighted scope inserted into the bladder for direct visualization of the bladder and the urethra. The status of the bladder wall can be appreciated, and evidence of infection, calculi, or tumors not evident on X ray or ultrasound, can be detected. Calculi can be fragmented and removed.

Renal Ultrasound

The renal ultrasound also demonstrates kidney function and is used to detect obstruction, hydronephrosis, and calculi. Because of its noninvasive nature, renal ultrasound is being more widely used in follow-up evaluation. An IVP is still considered necessary for a more exact initial assessment and a more accurate visualization of a problem encountered by ultrasound.

Urodynamic Studies

The rapidly expanding influence of urodynamic studies has shed light on neurogenic dysfunctions common to persons with SCI and has contributed significantly to progress in clinical management. The level of injury may not accurately reflect urinary tract function as both high and low pressure systems are found in patients with various levels of injury (Herschorn, Barkin, and Comisarow 1982). For example, one may erroneously assume that a person with paraplegia resulting in flaccid leg paralysis would experience a flaccid lower urinary tract also. In fact many such persons experience high pressure systems as revealed by urodynamic studies. Studies also monitor the effects of drugs used in treatment.

Urodynamic studies focus on the function of the mechanics involved in bladder filling, storing, and emptying in terms of:

- Pressure of urine within the system
- Flow rate of urine
- Muscular activity
- Resistance factors calculated from pressure and flow readings

Pressure, volume, and muscular activity measurements are determined electronically and recorded on a graph. These measurements and other observations of sensation and reflex activity, including response to selected drugs given during testing, assist in determining the exact classification of neurogenic bladder and sphincter dysfunctions.

The bladder may be thought of as a reservoir with one exit. Questions to ask are:

- Does it hold enough urine (storage)?
- Does it not hold enough urine?
- Does it empty?
- Does it empty enough?

A high pressure system (with overdistension and backflow or reflux) is directly related not only to the bladder's ability to store urine effectively and to initiate and sustain adequate bladder contractions for emptying, but also to resistance outflow (coordination and ability of sphincters to relax adequately) to allow emptying.

The *cystometrogram* is the main diagnostic test for determining the nature and extent of neurological impairment to the bladder. To document abnormalities of the urethra and its surrounding muscles that create the internal and external bladder sphincters, further studies, such as the *urethral pressure profile* and *electromyography*, are needed.

Cystometrogram (CMG). The CMG best assesses how the bladder responds to the filling and storing phase. The CMG measures:

- Bladder reactivity (the weakness or strength of the bladder wall contractions)
- Bladder capacity (the volume of urine the bladder holds)
- Evidence of reflux

The principles of the CMG are:

- As CO_2 gas (more rapidly absorbed) or fluid is instilled through an indwelling urinary catheter, the bladder reacts as if it were naturally filling with urine.
- When the gas or fluid volume is increased, the normal bladder will eventually respond by contracting to expel the fluid.
- Detrusor muscle action produces measurable increases in pressure within the bladder itself.

The normal bladder response is the ability to perceive "(1) temperature and entrance of fluid; (2) the point at which a desire to void is experienced; and (3) the stage at which pain or distress is first felt, as well as the point of severe pain beyond which no further bladder filling can be tolerated . . . until a massive contraction empties the bladder" (Chusid 1979: 270).

Full understanding of the abnormal results of cystometric testing requires a clear understanding of the concept of lesions involving upper motor neurons as contrasted with lesions involving lower motor neurons at the voiding center.

In a person with an upper motor neuron (spastic) bladder dysfunction, after spinal shock subsides, a cystometrogram will reveal many uncontrolled contractions in response to bladder filling. See Figure 18–4(A) (p. 367). Eventually, one contraction will be strong enough to expel some of the fluid. This usually occurs at a lower-than-normal bladder capacity (approximately 250 to 300 ml). A large residual amount of urine is often left. Many patients do not have either desire to void or a feeling of bladder fullness but an involuntary urinary stream may be elicited by various trigger methods. Care must be taken to avoid autonomic dysreflexia.

In a person with lower motor neuron (flaccid) paralysis of the bladder, a cystometrogram will show no uninhibited bladder contraction because the reflex arcs to the voiding center are damaged. See Figure 18–4(B). A person experiencing spinal shock will also demonstrate this flaccid bladder profile. No sensation or desire to void is present. The bladder cannot expel urine. Manual expression or catheterization is required to empty the bladder.

During cystometric tests insertion of warm or cold fluids may be used to test sensation. Insertion of ice-cold fluid into the bladder of a patient with a hyperreflexic motor neuron bladder will elicit a strong contraction causing expulsion of the solution. A patient with an areflexic motor neuron or bladder will have no response. This is referred to as the *ice water test*.

Alternatively, medications are sometimes used to assess bladder sensitivity and response to the drugs.

Urethral pressure profile. Urethral pressure profiles (UPP) are used to measure pressures along the length of the urethra. The test is performed by slowly removing a small catheter at the same time as fluid or gas is infused. Pressures recorded reflect pressures along the length of the urethra, indicating the nature of urine outflow as it exits from the bladder. The *Uroflow* tracks the speed and pattern with which the urine exits from the bladder.

Electromyography. Muscular activity measurement of the external urinary sphincter and rectal sphincter may be recorded simultaneously with the CMG by sphincter-perineal *electromyography* (EMG). Electrically sensitive rectal plugs and urethral catheter sensors are used to record electrical activity of the pelvic floor. Again, hyperactivity is suggestive of upper motor neuron damage; flaccidity, of lower motor neuron damage.

Rectal tone and pelvic muscle activity yields important information about sphincter activity. The sphincters relax during normal voiding, thus, the presence of activity impedes the flow of urine (detrusor-sphincter dyssynergia).

Voiding cystourethrography (VCU). The VCU is a very useful examination for visualizing the voiding cycle.

The bladder is filled with radiopaque contrast media to the point where emptying is initiated and the catheter is expelled. Fluoroscopy or a series of X rays are taken to show up the major impediments to emptying at the bladder neck and sphincter areas. It indicates whether the major obstruction to urine flow is at the bladder neck (internal sphincter), the external sphincter, or both. This helps determine whether an operative procedure is needed to lessen outflow resistance.

RESTORATIVE MANAGEMENT

The most important defense mechanism protecting the upper urinary tract is intact ureterovesical valves that prevent infection and reflux of urine up the ureter into the kidney. Damage to these valves is caused by overdistending the bladder as a result of increased intravesical pressure from high residuals, infrequent emptying of the bladder, infection, or obstruction to urinary outflow. Unchecked, damage can progress from *ureteritis* to dilation of the ureters (*hydroureter*) and can eventually ascend to the kidney and cause *pylonephritis* and *hydronephrosis*. Maintaining a low pressure system to protect these valves is the key to bladder management.

Maintaining Elimination during the Initial Postinjury Period

Although an intermittent catheterization program is the method of choice in the management of neurogenic bladder dysfunction in patients with SCI (see Box, Intermittent Catheterizations), it is almost always necessary to insert an indwelling catheter to establish continuous drainage for the initial 12-hour postinjury period. An indwelling catheter may be required for a prolonged period during the acute phase to monitor a seriously ill patient. See chapter 6.

Initiating Intermittent Catheterizations

An intermittent catheterization program is based on the concept of evacuating the bladder at regular intervals by inserting a straight (nonretaining) urethral catheter every few hours to drain the bladder of urine. For most patients with SCI, the ultimate goal of bladder retraining is to establish a reliable method of emptying and become catheter free.

INTERMITTENT CATHETERIZATIONS

Although bladder retraining continues to be a subject of much debate, during the past decade intermittent catheterization has gained worldwide acceptance as the preferred method of initial management (Lindan, Leffler, and Freehafer 1990; Gardener, Parsons, Machin, Galloway, and Krishnan 1986). Many patients suffering neurogenic bladder dysfunction due to SCI have achieved a catheter-free state with this method. Numerous investigators have found considerable reduction in persistent bladder infections and prevention of the many serious problems associated with any form of indwelling catheter. Other advantages include better patient acceptance, because freedom from an indwelling catheter promotes independence, improves personal hygiene, and eases sexual relations. Intermittent catheterization was first introduced by Sir Ludwig Guttman in 1949, following his work with large numbers of British veterans of World War II with SCI. Guttman used a scrupulous, sterile procedure performed only by physicians, but more recently a clean procedure, often performed by patients, has gained acceptance (Maynard and Dionko 1980; Barkin, Herschorn, and Comisarow 1982; University of Michigan Urology Associates 1988). However, for the most part, a sterile procedure is adopted when the patient is hospitalized to reduce the ever-present hazard of cross-contamination.

Many larger SCI centers in the United States have catheterization teams composed of a group of technicians often led by RNs or nursing assistants. Bladder management is their exclusive duty. Part of the rationale for this specialization is to eliminate any contact with the gross contamination encountered in general nursing care duties. The other aspect is mainly ease of training for fewer staff members. However, the patient population does not always support such an approach, and more and more centers consider repeated catheterizations an integral part of nursing care. Existing literature does not clearly correlate infection rates with categories of staff performing the catheterizations.

In terms of female nurses catheterizing male patients, there is no particular problem with this providing the nurse is adequately trained in the technique. Many patients feel that bowel accidents or procedures are far more distasteful or embarrassing than a "clean" medical procedure such as catheterization.

During spinal shock, the tone of all tissues, including blood vessels, is reduced and the pressure of a catheter in the urethra can produce ischemia and lead to formation of abscesses or fistulae very quickly. The presence of an indwelling catheter for a week or more is invariably associated with infection and a tendency toward bacterial urethritis and prostatitis in male patients (Pearman and England 1973). See Procedure 18–1 and Figure 18–4 for more information on indwelling catheter care.

Renewed interest is evident in *suprapubic* catheterization as an alternative in both the acute and rehabilitative phases of management to reduce the incidence of urethral complications (Lloyd, Kuhlemeier, Fine, and Stover 1986). Others feel it increases the risk of late bladder cancer. The suprapubic cystostomy is a direct opening made into the bladder through the abdomen. An indwellng catheter or an intermittent catheter program may then be used.

An indwelling suprapubic catheter may be selected as a temporary measure to bypass the urethra when strictures make urethral catheterization impossible, or during the course of treatment for ailments such as penoscrotal fistula, abscess, or epididymitis. Suprapubic drainage may also be selected as a permanent measure to avoid the use of a perineal catheter in women, for example.

It is possible to limit infection, and the use of fine-gauge, nonreactive silastic tubing decreases the chance of precipitating stone formation. Aspiration is necessary to empty the bladder satisfactorily and occasionally irrigation of the cystocatheter or advancing and retracting the tubing through the puncture site may be necessary to ensure unobstructed drainage (Donovan, Kiviat, and Clowers 1977).

As the suprapubic catheter introduces a route for ascending bacteria, care measures are similar to those needed with a regular indwelling catheter. The suprapubic catheter should be anchored to the abdomen with tape to prevent any direct trauma to the bladder or stoma.

Intermittent catheterization with a fine-bore suprapubic catheter (as opposed to a urethral catheter) may also reduce the incidence of infection (Noll, Russe, Kline, Botel, and Schreiter 1988).

Procedure 18–1 Care of a Patient Requiring a Continuous Drainage System

Purpose

To provide unobstructed drainage while avoiding trauma to the urethra and bladder neck and preventing infection.

Equipment and Supplies

- Size #14 or #16 (French) silicone indwelling catheter
- Standard sterile catheterization set
- Urinary collection system (tubing and bag)

Action

1. Select a catheter no larger than a size #16 (French). Do not inflate balloon beyond 10 cc.

2. Lubricate the catheter *liberally*.

3. Follow strict sterile technique when catheterizing patient. If a "no-touch" technique is practiced, after donning sterile gloves, use one set of forceps to hold the cotton balls for cleaning genital area and an additional set of forceps to manipulate catheter for insertion. Secure tip of the catheter with forceps; control end of the catheter by placing between third and fourth fingers.

4. If there is any difficulty passing the catheter, try a curve-tipped (Coudé) catheter directed anteriorly. It can be gently rotated to maneuver past the penoscrotal angle or circumnavigate any narrowing of urethra or resistance at bladder neck. Obstructing spastic external sphincter can usually be overcome with gentle, persistent pressure.

5. Secure catheter with tape. Tape catheter to inner thigh of a female; determine length of catheter by abducting and externally rotating leg before securing. Tape upward on abdomen of a male. If a patient is on a regular bed, tape catheter in a central position on the abdomen so that tubing can be placed to either side when patient is turned. If patient is on a Stryker frame, pad catheter tubing with gauze and place it just above iliac crest before turning to prone position. If patient is sitting, catheter can be taped more to side of the abdomen to promote drainage.

6. In early stages, while patient is on bedrest, secure catheter with a strip of lightweight paper or nonallergic tape. Secure in such a way that the tubing does not come into direct contact with the skin. Later, taping can be eliminated by using the leg bag straps to anchor catheter in position.

7. Coil excess tubing at level of the patient's bladder and secure the collection bag at a lower level. *Never* lift the drainage bag above level of patient's bladder when turning or transferring. Be alert for a solid column of urine in the drainage tubing indicating obstructed flow. Air bubbles should always be present. Low urine output may be another indication that urinary flow is obstructed. Catheter may simply need to be changed or if continual obstruction is a problem, bladder irrigations may be necessary. Routine irrigation of catheters is not recommended.

8. Clean entire perineal area, particularly external urinary meatus. Gently wash the perineum with soapy water twice daily. Rinse and dry well. Avoid use of powders and lotions in the perineal area. These tend to become trapped in the skin folds.

Rationale

Avoid larger sizes that dilate the urethra and sphincters unnecessarily.

To minimize urethral trauma, especially when patient is without sensory warning mechanisms. Also, male patient, because of the longer urethra, requires additional lubricant.

This "no-touch" technique is recommended to minimize the risk of introducing infection. There is a risk of contaminating the sterile glove when cleaning, even though forceps are used.

To avoid urethral trauma, *never* force introduction of a catheter; notify the physician if any difficulty arises.

Taping prevents any pulling on the urethral mucosa or the bladder neck. When the penis rests in a downward position, there is a sharp anatomical angulation at the penoscrotal junction. If the catheter is taped on the thigh, excessive pressure causes irritaiton and greatly increases the risk of penoscrotal fistula. Taping the catheter upward onto the abdomen straightens the urethra at the penoscrotal angulation, relieves undue pressure, and reduces risk of complications. See Figure 18–4.

This tape is sufficient and less traumatic to newly desensitized skin.

To provide continual gravity-assisted drainage to promote constant urinary outflow.

To prevent accumulation of bacteria at the point where catheter enters body. Because of its proximity to the bladder, this is a significant site of possible infection.

(Procedure continues)

Procedure 18–1   Care of a Patient Requiring a Continuous Drainage System (continued)

Action

9. Observe entire perineal area, including gluteal fold, for reddened, irritated areas. Clean and dry. Directing the airstream from a hairdryer set on cool may sufficiently dry area. Try to alleviate cause. If you suspect that soap is irritating, clean with normal saline instead.

10. If infection is suspected, swab area for a culture and apply appropriate topical antibiotics as ordered by physician. Crusted secretions around the meatal opening can be removed with hydrogen peroxide. Neomycin ointment may be applied to meatal opening twice daily as a prophylactic measure.

11. Care for the urinary collection system. When patient is on bedrest, change urine collection bag only when catheter is changed unless it is accidentally contaminated or leaking. Sediment or odor indicates need for a change. To obtain a urine specimen from indwelling catheter, swab puncture area distal to the branch of the Y with alcohol and aspirate the urine with needle and syringe.

12. Change catheter routinely every 2 to 3 weeks. To check for crystal formation, roll catheter between fingers. If there is grit in the catheter, change it and report it to physician.

13. Provide adequate fluid intake. Generally 2500 to 4000 ml every 24 hours is recommended, but in acute stage, fluid intake may be restricted for other priorities.

14. Observe for redness or swelling of the scrotum.

Rationale

When female patient is in supine position cleansing solutions tend to run down and accumulate in gluteal fold. Be sure to check area thoroughly. It is necessary to turn patient to do so. It cannot be overstressed that reddened areas on desensitized skin with compromised circulation will rapidly break down unless dealt with immediately.

Even though modern drainage tubing and collection bags incorporate drip chambers, one-way flutter valves, and vents that have drastically reduced possibility of urinary backflow and contamination when emptying, this equipment is still a major source of ascending infection. Any opening of system increases the risk of infection.

Rubber catheters will deteriorate, absorb fluid, and swell. Catheter should be free of debris inside and out when removed.

Risk of epididymitis is increased.

To ensure success, the principles of an intermittent catheterization program must be clearly understood:

- Avoid overdistension of the bladder. Overstretching the bladder wall ruptures detrusor muscle cells. Resultant fibrosis, associated with loss of contractility, may permanently impair bladder tone and function. Overdistension significantly decreases the blood supply to the urethra, bladder, ureters, and kidneys and weakens resistance to infection. Furthermore, the increased pressure of chronic overdistension causes ureterovesical reflux allowing ascending infection to infiltrate the ureters and kidneys: Preservation of the upper urinary tract is vital to life. Prevention of overdistension is thought to be the key to preventing urinary tract infection.
- The bladder must be emptied completely and frequently to reduce the residual medium in which bacteria may multiply rapidly.
- The catheter must be inserted with the utmost care to prevent urethral trauma.

- Early initiation of intermittent catheterization is believed to accomplish faster retraining results and reduces the inevitable infections associated with an indwelling catheter. One to 3 months after injury is a reasonable time to estimate for return of detrusor activity in patients on an intermittent program.

Keeping these principles firmly in mind, begin intermittent catheterization programs as outlined in Procedure 18–2. See also Table 18–3.

Maintaining an Intermittent Catheterization Program

While maintaining an intermittent catheterization program, a number of techniques are used to induce bladder emptying (detailed in next section). Whatever techniques are selected, integrated goals strive toward maintaining

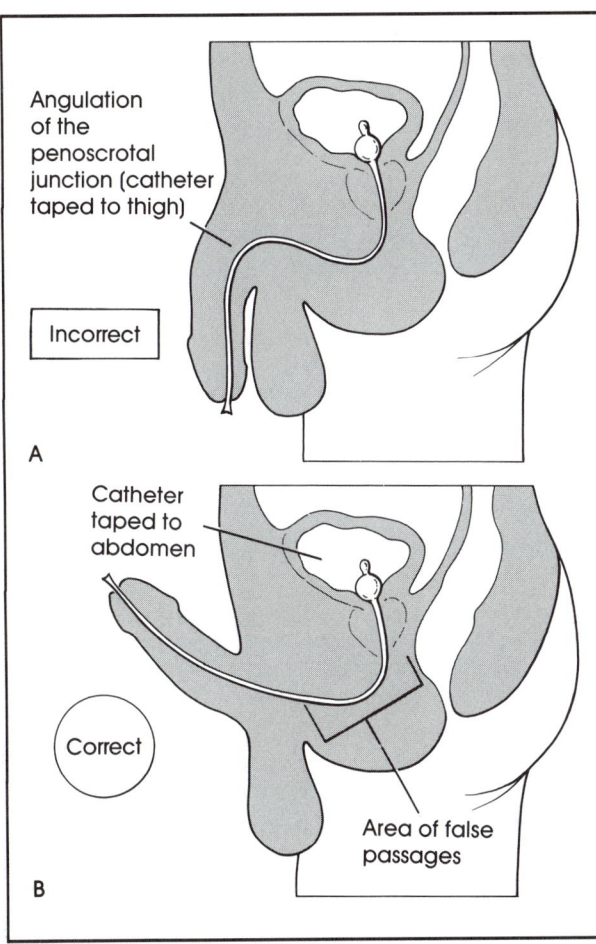

Angulation
of the
penoscrotal
junction (catheter
taped to thigh)

Incorrect

A

Catheter
taped to
abdomen

Correct

Area of false
passages

B

FIGURE 18–4   Positioning an indwelling catheter to the abdomen of a male patient straightens the angulation of the penoscrotal junction and reduces pressure exerted by the catheter.

tant during bladder retraining (Pearman and England 1973). A drinking pattern is necessary to develop the desired relationship between timing and amount of fluid intake, and timing and amount of voiding or catheterization volumes. Intake should be maintained at approximately 2000 ml/day and periods of excessive intake or no intake at all should be avoided. Once established, recording intake is not necessary; concentrate on output patterns for more accuracy.

With intense rehabilitation activities, it is difficult to regulate hourly intake; because patients must avoid large amounts of fluid at any one time, it is helpful to have drinks available during physical therapy sessions.

During the day, fluids accumulate in the dependent areas of the body. When the patient lies down at night these fluids are reabsorbed and produce a dramatic increase in output, even when fluids are restricted during the evening hours. It may be helpful if the patient is in bed early, by 2100 hours, and a catheterization is done at 2400 hours, for example. Typically the early morning catheter volumes are high and the last to be discontinued (Ozer 1988, p. 58).

Avoid excesses of caffeine-containing drinks and carbonated and alcoholic beverages, which tend to irritate the bladder.

a *balanced bladder* while encouraging a good fluid intake. A balanced bladder exists when regular emptying occurs without a high pressure of urine remaining in the bladder (intravesicular pressure). Less than approximately 100 ml of residual volume remaining after bladder emptying is generally acceptable (Ozer 1988: 58). However, assessment does not depend on the actual residual volume alone, but must include consideration of the relationship of residual volume to the bladder capacity or total volume of urine stored in the bladder. Low residual urine alone is not by itself a predictor of an acceptable state—for example, sometimes a high pressure bladder with upper tract deterioration can have negligible residuals.

The information in this section is summarized in Table 18–4.

The fact that the detrusor muscle responds with more powerful contractions when the bladder is full is impor-

---

A BALANCED BLADDER

A state of balance is expressed in percentages or ratios. The goal is a minimum requirement of 5:1 ratio, 5 parts urine voided or expressed to 1 part residual. In other words the residual is 20% of the total volume of urine in the bladder. A normal bladder residual is 0 ml. For example, when a patient voids or expresses 375 ml urine, a postvoid residual of 75 ml is considered acceptable. The bladder is balanced:

$$\frac{375 \text{ ml voided/expressed}}{75 \text{ ml residual}} = \text{ratio 5:1 or 20\%}$$

However, if a patient voids or expresses 225 ml urine, a postvoid residual of 75 ml would be considered unacceptable, despite the fact that the actual volume of residual is the same in both cases. In this case, the bladder is unbalanced:

$$\frac{225 \text{ ml voided/expressed}}{75 \text{ ml residual}} = \text{ratio 3:1 or 33\%}$$

Procedure 18–2   Beginning an Intermittent Catheterization Program

Purpose

For most patients with SCI, to become catheter free. During the intermittent catheterization program goals of management are (1) to prevent overdistension of the bladder; (2) to prevent introduction of infection; and (3) to control infection by complete and frequent emptying of the bladder.

Action	Rationale
1. Assess general condition of the patient.	To determine if it is possible to begin intermittent catheterization when patient: • Has stable blood pressure, pulse, and respiratory rate and a normal body temperature • Produces adequate amounts of normal urine consistently (approximately 60 ml/hr over a 24-hour period) • Is free from associated trauma or preexisting conditions that would make repeated catheterizations difficult and traumatize the urethra Intermittent catheterizations are contraindicated when: • Monitoring of hourly urinary output is required • Natural or forced diuresis is present
2. Regulate fluid intake to total of approximately 200 ml/24 hr. Encourage patient to follow a regulated drinking pattern adjusted to maintain desired output.	This avoids large amounts of urine from overdistending the bladder. Unregulated fluid intake causes fluctuating voiding responses and difficulty in detecting and controlling bladder fullness. Regulating fluid intake becomes a major patient responsibility as rehabilitation progresses.
3. Schedule catheterizations. Begin every 4 hours around the clock. Remove the indwelling catheter in the early morning hours. A convenient schedule to start with is 1000, 1400, 1800, 2200, 0200, and 0600 hours. Adjust times to maintain catheter volumes of 400 to 500 cc.	This facilitates close observation of patient throughout the day. Try to avoid catheterizations when the ward is particularly busy, such as mealtime or change of shift.
4. Use a small, flexible catheter, a size #12 or #14 (French) or Coudé if necessary.	This prevents urethral dilation and trauma.
5. Perform catheterizations. Follow a strict sterile technique. Insert catheter just far enough into the bladder to get urine to flow.	The technique in Procedure 18–1 (step 3) may be used. Disposable kits for males and females are available.
6. Withdraw the catheter slowly and apply a firm, continuous downward pressure over the suprapubic area.	This ensures complete bladder emptying and prevents air from entering the bladder through the catheter. However, if too much force is used, it may cause backflow into the upper tracts.
7. Observe the patient closely for overdistension. Initially check the abdomen for palpable distension every 1 to 2 hours. Catheterize immediately if distension is suspected.	This minimizes overdistension of bladder with subsequent loss of bladder tone and susceptibility to infection.
8. Maintain bladder capacity of less than 500 ml. If the volume is greater than 500 ml reevaluate intake regulation and frequency of catheterizations. If diuresis is present, resume continuous drainage.	The volume of urine obtained at any catheterization should not exceed 500 ml. If it does consistently, contact the physician to reevaluate the situation. No more than 4 to 6 catheterizations during a 24-hour period are recommended, but intervals may vary from 2 to 8 hours. If, despite controlled intake, the volume is persistently greater than 500 ml at each catheterization, diuresis should be suspected. This is common during the first week after injury. Delay the intermittent catheterizations temporarily.
9. When intravenous fluids are discontinued, schedule catheterizations at 6-hour intervals. Maintain bladder capacity at approximately 450 ml. If bladder capacity exceeds this volume, resume 4-hour schedule.	If complications are not present, regulating oral intake should control bladder capacity. Patterns of urine formation may dictate a unique pattern of timing for catheterizations.
10. Record intake and output initially; then only output as pattern becomes stable.	Conventional fluid charts, which are tallied at the change of each shift, do not lend themselves to recording an intermittent catheterization program. Table 18–3 is an example of a chart record that may be used throughout the program.

TABLE 18–3 An Intermittent Catheterization Program Sample Chart Record

A numerical recording of fluid intake and output

- The *time* column permits a maximum of six separate entries, enough spaces to accommodate recording of intermittent catheterizations performed every 4 hours over a 24-hour period (Example 1). When catheterizations are reduced, for example, to every 6 hours as shown in Example 2, record data in the first four consecutive spaces.

- Calculate fluid intake for the time interval between catheterizations, rather than the standard practice from shift to shift. Enter fluid intake in the second column at the beginning; otherwise omit. Concentrate on output.

- Next record the amount of urine voided between or before catheterizations. This amount refers to output obtained when voiding is spontaneous or is induced by trigger techniques or straining to void.

- Use the Manual Techniques column to record the amount of urine expressed manually.

- The urinary output obtained via catheter is the residual volume of urine obtained.

- Total the urinary output from all sources.

DATE	TIME	INTAKE (optional)	VOIDED	MANUAL TECHNIQUES	CATHETER (Residual)	TOTAL OUTPUT	SPECIMENS	COMMENTS
		Example: q 4 h	*program*					
Example 1	TOTAL							
	0200	400	—	—	300	300	Admission	
Sept. 10, 1990	0600	400	—	—	300	300	urinalysis	
	1000	500	—	—	300	300	C & S	
	1400	500	—	—	500	500	taken	
	1800	300	—	—	350	350		
	2200	300	—	—	350	350		
	TOTAL	2400				2100		

DATE	TIME	INTAKE	VOIDED	MANUAL	CATHETER	TOTAL	SPECIMENS	COMMENTS
		Example: q 6 h	*program*					
Example 2	TOTAL							
	0600	280	—	200	250	450		Incontinent
Oct. 1, 1990	1200	800	50	250	100	400		
	1800	750	300	200	200	700		See nursing
	2400	280	400	—	100	500		notes.
	TOTAL	2110				1950		

Techniques to Induce Voiding

During the recovery phase from spinal shock continual assessment is necessary in order to begin appropriate manual techniques to elicit a voiding response. Intermittent catheterizations, by allowing filling and emptying of the bladder, facilitate manual techniques because they stimulate existing spinal cord reflexes and assist in maintaining bladder tone.

The manual techniques are *trigger voiding, straining to void,* and *manual expressions (Credé maneuver).* A fourth technique, *anal sphincter stretch,* is specifically practiced to overcome the problem of detrusor-sphincter dyssynergia and will be described later in this section.

Trigger Voiding

A number of maneuvers are used to stimulate so-called trigger areas by eliciting a strong reflex or spasm in the detrusor muscle of the bladder, which expels urine and efficiently empties the bladder. The reflex contractions that occur spontaneously from the filling of the bladder usually do not empty the bladder completely. The patient finds a "trigger point" to augment the voiding contraction (Burke and Murray 1975). See Procedure 18–3.

TABLE 18–4 Maintaining an Intermittent Catheterization Program: A Summary of Information

Action	Rationale
1. Establish a pattern of regulated fluid intake. An intake record is useful in the beginning to encourage a pattern. Further monitoring is not usually necessary. Concentrate on output volumes.	This promotes more effective bladder emptying. Complete patient and family health education regarding regulation of fluids and avoidance of fluids that irritate the bladder.

2. Introduce appropriate manual techniques to induce voiding.	For most spinal cord injured patients these techniques are used to achieve a catheter-free state.
	Using these voiding techniques emphasizes the need for:
	  • Continual assessment to detect the passing of spinal shock (when reflex activity returns)
	  • Knowledge of the characteristics of the neurogenic bladder dysfunction exhibited
	  • Manual skills to use voiding techniques correctly
	
	Perform, or, when appropriate, teach the patient to perform, the following techniques:
	  • Trigger mechanisms
	  • Straining to void (a Valsalva maneuver)
	  • Manual expression (Credé maneuver)
	  • Anal stretch technique
	
	Also when appropriate teach the patient (and possibly the family) to perform catheterizations.

3. Help the patient achieve a "balanced bladder." (Note Box in this chapter.)	Continual assessment is needed to prevent overdistension and ensure complete emptying of the bladder. Reduce frequency of catheterizations depending on amount of residual volumes of urine. • Maintain bladder capacity of 300 to 400 ml using combined techniques of catheterizations and maneuvers to induce voiding.

4. Evaluate effectiveness of program.	Observe for return of neurological function and for kidney function.
	
	Compare serial diagnostic tests with baseline data:
	  • Neurological examination
	  • Urinalysis (regularly)
	  • Urine for culture and sensitivity as indicated
	  • Blood urea nitrogen and serum creatinine levels
	  • Intravenous pyelogram
	  • Urodynamic studies
	
	Be alert for infection (note early signs of elevated systemic temperature and urinary pH above 6).
	Detect high residual urine volumes (over 2- to 3-month period) and collaborate with physician to diagnose specific problem.

Trigger voiding is successful only when the reflex arcs to the sacral voiding center are intact. It is of no use if the patient has an areflexic bladder.

Straining to Void

When straining to void (a Valsalva maneuver) the patient strains as if attempting to have a bowel movement by taking a deep breath and bearing down. Straining requires strong abdominal muscles. As these muscles are innervated by the T_{6-12} cord segments, patients with injury sustained at or above the lower thoracic vertebrae will not find this technique helpful for bladder evacuation. See Procedure 18–4.

Straining to void is used only by persons with areflexic (lower motor neuron lesion) bladders. It may or may not be helpful.

Manual Expression (Credé Maneuver)

This controversial maneuver involves application of strong external pressure over and around the bladder so that pressure within the bladder builds and overcomes the resistance of the bladder neck and urinary sphincters. Urine is literally forced to pass. Manual expression is used when a flaccid bladder exists and only after a VCU confirms the absence of ureterovesical reflex during the expression. *Use with*

Procedure 18–3 Trigger Voiding

Purpose

To stimulate effective reflex bladder emptying.

Action

1. Observe for leg spasms; reflex erections, which commonly occur during catheterizations; or a positive bulbocavernosus reflex to indicate that trigger voiding attempts may be successful.

2. Ensure that patient is in a comfortable position. If in bed, flex patient's hips slightly and elevate the head of the bed if possible.

3. Firmly tap, stroke, or gently pinch the lower abdomen and inner thigh. Alternatively gently pull on the pubic hair, stimulate the rectum, or apply gentle suprapubic pressure.

4. If successful, trigger mechanisms will start the urinary stream within a minute or so.

5. Once the best trigger point or points are located, *show* the patient the exact site.

6. Record the location and effectiveness of mechanisms used.

Rationale

Reflex voiding is one of the last functions to return as spinal shock passes in an ascending manner. If the bulbocavernosus reflex is not present do not frustrate patient by attempting trigger voiding.

This position facilitates voiding and reduces the chance of causing leg spasms. The abdomen must be relaxed for stimulation to reach the bladder.

Of these methods, tapping is probably the most successful, and most patients with quadriplegia will eventually be able to perform the technique themselves.

Due to lack of sensation the patient will be unable to feel the trigger point.

Procedure 18–4 Instructing the Patient to Strain to Void

Purpose

To use the abdominal muscles to exert pressure on the bladder for more effective emptying. This is a potentially dangerous technique, if obstruction forces urine backflow into the upper tracts during straining. It is contraindicated for people with hyperreflexic bladders because the outflow sphincters tend to tighten reflexively.

Action

1. Select patients with strong abdominal muscles who can successfully and safely try this technique. Proceed with *caution.* Any tightness of the internal sphincter or malalignment of the bladder and urethra could create obstruction and cause backflow of urine.

2. When about to void, instruct patient to take a deep breath, hold it, and bear down. Ask patient to strain throughout the voiding process until the bladder is empty. The patient may rest for a minute or so and repeat technique if necessary.

3. Warn patient that hyperventilation or a bowel movement may occur.

Rationale

Patients with any history of coronary artery disease should avoid this technique. This Valsalva maneuver, or holding the breath against a closed epiglottis, should not be used when patient is on bedrest as it is associated with increased incidence of deep vein thrombosis (see Chapter 16).

This enhances bladder emptying.

Procedure 18–5 Manual Expression (Credé Maneuver)

Purpose

To empty the bladder as completely as possible.

Action	Rationale
1. Select patients with a flaccid bladder who will be able to use this technique safely. Safety is determined by VCU while this technique is used to confirm that ureterovesical reflux does not occur.	This technique is most successful when patient is free from resistance imposed by preserved abdominal muscles and is free from urinary outlet obstruction (as a result of a mixed neurogenic bladder or from preexisting disease). Avoid the use of manual expression for patients with spastic bladder because ureterovesical reflux may occur if the external sphincter is in spasm and contracts, thus blocking urinary outflow.
2. Assess the abdomen to detect overdistension. If overdistension is suspected, perform a straight catheterization. Do not proceed with manual expression.	To avoid the risk of manual pressure forcing urine into the upper urinary tract.
3. If possible have patient sit on the toilet, lean forward, and perform this technique.	To achieve the best angle at which to apply pressure. Since a flaccid type of bladder exists with trauma to the sacral portion of the cord, patients will have good upper extremity strength and transfer potential, so independence in performing manual expression is usually achieved.
4. Ask patient to strain to void (optional).	These techniques used together may be helpful for some patients with partially preserved abdominal muscles.
5. To perform a manual expression, place one hand on top of the other or use a closed fist to apply firm pressure over the bladder. Press downward toward the pubic arch and repeat several times until the urine is passed. In the early stages avoid undue exertion of pressure on a fracture site of the lower spine. If a body cast is required, a "window" is needed in the suprapubic area to allow manual expression of the bladder.	Manual expression requires considerable strength and is a potentially dangerous technique. If the pressure exerted is too vigorous or is applied in the wrong direction, urine may be forced back up the ureters, thereby damaging the ureterovesical valves and threatening the entire upper urinary tract (Smith et al. 1972). This is especially true if the technique is performed while the patient is supine or if the bladder is full.

extreme caution. An increased incidence of hernias and hemorrhoids may be noted. It is dangerous to express vigorously patients with hyper-reflexic bladders; the risk of reflux is high. See Procedure 18–5.

Reducing Frequency of Intermittent Catheterizations

As output is obtained from the use of various manual techniques previously described or spontaneous voiding occurs, the number of catheterizations per day may be reduced. Whatever the combination of methods used, adhere to the principles of maintaining bladder capacity at 300 to 400 ml, avoiding overdistension, and ensuring complete emptying of the bladder. The male patient will need to wear an external collection device and the female patient, protective pads.

Manual techniques or spontaneous emptying should be attempted between and before scheduled catheterizations. For example, if catheterizations are scheduled for 0800 and 1400 hours, trigger voiding should be performed just before 0800, again at 1100, and just before 1400 hours. Eventually trigger voiding alone will be effective enough to empty the bladder at timed intervals and replace catheterizations.

- As residual urine volumes decrease, reduce the frequency of intermittent catheterizations.
- When the catheter volumes are less than 100 ml for 2 days, discontinue the formal catheterization program, but catheterization checks should be performed regularly until adequate evacuation is ensured.
- When adjusting the number of catheterizations, monitor the patient's tolerance and response. Again, adhere to the principles of avoiding overdistension and ensuring complete emptying of the bladder. Check for palpable bladder distension, especially during the night, when a diaresis from reabsorption of fluid (from dependent edema) occurs. This can be achieved at routine turning times without excessively disturbing the patient. It may be necessary to "tap" or manually express the patient every 2 hours. The urine output may double during the night when the patient resumes the supine position.

- Observe the patient with quadriplegia closely. Many are unable to tolerate 3 hours without voiding and may experience nausea, headache, chills, or signs of autonomic dysreflexia should voiding techniques fail. Catheterize immediately in these situations.
- Catheterization should be rescheduled taking into account patient preferences, planned therapy sessions, and urine volumes.
- To assess the degree of bladder emptying accurately, obtain postvoid residuals immediately following spontaneous voiding or expression, before the bladder starts to fill with urine again, otherwise volumes obtained are not accurate.
- Should manual techniques begin to fail and the residual urine volume increase, check the patient's drinking pattern and types of fluids taken and be alert for any signs of bladder infection. Bowel irregularity can also play havoc with bladder function and schedules.
- Observe patients carefully on return from day and weekend passes. Although early outings are most valuable, problems related to bowel and bladder care tend to increase during them.

It must be stressed that the preceding information is a *general* guideline. Assess the program in terms of helping the patient achieve a balanced bladder.

Established Patterns of Dysfunctions and Approaches to Management

An unbalanced bladder with high residual urine volumes may persist, manifested by a constant, dribbling incontinence or by an inability to empty the bladder despite using various techniques. Recurrent infection is common, and for those with injury above T_6, obstruction may lead to repeated signs of autonomic dysreflexia.

Incontinence and/or urinary retention are caused by various coexisting bladder and sphincter dysfunctions. Imperfect emptying may be due to poorly coordinated, weak, or irritable expulsion forces (bladder detrusor muscle contractions) poorly balanced against spasticity of the external urethral sphincter and muscles of the pelvic floor. Obstruction associated with tightness of the bladder neck around the internal sphincter is common. Lack of all reflex activity may result in overflow incontinence.

For the patient with a spastic bladder, *detrusor-sphincter dyssynergia* represents a major obstacle to bladder management. This occurs when the detrusor muscle and the external urethral sphincter contract at the same time. (Urinary flow is interrupted or completely blocked when unable to overcome the resistance encountered.) The expulsion action of the detrusor muscle is blocked when it is unable to overcome the resistance of the contracted sphincter. One action counteracts the other. A combined cystometrogram (CMG) and electromyelogram (EMG) is valuable for evaluation of this condition. For some it may be possible to overcome the dyssynergia, empty the bladder completely, and maintain continence between voidings by the use of the *anal sphincter stretch technique* (Wu, Nanninga and Hamilton 1986; Wyndaele 1987a). The external anal and urethral sphincters relax when manual distension of the anal sphincter is sustained. See Procedure 18–6.

Common patterns of dysfunctions are outlined in Table 18–5. Drug therapy and surgical measures as well as other techniques can overcome these difficulties with varying degrees of success (Johnson 1980; Ozer 1988; Wyndaele 1987b; Fam, Sarkarati, and Yalto 1988).

Pharmacological Treatment
Pharmacological treatment may be used in conjunction with or instead of surgery. The intent is to establish as normal a urinary tract function as possible by aiding two actions—bladder *storage* and bladder *emptying*. This treatment maintains renal function, keeping the person dry between bladder emptyings and establishes a reliable pattern. This section is based on the interpretation of Ozer 1988.

Bladder *storage* is improved when medications increase detrusor stability and enhance as normal sphincter activity as possible. Anticholinergic drugs inhibit bladder contractility. Alpha-adrenergic agents or beta antagonists are prescribed to increase outlet resistance which holds urine in the bladder.

To facilitate bladder *emptying*, drugs that relax tight sphincters are used: at the level of the smooth muscle internal sphincter alpha-adrenergic antagonists and at the striated external sphincter, antispasticity drugs. Figure 18–5 explains drug actions further.

Surgical Interventions
Surgical interventions are considered when there is evidence of an obstruction at the bladder neck and/or the level of the external sphincter (usually following unresponsiveness to drug therapy or failure of permanent intermittent catheterizations, for whatever reason. Bladder outlet obstruction occurs in 30% to 40% of all persons with SCI, and in 50% of this group surgery must be repeated (Fam, Sarkarati, and Yalto 1988).

Bladder outlet obstruction is characterized by difficulty in maintaining a urinary stream, persistent high residuals, severe bouts of autonomic dysreflexia, persistent urinary tract infection, evidence of obstruction on cystometry and electromyography, and radiographic evidence of reflux.

Transurethral operations performed on male patients with SCI include transurethral prostatic resection around

Procedure 18–6 Teaching a Patient the Anal Sphincter Stretch Technique

Purpose

To overcome the problem of detrusor-sphincter dyssynergia. Although a staff member can perform this technique, the patient must accomplish it to provide a workable solution to this problem.

Action	Rationale
1. Collaborate with occupational therapist and possibly physical therapist to assess toilet transfer ability, balance, and hand function. Patients must demonstrate capabilities in each of these areas to be able to use this technique.	This technique is best accomplished when patient is able to perform a toilet transfer and maintain adequate balance. Adequate hand function is also needed. For this reason it is much easier for people with paraplegia, although selected quadriplegic people can manage the technique by using an adapted aid for finger insertion (Donovan, Clowers, Kiviat, and Marci 1977).
2. Instruct the patient to: • Bend forward on the toilet • Place one gloved hand behind the buttocks • Gently insert one or two gloved fingers just far enough in to stretch the anal sphincter • Pull in the posterior direction or spread the fingers apart	Warn patient that too vigorous stimulation of the rectal mucosa may result in a bowel movement and traumatize the rectum.
3. Have patient strain while voiding (optional).	Some patients find this helpful to aid in the opening of the bladder neck.
4. Have patient with high paraplegia try a corset.	Greater intraabdominal pressure may help some patients to void.

the internal sphincter at the bladder neck and external sphincterotomy. Second operations are sometimes needed to increase results. Detrusor-sphincter dyssynergia is the most important reason for surgical intervention for those with spastic bladder. Transurethral resection of the bladder neck may be selected for those with flaccid bladder when straining to void or manual expressions are not successful due to tightness of the internal sphincter (when sympathetic tone from the undamaged thoracolumbar cord is preserved).

Although surgical intervention is quite successful in relieving bladder outlet obstruction, it can also be associated with temporary loss of erection ability. It may also cause total incontinence, which necessitates external catheter drainage that was not previously needed. The patient must be fully aware of the possibility of these consequences, which are often a matter of great concern. Discussion with the surgeon and the sexual health counselor is appropriate. See Chapter 10.

MAINTENANCE MANAGEMENT

External Urine-Collection System Care

Many patients with SCI can ultimately become catheter free. However, even though adequate spontaneous voiding can be achieved, inability to predict or control urinary flow may necessitate some method of protection against incontinence.

A person with a spastic bladder may experience an accidental triggering of a voiding response from general physical activity, such as during transfers, or even the slight irritation from a piece of clothing. A person with a flaccid bladder may accidentally induce voiding by increasing intraabdominal pressure. This can result from bending forward during the course of daily activities or even laughing. For some people, constant dribbling of urine can be a problem. For others, even though an urge to void can be appreciated, the urgency may be so great that it is often impossible for them to reach appropriate facilities in time.

There are some fairly successful external catheter (condom) drainage devices available to men. No satisfactory device has yet been developed for women, who must therefore rely on experimentation with new products and absorbent padding.

External Catheter Drainage Device

A wide variety of condoms and drainage systems are used. However, whatever system is selected, it must be applied and cared for to ensure that:

- An unrestricted drainage system is provided.
- The penile skin is free from the effects of pressure and chemical irritation.

TABLE 18–5 Established Patterns of Voiding Dysfunctions

	Characteristics	Management Techniques	Pharmacological Treatment	Surgical Interventions
Upper Motor Neuron (Spastic) Profile *Bladder (Power) Profile* Bladder (detrusor) hyperreflexia • Hyperactivity of the detrusor muscle is often associated with ineffective emptying power. • Bladder contractions are often reduced in magnitude and interrupted by spasmodic sphincter contractions. • Combinations of spastic bladder function and altered sphincter functions occur. *Sphincter (Resistance) Profile* Detrusor-sphincter dyssynergia Unlike normal relaxation during bladder contraction, sphincter activity may be either sustained or intermittent in relation to bladder contraction (Ozer 1988: 41). When resistance overcomes the power of the bladder to expel urine, urinary retention occurs.	• Inability to void • Unbalanced bladder with persistent high-volume residuals • Incontinence (dribbling) • Persistent urinary infection • Evidence of abnormal activity, high pressure urine within the system, and/or obstruction on urodynamic studies • Radiological evidence of reflux in the upper urinary tract	• Intermittent catheterizations so as to achieve a balanced bladder. • Trigger voiding to stimulate reflex bladder emptying. • When a low pressure system is achieved (which may or may not require pharmaceutical and/or surgical interventions), condom drainage to manage incontinence is the choice for most men; absorbent padding for women seems to be the most reliable method until a collection system is refined. • For some, especially women, an indwelling catheter. • Regular follow-up care for life to detect high pressure within urinary system and other complications.	• Administer cholinergic (parasympathomimetic) agent to strengthen bladder contractions to initiate and sustain bladder emptying. • Administer an anticholinergic (sympathomimetic) agent to diminish frequency of uninhibited bladder spasms. • Drugs that interfere with the autonomic nervous system tend to produce side effects associated with fluid retention; therefore watch for blurred vision, dry mouth, constipation, increased heart rate, and sometimes drowsiness. Contraindicated often with elderly patients and those with glaucoma or heart disease.	• Although this is not developed fully, enlarging the bladder with a loop of bowel will someday provide a reliable means to increase bladder capacity and improve storage capabilities (Becker et al. 1989). • Surgical implants to electrically stimulate the sacral roots (reflex voiding cener), following a rhizotomy to create a LMN bladder, have been experimentally successful to keep women continent. (Men lose erection capability.) (Madersbacher et al. 1989) • Surgical interventions aim to lower urethral resistance. The timing postinjury and the degree of surgery performed is variable. Surgery is considered when the patient is unresponsive to nonsurgical management.
Dyssynergia of the smooth muscle of the bladder neck (internal sphincter) • Lack of coordination between the detrusor and smooth muscle of the bladder neck. • Delayed opening of the bladder neck; passive bladder neck opening with extensive injury to the thoracolumbar cord (causing sympathetic neural damage). • May or may not be associated with dyssynergia of the striated external sphincter.			• Administer sympathetic blocking agent, such as phenoxybenzamine hydrochloride (Minipress), to help relax the smooth muscle of the internal sphincter.	• Bladder neck resection around the internal sphincter. • Transurethral prostatic resection around the internal sphincter (in the male).
Dyssynergia of the striated muscle of the external sphincter • Spasmodic activity of the external sphincter and muscles of the pelvic floor. • Involvement may vary from a mild degree of striated sphincter dyssynergia despite some voluntary control, to severe enough to cause complete obstruction.		• Assist and instruct the patient to perform the anal sphincter stretch technique (to influence the external sphincter muscle simultaneously to relax as bladder contracts, decrease resistance to urinary flow, and allow voiding).	• Administer skeletal muscle relaxant, such as diazepam (Valium), to suppress spasms of the striated external sphincter and decrease resistance to urinary outflow. The tendency of these drugs to be addictive outweighs their benefits, which are also controversial. Watch closely for side effects, especially drowsiness.	• External sphincterotomy.

(Table continues)

TABLE 18–5   Established Patterns of Voiding Dysfunctions (continued)

	Characteristics	Management Techniques	Pharmacological Techniques	Surgical Interventions
Lower Motor Neuron (Flaccid) Profile				
Bladder (Power) Profile				
Bladder (detrusor) hyporeflexia • Flaccidity of the bladder; loss of tone; malalignment is common (acute angulation of the bladder in relation to the urethra results in varying degrees of obstruction). *Sphincter (Resistance) Profile* Nonrelaxing smooth muscle (internal) sphincter • Frequent retention of internal smooth muscle sphincter innervation from the undamaged thoracolumbar cord (which may or may not provide continence/obstruction). Relaxed smooth muscle (internal) sphincter combined with an areflexic, flaccid bladder and a denervated external sphincter • The patient is subject to incontinence whenever abdominal pressure is increased. Nonrelaxing striated (external) sphincter • A lack of relaxation of the urethral sphincter due to continued or increased electrical activity may cause problems with emptying. • Combinations of areflexic bladder and altered sphincter activity can occur.	• Inability to void • Overflow incontinence • Stress incontinence • Unbalanced bladder with persistent high-volume residuals • Persistent urinary infection • Evidence of abnormal activity on urodynamic studies, high pressure within the system, with or without obstruction • Radiographic evidence of reflux to upper tracts	• Permanent practice of intermittent catheterizations is the treatment of choice. • Selected patients may have success with straining to void or manual expression of urine. • Aggressive follow up evaluation required to detect high pressure system, which usually occurs without abnormal signs in the person's general bladder routine.	• Generally unresponsive to drug therapy.	• Surgical interventions not generally indicated. • External sphincterotomy.

• A reliable, convenient, and economical system is established.

An external catheter drainage system basically consists of a condom, attached to tubing which is inserted into a leg bag or, when the patient is in bed, a standard drainage system. See Figure 18–6.

An appliance can be made from any condom plus latex tubing and a leg bag. Several commercial styles are also available. In a constantly changing market, it is best to consult with local medical/surgical supply dealers and refer to *Accent* magazine and the *ARN Journal* for updated information. See Resources. Newer products are generally more expensive and tend to favor stiffer condoms that are less easily twisted, disposable supplies, and preassembly.

The condom can be secured by elastic tape, or by using a type of skin adhesive, or both. Adhesives used are surgical glues, cements, or sprays, similar to those used for colostomy care.

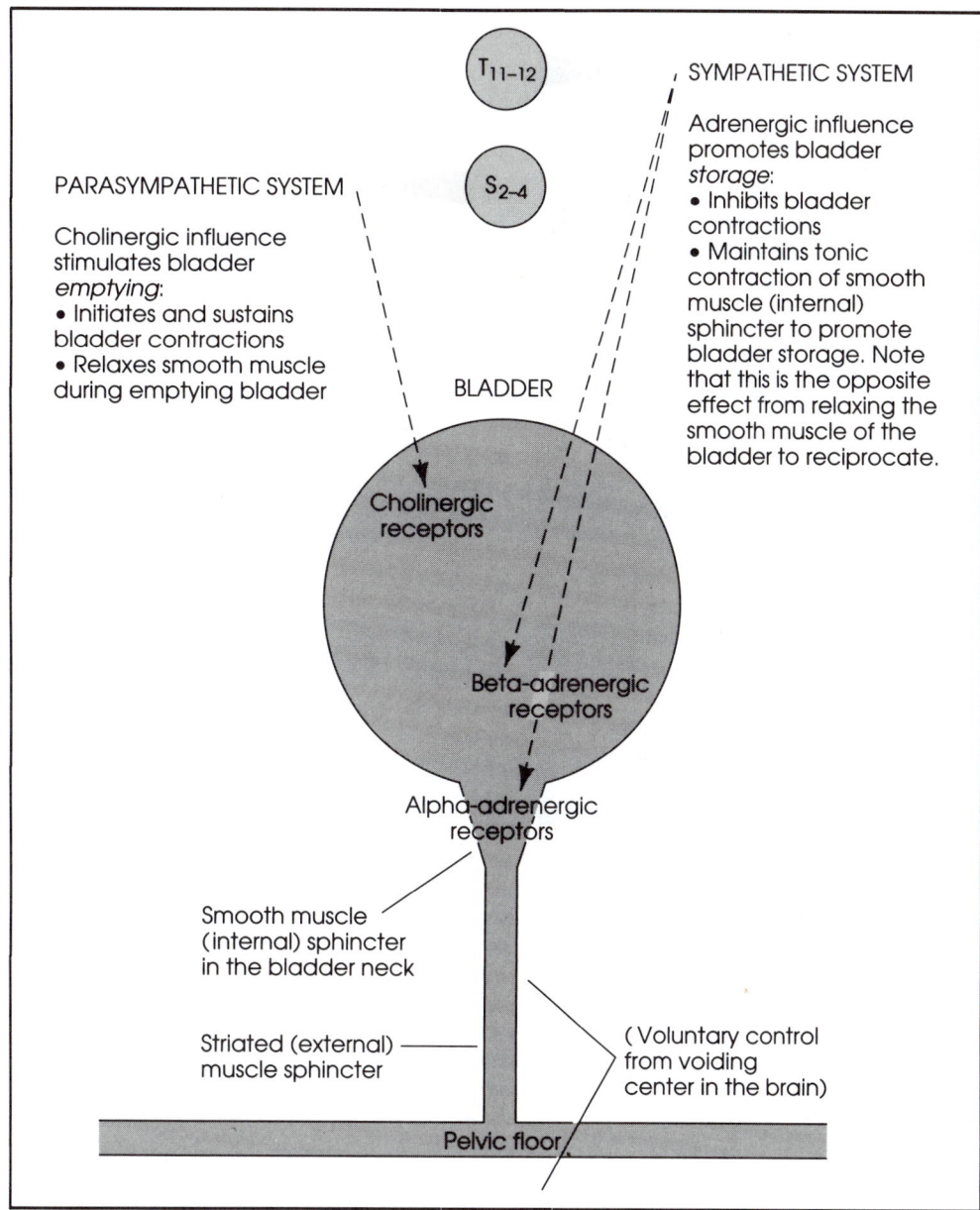

FIGURE 18–5   The autonomic nervous system and bladder control: pharmacological treatment

Condoms are available in small and large sizes. Occasionally however, a man may have a penis that is too short or retracted to make condom drainage a feasible, or even possible, method of management. The use of permanent intermittent catheterizations in conjunction with medications to achieve dryness may be considered as an alternative.

The problem of long-term exposure of the penile skin to continuous moisture, medical adhesives, and rubber chemicals predisposes the patient to skin breakdown. Good personal hygiene to ensure cleanliness and drying or airing of the genital area are imperative to avoid complications (Lawson and Cook 1977). See Procedure 18–7.

It is one skill to apply a condom; another to get it to stay on; and yet quite another to avoid complications. This seemingly simple procedure requires meticulous care, individual adaptation, and almost always some experimentation to develop a reliable system. During this time much support, encouragement, explicit instructions, and help with problem solving are needed.

Protective Absorbent Padding

There is no effective external collection device to handle the problem of incontinence in women. Vaginal inserts with an attached intravulvular cup, to collect and divert the urine into tubing and a leg bag, have variable success in

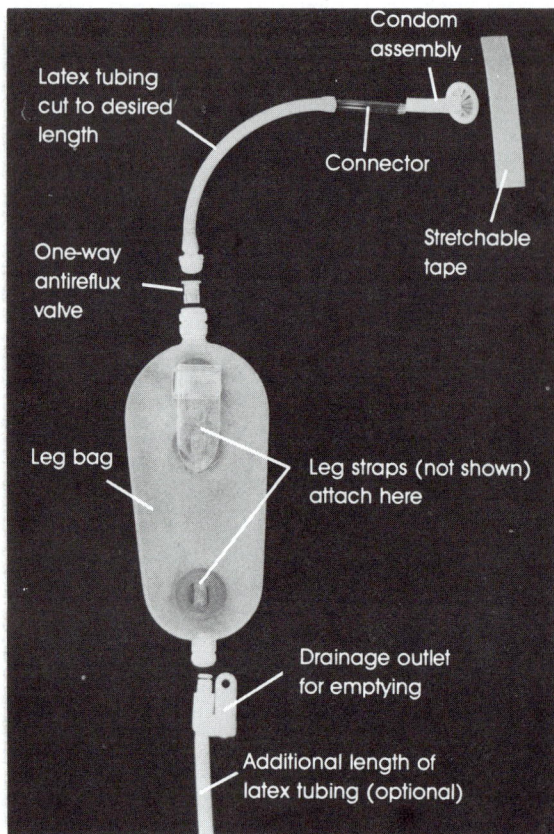

FIGURE 18–6   An external catheter (condom) drainage system.

practice. The use of sanitary napkins or disposable toddler-size diapers secured with plastic panties is a workable alternative. (Do not unfold the diapers, just place between the legs.) However, these pads are unable to absorb much urine, and every time the woman changes position the pads seem to need adjusting. Plastic panties can be fashioned with side snap or Velcro openings; these panties can be made at home or purchased. The woman with quadriplegia has the most difficulty changing pads as it is time consuming and/or requires assistance from others. Many women equate the use of absorbent padding with diapering and find it distasteful. It is important not to reinforce this idea by using the word *diaper*.

Although beset with a number of practical problems, the correct use of external padding is desirable to prevent infection of the upper urinary tract. General measures include prompt changing of wet pads with careful and frequent skin inspection and maintaining as dilute a urine as possible. Sleeping without plastic panties (just absorbent pads on a waterproof surface) helps dry the skin and prevent maceration. Daily bathing is the best way to ensure complete cleanliness and freedom from odor.

Intermittent catheterizations with the use of medication to obtain desired retention of urine may be an alternative.

Again, quadriplegic women with limited hand function will likely not be able to self-catheterize, find it too time consuming, and/or require assistance from others. Many resort to an indwelling catheter to overcome these problems. Fortunately, an indwelling catheter poses fewer complications in women than men because the female urethra is shorter and without angulation.

However, eventually there can be incontinence around the catheter related to a wide-bore urethra and urethral erosion. As more follow-up studies become available, it appears that an indwelling catheter is not as safe and effective as once thought in terms of urethral, bladder, and upper urinary tract functions (McGuire and Savastano 1986). A possible alternative is an early augmentation cystoplasty or a rhizotomy with the creation of a continent abdominal stoma to provide a means for easy catheterizations, which a woman with C_6 to C_7 quadriplegia can often manage herself.

Long-Term Indwelling Catheter Care

During the phase of recovery from spinal shock, it may become quickly evident that a patient needs a permanent indwelling catheter. For example, there may be preexisting bladder complications. For others, a bladder reconditioning program may be deemed unsuccessful after a period of time. The woman with quadriplegia may present the classic problem: incontinence between catheterizations that cannot be controlled or intermittent catheterizations that are just too cumbersome. In these situations, an indwelling catheter may be the only practical option.

The ultimate goal of an indwelling catheter is to provide unobstructed drainage while avoiding infection and trauma to the urethra and bladder neck. Infection and trauma predispose the person to a host of other complications. Despite the potential hazards, an indwelling catheter is the method of choice for long-term bladder management for some patients with SCI. With diligent care, complications can be minimized. See Procedure 18–8.

Provision of adequate fluid and dietary intake, activity, maintaining an acidic urine, and compliance with medications are other key factors in avoiding problems of the urinary tract when a catheter is in place.

SPECIFIC MANAGEMENT OF URINARY COMPLICATIONS

Infection

Although considerably reduced in incidence, the high risk of developing acute, chronic, and recurrent episodes of

Procedure 18–7   Application of an External Catheter (Condom) Drainage System

Purpose

To provide a reliable, convenient, and economical system of unrestricted urine drainage without leakage or skin problems.

Equipment

- Basin, soap and water, wash cloths, and a towel
- Skin Preparation* and/or tincture of benzoin (optional)
- Skin adhesive
- Stretchable tape (optional)
- Blunt-tipped scissors

- Preassembled condom drainage system (Figure 18–7) including a condom or condom assembly; 2-inch plastic connector; latex rubber tubing cut to the desired length (to reach from the condom tip to the leg bag); a leg bag with straps (or standard collection bag)

Action

1. Wash hands

2. Thoroughly wash genital area with soap, rinse with clear water, and dry well. If necessary, retract penile foreskin to clean. Leave area open to air (about 30 minutes daily). Then if patient is uncircumcised, pull foreskin toward head of penis before applying condom.

3. Apply adhesives if necessary.

   - Before using any adhesives on penile skin, perform a patch test on inner thigh.

   - Protect pubic hair with a paper towel (simply tear a small hole in center and place over penis).

   - Spray Skin Preparation* on shaft of penis (optional). Allow 30 seconds to dry and become tacky before proceeding.

   - Apply tincture of benzoin (optional) or a skin adhesive to penile shaft. (It may be easier for some to paint shaft near head of penis first and begin applying condom before putting cement over whole shaft.) Paint 1 to 4 inches of shaft of penis. Do not apply skin cement over reddened areas.

4. Before applying condom, unroll slightly to leave 3/4 to 1 inch free space between end of condom and tip of penis.

5. Unroll condom sheath slowly onto penis.

6. Clip off ring at top of condom with blunt-tipped scissors.

Rationale

This minimizes risk of cross-contamination.

This minimizes the accumulative effects of chemical irritants, bacteria, and moisture, which render the skin more susceptible to pressure and excoriation. Allowing the penile skin to dry is single most important defense against skin excoriation. Avoid using petroleum-based preparations to protect skin as they tend to interact with condom material. Powders tend to cake and be messy.

When necessary to remove condom every few hours, as during an intermittent catheterization regime, taping may be quite sufficent. However, most active patients need skin adhesives and sometimes additional tape.

To check for an allergic response to any chemicals.

Adhesives are difficult to remove from pubic hair and add to infection potential. Clipping pubic hair around base of penis is also helpful.

Skin Preparation* dries as a plastic film to provide a waterproof seal. It peels off easily and helps protect delicate skin (especially in early stages when skin tolerance is building). It may be used by itself or skin adhesive may be applied on top. If, during a retraining period, condom will be removed frequently for intermittent catheterizations, Skin Preparation* and taping may be sufficient and least irritating. There is an external condom-style device with removable tip for intermittent catheterizations (without removing sheath from penis).

This is a matter of personal preference. Generally, the more coverage, the more confident patient feels about avoiding accidental removal. Skin Prepration* or tincture of benzoin is not usually necessary once skin has toughened (6 to 12 months after injury).

This prevents plastic insert or end of reinforced condom tip from causing pressure or irritation on penis. If too much space is left, condom tends to twist, blocking urine drainage. This also prevents backflow of urine inside the condom.

Unrolling slowly helps avoid trapping air bubbles under condom. Bubbles can be pressed out with finger.

This prevents pressure from ring on the thigh and scrotum. Use blunt-tipped scissors to avoid scraping skin.

(Procedure continues)

---

*This aerosol adhesive, made by Dow Corning, is universally recommended (Nanninga and Rosen 1975; Bransbury 1979) because it is hypoallergenic and easy to remove, which reduces trauma to the skin. Unfortunately it is relatively expensive.

Procedure 18–7   Application of an External Catheter (Condom) Drainage System (continued)

Action

7. Spiral 1/2 inch stretchable adhesive tape around penis over condom (not on skin) (optional, avoid if possible). Do *not* stretch tape tight. Fold tape end back on itself to make a tab.

8. Assess circulation to penis now and, most important, within half-hour of application. Look for penile swelling or change in color.

9. Select appropriate drainage system. Use a standard collection bag when patient is in bed (while in hospital); use a leg bag assembly when patient is up.

10. Connect condom assembly to drainage system.

   - Insert connector between condom and rubber tubing leading to leg bag.

   - If a standard collection bag is used while patient is in bed (mostly for night drainage) ensure gravity-assisted flow of urine. Check that all connections are secure.

11. Attach rubber tubing to leg bag; secure leg bag to inner calf with soft, pliable straps and adjustable buttons or Velcro closure.

   - Do not attach straps too tightly.

   - Position drainage tubing carefully.

   - Do not cut tubing too long or too short. It should just reach between condom and leg bag when patient is sitting.

12. Change condom drainage system daily, or at least every other day.

13. Inspect skin when the condom is changed. Be alert for inflammation of glans penis, skin excoriation, ulceration, or flaking. Should this occur:

   - Air the area.

   - Do not apply adhesives directly.

   - Leave condom off overnight. A urinal (preferably one with flattened sides as opposed to rounded urinal) may be propped against patient to handle incontinence. If extremity spasms cause urinal to tip, absorbent padding may be used (even placed in a shower cap!).

   - Obtain a swab of area for culture and sensitivity if infection is suspected and apply topical antibiotic ointment as ordered.

Rationale

This reduces risk of condom peeling off. Spiral application of stretchable tape allows for relflex penile erection and adequate circulation. The greatest danger in using tape is applying it too tightly, which is in effect like applying a tourniquet. This constriction of penis reduces circulation and can lead to severe problems. Always use stretchable tape, never plain adhesive, silk, or paper tape. Tape tab facilitates removal.

To fit correctly, a condom must be applied snugly enough to prevent leakage but not so tightly to impair circulation. One key point to remember is to allow for reflex erections. Often manipulation of penis required when applying the condom results in a reflex erection. If erection occurs, wait for it to subside before applying tape.

Avoid using a leg bag assembly when patient is in bed because it is difficult to achieve a gravity-assisted flow of urine. For this reason, always connect condom assembly to a standard collection bag when patient returns to bed. When at home a length of tubing draining into a variety of containers can be used as an alternative to more expensive collection bags.

This prevents leakage.

It should be emphasized that function of tape and/or adhesive is to provide a watertight seal; correct placement and security of leg bag keep condom from pulling off.

This will create a tourniquet effect and obstruct circulation.

Any twisting will obstruct drainage.

Tubing cut too long will aggravate twisting; cut too short it will cause pulling pressure on the condom.

This maintains cleanliness, eliminates odor and reduces accumulation of bacteria at external urinary meatus. Changing system is most convenient and best accomplished during bathing or showering.

Patient may develop contact dermatitis or allergic responses at any time. If these measures are not successful, intermittent catheterization or use of indwelling catheter may have to be resumed temporarily. Constant irritation or inflammation of foreskin may necessitate circumcision for long-term management.

(Procedure continues)

Procedure 18–7   Application of an External Catheter (Condom) Drainage System (continued)

Action

14. Care for reusable leg bag assembly:

- Label each bag with patient's name.
- Thoroughly wash with lathering antiseptic soap and rinse. A syringe or small funnel will make pouring into the bag easier.
- Check tubing and connectors every few days for mineral buildup from the urine. Soaking in a 25% acetic acid (vinegar) solution in water overnight is the most effective method of removing these accumulations. If crusting is still evident, discard equipment.
- Located at the top of the leg bag is a flutter valve to prevent reflux of urine into tubing. To check patency of this valve, invert bag. If fluid leaks down tubing, discard bag.

Rationale

Although care and cleaning or supervision of leg bag and equipment is eventually within the patient's capability, in an acute setting disposable equipment, though expensive, is more convenient. Leg bags do not stand up well to usual methods of hospital sterilization.

This decreases risk of cross-contamination.

---

urinary tract infection following SCI remains, regardless of the method used for emptying the bladder. Although acute infections may be managed effectively, chronic and recurrent infections present difficult and complex problems. Areas of controversy about urinary infection include:

- How to define and diagnose it
- How frequently it occurs
- How important it is
- How best to prevent it
- When and how to treat it

Approaches to these problems tend to be based on institutional and personal professional preferences rather than scientific data (Gribble 1989). Despite the widespread use of intermittent catheterizations, improved control of infections with more effective antibiotics, more exact diagnosis of lower tract function with urodynamic studies, improvements in long-term surveillance and advancements in treating the closely related complication of calculi, clinical management problems still exist (Lloyd 1986).

Most such individuals have bacteria in their urine (bacteriuria) most of the time; acute illness (symptomatic bacteriuria) occurs less frequently (Gribble 1989). Over time, however, the urinary bladder somehow establishes a local relationship with these bacteria and, in the absence of high residual urines or reflux, their growth is partially controlled by and is confined to the bladder. There are no systemic effects (Burke and Murray 1975). A very confusing question persists. What constitutes a bladder infection that must be treated? In other words, what degree of bacteriuria is acceptable? From a review of the literature, it is difficult to compare results and identify the most successful techniques used for bladder care because the variables are so great. For

example, prophylactic use of urinary antiseptics, antibiotics, and local irrigating solutions varies greatly, and the frequency and method of obtaining culture specimens to monitor infection also differ.

Monitor patients at risk of developing bladder infection, and inhibit bacterial growth by preventing overdistension of the bladder and ensuring regular, and reliable emptying. Management involves controlling infection to preserve upper urinary tract function and avoid systemic involvement.

Management

1. Be alert for signs of urinary infection. More subtle complaints often heard from patients include feeling generally unwell; sensations of incomplete bladder emptying or discomfort in the kidney regions; increases in residual urine volume patterns; leakage around an indwelling catheter; increased abdominal and leg spasticity; and an unusual increase in autonomic dysreflexia signs in an individual with SCI above T_6 (Dwyer 1985).

An *upper urinary tract* infection is indicated by the following:

- A systemic illness with pyrexia
- An oral temperature of 37.5°C (99.5°F) or a rectal temperature of 38°C (about 100°F) for more than 8 hours. In the male, high fevers can often be encountered in acute epididymitis, and acute prostatitis. (An examination of scrotal contents is essential.) In the female most septic states are renal in origin.

The following may also be present with an upper urinary tract infection, but may indicate only *lower urinary tract* involvement.

Procedure 18–8   Long-Term Indwelling Cathether Care

Purpose

To provide unobstructed drainage while avoiding trauma to the urethra and bladder neck and preventing infection. Trauma and infection predispose the patient to subsequent (often severe) complications.

Action

1. Introduce silastic (silicone) or silicone-treated catheter.

2. For general use select catheter no larger than a size #16 (French) for males, and no larger than size #18 (French) for females. Balloons should not be inflated beyond 10 cm.

3. Insert and secure catheter with tape as outlined in Procedure 18–1.
   - Use an antiseptic lubricant as ordered by physician.

   - Particularly when catheterizing men, anticipate difficulty in passing catheter if external sphincter goes into spasm on contact with catheter. Maintain gentle pressure on catheter, and often sphincter will relax in a few minutes and allow catheter to pass.
   - Use nonallergic tape to secure catheter.
   - Check for pressure areas, even inside a woman's labia, and alter taping of the catheter from side to side.

4. Use leg bag assembly when the person is up in a wheelchair. Insert a connector between catheter and length of rubber tubing leading to leg bag. Swab all connections with alcohol before insertion.

5. Use standard drainage system when the person is in bed.

6. Care for urinary collection system:
   - Maintain sterile technique when changing from standard collection system, which patient needs at night or while resting in bed, to leg bag assembly, which is used when patient is up. When system is not in use, protect tips of tubing with sterile caps. These may be soaked in alcohol at bedside. Swab end of catheter and all tubings with alcohol before connecting.

   - Discard plastic disposable systems every 24 hours when alternating between leg bag and standard urinary collection systems. At home a chlorine bleach solution works well to disinfect bags and tubing.

   - If drainage system remains closed, that is, if the patient is on bedrest for a few days, do not change standard collection system unless you change catheter.

Rationale

The development of these newer catheters has introduced into long-term bladder management the principle of a smoother, nonadherent or noncling surface designed to reduce urethral irritation and discourage crystal and, therefore, calculi formation.

If urine bypasses catheter, it is usually due to bladder spasm. Selection of a larger catheter or larger balloon will not solve problem. An increased incidence of spasms is an indication of irritation from a noxious focus, and there should be a thorough investigation into cause. Often leakage can be early sign of bladder infection. If infection is not apparent, physician may order medication to subdue bladder irritability.

Lower portion of urethra itself, especially in patients who are permanently catheterized, tends to harbor bacteria that may be pushed back into bladder when catheter is introduced.
In long-term management, bladder spasms are not uncommon.

This minimizes the risk of building pressure areas. Sometimes leg spasms can produce rubbing or pulling on a woman's catheter.

The physically active patient, who is mobilized early, may greatly appreciate use of a leg bag within 1 to 2 weeks after injury. Although most nurses are thoroughly familiar with precautions necessary for indwelling catheter connected to a standard closed drainage system, leg bag assembly requires further care to minimize risk of infection.

This promotes gravity-assisted drainage, which is difficult to achieve when patient wears leg bag in bed. This minimizes risk of infection.

Leg bags are available in disposable plastic or reusable rubber designs similar to those used for condom drainage. Disposable bags are recommended for hospital use, to reduce risk of cross-contamination. It is always important to explain these extra precautions to patients, so when it is time to prepare for transfer or for home, they will be receptive to different techniques.

This also minimizes risk of infection.

(Procedure continues)

Procedure 18–8 Long-Term Indwelling Cathether Care (continued)

Action	Rationale
• Clean rubber reusable leg bag assembly. Thoroughly wash with lathering soap; rinse with aid of a syringe, funnel, or gooseneck tap; soak overnight in 25% acetic acid (vinegar) solution to remove accumulations.	Reusable leg bags do not stand up well to usual methods of sterilization. Cared for in the described manner, leg bag assemblies should last about 4 months.
• Label equipment with patient's name; order two complete leg bag assemblies, and alternate use.	
7. Clean perineal area with soap, particularly external urinary meatus, and rinse with clear water twice daily. Dry thoroughly; do not use powders or lotions. Remove crusted secretions around meatus with hydrogen peroxide; apply neomycin ointment (as ordered by physician) prophylactically. If infection is suspected, obtain a swab for culture and sensitivity. Tub bathing or showering with catheter in situ is acceptable.	Because of its close proximity to the bladder, the external urinary meatus is a significant potential source of infection. Powders, lotions, and strong soaps can become trapped in folds and irritate the skin.
8. Change catheter routinely:	
• Change silicone catheters every 2 to 3 weeks.	Rubber catheters will deteriorate in this time; rough surface may precipitate crystal formation.
• Roll catheter between fingers to check for grit, which indicates need for an immediate change. Watch for contact allergy when in use, and note any bubbling, peeling or cracking of catheter, which indicates need for an immediate change.	These firmer catheters with noncling, nonadherent surfaces are designed to discourage crystal formation so routine changes can be safely delayed. Even though these new catheters are considered nonreactive with human tissue, some patients still develop contact allergy and are unable to tolerate them.
9. Encourage maintenance of urine output of 3000 ml/24 hours if possible. (If this is not achieved during hospitalization, it is rarely achieved later.) Avoid excessive intake of caffeine and carbonated drinks.	Adequate fluids reduce debris and risk of bladder calculi formation. Some fluids are very irritating to the bladder.

- A white blood cell count greater than 10,000/cu mm
- Presence of one or two pathogenic organisms in the urine greater than 100,000 org/ml
- Presence of 20 or more pus cells in the urine as measured by urinalysis
- A low urinary output of concentrated, cloudy, or foul-smelling urine

2. Minimize the risk of overdistension. Assist patient to empty the bladder frequently and completely to remove multiplying bacteria. Ensure that the patient is taught, understands, and demonstrates competence in bladder management techniques before supervision is withdrawn. If the patient has an indwelling catheter, see that unobstructed, gravity-assisted drainage is constantly maintained.

3. Prevent introduction of bacteria into the urethra and bladder. Emphasize personal cleanliness, especially in the groin area, and the importance of handwashing for individuals and staff (Fawcett 1986; Sanderson and Rawal 1987). Follow strict aseptic technique when catheterizing and when caring for sterile drainage equipment, and ensure adequate and regular disinfection of external catheter (condom) drainage equipment. Select appropriate types and sizes of catheters to minimize urethral irritation, which predisposes the patient to infection.

4. Administer prophylactic medications as ordered. Methenamine mandelate (Mandelamine) is a urinary antiseptic, and vitamin C (ascorbic acid) is an acidifying agent that retards bacterial growth. These maintenance drugs are usually well tolerated but controversial in their actual value (Lloyd 1986). Prophylactic use of antibiotics is not recommended. Cautious and specific use is necessary to avoid developing resistance to a drug that may be badly needed in the long-term management ahead.

5. Observe and record the pH, volume, and nature of urinary output. Unusually high residuals, frequency or increased incontinence, and bypassing of urine around an indwelling catheter may also be less obvious signs of early infection.

6. Monitor urinalysis specimens. As an indicator of infection, be alert for alkalotic urine (pH above 7.5 or 8). A pH above 6 is considered significant when a patient is maintained on methanamine mandelate (Mandelamine). An increase in SG above the normal range of 1.010 to 1.025 for concentrated urine and the presence of more than 20

pus cells on microscopic examination are also considered significant.

7. Monitor urine culture and sensitivity reports. A urine culture should be obtained immediately at the onset of a suspected infection. Specimens are examined qualitatively for kinds of bacteria, and quantitatively for the maximum number of bacteria per ml of urine. After incubation a colony count is taken. A colony is 1000 organisms. A colony count of 10,000/ml, that is, 100,000 (10^5) organisms/ml, is generally considered a significant growth indicating a probably urinary infection. Once organisms are identified, they are tested for susceptibility or sensitivity to specific antibiotics. Common organisms causing urinary tract infections are E. coli, Klebsiella, proteus mirabilis, serratia marcescens, staphylococcus aures (Bhatt, Cid, and Maiman 1987). Criteria for significant bacteria on intermittent catheterizations are not clear. Some studies have shown that healthy females using intermittent catheterizations normally have bacteria present. Requesting sensitivities on all organisms may be prudent.

8. Observe the systemic signs of upper urinary tract infection including systemic illness manifested by general malaise, loss of appetite, chills, tremors, nausea, and vomiting; disturbance in voiding patterns; and additional signs of painful catheterization or dysuria in patients with preserved sensation.

9. Administer antibiotics as ordered. The physician should be notified of culture results as soon as possible to order the specific drug to which the organism is sensitive. If an indwelling catheter is in place, change it when antibiotics are begun.

10. Administer antipyretics and analgesics as ordered to control symptoms. Use sparingly so that useful information about a persistent fever is not obscured.

11. Encourage a regulated fluid intake to achieve an output of 1500 to 1800 ml for a patient on intermittent catheterizations. For a patient with an indwelling catheter at least 3000 ml is desirable.

12. Ensure adequate bladder emptying. Intermittent catheterizations are not contraindicated in the presence of infection. In fact, the physician may wish to resume a 4-hour schedule during the course of the infection to minimize the risk of urinary stasis and overdistension. In patients with septicemia, it is preferable to stop intermittent catheterization and place an indwelling catheter until the episode is over.

13. Be aware of possible ascending infection to the upper urinary tract caused occasionally by reflux of urine into the ureter and kidney resulting in pylonephritis. Observe for a high, spiked fever, usually over 40°C (104°F), severe chills, with loin pain or tenderness. Clinical signs and symptoms tend to be more severe and slower to respond to drug therapy. Be alert for presence of casts, protein, or occult blood in the urine, indicating kidney infiltration or impairment; elevated BUN and serum creatinine; and, in the later stages, evidence of dilation of the ureters or hydronephrosis on an IVP examination.

14. Watch for signs of septic shock. Bacteremia or sepsis is a rare complication of urinary tract or other systemic infection whereby gram-negative bacteria are released into the bloodstream and cause production of fatal endotoxins. Observe for sudden onset of signs and symptoms of respiratory distress, a decrease in level of consciousness, and other signs of central nervous system depression, such as a fall in blood pressure, pulse, and urinary output. It may be necessary to initiate advanced life-support measures. Make every effort to locate the entry source of the bacteria and eradicate or control the cause. Treatment usually consists of massive doses of IV antibiotics and corticosteroids and blood volume replacement.

15. Provide health education with a preventive focus.

Expected Outcomes

Evaluate the effectiveness of treatment according to level of outcome criteria reached:

- Bladder capacity so regulated as not to exceed 500 ml at any given time without evidence of retention or increased bouts of incontinence
- Clear urine of normal color and odor, free from infective organisms
- Urinary pH, SG, and microscopic examination within normal limits for patient
- BUN and serum creatinine levels within normal range
- Patient comfortable without signs or symptoms of systemic illness and body temperature within normal limits for patient
- Diagnostic tests (urodynamic studies) without evidence of reflux, dilation of upper tract, or deterioration when compared with baseline data obtained immediately after injury
- Individual activity involved with preventive care and problem solving

Calculi

Although the formation of urinary calculi or renal stones may be considered a more long-term complication, effective prevention of infection (associated with calculi formation) must begin during the acute stage. In addition to neurogenic dysfunction, multiple factors predispose patients to renal stone formation, including hereditary tendencies, metabolic imbalances, urinary stasis, and urinary infection or presence of a foreign body. Stones form when the constituent of the stone is highly concentrated or when inorganic substances in the urine precipitate around a nidus or nucleus. This central focal point may be bacteria, urinary crystals, or a foreign body such as the balloon on an indwelling catheter.

Patients with SCI initially experience hypercaluria when calcium is mobilized from the bones and concentrates in the urine as a result of paralysis and immobilization. About 90% of stones contain calcium or magnesium in combination with mineral salts and other substances. The patient is also prone to urinary stasis, mucosa inflammation of the bladder wall, and chronic infected urine. These factors place the paralyzed person at much greater risk of developing calculous uropathy, particularly when the patient has an indwelling catheter (Kohli and Lamid 1986; DeVivio and Fine 1986).

It should be pointed out that early mobilization, better control of infection, and intermittent catheterizations have greatly reduced the incidence of renal calculi formation.

Management

1. Reduce the risk of calculi formation. Take measures to prevent or control urinary infection as previously outlined and maintain unobstructed drainage to reduce stasis of urine. *Bladder calculi associated with urinary tract infection are most common.*

2. Maintain acidic urine by administering urinary antiseptics and ascorbic acid as ordered. A low urinary pH (around 5) discourages aggregation of calcium salts, which form best in alkaline urine. The patient may need to be taught how to check urinary pH routinely. If the pH is greater than 6 the physician should be notified and medications adjusted.

3. Maintain adequate urinary output of 1500 to 1800 ml/day, or up to 3000 ml/day if the patient has an indwelling catheter. A high fluid intake dilutes the urine, which then has a better "washout" effect. "Eggshell" calculi tend to form around the balloon of an indwelling catheter where the urine is most stagnant at the base of the bladder.

4. Change the indwelling catheter at regular intervals (the latex catheter every 1 to 2 weeks; the silicone catheter every 4 to 6 weeks). Check for grit in the tubing or catheter and report findings.

5. Encourage as much activity as possible, to combat skeletal calcium loss from immobilization. This is a most important measure. The restriction of milk and dairy products to reduce calcium intake is not as controversial as in the past. A normal but not excessive intake is recommended.

6. Recognize that stones may exist when urine bypasses an indwelling catheter or there is a general increase in spasticity or profuse sweating. Also watch for hematuria. The classic renal colic pain will not exist in a person without sensation, but referred pain and other signs may occur depending on the level of injury.

7. Observe abnormal results of diagnostic tests. Note the presence of red or white blood cells, crystals, or casts in the urinalysis. A positive urine culture, particularly of a proteus species, can produce urea-splitting organisms that are more apt to create "infection stones." The majority of calculi are detected by X ray, on plain abdominal films.

8. Assist the person to maintain unobstructed urinary outflow. Small stones may pass through the catheter or irrigation may be needed and ordered specifically. Surgical intervention by transurethral crushing and removal may be required. Newer methods of treating calculi such as shockwave lithotripsy (Lazare, Saltzman, and Sotolono 1988) sometimes combined with urase inhibitors and various buffered bladder irrigation solutions avoid repeated major surgery. Untreated stones generally lead to septic and renal complications (Lloyd 1986).

9. Urge regular follow-up care. Calculi have a tendency to recur. This must be monitored by a physician every 3 to 6 months.

Expected Outcomes

Evaluate effectiveness of treatment according to level of outcome criteria reached:

- Clear urine of normal color and volume, free from sediment and without evidence of dehydration or hematuria
- Acidic urinary pH of around 5
- Urine free from infective organisms, particularly *Proteus* or urea-splitting organisms.
- Continuous, unobstructed drainage from indwelling catheter without urine bypassing
- Adequate bladder emptying for those on intermittent catheterizations
- Good systemic health without chills, profuse sweating, increased spasticity, or referred renal colic pain
- Person active and participating with preventive measures and with follow-up care

Autonomic Dysreflexia (Hyperreflexia)

Autonomic dysreflexia is frequently precipitated by an overdistended bladder or urinary complications. It is commonly encountered during routine bladder care. Therefore, everyone—individuals, families, and caregivers—must be familiar with the onset of autonomic dysreflexia. Symptoms can quickly progress to dangerous or even fatal levels, thereby creating a medical emergency. A person is more prone to developing autonomic dysreflexia during the first year after injury, but a danger persists throughout life. This condition occurs when the injury is sustained at the T_{4-6} levels or higher and control from the higher nervous system centers is impaired. The incidence of autonomic dysreflexia can be diminished by a modified sphincterotomy (Barton, Khonsari, Vazari,

Byrne, Gordon, and Friis 1986). To review the mechanism of autonomic dysreflexia and interventions related to bladder management in detail, see Chapter 16. Health education must stress the relationship between bladder problems and onset of this complication.

HEALTH EDUCATION AND SKILLS

It is quite possible to begin education and introduce self-care skills within the first few weeks of injury. However, most patients approach such activities as physical therapy much more enthusiastically than the mundane tasks required for bladder care. Aversion—feelings that any of us might experience if we had lost bladder control—may surface quickly. Frustration levels are reached easily because these tasks, unlike gross motor activity, create rather than relieve anxiety.

Although obstacles can be encountered with psychosocial adjustments to SCI, early involvement gives patients some control and reinforces the idea that they will eventually be responsible for their own care. Perhaps the greatest incentive for achieving independence with bladder care is the early opportunity of a day or weekend pass. It is important for both the patient and the care givers to realize that bladder rehabilitation usually takes weeks, even months to accomplish. The person often becomes discouraged by continued incontinence and needs much encouragement to continue the program. Individuals gain motivation as they realize that bladder care is an integral part of reaching independence.

Interdisciplinary collaboration helps to meet individual needs. The marriage of skills required goes far beyond arranging convenient times to work with the patient. For example, it is far more meaningful for patients to learn how to apply condom drainage during morning care on the ward than for them to get dressed and go "down to O.T." to learn about it. Another distinct advantage of performing activities at the bedside is the facilitation of more thorough interdisciplinary communication about current progress or related problems.

Basically nursing responsibilities involve teaching patients the essential anatomy and function of the urinary tract in relation to their disability; the importance of fluid and dietary management; appropriate techniques to empty bladder; skin care; and how to prevent, recognize, and treat bladder infection and other complications. Care givers must be thoroughly familiar with application and care of all types of urinary drainage systems. Whether physical limitations allow patients to perform the task themselves or whether their responsibility is instructing others in doing so, patients will need to know this information.

The occupational therapist's responsibilities include assessing hand function and upper body strength and coordination, as well as transfer abilities, degree of balance when sitting, accessibility of toilet, and appropriateness of clothing; adapting or fabricating equipment for the patient's individual use such as a mirror-light system to see the urethra; suggesting alternative positions; altering clothing for easier removal or exposure of the perineal area; providing resources for available supplies; and instructing patients and families when appropriate. Eventually home assessment will be necessary.

To ensure optimum bladder management, the selected self-care skills should not impose an unnecessary burden on patients or families or curtail work, school, or social life. Above all, the techniques involved must be reliable and personally acceptable to patients if they are expected to become totally responsible for carrying on successfully.

Persons with Paraplegia

Persons with uncomplicated paraplegia generally have the physical potential for independence with all aspects of bladder care, and many progress very quickly. Preserved upper body strength and hand function improve tolerance, balance, transfer techniques, and ability to perform procedures. However, during the first 6 months after injury the required orthopedic thoracolumbar appliances may hamper ability to void by restricting access to the suprapubic area and preventing bending forward on the toilet.

Self-catheterization is probably the must difficult technique to learn, but most persons with paraplegia are able to accomplish this. Even if catheterizations are required for only a few months during the bladder retraining period, most people find self-catheterization convenient, especially when planning activities outside the hospital. Self-catheterization should be encouraged as soon as possible in the acute setting to promote independence and reduce the hazards of cross-contamination. See Procedure 18–9.

Persons with Quadriplegia

Persons with quadriplegia vary greatly in their abilities to become independent. Many of them are able to induce voiding by using trigger techniques and can apply and empty condom drainage systems by using aids and adaptive devices. See Figure 18–7. Some may master catheterizing themselves. Review Procedure 18–9.

The person sustaining injury from C_{1-4} will be totally dependent on others for all aspects of bladder care. Persons with C_5 to T_1 lesions may become independent with adaptive aids for condom application, leg bag assembly and emptying, and trigger methods to induce voiding. Others may find it too time consuming. Selected

Procedure 18–9 Teaching Self-Catheterization

Purpose

To empty the bladder regularly and completely. The ultimate goal of an intermittent catheterization regime for many patients with SCI is to become catheter free. For those with lower motor neuron neurogenic bladder dysfunction, lifelong practice of intermittent catheterizations is the treatment of choice.

When teaching this procedure to a patient it is vital to reinforce the following concepts (U. Michigan Urology Assoc. 1986):

- The importance of regular and frequent emptying to prevent overdistension of the bladder, which weakens its resistance to infection.
- The necessity of performing catheterizations on time to control bacterial growth in the bladder. Stress that the washout effect of frequently emptying the bladder to remove multiplying bacteria, rather than the sterility or cleanliness of the technique used, is the major defense against infection. Complete bladder emptying is also important to inhibit the growth of bacteria.

Part A: Female Patient

Equipment and Supplies

- Catheter: a short metal catheter with a slightly curved, nondilating tip, or a 6-inch plastic disposable catheter (preferred); a size #12 or #14 (French) catheter of red rubber or clear plastic may be used
- Sterile towel (for use in hospital only)
- Waterproof pad (if performed in bed)
- Antiseptic wipes for hand washing (while in hospital)
- Antiseptic wipes or cotton balls for cleaning perineum (while in hospital)
- Water-soluble lubricant (optional)
- Collecting device for measuring urine (during early stages); a large plastic or paper cup (500 to 1000 ml), kidney basin, or bedpan may be used
- Mirror (first few times only)
- Washcloth and towel for genital hygiene following procedure
- Covered container with antiseptic solution for storing reusable catheters (while in hospital)
- Self-sealing storage bag or container (for home use)

Action

1. Before teaching actual technique, explain principles (concepts) supporting intermittent catheterization.

2. Help patient assemble equipment. Show most convenient arrangement by using a table beside bed or toilet. (When in hospital, cover table with a sterile towel.)

3. Have patient assume a well-balanced, comfortable position in bed. Position patient at a 60-degree angle with knees spread apart (possibly supported with pillows) and heels placed together (frog position). Place waterproof pad under buttocks. Or have patient sit on toilet or forward in wheelchair. When on toilet (or balanced forward in wheelchair) a rigid device to spread the legs may be used if maintaining correct position is difficult due to spasms.

4. Ask patient to wash hands. When in hospital, antiseptic wipes are recommended. At home, hand washing with mild soap and water is sufficient.

5. Show patient how to open sterile towel, catheter package, or container and to apply lubricant to catheter tip (optional).

6. Clean inner labia and urethral opening with downward strokes, from pubic area to anus, using an antiseptic towelette or cotton balls soaked in antiseptic solution or normal saline, if antiseptic is too irritating.

7. Instruct patient to:
   - Spread labia using her nondominant hand.

Rationale

It is usually easier to begin teaching with patient in bed. This position improves vision of perineum and eases catheter insertion and drainage.

This minimizes risk of cross-infection and is convenient.

Use of lubricant is optional because of natural secretions in female urethra. However, until patient is proficient with self-catheterization, use lubricant to minimize risk of trauma.

While in hospital, added precaution of cleaning perineum is preferred to reduce risk of infection. At home, antiseptic cleaning is unnecessary.

This leaves dominant hand free to manipulate the catheter.

(Procedure continues)

Procedure 18–9   Teaching Self-Catheterization (continued)

Action	Rationale

Action

- Using her third finger, locate urethral opening just below clitoris (which is easier to feel) and above vagina.
- Lift third finger off opening while keeping other fingers in place.
- Grasp catheter 1 to 3 inches from tip.
- Gently insert into urinary opening (about 2 inches) until urine flows.

Be sure to tell woman to insert catheter in an upward motion to follow natural anatomical curve. (Aim at umbilicus, but variable.) If resistance is met, taking a few deep breaths may help overcome sphincter spasm. If urine flow stops abruptly, rotate catheter 180 degrees.

8. Remind patient to check that end of catheter is in the collection container.

9. Instruct patient to remove catheter slowly. Show patient how to press gently downward on bladder (manual expression or Credé maneuver) during removal of catheter.

10. Remind patient to pinch catheter or place finger over open end before removing.

11. Encourage patient to wipe herself well with a damp washcloth and dry perineal area.

12. Teach patient to measure and recond urinary output on a bladder retraining flow chart.

13. Teach patient how to care for equipment:

- If the catheter is a reusable metal one, patient should run tap water through it and store it in a covered container in a mild antiseptic solution, while in hospital. Solution should be changed twice weekly, at which time metal catheter could be sterilized as an added precaution. At home, a reusable catheter can be stored in containers such as a paper towel, a plastic toothbrush case, a cosmetic bag, or a self-sealing plastic bag. No solution is necessary. The home care of standard red rubber catheters is discussed in Part B.
- Disposable catheters should be discarded after each use.

Rationale

Use a mirror (for first few times) to show her anatomical structures. *Feeling* for urinary opening becomes the easier and more reliable method.

The firm plastic or metal catheters are easier to direct; a soft, pliable catheter may have to be held nearer tip.

To avoid catheter from lodging up against bladder wall, a length of IV tubing can be used as an extension if needed.

This ensures complete emptying of bladder.

This avoids wetting clothes or bedding from urine left inside catheter.

This will remove any irritating solutions, lubricant, or urine that might make the skin more susceptible to the effects of pressure and excoriation.

Recording progress is essential during early stages of intermittent catheterization program. It is also wise to monitor urinary output for a few weeks after discharge. Measurement of residual urine is a valuable diagnostic aid throughout life for patient with a neurogenic bladder dysfunction.

Part B: Male Patient

Goals

The methods and goals of self-catheterization for male patients are similar to those for female patients.

Equipment

- Catheter: a soft, pliable size #12 or #14 (French) catheter, of red rubber or clear plastic; feeding tubes may be used for children
- Sterile towel or waterproof pads for lap (for use in hospital only)
- Antiseptic wipes for hand washing (while in hospital)
- Antiseptic solution for cleaning penis (while in hospital)
- Water-soluble lubricant
- Collecting and measuring device (during early stages)
- Washcloth and towel for genital hygiene following procedure
- Storage bag or container (for home use)
- For a sterile procedure, disposable catheter kits or, when at home, forceps and sterile 4 × 4 inch gauze may be used.

(Procedure continues)

Procedure 18–9   Teaching Self-Catheterization (continued)

Action	Rationale
1. Help patient assemble and arrange equipment. A urinal can be hooked in a variety of places for convenient collection and measurement.	
2. Have patient assume a comfortable, well-balanced sitting position in bed or wheelchair or on toilet.	During early stages a person with paraplegia is able to assist a staff member with sterile intermittent catheterization program as soon as he is able to sit at a 45-degree angle in bed. At first patient may assist nurse with steps involved in sterile procedure. Then as mobility and strength increase and transferring to toilet is possible, procedure can be modified.
3. Remind patient to use manual techniques to induce voiding before catheterizing.	Patient with an upper motor neuron bladder dysfunction may successfully use trigger voiding, manual expression, straining to void, or anal stretch technique. Those with lower motor neuron dysfunctions may plan on lifelong use of intermittent catheterizations.
4. Ask patient to wash hands well with an antiseptic soap. Penis may also be cleaned with an antiseptic solution or washed with soap and water. If patient is uncircumcised, instruct him to pull back foreskin before cleaning. A sterile towel or disposable pad may be placed over the lap. At home, good personal hygiene is essential to prevent gross contamination. Washing hands and penis with a mild soap and water is usually sufficient.	This reduces risks of cross-contamination and hospital-induced infection.
5. Show patient how to open the catheter package (almost completely) and generously lubricate the tip and almost entire length of catheter with water-soluble jelly.	Unlike female urethra, male urethra lacks natural secretions. Lots of lubricant is needed to minimize risk of trauma to long urethra.
6. Instruct patient:	
• To hold penis, with nondominant hand, in an upward position (at a 60-degree angle to things) and apply a slight stretch.	It is easier to manipulate catheter with dominant hand.
• To grasp catheter firmly about 3 inches from tip and slowly and gently insert it about 6 inches until urine flows.	
• To maintain a continuous gentle pressure on catheter; taking a few deep breaths or slightly twisting the catheter will help overcome resistance.	Slight resistances are normally encountered at internal and external urethral sphincters. With upper motor neuron dysfunction stronger resistance from sphincter spasms is common. Stop and wait for spasm to pass.
• Never use force to overcome a major resistance.	
7. Remind patient to direct catheter end toward collection container.	
8. Instruct patient to remove catheter slowly. Show him how to press gently downward on bladder (manual expression or Credé maneuver) during removal of catheter.	This ensures complete emptying of bladder.
9. Encourage patient to clean and dry genital area thoroughly.	This will remove any irritating solutions, lubricant, or urine that might render skin more susceptible to effects of pressure and excoriation.
10. Teach patient to measure and record urinary output on a bladder retraining flow chart. Be sure to include any output obtained from manual techniques to induce voiding.	Recording progress is essential during early stages of an intermittent catheterization program. It is also wise to monitor urinary output for a few weeks after discharge. Measurement of residual urine is a valuable diagnostic aid throughout life for patient with a neurogenic bladder dysfunction.

(Procedure continues)

Procedure 18–9   Teaching Self-Catheterization (continued)

Action	Rationale
11. Teach patient how to care for equipment:	
• While in hospital, a fresh sterile catheter should be used each time.	
• For home use, a variety of carrying containers (similar to those used by women) can be used for catheter storage. Following each use, run tap water through catheter. Red rubber catheters can be boiled (for 10 minutes) once weekly to sterilize. Sterile catheters can be stored in the refrigerator in individual plastic self-sealing bags along with lubricant for convenient future use.	Risk of cross-contamination is considerably less at home. Storage in refrigerator helps retard bacterial growth. This procedure will keep catheters soft, pliable, and free of debris. With care, a dozen catheters will last about a year. Disposable catheter sets designed specifically for intermittent catheterization, although more expensive, are an attractive alternative.
Warn the patient to discard a rubber catheter when it becomes brittle or is deteriorating.	

persons with injury to the lower cervical region (C_6–T_1) may use adaptive aids to self-catheterize and to perform an anal-stretch technique if detrusor-sphincter dyssynergia is a problem.

For the person with low quadriplegia (C_5–T_1) the greatest loss of muscle power is in the hand with varied limited movements of the shoulder, elbow, and wrist depending on the level of injury. Those with adequate hand control may not require adaptive aids. Some may use natural tenodesis or pressure of the palms together; others may need orthoses (specifically the flexor-hinge point) to create a pincer grasp. Generally when the flexor-hinge splint is needed to achieve some of these skills it meets with better success and patient acceptance later in the rehabilitation period. See Chapter 22 for discussion of splinting.

The natural progression of skills to be learned is generally as follows:

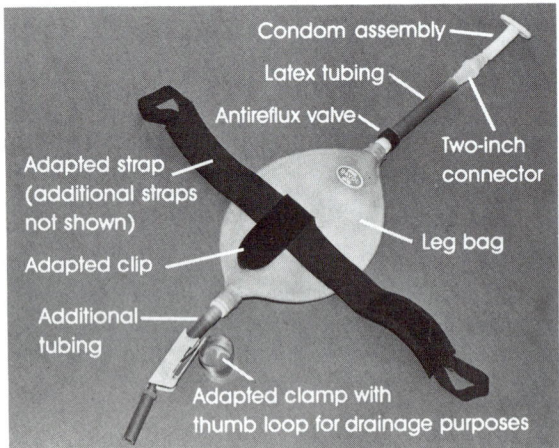

FIGURE 18–7   A condom drainage system adapted for independent use.

• *Trigger voiding* can be achieved by the use of the ulnar side of the hand for tapping. Tell the patient where the most effective spots are. Suprapubic tapping is easiest when sitting at 45 degrees in bed or up in the wheelchair. It is difficult to move arms against gravity while lying in bed.

• If the patient has adequate hand control, *condom application* can be attempted next. (The skills required to manage and empty the leg bag may be easier, but balance and ability to resume an upright position is also necessary and this is most difficult in the early stages.) A plastic mirror, adapted glue and spray cans, and a groin shield are necessary equipment. Different ways of using hand control is also possible. See Figure 18–8.

• *Leg bag assembly and emptying* is possible with the aid of adapted straps and clips. The leg bag may be emptied into the toilet or into a urinal or other container.

Intermittent *self-catheterization* is possible for selected persons with injury at the C_6 to T_1 cord segments (Ford and Duckworth 1987). The sterile insertion procedure required for an indwelling catheter is not possible, but a sterile procedure for irrigation is. This is a most complex task requiring much time, patience, and individualized adaptation during the final stages of rehabilitation.

The method to follow when teaching a patient to use the *anal stretch technique* to overcome detrusor-sphincter dyssynergia has been described previously. Persons with C_{6-7} quadriplegia, who are able to transfer to the toilet and maintain adequate balance, may use an adaptive aid made for finger insertion to provide adequate stretch.

Adaptation and aids for the toilet are described in Chapter 19.

When persons are discharged to the home setting they must be fully aware of their individlized bladder programs, from care of equipment in the home to prevention of complications and recognition and initiation of early treatment (Hammond, Umlauf, Matteson and Perduta-Fulginiti 1989). Some excellent and creative literature for patient and family education is described in the Resources. Reassure the person that it is unwise to make long-term choices until techniques are tried at home and are shown to be practical. When discharged, however, the person must have *a resource person* to contact. This may be the urologist, the public health nurse, the family practitioner, or a rehabilitative outpatient service. If the person has doubts or difficulties, a simple telephone call may solve both large and small problems.

LONG-TERM IMPLICATIONS

Precise urinary management is essential throughout life to preserve the delicate and precious function of the upper urinary tract. Even though bladder emptying may appear to be well- and safely established, over time deterioration may occur because of:

- Changing neuronal activity in isolated cord segments or late complications, such as syringomyelia
- Anatomical/structural changes usually related to chronic infection and calculi formation

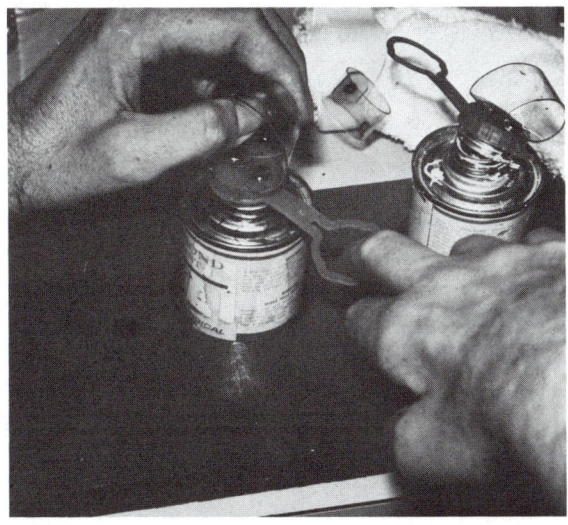

A

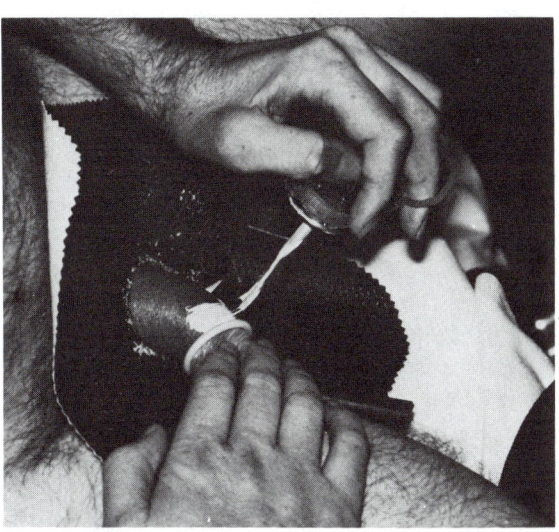

B

C

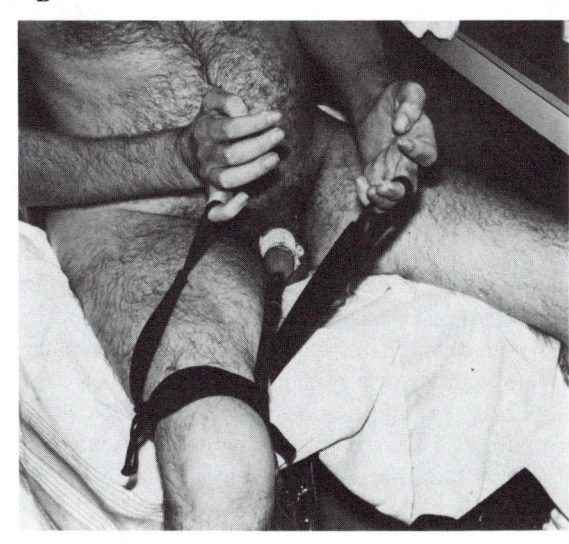

D

FIGURE 18–8 A person with low quadriplegia demonstrates independence with condom application (**A**) by using an adapted skin cement can; (**B**) by using a groin shield; (**C**) by using blunt-tipped scissors to clip the collar off the condom; (**D**) by using adapted leg straps.

- Obstructive changes if a man develops an enlarged prostate
- The natural process of aging
- Hypertension, a late hazard that should be controlled

Serious upper urinary tract involvement can occur, especially when a person is catheter free and without symptoms (Nanninga and Rosen 1975). In fact, long-term surveillance is needed for persons without any obvious symptoms (Ozer and Shannon 1991).

Clinicians/researchers are giving screening procedures close attention and recommend various combinations of diagnostic procedures, shown also to be cost effective (Morcos and Thomas 1988; Tuel, Meythaler, Cross, and McLaughlin 1990; Badner, Witcher and Resnick 1990).

The trend is now toward noninvasive techniques, with less X ray exposure, and away from cumbersome procedures to clear the bowel. More convenient procedures and less disruption to the daily lives of spinal cord injured persons should encourage regular checkups for many of them, but the psychological issues preventing some people from participating are very difficult to manage. As Dwyer (1985) emphasizes, a person who has not adapted to life in a wheelchair often reacts by neglecting personal health. By neglecting bladder care, resultant infections with ensuing complications are virtually inevitable. The invasion of privacy and the loss of control over such personal body functions can also be deterrent factors. To increase awareness of the serious risks and to encourage people to minimize them, introduce peer consultation services or peer influences, and explore creative ways to mainstream disabled people. Typically solutions to these issues lag behind technological advancements but challenges in life care planning are a natural continuation of rehabilitation. See Chapter 33.

Although some generalizations are possible, after the formal rehabilitation period, the individual directs the need and timing of evaluations. Hypocompliance is a significant problem (Hackler, Hall, and Zampieri 1989). Urinalysis and culture and sensitivity specimens, and residual volumes may need to be checked every few weeks or months. Annual examinations combining IVP or ultrasound and urodynamics have proven most useful in evaluating bladder and sphincter dysfunction and in the search for ureterovesical reflux (Wyndaele 1987b), which is most likely to develop 1 to 2 years postinjury, more frequently in persons who have a complete upper motor neuron injury (Lamid 1988). Renal ultrasound of the kidneys appears to be a reliable, cheaper, and safer (noninvasive) alternative to an annual IVP but does not replace the use of an IVP for initial evaluation (Morcos and Thomas 1988). Renal scintillation procedures, basically a computerized record of individual kidney function generated by a special camera that detects the uptake of a radiopharmaceutical at various intervals, have also been used as effective screening and monitoring tools (Lloyd 1986). Both ultrasound and scintillation procedures

are combined with plain abdominal X rays to detect calculi, for example. Small bladder calculi can only be seen during cystoscopy, however.

Urinary tract infection continues to be a common problem. Several ways to reduce this problem are (Cardenas and Mayo 1987):

- Self-catheterizations as opposed to catheterization by others
- Intermittent catheterizations as opposed to indwelling
- Surgical interventions to decrease urethral resistance, primarily the external sphincterotomy

Obstruction is a closely related major problem, whether due to infection, calculi, neurophysiological changes within the bladder and sphincters, or other physical changes, most notably an enlarged prostate gland in the male. To prevent kidney function damage, urine must be stored and expelled within a low pressure system. Pressure measurements above 40 mmHg or above 80 cm H_2O, as evidenced on urodynamic studies, are alarms indicating that the upper urinary tract is in danger of damage by reflux.

For women, great concern remains over the continued risks associated with a permanent indwelling catheter. Because prolonged indwelling catheters can lead to squamous metaplasia and squamous cell cancer, close follow-up with cystologies, cystoscopy, and bladder biopsies is required (Fam, Sarkarati, and Yallo 1988).

The increased risk of *cancer* associated with chronic inflammation/irritation from recurrent infection is a threat for all persons with SCI. Bejany, Lockhart, and Rhamy (1987) estimate that approximately 2% of the total SCI population is affected and that ultrasonography and computerized tomography of the abdomen and pelvis should be included in the care of persons with recurrent infection, calculi, and hematuria.

When assessing a person who has had neurogenic bladder dysfunction for some time, always be alert for signs of infection and calculi. Anticipate a low-grade bacteruria without symptomatic infection. Immediate postinjury (baseline) data and accumulated data for comparison are essential for identifying trends and spotting actual or potential problems.

Some regional rehabilitation centers coordinate services with local resources to minimize time, inconvenience, and expense to the disabled person. Tests can be done locally and results relayed to the centers for interpretation. Other centers are developing outreach programs for people in rural areas. However achieved, follow-up services are vital for well-being.

Specialized medical evaluation is encouraged because improved diagnostic procedures give more exact direction to management techniques and can result in better-designed urinary products, newer and better drugs, and more refined surgical advancements. For example, future development of a technique to enlarge the small spastic bladder (cystoplasty) with a loop of bowel holds promise to allow persons to catheterize themselves rather than depend on a problematic external drainage system.

Lifetime health care services that include expert medical surveillance are advocated, but such specialized care is not yet widely available. Many problems remain to be overcome, including economic and geographical barriers and to limitations of health care professionals who may rarely see a person with SCI. Although the need for long-term follow up is universally recognized, there is no consensus as to what needs to be done and how often. Nevertheless, care for life is essential, and improved continuing care leads to better health and longer survival. See Chapter 33.

REFERENCES

Barkin, M., Herschorn, S., and Comisarow, R. 1982. The urological care of the spinal cord injured patient. In *Early Management of Spinal Cord Injury*. Ed. C. Tator. New York: Raven Press, pp. 273–278.

Barton, C., Khonsari, F., Vazari, N., Byrne, C., Gordon, S., and Friis, R. 1986. The effect of modified transurethral sphincterotomy on autonomic dysreflexia. *Journal of Urology* 135 (1); 83–85.

Becker, E. F., et al. 1989. High pressure neurogenic bladder after spinal cord injury manage by augmentation enterocystoplasty. *American Urological 83rd annual Meeting Journal Part 2*, 139 (4). (*Journal of Urology.*) *Following surgery all patients remained continent on intermittent catheterization with upper urinary tract stability or improvement and without bouts of autonomic dysreflexia. Enlarging the capacity of a small spastic bladder with a remodeled portion of the bowel proved effective in 12 patients.*

Bejany, E., Lockhart, J., and Rhamy, R. 1987. Malignant vesicle tumors following spinal cord injury. *Journal of Urology*, 138 (6): 1390–1392.

Bhatt, K., Cid, E., and Maiman D. 1987. Bacteremia in the spinal cord injured population. *American Journal of Paraplegia* 10 (1): 11–14. *Stresses the importance of preventive care for patients with underlying risk factors of poor nutrition, respirator dependency, indwelling catheters, and manipulative procedures. The most common sources of contamination were the genitourinary system and the respiratory system.*

Boner, D., Witcher, M., and Resnick, M. 1990. Application of office ultrasound in the management of the SCI patient. *Journal of Urology* 143 (5): 969–972.

Bransbury, A. 1979. Allergy to rubber condom urinals and medical adhesives in male spinal injury patients. *Contact Dermatitis* 5 (5): 317–322. *Describes several products, cites common problems; recommends ideal qualities to look for when selecting adhesives for condom application.*

Burke, D., and Murray, D. 1975. *Handbook of Spinal Cord Medicine*. London and Basingstoke: Macmillan Press. *Concise overview of neurogenic bladder dysfunction, bladder training, and potential complications. Excellent introductory resource.*

Cardenas, D., Kelly, E., Krieger, J., and Chapman, W. 1988. Residual urine volumes in patients with spinal cord injury: Measurement with a portable ultrasound instrument. *Archives of Physical Medicine and Rehabilitation* 69 (7): 514–516.

Cardenas, D. D., and Mayo, M. E. 1987. Bacteriuria with fever after spinal cord injury. *Archives of Physical Medicine and Rehabilitation* 68 (5, Pt. 1): 291–293.

Chusid, J. 1979. *Correlative Neuroanatomy and Functional Neurology*. Los Altos, CA: Lange Medical Publications, Chapter 20. *Helpful illustrated section on the diagnosis and pathophysiology of neurogenic bladder dysfunction.*

Dailey, J., and Michael, R. 1977. Non-sterile self-intermittent catheterization for male quadriplegic patients. *American Journal of Occupational Therapy* 31 (2): 86–89. *An illustrated guide for a patient with C_{6-7} quadriplegia; assessment, procedure, and adaptive aids described.*

DeVivio, M. J., and Fine, P. R. 1986. Predicting renal calculus occurrence in spinal cord injury patients. *Archives of Physical Medicine and Rehabilitation* 67 (10): 722–725.

Donovan, W. 1977. A finger device for obtaining satisfactory voiding in spinal cord-injured patients. *American Journal of Occupational Therapy* 31 (2): 107–108. *Fabricated device that enables C_7 quadriplegic patients to perform anal stretch technique to overcome detrusor-sphincter dyssynergia.*

Donovan, W., Clowers, D., Kiviat, M., and Macri, D. 1977. Anal sphincter stretch: A technique to overcome detrusor-sphincter dyssynergia. *Archives of Physical Medicine and Rehabilitation* 58 (July): 320–324. *An updated review of this technique, which illustrates methods, describes criteria for selection of patients, and examines results; includes introduction of a simple finger prosthesis for independent use by selected quadriplegic patients.*

Donovan, W., Kiviat, M., and Clowers, D. 1977. Intermittent bladder emptying via urethral catheterization or suprapubic cystocath: A comparison study. *Archives of Physical Medicine and Rehabilitation* 58 (July): 291–296. *A study primarily undertaken to determine infection rates; includes helpful information on procedures and equipment.*

Dwyer, L. 1985. Bladder and bowel dysfunction. In *Nursing Spinal Cord Injuries*. Ed. N. M. Woll. Totowa, NJ: Rowman & Allanheld Publisher, pp. 27–36.

Fam, B. A., Sarkarati, M., and Yallo, S. V. 1988. Spinal Cord Injury. In *Neurourology and Urodynamics: Principles and Practice*. Eds. S. V. Yalla, E. J. McGuire, A. Elbadowi, and J. G. Blaivis. New York: Macmillan.

Fawcett, S. 1986. A study of the skin flora of spinal cord injured patients. *Journal of Hospital Infections* 8 (2): 149–158. *The perinea, groin, penile shafts and urethras of spinal cord injured patients, as compared to healthy subjects, were heavily colonized by a wide range of drug-resistant, gram-negative bacilli within 2 to 3 days of admission. Serratia marcecens and Klebsiella pneumoniae are predominant on the skin and are directly related to urinary tract infections.*

Felder, L. 1979. Neurogenic bladder dysfunction. *Journal of Neurosurgical Nursing* 11 (2): 94–104. *Comprehensive overview of all types of neurogenic bladder dysfunctions as a result of brain and spinal cord damage; includes chart to correlate classification, signs and symptoms, sensation, and principles of nursing management.*

Ford, R. D., and Duckworth, B. 1987. *Physical Management of the Quadriplegic Patient.* 2d ed. Philadelphia: V. A. Davis. *Extensive photostory presentation to reflect up-to-date management techniques and philosophies. Contains helpful materials on bladder and bowel management including self-catheterization and toilet transfers, among many other topics.*

French, R. 1980. *Guide to Diagnostic Procedures.* 5th ed. New York: McGraw-Hill, Chapter 6. *Tests for specific kidney function and related nursing care.*

Gardener, B., Parsons, K., Machin, D., Galloway, A., and Krishnan, K. 1986. The urological management of spinal cord damaged patients: A clinical algorithm. *Paraplegia* 24: 138–147. *A simple computer program based on these charts is available.*

Gribble, L. 1989. Urinary tract infection in spinal cord injured persons. In *Proceedings: Spinal Cord Injury Research Symposium (Canada),* Vancouver, BC. (Abstracts available from British Columbia Paraplegic Association, 780 S.W. Marine Drive, Vancouver, BC. Canada V6P5Y7).

Hackler, R., Hall, M., and Zampieri, T. 1989. Bladder hypocompliance in the SCI population. *Journal of Urology.* 141 (6): 1390–1393.

Hammond, M. C., Umlauf, R. L., Matteson, B., and Perduta-Fulginiti, F. (Eds.). 1989. *Yes, You Can! A Guide to Self-Care for Persons with Spinal Cord Injury.* Washington, DC.: Paralyzed Veterans of America (PVA). *Chapter 6 presents an exceptional overview of bladder management and concerns. Explains diagnostic tests and contains explicit information on recognition of infections and actions to take.*

Herschorn, S., Barkin, M., and Comisarow, R. H. 1982. Value of urodynamic studies in the management of neurogenic vesical dysfunction in spinal cord injured patients. In *Early Management of Acute Spinal Cord Injury.* Ed. C. Tator. New York: Raven Press, pp. 279–289.

Hirsch, D. 1979. Do condom catheter collection systems cause urinary tract infections? *Journal of American Medical Association* 242 (4): 340–341. *A study that concludes that the use of condom drainage does not increase the risk of upper urinary tract infection if the patient is cooperative with personal care.*

Johnson, J. 1980. Rehabilitative aspects of neurologic bladder dysfunction. *Nursing Clinics of North America* 15 (2): 293–307. *Comprehensive review of neurogenic bladder dysfunction emphasizing nursing assessment and intervention in conjunction with drug therapy, intermittent catheterization, and surgical measures to maintain optimal urinary function.*

Kohli, A., and Lamid, S. 1986. Risk factors for renal stone formation in patients with spinal cord injury. *British Journal of Urology* 58 (6): 588–591.

Lamid, S. 1988. Long-term follow-up of spinal cord injury patients with vesicoureteral reflux. *Paraplegia* 26 (1): 27–34.

Lawson, S., and Cook, J. 1977. Condom urinals. *Nursing Mirror* (Dec.): 19–21. *Practical overview of condom application techniques and precautions.*

Lazare, J. N., Saltzman, B., and Sotolono, J. 1988. Extracorporeal shock wave lithotripsy treatment of spinal cord injury patients. *Journal of Urology* 140 (2): 266–269.

Lindan, R., Leffler, E., and Freehafer, A. 1990. The team approach to urinary bladder management in SCI patients: A 26-year retrospective study. *Paraplegia* 28 (5): 314–317.

Lloyd, L. K. 1986. New trends in urologic management of SCI patients. *Central Nervous System Trauma* 3 (1): 3–12.

Lloyd, L., Kuhlemeier, K., Fine, P., and Stover, S. 1986. Urological neurology and urodynamics. Initial bladder management in spinal cord injury: Does it make a difference? *Journal of Urology* 135 (Mar.).

Madersbacher, H. 1989. Sacral posterior root rhizotomy together with implantation of the sacral anterior root stimulator (Brindley) for control of an unbalanced reflex bladder with uncontrollable incontinence. In *Proceedings from American Urological 83rd Annual Meeting Journal Part 2,* 139 (4). *(Journal of Urology). The creation of a lower motor neuron bladder by cutting of the posterior root (rhizotomy) and implantation of a sacral anterior root stimulator was considered very successful for 28 women. (Men were unable to produce a reflex erection following.) Questions unanswered are: Will electrostimulation last throughout life? and Will the materials used for the implant fatigue with time? An Austrian perspective.*

Maynard, F., and Dionko, A. 1980. Clean intermittent catheterization in the management of the neurogenic bladder of traumatic spinal cord injured patients: A critical review. *Abstracts Digest Sixth Annual Scientific Meeting, American Spinal Injury Association,* May 8–11, New Orleans. *Report on extensive follow-up, which concludes that clean technique is safe and satisfactory with the added advantages of patient acceptance and compliance. Stress the need for careful follow-up similar to other methods for management of neurogenic bladder dysfunction.*

McGuire, F., and Savastano, J. 1986. Comparative urological outcome in women with SCI. *Journal of Urology* 135 (4): 730–731.

Mohler, J., Ellison, M., and Flanigan, R. 1986. The evaluation of creatinine clearance in spinal cord injury patients. *Journal of Urology* 136 (2): 366–369.

Morcos, S. K., and Thomas, D. G. 1988. A comparison of real time ultrasonography with intravenous urography in the follow-up of patients with spinal cord injury. *Clinical Radiology* 39 (1): 49–50.

Nanninga, J., and Rosen, J. 1975. Problems associated with the use of external urinary collectors in the male paraplegic. *International Journal of Paraplegia* 13: 56–61. *Cites complications of inflammation of the penis, skin breakdown, and urethral fistula with some recommendations for management.*

Noll, F., Russe, O., Kline, E., Botel, U., and Schreiter, F. 1988. Intermittent catheterization versus percutaneous suprapubic cystostomy in the early management of traumatic spinal cord lesions. *Paraplegia* 26 (1): 4–9.

Ozer, M. M. 1988. *Management of Persons with Spinal Cord Injury.* New York: Demos Publications. *An excellent interdisciplinary, introductory guide providing a synopsis of major issues of spinal cord injury across the life span. A rehabilitative focus.*

Ozer, M., and Shannon, S. 1991. Renal sonography in asymptomatic persons with SCI: A cost-effective analysis. *Archives of Physical Medicine and Rehabilitation.* 72 (1): 35–37.

Pearman, J., and England, E. 1973. *The Urological Management of the Patient Following Spinal Cord Injury.* Springfield, IL: Charles Thomas. *Includes normal bladder function; neurogenic dysfunctions, diagnosis and treatment throughout all phases of care, and guidelines for procedures. An Australian perspective primarily.*

Sanderson, P. J., and Rawal, P. 1987. Contamination of the environment of spinal cord injured patients by organisms causing urinary tract infection. *Journal of Hospital Infections* 10 (2): 173–178. *Contamination of bedding, towels, and other items found in patients' rooms were tested. The need to confirm and expand handwashing by patients and staff is recommended.*

Smith, P., et al. 1972. Manual expression of the bladder following spinal cord injury. *International Journal of Paraplegia* 9: 213–218. *Provides cautionary implications for nursing practice when using manual techniques (Credé maneuver) to empty bladder; cites complication of dilation of upper urinary tract among others.*

Stark, L. 1980. BUN/creatinine—keys to kidney function. *Nursing* 5: 33–38. *Explains how to interpret laboratory findings and relate information to nursing care.*

Tuel, S., Meythaler, J., Cross, L., and McLaughlin, S. 1990. Cost-effective screening by nursing staff for urinary tract infection in the SCI patient. *American Journal for Physical Medicine and Rehabilitation* 69 (3): 128–131.

University of Michigan Urology Associates. 1986. *Intermittent self-catheterization* (Available from A. A. Traubman Health Care Center, Room 2325, Box 0330, 1500 East Medical Center Drive, Ann Arbor, MI 48106–0330.) *Exceptionally well designed pamphlets for both males and females stressing the importance of regularly emptying the bladder despite difficulties maintaining clean techniques when at home.*

Winter, C., and Morel, A. 1977. *Nursing Care of Patients with Urologic Disease*. 4th ed. St. Louis: C. V. Mosby. *Comprehensive text, which contains helpful information on neurogenic bladder disease in Chapter 17; discusses acute stage recovery from spinal shock, and retraining following SCI. Also contains helpful information on infectious neuropathy and neurogenic bladder disease.*

Wu, Y. C., Nanninga, J. B., and Hamilton, B. B. 1986. Inhibition of internal urethral sphincter and sacral reflex by anal stretch in spinal cord injured patients. *Archives of Physical Medicine and Rehabilitation* 67 (2): 135–136.

Wyndaele, J. J. 1987a. Urethral sphincter dyssynergia in spinal cord injury. *Paraplegia* 25 (1): 10–15.

———. 1987b. Urology in spinal cord injured patients. *Paraplegia* 25: 267–269. Describes advances in genitourinary care citing the renewed interest in the suprapubic catheter for acute management.

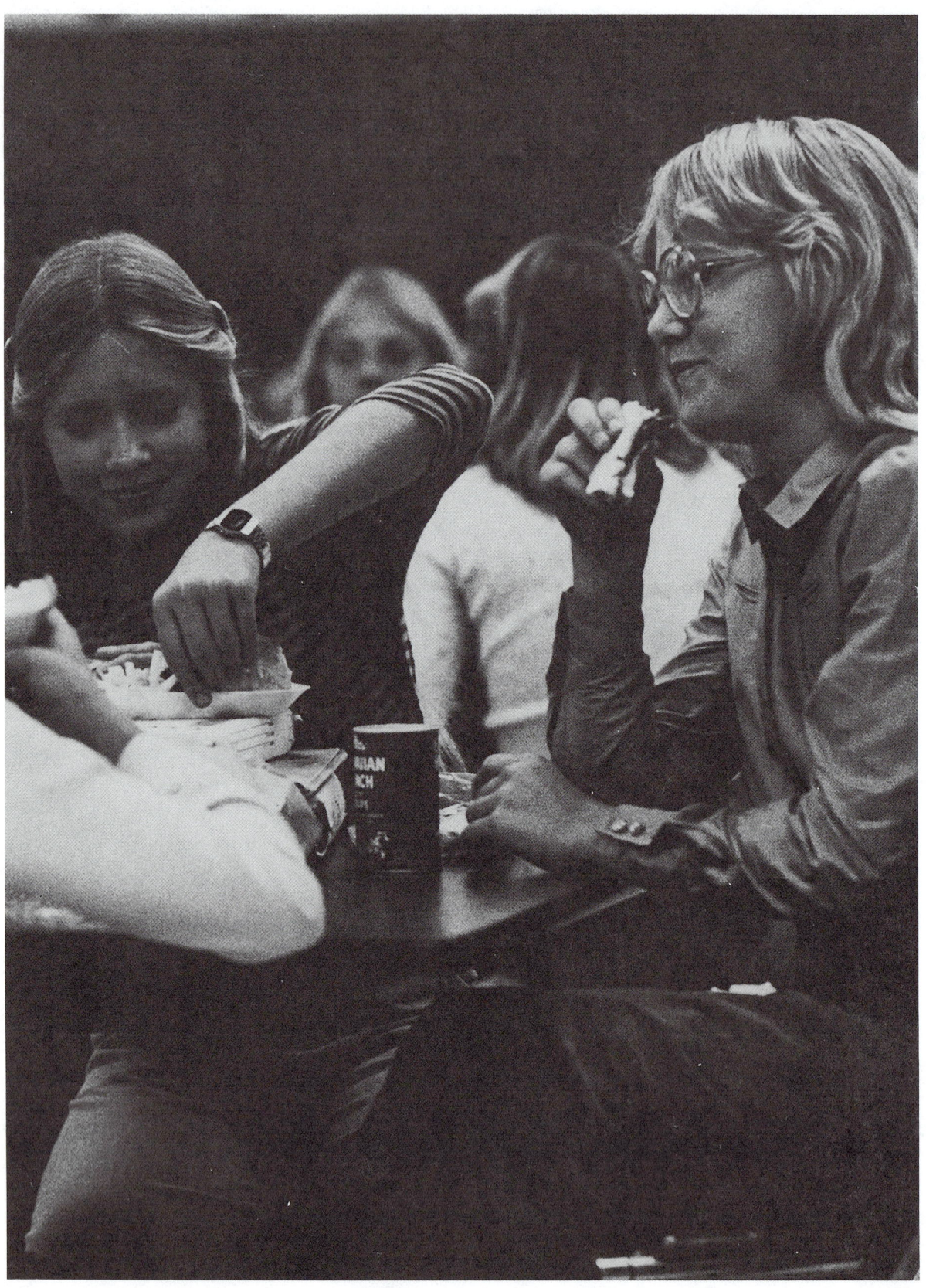

CHAPTER
— 19 —

Reestablishing Bowel Control

Chapter Outline

Health Care Objectives

- To identify health care goals of reestablishing bowel control following SCI
- To understand normal bowel function and correlate dysfunctions of bowel control with level of injury
- To discuss the relevance of other factors that influence resuming bowel control
- To describe a comprehensive assessment, management, and education plan
- To describe long-term implications associated with neurogenic bowel dysfunction

A good bowel management program, so often relegated to a minor role, is as important as any other aspect of care for patients with spinal cord injuries (SCI). Devising reliable methods to regulate a bowel program involves understanding the significance of a preinjury pattern of bowel habits; the current nutritional, emotional, physical, and functional status; and the type of neurogenic bowel dysfunction exhibited, together with knowledge and appropriate skills to stimulate defecation.

A *bowel program* provides a reliable method for stimulating a bowel evacuation to take the place of the normal response, which is to defecate when the urge is felt. With complete loss of sensation and movement following SCI, voluntary expulsion and normal control over bowel activity is no longer possible. Once established, a good bowel program regulates bowel movements; avoids accidents; and prevents constipation, diarrhea, and resulting complications. A bowel program sometimes takes months to establish and requires careful management to maintain. The goals of the health care team are:

- To ensure regular and complete evacuation to preserve bowel function (without overstretching the bowel)
- To devise a reliable and convenient bowel program that patients will be able to perform or teach others how to manage. Aim for a program *no longer than 30 minutes.*
- To assist the patient with appropriate modifications of the home bathroom and securing ongoing supplies.

BOWEL DYSFUNCTION AFTER SPINAL CORD INJURY

The Large Intestine

The large intestine or colon extends from the *ileocecal valve* (which connects to the small intestine) to the *anus*. See Figure 19–1. The *cecum*, a pouchlike structure located in the right lower quadrant of the abdomen, forms the beginning of the large intestine. The *appendix* is a short outgrowth attached to the cecum. The colon then basically consists of three straight portions—the ascending, transverse, and descending sections—arranged around the abdominal perimeter. The descending colon continues downward to the pelvic brim ending in an S-shaped segment called the *sigmoid colon*. The sigmoid colon leads to a short section of bowel called the *rectum*, which terminates the intestinal tract at the anus. Two sphincters control the anal canal. The *internal anal sphincter* is a thickened portion of circular muscle surrounding the canal just inside the anus. This sphincter remains tonically contracted to

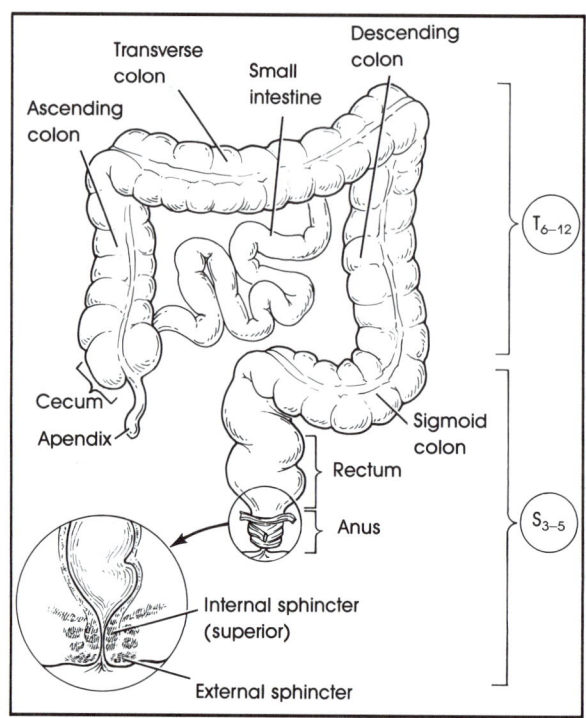

FIGURE 19–1 The large intestine: the thoracic and sacral cord segments innervate the abdominal musculature and rectal sphincters.

maintain continence. The *external anal sphincter* is the visible portion of the anus. The *levator ani* muscles also act as a sphincter of the intestine and support the rectum and pelvic floor. The unique feature of the two latter structures is the ability to contract and relax voluntarily to control bowel evacuations.

The primary functions of the large intestine are to complete the digestive process by absorbing water and electrolytes from the undigested residue and to store fecal matter until it can be expelled. The proximal half of the large intestine is concerned mainly with absorption; the distal half with storage.

Motility in the large intestine is normally sluggish and includes mixing movements to aid in digestion and propulsive movements to push fecal matter toward the anus. Circular constrictions of each pocket of the large bowel (*haustral contractions*) cause further mechanical breakdown of contents to promote absorption. Unlike the continual peristaltic movements of the small intestine (described as bowel sounds), strong peristaltic movements, called *mass movements*, occur a few times each day and push the fecal material large distances in a few seconds. Such a mass movement frequently occurs following a meal when the filling of the stomach and duodenum increases the activity of the entire colon. This action is referred to as the *gastrocolic reflex* and is generally strongest following the first meal of the day—an important fact to remember when initiating bowel retraining. Eventually, when the rectum is distended with feces, the urge to defecate is felt. The residue from any given meal is normally eliminated in 24 to 48 hours.

Neural Control of Bowel Function

The nerve supply to the large intestine includes an *intrinsic component* (located entirely within the bowel); *autonomic nervous stimulation*; and, similar to mechanisms involved in voiding, an element of *central nervous system* innervation to control the actual act of defecation.

Intrinsic control is achieved by networks of nerve fibers within the walls of the large bowel that respond to local stimulations. When the bowel becomes overdistended with fecal material peristalsis is stimulated. Because of this intrinsic factor, it is difficult to interrupt nervous stimulation, so bowel function is maintained even after severe injury to the autonomic nervous system.

The autonomic nervous system provides both parasympathetic and sympathetic stimulation to the bowel. Parasympathetic fibers emerge from the vagus nerve and sacral (S_{2-4}) outflow to terminate in the colon, rectum, and internal and external anal sphincters. Sympathetic fibers emerge from the lower thoracolumbar (T_6-L_3) outflow to innervate the same areas. The parasympathetic influence is more important to daily regularity. Parasympathetic stimulation increases motility and peristalsis, maintains tone, stimulates secretions, and usually relaxes sphincter activity; sympathetic stimulation provides antagonistic control to decrease motility, slow peristalsis, inhibit secretions, and generally contract sphincters (Chusid 1979; Guyton, 1976).

Defecation is controlled by communications from the brain, via the sacral spinal cord (S_{3-4}), to the external anal sphincter. When sufficient stool enters the rectum, the urge to defecate is felt, and if it is convenient to do so, voluntary relaxation of the external anal sphincter allows stool to be passed. If it is inappropriate to defecate, however, the external anal sphincter is kept tonically contracted until the defecation reflex is suppressed and disappears for several hours. At an appropriate time the person can stimulate the defecation reflex by abdominal straining, but this is not usually as effective as a natural reflex.

Actual elimination of stool may be aided by straining the abdominal muscles. This is accomplished by a *Valsalva maneuver* when the person takes a deep breath and attempts to exhale against a closed glottis while at the same time tightening the abdominal muscles. This action may be described as "bearing down" and requires intact innervation to the lower thoracic cord (T_{6-12}) to stimulate these accessory muscles. The actual increase in intraabdominal pressure forces stool into the rectum.

In summary, the complex mechanisms of defecation require the combined action of the intrinsic and spinal (autonomic) reflexes, aided by voluntary actions. See Figure 19–2.

Loss of Bowel Control after Injury

The location and completeness of cord injury determines the extent to which control of defecation is altered. Ba-

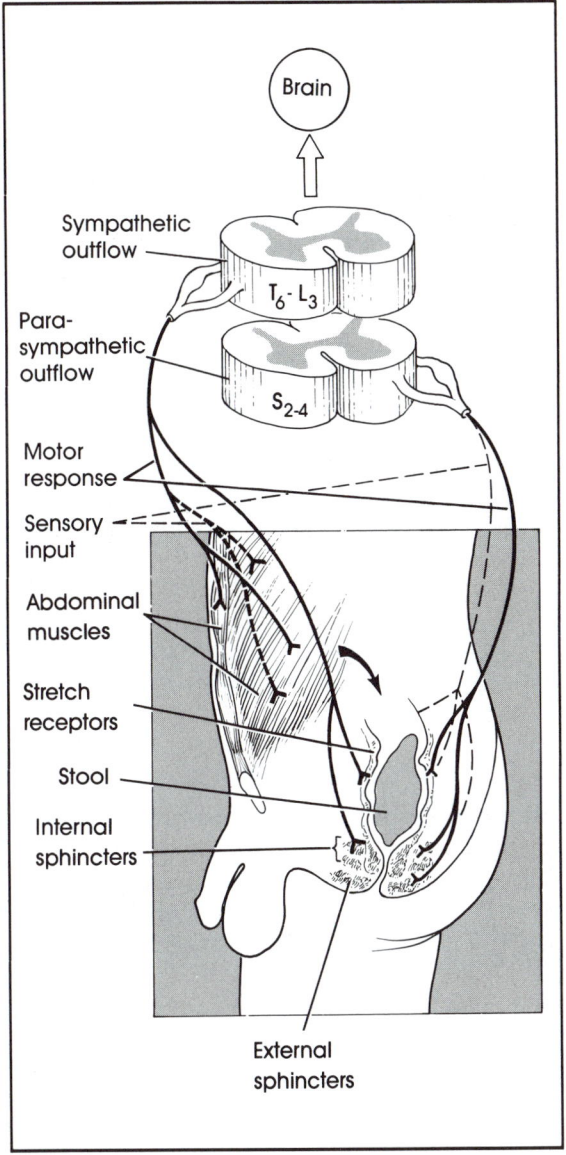

FIGURE 19–2 An upper motor neuron (UMN) lesion results in a spastic bowel function with injury at T_6–L_3 or above; injury to the spinal (autonomic) reflex center (S_{2-4}) will result in a lower motor neuron (LMN) lesion and flaccid bowel function.

sically SCI can damage either the upper motor neurons, located above the defecation reflex center in the sacral cord, or the lower motor neurons, which destroy the defecation reflex center (Connell 1967; Frankel 1967; Devroede et al. 1979; Guttman 1976). In either case voluntary control is impaired or lost due to interrupted communication with the brain.

Tests that determine perineal sensation and activity may help determine the type of neurogenic bowel dysfunction following injury.

If the patient can appreciate any sensation in the *saddle area* of the perineum, it indicates that some sensory function remains at the sacral spinal level. Any ability to sense the urge to defecate will help establish bowel control. This is most valuable information for the patient with an incomplete injury, such as a central cord injury or sacral sparing. Sensation will be absent in patients with a complete injury.

A *positive bulbocavernosus reflex* indicates that the reflex activity of the sacral cord is intact. This reflex causes a palpable and visible contracture of the anal sphincter when pressure is applied to the glans penis or clitoris. The bulbocavernosus reflex is usually present very soon after injury, before spinal shock fully subsides. It indicates an upper motor neuron bowel dysfunction.

The *anal reflex, or anal wink*, if present, also indicates an upper motor neuron bowel dysfunction. This reflex causes a visible contraction of the external anal sphincter in response to a pinprick.

Although techniques involved in the management of each are similar, the patient with upper motor neuron damage is a little easier to regulate. Note that neural damage alone does not dictate bowel habits; coping abilities, dietary intake, activity, and medication are some important variables to consider when attempting to regulate bowel activity.

Upper Motor Neuron Damage

Upper motor neuron damage occurs when injury to the cord is sustained above the conus medullaris (Figure 19–3) and the *reflex defecation center remains intact*. As this sacral portion of the cord (specifically S_{2-4} segments) corresponds to the T_{12}–L_1 vertebrae, the patient sustaining a thoracic or cervical fracture will probably experience an upper motor neuron injury. This causes *spastic* paralysis of the bowel with inability to control defecation. Reflex activity is uninhibited. Ascending sensory signals are interrupted and the patient is unable to feel the normal urge to defecate; descending motor signals are interrupted blocking the normal control of external anal sphincter activity. (Fortunately, the spastic contraction of this sphincter discourages leakage of stool.)

The rectal colon appears to function in a similar manner to the bladder; abnormal storage problems and external

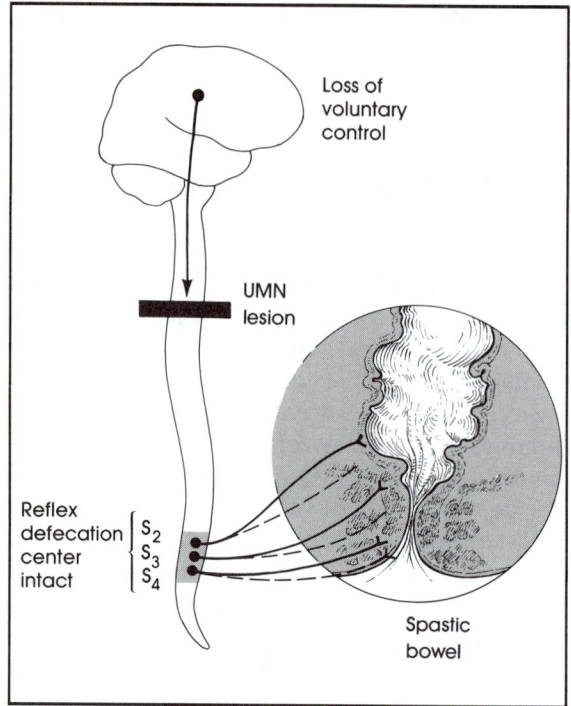

FIGURE 19–3 An upper motor neuron (UMN) lesion results in spastic bowel function. With spasticity of the rectal sphincters the anus remains closed; involuntary stools are less likely. As rectal filling proceeds, the sphincters are less able to contract. Automatic evacuation occurs.

sphincter dyssynergia may occur (Meshkinpour et al. 1983; Yarnell and Manofy 1984). That is, rectal contractions to expel stool are blocked by the external sphincter contracting at the same time. However, it is possible to establish a regular stimulation program to control bowel movements.

Lower Motor Neuron Damage

Lower motor neuron damage occurs when the injury is sustained directly to the sacral cord segments in the conus medullaris or the sacral nerve roots in the cauda equina. The *reflex defecation is damaged* directly. These injuries are generally associated with fractures of the lumbosacral spine below the T_{12} level. The lower motor neurons, which are responsible for the defecation reflex center, are destroyed, causing a *flaccid* paralysis. Loss of anal tone and the lack of tonic external sphincter contraction make defecation even more likely (Ozer 1988). See Figure 19–4. Even though intrinsic contractile responses remain, peristaltic movements are quite ineffective without the support of the spinal reflex. Fecal retention and oozing of stool through the flaccid sphincter are associated with lower motor neuron damage. As the final path-

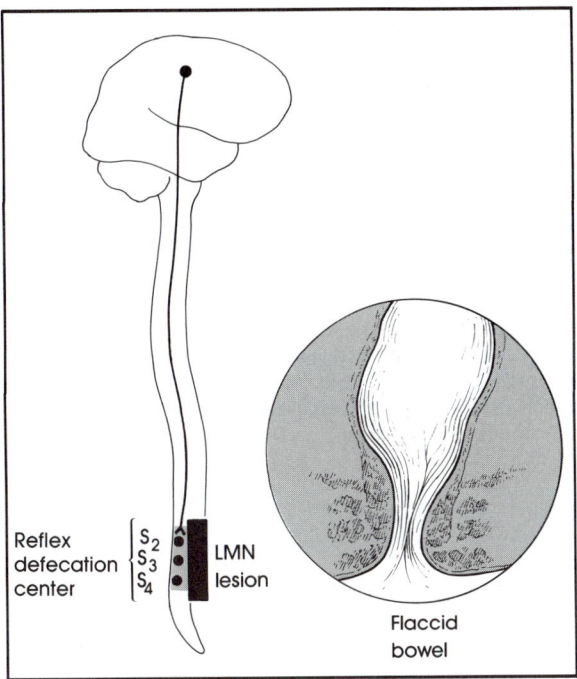

FIGURE 19–4 A lower motor neuron (LMN) lesion results in flaccid bowel function. (Damage to the reflex defecation center.)

way for sensory and motor signals is interrupted, the patient loses the ability to appreciate a normal urge to defecate and exercise voluntary control of the external anal sphincter. Table 19–1 summarizes the characteristics and management techniques involved with both types of neurogenic bowel dysfunction.

Other Factors Influencing Bowel Dysfunction

As the patient's general condition stabilizes, question the patient about past elimination patterns, nutritional and fluid intake, reaction to loss of bowel control, and any associated injuries that may negatively affect reestablishment of bowel control. If the patient's bowel habits were healthful, every effort should be made to duplicate them; if not, reeducation and modifications will be needed (Cannon 1980).

Associated Trauma

Associated abdominal injuries are not uncommon with multisystem trauma (outlined in Chapter 6). For example, a traumatic pancreatitis may cause early constipation and later diarrhea. If prolonged parenteral or enteral support is required for any reason, bowel-related problems, commonly diarrhea, may ensue. See Chapter 17.

Preinjury Elimination Patterns

Many patients are almost unaware of elimination patterns before injury. As bowel habits are a very personal and private concern, some patients may be embarrassed to discuss them. However, explaining the value of a bowel history to establish a program that will control incontinence usually overcomes this problem.

It is important to note the *frequency* of bowel movements. The definition of *normal* has a wide range. A daily bowel movement is not necessary for everyone; elimination may occur twice a day, every second day, or even every third day.

The *consistency* of the stool is much more important than the frequency of bowel movements. Therefore, ask about the nature and amount of stool. The time of day most convenient for defecation will help determine the most suitable time for a bowel program later on. It is also necessary to ask about anything that stimulates bowel action, such as exercise, hot drinks, fruits, or spicy foods; whether the patient is prone to constipation or diarrhea; and the use of laxatives, suppositories, and even enemas on a regular basis. Older patients may have preexisting bowel problems because gastrointestinal system motility generally slows with age. Occasionally preexisting bowel disease or complications may be evident.

Nutritional History

Nutritional and fluid intake is the single most important factor in achieving bowel control. Therefore it is imperative to take a detailed history assessing nutritional adequacy, food preferences, fiber content, fluid intake, cultural implications, and excessive intake of undesirable foods such as greasy ones or those high in calories but low in food value. For further discussion of nutritional data collection, see Chapter 17.

Reaction to Loss of Bowel Control

During the early stages the nurse must assume almost total responsibility for maintaining bowel elimination. This can be a most unpleasant and degrading experience for the patient, producing stressful feelings of helplessness, depression, or loss of sexuality. Nurses must make every effort to be sensitive to these feelings. As the rehabilitation process unfolds, self-care is encouraged. Again, adaptation to injury may elicit feelings of anger or depression, which may interfere with learning and coping abilities, and nurses may have to resume responsibility for the bowel program temporarily. See Chapter 9. Acknowledgment of feelings and concerns will help patients resume participation, which will increase the likelihood of a successful bowel program.

TABLE 19–1   Classifications of Neurogenic Bowel Dysfunction Following Spinal Cord Injury*

Upper Motor Neuron Dysfunction (Spastic Bowel Dysfunction)	Lower Motor Neuron Dysfunction (Flaccid Bowel Dysfunction)
Level of injury occurs above the reflex defecation center in the sacral cord.	Level of lesion damages the sacral cord involving the reflex defecation center.
Generally associated with fractures of the T_{12} vertebra (T_{11} cord segment) and above.	Generally associated with the lumbar and sacral spine (T_{12} cord segment and below).
Communication pathways between brain and reflex defecation center are interrupted; communication pathways between reflex defecation center and bowel are preserved (reflex activity recovers after passing of spinal shock). Patients are unaware of normal sensation to defecate, but may be able to identify some consistent signal that a bowel movement is imminent. Autonomic dysreflexia signs, such as sweating, increased spasticity, or headache, are not uncommon. Exercise, nutrition (fluid and fiber) management, and consistent timing are important.	Communication pathways between reflex defecation center and bowel are interrupted (loss of reflex activity); hence, communication pathways to the brain are interrupted. Patients are unaware of normal sensation to defecate and are less likely to experience a consistent signal that a bowel movement is imminent.
Bulbocavernosus and anal reflexes are positive.	Bulbocavernosus and anal reflexes are negative.
Spastic contraction of anal sphincter discourages leakage of stool, but involuntary evacuations will occur unless regulated.	Tendency toward fecal retention with oozing of stool through flaccid anal sphincter.
Evacuation may be planned for every 2 or 3 days.	Daily planned evacuation is necessary to minimize leakage of stool.
Medications and suppositories have slower than normal action but produce desired results. Once a pattern has been reestablished, it is generally possible to reduce medications.	Medications and suppositories tend to be less effective on a flaccid bowel.
Digital stimulation technique used to initate a reflex bowel evacuation. May or may not need glycerine suppository for long-term management.	Manual removal of stool is necessary. Bearing down (a Valsalva maneuver) will likely be helpful because patients have strong abdominal muscles and can force stool out. Digital stimulation is of no value because there is no reflex activity to stimulate.

*Note: An incomplete injury to the spinal cord results in varying degrees of preserved motor and/or sensory function below the level of cord injury sustained. For example, the patient may be aware of sensation to defecate but have limited or no control over bowel movements.

ASSESSMENT OF BOWEL DYSFUNCTION

Physical Assessment

Assessment of the Abdomen, Lower Bowel, and Rectal Area

Be familiar with the patient's history and physical assessment as recorded on the medical record and by communication with other team members. Awareness of previous bowel and nutritional health will help identify and evaluate potential problem areas. The physical examination should include assessment of the abdomen and assessment of the lower bowel and rectal area. See Procedures 19–1 and 19–2.

Examination of the Stool

A normal stool is softly formed and has a characteristic odor caused by the bacteria present in the large bowel to aid digestion. A normal stool is composed of 75% water and 25% solid materials, such as undigested roughage and other digestive wastes. Note any hard, dry stools that are difficult to pass or any loose, watery stools. During the first 4 weeks after injury, when gastric ulceration is most frequent, be alert for dark, tarry stools (melena).

Diagnostic Findings

An X-ray examination of the abdominal organs shows the condition of the intestinal pathways and the extent and locale of any distension. Orally administered contrast media or a contrast enema is rarely necessary (Paeslak 1966). To determine intestinal motility, espe-

Procedure 19–1   Assessment of the Abdomen

Purpose

To help determine the status of the patient's gastrointestinal system, especially to detect paralytic ileus and constipation.

Action	Rationale
1. Place patient supine and remove clothing or bed covers.	
2. Auscultate entire abdomen to listen for bowel sounds.	Complete auscultation before percussing and palpating the abdomen. These latter techniques tend to activate bowel sounds and therefore give a false impression.
• During the first 7 to 15 days after injury, be alert for occasional or absent bowel sounds.	Lack of bowel sounds indicates that paralytic ileus has not yet subsided. With the exception of manual removal of stool from rectum, it is dangerous to proceed with any laxatives, suppositories, or enemas if paralytic ileus is present.
• Note any hyperactive sounds in the small bowel.	These indicate impending diarrhea.
3. Inspect abdomen for distension. If distension is suspected, measure abdominal girth at level of umbilicus and obtain serial comparisons daily.	Always obtaining serial measurements at the umbilical level ensures more accurate comparisons of serial data.
4. Be alert for abdominal signs of constipation: • A dull sound on percussion of descending colon • Hardness or resistance of abdomen on palpation, especially on right side • Rigidity or hard stool felt in any bowel section • Referred pain, especially aggravated by assessment techniques • Increased leg spasms aggravated by assessment techniques	With neurogenic bowel dysfunction, there is a definite tendency toward constipation. These signs are caused by accumulation of fecal material, usually in the descending colon.

Procedure 19–2   Assessment of Lower Bowel and Rectal Area

Purpose

To help determine the type of neurogenic bowel that exists and to detect complications.

Action	Rationale
1. Observe external anal area for any skin excoriation and also for hemorrhoidal tissue.	Development of hemorrhoids is common for people with SCI. Causes and treatment are discussed in this chapter.
2. Use well-lubricated gloved finger to complete internal examination. Check for presence of stool in rectum. Sometimes internal hemorrhoids can be felt.	This minimizes irritation, or even trauma, to desensitized rectal area.
3. Check if patient can appreciate any sensation in *saddle* area of the perineum; also check status of *bulbocavernosus* and *anal* reflexes.	Tests that determine perineal sensation and reflex activity help determine type of neurogenic bowel dysfunction present. Their status of reflexes has implications for care. Table 19–1 summarizes types of neurogenic bowel dysfunction.

cially slowed function, radiopaque markers administered orally may be monitored as they pass through the intestinal tract (transit time).

The normal digestive flora in the bowel can be greatly reduced in patients requiring long-term administration of antibiotics.

Pseudomembranous colitis should be considered if diarrhea develops and does not respond to simple measures (Johnson and Balmaseda 1985).

Chemical and microscopic examination will determine the presence of occult blood or actual composition of the stool. If diarrhea is present a Gram's stain, stool culture, or stool for ova and parasites is useful to pinpoint the source of an infective process. A white blood cell count would also be included.

Observation of Activity Level and Functional Skills

Early activation is a most important consideration when promoting elimination. Regular turning of patients and range of motion exercises during the early phases are just as important as general physical activity when orthopedic stability allows. Eventually athletic activity is advised.

Because gravity assists bowel evacuation in the sitting position, thought must be given to toileting activities as mobility and strength are regained. Sitting tolerance, trunk balance, and ability to transfer to a commode or toilet will need to be assessed. In addition, the quadriplegic patient's hand function and ability to use arms need to be assessed before introducing self-care skills such as suppository insertion or digital stimulation. This usually requires the combined efforts of the patient, the nurse, and the occupational and physical therapists.

RESTORATIVE MANAGEMENT

Observe, on a daily basis, the effectiveness of the bowel program and collaborate with the physician to establish a reliable program for each patient. Patient cooperation is also needed to achieve this goal. A bowel program is a planned approach to avoid incontinence (Cannon 1980: 224). The objective is to produce a planned, predictable bowel movement. In other words, a fixed time pattern—the same time each day, every other day, or every third day—takes the place of normal voluntary control to avoid accidents. An individualized bowel program is based on a thorough assessment and knowledge of the type of neurogenic bowel dysfunction exhibited. The patient's general state of health, altered physiology of the lower gastrointestinal tract, activity, functional skills, and ability or willingness to participate

in the program are all aspects that must be taken into account.

Measures discussed in this general section describe methods to promote bowel elimination while the patient is on bedrest or during early mobilization. As the rehabilitation period progresses, the patient's participation must dramatically increase to ensure success. Careful consideration must also be given to the convenience and practicality of the program designed for use at home.

Assisting with Early Bowel Evacuation after Injury

When strong bowel sounds have returned, the patient may begin with clear fluids and progress from a light to a full diet. A minimum fluid intake of 2000 ml per day is recommended. Oral intake is usually possible on the second or third day after injury, unless prolonged paralytic ileus or other complications have set in. As most patients will be suffering from spinal shock at this time, a flaccid bowel can be expected.

Procedure 19–3 outlines certain measures, which, if initiated early, can avert serious problems. However, due to frequent paralytic ileus, immobilization, and lack of oral intake, it is not unusual for the patient to be without a substantial bowel movement for 5 to 7 days immediately postinjury, which is acceptable.

Frequent enemas are not necessary during the early stages. Enemas cause dilation of the lower bowel; frequent dilation overstretches the bowel musculature and causes loss of bowel tone. This is the complete opposite of the desired effect.

Administering Medications

Laxatives are greatly abused by the general public and health professional alike, and there are many erroneous ideas concerning constipation. However, during the acute postinjury period, laxatives are essential to maintain bowel elimination for most patients.

Medications helpful in establishing bowel programs include bulk-forming laxatives, stool softeners (emollient laxatives), and stimulant laxatives (Mathews and Carlson 1987). Harsh cathartics should be avoided. There is a wide and confusing variety of laxatives but little rationale to support their use and insufficient data to compare their properties. It is difficult to recommend exact medications and effective dosages, but a few general concepts are useful:

- Carefully consider the effect of medications and their action time. The paralyzed bowel is insensitive and seems to take approximately 24 hours longer to respond than a normal bowel. Increasing the dosages at

Procedure 19–3   Assisting With Early Bowel Evacuation

Purpose

To eliminate fecal material from the bowel and prevent constipation.

Action	Rationale
1. Position patient on right side if possible. If a special bed is in use, place bed flat and manually logroll patient. Alternate positions are:	This position is preferable to provide gravity-assisted evacuation.
• Supine with knees flexed and supported with pillows	Although bowel evacuation is possible in supine position on a turning frame, prone position allows better access to rectal area and therefore minimizes risk of inadvertent trauma to desensitized area.
• Prone, if patient is on a turning frame	
2. Protect bed linen with soft waterproofed pads. *Never use bedpan.*	This avoids any possible pressure or trauma to skin.
3. Insert a well-lubricated gloved finger into rectum. Gently and slowly remove fecal material.	Generous lubrication minimizes risk of trauma for patient without rectal sensation.
4. Note amount and *consistency* of stool.	
5. If stool is not too hard (and it usually is not within a few days of injury), administer a small-volume commercially prepared enema, with aid of an ordinary, well-lubricated rectal tube attached to nozzle.	Placement of enema must be high in bowel, as lack of sphincter tone makes it impossible for patient to "hold" fluid. This method is usually effective.
6. If stool is dry and hardened, or if impaction higher in the bowel is suspected, administer an oil retention enema.	When stool is softened and dislodged, it can be more easily removed from rectum.
7. Give oral laxatives as needed. Start with mild stimulant laxative on third or fourth evening after injury.	This controls stool consistency and stimulates peristalsis.

the regular suggested time interval often results in unpleasant cumulative reactions that are difficult to control. Generally, start out with the minimum recommended dosages and gradually increase until effective.

- Plan bowel evacuation to coincide with peak effectiveness of oral medications.
- Remember adequate fluid intake is essential for bulk-forming laxatives and stool softeners to work. If intake is not sufficient they will cause constipation.
- Should medications need adjusting, change only one element of the bowel program at a time and allow sufficient time to evaluate results (at least 3 days).
- Some stimulant or irritant laxatives can cause harsh side effects, such as signs and symptoms of autonomic dysreflexia; others, such as osmotic agents, may cause electrolyte imbalance. Side effects of all medications may be hard to detect, especially in quadriplegic patients, who cannot feel cramps due to lack of sensation but may experience nausea and general malaise.
- Laxatives tend to lose their effectiveness when used on a long-term basis. Dietary control and good fluid intake must take their place. Sticking to regular evacuation times is most important. Generally the need for medication decreases as activity increases. For long-term management, strong stimulant medications are best avoided.
- Plan for decreasing dosages.

Maintaining High Fluid Intake

Keeping the formation of stool soft requires a daily intake of 2000 to 3000 ml. This intake must be regulated according to the requirements of the bladder program With a diet high in fiber and/or when stool softeners or bulk-producing laxatives are used, a *high fluid intake is mandatory* to prevent cramping constipation. Stools will become elastic if these laxative dosages are too high or, more commonly, if fluid intake is too low.

Encouraging Intake of High-Fiber Foods

Dietary fiber is a complex carbohydrate that is not completely broken down by the digestive process. Fiber not only adds bulk to the stool but also promotes normal peristalsis. Table 19–2 contains a recommended high-fiber diet (minimum of 25 g dietary fiber per day).

TABLE 19–2 Shaughnessy Hospital High-Fiber Diet

Patient's Name: Dietitian:

Date: Phone:

General Instructions

1. This diet is based on Canada's Daily Food Guide.
2. At least three regular meals each day are important to establish good bowel habits and to prevent constipation.
3. Whole grain cereals and breads, sources highest in dietary fiber, must be used in place of refined cereals and breads.
4. Fruits and vegetables, cooked or raw, must be used in liberal amounts. Prunes and figs contain substances that are natural laxatives, and their use is recommended.
5. Normal amounts of liquids must be consumed each day (approximately 6 to 8 cups).
6. Excess use of concentrated sweets must be avoided.
7. Milk and milk products should be consumed as recommended by the Daily Food Guide.

Foods to Emphasize

1. All unrefined foods.

   Breads—whole grain breads, e.g., 100% whole wheat bread and bran muffins

   Cereals—coarse whole grain and bran cereals, e.g., granola, all bran, and bran buds. (2/3 cup contains 15.8–17 grams of fiber.)

   Cookies—made from coarse whole grain flours and/or fruit and nut filled, e.g., graham wafers, digestives, or oatmeal.

   Fruit—preferably raw and dried fruits. The skins of apples, peaches, and pears should be eaten. Blackberries and strawberries are good sources of fiber, too.

   Nuts and seeds.

   Soups—preferably made with fresh coarse vegetables and whole grains, e.g., barley, corn, dried peas, brown rice.

   Vegetables—preferably raw and green, leafy, e.g., carrot sticks, all salad greens, and tomatoes; potato with skin. (Cooked peas, corn, broccoli, and spinach contain 4–6.3 g of fiber for an average serving.)

2. Fats such as butter, cream, gravies, margarine, oils, salad dressings, and sauces should be included in appropriate amounts.

Foods to Restrict

1. All highly refined foods.

   Breads—white bread, refined melba toast.

   Cereals—cream of wheat, puffed rice. (1 cup of Rice Krispies contains 0.1 grams of fiber.)

   Cookies—arrowroots, social teas, plain sugar.

   Sweets—candies, rich desserts, honey, jam, jellies, and syrups.

2. Excessive amounts of fried foods.

3. Excessive use of seasonings and spices.

Suggested Meal Pattern

Refer to the lists of Foods to Emphasize and Foods to Restrict so that you can vary your menu daily.

Breakfast	*Lunch*	*Supper*
Fruit	Egg, cheese,* meat, or meat alternate	Egg, cheese,* meat or meat alternate
Whole grain cereal and/or bread	Whole grain bread and/or potato	Whole grain bread and/or potato
Fat	Fat	Fat
If desired, egg, cheese, meat, or meat alternative	Vegetable	Vegetable
	Fruit	Fruit
Milk	Milk	Milk
Beverage	Beverage	Beverage

(Table continues)

TABLE 19–2 Shaughnessy Hospital High-Fiber Diet (continued)

Between-meal nourishment, if desired, may be selected from any of the foods listed under Foods to Emphasize.

Your friends and family want to bring some food for you? Please ask them to select among the items below. These foods are nutritious and also contribute to increasing your fiber intake.

1. Fresh fruits: apples, peaches, pears, bananas, oranges, plums.

2. Nuts and seeds: dried fruits such as prunes, raisins, dates, and apricots; trail mix (mixture of dried fruits and nuts).

3. Granola bars.

4. Date square; banana/carrot/nut/dried fruit loaves; peanut butter and oatmeal cookies; fruit crisps; cinnamon rolls made with whole wheat flour; bran muffin; muffins made with dried fruits or nuts or whole wheat flour. Rye and wheat snacks are good too.

*An additional iron source must be chosen when cheese is substituted for egg, meat, or meat alternate.
Source: Shaughnessy Hospital, Vancouver, B.C.

Fiber aids in stool formation by absorbing many times its own weight in water. This makes a larger and softer stool that is more stimulating to the rectal wall, is more easily passed, and thus helps prevent constipation. In North America many foods are prepared with refined flour and sugar, which are low in fiber. A diet restricted in fiber will result in formation of very firm, often dehydrated stools that are difficult for the bowel to pass. Natural elimination is also assisted by a high intake of dietary fiber because it stimulates the muscle lining of the colon to move stools along.

The chief sources of fiber are the *bran* of whole grain breads and cereals and the *cellulose* of fresh raw fruits and vegetables with skins and seeds. Nuts are another good source.

To avoid cramping or discomfort, natural laxative foods must be introduced *gradually*. It is wise to start with cereal or cereal products and then increase the amounts of cooked fruits and vegetables before introducing raw ones. Unprocessed bran may also be added. Generally, one to two ounces daily will be sufficient for an adult. Bran can be sprinkled on cereals, taken in yogurt, used in baking, or added to casseroles and sauces. Prune juice and orange juice are well-known natural laxatives. One or two tablespoons of a fruit laxative (a mixture of one-third each dates, prunes, and figs, blended with a little water) may also be given.

Eating at regular times and incorporating many high-fiber foods in the diet will help the patient attain the goal of more predictable, natural bowel training. Dietary measures to control stool consistency, maintain bowel tone, and prevent constipation are of great value to maintain a healthful, long-term bowel management program (Meiners 1976; Ozer 1988).

Promoting Physical Activity

Encourage as much activity as orthopedic stability will allow. Inactivity reduces food needs and slows muscular and physiological responses. When patients are on bedrest, vigorous exercises to unaffected limbs and range of motion exercises to paralyzed limbs help prevent sluggish bowel activity that leads to constipation. Encouraging patients with such skills as feeding, dressing, grooming, and pushing their own wheelchairs promotes rehabilitation activities that also improve general bowel function.

Selecting Consistent Time for Evacuation

Planning a consistent time for evacuation each day is vital to successful bowel retraining. Unless the same hour is used each time, defecation will take longer to stimulate and constipation may occur more easily.

To begin with in an acute setting, a bowel program established every other morning is usually sufficient and most convenient. To take advantage of the *gastrocolic reflex*, plan bowel stimulation 30 to 60 minutes after breakfast or dinner—whichever suits the patient better.

As the rehabilitation period progresses it is wise to review the timing of the bowel program to consider preinjury habits and home schedule. During rehabilitation, the patient will begin to realize how difficult it is to stick to a rigid schedule. There are times when establishing bowel control must take priority over early morning therapy class or evening recreational activities. When changing the bowel routine from a morning to an evening schedule, it will take 2 or 3 weeks to reestablish regularity.

408

Providing Privacy

Privacy is an important issue in developing a bowel regulation plan. Bowel procedures are distasteful and stressful to most patients and heighten feelings of asexuality, regression, and helplessness. Patients are most aware of the sounds and odors created when they are on bedrest and other people are around in the room. To minimize the patient's embarrassment:

- Place a few drops of a strong liquid deodorizer on a paper towel at the bedside.
- Turn the radio up.
- Drape the patient fully.
- Pin the curtains closed to avoid interruptions.

It is hard to believe that some care givers insist on "getting the bowel record straight" during visiting hours and are insensitive to this invasion of the patient's privacy. At a summer camp for disabled adults, to be aware of the bowel functions of the "camper" population, a nurse posted a sign in the corridor asking the counselors to check on and record the campers' "performance." During the night the list was replaced with graphic details of the counselors' bowel habits—the nurse's at the top of the list! Message received.

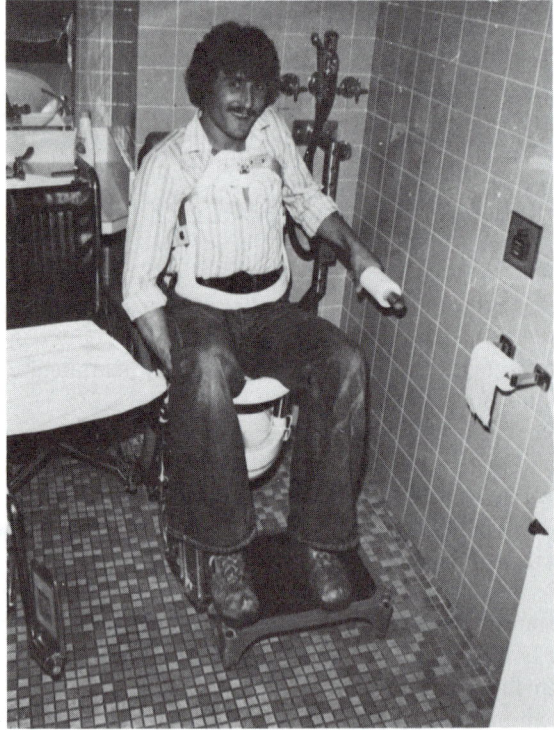

FIGURE 19–5 A paraplegic patient performs a toilet transfer. Note the padded *raised* toilet seat (allowing easier access to the rectal area), the grab bar, and footstool used as aids.

Family members may also be a source of embarrassment for the patient. Many patients cannot accept having a family member, particularly a spouse, learn about such procedures. This should not be pushed for the sake of gaining independence in the home. If this is so, whenever possible make alternate arrangements for care if the patient will not be able to manage independently.

Positioning the Patient

Methods to position patients in bed are described in Chapter 20. In general, having the patient positioned on the left side promotes absorption of suppositories or enemas by using gravity to assist the anatomical structure of the sigmoid colon; conversely, positioning the patient on the right side aids in evacuation of stool.

The sitting position takes the most advantage of gravity assistance in bowel evacuation and the patient who can sit on the toilet in the bathroom gains privacy. *Initiate toilet transfers* (see Figure 19–5) when spinal stability is achieved or protected adequately with braces, and when balance and tolerance are adequate to allow completion of the procedure (30 to 60 minutes). This generally means the patient can tolerate 2 to 4 hours up in the wheelchair. Bowel procedures can be exhausting, especially for the quadriplegic patient who has an initial tendency to faint with the additional stress of these procedures. Collaborate with therapists to determine transfer capabilities and to determine use of aids in the bathroom.

Care must be taken when placing the patient on the toilet. It is important not to part the buttocks, which will cause tension on the cleft of the gluteal crease. On the other hand the buttocks must not be compressed, which would inhibit evacuation (Ford and Duckworth 1987). Especially for the heavier patient, placement of a towel underneath the thighs helps to transfer the patient to the toilet, because the towel makes it easier to grip and control the patient. Also be cautious on bathroom floors that may become wet, slippery, and unsafe.

A *raised toilet seat* improves access to the anal area for suppository insertion, digital stimulation, or manual evacuation of stool. It also makes transfers easier because of the compatible height with the wheelchair. Commode chairs or a shower chair that doubles as a commode chair can also be used, but generally they are not as sturdy; good arm, foot, and back supports are essential for *safety* and *comfort*. If the commode has castors, it can be wheeled over the toilet, but reliable brakes are essential. Some models have side openings that improve access to the perineal area.

To protect the patient's skin, the toilet seat must be *padded*. Padded backrests are also available. Powdering the seat will prevent the patient from sticking. Patients must not remain sitting too long, especially patients who are thin and without sensation. Decreased circulation can cause both pressure areas and hemorrhoids.

To aid with balance, a *footstool* is needed because of the added height of the toilet seat. Grab bars are also useful for assisting with transfers and maintaining balance.

Be constantly aware of *safety*. Using the toilet for bowel elimination is desirable but not always practical. Tolerance must be developed. If balance is poor or spasms may cause a loss of position, additional stability can be attained by securing the patient to the backrest or commode with a safety buzzer or some other way to notify staff quickly and easily in the event that problems develop.

Other Factors That Facilitate Bowel Evacuation

Patients who have strong abdominal muscles (innervated from T_{6-12}) can bear down (Valsalva maneuver) to initiate defecation. This technique is contraindicated for patients with cardiac problems. Clockwise massage of the abdomen may stimulate stool evacuation. Also to increase intraabdominal pressure, instruct patients to lean forward if their balance is sufficient and movement is not restricted by braces.

In general, use any stimulating agents, such as hot liquids, that have been helpful to the patient in the past, and avoid things that have led to constipation.

Stimulation Techniques

Although many measures, such as nutritional management and maintaining physical activity, are common to all patients with SCI, actual stimulation techniques differ slightly. The following information is partially based on the work of Emerick (1979) and Cannon (1980).

Upper Motor Neuron Dysfunction
To determine the passing of spinal shock, which indicates a transition from a flaccid to a more spastic bowel, carefully observe patients with fracture sites above the T_{12} vertebra for leg spasms; reflex erections, especially during catheterizations; and a positive bulbocavernosus or anal wink reflex. If these signs are present, an upper motor neuron dysfunction is indicated and the techniques given in Procedure 19–4 apply.

Lower Motor Neuron Dysfunction
When the patient exhibits a flaccid paralysis of the extremities and/or the bulbocavernosus and anal wink reflexes are absent, a lower motor neuron dysfunction exists. This may be temporary, as in spinal shock; or permanent, when the patient has a conus medullaris or cauda equina injury (generally associated with fractures at or below the T_{12}–L_1 vertebrae). See Procedure 19–5 for special techniques.

For all patients it is important to note any return of sensation, sometimes experienced when a catheter is passed or during perineal care. An incomplete injury may exist and ability to feel is valuable in bowel management.

Recording

Accurate and comprehensive recording of bowel program results is often difficult in an acute care setting. Standard clinical records provide only a small space to check whether bowel movements have occurred, and collected data frequently become lost when charted in the nurse's notes. To meet this need, a clinical sheet may be devised or adapted. Note, however, that from the legal point of view, it is unwise to add forms without appropriate consent.

Many rehabilitation centers have developed bowel program records to include information about medication, stimulation techniques, facilities used, stool consistency, and results obtained. See Figure 19–6. Detailed records may be necessary only during the beginning stages of retraining or for problem solving. Asking the patient to keep the menu and record nutritional intake for a few days often helps detect causes of problems.

Evaluation

Patient involvement in continual evaluation is essential to a successful program. Evaluation encompasses the rehabilitation/education process. Anxiety and stress levels, cognitive abilities, and coping strategies will give direction to the process. Usually ensuring the patients' understanding will help them cooperate. Keep patients well informed about their progress, any necessary adjustments to the program, and the reason for change. Explain the relationship between fluid and dietary intake and stool consistency; and between physical exercise and bowel motility. Provide information about medications and suppositories, including action time (the time between intake or insertion and bowel movement), dosage, side effects, and changes necessary.

Common problems are deliberate constipation to avoid bowel procedures, unpalatable laxatives, and bowel programs that are impractical because they are too time consuming. Aim for a program of 30 minutes.

A successful bowel program will result in:

- An adequate amount of softly formed stool
- Stimulation of defecation at regular and predicted intervals to ensure adequate bowel elimination
- Freedom from bouts of constipation and diarrhea

SPECIFIC MANAGEMENT OF COMPLICATIONS

Constipation

Constipation may be described as difficult or infrequent passing of hard stools. The longer the stool is retained in the

Procedure 19–4   Stimulation of the Defecation Reflex for a Patient with Upper Motor Neuron Dysfunction (Digital Stimulation Technique)

Purpose

To evacuate stool adequately from the lower bowel, using suppositories and the digital stimulation technique. Eventually it is desirable to use digital stimulation alone to produce reflex elimination.

Action	Rationale
1. Stimulate defecation reflex at a planned time, usually every other day:	
• Insert suppository against rectal mucosa.	*Contact with rectal mucosa is essential for absorption;* this is not possible if suppository is directly inserted into stool.
• Insert suppository 15 to 30 minutes ahead of planned evacuation time, usually just before breakfast.	This takes advantage of the gastrocolic reflex, which naturally stimulates defecation.
• Try glycerine suppository first (medium strength). If it is ineffective, try stronger bisacodyl (Dulcolax) suppository, but watch for signs of autonomic dysreflexia.	Starting with weaker medication can prevent undesirable cumulative effects.
2. Ask patient to:	
• Attempt evacuation on toilet if possible.	These measures assist with defecation.
• Bear down (Valsalva maneuver) if abdominal muscles are strong.	Do not teach Valsalva maneuver if patient has a cardiac problem.
• Massage abdomen in clockwise manner.	
• Lean forward, if possible.	
3. If no bowel movement has occurred within 15 to 30 minutes, attempt *digital stimulation* (National Rehabilitation Hospital, 1988):	
• Glove, lubricate, and *gently* insert index finger 1/2 to 1 inch (or to first finger joint) into the rectum.	Generous lubrication minimizes risk of traumatizing rectum. Digital stimulation is contraindicated if any rectal bleeding or hemorrhoids are present. Digital stimulation stretches and relaxes anal sphincters. Again, bearing down and abdominal massage may be helpful. This is essential to empty the bowel completely and prevent accidents.
• Gently move finger in circular motion (approximately 5 circles) until internal sphincter relaxes. (Simple insertion may be enough for one patient; a full massage may be necessary for another.)	
• Do not stimulate for more than 1 minute.	
• Stop if severe spasms of the anal sphincter occur or if signs of autonomic dysreflexia appear.	
• Once sphincter is relaxed, allow stool to pass. Repeat in 5 minutes to ensure that all stool has passed.	
4. If no results in 1 hour (after digital stimulation every 15 minutes), repeat suppository.	
5. If no bowel movement has occurred, repeat entire procedure next day. If this is not successful, take measures to treat constipation.	Assessment and interventions to alleviate constipation are detailed in this chapter.
6. Evaluate timing of the program.	To begin program some may prefer a daily evacuation until a reliable bowel pattern is identified. A consistent pattern of a large, soft stool one day and a small, soft stool the next signals that an every-other-day program would be appropriate. If stool consistency remains soft, an every-third-day program may be attempted. Twice weekly may be sufficient for some, but not good if patient develops lethargy, poor appetite, or autonomic dysreflexia during evacuation.

Procedure 19–5   Evacuation Methods Used for a Patient with Lower Motor Neuron Dysfunction

Purpose

To evacuate stool adequately from the lower bowel using suppositories and manual removal.

Action	Rationale
1. Time program according to patient's activity. While patients are on bedrest every other day is usually sufficient, but when mobilization begins, a daily bowel program is recommended.	When patient is active any stool in rectum may be expelled whenever the intraabdominal pressure is increased (e.g., during transfers). Accidents can be prevented by evacuating any stool in rectum before periods of activity. In addition, though, a major evacuation should be carried out daily.
2. Ask patient to: • Transfer to toilet, if possible • Bear down (Valsalva maneuver) • Massage the abdomen • Lean forward, if possible	These measures are all helpful to initiate defecation. Strong abdominal muscles and measures to increase intraabdominal pressure help force stool through flaccid anal sphincters.
3. If these measures are ineffective, manually remove stool from rectum with generously lubricated gloved finger.	This must be done with caution to avoid trauma to the desensitized rectum.
4. After removing stool from lower rectum, insert a strong stimulant suppository (such as bisacodyl or senna preparations) as high as possible against rectal wall.	This stimulates colon (via intrinsic or local reflexes) to empty stool into rectum, where it can be expelled or removed manually.
5. Examine stool consistency.	Stool consistency is a vital factor for these patients, as loose stools leak through a flaccid anal sphincter and hard stools are difficult to remove.
6. If these techniques are ineffective, repeat entire procedure next day. If this is not successful, take measures to treat constipation.	

colon, the drier it becomes, because water is continually absorbed by the colon. Constipation is the most common complication encountered with neurogenic bowel dysfunction. Interrupted defecation mechanisms result in sluggish movement of fecal material through the bowel. This may be aggravated by insufficient bulk in the diet, low fluid intake, inactivity, immobilization, and inconsistent bowel management techniques.

Progressive accumulation of feces may result in *impaction*—a mass of stool that blocks the bowel. Signs and symptoms of impaction are similar to those of constipation. The two conditions will be discussed together.

Goals of care are to assist patients with evacuation of constipated stool or relieve impaction and to evaluate and adjust bowel program to prevent recurrence.

Closely observe patients most at risk of developing constipation—the elderly; those with preexisting difficulties; and, especially, those with lower motor neuron bowel dysfunction. Lower motor neuron loss makes regulation more difficult to achieve. The destruction of the sacral segments or roots causes loss of spinal reflex activity and, in turn, an atonic bowel with diminished propulsive forces and tone. The colon does not automatically respond to distension of

its walls with feces, and peristalsis is not stimulated as it is for patients with higher cord injuries.

Management

1.   Look for signs and symptoms of constipation, such as loss of appetite, abdominal discomfort or referred pain (quadriplegic patients may feel unusually irritable or experience headache or diaphoresis, nausea, and even vomiting), and a hard or distended abdomen. If the patient is continually oozing liquid or loose stool, impaction is a possible cause.

2.   Check the bowel program record for number of days since the last bowel movement, the quantity of stool produced, and fecal consistency. Be sure to check this information with the patient; some will insist they are constipated if only one day has been missed.

3.   Institute vigorous treatment if no bowel movement has occurred for 4 or 5 days. The sooner interventions are started, the more effective they will be. Emerick (1979) suggests some of the following measures. Perform a rectal examination to determine presence of stool in the lower bowel. Gently break up and manually remove any stool in the rectum. If the patient is oozing stool around an impacted

BOWEL TRAINING PROGRAM RECORD

BOWEL TRAINING PROGRAM COMPONENTS

DIETARY ADJUNCTS:
HIGH FIBER DIET

FLUIDS:
2,000 cc / 24 hrs.

POSITION:
ON TOILET

FREQUENCY:
Q o EVE

TIME OF DAY:
2000

STIMULI:
DIGITAL STIMULATION

DIAGNOSIS: *C₇ QUAD*

PRIMARY NURSE: *PAT COVINGTON, RN*

MEDICATIONS:
PERICOLACE 100 mg PO BID
DULCOLAX SUPP. PR c̄ BOWEL PROGRAM

DATE	START TIME	MANUAL CHECK	STIMULI	RESULTS	RESULT TIME	POSITION	HEMOCCULT GUAIAC +/-	EPISODE OF INCONT.	COMMENTS/INITIALS
6-29-89	2000	SF	DULCOLAX DIGSTIM	LF	2100	OVER TOILET	∅	NO	PT. INSERTED SUPPOSITORY — P.C.

SIGNATURES

Pat Covington RN

KEY: FOR MANUAL CHECK, RESULTS, AND
INCONTINENCE COLUMNS.

Stool Amount
L = Large
M = Moderate
S = Small

Stool Consistency
L = Liquid
H = Hard
F = Formed
S = Soft

FIGURE 19–6 Bowel training program record. (Courtesy of National Rehabilitation Hospital, Washington, DC, © 1989)

fecal mass, it may be possible to feel such a mass and proceed with manual removal. A mineral oil retention enema may be used before manual removal of stool to soften the fecal mass or a small-volume cleansing enema may be placed high in the bowel using a rectal tube following the procedure. Throughout these procedures be constantly alert for the onset of *autonomic dysreflexia* in the high paraplegic and quadriplegic patient.

4. Administer a stimulant laxative if impaction is located above the rectum. Medication, such as large doses of senna (Senokot) tablets—four tablets twice a day for 1 or 2 days—is usually well tolerated and effective in moving stool to the rectum where it can be expelled or manually removed.

5. Ensure the bowel is empty before restarting the program. Reassess the effectiveness of diet, fluids, medications or suppositories, activity, time of planned evacuation, and stimulation techniques used, and initiate appropriate changes. Remember to alter only one aspect of the bowel program at a time and observe for at least 1 day to allow accurate evaluation.

6. Pain, tension, surgical intervention, and emotional upsets may slow bowel activity. Identify the relationship of these additional stresses to bowel elimination and initiate appropriate interventions to relieve the case.

7. Evaluate the program daily until regularity is achieved.

Expected Outcomes

Evaluate effectiveness of treatment according to level of outcome criteria reached:

- Patient satisfied and actively involved in plan; has a preventive focus and problem-solving skills
- Bowel movement of normal color, amount, and consistency at planned evacuation times (at least twice a week)
- Daily bowel movement of adequate formed stool for those with lower motor neuron bowel dysfunction
- Good appetite
- Abdomen soft and flat without evidence of discomfort, referred pain, or distension
- No signs or symptoms of autonomic dysreflexia

Diarrhea

Diarrhea may be described as the frequent passing of watery stool. The frequency and, to a lesser extent, the fluidity of bowel movements is relative to the habits of each individual. For some, three bowel movements a day is quite normal. For patients with neurogenic bowel dysfunction, diarrhea usually reflects an upset in the gastrointestinal system rather than an infective process, although the latter possibility should not be ruled out. Diarrhea is often related to ingestion of different foods or alcohol; excessive use of laxatives; or possibly side effects of other medications, especially antibiotics. Anxiety and stress may also be contributing factors. The possibility of impaction must always be investigated. Diarrhea cannot be treated without determining the cause.

Goals of care are to initiate early corrective treatment, to prevent skin breakdown of perineal area, and to evaluate and adjust bowel program to prevent recurrence.

Management

1. Discuss patient concerns and cooperation with plan; reinforce teaching; and encourage active participation (Rehabilitation Nursing 1987).

2. Take measures to avoid diarrhea. Foods and fluids that stimulated diarrhea in the past will do so after injury. Spicy foods and too many fruit juices can interrupt a well-regulated bowel program. If constipation is suspected, refrain from increasing laxatives too quickly and always begin with minimal dosages. Remember cautious adjustments to the bowel program will prevent accumulation of undesired effects that are difficult to control. Closely observe patients with preexisting tendencies to develop diarrhea.

3. Carefully observe the patient's drug profile. Many antibiotics and certain antacids have side effects that can contribute to diarrhea and may need to be discontinued. Antibiotics may also result in *pseudocolitis* by destroying natural bacteria in the bowel.

4. Avoid harsh laxatives at all costs. Strong cathartics such as castor oil are routinely used before certain X-ray procedures, such as the intravenous pyelogram. Although the bowel must be cleared to visualize the urinary tract, this type of routine should be modified for patients with SCI. For example, you might schedule the diagnostic procedure after a routine bowel evacuation. Otherwise uncontrolled diarrhea, with all its other ramifications and patient discomforts, may persist for 1 or 2 weeks.

5. Determine whether the patient is impacted. Check the bowel program record for previous signs of constipation. Perform a rectal examination to determine if a fecal mass is blocking normal passage of stool. If such a mass cannot be felt rectally, palpate the abdomen over the area of the large intestine to feel any hardened areas. Abdominal distension, discomfort, or referred pain with loss of appetite or nausea and vomiting may also be present. Collaborate with the physician to follow measures for relief of impaction. Remember that with neurogenic bowel dysfunction, diarrhea, resulting from liquid stool oozing past the blockage of fecal matter, is a common sign of impaction.

6. Determine whether diarrhea is the result of an infective process. Observe for systemic signs of a fever. Stool may be an abnormal color or foul smelling. Obtain stool specimens as ordered for culture, ova, and parasites. A complete blood count and differential may show abnormality. In bacterial infection, the white blood cell count will be elevated. In extremely rare cases septicemia—characterized by a de-

crease in consciousness level, persistent high fever, and signs of hypovelemic shock—may ensue. Follow interventions as ordered by physician and take measures to isolate the patient to stop spread of infection.

7. Replace fluid and electrolyte loss if patient has become dehydrated. Watch for decreased amounts of concentrated urine or dryness of skin and mucous membranes. The patient may have to return temporarily to a 4-hour intermittent catheterization schedule to compensate for a higher fluid intake. Drinks, for example, Gatorade, and broths are recommended for their high sodium and potassium content. Milk, fruits, and high-roughage foods should be avoided for a few days. Plain yogurt is good to restore normal bowel flora.

8. Administer prescribed drugs if diarrhea persists. Lomotil or kaolin with pectin may decrease gastric mobility and fluid loss.

9. Ensure the bowel is empty before restarting the program. Reassess the effectiveness of diet, fluids, medications or suppositories, activity, time of planned evacuation, and stimulation techniques, and initiate appropriate changes. Remember to alter only one aspect of the bowel program at a time and observe for at least 1 day to allow accurate evaluation.

10. Evaluate program daily until regularity is achieved.

Expected Outcomes

Evaluate effectiveness of treatment according to level of outcome reached:

- Bowel movement of normal color, odor, and consistency at planned evacuation times
- Stool cultures negative
- CBC and electrolytes within normal limits
- General condition satisfactory without evidence of infection, dehydration, or loss of appetite
- Abdomen soft and flat without evidence of distension or firmness
- Patient satisfied and actively involved with plan with a preventive focus

Hemorrhoids

Hemorrhoids are varicosities of the veins around the rectal and anal areas. These dilated blood vessels may occur outside the anal sphincter or within the sphincter but beneath the mucous membranes. In the general population straining with constipated stool is a common cause. For patients with SCI a number of additional factors may impair venous circulation from the rectal area. Changes in the autonomic nervous system tend to produce a general passive state of vasodilation, which hampers venous return to the heart. Lack of position change, extended time periods spent on the toilet, and, occasionally, rough manual stimulation of the bowel will cause local trauma to the rectal area. Bowel

irregularity and sometimes preexisting tendencies will aggravate the situation.

Goals of care are to alleviate the cause, to heal the affected areas and arrest any bleeding, to prevent secondary infection, and to minimize risk of recurrence.

Management

1. Promote circulation to the rectal area. Ensure pressure relief by position changes every half-hour when the patient is up in the wheelchair. Do not let patients sit on the toilet too long during a bowel program. The entire body weight against the toilet seat can rapidly diminish circulation to the area. Pressure relief lifts are a good idea if the patient is able to perform them. One hour should be the maximum toilet time.

2. Closely observe patients who are at additional risk: those with preexisting occurrence; those who tend to become constipated; and, especially, those with lower motor neuron damage. The degree of vasodilation tends to be greater with flaccid paralysis, and these patients require more manual manipulation of the rectal area to evacuate stool. Generously lubricating the gloved finger will minimize trauma to the rectal wall. When patients are learning manual techniques, too vigorous stimulation may be a problem if they become frustrated or angry. Emphasize the importance of gloving (or use of finger cot) for added protection, even if in a hurry and stool evacuation is frequent.

3. Observe stool and cleaning tissue for blood—a most common sign of internal hemorrhoids. (External hemorrhoids are easily identified). Although pain and itching may not be felt, an increase in leg spasticity in patients with higher injuries may be a clue.

4. Stop or proceed very gently with bowel procedures. It may be possible to reinsert external hemorrhoids with the use of a lubricant when the patient has returned to bed. Warm daily baths may also help to promote circulation. Ice packs should be used cautiously, as they can easily burn the skin.

5. Administer anti-inflammatory suppositories or topical ointments as ordered. Occasionally the physician may incise or inject the hemorrhoidal tissue. In rare instances anal fissures or fistulas may develop (Taylor, Berni, and Hornig 1973).

6. Clean and dry the rectal area thoroughly following each bowel movement or every 8 hours to prevent secondary infection.

7. Reassess the effectiveness of the bowel program. Take measures to avoid constipation. Collaborate with the dietitian to alter diet and add stool softeners to bowel medications (as ordered) to produce a softer stool if necessary.

Expected Outcomes

Evaluate effectiveness of treatment according to level of outcome criteria reached:

- No evidence of external hemorrhoids or rectal bleeding
- Bowel program well established
- No evidence of aggravated leg spasticity in those with higher injuries
- Person actively participating in management with a preventive focus and problem-solving skills

Autonomic Dysreflexia

Autonomic dysreflexia or *hyperreflexia* is mainly characterized by a sudden, severe headache secondary to an uncontrolled elevation of blood pressure, which, if untreated, may progress to fatal complications, such as cerebral hemorrhage or myocardial infarction. As signs and symptoms may be precipitated by routine bowel evacuations, individuals and staff, particularly assistants who are involved in bowel care, should be familiar with its onset and treatment to avoid a medical emergency. Chapter 16 outlines this pathophysiology in detail. Although the most frequent source of abnormal stimuli is bladder overdistension, rectal stimulation and a blocked bowel are also common causes. Autonomic dysreflexia can be an isolated incident precipitated by a full bowel or may recur during routine bowel procedures.

HEALTH EDUCATION AND DAILY LIVING SKILLS (DLS)

Patients must be taught principles of good bowel management. To achieve regularity and control stool consistency, emphasis is placed on maintenance of a high fluid intake, a high-fiber diet, and as much physical activity as possible. Prolonged use of laxatives irritates the bowel, which results in decreased tone; the laxatives then become less and less effective (Virginia SCI Manual 1988).

A mechanical approach offers the most effective bowel control, that is, without stimulant laxatives and without irritant contact suppositories (Cornell, Campion, Bacero, Fracier, Kjellstrom, and Purdy 1973). Advantages include:

- Less time required for evacuation to occur after stimulation
- Less chance that evacuation will not occur after stimulation
- Less chance of accidental evacuation

Persons with Paraplegia

Persons with paraplegia are generally physically capable of becoming totally independent with all aspects of bowel care. Good arm function and upper body strength enable the person to perform toilet transfers and cope with supposito-

ries, digital stimulation, and manual extraction of stool with relative ease. Occupational therapists can help organize bowel equipment and, following a home assessment, recommend bathroom alterations. Often only additional hand rails are needed; a padded, raised toilet seat may not be necessary. Ongoing arrangements for equipment and supplies must be included. Disposable, plastic sandwich bags are good substitutes for gloves.

Persons with Quadriplegia

Bowel care is much more difficult for quadriplegic persons because of poor dexterity, weak arms, and difficulty balancing on the toilet (see Ford and Duckworth 1987).

For independent bowel care, a person must be able to transfer to the toilet or commode or assume a side-lying position in bed. Equipment may be needed for digital stimulation. A loop attached to a wrist device and tension applied to isolate the middle finger for insertion or a smooth plastic digital stimulator may be necessary. Some people will require suppository inserters. Handles can be individually designed for optimal angle insertion, or a compression ejector device may be needed. Some wrist strength or wrist splinting to maneuver most devices is required. Arm placement must, of course, be adequate to reach the rectal area.

Following bowel procedures, cleanliness must be considered. Initial cleansing with toilet paper may require the use of an adaptive holder. Most people will probably need to return to bed to wash the perineal area, or they may take a shower if convenient. The buttocks should be washed with mild soap and water and thoroughly dried to prevent odor and skin breakdown. At home, a rectangular plastic storage unit, with legs, may be more stable to manage than a regular wash basin. Close collaboration with therapists is essential to teach this independent living skill, and home bathroom renovations, often using a commode, will likely be more extensive. Obviously, resources to obtain equipment and supplies must be included also.

The very high quadriplegic person (C_{1-4}) will be unable to maintain a safe balance when on the toilet and to proceed with manual skills. Such people will require assisstance but need to be able to supervise others.

LONG-TERM IMPLICATIONS

When assessing a person who has been paralyzed for some time, keep in mind that planned and regular evacuation is a realistic goal, although there is always a tendency toward constipation. Should problems occur, nothing but a multifaceted assessment will identify the problems accurately. Based on that assessment, help persons continue with desirable components of current practice, provide appropriate intervention, or refer to other resources, such as a nutritional counselor or rehabilitative facility, to update their skills. Be alert with the person who has bouts of constipation. Underlying depression, inactivity, or lack of social or vocational opportunities may be major contributing factors.

It is wise to follow the patient very closely for the first month following discharge from a rehabilitation facility, for this is when bowel accidents are most likely to occur. If the bowel program was well established in the hospital, reassure them that it will probably settle down as they adjust to home life and routines become more established. Many people with SCI agree that fear of having a bowel accident or failure to achieve bowel management can lead to social isolation.

In severe situations, enterostomies have been performed to manage complications such as bowel tumors, prolapse, or fecal contamination of pressure ulcers. Bowel care is considerably more convenient (Frisbie, Tun, and Nauyen 1986).

REFERENCES

Cannon, B. 1980. Bowel function. In *Comprehensive Rehabilitation Nursing*. Eds. N. Martin, N. Holt, and D. Hicks. New York: McGraw-Hill, pp. 223–241. *Normal and altered function of neurogenic bowel disease, assessment, management, and common complications. Highly recommended.*

Chusid, J. 1979. *Correlative Neuroanatomy and Functional Neurology*. 17th ed. Los Altos, CA: Lange Medical Publications. Chapter 6. *Describes physiology and effects of the autonomic nervous system on the gastrointestinal system and defecation.*

Connell, A. 1967. The physiology and pathophysiology of constipation. *International Journal of Paraplegia* 4 (Feb.): 244–250. *Review of normal and altered bowel habits and defecation patterns following SCI.*

Cornell, S., Campion, L., Bacero, S., Frazier, J., Kjellstrom, M., and Purdy, S. 1973. Comparison of three bowel management programs during rehabilitation of spinal cord injured patients. *Nursing Research* 22 (4): 321–328.

Devroede, G., et al. 1979. Traumatic constipation. *Gastroenterology* 77: 1258–1267. *Examines four ambulatory patients with trauma to the lumbar spine resulting in chronic constipation; includes detailed explanation of diagnostic aids—marker studies to measure transit time in the bowel and rectal pressure and reflex studies.*

Emerick, C. 1979. Nursing management of the neurogenic bowel. *Association of Rehabilitation Nurses Journal* 4 (Jan.–Feb.): 15–16. *Excellent reference on altered physiology, the effects of diet and medications on a bowel program, and related nursing care.*

Ford, R. D., and Duckworth, B. 1987. *Physical Management for the Quadriplegic Patient*. Philadelphia: F. A. Davis. *An excellent pictoral guide to bowel management adapted to functional abilities and for home use. Suppository aids, methods, and position for insertion; equipment for digital stimulation; and positions and methods of cleansing are thoroughly presented.*

Frankel, H. 1967. Bowel training. *International Journal of Paraplegia* 4 (Feb.): 254–258. *Principles of bowel management during and after spinal shock.*

Frisbie, J., Tun, C., and Nauyen, C. 1986. Effect of enterostomy on quality of life in SCI patients. *American Journal of Paraplegia*. 9 (1–2): 3–5.

Guttman, L. 1976. *Spinal Cord Injuries Comprehensive Management and Research*. 2d ed. London: Blackwell Scientific Publications. *A classic, multifaceted reference text on spinal cord injuries.*

Guyton, A. 1976. *Textbook of Medical Physiology*. 5th ed. Philadelphia: W. B. Saunders. *Classic text detailing neuroanatomy and physiology, including that of the gastrointestinal system and functional disorders.*

Johnson, D. K., and Balmaseda, M. T. 1985. Pseudomembranous colitis in spinal cord injury. *Archives of Physical Medicine and Rehabilitation* 66: 394–396.

Mathews, D., and Carlson, D. 1987. *Spinal Cord Injury: A Guide to Rehabilitation Nursing*. Chicago, IL: Rehabilitation Institute of Chicago.

Meiners, C. 1976. *How to be Healthier Through Proper Nutrition*. Published by the National Paraplegia Foundation and the NPF Allied Health Committee. Available from the National Spinal Cord Injury Foundation. *General nutritional information related to specific needs of people with SCI; includes detailed information on dietary fiber, sources, and recommended intake.*

Meshkinpour, H., et al. 1983. Colonic compliance in patients with spinal cord injury. *Archives of Physical Medicine and Rehabilitation* 64: 111–112.

National Rehabilitation Hospital. 1988. *Policies and Procedures—Bowel Management for Neurogenic Bowel Dysfunction*. No. 102.001. Washington, DC: National Rehabilitation Hospital.

Ozer, M. N. 1988. *Management of Persons with Spinal Cord Injury*. New York: Demos Publications, pp. 43–46, 59–60.

Paeslak, V. 1966. Disorders of bowel function in spinal lesions. *International Journal of Paraplegia* 4: 250–254. *Neural and functional pathology; physical assessment skills; and bowel-training techniques.*

Rehabilitation Nursing Foundation. 1987. *Rehabilitation Nursing: Concepts and Practice—A Core Curriculum*. 2nd ed. Skokie, IL: Author, pp. 177–187.

Taylor, N., Berni, R., and Hornig, M. 1973. Neurogenic Bowel Management. *American Family Physician* 7 (5): 126–128.

Virginia Spinal Cord Injury Care and Teaching Manual. 1988. The Virginia Spinal Cord Injury System, University of Virginia Center and Virginia Dept. of Rehabilitation Services, Woodrow Wilson Rehabilitation Center, Box W-279, Fisherville, VA 22939. *Concise and clear presentation, including factors to consider when setting up and maintaining a bowel program, helpful tips, aids, medication, and problem solving.*

Yarnell, S. Z., and Manofy, E. 1984. Dyssynergic bowel (abstract). *Archives of Physical Medicine Rehabilitation* 65: 632.

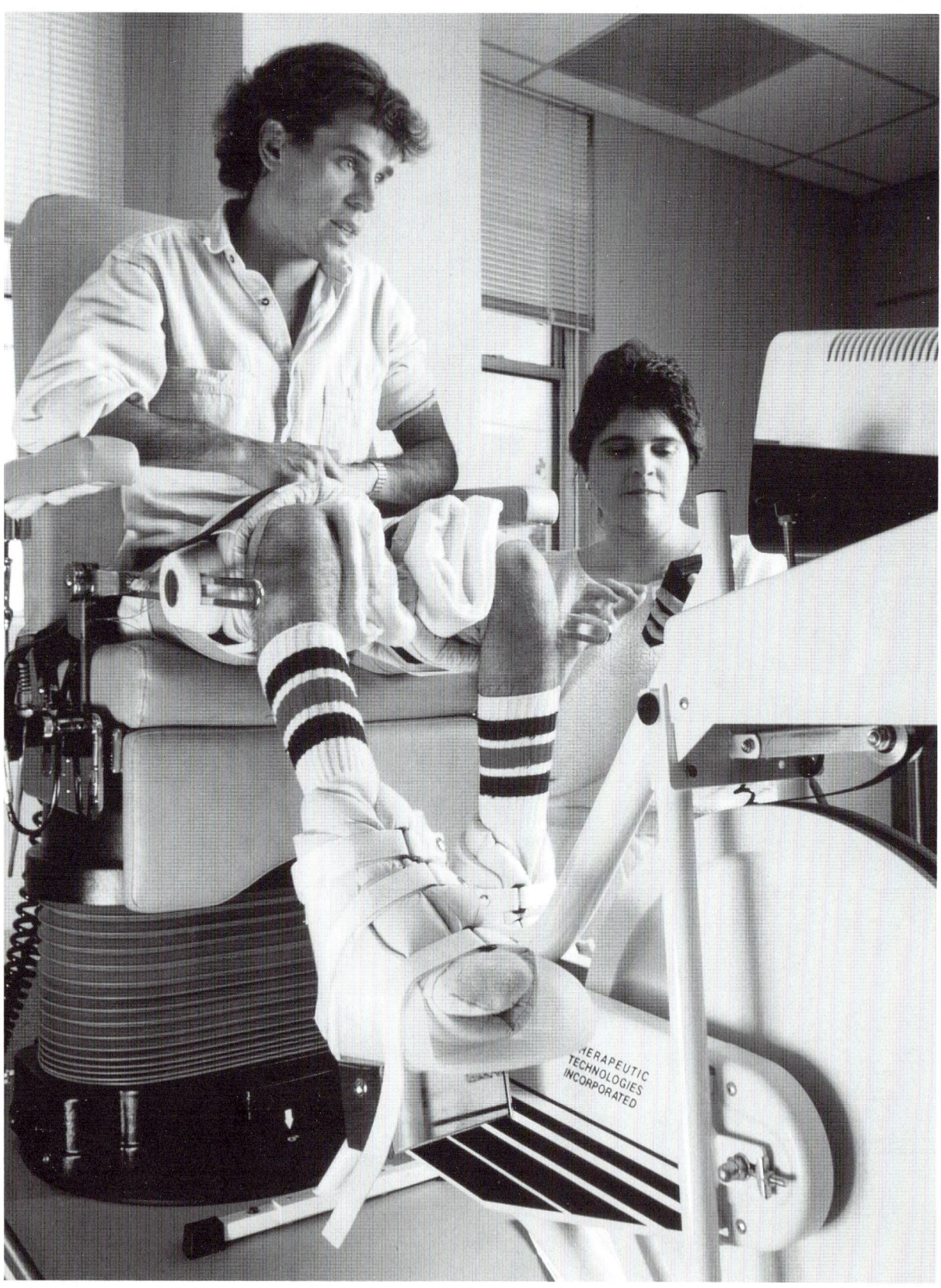

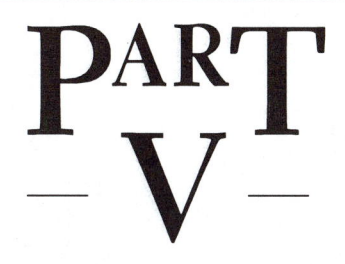

PART V

REESTABLISHING MOBILITY AND INDEPENDENCE

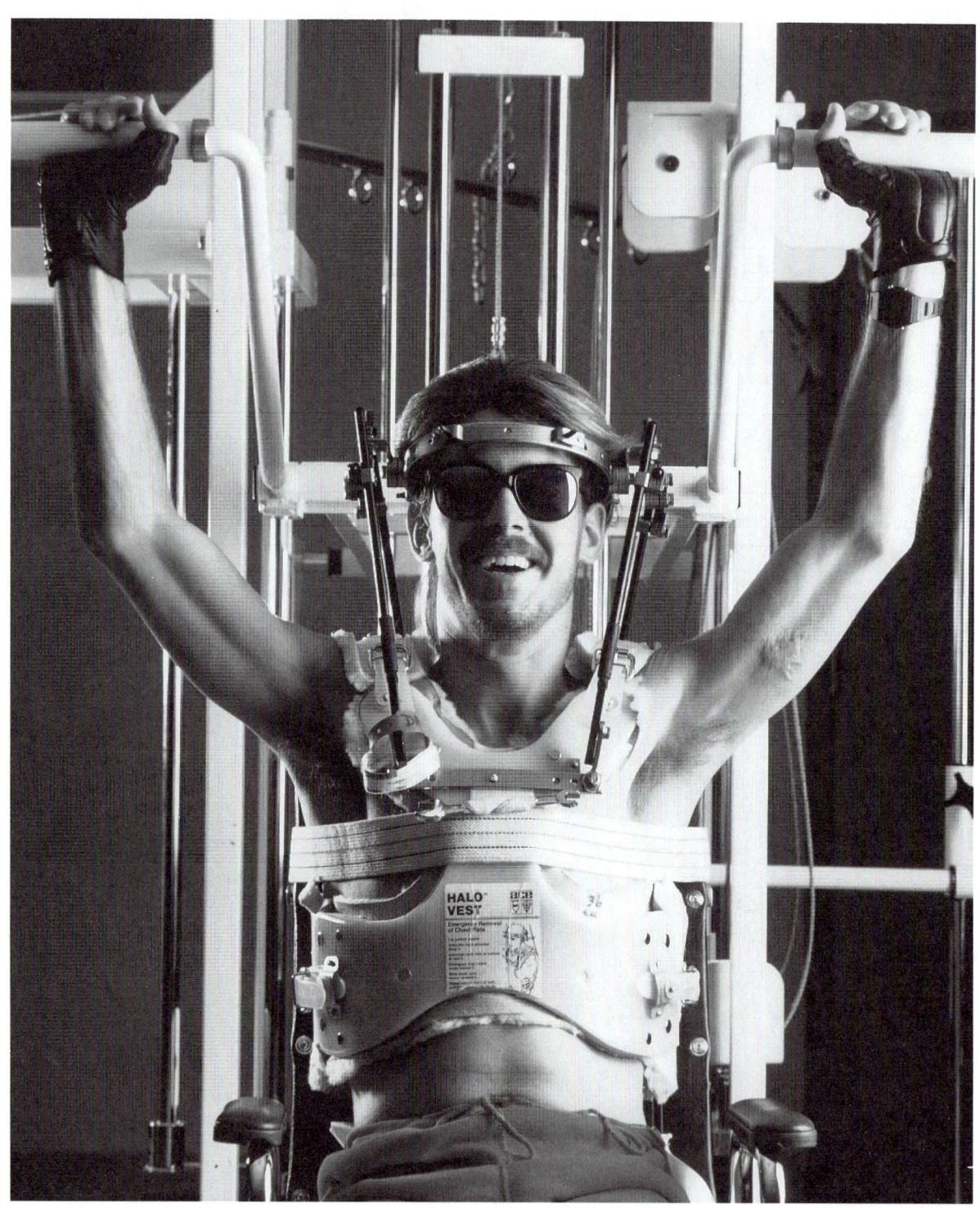

CHAPTER
— 20 —

Maintaining
Skeletal System Integrity

Chapter Outline

Health Care Objectives

- To prevent further neurological damage and/or facilitate potential functional return
- To provide complete stability to the injured spine, ensuring early and adequate immobilization of the spine throughout the acute phase to prevent long-term complications
- To maintain correct body alignment and ensure adequate position change, preventing skin breakdown, muscle fatigue, contractures, and nerve or joint damage and minimizing patient discomfort and spasticity

Considerable advancements in both surgical and nonsurgical management techniques have allowed earlier general mobilization of the patient while still protecting and immobilizing the spine. These advances have greatly reduced both the formerly lengthy periods of bedrest and the accompanying hazards of physical immobilization and psychological isolation. This means a shorter period of hospitalization and earlier return to community life.

ASSESSMENT OF THE SKELETAL SYSTEM

Assessment of the skeletal system begins with a review of the patient's history to note any preexisting factors that would, in addition to the SCI, influence skeletal system integrity. See Chapter 4. Preexisting conditions or abnormal findings necessitate additional precautions and modifications to the care plan.

In-depth assessment of skeletal system integrity depends largely on radiological findings. During the remobilization period, X-ray evaluation is used at specific intervals to monitor spinal stability, evaluate the degree of healing, and detect evidence of any developing malalignment. This information can also predict what degree of stress the patient will safely tolerate with increased physical activity, and ascertain when less rigid orthoses are required.

GENERAL MANAGEMENT

Spinal immobilization and/or stabilization may be achieved by *bedrest* (with or without traction); by the use of *orthoses*; and by *surgical intervention*. These techniques are often used in combination.

Immobilizing the Patient with Bedrest

Maintaining Correct Alignment
Measures to ensure correct positioning help make the patient comfortable, enhance respiration, promote circulation, prevent gravitational edema, and preserve muscle function by preventing contractures. While the patient is in bed the side-lying, supine, prone, and sitting positions may be assumed as indicated; each has specific advantages.

Immediately after injury patients require a *change of position every 2 hours* around the clock. *Minor position changes are often required more frequently.* Techniques need to be modified and the schedule adjusted to meet individual needs and as tolerance for selected positions increases. Eventually self-turns can be taught to patients

with sufficient strength and mobility. Chapter 21 details this ongoing process.

Side-lying position. The side-lying position is used to minimize risk of aspiration during mealtime; mobilize secretions from dependent areas of the lung; relieve pressure on the sacral area; and decrease spasticity. Care must be taken to avoid undue curvature of the cervical or thoracic spine, to protect bony prominences and the nerve plexus in the shoulder, and to support and separate skin surfaces of the extremities. See Table 20–1 for a summary of potential problems and measures associated with this position.

Supine position. The supine position is desirable for many general nursing functions such as bathing or catheterizations. Because this position is assumed so frequently, it is better to *schedule turns from side to side (and not from side to back to side) to avoid the patient spending prolonged periods of time on the back.* Patients with limited neck movement will need prism glasses to see and observe activities around them. Take measures to avoid rotation of the neck, support natural body curvatures, protect the sacral area and heels from pressure areas, and support feet to prevent foot drop. See Table 20–2 for a summary of potential problems and measures associated with this position.

Prone position. The prone position is especially valuable to counteract prolonged periods of hip flexion and to provide pressure relief for the buttocks following long periods of sitting in a wheelchair.

Check with the physician before placing the patient in the prone position and check again when different orthoses are used. For example, a patient in a halo may tolerate the prone position well, but when the brace is removed and replaced by a less protective neck brace, the position may be quite unsafe. Check with the physician when thoracolumbar braces are removed. Rotational movements may still need to be restricted.

Many patients are apprehensive about trying this position because they fear difficulties with breathing or discomfort. For this reason, it is advisable to try the prone position during the day before attempting to include it in the night routine. Building a tolerance for proning can eventually allow undisturbed rest in that position throughout the night.

Take care to avoid undue curvature of the cervical or thoracic spine; to position arms comfortably; to protect male genitalia, iliac crest bone, and knees; and to prevent foot drop. See Table 20–3 for a summary of possible problems and supportive measures associated with the prone position.

Sitting position. Patients with cervical injuries, once braced, are encouraged to sit in bed as tolerated. Orthopedic surgeons will specifically order the sitting position for patients with thoracic and lumbar injuries. (Elevation of the head of the bed will be stipulated from 30 to 90 degrees.) Sitting is limited mostly to mealtimes or short periods of 20 to 30 minutes, because it increases the load on the healing spinal fracture site and causes excess pressure on the but-

TABLE 20–1   Side-Lying (Lateral) Position

Potential Problems	Supportive Measures for Patients with Cervical Injuries	Supportive Measures for Patients with Thoracic or Lumbar Injuries
Excessive lateral neck flexion; fatigue of sternocleidomastoid muscles (which aid respiration)	One-inch foam pad or small, flat pillow placed under head of newly injured patients	Regular pillow under head (high thoracic injured patients may be more comfortable with a small pillow)
Pressure area on ear	Soft protective padding surrounding ears	
Pressure on and pain in dependent shoulder	Grasp scapula and move shoulder through to avoid pressure on nerve plexus	
Loss of correct position; subsequent malalignment of spine and limbs contributing to discomfort and extremity spasticity	Rolled pillow positioned securely behind back	Rolled pillow positioned securely behind back
Skin excoriation under arms; limited chest expansion; compromised circulation to and gravitational edema in paralyzed arms; and internal rotation and adduction of the shoulder with contractures of arm musculature	Pillow under top arm and bottom forearm to support them in good alignment*	Pillow under arms to support in position of comfort
Hip internally rotated and adducted; loss of correct positioning contributing to back discomfort and extremity spasms	Pillows placed lengthwise between legs to maintain good alignment, balance, and comfort	Pillows placed lengthwise between legs to maintain good alignment, balance, and comfort
Foot drop, which complicates sitting in wheelchair, is universal	Support feet in 90° position	Support feet in 90° position
Pressure areas developing over bony prominences	Padding to separate ankles	Padding to separate ankles

*For most quadriplegic patients position arms in extension to avoid flexion contractures of the elbow. If the patient has a high-level cervical injury with no arm movement, alternate flexion and extension positions to avoid contractures (illustrated in Figure 6–4).

tocks. The position is also difficult to maintain for any length of time without slipping down the bed.

Take measures to maintain the patient's balance; prevent rotational trunk movement; protect the sacral skin; and, above all for the patient with paraplegia, avoid undue pressure on or curvature of the lumbar and thoracic spine. See Table 20–4 for a summary of potential problems and supportive measures associated with this position.

Foot and ankle positioning.   Several devices for the ankle and foot may be used to:

- Relieve pressure on the bony prominences (heel and ankles)
- Maintain the foot in dorsiflexion to prevent contracture at the ankle

The Multipodis Boot,* for example, offers good pressure relief and good alignment when active contracture preven-

*Multipodis Boots, L'Nard Multipodis Splint System, 12201 28th St. North, St. Petersburg, FL 33716.

tion can increase functional capabilities. However, these and other similar devices should not be used if the fit is poor because of the risk of increasing pressure points. If the device cannot be placed on the foot correctly according to the manufacturer's guidelines, do not use it. *Edema, large-size foot, spasticity, and bandages* may preclude use. High-top sneakers, a size larger than normal, may be an alternative.

Support the legs and feet in such a way that external rotation is prevented, perhaps by a small roll at the lateral side of the ankles. Also when the patient is side-lying, place a pillow between the knees and boots themselves to maintain correct alignment.

Special Immobilization Beds
Therapeutic immobilization beds may be of benefit in both acute and chronic situations. The motorized RotoRest Treatment Table may be used when the spine is unstable and is especially useful for the cervical injured patient with multiple trauma. It very gradually, but continually, rotates the patient from side to side in a cradlelike fashion, allevi-

TABLE 20–2 Supine Position

Potential Problems	Supportive Measures for Patients with Cervical Injuries	Supportive Measures for Patients with Thoracic or Lumbar Injuries
Excessive flexion or extension of the head and neck exerting undesirable pressure on injury site	One-inch foam pad or small flat pillow placed under head of newly injured patient	Pillow of suitable thickness placed under head
Flexion of lumbar curvature with undue pressure contributing to back pain and possibly increased neurological deficit		Hyperextension padding (as ordered) to support lumbar curvature and promote reduction of injured spine
Compromises of circulation; gravitational edema of forearms and hands; and elbow contractures	Pillows elevating forearms and hands*	Support not required except as comfort measure
Hyperextension of knees; impaired circulation; and tension on the lower spine	Small pillow or padding under lower thigh to flex legs slightly (optional if full-length padding is used on bed)	Small pillow or padding under lower thigh to flex legs slightly (optional if full-length padding is used on bed)
Foot drop	Pillows or padding and footboard to flex feet at a 90° angle	Pillows or padding and footboard to flex feet at a 90° angle

*Position most quadriplegic patients with arms extended to avoid flexion contractures of the elbow. If the patient has high-level cervical injury and *no* arm movement, alternate flexion and extension positions to avoid contractures in either direction.

TABLE 20–3 Prone Position

Potential Problems	Supportive Measures for Patients with Cervical Injuries	Supportive Measures for Patients with Thoracic or Lumbar Injuries
Rotation, flexion, or extension of an unstable neck fracture site with subsequent interruption of bony healing and possible loss of function	Padding to support the chin and forehead and allow a "breathing space"	
Loosening of brace with loss of immobilization resulting in interrupted bony healing and possible loss of function	One or two pillows to support chest and relieve pressure on bars of the halo brace	
Hyperextension of lumbar curve; undue pressure on iliac crests and male genitalia; pressure on female breasts; and difficulty breathing	Pillow placed under abdomen	Pillow placed under abdomen
Hyperextension of knees, undue pressure on knees and toes, and foot drop	Pillow placed under lower legs to flex legs slightly, relieve pressure on knees, and promote plantar flexion	Pillow placed under lower legs to flex legs slightly, relieve pressure on knees, and promote plantar flexion
Brachial plexus damage and impaired circulation	Place arms in comfortable position alleviating pressure on shoulders	Place arms in comfortable position alleviating pressure on shoulders
Undue pressure on toes; foot drop	Position feet between mattress and footboard	Position feet between mattress and footboard

*Turning the patient prone can be simplified with the following techniques. Move the patient to the side of the bed in the supine position, and arrange pillows in the desired position beside the patient. Prepare the patient for turning prone by placing the opposite arm and leg across the body; if turning the patient toward the left, position the right arm and right leg. Tuck the left arm down by the patient's side or place above the head. Finally, logroll the patient toward the pillows.

TABLE 20–4   Sitting Position in Bed*

Potential Problems	Supportive Measures for Patients with Cervical Injuries	Supportive Measures for Patients with Thoracic or Lumbar Injuries
Loss of neck immobilization with interrupted healing of the bone and possible decrease in function	Position neck orthosis before attempting to sit up	
Loss of position; possibility of falling	Pillows placed at patient's sides to maintain balance	
Shoulder pain; impaired circulation; gravitational edema of forearms and hands	Pillows placed under arms for support	
Strain on fracture site of lower spine	Padding under knees not necessary	Pillow placed under knees to relieve pull on lower spine; eventually long sitting (without supports) allowed
Pressure area on sacrum and heels; foot drop	Padding under ankles to relieve pressure on heels; footboard to maintain plantar flexion	Padding under ankles to relieve pressure on heels; footboard to maintain plantar flexion

*Limit initial time periods in this position, check pressure points frequently.

ating the need for manual turning. Decreased pulmonary, urinary, and venous stasis complications have been observed (Green, Green, and Klose 1980). However, the continual motion can be associated with diarrhea, and skin breakdown can still occur from various factors, especially if the patient is not turned manually for skin inspection and care. The Stoke-Eggerton bed is also motorized and turns the patient from side to side by operating longitudinal sections of the mattress (Rogers 1978–1979).

The most widely used turning frame is the Wedge-Stryker frame, noted for its "pie" shape formed by the anterior and posterior frames for added protection against movement of the spine when turning (Figure 20–1).

The Wedge-Stryker frame is most suitable for patients with uncomplicated low cervical or thoracic or lumbar injuries. It is unsuitable for obese patients (check the manufacturer's recommended weight limit—usually not over 200 pounds); unconscious patients; or patients with respiratory complications or severe restlessness from head injury, a psychiatric condition, or alcoholic/drug-related state.

It is convenient to move the frame freely around the ward to encourage socialization. Detachable traction devices, arm boards, and footboards are available. Height and weight adjustments can be made. Its greatest disadvantage is that the patient may not be able to tolerate the prone position and the frame does not allow for a side-lying position.

Secure all tubing just before and after each turn. Stop to visualize the exact route the IV tubing will follow. Should the IV bag be passed under the frame or over the top? Be sure the catheter bag is placed on the side toward which the patient is turning.

Position the patient in basic alignment and schedule turns every 2 hours. It is possible to adjust the time to 3 hours prone and one hour supine or vice versa for special needs. A one-inch continuous foam mattress can be designed to cover both anterior and posterior canvases. A full-length sheepskin is an important adjunct. Padding of this thickness eliminates the need for numerous smaller pads, which tend to be misplaced or slip.

The *prone* position allows for maximum hand activities involved with self-care such as personal hygiene, reading, or writing. Eating is much easier although the patient may need straws and assistance with cutting meat. Bowel procedures should also be performed while prone. Removing a canvas strip to insert a bedpan is most dangerous, especially

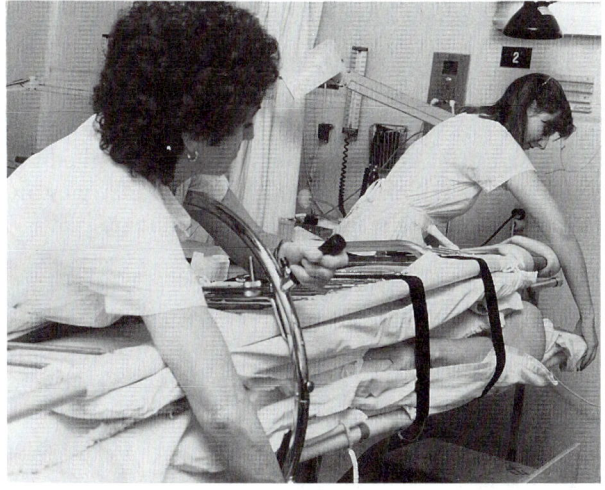

FIGURE 20–1   The Wedge-Stryker frame.

for lumbosacral injuries. The prone position improves visualization of the anal area, which is essential when using manual evacuation techniques. While prone:

- *Head/neck.* Traction and a cervical face piece can be added for patients with cervical injuries. Be sure the forehead and the chin are well protected to prevent skin breakdown. Additional foam pads with soft coverings are usually necessary. Countertraction is possible by tilting the head of the bed up.
- *Trunk.* If smaller pads are to be used, one- or two-inch narrow foam pads are best. They may be positioned between the shoulder and just above the nipple line; across the abdomen below the diaphragm and above the pubis; and above the knees and just above the ankles. This padding helps relieve pressure on the clavicle, ease body weight pressing on female breasts, enhance lung capacity, bridge the male genitalia, and relieve pressure on knees. It is also believed to be less fatiguing on back muscles.

  For the male patient an indwelling catheter can be padded with gauze and taped just above the iliac crest to promote drainage and avoid any pressure on the abdomen. Again, if sheepskin is used it is not necessary to add additional foam pads. If not, a one-inch foam pad can cover the iliac crests and, along with another pad on the thighs, will bridge the genital area.
- *Extremities.* Check the point at which the front of the shoulders touch the frame. This is especially important for patients with cervical injuries; those without sensation will be unable to feel numbness, tingling, or weakness in the arm indicating pressure on the brachial plexus. To avoid pressure on this area the arm boards should be elevated to the level of the frame and should be padded with pillows or foam and comfortable for the patient; the patient's arms should be extended upward or outward.

The CircOlectric Bed should be avoided during initial management because it may cause excessive axial loading on the fracture site and postural hypotension due to a rapid progression to the upright position. A variety of air-fluidized and low air-loss flotation beds are available for pressure management once the spine is stable (Yoshimura 1989).

Cervical Traction

Skeletal traction in the treatment of cervical spine injuries is universal. Realignment of the spinal canal not only corrects the mechanical damage but also protects the cord and nerve roots from further compression. Skeletal traction may be used to achieve both reduction and immobilization of the fracture.

Various types of skull traction devices, tongs or calipers, may be used. See Table 20–5 and Procedure 20–1. The

halo ring can also be used as an immediate skull traction device with the support vest being attached at a later date.

When cervical traction is in place, care includes the following:

- Maintain a constant traction force at all times. Ensure that weights hang freely and do not touch the floor. check this especially during postural drainage and chest physical therapy. Also check that the knot on the traction rope tied to the skull fixation device is clear of the traction pulley or traction collar. If not, move the patient down in bed using a four-person lift with the patient in a supine position. If this is a continual problem, check with the physician to see if countertraction can be applied by raising the head of the bed.

  If the tongs should be accidentally dislodged, immediately immobilize the head and neck by hand. Maintain a gentle, but firm, pressure on the jaw and occiput and summon the physician immediately. Application of a collar with sandbags will assist with immobilization. It is difficult to apply halter traction without manipulating the neck, and therefore this procedure presents too much risk. To prevent infection, clean and dress the original tong sights and look for leakage of cerebrospinal fluid (a clear, yellowish fluid that will leave rings on the bed linen and test positively for sugar on a reagent paper strip). A specimen of any fluid leakage should be collected for laboratory identification.
- Clean insertion sites regularly every 4 to 8 hours. See Procedure 20–2.
- Turn and position the patient every 2 hours. The person at the patient's head must reach around the traction device and place one or both forearms just behind the skull tongs with extended hands reaching the patient's shoulders. (In other words the elbows are placed flat along the bed.) If it is too difficult to place your arm or will be too difficult to remove your arm once the patient is turned, simply use one hand to guide the head and neck and extend the other arm and hand to the patient's shoulder to ensure alignment. Before turning times, explain the procedure carefully, as patients tend to be extremely apprehensive during this time.

MANAGEMENT WITH ORTHOSES

Orthoses are externally applied support systems (either braces or splints) that exert mechanical forces on the body at prescribed points. Spinal orthoses frequently apply forces to the head or torso at some distance from the spine itself to limit movement and control position.

TABLE 20–5 Skull Traction Devices

Type	Description	Preparation for Application	Special Equipment
Crutchfield tongs	Small skull calipers that fit to the top of the head, just behind the hairline	Requires localized shave preparation and scalp incisions	Requires drill for application; tightening screw device attached directly to tongs for individual adjustment
Cone-Barton tongs	Larger skull calipers that fit to the side of the head, just above the ear, with pointed pins that insert directly into the skull	Requires localized shave preparation	A wrench (not interchangeable) accompanies each set of tongs to fit tightening device
Vinke tongs	Large skull tongs that fit to the side of the head, again just above the ear, with an interlocking device between the inner and outer tables of the skull for maximum stability; prevention of slipping or dislodging is the primary feature of these tongs	Requires localized shave preparation and scalp incisions	Specialized Vinke drill accompanies tongs for application
Gardner-Wells tongs	Large tongs that fit to the head just above the ear that feature large side knobs to grasp for insertion; Gardner-Wells tongs do not actually penetrate the skull; may be inserted by skilled paramedical personnel at the accident site	No shave preparation or incisions necessary	No drills or other equipment necessary

Orthoses are named for the parts of the body they support as opposed to the parts they cover. Treatment focuses on achieving desirable position and limiting movement so that the spinal fracture site can heal in good alignment, preventing long-term complications such as scoliosis or muscle contractures.

In the immediate postinjury phase rigid immobilization is warranted in the presence of serious instability. As rehabilitation progresses, callus formation will eventually heal the bony injury, and less rigid external support will be required to maintain alignment. While surgical intervention may realign the vertebral column, bone growth is still required to complete healing. For this reason orthoses may still be required during the postoperative period. Rigid immobilization of a fractured spine is usually necessary for the first 3 months after injury, and a less rigid support is needed for the next 2 to 3 months.

The *orthotist* works in close collaboration with the treatment team, particularly the orthopedic surgeon, to provide effective and comfortable support to the damaged skeletal system. The orthotist measures, designs, and fabricates a variety of braces and may modify commercially produced braces. However, correct application is essential to provide their fullest benefit. This, and meticulous care of the skin at points where the brace applies force to the body surface, are major concerns. If the contact force exceeds capillary pressure, blanching, then redness, and later ischemia will occur. Such pressure will normally cause extreme pain, but if the brace covers an area of the body that is without sensation, conscientious skin care must compensate.

When the patient requires an orthotic device, be familiar with:

- The appearance and function of orthoses
- The method of application (or donning)
- Specific safety precautions and procedures
- The contact points on the body where the brace exerts the greatest pressure
- The degree of physical activity allowed
- Measures for removing the brace

There are three broad categories of cervical orthoses: those that provide rigid immobilization (the halo apparatus); those that provide moderate immobilization; and orthopedic collars that limit neck movements minimally.

Thoracolumbar orthoses include two categories: standard hyperextension braces (such as the Jewett), and individualized trunk supports (such as body jackets or casts).

Procedure 20–1   Application of Skull Traction Devices

Purpose

To produce cervical traction by simply maintaining alignment or, with additional weights added, reducing the fracture.

Equipment

- Immobilization bed of choice with traction setup
- Rope
- Selected weights
- Cardiac monitor (optional)
- Nasogastric tube (optional)

- Local anesthetic such as 1% lidocaine hydrochloride with a variety of syringes and needles
- Sterilized tray including appropriate devices, drills (optional), and specialized equipment (see Table 14–5)
- Razor and shaving equipment (optional)
- Sterile gloves for physician (optional)

Action	Rationale
1. Explain procedure to patient. Obtain consent. Give presedation as ordered. Reassure patient and communicate throughout procedure.	This is a painful procedure and can be frightening, especially when the skull is penetrated.
2. Place patient on the immobilization bed of choice and assemble appropriate traction equipment.	Compatible cervical traction units come with specialized beds. There are traction setups, with two supporting poles at either side and a crossbar with sliding pulley apparatus, that fit many regular beds or emergency stretcher beds.
3. Assess neurovital signs for baseline data.	Throughout the procedure, inquire about any changes in sensation, or movement, or pain. Inadvertent movement of the neck causes further deterioration.
4. Provide continuous cardiac monitoring during procedure for severely traumatized, fatigued, and older patients.	The added stress of inserting skull traction devices may precipitate pulse irregularities, cardiac dysrhythmias, and fainting.
5. If necessary, insert a nasogastric tube to evacuate stomach contents before proceeding.	The stress of this procedure can precipitate aspiration if the newly injured patient has recently eaten.
6. In most instances, assist physician to shave area surrounding tong insertion sites.	This minimizes risk of infection spreading to inner table of skull.
7. Clean insertion sites with antiseptic solution.	
8. In most instances, assist physician to infiltrate insertion sites with local anesthetic.	
9. When necessary, assist physician with scalpel incisions, drill penetration, and tong insertion.	
10. Secure selected weights, thread through a pulley or traction device, and tie to skull tongs or calipers to produce traction.	Traction may be held in a neutral, extension, or flexion position to counteract the mechanism of injury. Traction begins from 5 to 50 lb depending on the bony level of injury involved.
11. Ensure that weights hang freely and do not touch floor. Also the knot on traction rope tied to skull fixation device must be clear of pulley or traction collar.	This establishes a constant traction pull.
12. Reassess neurovital signs.	To ascertain neurological status.
13. Following the procedure, assist with positioning patient for X-ray evaluation.	This helps to determine alignment and traction force. If closed reduction is being attempted serial clinical and X-ray evaluation is needed. Additional weights are added in 5-lb increments after 15-minute intervals. The maximum amount of weight usually varies.
14. Anticipate discomfort at insertion sites, headaches, and neck discomfort. Give analgesic as ordered.	The patient needs to be continually evaluated for pain tolerance, especially if traction forces are increased.

Procedure 20–2 Tong Site Care

Purpose

To maintain cleanliness and prevent infection at tong insertion sites.

Equipment

- Face mask and sterile gloves
- Sterile dressing tray
- Package of sterile cotton-tipped applicators

- Hydrogen peroxide
- Bacteriostatic solution

Action	Rationale
1. Set up small dressing tray with sterile cotton-tipped applicators and small containers of sterile cleaning solution (hydrogen peroxide) and bacteriostatic solution (tincture of Savlon 1:30). Use mask and gloves.	
2. Remove gauze wrapped around tong site.	
3. Observe condition of tissue surrounding each tong site, looking for any redness, swelling, skin tension, tenderness, or pruritis.	These signs may indicate infection.
4. Clean each tong site with a sterile applicator dipped in hydrogen peroxide. Clean in one sweeping motion around tong site; discard swab. Gently repeat until site is clean. Do not dab or prod with swab, even to remove crusting. This additional trauma is a major cause of tong site infection because it increases irritation.	Serous crusting is common. 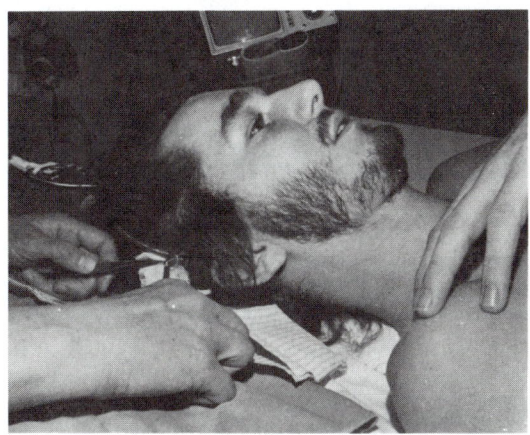
5. If excessive discharge is evident, apply a nonocclusive bacteriostatic solution (with or without dressings). A 2 × 2 inch gauze unfolded then refolded lengthwise and tied around the tong will stay in place best.	Sprays or ointments may cake around insertion sites and increase risk of infection.
6. If drainage is present obtain a wound culture.	Infection may be present and a course of antibiotics may be necessary. If infection cannot be controlled, traction device may have to be removed and reinserted to prevent more serious complications of abscess formation or osteomyelitis.
7. Wash patient's hair weekly or more often with a liquid antibacterial soap.	Bathrooms large enough for beds and equipped with long hose spray attachments are ideal.

Rigid Immobilization: The Halo Apparatus*

The use of the halo device has virtually revolutionized the care of the quadriplegic patient, replacing skeletal traction, turning frames, and prolonged periods of bedrest formerly used to immobilize the cervical spine during bony healing (Nickel 1977). The purpose of the halo brace is to immobilize the cervical spine rigidly. Contraindications for its use include severe respiratory problems, chest injuries, or burns on the trunk or abdomen. Many brands and varieties of halo devices are available but all include three basic parts (Figure 20–2):

*This section was written with Corrine Koehler, R.N., C.R.R.N., Craig Hospital, Englewood, CO.

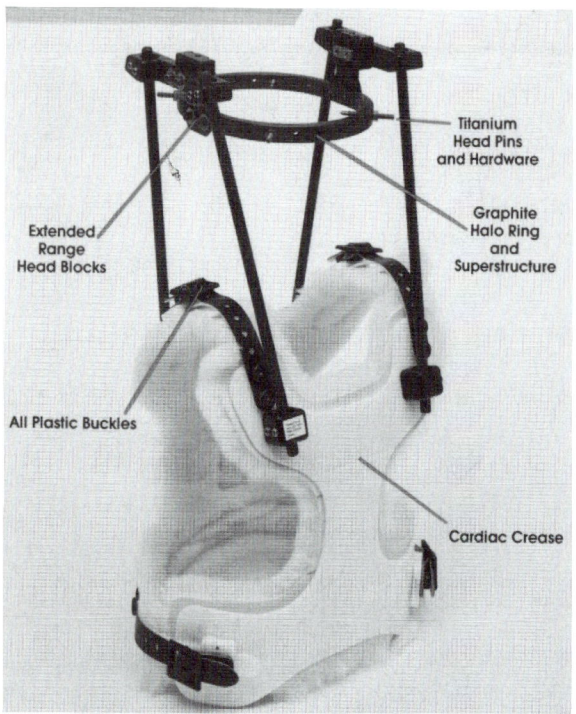

FIGURE 20–2 The newer P.M.T. (Progress Mankind Technology) is MRI compatible with a graphite halo system and provides, according to the manufacturer's literature (1988), artifact-free images; enhanced patient safety; high resistance, electrically isolated graphite ring; minimal potential for current loop generation; easy adjustability without loss of traction; stability and reliability. PMT Corporation, 1500 Park Road, Chanhassen, MN 55317.

1. The halo *ring* goes around the head and has four skull pins, which are threaded through the ring and into the skull. The pins are the main point of fixation of the brace and penetrate the bone about one-eighth of an inch. When in place, only the pins touch the skull.

2. The halo *vest* is made of plastic with an anterior and a posterior plate and lined with sheepskin. When the vest is secured around the patient's chest, it provides a stable force to which the hardware is attached.

3. The *superstructure (hardware)* is an array of rods, bolts, nuts, and screws that connect the vest to the ring. When the hardware is tightened into place, immobility of the cervical spine is achieved. The weight of the entire apparatus, about 8 to 10 pounds, is designed to be distributed around the circumference of the chest and not borne by the neck and shoulder muscle groups.

Method of Application

Incorporate information in Procedure 20–3 into preparation and teaching for *application* of the halo orthosis. Except for the skull pins being inserted, application is relatively painless but usually frightening. Emphasize that the skull pins do not penetrate the brain, a common fear of patients. Following application of the ring, the vest is buckled into position at the shoulders, the sides, and the waist. An assortment of hardware is then adjusted to connect the ring to the vest.

General Considerations

One of the most critical elements when caring for a patient in halo bracing is management of cardiopulmonary arrest, should it occur. The unique and individual manner that the anterior vest can be removed to allow access to the chest for effective cardiac compressions must be noted as each manufacturer uses a different style vest and method for design (Koehler 1980). Identify and investigate the exact method and size of wrench necessary to remove the anterior vest at the time of application or admission. Practice safety precautions as outlined in Procedure 20–3.

In an emergency situation, after the anterior bolts are removed, the side straps and shoulder straps are unbuckled and the vest lifted from the chest, as in Procedure 20–4. It is not necessary to loosen any other hardware for vest removal; therefore, cervical spine manipulation is minimal.

Some manufacturers have designed a cardiac crease (the "living hinge" concept) to provide chest access for CPR. The vest has a crease line in the anterior vest plastic. When the side straps are released, the lower portion of the vest can be bent up, exposing the chest for CPR. It is necessary to evaluate each individual patient with this type of halo vest to assure that the crease line is above the sternum level used for accurate chest compressions. Even if the crease line allows proper hand placement, it may be advantageous to continue with anterior vest removal as defibrillation may be required.

The defibrillator can be used, but the paddles must not come into contact with any metal at any time. Remember that the upright hardware does not come off with the anterior vest removal and remains around the patient's head, face, and neck areas.

Following any procedure involving removal of the front vest, reapplication by the attending physician and radiological reassessment of alignment are necessary.

Because the halo brace is in place for many weeks, patients' questions about the daily care of the brace must be addressed (Browner and Mattingly 1986) and steps taken to reduce apprehension and put expectations into perspective. Be consistent as a team in saying when the halo is coming off. Radiology findings and medical clinical judgment determine an exact appropriate removal date. Choose words carefully when communicating with patients to prevent misinterpretation. People tend to hear what they want to believe. For instance, "We use the halo to heal your neck" can lead patients to think they will be able to walk again without difficulty! Remember that the halo stabilizes and maintains alignment of the cervical spine.

Patients have difficulty imagining what is possible after the halo is removed. Tell patients what specific movements

Procedure 20–3   Application of the Halo-Thoracic Brace (Ring and Vest)

Purpose

To provide rigid immobilization of the cervical spine.

Special Concerns

Throughout the procedure the nurse's role is to communicate with and reassure the patient. Assess pain tolerance and inquire about changes in movement or sensation to detect risk of neurological deterioration.

Equipment (sterile procedure)

- Local anesthetic such as 1% lidocaine hydrochloride without epinephrine.
- Two (2) 10 cc syringes with 22 ga. x 1 1/4″ needles. This allows 5 cc anesthetic at each skull pin site.
- Gauze pads, forceps, razors, and antiseptic solution for preparing pin sites.
- Sterile gloves for physician.
- Sterile tray to include:

  - Halo rings in several sizes.

  - Four (4) skull pins. *Use new skull pins each application. Skull pins are never reused.*

  - Four (4) positioning pins and discs.

  - Four (4) skull pin locks.

  - Three (3) 7/16″ bolts with washers (to secure upright hardware to halo ring).

- Variety of halo tools necessary for adjustments (Figure **A**)

  - Two (2) torque screwdrivers for tightening skull pins.

  - Allen, or **L**-shaped, wrenches to fit smaller sockets.

  - Regular wrenches to fit larger bolts on connecting hardware between ring and vest (common sizes: 7/16″, 1/2″, 9/16″).

  - Four (4) skull pin plastic protectors.

  - Sandbags (optional).

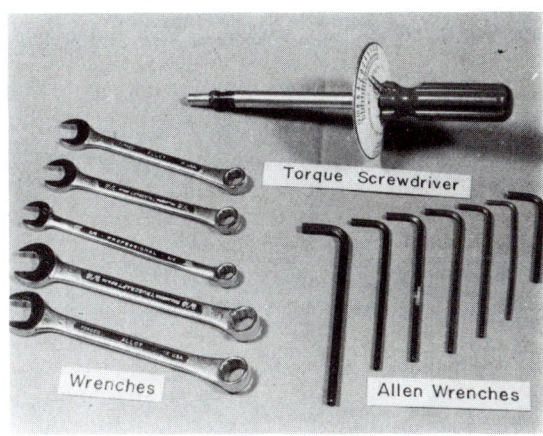

A

Action

Rationale

Preparation and Selection of Equipment

1. Collaborate with physician to assess patient's general condition, particularly respiratory status.

2. Check neurovital signs and record for baseline data.

3. Obtain patient consent.

4. Obtain/order vest and ring.

   - To order correct vest size, measure chest circumference at level of xiphoid process.

   - To order correct ring size, measure head circumference by placing tape measure around head 1/2″ above top of ears and 1/2″ above eyebrows.

5. Plan for individual adjustments. Note any irregular shape or bony protuberances of chest, back, and head. Cut vest edges accordingly and cover cut edges with foam tape.

6. Plan time (about 30 minutes) and schedule procedure room. Explain procedure to patient. Give pre-sedation as ordered.

The halo vest limits accessibility to the chest. It may be necessary to delay application of halo vest if frequent clapping and vibration are necessary to free lungs of secretions or if patient risks developing cardiopulmonary problems.

Halo rings and vests (plastic with natural or synthetic sheepskin liners) are available in a variety of sizes.

The plastic vest may be shaped to the individual to prevent undue pressure that might cause skin breakdown. To allow for the enlarging uterus with advanced pregnancy, the anterior vest edge can be cut. For additional comfort, apply a posterior halo vest a size larger than the front vest. This allows for appropriate sizing at the shoulders while providing additional width at the abdomen.

(Procedure continues)

Procedure 20–3   Application of the Halo-Thoracic Brace (Ring and Vest) (continued)

Action

7. Shave small posterior patches and clean scalp around each of four pin site areas with antiseptic solution. A 2″ square above and behind each ear is shaved.

8. Position patient supine on a firm bed or stretcher with head just beyond edge. The head *must* be supported by an assistant's hands or a 4″ wide board placed under head and back. *Note:* A cervical collar may be placed on patient during all positioning moves before halo vest application.

Application of Halo Ring

9. Select halo ring that will allow $1\frac{1}{2}$ cm clearance all around head.

10. Assist physician to infiltrate each of four pin sites with local anesthetic. Assure local anesthesia before proceeding.

11. Tighten positioning discs to secure ring temporarily to head. Posteriorily, ring is placed 1/4″ to 1/2″ above ear (not touching pinnae, which are very sensitive) and anteriorily, just above eyebrows.

12. When desired position is achieved, physician will don sterile gloves and screw each pin through ring and into skin. Anterior pins should *avoid the temporalis region. It is helpful to have the patient close eyes tightly while inserting anterior pins to draw forehead skin down.*

13. Provide torque screwdrivers to tighten pins, ideally used by two operators tightening opposite pins simultaneously. Final tension should reach 5.5 to 6 kg/cm in adult (as measured by dial on torque screwdriver). Guard against facial injury if any of the tools slip.

14. Tighten skull pin locks after skull pins are at desired tension. Place plastic skull pin protectors on skull pin tips. At this point bail traction may be applied (Figure **B**) and the vest donned at a later date.

Rationale

Minimize risk of infection, allow for easy visualization of posterior pin sites, and prevent hair from twisting around skull pins during application and removal.

To maintain skeletal alignment and guard against inadvertent movement of neck. Patient is positioned so that there is free access to the circumference of the head for ring placement.

It is important for skull pins to be at a 90° angle to skull. If halo ring is positioned too high on head, pins may skid up on skull.

Pins placed in temporalis region:
- Make mastication difficult and painful
- Can be difficult to maintain pin torque
- May leave large scars

The ring is held in place by uniform pressure on each pin (about 6-inch pounds of pressure per pin site).

Skull pin locks prevent pins from working loose. Pin protectors alert staff/family to skull pins.

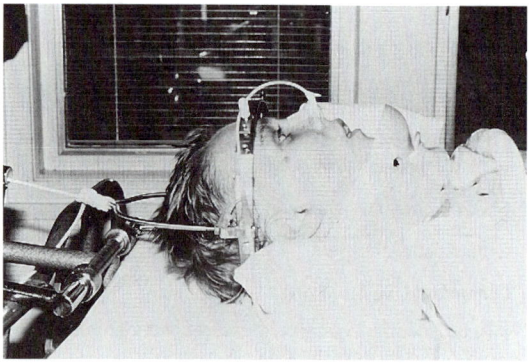

B

Application of the Halo Vest

15. Assist to assemble vest and sheepskin liners.

16. Position posterior vest on patient. Patient can be lifted as a unit up and into the vest or patient can be logrolled into vest. *It is important for staff to maintain cervical spine alignment during this procedure. All staff should work at the direction of the physician as to timing of lift/logroll.*

(Procedure continues)

Procedure 20–3   Application of the Halo-Thoracic Brace (Ring and Vest) (continued)

Action	Rationale
17. Position anterior vest on patient and buckle all straps.	Make certain that vest is positioned as low and snug over shoulders as possible to prevent vest from riding up when upright.
18. Loosely attached metal hardware to connect vest and ring. When proper alignment is achieved, all nuts and bolts are tightened.	Work carefully around hardware with metal wrenches as metal on metal is noisy and distressing to the patient.
19. Assure that patient can swallow without difficulty. Instruct patients to use a straw for drinking and to chew small bits of food thoroughly.	Cervical hyperextension can create difficulty in swallowing and potential choking. It may be necessary to readjust hardware.
20. Following procedure, assist with positioning patient for radiological evaluation.	A cervical spine X ray to determine alignment or a skull X ray to check depth of skull pins may be ordered.
21. Recheck neurovital signs and compare to baseline data.	Look for any signs of deterioration that may be caused by changes in cervical spine position.

Safety Precautions

22. Check that it is possible to perform the *subdiaphragmatic abdominal thrust (Heimlich maneuver)* with the halo brace in place. Place one hand against the abdomen, in the midline slightly above the navel and well below the tip of the xiphoid, and place the second hand directly on top of the first. Press hands into abdomen with a quick upward thrust. If the bottom edge of the vest extends so far down on the patient's body that proper hand placement is not possible, the bottom edge of the vest can be cut with a cast cutter, about 1 inch up or until hand placement is possible. Cover all vest edges with foam tape to prevent rough edges from coming in contact with the skin.

23. Be alert for the following problems and notify physician to make corrective adjustments if:

   • Discomfort persists for more than 24 to 48 hours

   Patients may have headaches for a day or two, which can usually be relieved with mild analgesics. Once established, the halo is surprisingly comfortable.

   • Persistent neck pain or swallowing difficulties occur

   These problems often indicate too much cervical hyperextension.

24. Provide information for potential emergency removal of anterior vest. Refer to Procedure 20–4 to start CPR.

   • *Mark appropriate anterior vest bolts with red fingernail polish to alert staff.*

   • *Tape wrench to fit bolts securely on anterior vest.*

   • *Attach self-adhesive label with emergency instructions to anterior vest. (See Procedure 20–4 for example of label.)*

25. Complete charting for patient in halo bracing should also include information on application, with measurements and ring and vest sizes, skull pin torque, and the removal procedure. The documentation of daily skin, hardware, and vest inspection as well as skull pin care can be incorporated on a daily nursing care flow sheet.

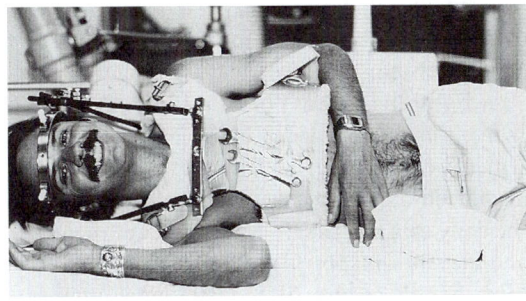

C

Procedure 20–4   Emergency Removal of the Anterior Halo Vest

Purpose

To give cardiopulmonary resuscitation.

Equipment

- Firm surface
- Wrench to fit anterior vest bolts

Action	Rationale
1. Position patient supine on firm surface.	Necessary position to perform CPR. A backboard must be placed under the patient—the plastic halo vest is *not* a substitute.
2. Open airway using jaw-thrust as in Procedure 5–2.	The hardware limits cervical extension and cervical alignment can be maintained with the jaw-thrust method.
3. Remove anterior vest bolts that connect hardware to vest.	A wrench to fit bolts should be taped to vest (and also in an obvious central location) at all times. *Anterior vest bolts can be marked with red fingernail polish on application/admission to alert all staff of appropriate bolts to remove in an emergency.*
4. Release both shoulder and side vest straps. Lift vest off of chest. Begin CPR.	Allows total access to chest for compressions and defibrillation.
5. For halo vest with living hinge feature, follow instructions on self-adhesive label* front of halo vest:	

Emergency Removal of "Breakaway" Halo Vest

- Lie patient supine.
- Undo side straps.
- Stabilize vest above "breakaway" line.
- Lift upwards and fold at "breakaway" line.
- Start CPR.

6. Anterior vest reapplied by physician following emergency. Cervical spine X rays may be ordered to check cervical spine alignment.

*Reprinted with permission: National Rehabilitation Hospital, Washington, DC.

and sensations are realistic to expect based on the level of injury. Side-to-side head movement can give a tremendous sense of freedom and independence to a quadriplegic person after being in a halo for 12 weeks.

An adapted call-bell system increases independence and safety. One system, the Leaf Switch** (Figure 20–3), can be placed near the patient's mouth. It is tongue-activated. If a patient objects to having the switch near the mouth, placement near the lower jaw is an alternative. Slight movement will activate the switch. Biting will destroy it.

The daily care of a patient in a halo requires meticulous *management of skull pins* to prevent infection and excessive scarring. See Procedure 20–5. Infection at a pin site can loosen the skull pin torque and require retorquing—a pain-

ful procedure—or actual reinsertion at another site. Infection can also leave large scars at the pin sites, and with the anterior pins in the forehead, patients are concerned with scars. The tightness of the skull pins should be checked by hand daily. If the skull pin lock or skull pin can be turned, the physician should be notified immediately.

Regular hair washing, at least weekly, is essential. Give a shampoo by placing the patient on a stretcher with the head extended over the edge of the stretcher to the edge of the sink. To prevent water from running down the patient's neck and under the vest, place plastic bags and towels around the neck, to assure that water does *not* drain onto the sheepskin. Be certain the patient is strapped safely on the stretcher. After shampooing, the skull pin sites should be cleansed as in Procedure 20–4. Use paper and plastic cups during the shampoo as metal utensils are noisy should

**Zygo Industries, Inc., P.O. Box 1008, Portland, OR 97207–1008.

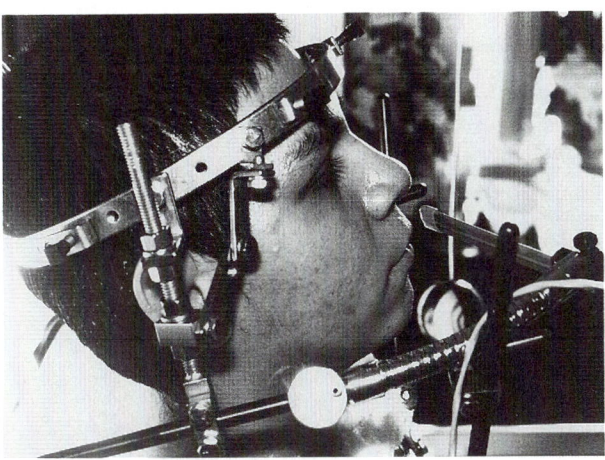

FIGURE 20–3   A Leaf Switch in place using a gooseneck adaptation attached to the hardware.

they accidentally bump against the hardware apparatus around the patient's head.

A big help for easy visualization of the posterior pin sites is to keep hair clipped short. When the halo ring is applied, the scalp is shaved at the posterior pin sites, and it is easy to see the pins. However, as patients may be wearing the halo for up to 12 weeks, hair will grow and obstruct the view.

Care of the Skin

Maintaining *skin integrity* under the halo vest is vital. Skin should be checked day and evening to assure that there is no skin pressure or breakdown. Maintaining cleanliness is also important. See Procedure 20–6.

There should be room under the vest to check the skin by hand without releasing the side and shoulder strap. A flashlight can facilitate viewing the posterior vest area (Figure 20–4). If necessary to see the skin completely or identify potential problem areas, a physician's order is obtained before releasing straps as vest position can be affected.

Keep the sheepskin or polyester lining as clean and dry as possible during the weeks it is in place. It is extremely difficult to dry sheepskin as it is sandwiched between the plastic vest and the patient's own body heat and moisture. Changing vest liners as they become soiled must be weighed against the risk of the potential of any cervical alignment change. See Procedure 20–7.

If a skin problem is suspected under the vest, a soft piece of cloth (a clean pillowcase works well) can be threaded through the vest and grasped at each end. By moving the cloth across the skin and under the vest and then pulling it out, any skin problem area that is draining can be identified. If a problem area is identified, the physician is to be notified for possible vest removal and wound dressing. Permeable clear membrane dressings (Op-site, or Tegaderm, for example) have been effectively used for open pressure sores under the halo vest as they can be left in place for 3 to 7 days. Small foam padding placed above and below endangered areas are effective in redistributing direct pressure. Potential sites for pressure areas include:

- Pin sites
- Scapula
- Clavicle
- Vertebral column (especially if patient is thin)
- Breast area (especially if breasts are large/pendulous)
- Rib cage

Procedure 20–5   Halo Pin Site Care

Purpose

To prevent infection of pin sites.

Equipment

- Sterile dressing tray with gloves
- Sterile cotton-tipped applicators
- Two sterile bowls or medicine cups

- Sterile normal saline
- Disinfectant solution (tincture of Savlon 1:30; Betadine)
- Flashlight

Action

1. Tightness of skull pins should be checked by hand daily. If skull pins can be turned, do not move patient and notify physician immediately (Garfin et al. 1986).

2. Set up small dressing tray with sterile, cotton-tipped applicators and small containers of sterile normal saline and sterile disinfectant solution.

Rationale

Actual tightening of skull pins is done by physician. Nickel (1977) warns that pins should be tightened only when they become loose. Routine tightening of pins will hasten erosions and penetrations. If, on tightening, a pin appears to be penetrating too deeply, or if there is excessive inflammation around pin site, the pin should be replaced in an adjacent location.

(Procedure continues)

Procedure 20–5 Halo Pin Site Care (continued)

3. Gently clean each pin site separately with sterile applicator dipped in disinfectant solution. Clean in one sweeping motion around pin site; discard applicator. Repeat until site is clean.

4. In the same manner repeat procedure with normal saline to remove disinfectant from skin.

5. Dry pin site with dry sterile applicator.

6. Repeat procedure for every pin site.

As skull pins are anchored to skull, prevention of osteomyelitis is important. Sprays or ointments may cake around pin sites and increase risk of infection.

Solutions left on skin will cause excoriation.

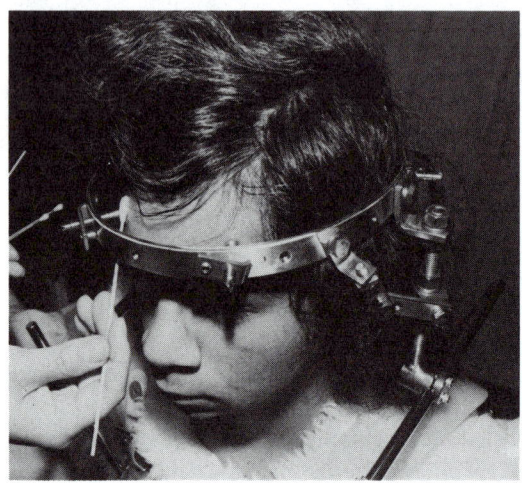

7. To remove any crusting, wrap gauze soaked in normal saline around pin site for 15 minutes to loosen. Repeat soaks until crust can easily be removed.

8. Observe condition of tissue around each pin site. Look for any redness, swelling, crusting, skin tension, tenderness, or pruritis. Use flashlight to visualize posterior pins.

9. Repeat procedure every morning and evening, or more frequently if pin sites are crusty or infected.

10. For complete visualization of posterior pin sites, it may be necessary to clip hair with scissors.

11. Shampoo patient's hair with antibacterial soap weekly, or as needed. Protect halo vest and sheepskin liner with plastic sheeting or plastic bags.

12. If drainage is present obtain a wound culture.

13. Check and tighten bolts on connecting framework and vest weekly. *Never* use bars, framework straps, or vest when turning or transferring patient.

Do not dab or prod crusts with applicator to remove. This additional trauma is a major cause of pin site infection from irritation. Also, removing crusts can be very painful if not soaked loose first!

These may indicate infection, loose pin, or pin skidding on skull.

CAUTION: Clip hair around sites *very carefully* to avoid cutting skin tags that sometimes form at pin sites!

Hair washing greatly minimizes risk of infection. Bathrooms large enough for beds and equipped with long hose spray attachments are ideal.

Infection may be present and a course of antibiotics may be necessary. If infection cannot be controlled, pins may have to be removed and reinserted to prevent more serious complications of abscess formation or osteomyelitis.

These measures protect brace from loosening that could jeopardize cervical alignment.
Note: Metal wrenches on metal hardware are noisy to patient!

---

* Arms (when rubbing against side buckles)
* All edges of brace

To prevent skin scrapes on patients' arms when wearing a halo, pieces of sheepskin may be taped across the buckles on each side of the halo vest. This is especially important when control is impaired. Similarly, all edges of the vest can be padded to prevent irritation and pressure.

To provide patient comfort and safety, specific padding while the patient is in bed is required. See Table 20–6. Any pressure on the halo ring can create intense pain at the skull pin sites. Similarly, *never* grasp the rods to help position or move the patient. Staff must also be cautious of the hardware so as not to injure themselves on protruding rods.

Procedure 20–6   Skin Care For Halo Vest Patient

Purpose

To maintain skin integrity and prevent skin breakdown.

Equipment

- Washcloths
- Basin of water
- Pillows to secure patient in position
- Flashlight

Action	Rationale
1. Check skin under vest daily. Use flashlight to facilitate view. Obtain physician order to release straps if necessary to see skin.	If straps are released, take care *not* to stress framework. Return buckle to previous location on strap (mark location with pen).
2. Use water without soap.	This prevents irritants from accumulating on skin. It is also unwise to use lotions or powders.
3. Wring washcloth out thoroughly so only damp.	This minimizes risk that the liner will get wet. A wet lining will become matted, is difficult to dry (may take several days to do so), and can cause skin problems.
4. Wash patient by reaching under the vest. Securely support patient with pillows.	Gentle handling prevents undue stress on patient and framework of brace.
5. Dry with soft cloth in same manner.	Towels are too bulky. A pillowcase works well.
6. Avoid food crumbs, tobacco, liquids from getting under vest.	A towel can be placed around neck and across front of vest during meals.
7. Observe skin for redness, indicating pressure. Relieve pressure areas with foam padding placed above and below red area.	Padding redistributes weight without direct pressure to area. Place pads between vest and sheepskin so that sheepskin is always next to skin.
8. Provide side-to-side weight shifts for halo patient in wheelchair.	Allows blood to flow to compressed tissue at sacrum and ischial areas.

Also, do not slide the patient up or down in bed. Halo vests and hardware do not slide! Lift the patient with a three-person lift to the desired position.

Activity

For the newly injured patient in halo brace, the three-person lift can be used to transfer from bed to wheelchair, and a full-length transfer board can be used to transfer from bed to bed or bed to tilt table.

When the three-person transfer is used, line up two persons of similar height to handle the trunk/vest area. Position staffs' arms under the patient's vest. Prevent staff arm injury by placing a pad on their arms where they contact the halo vest and hardware. Logroll the patient into the staff's arms and then gently lower the patient into the wheelchair that is being tilted back by a fourth staff person.

As soon as the patient can tolerate the upright sitting position, the sliding board transfer may be used for moving patients from bed to wheelchair and from wheelchair back to bed (Procedure 22–2). Those with physical potential

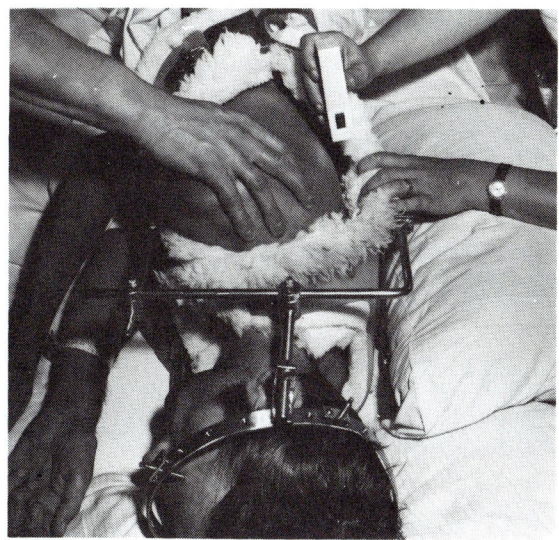

FIGURE 20–4 With the patient in a side-lying position a skin inspection is performed with the aid of a bright flashlight.

Procedure 20–7   Changing Halo-Vest Liners

Purpose
To protect the skin and prevent breakdown, and to maintain personal hygiene.

Equipment
- A *firm* stretcher, table, or bed
- Three pillows
- Two clean liners (anterior and posterior)
- Additional sheepskin pieces (optional)
- Water, soap, face cloth, and small towel

Action and Rationale

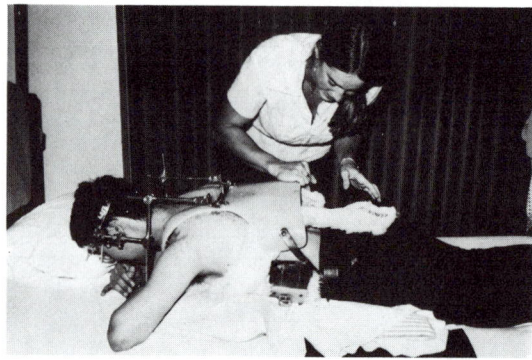

1. Position patient prone on a firm surface with one or two pillows under chest. Place a third pillow under lower legs to relieve pressure on feet. Front bars of brace must be well supported and well *balanced* to maintain alignment throughout procedure. See prone padding and positioning, Table 20–3.

2. Release side buckles *only*. This will maintain maximum support to neck.

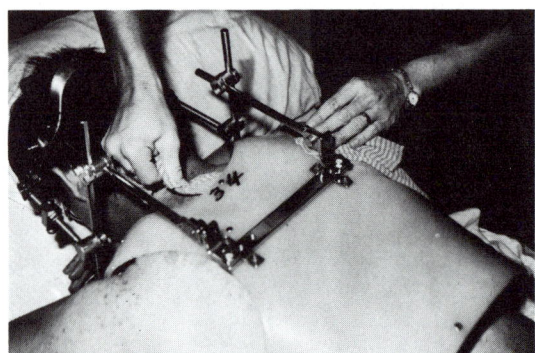

3. Beginning at the shoulders, loosen liner from vest by separating Velcro closures; roll liner downward to bottom of vest. This will move or lift vest as little as possible.

4. Inspect the skin and thoroughly wash and dry the back.

5. Slide a new liner into position under the vest. Once liner is in position, stick liner Velcro to vest Velcro. Ensure that a margin of sheepskin overlaps all edges of the vest. Overlapping is essential to provide adequate protection for the skin.

6. Tighten and buckle side closures in original position. Side closures must be secure before turning patient supine.

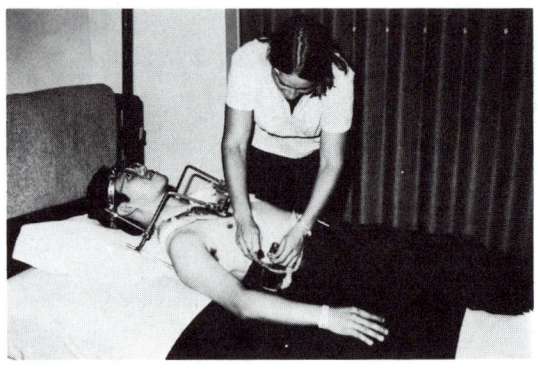

7. Position patient supine and change anterior liner in the same manner.

8. The liners must overlap underneath the side closures. If they do not, cut extra sheepskin 6 × 6 inch squares to cover this area. Squares smaller than 6 × 6 inches will not stay in place.

---

progress with rehabilitation activities, such as pressure relief measures (Figure 20–5). A safety strap, placed high across the vest, is a necessary precaution.

What to wear? Clothing can be modified to fit around the vest and hardware. Shirts or blouses must be one size larger than normally worn. Any top that buttons down the front is fine. Slits from the center of the shoulder to the nipple line at the front and the midportion of the back can be measured against the halo bars for an individual fit. Reinforce edges with bias tape and use Velcro or button and loop closures. For women, a maternity pattern with a yoke can be easily modified simply by sewing Velcro or snaps along the yoke instead of sewing down flat. Families are often eager to help and enjoy making these modifications. Scarves and bandanas can be worn around the neck for warmth, especially in the winter months, and they do not interfere with the hardware (Craig Hospital 1984).

Removal of the Halo Brace
The halo brace takes about 15 to 20 minutes to remove and does not require local anesthesia.

A soft cervical collar is applied before the removal procedure to prevent any excessive flexion and extension of the

TABLE 20–6 Padding for the Patient with a Halo*

Purpose

To provide protection for the joints; to relieve body weight on pressure joints; to accomplish comfort for the patient; and to provide protection from the equipment.

Equipment:

- Pillows
- Foam pads 6″ × 18″ × 3″

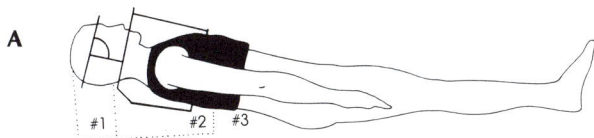

SUPINE

#1	HEAD	A soft pillow or small pad can be placed under the patient's head. *Avoid* direct pressure on the halo ring and head. The halo ring must remain off the mattress. There is to be no firm pressure under the neck area as this may cause hyperextension of the cervical spine.
#2	UNDER VEST	A pad is placed under the back vest hardware to prevent the hardware from puncturing tilt tables, mattresses, and linen and to keep weight off of the halo ring.
#3	BACK	Pad placed in low of back, above spinous processses, to provide elevation of the sacrum, relieve pressure on coccygeal area, relieve muscle tiredness in the back. Another pad is placed below tailbone, across buttocks.

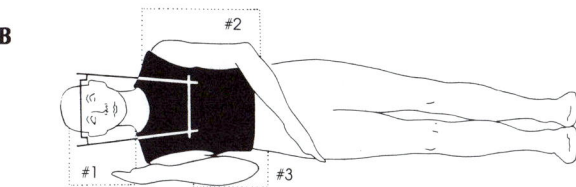

SIDE

#1	HEAD	A soft pillow or small pad can be placed under the patient's head. *Avoid* direct pressure on the halo ring and head. The halo ring must remain off the mattress. There is to be no firm pressure under the neck area as this may cause hyperextension of the cervical spine.
#2	BACK	A pillow is placed behind the patient to help maintain side position. Be sure bottom hip is pulled back to prevent patient from rolling backwards on sacrum.
#3	SIDE	A pad is placed lengthwise from the armpit to waist to maintain proper body alignment, for vest support and pressure equalization, and to prevent undue pain and pressure on the shoulder.

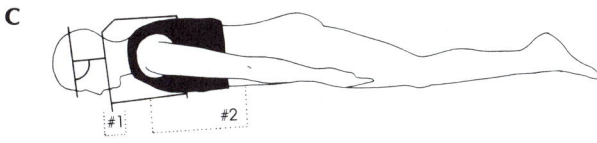

PRONE*

#1	UPRIGHT BARS	Positional padding folded in half is placed under the upright bars to elevate the patient's face. Be certain padding does not interfere with patient's breathing passages.
#2	CHEST	Place a pillow lengthwise under the chest for support and pressure equalization.

---

*Patients who were prone sleepers before injury usually have no problem with the prone position. Others are usually reluctant and not comfortable sleeping prone while in halo brace.
WARNING: Do *not* substitute folded towels or blankets for foam padding or pillows. These can be too firm and cause skin breakdown. Correctly position hips and lower extremities as described in text. (Source: Craig Hospital)

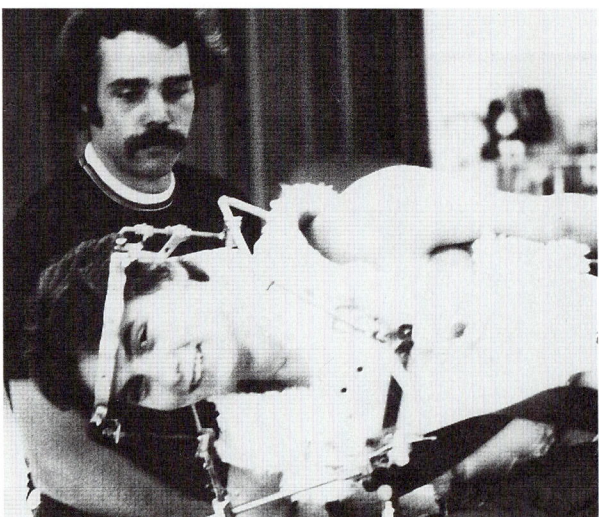

FIGURE 20–5 A patient doing side-weight shift with staff person in attendance.

cervical spine once the hardware is disconnected. The patient's head will seem heavy and wobbly; thus the collar provides a sense of security as well as safety. The hardware is then loosened and removed from the halo vest and ring. The noise may be distressing to the patient, thus it is important for wrench movements not to hit metal on metal more than necessary. The vest is removed by unbuckling the straps. A firmer cervical collar can replace the soft collar at this time.

The halo ring is removed last. It is important for a staff member to hold the ring in place during skull pin loosening so that the ring does not slide on the patient's head as the pins are released. Because many patients complain that the pins are being tightened rather than being loosened, it is important to tell the patient about this potential sensation *before* starting the procedure. This sensation is felt to be the result of the pins creating uneven pressure against the skull. This pin pressure discomfort disappears with 30 to 60 seconds once all pins are removed. It is advantageous to have two persons loosening opposite pins simultaneously for minimum discomfort to the patient.

Once the entire brace is removed, examine the skin for pressure areas from the vest. Clean the pin sites thoroughly with a disinfectant solution. A scab will form at the pin sites within 24 hours. Cleaning the pin sites should be continued until the scabs drop off in 5 to 7 days. After the scabs drop off, massage the pin sites to smooth out any puckering skin, which will decrease scarring. Take cervical spine X rays following halo removal to verify alignment.

The patient can have a shampoo after the scabs have formed at the pin sites. Remember that the patient may require additional padding under the head when in bed.

Without hardware to hold up the head and with tender neck muscles for 2 to 3 days following halo removal, a patient lying in the side position may require an additional pillow.

Semirigid Cervical Orthoses: The Guilford Brace

The Guilford brace is an example of a rigid cervical orthosis. These neck braces afford fairly good support limiting flexion and to a lesser extent extension and rotational movements. This type of orthosis is characterized by rigid struts between the chest plate and chin support anteriorly and between the back plate and occipital support posteriorly. See Figure 20–6. These posts are usually adjustable, and there are commonly two or four of them. Leather straps over the shoulders and around the chest connect the anterior and posterior structures.

The Guilford brace is described here because it is widely used, is a simple style, and is easy to apply. The circular support structure for the head spreads the pressure on the skin surface, increasing patient comfort, and the shoulder straps make alignment adjustments easy.

Method of Application

The initial application and fitting is usually completed by the orthotist. Following application observe for any swal-

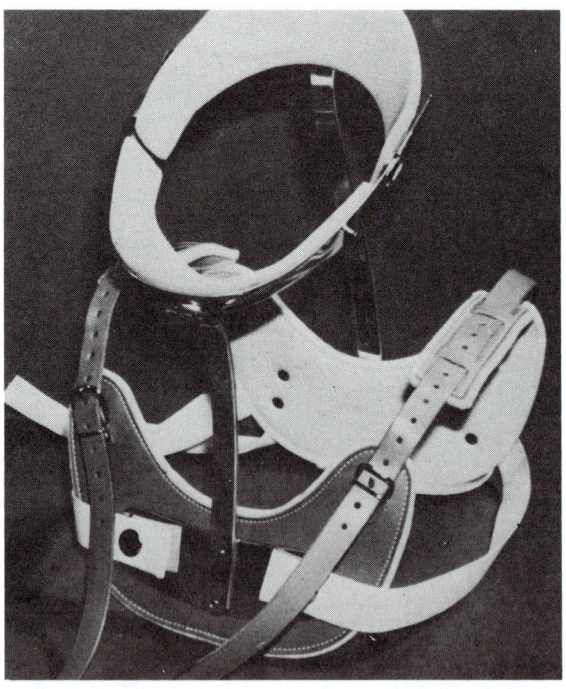

FIGURE 20–6 The Guilford brace is an example of a cervical orthosis that provides moderate support.

lowing difficulties. Adjustment may be necessary. Initial X-ray evaluation may be ordered to check alignment. See Procedure 20–8.

The brace is designed to support weight in the sitting or standing position and will cause uncomfortable pressure points otherwise. Therefore, the brace can generally be removed for short periods or at night when the patient is in the supine position. Prevent excessive flexion, extension, and rotation when the brace is removed, leaving the neck unprotected. Support the neck manually or with a soft collar when bathing or moving in bed. Instruct patients not to move their necks. An old brace can be

Procedure 20–8 Donning the Guilford Brace (an Example of a Rigid Cervicothoracic Device)

Purpose

To provide support by limiting flexion and, to a lesser extent, extension and rotation of the cervical spine.

Action	Rationale
1. Assemble brace and check to make sure that buckles and straps are not broken or worn.	This is a safety precaution to prevent accidental movement when brace is in place.
2. Always don (and remove) brace when patient is flat in bed.	Donning the brace before patient sits up protects against major forces causing neck movement. This principle also applies to removal.
3. Logroll patient to one side keeping neck rigid. Put on back plate of the brace so occipital support fits snugly to base of skull. Extend straps and make sure they are not twisted. Emphasis is placed on the back portion of the brace being placed correctly (evenly and straight) before attempting to put on the front.	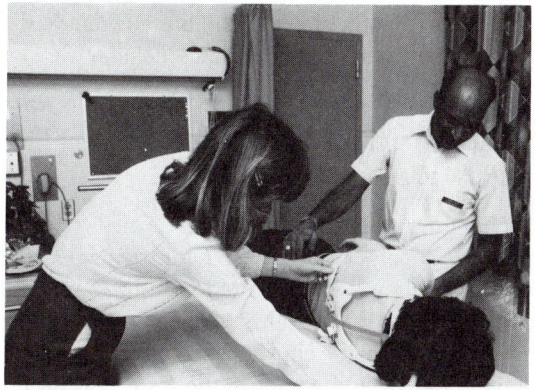
4. Return patient to supine position.	
5. Put on chest plate so that chin support fits correctly (snugly).	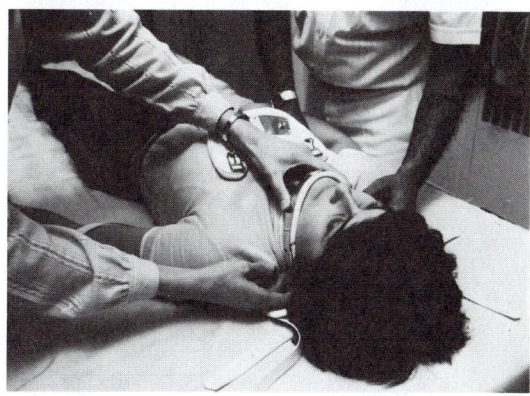
6. Secure under-the-arm and over-the-shoulder straps. Ensure that brace is snug and comfortable but not too tight.	The front and back pieces of the brace must fit securely to provide adequate support.
7. Mark straps with ink at the desired buckle closure.	Following adjustments, this ensures that correct position is then maintained.
8. Check the brace again, when the patient is sitting up 30° to 45° in bed, before transferring to the wheelchair.	With the change in posture, the shoulders tend to drop, and the desired pressure on the shoulder straps is lost.

worn while showering so that the good one remains dry. A soft collar must replace the brace during the night.

Care of the Skin

Points of greatest pressure on the skin are around the chin and occiput and under the straps and buckles, especially at the shoulders. Men can apply alcohol after shaving to toughen up the skin. For added protection, place the brace over a T-shirt. Examine the skin every 2 hours for a few days after application, then daily during morning and evening care. Daily bathing and, of course, turns or changes of position every 2 hours are needed to prevent general skin breakdown. It is dangerous to use the prone position.

Activity

When the fracture site requires this lesser degree of immobilization, the physical activity involved will be as full a program as the patient can tolerate, with occasional specified limitations.

Removal of the Brace

X-ray evaluation is required before the brace is removed. After it is removed, patients often wear a soft collar.

Limiting Neck Movement: The Cervical Collar

In its simplest form, the *soft cervical collar* is made of very soft foam with a polyethylene strip reinforcement with stockingette covering and Velcro posterior closures—a "neck warmer." See Figure 20–7. Whatever the construction, collars extend only from the chin and occiput to the shoulders and do not actually immobilize the neck. A cervical collar is applied whenever patients need a nonrigid support to remind them to be cautious with neck movements. (It is usually applied after removal of other braces or when no bony injury has occurred.)

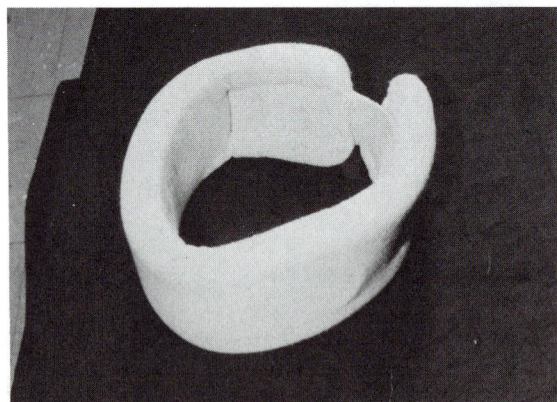

FIGURE 20–7 A soft collar is used when minimal cervical protection is desired.

Method of Application

Once the correct size and initial fitting has been completed (often by an occupational therapist) the collar can often be removed for short periods to provide nursing care. The same principles apply as when donning a neck brace: that is, major protection is needed during activity, so the collar should be removed and reapplied when the patient is in the supine position with the neck stabilized.

Care of the Skin

A cervical collar exerts greatest pressure on the skin at the chin, occiput, and collar bone. Examine and wash the skin under the collar every day.

Activity

Patients are generally allowed as much physical activity as they can tolerate.

Removal of the Collar

The soft collar is used primarily to provide some vertical support, which may reduce muscle spasm and neck ache. When discontinuing its use the physician will weight this comfort aspect against the possibility of contributing to muscle atrophy from disuse of neck muscles.

Thoracolumbar Orthoses

Fractures of the thoracolumbar spine are notoriously unstable. The physician will select a mode of management based on extent of neurological deficit, severity of spinal fracture, and general condition.

Immobilization with bedrest (with or without surgery to the spine) may be augmented by a brace to provide additional safety and comfort. Generally, a 6- to 8-week period of bedrest is required for soft-tissue healing and bony union. Following a sufficient period of bedrest, bracing is mandatory to provide spinal stability during gradual mobilization. When surgical reduction and internal fixation are carried out, bracing is still required but mobilization is usually more rapid.

The bracing is usually some type of individually molded body jacket, which can be removed for skin care, or removable hyperextension bracing. See Procedure 20–9. A permanently placed body cast may be applied when the patient has a low lumbar injury with preserved sensation over most of the torso.

Method of Application

Body jackets are generally individualized braces fabricated by the orthotist. This involves application of a plaster body cast that is later cut up each side (bivalved) and used as a body cradle or as a mold to make anterior and posterior shells of various sturdier plastics. The shells are lined with removable sheepskin and joined together by straps at the level of the chest and abdomen.

Procedure 20–9   Donning the Jewett Brace (an Example of a Hyperextension Thoracolumbar Orthosis)

Purpose

To provide support by maintaining hyperextension and preventing flexion of the thoracic and lumbar spine.

Action	Rationale
1. Assemble brace and check that side closure is sturdy.	This is a safety precaution to prevent accidental movement when brace is in place.
2. Select a sheepskin liner (optional) that overlaps borders of anterior frame.	Overlapping is necessary to protect skin adequately. However, if brace is worn over soft clothing, sheepskin liner may not be needed.
3. Always don (and then remove) brace while patient is supine.	This avoids movements when patient is active.
4. Place the anterior frame low over torso (part covered by bikini).	
5. Logroll patient to one side and close back strap.	

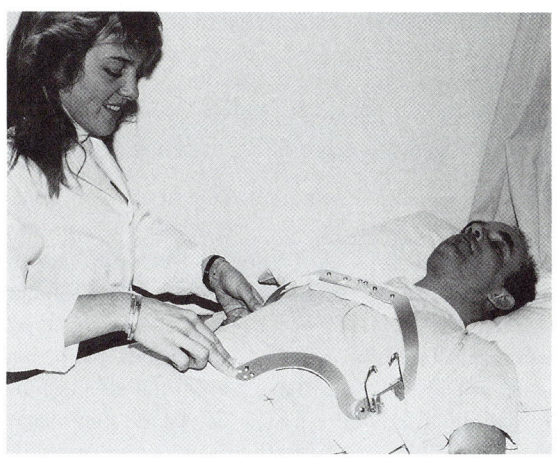 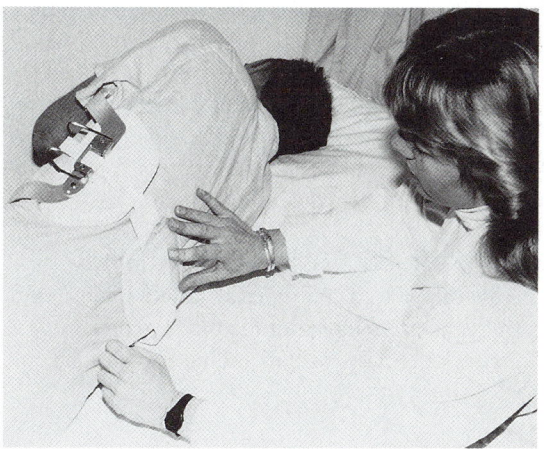

6. Ensure that brace fits snugly. It should be comfortable but not too tight.	
7. Check position of the brace when patient is sitting in wheelchair.	Braces have a tendency to ride up when sitting.

Commercially made three-point fixation braces, such as the Jewett hyperextension brace, afford less stability but are widely used because they are much less expensive and can be individually adjusted to hip and body length. The anterior frame should be lined with sheepskin initially, and later worn over soft clothing. A back strap with a side closure secures the brace at the waist. Following initial application and fitting, the physician may allow removal for daily hygiene and, eventually, at night while the patient is in the supine position. Prevent any flexion, extension, or rotation movements when the back is unprotected by the brace, and caution patients against attempting to move the trunk.

Care of the Skin

Examine the skin under the brace every 8 hours for 1 to 3 weeks after application and then daily, until the brace is discontinued. Closely observe the underarms, iliac crests, small of back, and under buckles and Velcro straps. Regular change of position is necessary to prevent general skin breakdown. Once the patient can tolerate a full program of activity, a substitute brace can be used when tub bathing. It is a good idea to have former patients donate their braces when they no longer require them.

Activity

Each stage of the progression of activity is specifically ordered for each patient, depending on clinical, surgical, and radiological findings, but the stages include:

- Bedrest in the recumbent position. (A longer period is required for conservative management.) During this time, the patient may use a self-propelling wheelchair-stretcher. The patient is positioned prone for propelling this equipment.

- Gradual mobilization over 7 days by elevating the head of the bed 45 degrees, flexing knees over the pillows placed lengthwise, and using the tilt table up to 70 degrees in physical therapy.
- Increased mobilization over 7 days by sitting in a wheelchair, assisting transfers at all times, avoiding trunk rotation, and avoiding long sitting.
- Full mobilization allowing all wheelchair activities, independent transferring, and using long sitting position for dressing.

The fracture site is evaluated regularly at the following intervals:

- Following application of the orthosis
- When the patient can tolerate a position of 70 degrees (with approximately 7 days of tilt table activity) (standing X rays)
- When the patient can tolerate a partial program of mobilization (7 days) (sitting X rays)
- After any accidental fall or with increased pain and spasm or neurological deterioration

Removal of the Orthosis

Radiological evaluation is continued at various intervals for 4 to 6 months before removal of the brace. The patient's clinical picture will be assessed, including any pain, before making a decision.

SURGICAL INTERVENTION*

Accurate evaluation and appropriate management of bony and ligamentous injuries of the spinal column are a most important aspect of acute care. See Chapter 4. Ultimate surgical management of SCI is best achieved by collaboration between an orthopedic surgeon and a neurosurgeon, and with the cooperation of a health care team that will select a total treatment approach that accommodates the patient's general condition, stabilizes the fracture site, and facilitates any potential neurological recovery. Early mobilization to prevent physiological and psychological complications associated with bedrest is a key consideration influencing this decision-making process.

There are no absolute indications for surgical stabilization of the spine. The possible gains must be weighed against the risks of operating on patients who often have

multiple trauma and autonomic dysfunction with respiratory and cardiovascular instability (Meyer 1989). However, *general* conditions warrant surgical treatment in the acute and early stages as vertebral column injuries that cause severe fracture dislocations, facet-locking dislocations, or grossly unstable fractures, especially when the neurological injury is incomplete. Other indications for operative intervention are failure to achieve adequate alignment by closed techniques and bone fragments in the spinal canal. Progressive neurological deterioration is often considered an absolute indication for surgical intervention in selected patients.

Cervical Spine Surgery

Operative treatment of an unstable cervical spine injury has two main objectives:

- To decompress the spinal canal by removing all bony and soft tissue elements that are pressing against the spinal cord
- To obtain immediate stability so that the patient can be mobilized and begin early rehabilitation

In general, decompression is of benefit even in severe cervical cord injuries. In incomplete injuries, decompression of the spinal canal affords the best environment for spinal cord recovery. In complete SCI, decompression may be indicated to allow for recovery of a single nerve root level. In the cervical spine, recovery of one additional nerve root is significant because it may have a profound effect on the patient's ability to function independently. *Decompression* is most commonly achieved by the surgical removal of the fractured vertebral body (a corpectomy) via an anterior approach.

Stabilization of the cervical spine is most commonly achieved via a posterior approach using wires and bone grafts. Graft sources are the iliac crest, fibula, or tibia. Wiring is secured in the strong, large spinous processes of the cervical spine. This technique usually provides immediate stability such that the patient is only required to wear a semirigid brace after surgery. If the degree of bony injury or medical condition precludes surgical stabilization, a halo vest is used because it is the most rigid orthosis for maintaining alignment of an unstable spine until healing has occurred. Newer methods of stabilizing the cervical spine use anterior and posterior plates and screws.

Thoracolumbar Spine Surgery

Determining the degree of stability and necessity of surgery is complex. Stability may be determined based on the degree of disruption of the anterior, middle, and posterior columns of the spine as detailed in Chapter 4. Fractures of the upper thoracic spine tend to be initially stable because of the protective rib cage. But although bony damage may

*This section was contributed by James S. Keene, M.D., Associate Professor of Orthopedics, University of Wisconsin, and codirector of the University of Wisconsin Spine Injury Center, Madison, Wisconsin, and Thomas A. Zdeblick, M.D., Assistant Professor, Division of Orthopedic Surgery, University of Wisconsin.

be minimal, ligamentous damage tends to be extensive. When natural healing occurs, torn ligaments are replaced with fibrous tissue, which is often not as strong as the original, and late spinal instability may then occur (Ozer 1988). Early operative treatment may prevent this, but on the other hand, spontaneous healing may result in a more stable union. Injuries to the thoracolumbar junction are much more likely to be severe and unstable. Indications for surgery are less controversial.

Back surgery generally requires instrumentation. *Harrington rods*, for example, are steel instruments that are as thick and long as pencils with cleats at each end. The rods are embedded in the neural arch and the cleats are ideally attached to the strong pedicles one to three levels above and below the fracture site. Generally a local fusion is performed at the same time.

Operative treatment of the unstable thoracolumbar spine is predicated on the anatomic structures disrupted and the biomechanical forces produced by the instrumentation used (Torg et al. 1986; Keene 1987). For example, *forward flexion injuries (wedge compression fractures)* are usually stable injuries because the middle and posterior columns have not been disrupted. Operative treatment may not be indicated. However, when there is severe compression of the vertebral body, or in cases of multiple contiguous compression fractures, disruption of the posterior column occurs. Instrumentation that permits distraction (a force to push apart or separate) of the anterior column, and compression (a force to draw together) of the posterior column of the spine, appears to be the best method of stabilization to avoid the potential for progression of the kyphotic deformity. When Harrington instrumentation is used, the distraction rod restores the height of the compressed vertebra, and the compression rod supplies the posterior mechanical hinge that has been disrupted.

Flexion-axial compression injuries (burst fractures) also can be classified as stable and unstable injuries (McAfee, Yua, and Lasda 1982). In stable burst fractures, the facet joints of the posterior column remain intact. With acutely unstable burst fractures, the posterior column has sustained injury, particularly the facet-joint capsules, in addition to the anterior and middle columns. If this injury is operatively treated and internally stabilized, bilateral distraction instrumentation should be used. Bilateral distraction instrumentation will stabilize the spine and, to varying degrees, reduce the retropulsed, posterior wall of the vertebral body. Compression instrumentation produces a component of anterior axial compression and requires an intact posterior wall of the vertebral body (the axis of rotation) for it to be effective (Torg et al. 1986). Therefore, use of this instrumentation by itself for burst fractures does not appear to be biomechanically sound.

More recently, pedicle screw fixation devices have been used for the treatment of thoracolumbar burst fractures. The advantages of this method are not only one level above

and below the fractured vertebra are stabilized and fused. Newer fixator systems can apply both distraction and lordosis to reduce the deformity and have rigidity which promotes fracture healing, but their clinical use is just beginning.

There are two main types of *flexion-distraction injuries*. In the first type, chance fractures, the flexion axis is anterior to the anterior longitudinal ligament. This injury does not require operative treatment when there is minimal angulation and displacement at the fracture site. In the second type, the flexion axis is posterior to the anterior longitudinal ligament. This results in varying degrees of anterior compression of the vertebral body (anterior column) and disruption of the bony and/or ligamentous components of the middle and posterior columns. Operative treatment of this injury is called for if the posterior anatomic hinge has been disrupted. Because distraction instrumentation does not provide a posterior mechanical hinge, bilateral compression rods are the instrumentation of choice (Keene et al. 1986; Torg et al. 1986). If, however, there is moderate to severe anterior compression of the vertebral body, the combination of distraction and compression instrumentation is preferred.

Fracture-dislocations involve various components of the other injuries. Operative treatment of this injury requires reduction of the deformity with distraction instrumentation and maintenance of the reduction with compression instrumentation. The loss of any anatomic hinge that occurs with this injury precludes the use of bilateral distraction instrumentation.

Many studies of the results of spinal instrumentation indicate that anatomic reductions result in a much lower incidence and severity of subsequent back pain than is observed with nonanatomic reductions. However, only McAfee, Yuan, and Lasda (1982) and Keene and associates (1986) have analyzed the quality of reductions achieved with respect to both type of injury and the method of instrumentation. Keen and associates (1986) found that compression combined with distraction instrumentation provided the best percent correction in angle of deformity and displacement over all categories of injuries. However, the best percent corrections achieved in burst fractures and flexion-distraction injuries were obtained with bilateral distraction and bilateral compression instrumentation, respectively. The study also found that fractures instrumented within 6 weeks of injury had significantly better corrections than those instrumented after a longer interval.

Preoperative and Postoperative Care

Preparation. In addition to the general preoperative teaching and preparation required for any surgical patient, it is important to ensure that both the patient and the family have realistic expectations of the pending operation. Assess their understanding of the expected outcome after they have spoken with the surgeon, reinforce explanation that bone structures can be repaired but the spinal cord cannot, clarify concerns, and refer misconceptions appropriately. Realization that surgery is not a cure is a frequent postoperative disappointment.

Postoperative care. General postoperative care includes observing for excessive blood loss and monitoring for reactions to anesthetic gases, drugs, transfusions, and fluid replacement. Assess vital signs remembering that patients with quadriplegia generally have a lowered blood pressure (90/60 mmHg). To detect blood loss, scrutinize blood values carefully, especially watching for a lowered hematocrit. (See Chapter 6 for review of neural control of blood pressure and dysfunctions following SCI. Hemorrhagic versus spinal shock is also described.)

If the anterior approach has been used for a cervical operation, closely assess respirations. Distress may be caused by neck edema at the operative site.

Be familiar with the patient's preoperative *neurological status* to establish baseline data. During the immediate postoperative period, frequent (hourly) serial neurological assessment should be completed. (Chapter 4 reviews this process.) Any deterioration may be related to cord edema or hemorrhage at the operative site.

Prevention of secondary complications. All the general measures to protect patients from the hazards of immobility very much apply after surgery. Reliable turning and correct positioning must be carried out. However, during the first 4 to 8 hours, patients may be kept supine to promote blood coagulation by increasing pressure on posterior cervical or thoracolumbar incisions. Special assistance to help patients with quadriplegia keep the chest clear from retained secretions is important. Also follow protocols to prevent formation of a deep vein thrombosis as described in Chapter 16. Surgery further increases risk for paralyzed patients. If anticoagulant therapy is used, anticipate an added risk of hemorrhage from the operative site.

Alleviating pain. Assess the level of pain and anxiety, which are often related to movement and turning of the patients in bed. Small doses of intravenous analgesics and antispasticity medications are generally sufficient to relieve pain, muscle spasm, and tension. Try to anticipate needs; for example, medicate before physical therapy treatments.

Recovery period. Because of interference with the responses from the central and autonomic nervous systems, postoperative reactions of paralyzed patients tend to be more pronounced than those of other patients. When added to existing respiratory or circulatory problems, these heightened reactions can slow postoperative recovery.

Gradually, within a few days or weeks following surgery, patients are mobilized. To promote maximum healing of the spine and supporting ligaments, orthotic devices are frequently used to provide additional support and protection (approximately a 3-month period required), minimize pain, and avoid late complications of spinal instability. Careful clinical monitoring and serial flexion-extension X rays are used to evaluate the healing process, which gives direction to the amount and types of increased physical activity recommended.

LONG-TERM IMPLICATIONS

When assessing a person who has been spinal cord injured for a while, the healthy and active disabled person will probably be able to maintain good body posture without evidence of contractures. Continued use of the *prone* position, especially as a natural sleeping position, is well advised as a preventive measure to combat hip and knee contractures and relieve pressure on the buttocks to avoid skin breakdown.

However, difficulty maintaining an erect position in the wheelchair and spinal curvatures may become evident relatively quickly following injury. This is especially true for those sustaining thoracolumbar fractures and for children still growing. Problems are often related to inadequate or late stabilization and undetected problems (see Chapter 4) during the acute stage, and perhaps difficulty with extensive fracture site, too much or too stressful activity too soon, or premature removal of orthoses.

Chronic Posttraumatic Instability*

Chronic posttraumatic instability can occur with all types of spine fractures. It may present with or without fairly obvious progressive *kyphosis*. Diagnosis should be considered with a positive instability test. The weight-bearing thoracolumbar spine is prone to problems.

Late, postfracture *kyphosis*, often following laminectomy, may cause chronic pain, progressive neural deficits, and incomplete rehabilitation. However, posttraumatic instability due to posterior ligaments (flexion-distraction) injuries may be difficult to recognize. Reports in the literature have not specifically addressed the problem of chronic instability that occurs without progressive kyphosis, nor identified the types of injuries that produce chronic painful instability (Malcolm, Bradford, and Winter 1981; Roberson and Whitesides 1985). In a recent study (Keene, Lash, and Kling 1988), the types of injuries that result in chronic instability were evaluated.

This study's results suggest that the surgical management of chronic posttraumatic instability are influenced by the type of injury, time to surgery, and method of instrumentation.

In summary, the bad prognostic signs for successful surgery in these patients include: (1) wedge-compression fractures, especially multiple fractures involving consecutive levels and (2) the presence of a progressive kyphotic deformity. Compression instrumentation produces good results,

*This section was contributed by J. Keene, M.D.

especially in flexion-distraction injuries, but good results should not be expected following late stabilization of wedge-compression fractures, regardless of the type of surgical treatment rendered.

Noncontiguous spinal injuries are common and are associated with late complications (Figure 20–8). Patients with fractures at one level should have radiographic examination of the entire spine (Chapter 4). If noncontiguous fractures are evident on the standard radiographs, all levels of injury should be thoroughly evaluated with computed tomography. If the minor level is unstable or there is doubt concerning its stability, it should be reduced and internally stabilized. With Harrington instrumentation, this method of treatment may require instrumentation of very long segments of the spine and severely restrict motion. Thus, short segmental fusions and interpedicular screw fixation, or short fusions that only encompass the unstable segments and removal of the Harrington rods after the fusions are solid, may prevent deformities and enhance subsequent mobility of the spine.

Immobilization Hypercalcemia

Immobilization hypercalcemia is not a common complication of SCI, but its incidence is greatest in adolescent males with complete cervical cord injuries when dehydration and prolonged periods of immobilization are experienced (Kaplan et al. 1978; Berczeller and Bezkor 1986). During this time, bone formation is essentially decreased while the rate of calcium absorption remains elevated. The exact mechanism of this endocrine imbalance is not known.

Major symptoms include anorexia, nausea, and headache, which can easily be misinterpreted as nonspecific complaints of SCI. Diagnosis is confirmed by laboratory tests indicating increased levels of calcium in the blood and urine. Treatment is aimed at lowering serum calcium and includes vigorous hydration, calcitonin, and steroids (Maynard 1986). Hypercalcemia is thought to be self-limiting but may last more than a year without corrective treatment.

Heterotopic Bone Formation

Heterotopic bone formation, or more specifically *para-articular heterotopic ossification*, is misplacement, or an abnormal deposit, of new bone formation around joints

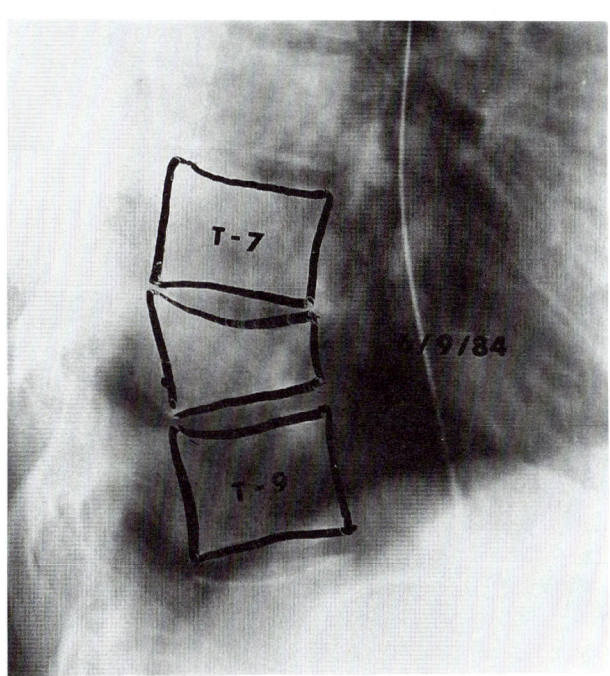

A

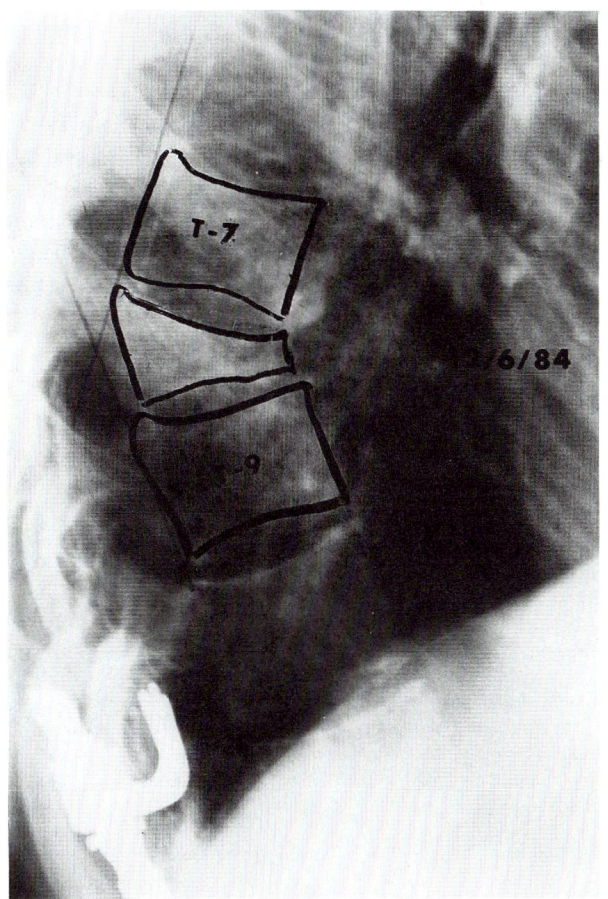

B

FIGURE 20–8   Initial lateral radiograph (**A**) demonstrating noncontiguous, T_8 compression in a patient with an L_1 burst fracture that was operatively treated with bilateral distraction instrumentation which extended from T_{10} to L_3. Six months after injury the burst fracture had healed, but a lateral radiograph of the thoracic spine (Figure **B**) demonstrated that anterior compression of T_8 had increased from 21% to 63% and the angle of deformity (kyphosis) from 14° to 30°.

of paralyzed limbs. The etiology is completely unknown, but it has been reported in approximately 15% to 20% of all patients with SCI (Freehafer 1977). It is more common in higher level injuries, often involving the hip, knee, elbow, or shoulder joints. Completeness of injury; older age; and the presence of pressure sores and spasticity are suggested risk factors that appear to be additive (Santosh, Hamilton, Heinemann, and Betts 1989). Calcification, which evolves into mature bone formation, causes swelling, stiffness, and limited function of involved joints. The process may last for a period of months and occurs in various stages (Egan and Stack 1985). Onset is usually within one year after injury.

Note characteristic signs: localized redness, swelling, or stiffness of joints, swelling of the involved extremity, systemic temperature elevation, and possibly discomfort or referred pain. Also the serum phosphatase and erythrocyte sedimentation rate (ESR) will remain elevated. Radiological evaluation and bone scanning will reveal bone formation and confirm diagnosis. Serial evaluations will monitor rate of bone formation.

Activation as soon as possible is the treatment of choice, providing gentle range of motion exercises at frequent intervals. Sitting with the hips and knees bent is desirable. Bedrest may cause stiff joints, which may eventually render sitting impossible. Fortunately, many patients respond satisfactorily with minor limitation of motion. Disodium editronate diphosphonate is a drug used to prevent mineralization, which may also be given prophylactically (Berczeller and Bezkor 1986). Eventually, however, when bone formation is mature, surgical removal may be necessary.

Joint Immobility (Ankylosis)

Although many patients with heterotopic bone formation are able to complete a rehabilitation program, if ossification progresses it may cause joint immobility (ankylosis), which may lead to severe loss of function or prevent sitting in a wheelchair. Surgical removal may be necessary, but unless undertaken when bone is mature (1 to 2 years) there is a definite incidence of recurrence (Stauffer 1977).

Pathological Fractures (Long Bones)

Pathological fractures of the long bones are associated with osteoporotic changes accompanying paralysis (Berczeller and Bezkor 1986). This increase in porosity and softness of the bones is related to disuse and is not sufficiently advanced until at least a year after injury to cause problems. Then a minor trauma, such as a careless transfer or a fall from a wheelchair, can cause a fracture, commonly in the leg bones. Observe for any localized swelling, abnormal alignment or mobility, creptitus, and possibly increased spasm.

Most of the time individuals will hear a crack and be well aware of the break. Long bone fractures, in both acute and chronic situations, may require surgical fixation to reduce complications and increase functional level.

REFERENCES

Berczeller, P., and Bezkor, M. 1986. *Medical Complications of Quadriplegia.* Chicago: Year Book Medical Publishers.

Browner, C., and Mattingly, G. 1986. Why Me? A patient education booklet designed for the ambulatory patient in halo brace. Distributed by Ace Medical Company, Los Angeles, CA.

Craig Hospital, 1984. *A viable way to involve patients with cervical injuries in an active rehabilitation program.* Denver, CO: Craig Hospital Literature, RMRSCI, Inc. *Describes development and implementation of a halo protocol and systematic follow-up procedure for patients in halo bracing.*

Egan, J., and Stack, J. 1985. In *Nursing Spinal Cord Injuries.* Ed. N. M. Woll. Totowa, NJ: Rowman & Allanheld. *Valuable text based on nurse practitioner program at the Veterans' Administration Medical Center and California State University, Long Beach. Includes in-depth section on nursing patients with para-articular ossification.*

Freehafer, A. 1977. Long-term management of lumbar paraplegia. In *The Total Care of Spinal Cord Injuries.* Eds. D. Pierce and V. Nickel. Boston: Little, Brown, pp. 135–164. *Multifaceted overview of management principles and potential complications.*

Garfin, S., et al. 1986. Complications in the use of the halo fixation device. *Journal of Bone and Joint Surgery.* 68-A (3): 320–325. *Medical records of 179 patients reviewed to identify complications related to the halo device. Discusses complications of pin loosening and pin-site infection in detail.*

Green, B. A., Green, K. L., and Klose, K. J. 1980. Kinetic nursing for spinal cord injury patients. *Paraplegia* 18 (3): 181–186. *Reviews 105 patients over a 42-month period treated on the RotoRest Treatment Table. Observed reduced occurrence of complications in pulmonary, cardiovascular, skin, musculoskeletal, nervous, gastrointestinal and genitourinary systems while maintaining spinal stability during mobilization.*

Kaplan, P., et al. 1978. Calcium balance in paraplegic patients: Influence of injury duration and ambulation. *Archives of Physical Medicine and Rehabilitation* 59 (Oct.): 447–450. *Research indicates that hypercalciuria (negative calcium balance) is significantly decreased with early ambulation; includes review of calcium metabolic balance determination studies and previous clinical and experimental data. Extensive bibliography.*

Keene, J. S. 1987. Thoracolumbar fractures in winter sports. *Clinical Orthopedics* 216: 39–49.

Keene, J. S., Lash, E. J., Kling, T. F., Jr. 1988. Undetected post-traumatic instability of "stable" thoracolumbar fractures. *Journal of Trauma* 2 (3): 202–211.

Keene, J. S., Wackitz, D. L., Drummond, D. S., et al. 1986. Compression-distraction instrumentation on unstable thoracolumbar fractures: Anatomic results obtained with each type of injury and method of instrumentation. *Spine* 11: 895–902.

Koehler, C. 1980. RMRSCIS halo protocol and halo vest nursing management. *SCI News Briefs*, 2 (10). December. *Reports a study of 17 halo patients followed on the halo protocol to monitor appropriate healing of cervical spine and preventing further neurological loss. Describes procedure for emergency removal of anterior vest.*

McAfee, P. C., Yuan, H. A., and Lasda, N. A. 1982. The unstable burst fracture. *Spine* 7: 365.

Malcolm, B. W., Bradford, D. S., and Winter, R. B. et al. 1981. Post-traumatic kyphosis. *Journal of Bone and Joint Surgery* 63-A: 891–899.

Maynard, F. M. 1986. Immobilization hypercalcemia following spinal cord injury. *Archives of Physical Medicine and Rehabilitation* 67 (1): 41–44.

Meyer, P. R. (Ed.). 1989. *Surgery of Spine Trauma.* New York: Churchill Livingstone. *Expertly illustrated material on numerous sequelae of SCI renders this text a valuable resource for the entire interdisciplinary team. Focus on acute stabilization of multisystem trauma and the skeletal system.*

Nickel, V. 1977. The halo. In *Spinal Disorders, Diagnosis and Treatment.* Eds. D. Ruge and L. Wiltse. Philadelphia: Lea and Febiger.

Ozer, M. 1988. *The Management of Persons with Spinal Cord Injury.* New York: Demos Publications.

Roberson, J. R., and Whitesides, T. E. 1985. Surgical reconstruction of late post-traumatic thoracolumbar kyphosis. *Spine* 10: 307–312.

Rogers, E. 1978–1979. Nursing management in relation to beds within the national spinal injuries center for the prevention of pressure sores. *International Journal of Paraplegia* 16: 147–153. *Focus on nursing management of the patient on a Stoke-Eggerton turning and tilting electrical bed; includes step-by-step procedure for operating bed and instructions for positioning and manually lifting a patient.*

Santosh, L., Hamilton, B. B., Heinemann, A., and Betts, H. B. 1989. Risk factors for heterotopic ossification in spinal cord injury. *Archives of Physical Medicine and Rehabilitation* 70 (May): 387–390.

Stauffer, E. 1977. Long-term management of quadriplegia. In *The Total Care of Spinal Cord Injuries.* Eds. D. Pierce and V. Nickel. Boston: Little, Brown, pp. 81–102. *Multifaceted review of ongoing assessment, principles of management, functional goals of rehabilitation, and potential problems.*

Torg, J. S., Pavlov, H., Genuario, S. E., Sennett, B., Wisneski, R. J., Robie, B. H., Jahre, C. 1986. Neuropraxia of the cervical spinal cord with transient quadriplegia. *Journal of Bone and Joint Surgery* 68-A: 1354–1370.

Yoshimura, T. 1989. Nursing management. In *Management of High Quadriplegia.* Ed. G. Whiteneck. New York: Demos Publications pp. 61–75.

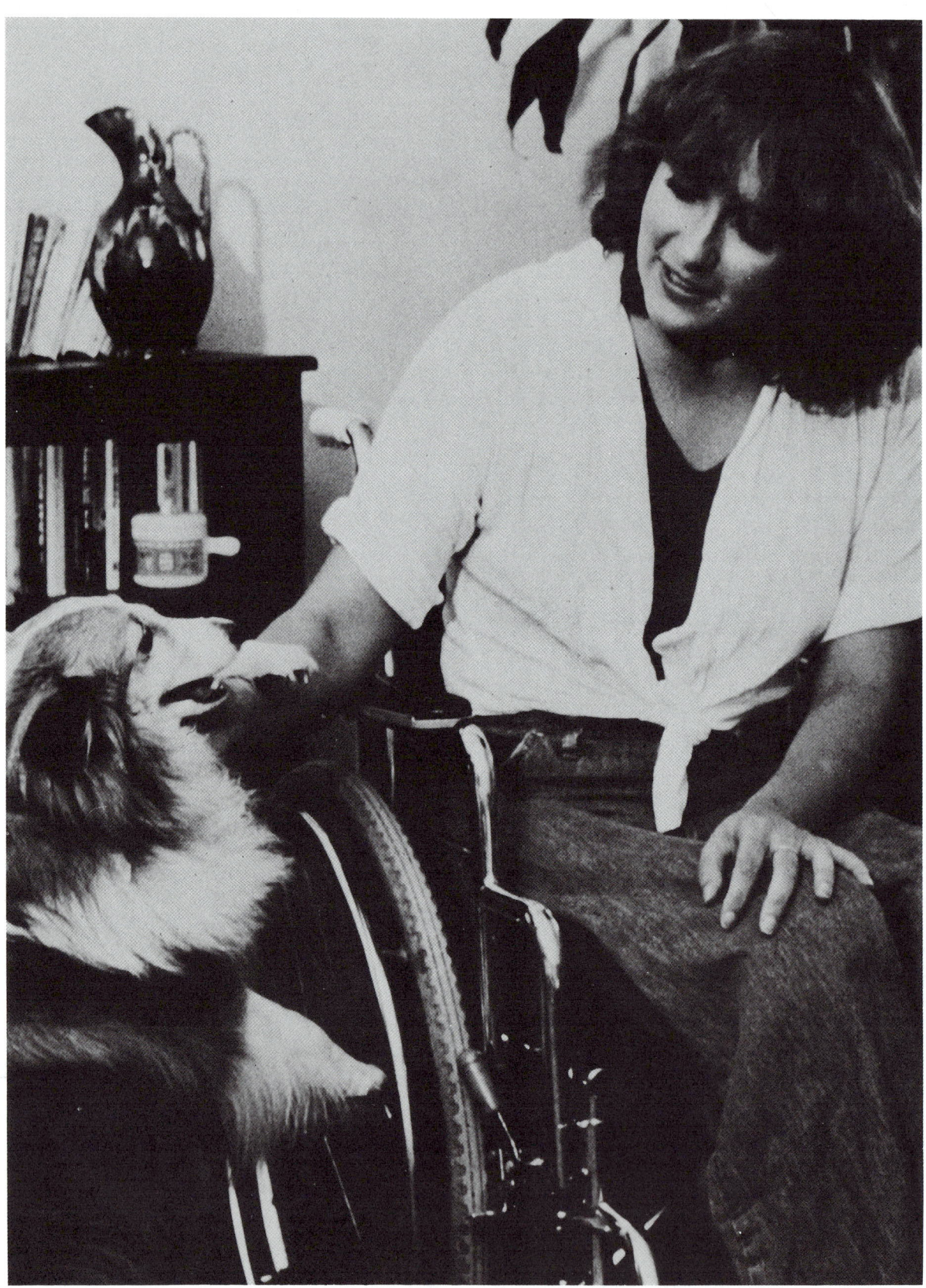

CHAPTER
– 21 –

Maintaining Protective Functions of the Skin*

Chapter Outline

*This chapter was developed with D. Sue Briggs R.N., M.S.N.,
C.R.R.N., Assistant Director of Nursing; Lois A. Schaetzle, R.N.,
M.S., C.R.R.N.; Kelly Cox Watkins, R.N., M.S.; and Linda J. Todd,
R.N., C.R.R.N., Spinal Cord Injury Service, Craig Hospital,
Englewood, CO.

Health Care Objectives

- To identify health care goals for maintaining protective functions of the skin following spinal cord injury
- To describe general functions of the skin, neural control, and dysfunctions following spinal cord injury
- To avoid prolonged pressure, shearing forces, or local injury to the skin that cause skin breakdown
- To minimize secondary factors contributing to skin breakdown
- To design and implement an effective plan to meet individual needs
- To provide education that promotes understanding, responsibility for self-care, and compliance with skin care regimens
- To describe long-term implications associated with care of the skin

No single complications of spinal cord injury (SCI) is as potentially preventable, as difficult to manage, or as much of a deterrent to the progress of a total rehabilitation program as skin breakdown. The process by which it occurs is fast and insidious. Efforts to prevent it must be planned and constant (Thomas 1977).

Holistic care, combining basic knowledge of the integumentary system and numerous manual and teaching skills, is essential for patients who must eventually assume responsibility for skin care.

THE COMPROMISED INTEGUMENTARY SYSTEM FOLLOWING SPINAL CORD INJURY

Structure and Function of the Integumentary System

The skin and its accessory structures—the hair, nails, and skin glands—comprise the *integumentary system*. The skin is the body's largest and one of its most important organs. Skin functions are crucial to survival.

The skin is a thin, relatively flat organ classified as a membrane—the cutaneous membrane. Two main layers compose it: an outer, thinner layer called the epidermis and an inner, thicker layer named the dermis. Under the dermis lies a layer of connective tissue called subcutaneous tissue or superficial fascia.

The skin functions as protector, a temperature regulator, and a multiple sensing device. In addition, the skin excretes fluid and electrolytes, stores fat, and synthesizes Vitamin D.

The keratinized, stratified, squamous epithelial tissue that composes the epidermis makes it a formidable barrier. It protects underlying tissues against invasion by unconquerable hordes of microorganisms, bars entry of most chemicals, and minimizes mechanical injury of underlying structures.

The skin plays an important role in maintaining homeostasis of body temperature. Briefly, if body temperature rises above normal, blood vessels in the dermis dilate and sweat secretion increases. More heat is, therefore, lost by radiation from the larger volume of blood in the skin and by evaporation of sweat on the skin's surface. If blood temperature decreases below normal, skin blood vessels constrict and sweat secretion decreases.

Millions of microscopic sense organs lie in the dermis of all skin areas. They serve as antennas that detect stimuli which lead to sensations of heat, cold, pressure, and pain (Anthony and Thiebodeau 1983). The entire skin surface of the body receives innervation from the central and autonomic nervous systems. Cutaneous distribution of this innervation is organized in *dermatomes*. Each section or level of the body is supplied by a cranial or spinal nerve (Figure 21–1).

The central nervous system (in communication with the peripheral nervous system) provides sensory appreciation and motor control to each dermatome. The autonomic nervous system helps control body homeostasis, which helps to maintain healthy skin and protects the skin from the environment by reflex activity. In response to sensory stimuli, a person moves to avoid unpleasant or painful sensations. Actions may be as simple and automatic as withdrawing a hand from a hot stove; or may require more complex actions, such as adjusting to a more comfortable position or changing clothes to suit outside temperatures. Related anatomy and physiology are described in Chapter 4.

Changes in the Integumentary System Following Spinal Cord Injury

People with SCI lose voluntary motor ability and sensory appreciation below the level of injury. SCI may also cause autonomic nervous system mechanisms to operate poorly, altering body homeostasis and circulation. Reflex activity may be preserved and become hyperactive or may be absent. The lack of sensory warning mechanisms, inability to move freely, and circulatory changes in people with SCI pose major threats to the integumentary system. The actual surface area (dermatome) susceptible to skin breakdown correlates with the level of injury.

Factors That Disrupt Skin Integrity

The cells of the integumentary system, like all cells, require constant oxygenation, nourishment, and elimination of waste products to remain functional. This is achieved only by good blood flow to all areas of the skin. Any prolonged blockage quickly causes skin breakdown. The degree of breakdown is primarily related to the amount and duration of force, but other factors also play a role.

Primary Factors
Primary factors that predispose any patient to potential disruption of skin integrity are:

- excessive *pressure*
- *shearing* forces
- localized *trauma*

Obstruction of capillary flow and accompanying ischemia are widely recognized as the mechanisms responsible for skin breakdown or ulcer formation. Direct pressure and shearing forces can cause this obstruction. Trauma or other local irritations can also contribute, but by mechanical forces to the epidermis rather than by ischemia (Mikulic 1980).

Pressure. *Pressure area, pressure sore,* and *pressure ulcer* are the accepted terms for skin breakdown. Preventive and

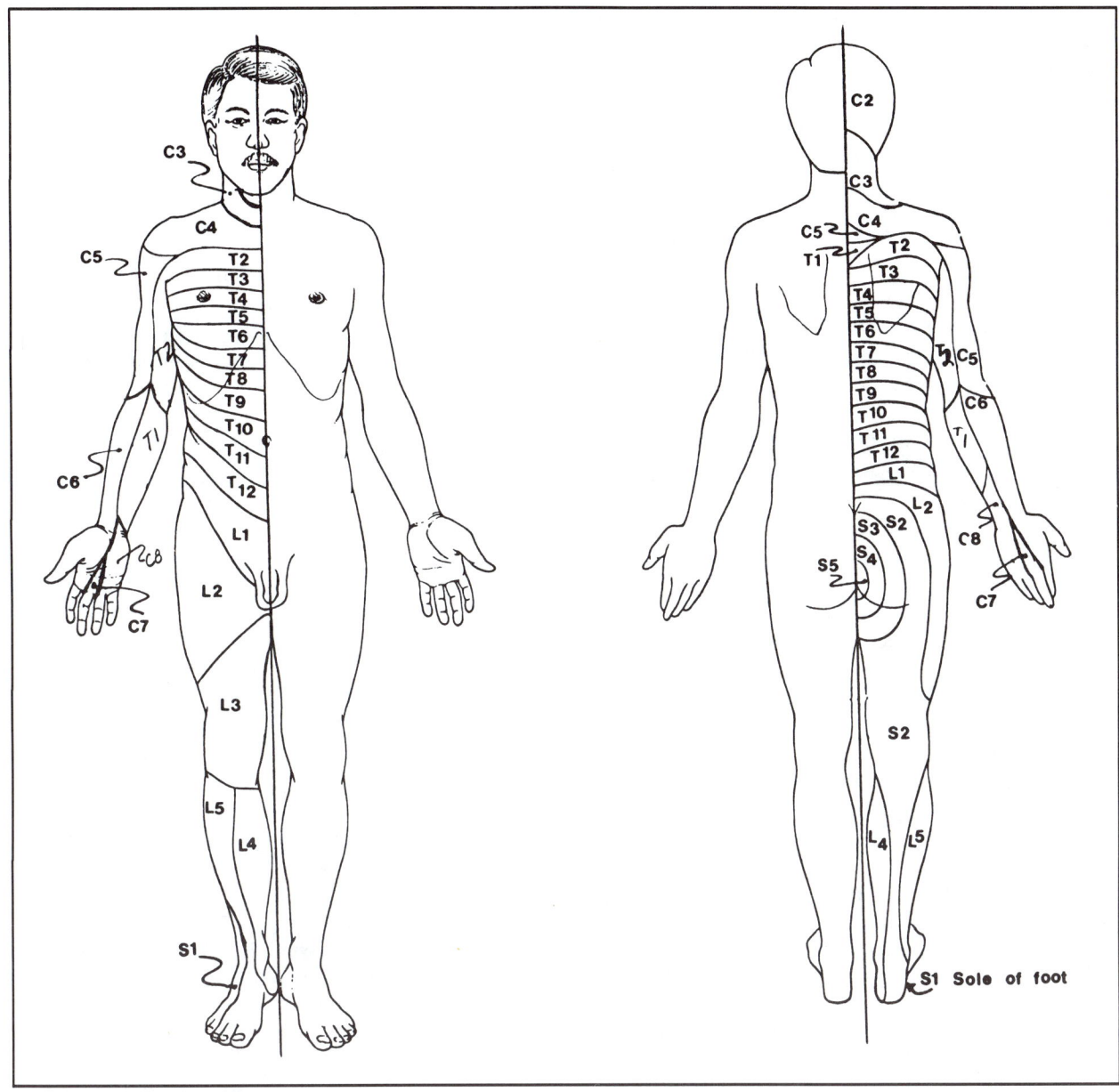

FIGURE 21–1 Sensory level dermatomes. (Source: Craig Hospital, Englewood, CO.)

restorative measures must adequately address the cause—pressure (Mikulic 1980).

Pressure develops through lack of movement of body weight. To avoid pressure, healthy people continually move their bodies in response to sensory stimuli, even during sleep. Areas of increased pressure may occur anywhere on the body, but pressure is most concentrated between bones and skin surfaces that support body weight. When soft tissue is compressed between a bone and another hard surface, such as a bed, wheelchair, or brace, blood is squeezed out of underlying tissue and the circulation is blocked. Altering position changes the pressure points.

The skin becomes red as a result of transient pressure, but this disappears when the pressure is removed. Relief of pressure following prolonged soft tissue compression results in a cellular reaction of edema and inflammation. If pressure is not relieved, sustained ischemia destroys cellular metabolism, which may lead to necrosis of fat, fibrous tissue, muscle, and even bone. Extensive involvement and undermining of deep fascia, muscle, bone periosteum, and nearby joint structures are evident. Large amounts of fluid and protein are lost from the wound. During this stage, the patient may have multiple areas of skin breakdown and may develop dehydration, anemia, and toxicity, which can cause death.

There is a definite relationship between the duration and amount of pressure and the development of pressure sores. Usual pressures from body weight cause microscopic ischemic changes in capillary blood flow in less than 30 minutes. However, there is a critical interval of between 1 and 2 hours before pathological changes occur in both normal and denervated tissue. These changes are reversible if pressure is relieved every 2 hours (Burke and Murray 1975). If the pressure force is greater than that caused by normal body weight, such as can be caused by wrinkles in the bed linen or an ill-fitting brace, irreversible changes can occur more quickly.

Shearing Forces. Although not as great a factor as pressure, *shearing forces* can block blood flow significantly. Shearing forces occur when tissues rub or are pulled rather than compressed against each other. The forces of pulling and sliding stretch blood vessels and tear the inelastic soft tissue, resulting in necrosis and frequently, *sacral slits* (Benda 1983). For instance, when a patient slumps in a chair or bed, the soft tissues are pulled out of shape when the skin sticks to the chair back or mattress while the weight of the body slides to the foot of the chair or bed.

Localized Trauma. When skin nutrition and blood supply are compromised in a local area by trauma or entrapment of moisture and heat, tissue resistance is decreased. The area then becomes more susceptible to pressure forces and skin breakdown. Infection occurs more easily and takes longer to heal.

Traumas, such as cuts or bruising, and other forces, such as friction, may abrade the skin and interrupt blood flow. Friction may occur when a patient is slid rather than lifted up in bed or when bare skin comes into contact with a transfer board. Spasticity may be another source of friction.

Entrapment of localized moisture and heat also contribute to skin breakdown and excoriation. Possible sources of moisture are perspiration, stool, or urine. Prolonged wetness can lead to loss of layers of skin. The increased use of plastic incontinence padding and plastic or foam wheelchair cushions and mattresses may also impede dissipation of moisture and heat.

Secondary Factors

Several secondary factors can significantly contribute to potential skin breakdown for people with SCI. Risks include (Benda 1983):

- Sensory deficits
- Motor impairment, resulting in decreased ability to relieve pressure
- Decreased level of awareness, as with prescribed medications or substance abuse
- Nutritional deficits, such as dehydration, anemia, and weight management difficulties
- Musculoskeletal problems, primarily spasticity, leading to positioning difficulties
- Cardiovascular problems, such as spinal shock and dependent edema, particularly of the lower extremities
- Infections
- Aging
- Psychosocial factors

Other associated negative factors include stress, smoking, incontinence, and lack of activity (Feustel 1982). Medications, especially drugs resulting in immunosuppression and coagulation abnormalities, also affect wound healing (Peacock 1984).

ASSESSMENT

To understand the actual and potential problems that people with SCI may experience requires a thorough assessment of the historical, physiological, mechanical, and psychosocial factors involved. Specific assessment tools that rate contributing primary and secondary factors can help determine the patients' relative risk for developing pressure areas and also aid in diagnosis, planning, and evaluation (Kozier and Erb 1991).

History

Assessment includes a thorough interview with the patient and family or significant other. Information such as the patient's skin type, age, medications, life-style, and any preexisting conditions help identify risk factors associated with skin breakdown.

How recently the patient was injured and at what level injury was sustained greatly influence the patient's susceptibility to skin problems. Newly injured patients are probably unaware of the tremendous importance of skin care and the risk factors associated with skin breakdown. Rehabilitated patients are usually educated in proper skin management, but may experience new problems due to changes in life-style, equipment, or general physical health.

Higher-level SCI patients have more risk factors and pressure point areas to monitor than patients who have a lower-level injury.

Age

A patient's age can indicate potential risk factors, particularly advanced age. In the course of normal aging, the skin tends to become thin, wrinkled, dry, and occasionally scaly. The skin structures and subcutaneous fat are supported by an underlying network of collagen and other elastic fibers that give the skin its characteristic flexibility, elasticity, and strength. Changes in the skin due to aging—atrophy of all skin layers, decreased vascularity, and decreased elasticity—lead to loss of skin water, reduced sweating, decreased oil production, loss of hair, and pigmentation changes. Hair becomes grayer, and the skin has a more mottled appearance (Spence and Mason 1983).

Dermatitis often stems from frequent soap-and-water bathing, which is poorly tolerated by the fragile skin of the elderly and leads to the common problems of dryness and eczema. The vulvae and vaginal mucosa are particularly susceptible.

Personal Profile

Assess whether the patient has *normal*, *oily*, or *dry* skin. Dry skin is particularly troublesome because it is inelastic and tends to crack, thus forming sites for ulceration. People with fair skin, especially those with red hair, generally have extremely sensitive skin.

Note any *preexisting* skin complications. Occasionally, a dermatological disorder such as eczema, or a circulation-related condition, such as diabetes, may be present.

A *medication* history is vital, particularly if the patient has a known allergy to any of the systemic or topically applied drugs used for a variety of disorders. Side effects of many medications may be skin dryness, pruritus, or rashes.

Ask patients about their personal *hygiene* routine. How often do they bathe and shampoo? Do they routinely inspect their skin? Do they use a hand mirror to self-inspect, or does someone else inspect the skin for them? Assess for cleanliness; however, it is important to understand how much time and attention are currently spent on routine hygiene.

Identify the patient's current *bowel* and *bladder management programs*. Does the patient have any control of these functions? If not, is the patient having involuntary bowel movements frequently? What kind of bladder management is being used? Is the patient on an intermittent catheterization schedule? Does the patient wear an external collector, or is there a urethral or suprapubic catheter in place? Indwelling catheters and external collectors can create pressure areas that will lead to skin breakdown if not secured properly. Ask whether the patient is experiencing difficulty in keeping dry. Excoriation from incontinence is a common problem that, if not properly managed, can lead to even greater skin problems.

Poor *nutrition* is a major risk factor in the development of skin breakdown. Malnutrition and significant weight loss are common following trauma. Anorexia, dehydration, or repeated infections may result in continued malnutrition, and protein deficiency is considered to be significant factor in pressure sore development. When cellular metabolism is decreased, tissue resistance is lowered, and the body becomes more susceptible to forces of pressure. Ask patients about their general nutrition and dietary habits. Have they experienced any recent weight gain or loss?

Physical Assessment

In-depth physical assessment is a major nursing responsibility. Assessment must encompass inspection of the skin, assessment of cardiovascular status (Chapter 16) and nutritional status (Chapter 17), detailed observation during general illness, and assessment of functional equipment and clothing.

Inspection of Skin

Meticulous inspection of the skin is crucial in the prevention of pressure sores. Begin the skin assessment from head to toe and note any of the following observations:

- Redness or erythema
- Warmth/temperature to touch
- Elasticity/skin turgor
- Dryness
- Moisture
- Capillary refill/skin color
- Edema
- Hardness
- General cleanliness/skin folds
- Skin disruptions such as rash, excoriations, scrapes, cuts, or bruising that would render a particular area more susceptible to skin breakdown

Give special attention to weight-bearing bony prominences. As soft tissue pressure is greatest over bony prominences that support body weight, changes in body position change the areas endangered. Recognize the areas of the body that need special attention for skin care. Figure 21–2 illustrates areas most susceptible to pressure formation in the supine, side-lying, prone, and sitting positions. Signs indicative of too much or prolonged pressure begin with a reddened area. No damage has occurred if the redness fades within 15 minutes after the pressure is removed. A *pressure sore* is first manifested by a reddened area that does not disappear within 30 minutes or so after pressure is removed. Edema, inflammation, or blistering over a bony prominence may occur (see Table 21–1). If pressure is not relieved, a superficial *pressure* area forms. The measures suggested in this chapter, especially pressure relief, prevent or reverse the process at this stage.

During the early stages, skin inspection must be performed following each turn in bed and on return to bed from the wheelchair. Also examine the skin carefully when a patient returns to the ward from diagnostic or radiological tests or operative procedures. These activities often necessitate positioning the patient on a hard surface, which increases pressure on bony prominences. As skin and wheelchair tolerance builds, skin inspection may be performed each morning before getting up and each night when returning to bed. This must become an integral part of the person's daily life.

Skin assessment techniques combine visual observation and palpation for increased temperature in localized areas. The latter skill is particularly helpful for detecting hyperemic responses in dark-skinned patients when visual inspection is difficult. Be sure to use the back of the hand, which is more sensitive than the fingertips to temperature changes. Good lighting is important. A bright flashlight should be used during the night shift and when checking under braces.

Any assault on the patient's overall health increases the risk of skin breakdown. During illness, monitor the patient closely.

The *febrile state* associated with infection increases oxygen demands at a cellular level. Failure to meet nutritional and caloric needs will cause cellular deficiency. This will

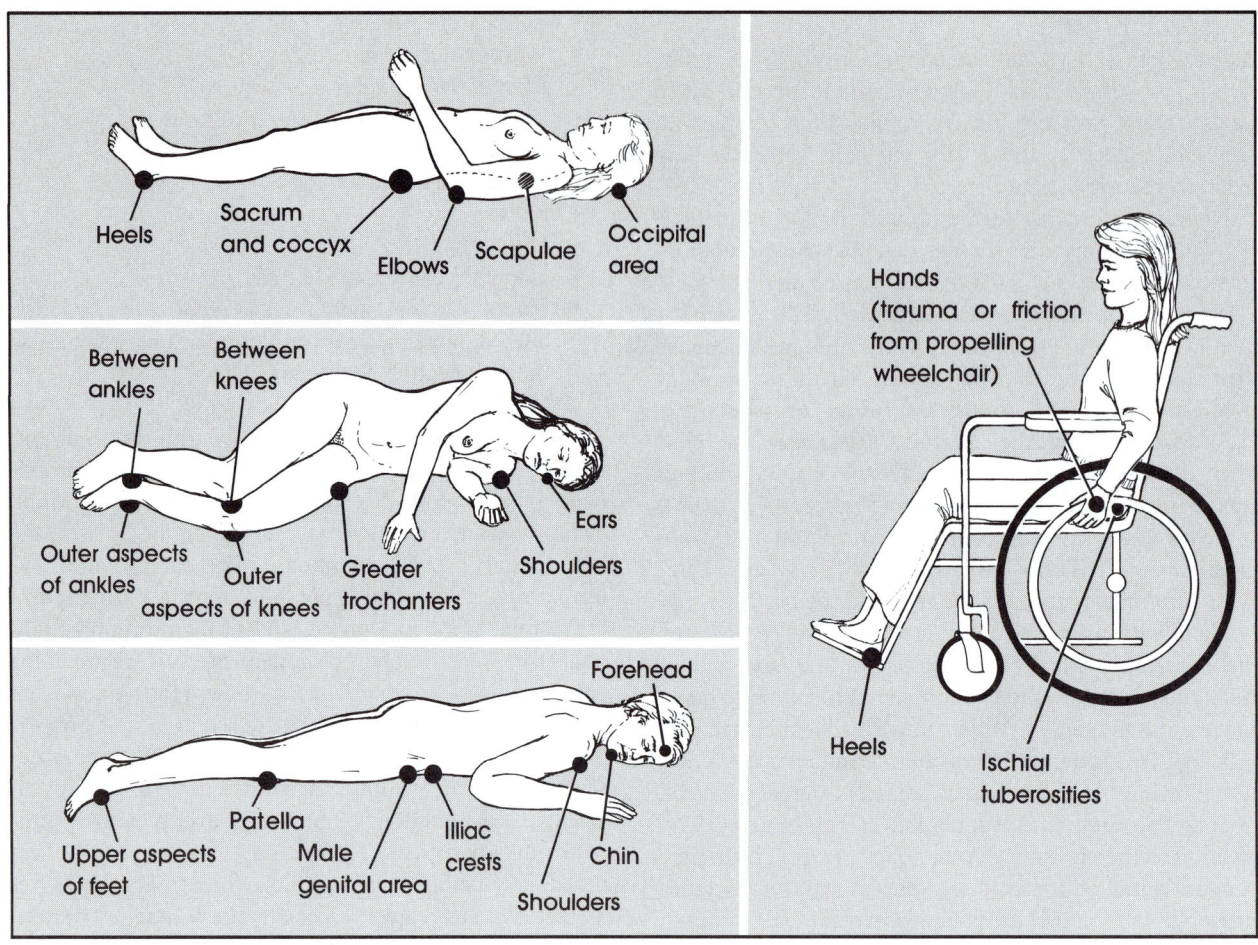

FIGURE 21–2   Points on the body susceptible to pressure vary when different positions are assumed.

make the body more susceptible to the effects of pressure, and skin breakdown will occur more easily.

Assessment of Clothing and Functional Equipment

Check that clothing fits properly. Tight, ill-fitting blue jeans are a notorious cause of skin breakdown. Seams, pockets with rivets, buckles, zippers, and wrinkles can all cause pressure and threaten skin integrity. Soft, loose-fitting clothes of wash-and-wear fabrics are ideal. Ill-fitting clothing can cause pressure areas and edema. Cotton underwear is most absorbent. Avoid all nylon clothes as they tend to hold perspiration against the skin. Brightly colored warm-up suits are a convenient choice during early rehabilitation. Blouses and shirts can be loose fitting or cut to fit around the bars of the halo device. Shoes must also be checked to ensure a comfortable fit. Additional assessment is necessary when a patient is wearing a variety of immobilization devices or splints. Examine the skin carefully where the orthotic device exerts the greatest pressure on the skin. Table 21–2 summarizes pressure points exerted by a variety of orthoses. Wheelchairs that are too narrow

for a patient who has gained weight, that have broken parts, and that have improperly fitted and/or worn out cushions are also culprits.

Psychosocial Assessment

The patient's ability to maintain the integrity of the skin does not appear to be directly related to the level of injury, which suggests that psychosocial variables are important in skin care.

One study revealed that maintaining the skin integrity was not so much a function of mechanical aids, intellect, or achievement as of patient attitudes (Anderson and Andberg 1979). Quadriplegic patients who accepted responsibility for skin care and achieved satisfaction from activities in life were less likely to develop pressure sores than paraplegic patients who did not accept responsibility Acceptance of responsibility for one's body is indeed a prerequisite for adaptation to the many physical changes SCI entails and affects the incidence of pressure sores (Trieschmann 1988). Also, if people with paraplegia—who are considerably more self-reliant than people with quadriplegia, who need assis-

TABLE 21-1   Characteristics of a Newly Developed Pressure Area

Reddened area

Reactive hyperemia appears as the first sign of a pressure area

Localized warmth (identified by palpation)

Hardened area (identified by palpation)

Localized area of edema or blistering

Bluish discoloration

Small open area

Ulceration of epidermis; possible inflammatory reaction affecting underlying soft tissue

With removal of pressure, healing will occur in 48 to 72 hours

tance with skin checks—are depressed or unmotivated, no one else assumes this responsibility. See Chapter 9.

Find out what patients actually know about skin care. Do they understand the integumentary system? Are they aware of risk factors? Do they know how to inspect and care for their skin properly? Also explore their attitudes toward preventive skin care. Attitudes, feelings, and knowledge all significantly affect the patient's compliance with a skin care program.

Further research is needed to find ways to help patients comply with essential skin care regimens. Judging from the high incidence of pressure sores following discharge (as high as 80% of all patients (Gosnell 1973), prevention is a worthy goal (Graitcer and Maynard 1990). See also Chapters 2 and 33 for further discussions about issues surrounding prevention of secondary disabilities.

PREVENTIVE MANAGEMENT: PLANNING AND IMPLEMENTATION

General Health and Well-Being

Although acute skin care management begins as a professional responsibility, the key to continuing success, often difficult to achieve, is to encourage the patient and/or family to assume responsibility. Most care givers have seen large, open pressure sores but most patients have not. Patients thus do not comprehend the serious implications of poor skin care. Provide comprehensive education about skin care because it must become an important daily routine. Incorporate management strategies described in Part III of this text to enhance learning and cooperation; also see Part V for how to promote an active life-style.

Maintaining adequate *nutrition* is essential in the prevention and healing of skin breakdown. Overweight or underweight patients are more susceptible to pressure sores. Excess weight exerts more pressure on the areas of skin tissue over bony prominences. Underweight patients have a thinner layer of fat below the skin to protect from pressure.

Dietary proteins are vital for the building and repair of skin cells. Many vitamins, including vitamins A and C, have specific functions in the synthesis and maintenance of healthy skin tissue. Adequate fluid intake of 2000 to 3000 ml per day (adjusted to bladder management requirements) also maintains healthy skin and prevents dehydration. Review Chapter 17 for management of nutritional needs.

TABLE 21-2   Pressure Points Created by Commonly Used Orthotic Devices

Halo-Thoracic Brace

- Pin sites and skin underneath circumference of halo ring
- Shoulders (especially top)
- Underarms
- Rib cage
- All edges of the brace and underneath the side buckle area

Cervical Brace

- Occiput
- Chin and jaw line
- Underarms
- Sternum
- Spine
- Underneath all edges of brace, straps, and buckles

Thoracic Brace

- Upper trunk and underarms
- Iliac crests
- Spine
- Underneath edges of brace, buckles, and straps

Hand Splints

- Palms
- Wrist bones
- Underneath straps and buckles

KAFOs (Knee-Ankle-Foot Orthoses) or AFOs (Ankle-Foot Orthoses) (Collaborate with physical therapist to observe)

- Groin area
- Hinge sites
- Heels and toes (tend to curl up in shoes)

Cardiovascular health is essential to ensure cellular oxygenation and nutrition. Chapter 17 presents ways to prevent or control postural hypotension and gravitational edema by passive and active range of motion exercises, graded mobility programs, and application of elastic stockings and abdominal binders that improve systemic circulation.

Hygiene

Good personal hygiene is fundamental to maintaining protective functions of the skin and preventing skin breakdown. Giving encouragement for the smallest signs of interest in appearance also helps patients take more steps toward increasing self-esteem, accepting responsibility for their own bodies, and eventually achieving independence.

Bathing

Bathing is refreshing and promotes normal skin functioning by removing contaminants and dead skin. Establish frequency according to need by considering general skin type, age, amount of exercise, body odor, and habits before injury. For example, patients with quadriplegia experience profuse sweating above the level of injury, which may necessitate more frequent bathing, and active patients engaged in strenuous physical therapy will require daily showering to prevent body odor. Provide daily care to face, hands, underarms, and the groin area. Also be sure to clean and dry the skin following bowel or bladder procedures. This usually involves turning the patient, as the perineum is best exposed in the supine position and the buttocks (which must be separated) in the side-lying position. *Promptly* attend to the patient who is incontinent. An opportune time to perform skin inspection is during bathing.

To minimize excessive drying and skin irritation, generally select a mild soap without perfume or detergents; use tepid (not hot) water; and allow skin to toughen naturally. Do not apply lotions or alcohol rubs routinely. Creams or lotions are necessary only if the skin becomes dry and scaly (to prevent cracking or bleeding). Be especially careful in checking the lower limbs, where skin tends to become dry due to autonomic nervous system dysfunction and lack of sweat production.

Moisture softens the skin, so wet skin is more susceptible to breakdown. Always dry the patient thoroughly, especially between the toes and in the groin area. Remember that plastic-backed or waterproof pads trap moisture and heat. If absolutely necessary, use one pad correctly placed. Avoid using several pads that will become bunched underneath the patient. If the patient is sweating profusely, as is common with quadriplegia, terry towels placed about the neck and shoulders will absorb the moisture. Complete linen changes may be needed with each 2-hourly turn.

Tub bathing should begin as soon as possible. One extremely valuable aid for early care is a combination *bath stretcher-tub unit*. The model described here, and illustrated in Figure 21–3, was originally designed in Sweden to bathe dependent patients. It is particularly well suited for patients with SCI because spinal immobility can be maintained. The unit consists of a portable stretcher base, a stretcher platform, and a large tub with a submersible support structure that receives the stretcher platform. The patient is transferred to the portable stretcher unit at the bedside (a three-person lift is used) and transported to the tub. For a patient with a thoracolumbar fracture, who must remain flat, the stretcher may be swung around so that the feet are elevated or a spray attachment can be used. Pneumatic controls allow for ease of operation by one staff member. Other valuable features of this unit include: water temperature control, a disinfectant spray device, and soft, waterproof padding for the stretcher.

Wheelchair-accessible showers, with hand-held shower heads, are convenient for patients and staff. Shower (waterproof) wheelchairs are widely used also. Independent skills for washing can be introduced very early. Once specific activity orders have been outlined by the physician—mainly the degree of elevation in bed and type of movements and transfers allowed—closely collaborate with the occupational therapist to begin a self-care regime. Generally, the occupational therapist is responsible for assessing the patient's physical potential, establishing realistic goals, advising on positioning that allows the patient the greatest ease, selecting appropriate aids, and initiating progressions in self-care skills. The nurse must integrate these skills into daily care, reinforce the lessons of the occupational therapist, monitor patient response, and communicate any problems to the occupational therapist. Warn the patient about excessively hot water causing burns to desensitized skin, and always test the water temperature with a bath thermometer beforehand. A temperature control device on a shower control is useful (especially during training when patients are learning to control hand and arm movements).

For the patient with a thoracic or lumbar injury, upper extremity washing can be introduced while on bedrest as soon as the patient is physically stable. Bathing in a stretcher-tub unit is usually permissible as soon as any surgical incisions are healed. Lower extremity washing can be introduced when the patient is allowed to sit at a 45- to 60-degree angle in bed. Place pillows under the knees to avoid a pulling strain on the back. As wheelchair sitting tolerance increases, teach the patient to transfer to a shower chair for hygiene care. When long sitting is allowed and the patient can perform good lifting maneuvers, transfers to an ordinary bathtub can begin (Figure 21–4).

For the patient with a *cervical injury*, upper extremity washing can be introduced when the patient is comfortable sitting at a 45-degree angle in bed. Use a bath mitt. Consult with the occupational therapist about using other aids, and adapt positioning for individual needs. Lower extremity washing may be possible when the patient is able to balance well in long sitting.

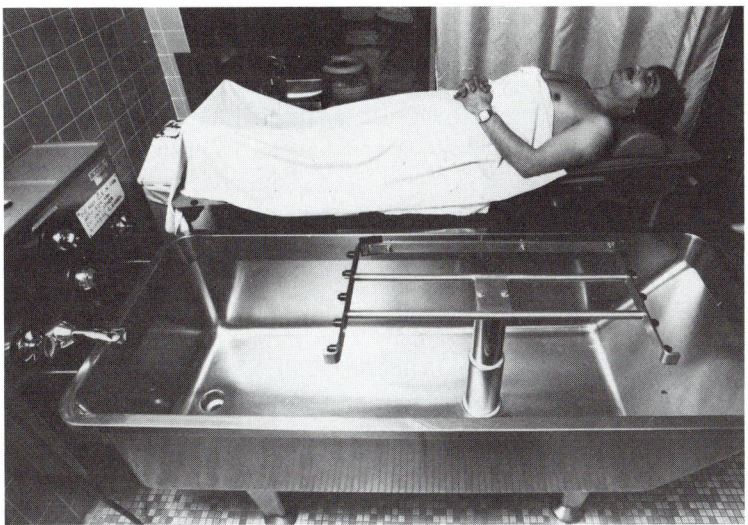

FIGURE 21–3 A combination bath stretcher-tub unit: The mobile stretcher is wheeled to the bedside to receive the patient and then returned to the tub. The platform is separated from the mobile base, moved over the tub, and anchored on a submersible frame, which is lowered into the tub by pneumatic controls. The head of the stretcher automatically elevates 30 degrees as the platform is lowered.

Throughout the mobilization program, many bathing activities can only be performed with the added protection of a brace. When leather portions of the brace get wet, they obviously cannot be worn for the remainder of the day. Encourage former patients to contribute no longer needed orthotic devices so that patients have extra bathing braces.

Grooming

Attending to personal appearance contributes significantly to a patient's self-image and comfort. Clean hair, a fresh shave, or a touch of makeup can mean a lot to the dependent patient. Close collaboration with the occupational therapist is essential to promote independence in grooming.

Encourage patients with *thoracic or lumbar injuries* in such grooming skills as brushing teeth and combing hair before mobilization has begun. As soon as patients can tolerate short periods in the wheelchair, they can complete all grooming activities at the sink. A lowered mirror, tilted forward, helps.

For the patient with a *cervical injury*, introduce grooming skills when the spine is considered stable (often just after the halo brace is applied) and the patient is comfortable sitting at a 60-degree angle in bed. When the patient is in the wheelchair and is comfortable in that position for an hour or more, grooming can be done at the sink (see Figure 21–5). When assisting patients, be sure to place them in a comfortable position free from interference from the bed or

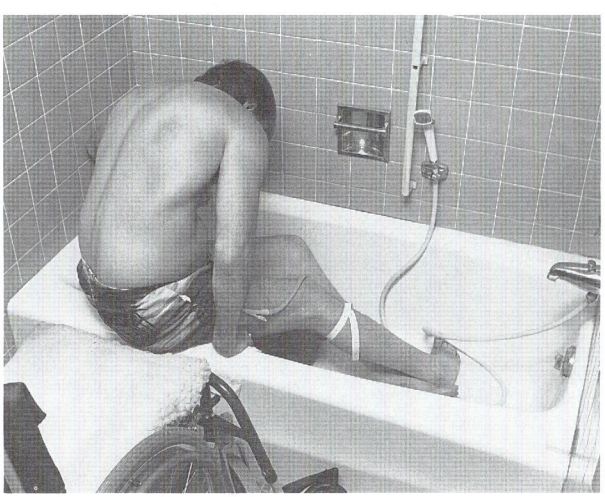
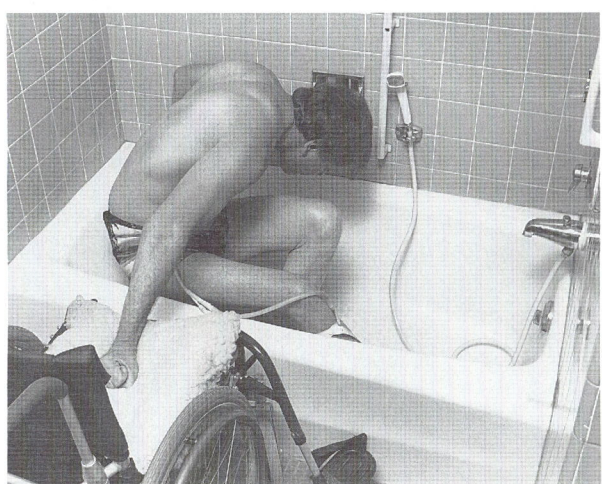

FIGURE 21–4 A person with paraplegia performs an independent transfer into the bathtub.

wheelchair. Individualized adaptive aids may include a padded toothbrush, comb, or hair brush, or a pocket splint to fit these items. Generally, an electric razor, perhaps with an adaptive holder, is easiest.

Maintaining *dental hygiene* can be awkward for the dependent patient. If the patient is on bedrest, take measures to prevent aspiration. Use the side-lying position; elevate or raise the head of the bed, if possible, and have a suction apparatus at hand. If the patient has difficulty expectorating into a kidney basin, apply continuous suction to the dependent side of the mouth, or use a straw to expel oral contents into the basin. Sometimes a toothbrush curved like a dental instrument, with a smaller brush area, is easier to maneuver. Use toothpaste and water sparingly; the mechanical action of brushing is more important. Flossing helps remove plaque. Naturally, dental hygiene is much easier if the patient can sit up.

Hair Care

Wash the hair weekly or as before injury. To avoid excessive drying, use a pH balanced commercial shampoo. If the patient has tong sites or pin sites, use an antibacterial liquid soap. Clean sites using established procedures immediately after washing hair. See Procedures 20–2 and 20–5. Weekly hair washing significantly minimizes risk of infection at insertion sites.

Foot Care

Patients with lower extremity paralysis may develop an excessive accumulation of hardened skin on the feet and hardened, thickened toenails. Cracks, cuts, calluses, and long toenails can lead to additional problems. Observe for cracking and maceration between the toes which may indicate a fungal infection. Feet should be washed and dried each day, paying particular attention to the areas between the toes. Soaking the feet or wrapping them in a warm, moist towel for 20 minutes once a week is sufficient to soften the skin. Gentle rubbing with a wash cloth will remove the hardened skin. Follow the foot soak with a lanolin-based lotion if skin appears dry or cracked. Carefully trim toenails straight across, preferably with clippers (clippers are a little easier to control should a spasm suddenly occur). Skin will sometimes adhere to the underside of the nail. If red areas develop at the corners of the nails, be aware that this could be the beginning of an infection.

Feet are also vulnerable to injury from bumping or dragging movements during transfer activity. The patient should wear shoes for added protection. A correct fit is essential to avoid pressure areas. Shoes often have to be purchased one size larger than normal to compensate for gravitational edema. Inexpensive tennis shoes are a good choice initially.

Feet are also prone to burns from hot water and car heaters. Feet must always be included in general skin inspection.

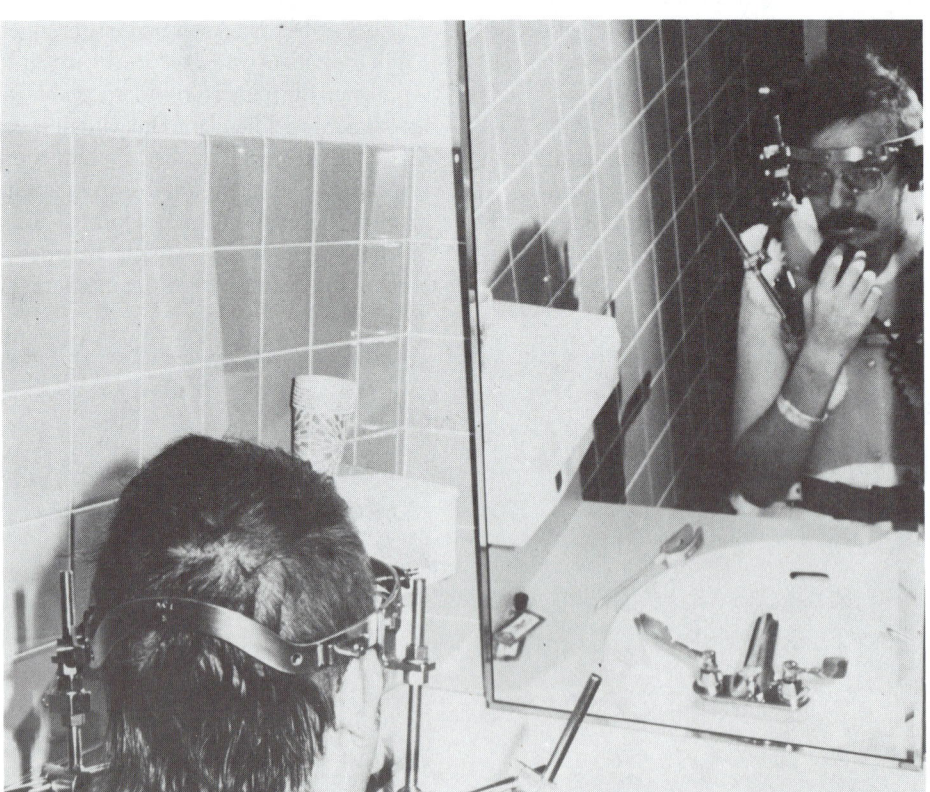

FIGURE 21–5 A quadriplegic person attending to personal hygiene while still in the halo apparatus.

Feminine Hygiene

Perineal care is a very important part of personal care for comfort and prevention of skin breakdown and bladder infections. The following information is partially based on the Virginia Spinal Cord Injury System (1988) and Ford and Duckworth (1987).

Daily care should include washing the outer perineum, labia, and area between the thighs with mild soap, rinsing well, and drying thoroughly. Perineal care should be done each morning and evening and after evacuation of urine or feces. This may be performed in bed (turn the patient to the side to separate the buttocks and clean the anal area) or on a toilet or commode. Teach the patient always to wash from front to back to prevent vaginal contamination from the rectal area.

Excoriation of the perineal area may be caused by frequent use of antiseptic solutions in an intermittent catheterization regime. To care for a woman on an intermittent catheterization program, clean with normal saline or sterile water, according to skin tolerance. Avoid harsher solutions. Squeeze excess cleaning solution out of cotton balls. This prevents the solution collecting in the gluteal crease and causing irritation. Turn the patient and dry area thoroughly following procedure. A woman with a urethral catheter should move the leg bag from one side to the other daily to avoid pressure on the labia minora.

A local infection, such as vaginitis or urethritis, may also cause skin irritation. Specific systemic or topical medication should be ordered by the physician to control the cause. Mild vinegar douching works well to curb mild but persistent vaginitis.

Tampons or sanitary pads may be used depending on personal preference, comfort, and ease with which a patient can independently insert tampons or place pads. Tampons are generally preferred for cleanliness.

Sanitary pads with double adhesive strips that stick to the underpants are best. A pad may be placed in the crotch of the underpants before pulling them up. A crotch flap, with a Velcro closure, made in a pair of stretchy underpants from leg opening to leg opening may be useful to some patients. Many women cannot tolerate the bulk and dampness of a normal sanitary pad. Larger dressings or commercial disposable diapers distribute the pressure and moisture.

Tampons or pads should be changed at least every 4 hours. During the menstrual cycle, the entire perineal area including the gluteal crease must be observed for skin irritation. Assist the woman to perform this task with a mirror.

Skin Inspection

Skin inspection to detect any developing pressure areas is one of the first crucial skills a patient must master. The totally dependent patient must learn to direct others with this care. When the patient is well informed, cooperation will likely improve.

The Anderson and Andberg study (1979) revealed that people with quadriplegia who actually performed skin inspection independently had fewer pressure sores than people with paraplegia who depended on others. This finding underscores the importance of patient involvement in successful care.

Patient education should begin within the first few hours after injury. Many patients are curious to know why they must be turned, a procedure they often view as uncomfortable or inconvenient at best. Therefore, introduce and reinforce the rationale behind pressure relief. (Note the term *pressure* is emphasized.)

Routine skin inspection must become a way of life for the patient. Table 21–3 outlines the steps for skin inspection. Any change in the skin is a sign of trouble. Inspection of the skin is, therefore, an early warning system.

Encourage patients to look at their own skin rather than rely on others to check for them. A mirror is an important aid to independence. If patients need help, instruct them to ask their care givers to hold the mirror so that the patients themselves can perform a skin check. A long-handled or adapted Plexiglas mirror may be needed. In collaboration with the occupational therapist, teach patients a variety of side-lying positions for checking skin (Figure 21–6). Arm placement and hand function must be considered. Additional mirrors strategically placed on the wall or bed may be needed.

Patients in braces may require partial or total assistance. Braces do not permit inspection of some parts of the skin, especially the back and buttocks. In the early stages of the treatment program, patients with paraplegia are not allowed excessive trunk rotation and cannot easily view the back until later in the program. Encourage independence when movements are no longer restricted.

Patients must also know under what conditions skin may be particularly vulnerable to breakdown. Patients need to be increasingly watchful during

- Periods of depression
- Illness and/or fever
- After drinking alcohol or using street drugs
- After a weight gain or loss
- After a change in spasticity
- When equipment, such as cushions, wheelchairs, or leg orthoses are changed or replaced

TABLE 21-3 Routine Skin Inspection

- Do it every morning and evening.
- Note any changes in the color of any skin area: reddened areas, bruised areas, blisters, and dry, chafed skin.
- Feel for any hardness or swelling—this is as important as looking.
- If there is a change in the appearance of the skin, *determine the cause* and *eliminate the cause*. All pressure on the affected area must be removed until it resumes a normal appearance.

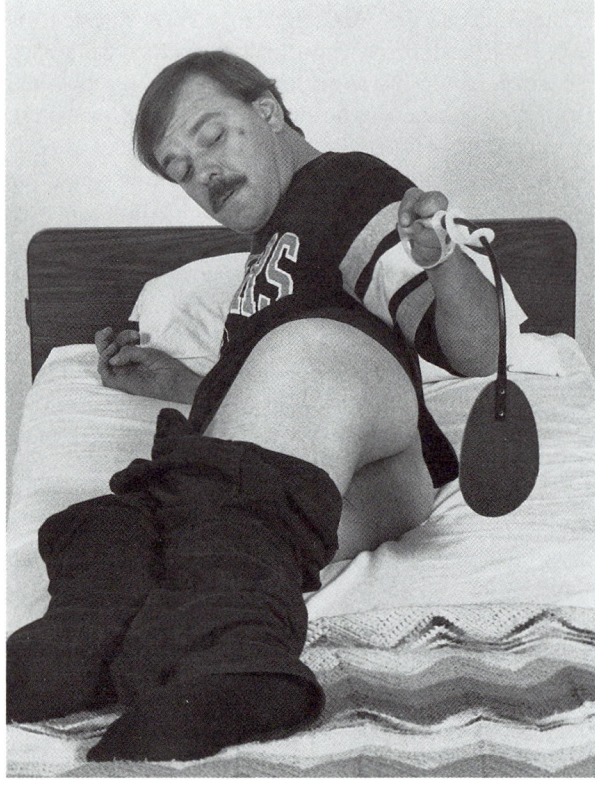

FIGURE 21-6 Self-inspection promotes compliance.

Pressure Relief in Bed

Numerous regimes have come and gone, but such time-honored and proven techniques as regular turning and bridging of bony prominences remain significant in prevention and treatment of pressure sores for patients in bed (King 1981). Although principles of turning and positioning are the same, modifications are necessary to protect the spinal fracture site during early phases of rehabilitation. See Chapter 20.

Bridging refers to supporting body weight so that a free space is created between a bony prominence and the bed. Small foam pads (3 × 6 × 18-inch upholstery foam) strategically positioned above and below bony prominences provide the best bridging effect. Proper bridging techniques for side-lying, supine, and prone positions are illustrated in Procedure 21-1. Padding may be adjusted to meet individual needs based on skin inspection. If necessary, pillows or pads may be covered with sheepskin. *Folded towels or blankets should not be substituted for foam pads or pillows, as they are too firm and may cause skin breakdown.*

Take special care when positioning to disperse pressure of body weight properly and maintain correct body alignment. Support extremities by following the body contour to avoid edema and muscle stretching or contracting.

In addition to proper positioning and bridging, patients must be turned regularly to relieve pressure when in bed. Establish a turning schedule that does not allow redness to appear on bony prominences. Patients usually require turning every 2 hours throughout the 24-hour period of initial bedrest. Depending on the patient's body type and tolerance, the turning schedule may be increased to every 2 to 5 hours, turning from side to back to side. The length of time between turns can be increased gradually by adding 30 minutes to the amount of time in a given position and then checking for redness. The only exception is lying prone. Patients can safely lie prone for up to 8 hours by using plump, firm pillows and small foam pads as illustrated in Procedure 21-1. Sleeping prone at night is recommended. Patients should be encouraged to sleep prone because

- Lying prone straightens the hips and helps prevent tightness of the hips and knees.
- The patient can have a restful 8 hours' sleep without interruption.

Relief of Pressure While Patient Is in Wheelchair

As soon as patients get up in a chair, they are taught to lift the weight off their buttocks to provide relief from pressure. They may perform the movement independently by pushing themselves up with their arms, commonly known as *pushup weight shift* (Figure 21-7), or by leaning over one side of the chair and then the other (Figure 21-8). The use of electric recliner wheelchairs for patients with C_6 or higher level injuries allows them to do weight shifts independently and be up on program sooner and for longer periods while building skin tolerance (Figure 21-9). Until pressure relief maneuvers become automatic, remind and encourage patients to establish their own routine every 15 minutes.

If patients are dependent for pressure relief measures, weight shifts must be performed by assistants. Procedure 21-2 illustrates assisted tilt-back weight shift.

Skin Tolerance

Although lifelong care is needed to protect the skin from pressure and other forces, skin tolerance can be increased. Develop skin tolerance by gradually increasing the time spent in one position followed by skin inspection to evaluate the process. For example, after any length of time in the wheelchair, the skin should blanch when touched, and pinkness or redness should disappear in 15 minutes or so. If it does, increase the time by 15 minutes and repeat the process. If the skin does not clear, keep the patient off the area and instruct or perform pressure relief maneuvers more frequently when next up. The same principles apply to the turning schedule, especially increasing tolerance to the desirable prone position.

As skin tolerance increases, it may be possible to remove some of the foam pads used in the prone, supine, and side-lying positions. Eliminating foam pads should be done very cautiously. Skin checks should be conducted within 15 minutes once a pad is removed.

Procedure 21–1   Distribution of Pressure When Lying Down

Part A   Side-Lying Position Padding

Purpose

To prevent pressure sores.

Side-Lying Position Padding

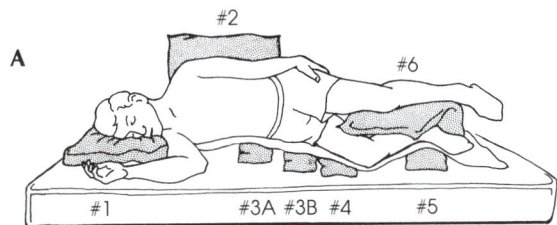

Pad #1	Head	A pillow or pad may be placed at a point of comfort for the patient.
Pad #2	Back	A pillow is placed behind the patient to help maintain side position. Be sure bottom hip is pulled back to prevent patient from rolling backwards on sacrum.
Pad #3A	Hips	Pad placed above the trochanter.
Pad #3B	Hips	Pad placed below the trochanter. When pads 3A and 3B are placed correctly, a flat hand can be slid between body and bed to be certain that pressure has been relieved. If pressure has not been relieved, an additional pad can be added under 3A and 3B.
Pad #4	Knees	A pad is placed above the head of the fibula.
Pad #5	Ankles	A pad is placed above the lateral malleolus to prevent skin breakdown.
Pad #6	Between lower legs	A pillow is placed lengthwise in front of bottom leg to prevent pressure on the head of the fibula and lateral malleolus. The top leg is placed forward on the pillow. Do not have legs directly on top of each other.

Part B   Supine Position Padding

Supine Position Padding

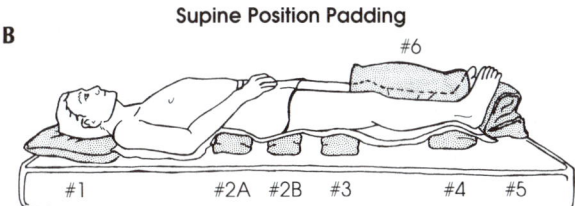

Pad #1	Head	A pillow or pad may be placed at a point of comfort for the patient. Do not use a pillow on cervical injuries.
Pad #2A	Back	Pad placed in low of back, above spinous processes, to provide elevation of the sacrum, relieve pressure on coccygeal area, relieve muscle tiredness in the back.
Pad #2B	Back	Pad is placed below tailbone, across buttocks. When pads 2A and 2B are placed correctly, a flat hand can be slid between body and bed to ascertain that pressure has been relieved. If pressure has not been relieved, an additional pad can be added under 2A and 2B.
Pad #3	Knees	The bend at the knee is a natural curvature. Use a pad *above* the popliteal space. It must *not* be *in* the popliteal space.
Pad #4	Ankles	At the back of the heel a small pad is necessary to relieve tension on the calf of the leg. Also, the heels must be off the bed to prevent skin breakdown.
Pad #5	Feet	A soft foot support is placed to allow simulation of weight bearing on the ball of the foot. Pads or pillows may be used in this area of support.
Pad #6	Between lower legs	A foam pad or pillow placed between the knees and ankles prevents possible breakdown at the head of the fibula and the lateral malleolus.

(Procedure continues)

Procedure 21–1 Distribution of Pressure When Lying Down (continued)

Part C   Prone Position Padding

Prone Position Padding

Pad #1	Head	A pillow or pad may be placed at a point of comfort for the patient.
Pad #2	Chest	This is an optional pad. A flat pillow or $\frac{1}{2}''$ thick foam pad can be placed across the chest to relieve pressure on the clavicle and to relieve pressure off the breasts of female patients.
Pad #3A	Above iliac spines	A pad is placed above iliac spines.
Pad #3B	Below iliac spines	A pad is placed below iliac spines. When pads 3A and 3B are properly placed, pressure is relieved: 1) on the bony iliac prominence, 2) on the suprapubic catheter, and 3) on the penis and scrotum of the male patient. These pads also allow for slight anterior flexion of the thigh and lessen abdominal breathing.
Pad #4	Knee	A pad is placed above the knees to maintain natural curvature of knee and relieve pressure on patellae.
Pad #5	Under lower legs	A pillow is placed crosswise under both lower legs. This pillow allows: 1) the lower leg and foot to be slightly flexed at the knee, 2) pressure relieved at patellae, 3) correct extension of muscle of the thigh, and 4) prevents foot-drop if feet do not extend over end of bed.
Pad #6	Between lower legs	A foam pad or pillow placed between the knees and ankles prevents possible breakdown at the head of the fibula and the lateral malleolus.

WARNING: Do *not* substitute folded towels or blankets for foam padding or pillows. These can be too firm and cause skin breakdown.
Source: Craig Hospital 1983. Reprinted with permission.

Equipment

Three main types of devices are used in the prevention and management of pressure sores: devices that assist with turning; devices that alter pressure intermittently; and devices that minimize pressure (King 1981). *Turning* devices are particularly suited for ease of skin care during the acute stage (Chapter 20). Numerous elaborate and sophisticated devices can alter pressure intermittently and minimize or equalize pressure. Flotation systems using air, water, or foam can significantly lower or reduce external pressure, thus decreasing capillary pressure. *However, although these devices may reduce pressure, they do not eliminate the need for turning and positioning, or, when used in the wheelchair, do not eliminate the clinical practice of pressure relief maneuvers.*

Wheelchair Cushion

The proper wheelchair cushion is crucial to a patient with SCI because it relieves pressure under the person while in the wheelchair and ultimately reduces the risk of pressure sores. No single cushion is optimal for all people with SCI. Objective measurements and clinical judgments are essential (Garber 1985).

Basically, wheelchair cushions are air-inflatable bladders, flotation devices, or gel pads. See Figure 21–10 for some examples of cushions. A variety of soft fabric, plastic, or vinyl covers facilitate sliding movements during transfers to protect the cushion.

- Air-inflatable cushions may be a simple air-inflated bladder, such as the Bye Bye Decubiti Cushion, or individually air-filled bladders secured to a single base, such as the RoHo Dry Flotation Cushion, which looks like an egg carton. Although some patients find these cushions lighter to manage, the somewhat unstable surface may cause balance problems, especially when transferring.
- Flotation cushions filled with water or air are another alternative. Water flotation cushions have a lower temperature than air. This may be an advantage, particularly in hot climates, as excessive heat is thought to render the skin more susceptible to soft tissue breakdown (Fisher, Szymke, and Kosiak 1978).
- Gel pads are most successfully used by patients with paraplegia, as they are heavy to move around. They also tend to sink, which makes transfer more difficult. They may be used in the wheelchair and then transferred to the bed to relieve pressure on the buttocks.

Interdisciplinary responsibilities in choosing wheelchair cushions vary greatly. Generally, the physical therapist and occupational therapist are primarily responsible for recommending the most appropriate wheelchair cushion for the patient.

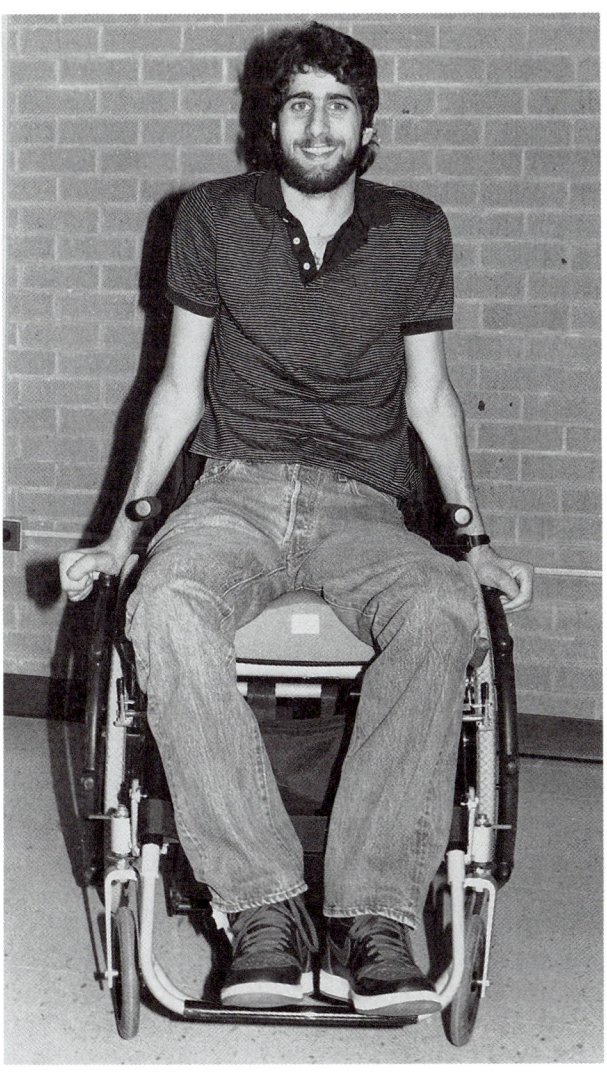

FIGURE 21–7 A quadriplegic person performs a pushup weight shift. Note his extended arms.

Some rehabilitation settings have positioning clinics to establish consistency in addressing patient posture, positioning, and equipment needs, as they relate to cushions. A positioning clinic can be beneficial to both newly injured patients, as well as to long-term injured individuals returning for reevaluation regarding seating and posture problems that cause skin breakdown (Craig 1988). Alterations in a patient's life-style, body build, or activity pattern may necessitate a change in cushion prescription; thus, periodic evaluation may be needed to prevent the development of pressure sores (Garber 1985).

Mattresses and Beds

The effects of increased pressure and shearing forces can be reduced in the spinal cord injured patient by using special mattresses and beds (Sklar 1985). Beds and mattresses range from simple to elaborate in cost, effectiveness, and ease of use. The most common types used to relieve pressure are:

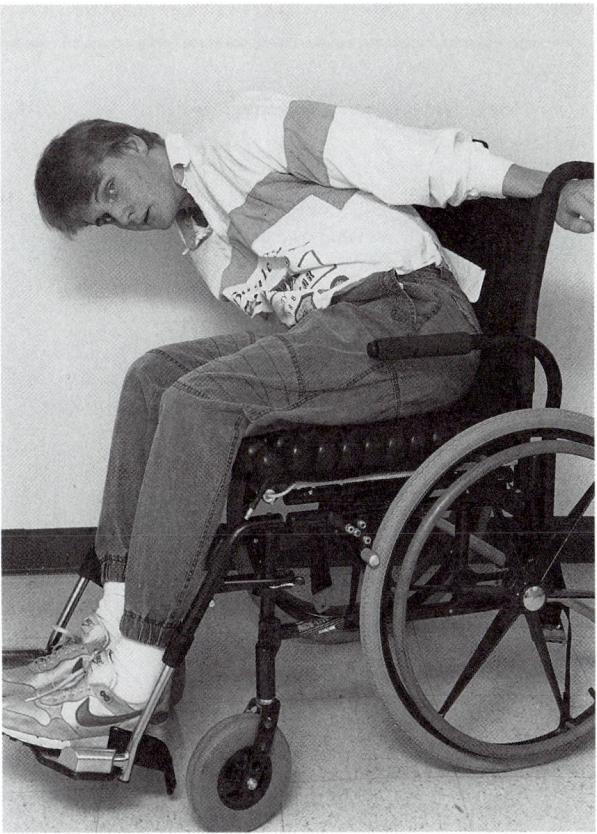

FIGURE 21–8 Leaning over in the wheelchair provides an alternative pressure relief movement.

- Alternating air pressure
- Water
- Gel pads
- Air
- Turning frames
- Air fluidized

Makleburst, Mondoux, and Sieggreen (1986) found that of six types tested, the Clinitron and Mediscus air fluidized

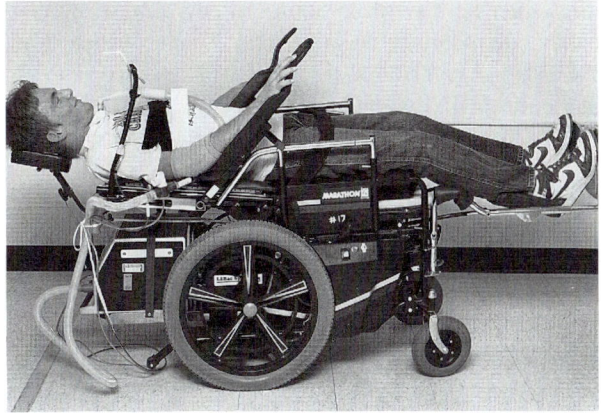

FIGURE 21–9 A person performs an independent weight shift with the recline feature on a power chair.

Procedure 21–2   Method to Provide Wheelchair Pressure Relief

Purpose

To provide relief for dependent quadriplegic patients by assisted weight shift.

Action

1. Assistant sits or stands behind wheelchair.

2. Lock brakes.

3. Tip wheelchair back to an angle of 30 degrees.

4. Hold 2 to 3 minutes.

5. Repeat procedure every 15 to 30 minutes while the patient is up.

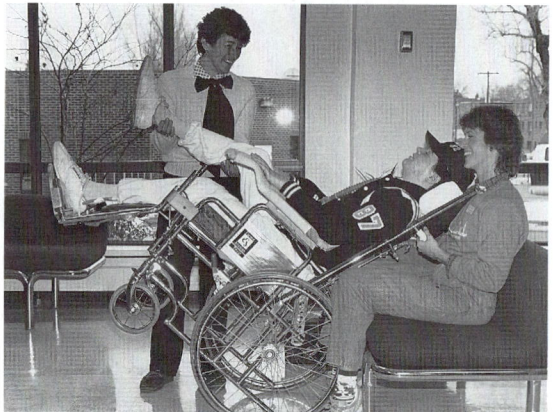

NOTE: In this procedure the leg is raised to allow the skin to breathe. This would also be done on the alternate leg.

beds and the Sof-Care bed cushion were most effective in relieving sacrum and trochanter pressure. However, bed and mattress selection must be evaluated individually. Simple, less costly devices are available and may be effective. For example, a simple, convoluted foam sheet (polyurethane), 2 inches thick, can help distribute body weight and reduce pressure.

Synthetic sheepskin is a popular, practical, and convenient aid. Synthetic sheepskin, preferably the full length of the bed, helps distribute pressure evenly, prevent shearing forces, reduce friction, eliminate wrinkles, dissipate heat, and absorb moisture. Smaller pieces *never* stay put. Synthetic sheepskin must be laundered regularly—about every 3 days, as it absorbs body perspiration, or more frequently if it becomes soiled with urine or fecal material. Strong detergents, hot water, or harsh drying cycles will harden and mat this material. To avoid trauma to the skin, the product must then be discarded. Some patients tend to develop contact dermatitis, especially in hot weather, when using sheepskin. A soft cotton or flannelette sheet placed on top of the sheepskin may be helpful.

A number of simple fluidized flotation systems are also available. For example, an air mattress (Figure 21–11) or commercial air mattresses filled with water to 60% to 70% of capacity have been used successfully as inexpensive pressure-dispersing devices (Kijeck and Jordan 1979).

Simple devices may also be needed for special circumstances—for example, for driving long distances or if the flu or some other temporary ailment confines the patient to bed for a few days. If a patient is at additional risk because of malnourishment or other secondary factors, then certainly consider more sophisticated flotation devices to prevent skin problems.

Protecting Skin from Injury

Special care must be taken when moving or transferring patients to avoid shearing or friction forces and minor skin injuries. When transferring patients, lift rather than drag. Always use good body mechanics and assure that there is adequate help for a safe, smooth transfer. Care givers should remove watches and jewelry to avoid injury. Care givers support the patient's body weight with the palms of their hands—not the fingertips. Never use the patient's trousers or other clothing to lift. Any tubings must be secured before the transfer—avoid touching the patient's skin. Before lifting the patient, check braces on the bed or chair and remove obstacles such as foot plates or chair armrest. Always inspect sheets

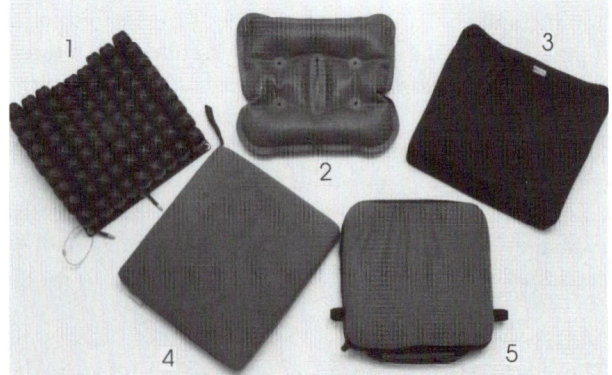

FIGURE 21–10   Commonly used cushins are: (1) RoHo Cushion, (2) BBD-Bye Bye Decubiti Cushion, (3) Jay Cushion, (4) Akros Cushion, (5) Vari-Lite Cushion.

and sheepskin for folds or wrinkles. Linen that is rough from excessive laundering should not be used. If the patient's bare skin will come in contact with the transfer board or toilet seat, the surface may be powdered to reduce friction.

One of the most dangerous problems for patients with SCI is the lack of sensory warning mechanisms to alert them to environmental hazards. Sitting or lying on objects can cause injury to the skin. Potential sources of injury are:

- Safety pins
- Curlers or bobby pins
- Buttons on mattresses
- Buttons on jeans or slacks; objects in pockets
- Catheter connectors
- Catheter clamps
- Tight pants over catheter tubing
- Broken hardware on equipment or braces

Extremes in temperature can also cause trauma to the skin. Burns can occur from heat, friction, chemicals, or tape. Possible sources of burns include:

- Sunburn
- Hot water, as in a bathtub or shower
- Hot water pipes
- Carrying hot foods or liquids on lap
- Kitchen stove during the cooking process
- Picking up or touching hot foods or drinks such as pizza or fried chicken
- Electrical appliances such as hair dryers or irons
- Electric blankets, hot water bottles, heating pads
- Sunlamps
- Cigarettes
- Sitting on hot objects such as rocks or concrete in the sun
- Automobiles—muffler, tailpipe, exhaust, car heater vents that are directed at the feet, seat belts, steering wheel, upholstery (any object that can get hot in a car)

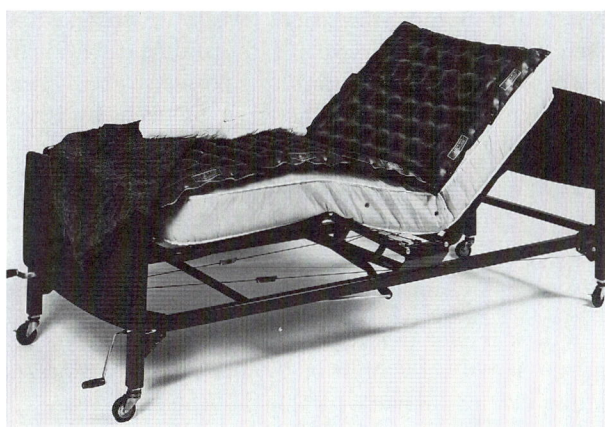

FIGURE 21–11 Bye Bye Decubiti Air Mattress Overlays convert any bed into a therapeutic flotation unit when used between the conventional mattress and pad. Available from Ken McRight Supplies, Tulsa, OK.

Friction burns can occur when skin surfaces rub against a hard surface, that is, from spasticity or prolonged sitting in bed at a 45 degree angle. Some *chemicals* such as disinfectants can cause burns, and *adhesive tape* can also cause burns. The nonallergic type is recommended for use.

Frostbite can occur as a result of exposure to a cold environment without enough protection. People with SCI should always dress warmly if they are going to be outside in cold weather. Ice packs are also a source of frostbite if they are not used properly.

Prolonged wetness can lead to skin breakdown. Possible sources of wetness are perspiration, stool, or urine. Chafing (excoriation) of the skin results from wetness. Bandaids may also cause an excessive accumulation of moisture under the protected area, which prolongs the healing process and can lead to loss of skin layers.

SPECIFIC INTERVENTIONS FOR MANAGEMENT OF PRESSURE AREAS

If any of the danger signs from pressure have already developed, immediately implement further preventive measures to reverse the underlying cause. As pressure sores are *always* caused by pressure, first relieve the pressure and then eliminate the sore. Assess the actual or protential impairment of skin integrity with an ulcer classfication system. See Table 21–4 (Sklar 1985).

The overall physiological status of the patient as well as the ulcer grade influence the healing process (Thomason 1988; Allen 1984). The stages of wound healing include vascular responses, cellular responses, epithelialization, and collagen formation. Care usually involves conservative treatment of Grades I, II, and III. A Grade IV ulcer generally requires surgical intervention.

Establishing specific ulcer care protocols is a difficult task because treatment plans must be individualized. Appropriate care is based on a complete assessment and the identified risk factors.

In an overview of pressure sore treatment Kozier and Erb (1991) stress the major principles of:

- Identification of invading (usually defective) organisms by judicious use of wound cultures
- Debridement (removal of foreign and contaminated or devitalized material from the pressure area)
- Promotion of healing by keeping area moist and preventing infection

Literally hundreds of skin care products are on the market. Categories of topical products and dressings as identified by Preston (1987) include:

- Liquid or gel film formers (to reduce irritation from tapes, dressings, or drainage)

- Transparent occlusive films (to allow for exchange of oxygen and moisture vapor while preventing invasion of organisms, works well on superficial pressure areas)
- Topical circulatory stimulants (to increase local blood flow and ease debridement)
- Wet-to-dry dressings (when placed in wound when wet and removed when dry, facilitate debridement)
- Moist-to-moist dressings (selected antiseptic solutions reduce contamination and retain protective moisture)
- Hydrocolloid and hydrogel products (may be used on top of other dressings to liquefy necrotic tissue and absorb drainage while retaining moisture)
- Exudate absorbers (used under other dressings to absorb waste fluid and cells)
- Enzymes (to digest moist necrotic tissue but less effective on dry eschar)

The use of topical agents should always be goal oriented, and continual assessment and evaluation of effectiveness of the treatment plan are essential.

Evaluation is an ongoing process in maintaining skin integrity. Patient acceptance of responsiblity in preventing skin breakdown must be evaluated as well as patient response to specific interventions. If the spinal cord injured patient does not comply with the skin care program, the patient and family can become burdened both financially and emotionally.

HEALTH EDUCATION

SCI patients need to know key concepts about managing their skin. Individual (and family) education must cover how pressure sores develop; how and when to inspect the skin; and how and when to perform pressure relief maneuvers, including turning and correct positioning in bed or in the wheelchair. Individuals should be taught the importance of general skin cleanliness, good personal hygiene, eating correctly, and maintaining good general circulation. In addition, individuals need to change their routines and habits. Teaching individuals to describe key concepts is frequently easier than actually changing routines and habits. Often a person can articulate the right information but does not make a commitment to change.

To change behavior, individuals need to perceive a pressure area as a potential threat. If applying the Health Belief Model (Rosenstock 1960) to skin care management, patients will act if they believe: (1) they are truly susceptible to pressure sores; (2) pressure sores will seriously affect them; (3) they can prevent pressure sores; (4) preventing pressure sores is less threatening than the pressure sores themselves.

Slides or pictures of pressure sores, testimonials, and discussion are good methods for instructing patients about the potential threat of skin breakdown. When viewing slides or pictures of skin sores, patients are often offended by the unpleasant appearance, but they begin to realize skin sores are a possible threat. Eventually, patients accept the reality of potential skin breakdown and are motivated to learn about prevention, monitoring, and problem solving.

Prevention

Maintaining optimal health is the key to prevention. Prevention also includes learning weight shifts, turning and padding when in bed, and awareness of environmental threats to skin integrity.

Monitoring and Problem Solving

People with SCI must learn how to monitor the condition of their skin by checking all bony prominences below the level of injury every morning and evening. Through regular skin inspection, problems can be discovered early and managed effectively, avoiding major skin problems.

People with SCI also must know how to deal with changes in skin condition. Key concepts to teach are: keep pressure off the problem area until the skin condition returns to normal, and determine why the problem happened. If a morning skin check reveals no problems but there is a problem in the evening, the person must evaluate the day's activities to determine the possible cause. Teach patients to determine why they have problems by asking questions such as:

- "Did I do enough weight shifts?"
- "Did I turn often enough?"
- "Is my cushion in good condition?"
- "Are my transfer techniques okay?"

If there is a red or bruised area or a small skin sore, the person should not sit or lie on the area until the redness or bruise fades or the sore is completely healed.

Teach patients with SCI about skin management through audiovisuals and classes, printed materials, and opportunities to demonstrate new skills. Continued reinforcement emphasizing the need for and methods of skin management, and encouraging responsibility for their own

TABLE 21-4   Ulcer Classification System

Ulcer Grade	Description
Grade I:	Erythema, induration, or ulceration of the dermis
Grade II:	Full thickness ulceration extending to subcutaneous fat
Grade III:	Ulceration through subcutaneous fat to deep fascia
Grade IV:	Penetrates deep fascia; necrosis involves all soft tissue; bone and joint structures involved

weight shifts and skin checks create opportunities for practice and the development of new habits.

LONG-TERM IMPLICATIONS

Management of a person with a pressure sore in the home must also encompass both physical and psychosocial aspects of care. If the patient is the homemaker, necessary bedrest may impose considerable difficulties. Support may be needed in the form of homemaking, child care, or other services. However, pressure relief is the primary goal; without it, the extent of the sore will increase and it will not heal, no matter what other treatment is used (King 1981).

Advanced pressure sore management is difficult with any patient. The additional risks run by patients with SCI mount up very quickly. Even before surgical intervention the wound must be debrided and free from infection; underlying conditions such as malnourishment must be reversed; and spasticity, if present, must be controlled. It may also be necessary to deal with self-destructive tendencies. Review Chapter 9.

Pressure sores may become life threatening. Their effects on self-image, body image, family and social relationships, sexuality, and vocational potential are difficult to quantify, but the cost is evident (Kijeck and Jordan 1979).

Disruption in skin integrity can lead to loss of time from work, loss of a limb, or ultimately loss of life. Thus, the importance of prevention is paramount.

REFERENCES

Allen, M. S. 1984. Nursing care of the spinal cord patient with recurrent pressure sores. *Journal of Rehabilitation Nursing* 9 (1): 34–36.

Anderson, T., and Andberg, M. 1979. Psychosocial factors associated with pressure sores. *Archives of Physical Medicine and Rehabilitation* 60: 341–346.

Anthony, C. P., and Thiebodeau, G. A. 1983. *Textbook of Anatomy and Physiology.* St. Louis: C. V. Mosby, pp. 76–82.

Benda, Shirley (Ed.). 1983. *Spinal Cord Injury Nursing Education— Suggested Content.* Chicago: American Spinal Injury Foundation, pp. 71–75.

Burke, D., and Murray, D. 1975. *Handbook of Spinal Cord Medicine,* Chapter 8. London and Basingstoke: Macmillan Press.

Craig Hospital. 1983. *Spinal Cord Injury Handbook.* Englewood, CO: Author.

— 1988. Wheelchair positioning clinic initiated. *Movin' On,* pp. 4–5. A brochure published by the author, Englewood, CO.

Feustel, D. E. 1982. Pressure sore prevention: Aye, there's the rub. *Nursing* 12 (4): 78–83.

Fisher, M., Szymke, T., and Kosiak, M. 1978. Wheelchair cushion effects on skin temperature. *Archives of Physical Medicine and Rehabilitation* 59 (Feb.): 68–72.

Ford, J. R., and Duckworth, B. 1987. *Physical Management of the Quadriplegic Patient.* 2d ed. Philadelphia: F. A. Davis.

Garber, Susan Lipton. 1985. Wheelchair cushions for spinal cord-injured individuals. *American Journal of Occupational Therapy* 39 (11).

Gosnell, D. 1973. An assessment tool to identify pressure sores. *Nursing Research* 22 (1): 55–59.

Graitcer, P., and Maynard, F. (Eds.). 1990. *First Colloquium on Preventing Secondary Disabilities Among People with Spinal Cord Injuries.* Atlanta: U.S. Department of Health and Human Services, Public Health Service, Centers for Disease Control.

Kijeck, J., and Jordan, M. 1979. Nursing strategies: Prevention and treatment of the pressure ulcer. In *Current Perspectives in Rehabilitation Nursing.* Eds. R. Murray and J. Kijeck. St. Louis: C. V. Mosby, pp. 84–96.

King, R. 1981. Assessment and management of soft tissue pressure. In *Comprehensive Rehabilitation Nursing.* Eds. N. Martin, H. Hold, and D. Hicks. New York: McGraw-Hill, pp. 242–268.

Kozier, B., and Erb, G. 1991. *Fundamentals of Nursing.* 4th ed. Menlo Park, CA: Addison-Wesley.

Makleburst, Mondoux, and Sieggreen 1986. Pressure relief characteristics of various support surfaces used in prevention and treatment of pressure ulcers. *Journal of Enterostomal Therapy* 13 (3): 85–89.

Mikulic, M. 1980. Treatment of pressure ulcers. *American Journal of Nursing* 80 (6): 1125–1128.

Peacock, E. E. 1984. *Wound Repair.* 3d ed. Philadelphia: W. B. Saunders.

Preston, K. M. 1987. Dermal ulcers: Simplifying a complex problem. *Rehabilitation Nursing* 12 (1): 17–21.

Rosenstock, I. M. 1960. What research in motivation suggests for public health. *American Journal of Public Health* 50: 295–302.

Sklar, C. G. 1985. Pressure ulcer management in the neurologically impaired patient. *Journal of Neurosurgical Nursing* 17 (1): 30–36.

Spence, A., and Mason, E. 1983. *Human Anatomy and Physiology.* 2d ed. Menlo Park, CA: Benjamin/Cummings.

Thomas, E. 1977. Nursing care of the patient with spinal cord injury. In *The Total Care of Spinal Cord Injuries.* Eds. D. Pierce and V. Nickel. Boston: Little, Brown, pp. 249–298.

Thomason, S. S. 1988. Protocol for pressure ulcer interventions. *SCI Nursing* 5 (3): 41–47.

Trieshmann, R. 1988. *Spinal Cord Injuries, Psychological, Social and Vocational Adjustment.* New York: Demos Publications, pp. 79–81.

Virginia Spinal Cord Injury System, University of Virginia Center, and Virginia Department of Rehabilitation Services. 1988. *Virginia Spinal Cord Injury Care and Teaching Manual.* Fisherville, VA: Woodrow Wilson Rehabilitation Center.

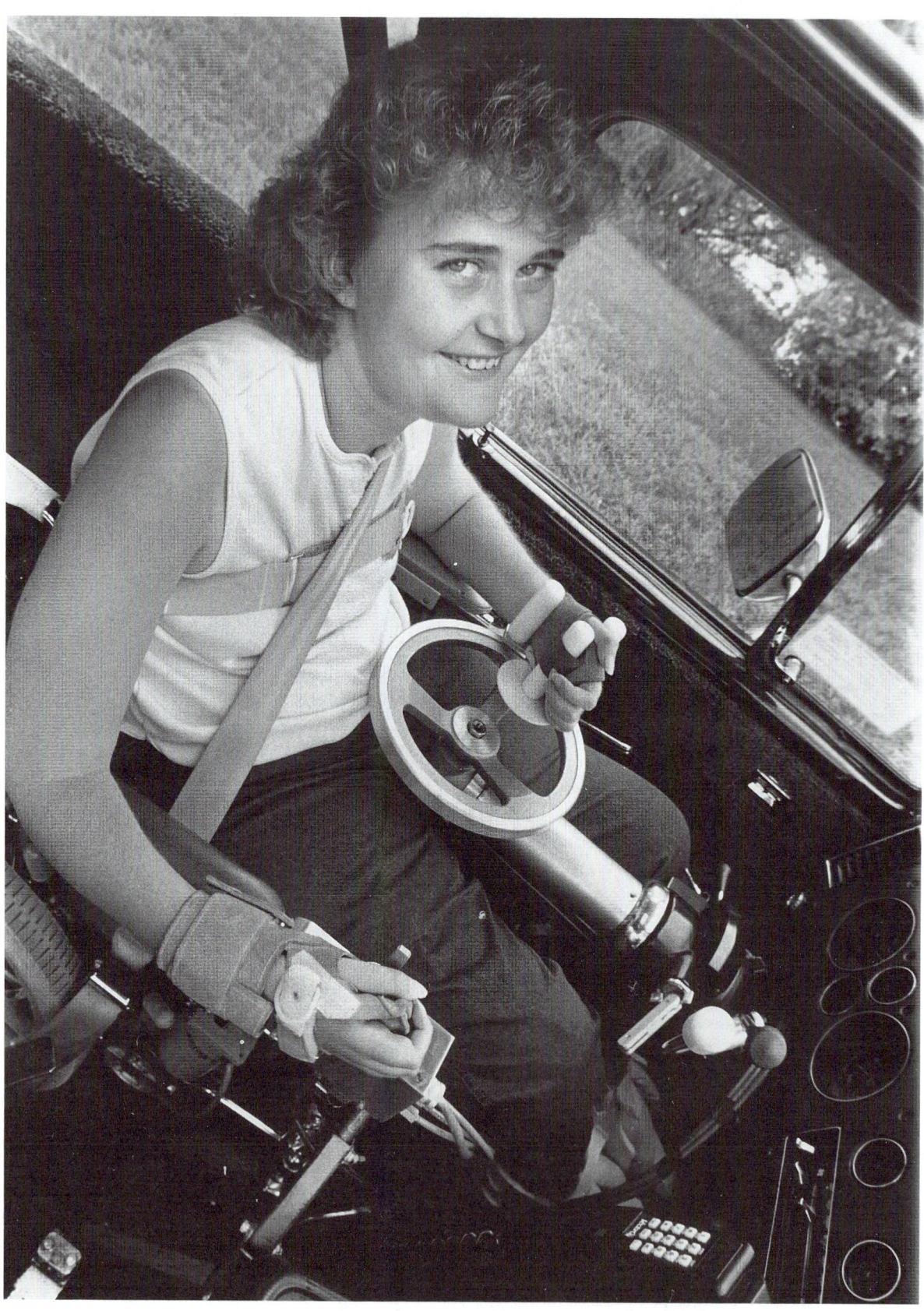

CHAPTER
— 22 —

Resuming Physical Activity and Daily Living Skills[*]

Chapter Outline

*This chapter was developed with assistance from S. P. Wasko, P.T.; D. Crowley, M.D.; S. Laughlin, B.S.R., M.B.A., former Senior Occupational Therapist; and D. Webster, B.S.R., Ph.D., former Senior Physical Therapist; Acute Spinal Cord Injury Unit, Shaughnessy Hospital, Vancouver, BC.

Health Care Objectives

- To enhance potential functional expectations related to the level of SCI sustained
- To prevent physical deterioration
- To promote optimal function by strengthening existing muscles and facilitating potential redevelopment of weak muscles
- To minimize discomfort, pain, and spasticity

- To develop DLS that individuals can realistically manage or teach others how to perform
- To teach individuals to understand the rationale of their treatment; to develop a positive attitude and to set their own goals; to learn the skills required to function at their maximum level of independence; and to teach others how to assist them when necessary

- To assist the disabled person in understanding potential environmental alterations that may enhance function at home and in the community
- To help individuals and families use community resources for assistance with personal care; homemaking services; and vocational, social, and recreational pursuits

Because all people with SCI suffer from some loss of strength and ability to move, an exercise program is essential to ensure that they regain maximum possible muscle function. Exercise is supplemented by measures such as correct positioning, turning, and provision of psychological support and encouragement. As the rehabilitation process evolves, physical capabilities are developed into more specific skills for accomplishing functional activities (Adkins 1985; Sargent and Braun 1986). Physical and occupational therapists select and teach appropriate activities and work closely with nurses to maintain safety and comfort while allowing patients to use the skills they have learned. Later in rehabilitation, this process may involve other disciplines, such as therapeutic recreational specialists and ultimately community-based exercise specialists to broaden the scope of treatment to include other community living skills, vocational pursuits, and recreational skills.

Fostering independence is as much the nurse's responsibility as the therapist's. For rehabilitation to be effective, techniques must be incorporated into daily activities and thus into daily care. The ready availability of therapists in patients' rooms during this time promotes application of functional activities and enhances sharing of professional expertise. This interaction is invaluable.

To gain maximum benefits from therapeutic programs that focus on development of functional living skills for community life, preventive and restorative measures must be comprehensive (Yarkony et al. 1987) and must begin within hours after injury.

ASSESSMENT ───────────────

Changes in Physical Capabilities after Spinal Cord Injury

Physical capabilities depend on the integrated functions of the nervous and musculoskeletal systems, modified by individual interests, desires, and inherent physical capabilities before injury. Following SCI, physiological damage is obvious and devastating. The individual must cope not only with motor and sensory loss, but also with skeletal immobi-

lization and physical exhaustion in response to the initial trauma. Generally, the higher the level of injury, the more profound the physical effects. Psychosocial factors associated with dramatic body image changes, compounded by accompanying physical fatigue, can suppress motivation considerably, and *motivation* is a key factor in resuming physical activity and achieving independence.

History

General Health before Injury
Patients who enjoyed good health, were well nourished, controlled their body weight, and exercised regularly before the injury can tolerate a planned activity program with greater stamina and more endurance. It is especially important to note any preexisting cardiopulmonary complications, which may be overt or subtle in nature. The degree of perceived fatigue following activity will dictate modifications in the exercise program.

Age
Muscle mass, strength, and coordination diminish in the course of normal aging. The older patient will probably tolerate less physical activity and will perform at a slower rate. The effect of aging must be assessed in the development of an exercise prescription.

Preexisting Neuromusculoskeletal Conditions
Preexisting neuromusculoskeletal conditions or disease may contribute to the extent of SCI and must be critically assessed as to the impact of the exercise prescription and the patient's tolerance for general activity. Program modifications must be considered and implemented based on the assessment of these conditions.

Associated Trauma
Patients with multiple trauma will need a specialized activity program. One of the most challenging associated traumas is *cognitive impairment*—either preexisting or as a result of the trauma causing SCI. Specific program modifications must be implemented as soon as possible (see Chapter 26) to adjust exercise prescription outcomes and maximize potentials within these constraints.

Preinjury Personality

It is imperative to assess the patient's preinjury personality. This information, obtained from an interdisciplinary perspective, will help the team understand how patients think and feel and will adapt to a physical activity program:

- Does the patient like himself or herself?
- Does the patient adapt easily?
- How has the patient previously dealt with challenges?
- Is the patient easily frustrated?
- Is the patient a private person?
- Is the patient very body conscious?
- Does the patient like to be independent?
- Are there influential social or cultural expectations?

By answering all these questions, the health care team can develop an individualized approach to self-care and problem solving.

Psychosocial Aspects

The emotions experienced during psychosocial adaptation to disability profoundly affect the patient's willingness to cooperate and readiness to learn. During the process of adaptation to loss, it often takes many long hours to break the cycles of depression and anger that inhibit motivation and prevent patients from totally involving themselves in planning and implementing a specific program. Emotional reactions tend to heighten when skills practiced since early childhood must be relearned. Patients with quadriplegia, for example, require tremendous energy and concentration to accomplish the simplest everyday task such as brushing teeth. Under these circumstances it is easy to become frustrated.

These feelings are normal reactions to an abnormal situation, and it requires an interdisciplinary team effort to help patients deal with them. Once patients have adapted to inevitable physical limitations, they learn alternative methods to gain mobility and independence with relative ease.

A supportive family is another significant factor in successful reactivation. Such a family can help meet the person's needs for love, belonging, and hope for the future, and it is encouraging when they take an active role in therapy programs. Other families may need more guidance in the form of gentle explanations of how and why the patient needs their support. Cultural expectations of members' roles also make a difference. The patients that do most poorly are generally those with no family support.

Although the family is significant, if it is not a viable resource, most persons belong to some other social network that can be tapped. Close friends can also help find ways of achieving rehabilitative goals. All resources must be creatively assessed to determine how they can be useful.

Physical Assessment

In-depth assessment of neuromusculoskeletal function involves close collaboration, primarily of the physician, the physical therapist, and the occupational therapist. Initially physicians and therapists are involved with detailed assessment to establish sound baseline data and further delineate diagnosis. Assessment is an ongoing process used to evaluate any change in neurological status, to monitor the patient's progress toward the goals of treatment, and to evaluate functional outcome of treatments. For this ongoing assessment, the physical therapist and occupational therapist use similar skills and techniques but focus on different aspects of physical activity and self-care. See Figures 22–1 and 22–2.

Although the nurse may not be directly responsible for the assessment, it is important to know the general terminology to improve communication with therapists, to appreciate the significance of their findings, and to understand implications for care.

Assessment of Muscle Strength

Manual muscle testing can determine the degree of weakness, loss, or return of muscle function. This skill involves isolating a muscle's function and then grading the weakness or strength present. See Chapter 4, especially Figure 4–21, Procedure 4–1, and Table 4–6. Accurate and serial manual muscle testing monitors progression or regression of a patient's function. As spinal shock passes, manual muscle testing for motor strength may be hampered, with spasticity affecting movements. The *quality* of controlled movements, not the *quantity* of strength or movement, evolves as the main issue (Schneider 1981). Detailed testing provides a sensitive test of any alteration in the neurological level. See Chapter 4.

Assessment of Range of Motion

All joints are assessed for any restriction in movement. Both *passive* movements (with the examiner moving the joint) and *active* movements (accomplished by patient strength alone) are measured. It is important to retain joint flexibility, increase muscle strength in nonparalyzed muscles, and prevent contractures in paralyzed muscles that will lead to loss of function.

Be aware of the causes of limitations in range of motion—particularly pretraumatic or associated traumatic injuries and *pain* and *spasticity*—to modify movements encountered during general care. The amount of pain the patient experiences often determines the amount of physical activity possible. During the acute stage, only pain-free activity is usually attempted. The presence of pain and the degree of spasticity affect the choice of positioning, the method of transfer, and the ability of the patient to perform active movements such as are involved with dressing or eating.

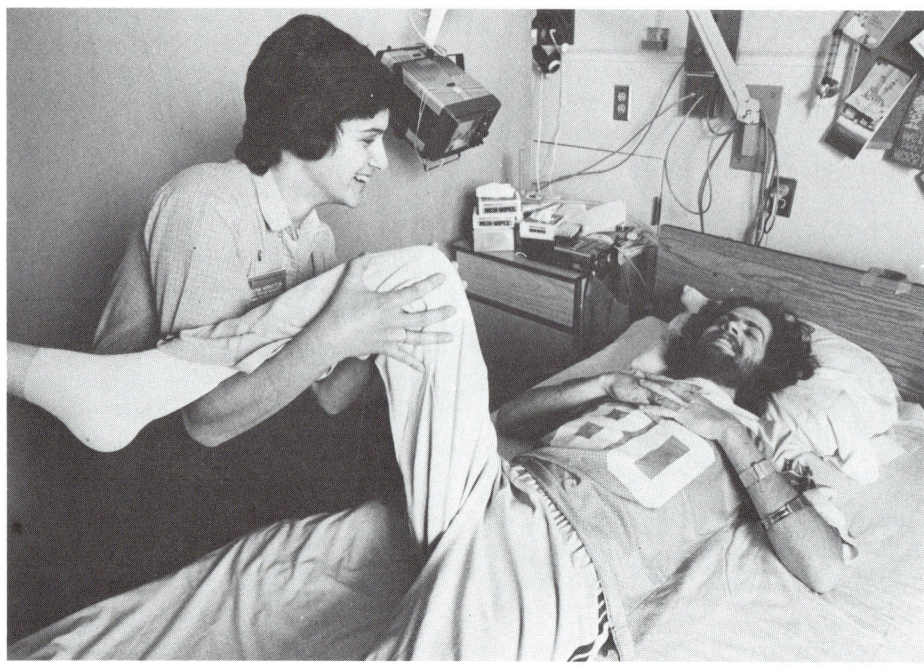

FIGURE 22–1   A physical therapist facilitates gross motor activity.

Assessment of Muscle Tone

Following SCI, muscles may become spastic (hypertonic) or flaccid (hypotonic) depending on the level of cord injury and the time elapsed since injury. The state of spinal shock,

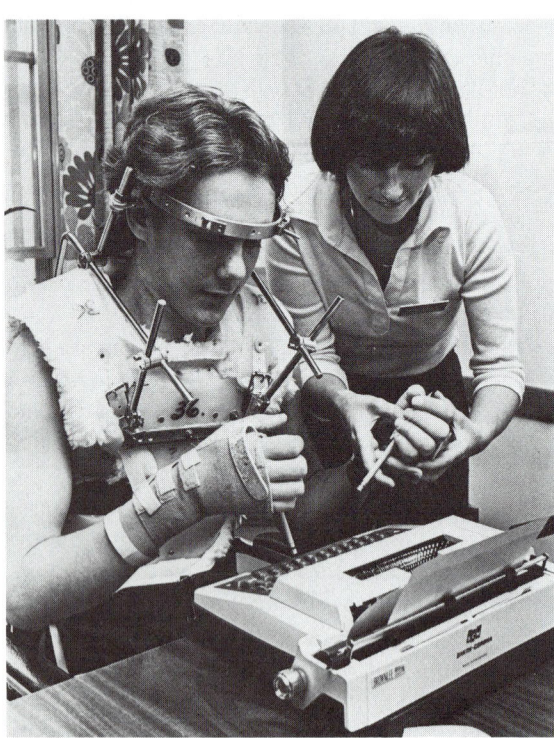

FIGURE 22–2   An occupational therapist develops potential fine motor activity.

in which all reflex activity below the level of injury is suppressed, usually lasts for several weeks or months after injury. Reflex activity is recorded as normal, hyperactive, or absent. After reflex activity returns, most patients develop some degree of spasticity, which will vary with each patient. The effect of changes in muscle tone on functional movements, balance, and body posture in various recumbent and sitting positions is of vital importance to a rehabilitation program.

Assessment of Sensation

Gross sensory testing is completed initially and repeated at intervals throughout the rehabilitation process to detect any improvement or deterioration in neurological function. Sensation is often illustrated schematically on diagrams (as shown in Figure 4–23). Sensation is described as normal, impaired (may be hypersensitive or hyposensitive), or absent; the description also includes information on levels of:

- Pain (appreciation of pinprick and application of deep pressure)
- Temperature (appreciation of hot and cold sensation)
- Touch (appreciation of light palpation of the examiner's hand)
- Vibration sense (awareness of vibrating object placed on the skin)
- Proprioception, that is, position sense (appreciation of where limbs are in space)

See Table 4–2 for further instructions on sensory testing.

Assessment of Body Build and Coordination

Good body awareness is a definite advantage for paralyzed people when it comes to moving their bodies in new ways, especially in transfers. Overweight or tall, thin people often have problems moving and positioning their bodies following SCI.

GENERAL MANAGEMENT

Care givers can do much to enhance the value of therapeutic sessions by promoting general health measures, particularly to minimize fatigue and pain. The condition of the patient's chest (and therefore respiratory reserves) directly determines how much physical activity the patient will tolerate. Vigorous chest treatments, turning, positioning, regular breathing exercises and resisted breathing programs (as well as encouragement to stop smoking) will improve ventilation and general circulation. Moreover, the well-rested and well-nourished patient who is free from bouts of constipation or bladder infections will sustain higher energy levels and tolerate more physical activity. It is also helpful if the patient is free of pain, so nurses should administer needed analgesics so that peak periods of pain relief will coincide with exercise times. Therapists should be informed of any changes in the patient's general condition, such as a physical setback or emotional upset, changes in nutritional intake, and any changes in routine schedules.

Continuity of care requires interdisciplinary education (Turney 1989), continuous communication of information, evaluation, and determination of appropriate approaches. Regular interdisciplinary team meetings, including the patient and family, are most valuable. Most important, everyone must understand the philosophy and terminology in use. In addition to verbal communication and the medical record, one helpful tool is the use of a large interdisciplinary care plan (Kardex) on which therapists can update information directly for nursing purposes. See Figure 22–3. Instructional bedside charts may also clarify the necessary detailed information flow.

Maintaining Joint Range of Motion

Exercises are performed to maintain or restore full joint range of motion, prevent muscle contractures, and stimulate the circulation. If joints do not receive adequate motion daily, stiffness and contractures will develop that interfere with functional ability. For example, shoulder stiffness decreases arm movement needed for eating and makes positioning more difficult for wheelchair transfers.

Exercises are commonly *active* (done alone), *active assisted* (patient needs help), or *passive* (patient is unable to participate).

The amount of range is determined by the structure of the joint and the length and tension of the muscle surrounding the joint. Range of movement is not the same for everyone, but depends on factors such as level of spinal fracture, age, body build, and the limitations imposed by disease, level of fracture, the presence of pain, and time interval since injury. Modifications in treatment will also be made based on these factors.

Frequency of exercises depends on the current status of joint flexibility, spasticity, and pain. (Range of motion exercises help decrease spasticity and prevent pain associated with contractures.) As mobility, strength, and independent skills increase, the need for range of motion exercises generally decreases.

The physical therapist is responsible for maintaining the full range of movement of all joints. If further range of movement exercises are to be performed by the nursing staff, the precautions and specific treatment required should be demonstrated by the physical therapist. The exercises outlined in Table 22–1 have been specifically selected to use as an *adjunct* to physical therapy treatment and do not include a complete selection of range of motion exercises.

During the acute stage the therapist performs range of motion exercises twice a day to maintain and restore muscle and joint function. Range of motion exercises should then be performed by the nursing staff, as needed, to make the patient comfortable, ensure a frequent change of position, and prevent circulatory stasis. These exercises require more skill than is commonly realized, and collaboration with the physical therapist is essential. Guidelines include:

- Avoid any movements that produce pain.
- Move only one extremity at a time.
- Do not force any movement. If spasticity occurs retain a firm hold and wait until it diminishes.
- For patients with lumbar fractures, do not flex the hip with the leg straight and do not flex the hip more than 90 degrees. (Pain may restrict flexion to 30 degrees at first.) These movements put a strain on the fracture.

Gradual Mobilization

Mobilization is introduced on a gradual basis to minimize the effects of postural hypotension and to carefully evaluate stress on the fracture site.

Adjustment to the upright position can be especially traumatic for patients with quadriplegia. Measures to minimize the effects of postural hypotension, to assist venous return, and to deal with hypotensive episodes are described in Chapter 16.

When the the patient can tolerate the upright position the physical therapist assesses the patient's readiness to transfer and perform the initial maneuver. This occurs

FIGURE 22–3 A large interdisciplinary Kardex form developed from a nursing history. Note: each discipline directly enters and updates pertinent information. (From Acute Spinal Cord Injury Unit, Shaughnessy Hospital, Vancouver, BC.)

ALLERGIES: None known		NAME:	Q. Smith
		S.I.N NO.:	202-139-049
		X-RAY NO:	TL 12394
		DATE OF INJURY:	Feb 1, 1982
		ADMISSION DATE:	Feb 1, 1982
		DIAGNOSIS:	Fracture dislocation C4-5 with complete quadriplegia
			C5 on right
			C6 on left
			M.V.A

TREATMENTS:

DATE	
Feb 7	Pinsite care q8h for Halo-ring
7	Phisohex washes to face, neck and shoulders B.i.D. for rash (am care and qhs)

SPECIMENS:

DATE	
Feb 1	Urinalysis / Urine C+S weekly

SPECIAL PROCEDURES/X-RAYS:

DATE	
Feb 1	Cervical spine, A/P & Lateral Chest X-ray
Feb 2	Cervical spine, chest X-ray (Intravenous pyelogram)
7	Cervical spine (post halo application) chest X-ray

OPERATIONS:

DATE	
Feb 1	Halo ring with 10 lbs traction
7	Application of Halo-thoracic vest

CONSULTANTS:

NEURO SURGERY:	G.B. Thompson
ORTHOPEDICS:	P. Kokan
UROLOGY:	Z. Perler
FAMILY PRACTITIONER:	P. Taylor

MEDICATIONS:

DATE	REORDER		DISC.
Feb 7		Darvon plain ī - īī po q4h for neck or arm pain	

BOWEL ROUTINE:

Fruit lax 1 tbsp.
Glycermid tabs ī } 0800
Glycerine supp. q 2 days

H.S. SEDATION:

PROBLEMS:
- Painful (L) arm
- Poor memory.
- Unrealistic hopes of recovery.
- Potential chest complications

GOALS: Reduce pain & Maintain range.

Regain orientation

Develop realistic expectations

Minimize risk conditions that aggravate quadriplegia

SPECIAL NEEDS/APPROACH:
a) avoid sudden movement & prolonged elevated position.
Assess need for analgesic prior to physical therapy

a) Use direct simple explanations.
Repeat when necessary for teaching

Be realistic & honest. Avoid giving false hope. Do not rush him. Support strengths.

Complete patient health education. Encourage to stop smoking.

OCCUPATIONAL THERAPY: TIME:
0900 - 1045   1400 - 1500   Individual
Hand class
PRINTING: Wear at night only   Long opponens splint for (L) hand
Short opponens splint for (R) hand

ADL Feeding-set-up. Use
A.D.L. splint and spoon. Able to use cup and eat finger foods with minimal assistance.
Grooming-uncap, squeeze toothpaste
Needs assistance in bed
Dressing - dependent

PHYSIOTHERAPY: TIME 1045
Individual treatment
1330
Introduction to mat & floor exercise
1500

I.V. THERAPY:		
INTAKE		q 4 h
OUTPUT		q 4 h
T.P.R.		9 am
B.P.		9 am

DIET: Full diet High pro/cho drinks T.I.D
Regulate intake = 2,000 ml
Teach drinking pattern

Daily Program Schedule
0745 - 0830 Breakfast
0900 - 1045 O.T. Introducing dressing in bed, grooming at sink next week
1045 Physical therapy (individual)
1145 Lounge for lunch
1230 Rest
1330 Physical therapy (group)
400 Occupational therapy (hand class)
1500 Physical therapy (individual treatment)
1700 Dinner

TURNING/POSITIONING:
Side to side q 2h
Introduce proning in afternoon
Night splints

BATH: Bed & Swedish Tub
q 3 days
DAY: Mon, Thurs, Sat
TIME: 0900

INTERMEDIATE PLAN:
1. Mobilize as tolerated
2. Guilford brace/soft collar in early May

BLADDER CARE: Intermittent catheterization q 4 h
If residual urine greater than 500 ml
Contact resident
TIME: 0200 - 0600 - 1000 - 1400 - 1800 - 2200

BOWEL CARE:
Check manually - daily
Glycerine supp. q 2 days (odd)
Position in bed

DISCHARGE PLAN:
- G.F. Strong Rehabilitation Center mid-May as in patient.
- Eventually home with parents
- Vocational Counselling

SOCIAL SERVICE:
FINANCIAL RESPONSIBILITY: Insurance
Corporation of B.C. providing full coverage
Canadian Paraplegic Association
C.P.A. J. Parker, Peer Counsellor

TIME: 9 am
NEXT OF KIN: Mr. and Mrs. R. Smith
NAME: J. Smith
AGE: 20
BIRTHDATE: 1900. 3/59
RELATIONSHIP: Parents
TELEPHONE NO.: 224-0896
RELIGION: Protestant
MARITAL STATUS: S☐ M☐ W☐ D☐
ADDRESS: 1234 - W.14 Ave. Vancouver
ROOM: 3/5-4

TABLE 22-1 Selected Passive Range of Motion Exercises

To maintain the comfort of the patient, it is important that the joints be moved either before or after each turn. The most practical method combines the movements of flexion, extension, abduction, adduction, and rotation. The exercise will be assisted or passive, depending on the patient's muscle strength. Use a firm but comfortable grip. Support the limbs at the joints. Perform the movement smoothly and rhythmically. Repeat three to five times every 2 hours. Range is done approximately 5 minutes for each limb.

Upper Limb Exercise

Support the patient at the wrist and above the elbow. Start with the arm down and out to the side, with the elbow straight and the palm down. Move it to place the palm on the opposite shoulder. Return to starting position.

Lower Limb Exercise

Support the patient under the knee and at the sole of the foot. Start with leg straight and in abduction. Flex the knee and the hip, move the leg up and across to place the heel on the opposite knee, and return it to the starting position.

Circulatory Exercise

To maintain adequate circulation, foot-pumping exercises should be performed during each shift. Grasp the patient above the ankle and around the sole of the foot. Keep the knee straight so that the calf muscle is stretched. Perform a firm up-and-down movement of the foot in a pedaling action. Repeat 40 to 50 times every 8 hours.

---

when the patient can sit upright in bed for 30 to 60 minutes or can tolerate daily sessions on the tilt table for a week or so without feeling faint or dizzy. See Figure 22–4.

Throughout this process of mobilization, close collaboration with the physician is necessary to evaluate spinal immobilization and stability (Phillips 1987). Methods of monitoring skeletal healing have been discussed in Chapter 20. For the first 7 to 10 days after injury there will be a certain amount of pain at the injury site due to fractured bones, torn ligaments, and local muscle spasm. However, any severe, shooting pain or prolonged discomfort on return to bed may indicate the spine is not stable enough to withstand the added stress of movement. The patient should remain in bed until the physician has evaluated the situation.

Muscle-Strengthening Activities

Not only can SCI result in total loss of muscle power, but disuse can also severely weaken muscles that remain intact. An individualized physical therapy program should be planned immediately on admission to develop functional mobility, that is, practical ways of getting around on an everyday basis. Treatment goals are to preserve strength and range of motion and to facilitate return of all weak but potentially active muscle groups. To compensate for lost muscle power, existing muscles must be strengthened to their maximum in order to achieve potential mobility and independence skills.

A *full physical therapy program* commences when the patient can tolerate being up most of the day. There are no restrictions on activity other than that of avoiding pain. All exercise is directed toward functional activities. Skills such as pressure relief maneuvers, transfers, and wheelchair management are examples of functional activities. Before this, the patient undertakes a *partial physical therapy program*. This program involves varying degrees of limited activity depending on patient tolerance to mobilization and restrictions of movement necessary to reduce stress on the healing spinal fracture site. For example, for persons with paraplegia, long sitting and lying prone would be restricted.

To promote functional exercise such as eating, transferring, and other self-care tasks, the nurse must be familiar with the general treatment programs and the specific restrictions for each patient. This information should always be taken into account when supervising, assisting, moving, or positioning patients during nursing care. The therapist

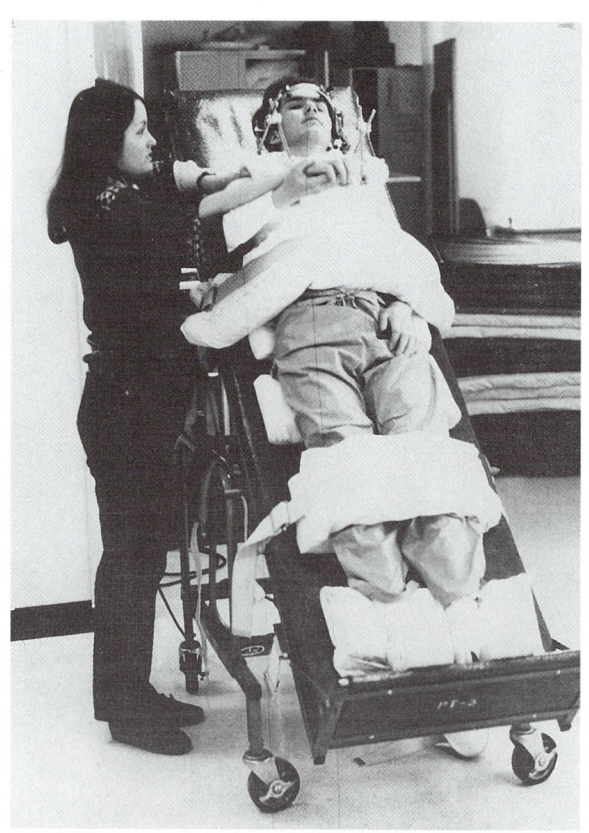

FIGURE 22–4 The tilt table is used to help a patient gradually build up tolerance to the upright position.

should inform the nurse of any changes in neuromuscular function and of progressions in treatment.

Active muscle-strengthening exercises are performed daily, progress gradually, and include general activities, mat activities, gait training, and swimming.

General Activities

In the early stages, particularly while the patient is in bed, the amount of activity directly depends on the amount of patient pain and fatigue. Some examples of general activities included in a physical therapy program are:

- Manual assistance or resistance, allowing the therapist to grade and control the movement
- Slings and springs to eliminate the effect of gravity and allow the patient to move a limb independently, even when it is very weak
- Weights and pulleys to provide resistant arm/leg exercises to improve and maintain normal strength and assist circulation
- Biofeedback (visual and auditory signals), which informs patients of the amount of muscle activity they are producing

Rehabilitation exercise equipment is becoming more available on the commercial market. Some equipment is suitable for a personal exercise program at home. Varying degrees of aerobic and circulatory benefits with a decrease in spasticity are reported by users along with psychological benefits. In fact, many of the products are designed by persons with disabilities. The Saratoga Cycle is an example of a well-researched, nonmotorized, accessible arm or leg aerobic exerciser for enhancing total body fitness for the paralyzed person. Passive motion exercisers offer continuous movement and operate on the principle of cross-lateral patterning (like walking) to enhance range of motion, but need to be used with caution in persons without sensation. Muscle and joint damage could occur, and monitoring by a licensed therapist is recommended. The Electric Passive Pedal Exerciser (EPPE) is particularly useful. The Flexaciser is a more sophisticated version. Partial or total funding may be possible through third-party payers for these aids.

The Freedom Machine is more suited to rehabilitation centers as it can accommodate up to four wheelchair users at a time. Originally designed for training competitive athletes, the Freedom Machine's innovative features allow numerous exercises using a variety of muscle-conditioning apparatuses, pulleys, and military and bench press units. See Resources for more information about exercise equipment.

Mat Activities

The purpose of mat work is to develop strength, balance, and coordination in preparation for other activities, such as transferring and dressing. Depending on the level of injury,

patients learn to balance in a sitting position, lift the buttocks to move around on the bed, roll over, get up into a sitting position from lying positions, and return to the wheelchair from the floor. Once the patient is up in a wheelchair, particular emphasis is placed on balance, strength, and coordination, which promote achievement of transfers; wheelchair management; and, for some, gait training at a very early stage.

Gait Training

Selected patients with low paraplegia and some pelvic control may achieve ambulation with the aid of crutches and knee-ankle-foot orthoses that provide rigid support to the knees and ankles. Braces may be modified later to suit individual needs, and crutches may or may not be needed. Whether to use this method of ambulation depends largely on patient motivation and preference, because it consumes a great deal of energy. Many patients prefer to combine methods of mobilization, using crutch walking for some occasions and the wheelchair for others.

Swimming

Pool therapy is psychologically and physically very beneficial to patients with all levels of injury. It is included in the treatment program depending on the patient's desire, bowel and bladder management, and orthopedic stability.

Transfer Activities

When spinal stability allows, therapists are very much involved with assessing the patient's readiness for transfer activities, performing initial transfers, teaching appropriate techniques, and selecting a wheelchair with various accessories and mobility aids (Ford and Duckworth 1987). Care givers then become active in performing, assisting, or supervising these transfers on a day-to-day basis.

To ensure safety and promote independence as the patient gains strength, sitting tolerance, and vertebral column stability, be aware of the exact amount and kind of assistance the patient requires. The patient, the family, the nurse, and the therapist must understand the methods of transfer and terminology used to describe these maneuvers. As the patient progresses, the helping roles change to encourage independence. Withdraw any assistance that is not needed. Patients with physical potential will naturally progress from dependent to assisted, to supervised, and finally to independent transfers.

Dependent Transfer

In dependent transfer the patient needs total assistance. This method usually requires two assistants and is usually necessary for a quadriplegic patient in a halo brace or any other patient who is difficult to move, such as obese patients or patients with multiple injuries.

Assisted Transfer

An assisted transfer is designed to allow patients to perform the maximum amount of the activity that they can on their own. Be prepared to assist and protect at all stages of the procedure. The method is the same as with the dependent transfer except that only one assistant is required. The patient generally uses a transfer board, and the footrests remain down in place.

Supervised Transfer

A supervised transfer requires only minimal or standby assistance. Stand in front of the patient. Help with balance if necessary, and ensure that the feet do not strike the chair as the patient puts them on the foot pedals. Help the patient lift the hips and slide into the chair as necessary. When returning to bed if long sitting in not allowed or is difficult, have the patient transfer the buttocks to the bed first, then lift the legs onto the bed while lowering the trunk. See Figure 22–5.

Independent Transfer

In an independent transfer the person does not require any assistance. The patient with paraplegia learns to transfer from wheelchair to bed, toilet, car, bath, and the floor and back independently. The patient usually accomplishes this within 4 to 6 weeks of being allowed up. The quadriplegic patient will require assistance with all transfers, at least until the halo brace is removed; then achievement of independence depends largely on level of injury sustained. For example, most persons with a C_5 injury will find it impossible to transfer independently; for those with C_6, it takes a lot of work.

Clinical proficiency at performing transfers requires formalized instruction followed by supervised practice sessions. Important aspects include skillful application of good body mechanics (see Figure 22–6), knowledge of transfer movements, and familiarization with the wheelchair and its accessories. The key points involved in general transfer techniques and alternative methods of transfer are discussed in Procedure 22–1.

To transfer a quadriplegic patient in a halo apparatus generally requires two assistants. Procedure 22–2 outlines this dependent transfer. The use of standard mechanical lifts is discouraged during the acute stage because of the undue curving pressure exerted on various parts of the spine. It is very difficult to prevent the lift from contact with the metal apparatus on the halo brace. Any pressure on these bars will loosen the orthoses. Procedure 22–3 shows how a transfer method for a quadriplegic person is simplified once spinal stability is achieved and spinal orthoses are removed (an active-assisted transfer).

To ensure safety as well as ease, many transfer techniques must be adapted to differing situations. Additional assistants

FIGURE 22–5 A paraplegic patient is supervised during an active-assisted transfer.

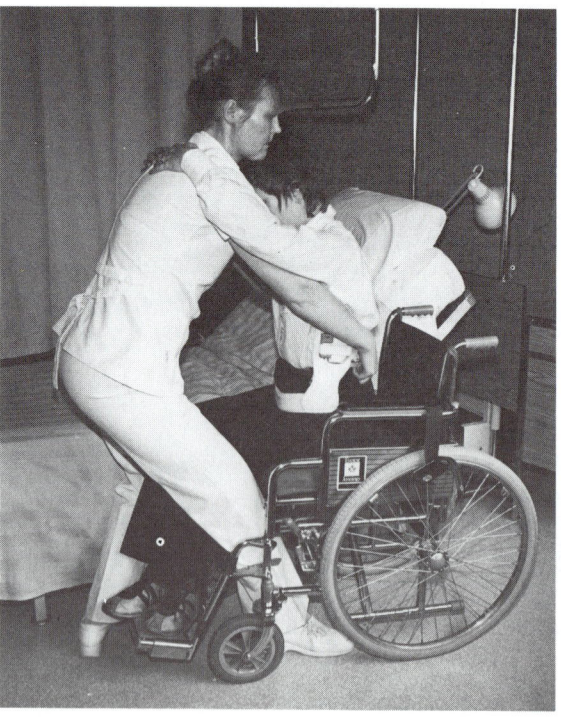

FIGURE 22–6 A nurse uses correct body mechanics: good posture with knees bent to absorb stress of patient's weight.

Procedure 22–1   Key Points In General Transfer Techniques

Purpose

To give key points in transfer techniques and to point out alternative methods suited for the patient with paraplegia or quadriplegia.

Action

Transfers make use of *sliding* or *lifting* techniques. A situation in which lifting techniques are necessary is transferring a patient (without protective clothing) to a commode or shower chair. These techniques may also be used in combination.

1. Prepare the patient by explaining the planned moves in advance; during transfer give short, clear directions of what to do next. To time moves, indicate when ready and perform moves together on the count of three.

2. On completion of transfer it is very important to clarify any areas of difficulty or concern.

3. During the early stages it may be necessary to *ease* patients to the sitting position.

- Roll patient on side (optional) and then raise the head of the bed 45°.

- Pull the patient forward and up to sitting position by slipping hands under patient's arms and placing over the scapula (**A**).

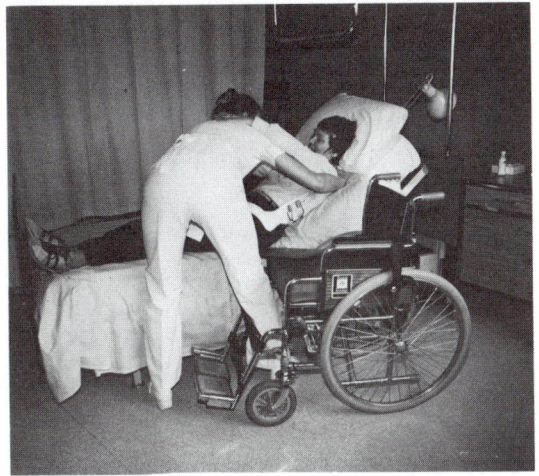

A

- Use your body weight to get patient's body in line.
- Simultaneously guide feet over edge of bed (**B**).
- When patient has a cervical injury, avoid pulling on the hands, arms, or shoulders.

4. It is important that the patient is dressed appropriately. Avoid pants with rigid seams or those that are tight fitting, especially jeans. Cotton track suits are ideal attire for early mobilization. It is possible to grasp patient's clothing to assist with sliding transfers, but *never* pull up on clothing to lift the patient. It is also important for patient to wear socks and shoes to provide additional protection for the feet when transferring (**C**).
Flat shoes with nonskid soles are a good choice.

5. Ensure that wheelchair is placed correctly at a 30° angle to bed.

- When getting patient out of bed, back wheelchair in alongside bed so that the front edge of chair is level with patient's hips.

Rationale

Sliding techniques are generally used during the early stages or when patients are unable to help with body movements; *lifting* techniques are taught as patient becomes more independent in transfers; they also provide additional protection to the skin.

This allows the patient to understand moves and be able to instruct others in the future.

This will help them to accommodate to the upright position and minimize discomfort.

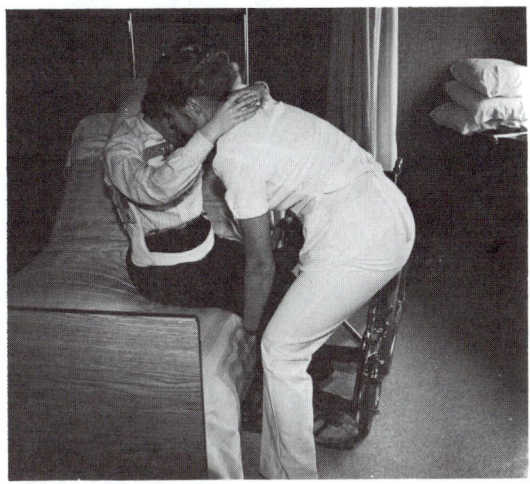

B

This gives long leverage and good mechanical advantage.

Pulling forces applied too soon will stress the cervical spine and cause pain.

It is necessary to protect the skin.

Pulling on pants can bruise the perineal area, create a split in the cleft of the buttocks, or blister or chafe the skin.

A size larger than normal may be necessary if gravitational edema is a problem. Open shoes on top with lacing or Velcro.

This eliminates unnecessary movement and lifting.

(Procedure continues)

Procedure 22–1   Key Points In General Transfer Techniques (continued)

Action	Rationale

Action

• When returning patient to bed, back wheelchair alongside bed and position front edge of the chair two-thirds up from foot of bed. Adjust bed height so it is the same as wheelchair height.

6. *Lock the bed brakes.* One feature that is particularly helpful on a regular hospital bed is the addition of small legs that come in contact with the floor only when the bed is adjusted to the lowest position. It is possible to remove the wheels from some beds. Always check mechanical safety of beds.

7. Set small front wheels of wheelchair facing *forward* to lengthen base of the chair and secure castor locks to maintain this position. *Lock the wheelchair brakes* (**D**).

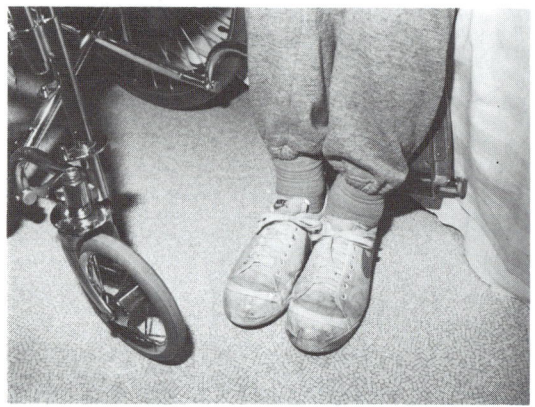

C

8. It is necessary to support the chest and buttocks and/or knees and feet.

• Slide buttocks forward.

• Place both feet on foot plate closest to bed (possible when castor locks provide secure base) or place feet on floor.

• Place the legs close to the bed for stability.

• Stabilize patient's feet and knees to prevent their sliding out of position. This is achieved by gripping your feet and knees on either side of the patient's. If this feels awkward, secure the lower extremities between your outer leg and the bed (**E**).

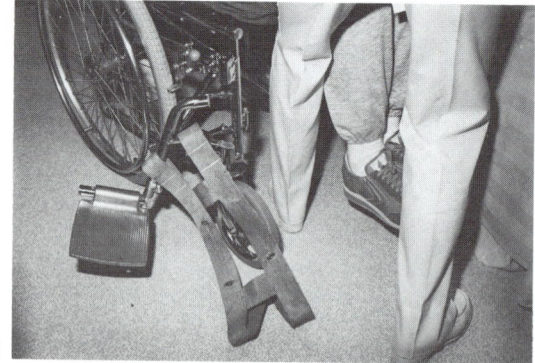

E

9. Protect the patient's buttocks from contact with wheel rim. With armrest removed, a protective device can be fitted to cover top of wheel.

10. If a straight, beveled transfer board is to be used, a 10-inch × 28-inch (with rounded corners to protect the skin) is a good size for maximum support (**F**).

Rationale

This places patient's buttocks in correct position for lying down.

This will eliminate any movement of the bed when patient's weight is shifted.
This offers maximum security as the weight of the bed is off the wheels.

This will stabilize wheelchair.

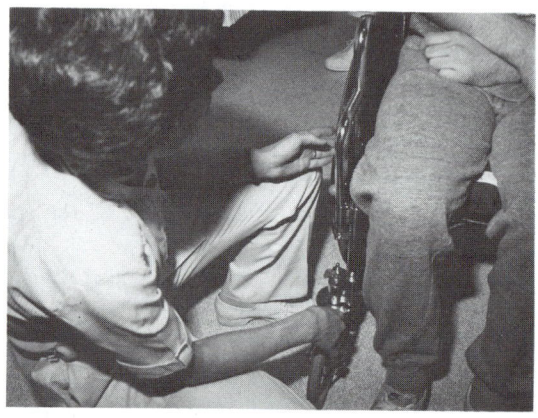

D

This ensures security of patient with paralyzed trunk musculature and/or paralyzed lower extremities.

This ensures that body weight is over the center of gravity and the buttocks will not come in contact with the wheel during the transfer.

This will control paralyzed lower extremities.

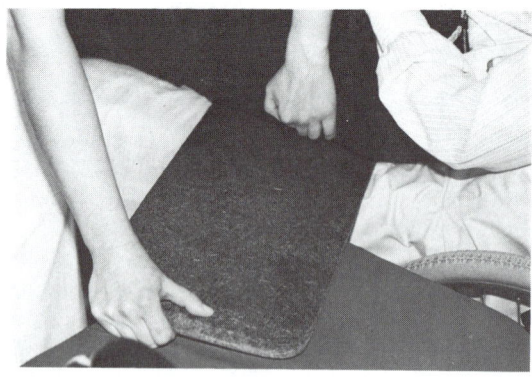

F

Make sure patient is well forward to avoid bumping the rim.

Procedure 22–2   Transferring a Quadriplegic Patient with a Halo Brace Using a Sliding Board

Part A: From the Bed to the Wheelchair

To prepare the patient for transfer:

A   Slide the patient toward the edge of the bed.

B   Position the transfer board.

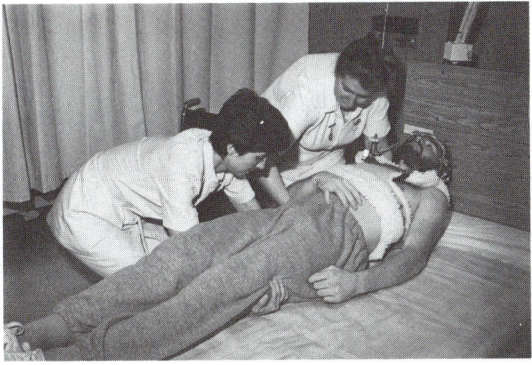

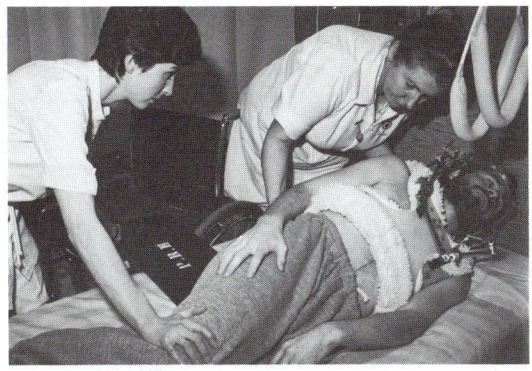

C   Position board to be free of wheel rim.

D   Ease to a well-balanced sitting position.

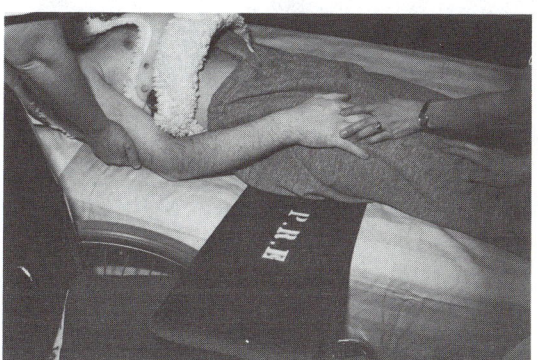

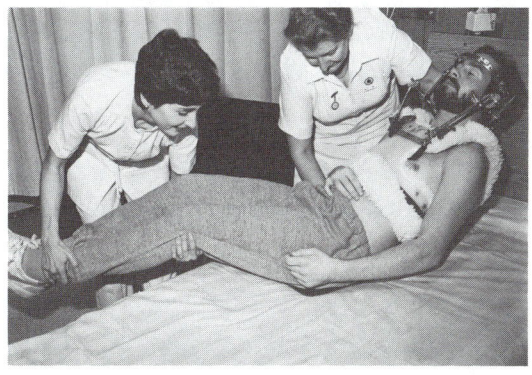

E   For this taller person, place the feet directly on the floor
for stability; otherwise feet may be balanced
on footplate.

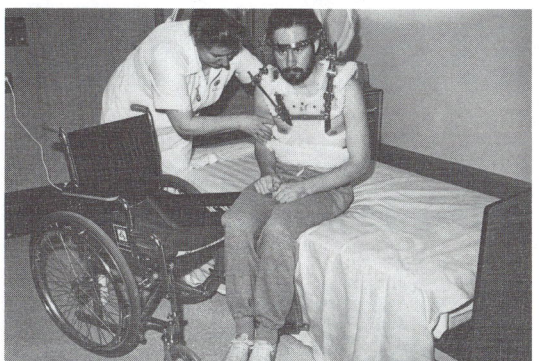

(Procedure continues)

Procedure 22–2 Transferring a Quadriplegic Patient with a Halo Brace Using a Sliding Board (continued)

Part A: From the Bed to the Wheelchair (continued)

To transfer the patient:

The assistant *at the front* simply stabilizes the patient's trunk and knees and guides the patient to the chair. Do not *lift*. This is the key to the success of this transfer technique. The assistant *at the back* gently slides the patient's buttocks along the transfer board to the chair.

F   Position the patient's body weight well forward and in opposite direction from move to provide good mechanical advantage.

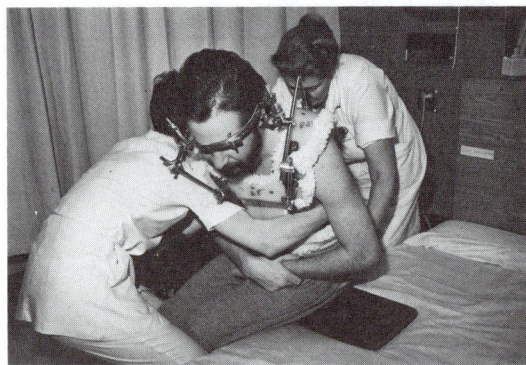

G   Position shoulder well away from the halo bars to protect both patient and self.

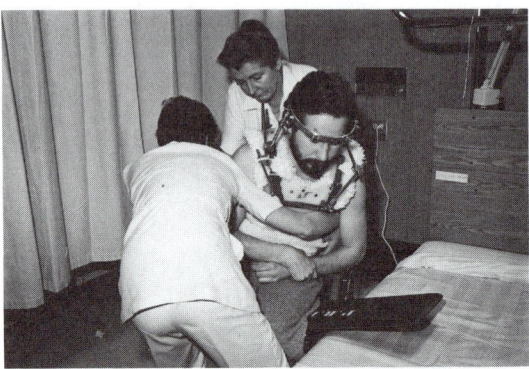

H   Remove the transfer board.

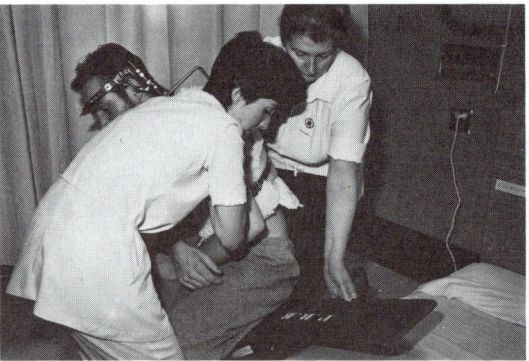

Part B: From the Wheelchair Back to Bed

To prepare the patient for transfer:

A   Place the wheelchair at the correct angle to the bed.

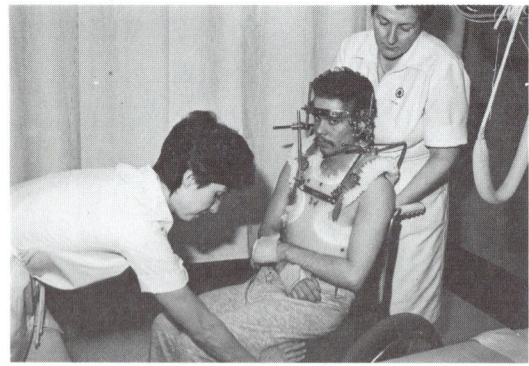

B   Position the transfer board while helping the patient lean to the opposite side of the chair.

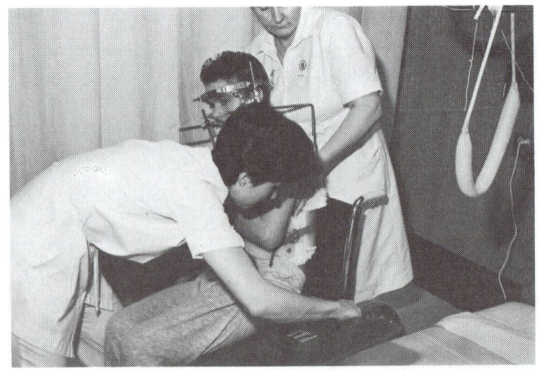

(Procedure continues)

Procedure 22–2 Transferring a Quadriplegic Patient with a Halo Brace Using a Sliding Board (continued)

Part B: From the Wheelchair Back to Bed (continued)

To transfer the patient:

C   Stabilize the patient in the sitting position.

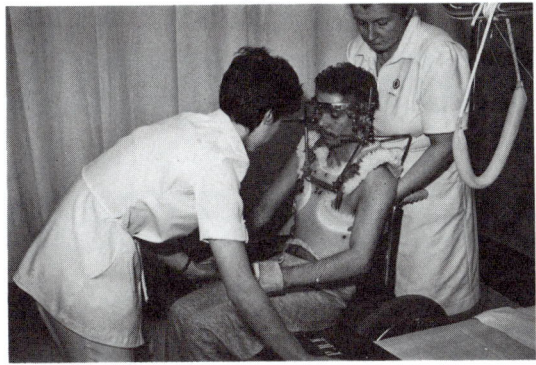

E   Lean well away from the halo bars.

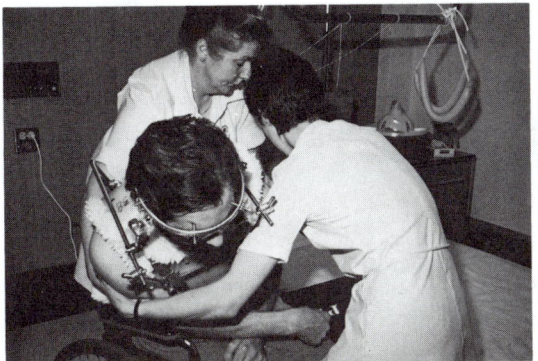

G and H   Together ease the patient to the recumbent position.

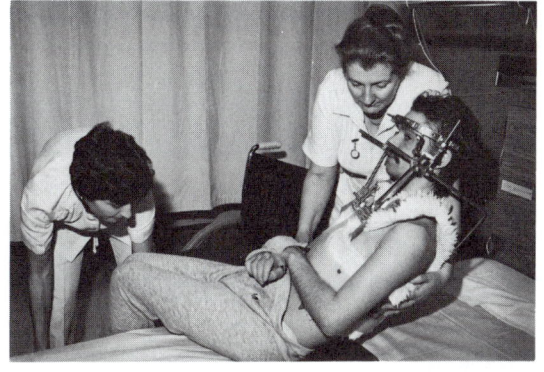

D   Pull patient's buttocks forward of wheel and onto the sliding board. Lean patient forward and in opposite direction of move. The front assistant guides, but does not lift, the patient's torso.

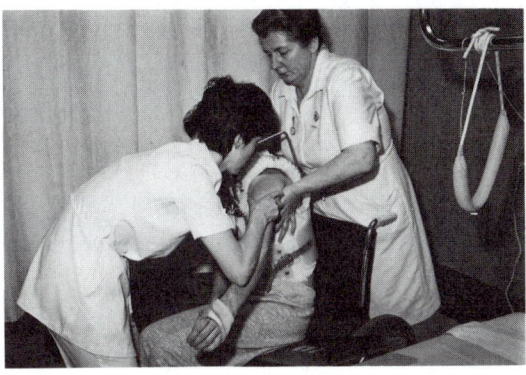

F   The assistant at the back, having the mechanical advantage, slides the patient's buttocks along the transfer board.

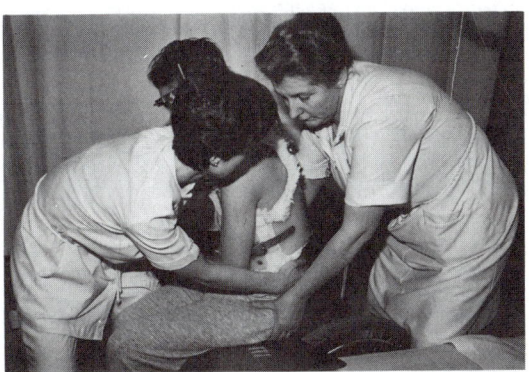

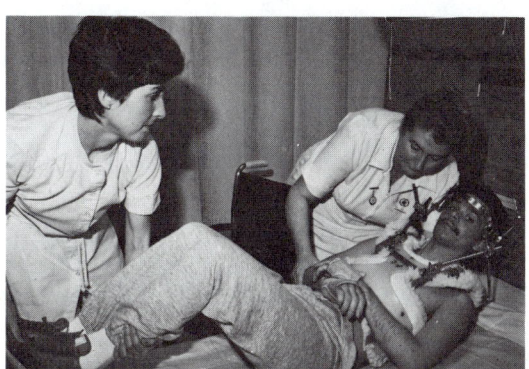

Prepared under the direction of Jack Ford, Director of Remedial Gymnastics; G. F. Strong Rehabilitation Centre, Vancouver, BC.

Procedure 22–3   Transferring a Quadriplegic Person From the Wheelchair to Bed Using a Sliding Board

To prepare the patient for transfer:

Ensure that the bed and chair are stabilized (the front castors of the wheelchair are locked into position) and that the chair is angled in the correct position to the bed.

A   Using good body mechanics, ease the patient to the front of the wheelchair.

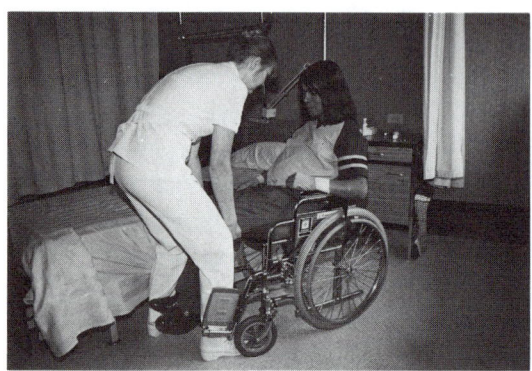

B   Position the transfer board.

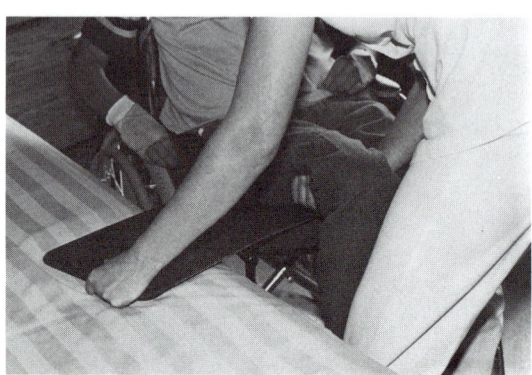

C   Position the shorter person's feet on the footplate; stabilize the patient's knees between your own; bend the patient with a stabilized spine completely forward to displace much of the patient's weight forward and gain mechanical advantage.

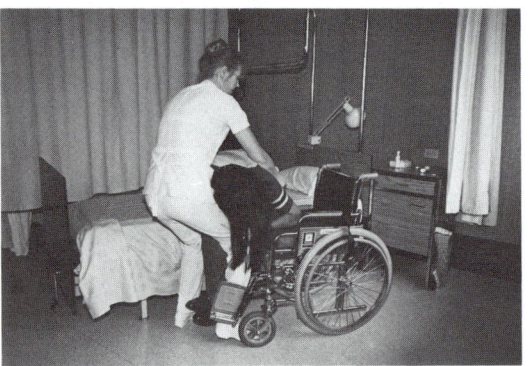

D   Slide and guide the patient's buttocks to the bed.

E   Achieve a balanced position before easing the patient to the recumbent position.

These techniques can be simply reversed to transfer the person from the bed to the wheelchair.

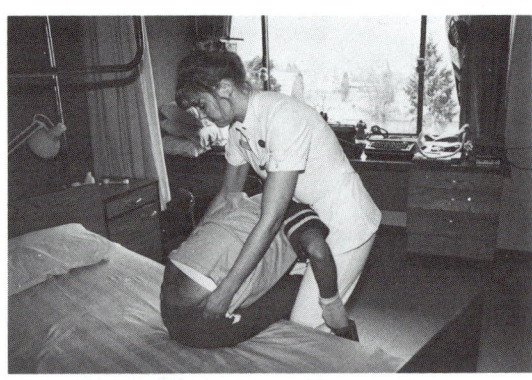

may be needed when transferring a patient in a small, confined area, as from wheelchair to toilet; when transferring a wet patient from the shower chair to the bed; or when transferring a fatigued patient from the toilet to the wheelchair after bowel disimpaction. Adaptations must also be made to accommodate differing size, weight, and coordination of both patient and assistant.

Especially for home use after the spine is stable, the no-sling lift by EasyPivot offers convenience with safety and security features (Figure 22–7). Designed by an engineer with quadriplegia, the principle of forward displacement of weight is used, just as in transfer techniques. Less strain is placed on assistants. The forward position allows for lowering of clothing for ease with toilet or commode transfers.

Correct Positioning in the Wheelchair*

The correct position in the wheelchair is as important to people with SCI as good posture is to the general population. Good habits adopted initially guard against pressure areas and progressive structural deformities (including

*The next 3 sections were contributed by S. P. Wasko, P.T.

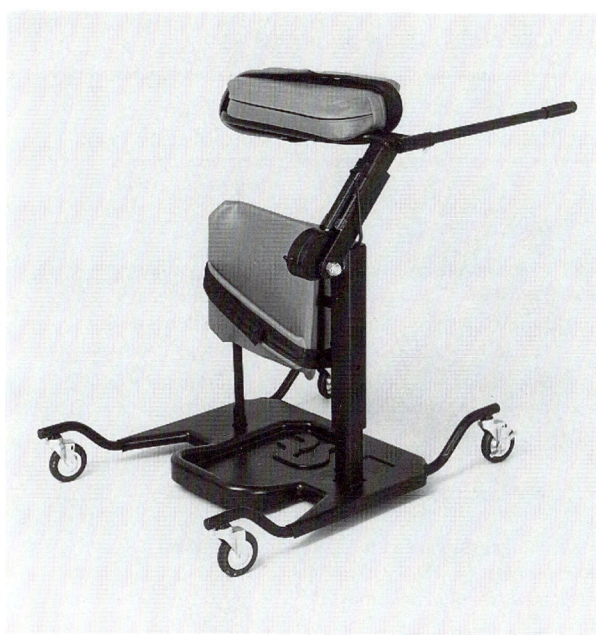

FIGURE 22–7 Chest pad and backstrap with knee supports allows disabled person to lean forward for transfers. Sturdy construction. Height adjustable. The EasyPivot lift is available from Rand-Scot, Inc., Fort Collins, CO.

respiratory compromise) and loss of functional abilities. These late complications are increasing as the SCI population ages. Chapter 33 describes some of the complexities that can be encountered with chronic seating difficulties.

Achieving the correct position in the wheelchair ensures a balanced position without slumped posture. Address the *pelvis* first. All other extremity positioning is dependent on the pelvis.

Correction of position may be necessary immediately following a transfer or when spasticity or gravitational forces have caused the patient to slip forward in the chair. A person will usually require repositioning more than once throughout the day. After securing the brakes and positioning and locking the small front wheels, several maneuvers can be used:

- An average-size patient requires one assistant behind the wheelchair. The patient should cross arms over the pubic bone, and the assistant's hands should pass under the patient's axilla and cross over the patient's hands. Lean the patient forward, squeeze the thorax, and pull back.
- The heavier patient may require one assistant in front. Grasp the patient's feet and knees between your own. Lean the patient's trunk forward, then simultaneously lift the patient's hips, and push with your knees.
- The very heavy patient or a patient with a halo brace may require two assistants. While the patient leans forward, the front assistant grasps the patient's shoulders and on the count of three, pushes on the patient's knees, while the back assistant lifts and slides the hips

back. See Figure 22–8. Alternatively, assistants using the same principles can work from each side of the chair.
- Persons with SCI C$_6$ or below have the potential physical ability to reposition themselves independently (by leaning forward and using arms to lift buttocks).

Table 22–2 summarizes proper positioning.

Wheelchair Management Skills

As soon as patients are up, the physical therapist begins to teach them how to perform, or teach others to perform, weelchair management skills. Individual programs are based largely on physical potential associated with level of injury sustained. Education includes basic maneuvers to wheel and position chair, negotiate obstacles, and handle the removable parts of the chair. Some patients can perform advanced activities such as balancing a chair on the back wheels (wheelie) in order to ascend and descend ramps or curbs. All patients and family members are taught dependent activities such as movement up and down stairs. Progress includes learning to cope with rougher ground and slopes out of doors. Formal instruction will be given to the patient and family in preparation for passes. However, all members of the staff should be familiar with the techniques

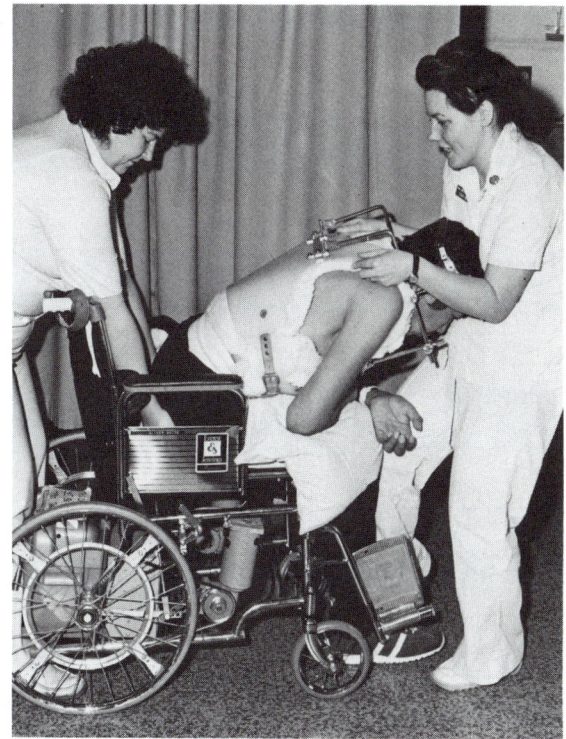

FIGURE 22–8 Two assistants correct the slumped position of a patient in the wheelchair.

TABLE 22-2 Proper Wheelchair Positioning: Some Complications and Possible Solutions

Body Part	Indications of Improper Seating	Complications	Possible Solutions
PELVIS			
Neutral*	—	—	—
Oblique	• One hip higher than the other • One shoulder higher than the other	• ↑ risk of pressure area on ischial tuberosities • Leads to scoliosis	• Reposition • Solid seat • Custom cushion • Proper seat belt
Rotation	• One knee sticking out farther than the other • One shoulder in front of the other	• Leads to scoliosis • ↓ efficiency in propelling manual wheelchair	• Proper seat belt • Reposition • Rigid pelvic stabilizer
Posterior pelvic tilt	• More than 3 or 4 finger spaces between the front of seat and the back of the knee • ↑ kyphosis	• ↑ risk of sacral pressure area • ↑ risk of pressure area on spinous process • Leads to structural deformity in spine • Respiratory compromise • ↓ in functional activities	• Seat belt • Wedge cushion • Tilt seat • Lumbar support
TRUNK			
Midline*	—	—	—
Scoliosis	• One shoulder higher than the other	• Structural deformity • ↑ pressure on ischial tuberosities that ↑ pressure areas	• Trunk supports
Leaning	• Person keeps falling to one side	• Jeopardize safety • ↓ in stability • ↓ in functional activities	• Chest strap • Trunk support
Kyphosis	• Forward head • Absence of lumbar lordosis	• Neck pain • Respiratory compromise	• Tilt seat • Lumbar support • Back support
ARMS			
Shoulder level*	—	—	—
Too much support	• Shrugged shoulders	• Neck pain • Pressure sore development	• Lower armrests • Increase cushion height
Inadequate support	• Dropped shoulders • Subluxation at glenohumeral joint	• Subluxation of glenohumeral joint • Pain • Leads to kyphosis	• Raise armrest height • Lower seat • Add arm troughs
HEAD			
Midline*	—	—	—
Inadequate support	• Head falling backward, forward, or to one side	• Pain • Compromise airway • Leads to deformity	• Head support

(Table continues)

TABLE 22–2   Proper Wheelchair Positioning: Some Complications and Possible Solutions (continued)

Body Part	Indications of Improper Seating	Complications	Possible Solutions
HIPS			
90 degrees*	—	—	—
Greater than 90 degrees	• Thighs overly abducted • Space between the sitting surface and the thighs • Knees hitting under table	• ↑ risk of pressure area over bony prominences	• Lower footrests
Less than 90 degrees	• Thighs abducted with legs internally rotated • Kyphosis • Pelvis tilted back	• ↑ risk of pressure sore on greater trochanter • Kyphosis	• Raise footrests • Solid seat • Abductor pommel support
THIGHS			
Even support*	—	—	—
Inadequate support	• Large space between seat upholstery and back of knees	• ↑ risk of pressure area on bony prominences	• Increase seat depth • Reposition • Seat belt (to hold back in chair) must be weighed against inhibiting pressure reliefs
Excessive support	• No space between seat upholstery and back of knee	• ↓ circulation to lower extremities • ↑ risk of pressure area on back of knee • Unable to twist in chair to reposition self	• Decrease seat depth • Add back cushion
FEET			
Midline*	—	—	—
External rotation	• Toes pointing outwardly	• Contributes to improper leg position • Leads to structural deformities	• Change tilt of footrest • Lower footrest • Alter heels on shoes
Internal rotation	• Toes pointing inwardly	• Contributes to improper leg position • Leads to structural deformities	• Straps to secure feet • Raise footrests

*Proper position

involved, so that they can reinforce the teaching process and assist patients when necessary, especially during evenings and weekends. Table 22–3 presents some commonly encountered maneuvers.

The Personal Wheelchair

A well-chosen personal wheelchair offers ease of mobility and promotes function, which translates into freedom and independence. Speed; maneuverability; ease of operation; durability; and cost, warranty, and service factors are important considerations. For proper posture and comfort when sitting, the chair must be the right size and style and equipped with the right features and accessories. The choice

in features and accessories allows the chair to fit the individual as opposed to making the individual fit the chair. Each feature and accessory must be evaluated to assure that it promotes mobility and function. General features include back rests, arm rests, foot rests, brakes, and front and rear wheels. There is a wide variety of choices and accessories within each category. See Table 22–4.

A person's neurological level of injury provides a key to potential physical functions and ultimately the wheelchair and accessories required to allow independent mobility. However, functional ability depends on many variables other than neurological status, such as motivation, age, and body build, strength, and weight. The majority of people who sustain SCI will require a wheelchair. The small

TABLE 22–3 Wheelchair Management Skills

- Tilting the Chair Backward

Grasp the handles. Keep close to body. Place one foot on the tipping lever. Tilt the chair back until in a balanced position. This technique gets the chair over small obstacles such as doorsteps.

- Ascending Curbs

Back the chair to within one foot of the curb. Tilt the chair back by stepping on the tipping lever. Pull the chair up the curb and wheel it back so that the front castors will be on the sidewalk when the chair is lowered. Alternatively, tilt the wheelchair back and place small wheels up on curb; simultaneously, roll the chair forward and lift up onto the curb.

- Descending Curbs

Facing the roadway, tip the chair back to balance on its back wheels. Roll the chair slowly over the curb and push forward before lowering the front castors. To maintain the patient's balance, support the front of the patient with one hand while lowering the front castors.

- Wheeling over Rough Ground

When negotiating rough or soft ground, tilt the chair back onto the two rear wheels. If the terrain is very difficult, it will be easier to pull the chair backward in the tipped position. In this position, the person in the chair is more secure and less likely to fall out.

- Wheeling down Slopes

Steep slopes may require that the chair be wheeled down the hill backward. If wheeling down forward, ensure the patient's balance in the chair with one hand over the patient's shoulder. If the slope levels abruptly, care must be taken not to snag the footrests when wheeling forward.

- Ascending Stairs

Tilt the chair back until balanced. Place one foot on the first step and one on the second. Pull the chair up the first step. Keep your arms straight. Mount the next step before proceeding. The patient can assist the lift by grasping the wheel rims and coordinating the pulling action, timing the "ready–lift" at each step.

- Descending Stairs

The same positions are used as for ascending stairs. Until confident, two assistants should be used. The front helper must be prepared to hold the chair if necessary, but don't attempt to lift, as the balance of the chair will be disrupted.

- Lifting the Wheelchair into a Car

To fold the chair, fold the footrests up and pull up on the seat. Secure brakes and tip the chair so that you can reach the far side. Grasp the front and the rear of the frame. Rock back, balancing chair on thighs. Hold armrests close to body. Swing and lift chair into trunk. If the chair has a fixed frame, remove the wheels and fold down the back of the chair.

minority who do not include individuals who have incomplete injuries and are ambulatory, and those who have very low paraplegia, who are also ambulatory.

Generally, persons with C_{1-5} quadriplegia need a power wheelchair for independent mobility. A strong person with C_6 quadriplegia may choose only a manual chair; another may wish to use a manual chair around home and a power chair outside; yet another, perhaps limited by excessive weight or decreased endurance, may need a power chair for all activities. Those with injuries below C_7 generally use manual chairs.

Table 22–5 presents a guide to functional considerations and Table 22–6 describes various specific options and rationale for personal wheelchair selection.

Throughout the acute period, needs change quite dramatically as body handling skills improve and strength rebuilds. Therefore, it is wise to wait, rather than rush into, expensive wheelchair investments. For example, persons with T_2 paraplegia initially may require a folding frame chair with swing-away footrests to get close enough to the bathtub to transfer independently. However, as they become more active, a rigid frame chair without removable footrests may be preferred.

In preparation for selecting a wheelchair for permanent use, take extreme care to assess functional expectations and personal preferences when educating consumers of choices that will best meet personal needs. Periodic reevaluation is necessary throughout life to ensure present needs are satisfied and that additional needs are addressed.

Assisting Quadriplegic Patients with Upper Extremity Activities

All care is directed toward maintaining a functional position of the hand and arm. See Figure 22–9. A functional position is one that will be useful for daily activities, such as holding and drinking from a cup. See Figure 22–10. A functional hand is essential for *all* self-care activities for the patient with quadriplegia.

Components of care required for upper extremities include correct positioning of hands, elbows, and shoulders; adequate range of motion exercises; and usually hand splinting to prevent contractures and deformities. See Figure 22–11. The occupational therapist is very much involved in assessing hand and arm function; providing appropriate hand splints and teaching method of application; and developing appropriate self-care techniques, which are then taught to the patient, staff, and family. The nurse assumes a large responsibility for maintaining correct positioning, providing adequate exercise, and applying and caring for splints on a day-to-day basis during the early stages. As rehabilitation progresses, encourage independence and withdraw any assistance that is not needed. As the patient is

TABLE 22–4   General Features of the Wheelchair

- Wheelchairs with standard or lightweight frames are a good choice for the active user. Rear tires and front castors made of hard rubber are best for indoor use and are easily maintained. Pneumatic tires may be desirable for a smoother ride outdoors.

- Swing-away detachable legrests are helpful for transfer maneuverability. Wheelchair armrests are also removable to facilitate lateral transferring. Armrests are also available in varying heights and widths. Removable desk arms, which are the most popular, allow proximity to the table or desk without being removed. A paraplegic person who does not require arm support, for example, may well prefer the smaller, sloping wrap-around version.

- Wheelchair seats and backs are available in varying lengths and widths. For the quadriplegic person, the back height must be low enough to allow free scapular movement, which is necessary for wheeling efficiency, but be high enough to provide adequate stability for the back. People with high cervical cord injuries need back extensions for head and neck support and for power mobility (see Figure 21–9).

- For wheelchair sports, elaborate and custom designs incorporate such features as extremely low backs, deeper seats, sloping side arms, different axle positions to throw more weight on the rear wheels, antitipping devices, and roll bars to prevent the footplates from gouging floors. (Note figures throughout Chapter 24.)

Some of the more common, often temporary, accessories that staff need to be familiar with during the acute period include: back extensions for head and neck support (**A**), projections of pegs installed on the drive rims of the large wheels to make pushing easier (**B**), a special pusher mitt, used by some people to gain more friction and protect the skin of the hand (**C**), front-wheel castor locks to stabilize the chair for lateral transfers (**D**), **H**-straps (**E**) to prevent the legs from falling backward (often caused by spasticity), and seat belts for trunk stability (**F**).

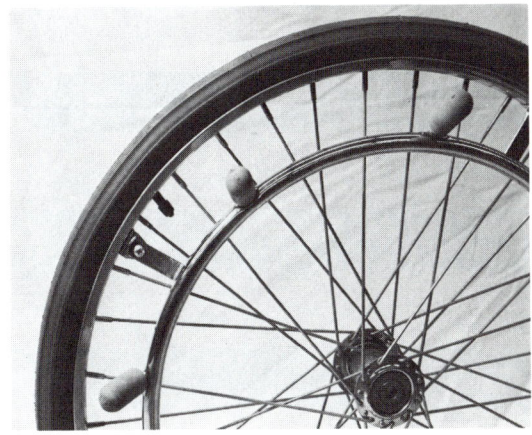

B

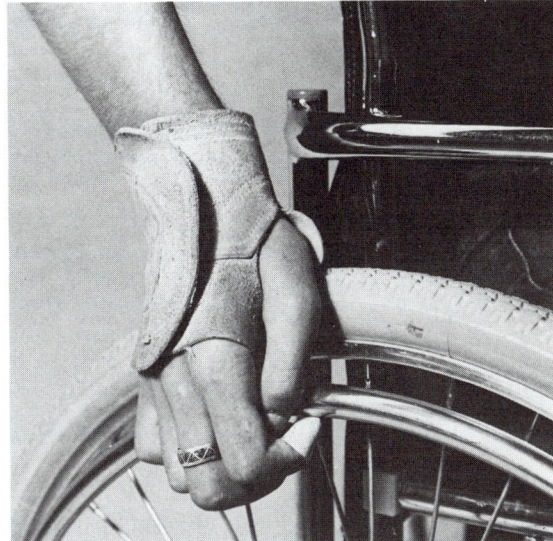

C

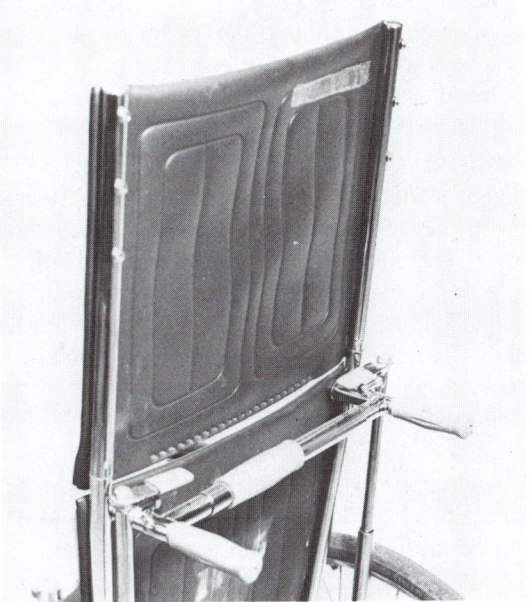

A

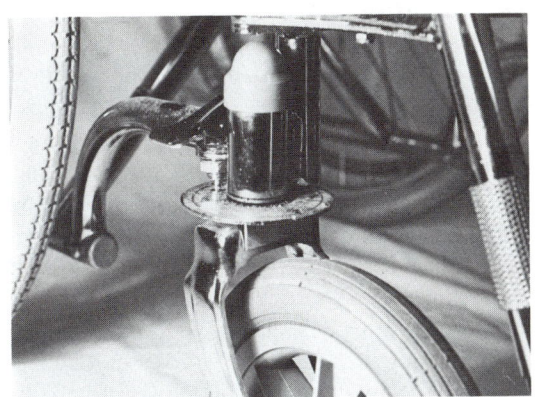

D

(Table continues)

TABLE 22–4   General Features of the Wheelchair (continued)

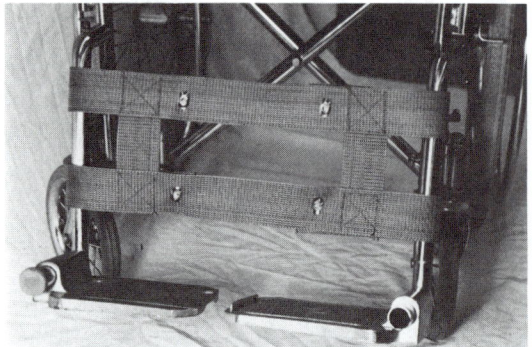

E

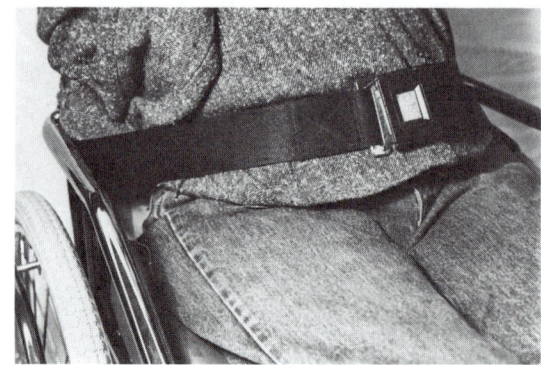

F

Source: J. Ford, *Wheelchair Handbook. A Guide to Selection, Cushions, Accessories and Maintenance,* Copyright, Canada, 1980, by G. F. Strong Rehabilitation Center, Vancouver, B.C., Canada.

able to participate more in self-care activities, muscles are strengthened and range of motion is maintained without specific exercises, and exact positioning becomes less important. Again, the patient, the nurse, the family, and the therapist must understand the terminology used to describe activities and be aware of the exact amount of assistance required by the patient.

Positioning and Range of Motion Exercises

Positioning and range of motion exercises are combined, since they must supplement each other if the overall program is to be successful. Figure 6–4 illustrates specific positioning of the upper extremities for patients with quadriplegia.

To the quadriplegic patient, wrist and thumb joint mobility are extremely important movements. For example, a flexible wrist is important for transfers. Patients can only support their weight when their shoulders and arms are extended in external rotation, the elbows are locked, and the wrists are bent into dorsiflexion or extension. Bending the wrist backward creates *tenodesis*. Tenodesis is the natural bending inward (flexion) of the fingers when the wrist is extended or bent backward. See Figure 22–12A. To simulate this action, cock your right wrist back with your left hand. If your right hand is relaxed, your fingers will automatically curl inward. Tenodesis is a key movement because it can be used to pick up objects when finger movement is absent. The hand must be trained to assume this position. Contractures of the fingers are actually encouraged. To assist tenodesis the web space between the

thumb and first two fingers must be maintained to enhance the grasp motion with the thumb in adduction. To release the grasp, patients simply relax the wrist. See Figure 22–12(B).

The occupational therapist is responsible for maintaining full range of motion in the hand. To promote tenodesis exercises:

- Increase wrist extension strength
- Maintain web space
- Allow finger flexion to shorten (never straighten the fingers when the wrist is extended as it will weaken tenodesis)

Splinting

If there is partial or total paralysis of the hand, temporary splints are needed and should be applied within 48 hours of injury. Generally splints should be worn all night and whenever the patient is resting to maintain a functional position. Splints stabilize flail joints and prevent contractures that cause deformity. These are referred to as *static* or *positioning splints.*

During the early stages the nurse's role involves correct application of positioning splints and meticulous care of the skin. Regardless of what type of splint is used, the nurse must check the skin for reddened areas every 2 hours and alert the occupational therapist if adjustments are necessary. Red marks most often occur when splints have been improperly applied or have slipped. Mark the corresponding area on the splint and reapply correctly. Remove splints if red marks persist and position the hand with other means—for exam-

TABLE 22–5 Potential Functional Status in Relation to Wheelchair Needs and Options

Level of Injury	Power Wheelchair			Manual Wheelchair	
	Use	Control Options	Accessory Options	Use	Accessory Options
C_{1-4}	• Independent mobility	• Tongue • Sip and puff • Chin (possibly for C_{1-2}) • Head (C_{3-4}) • Power tilt/recline	• Trunk supports • Head rest • Arm troughs • Seat belt • Chest strap • Ventilator tray	• Dependent mobility only (recommended for backup use; limited accessibility; or personal preference) • Cheaper	• Same as accessories for power wheelchair
C_5	• Independent mobility	• Hand controls most common	• Omit ventilator tray • Omit power tilt/recline if person can perform weight shifts	• Independent mobility for some (propelling lightweight chair over level terrain for short distances)	
C_6	• Full-time independent mobility or • Community mobility	• Hand control	• Omit tilt/recline	• Full-time or • Household mobility only	• Lightweight • Full to moderate back support • Friction rims (due to lack of grip) • Castor pin locks (to stabilize for transfers) • 8-inch castors (independent mobility on all terrain) • Swing-away footrests • Spoke guards (to prevent fingers from getting caught)
C_7-T_1	• Uncommon for this level of injury (and all levels below)			• Full-time independent mobility	• Lightweight • Moderate back height • Optional friction
T_{2-12}				• Full-time, independent mobility	• Lightweight • Lower backrest • Low mount brakes • 5-inch castors • Omit armrests • *Rigid* footrests • Crutch holder (for persons who ambulate with lower extremity braces) • Omit castor pin locks
L_{1-5} and S_{1-5}				• Full- or part-time • Sports	• As above • Very lightweight • Very low back • Rigid frame • Omit armrests and brakes

TABLE 22–6 Specific Wheelchair Features

Feature	Pros	Cons	Potential User
Armrest	• Provides arm support • Provides surface to push from when doing transfers	• Can interfere with propelling	• C_{1-5} • Any power wheelchair user • C_6 and below—questionable
Fixed full length	• Decreases overall width of wheelchair	• Cannot remove armrest to do side transfers	• Not very common
Removable	• Can remove for side transfers • When removed, decreases weight for lifting wheelchair	• Can get lost • Increases overall width of wheelchair if not wraparound type	• Any person using armrests
Desk length	• Can get close to tables or desks	• Limits hand placement for transfers • Harder to fit lap trays	• C_{1-5} • Any person using armrests who needs to get close to desks/tables
Full length	• Wide variety in hand placement for transfers • Adequate length to support lap tray/arm troughs	• Limits proximity to table or work station	• C_{1-5}
Height adjustable	• Can alter for proper arm support • Comfortable • Can accommodate for different cushion or seating system	• Increases cost of wheelchair	• Any person using armrests
Wraparound	• Decreases overall width of wheelchair	• Can decrease available seat width • Cannot use on recliner frame • May interfere with brackets for sling suspension	• Any person using armrests who wishes to decrease the width of the wheelchair
Tubular	• Can be easily swung out of the way for transfers	• Mud, dirt, and water can rub off on clothes • Some find it uncomfortable • Not as strong • Cannot fit lap trays	• Any level • Older people usually do not like it because it looks unsturdy.
Front Riggings	• Provide foot support	• Can increase overall length and limit accessibility	• All levels except those with bilateral amputations
Fixed	• Decreases weight • Makes wheelchair more stable	• Can make transfers difficult • Can be harder to transport in trunk because footrests cannot be removed	• Usually used with rigid frame wheelchairs • Most commonly associated with sports wheelchairs • T_6 and below

(Table continues)

TABLE 22–6 Specific Wheelchair Features (continued)

Feature	Pros	Cons	Potential User
Front riggings (cont.) *Swing away*	• Can get close to objects (tub, toilet), which makes transfers easier • Can remove to decrease weight	• Can get lost • Adds weight • Legs always in dependent position	• Any level • C_6 who must get close to objects to transfer
Elevating legrests	• Allows legs to be elevated for comfort or to decrease edema	• Increase cost • Increase weight • Increase turning radius	• Standard on reclining wheelchairs • Patients with edema
Backrest	• Provides back support and stability	• Can interfere with arm movement	• All levels
Low back	• Frees scapula for greater freedom of arm movement	• Limits back support • Can increase back pain and/or contribute to late spinal deformity	• T_6 and below • Sports wheelchairs
High back	• Provides good support	• Restricts arm movement	• High quads
Medium back	• Provides moderate support • Can free scapula for good arm movement	• Can restrict arm movement in very active persons	• C_{6-8} to T_6
Rear wheels	• Allows the person to push the wheelchair independently		• All levels
Pneumatic	• Smooth ride • Comfortable; provides the best shock absorption	• Requires maintenance • Can get flats • Unequal air pressure will cause pulling to one side • Hard to propel on carpets	• The majority of people who propel their own wheelchairs
Semipneumatic	• No maintenance • Moderate shock absorption	• Does not provide as much shock absorption as pneumatics	• Person who cannot or wishes not to do maintenance
Solid	• No maintenance • Easy to propel on carpets	• Minimal shock absorption	• A person who uses the chair indoors
High performance	• Excellent for sports • Smooth ride	• Wears out easily • Costly	• Those people actively involved in sports
Friction rims	• Provide better grip for those with limited strength	• Can cause burns if propelling fast	• C_{6-7} • C_8 (questionable)
Spoke guards	• Prohibits fingers from getting caught in the spokes • Decreases spoke damage from other wheelchairs during high contact sports	• Increases cost • Harder to clean out snow in winter	• Any level • $C_{5,6,7}$ who could easily get their fingers caught in the spokes
Quad pegs	• Provides surface to push against	• Can interfere with propelling	• C_5, weak C_6

(Table continues)

TABLE 22–6 Specific Wheelchair Features (continued)

Feature	Pros	Cons	Potential User
Front castors	—	—	• All levels
8-inch pneumatics	• Smooth ride • Will ride easily over small objects such as thresholds	• Hardest type to propel • Tires can go flat • Very hard to propel on carpets	• A person who travels over rough terrain
8" solid	• Will ride easily over small obstacles such as thresholds • No maintenance	• Hard to propel if person is weak	• A person who does not want maintenance • C_{6-8} who must propel over small obstacles
5" solid	• Easiest type to maneuver • Decreases turning radius	• No shock absorption • Can get stuck in small holes	• Used on sports wheelchairs • Used by person with limited strength • Mostly young active people with paraplegia
Castor pin locks	• Increases the stability of the wheelchair during transfers (needed for dependent transfers)	• Can become locked by accident • Increases cost	• C_{6-7} (typically) • T_{1-6} (sometimes) • T_6 and below (unusual)
Frame style *Folding*	• Ease in getting wheelchair in and out of the car • Folds for storage • More flexible over rough terrain	• Increases weight in respect to rigid frame • More movable parts with potential to break • Less energy efficient than rigid wheelchair	• C_6 and below • Typically used by quads who transfer independently and drive a car • Personal preference
Rigid	• Decreases overall weight • Ease in propelling • Fewer parts that could break, but those parts are more stressed and likely to break • One wheel may be left spinning on uneven ground	• Can be difficult for a person with quadriplegia to get in and out of a car • Must remove rear wheels to transport in standard cars • Takes up more room when folded in car	• C_6 and below • Personal preference • Sports wheelchairs
Rear axle *Single position*	• Low cost	• Zero adjustability • Cannot camber wheels to improve wheelchair's performance	• Backup manual wheelchair • Dependent mobility
Triple position	• Allows for some adjustability in the rear wheel, which will improve pushing	• Limited adjustability • Increases cost	• Individuals with limited funding • Usually older people who will not place as many demands on the wheelchair
Multiposition	• Very adjustable • Can camber the rear wheels to increase maneuverability • Can set the rear wheels to accommodate the person propelling the wheelchair	• Increases cost • Chair can tip backward if the chair is not set up properly	• Almost all persons with SCI who independently propel their chairs

(Table continues)

TABLE 22–6   Specific Wheelchair Features (continued)

Feature	Pros	Cons	Potential User
Rear axle (cont.) *Quick release*	• Easy to remove the rear wheels to make it lighter and more portable	• Must be secured or the rear wheel can fall off	• Almost always used on rigid chairs
Brakes *High mount*	• Easy to reach • Can attach brake extension handle	• Can get thumbs caught in brake while pushing	• C_{6-7} typically • Any level (personal preference)
Low mount	• Moves out of the way while propelling	• Must have good trunk control to access them	• People with mid- to low paraplegia
Accessories *Single leg strap*	• Prevents the legs from falling backward	• Must be removed to swing footrests away	• Any level
Heel loops	• Prevents feet from falling off the footrest	• Legs may spasm out of loops	• Any level; not generally recommended
Seat belt	• Safety • Prevents from sliding forward	• High tendency to be mounted incorrectly	• C_{1-4} • C_{5-6}; variable
Side guards	• Keeps clothes from getting dirty • Helps prevent hips from hitting the wheels	• Can interfere with transfers	• Any level who independently propels a manual wheelchair

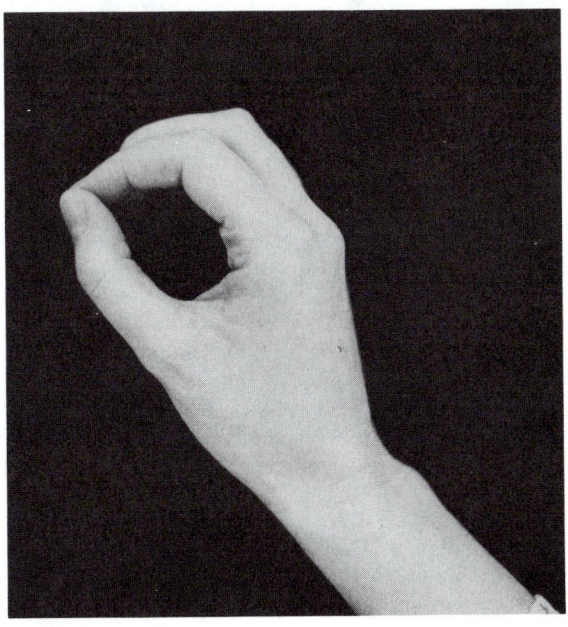

FIGURE 22–9   A functional position of a normal hand.

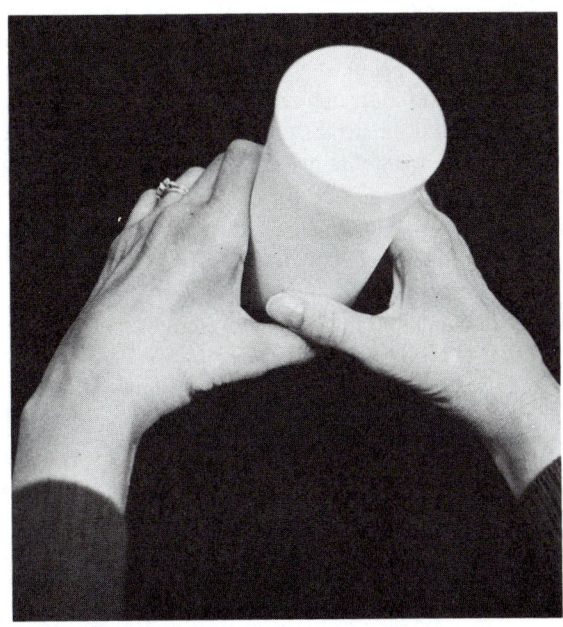

FIGURE 22–10   A functional hand position for the person with quadriplegia.

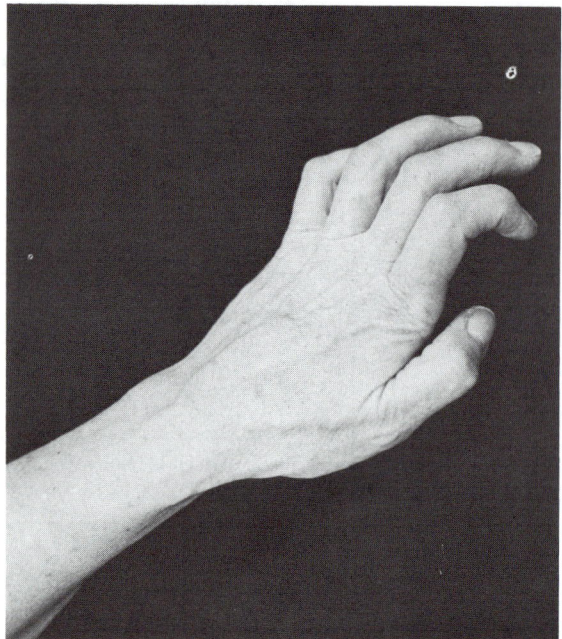

FIGURE 22–11   A nonfunctional contracted hand results from lack of positioning and inadequate exercise. Note the tight flexion of the thumb; the web space is lost.

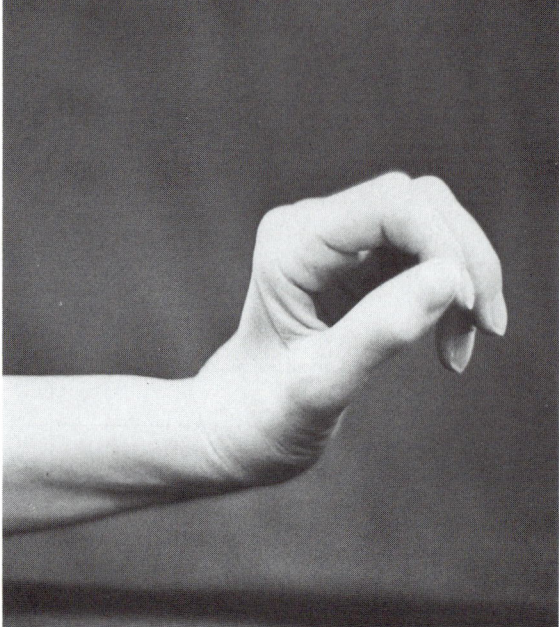

A

B

FIGURE 22–12   (A) Tenodesis, the natural flexion when the wrist is extended, is a valuable maneuver that enables quadriplegic persons, with active wrist extensors, to grasp objects even when active finger movement is absent. The hand must be aided to assume this position. (B) When the flexible wrist is relaxed, the fingers open.

ple, a foam roll—until the splint can be modified by the occupational therapist.

When hand swelling subsides, the occupational therapist will design and fabricate an appropriate permanent positioning splint. Such splints are made from thermal plastic (molded directly on the patient for precise fit) or padded metal supports. Generally *opponens* splints are used to keep the thumb in opposition to the first two fingers, maintain the web space, and slightly flex the fingers. Depending on wrist movement, *short* or *long* opponens splints may be used; the long opponens splint is necessary to support a flaccid wrist; the short opponens splint is used when there is good wrist movement. See Figure 22–13. Splints may be removed for range of motion exercises, hygiene, wheelchair activities, or as directed by the occupational therapist. Positioning splints are worn all night.

As the patient progresses, *dynamic splints* may be used to enhance a pincher grasp and actually assist the patient with independent activities. The thumb is used as a stable post, and the first two fingers act together to oppose the thumb. This allows the patient to pick up, hold, and release light objects in a limited but useful way. The power of the pincher grasp is directly related to the strength of the wrist extensor muscles. The purpose of dynamic splinting is to convert the motion or ability to extend or dorsiflex the wrist into activation of the orthoses to support the pincher grasp. See Figure 22–14. Dynamic splints may range from a simple short opponens splint, used when the patient has good wrist extensor movement, to externally powered hand

splints, which may be activated by shoulder movements when wrist extensor movement is absent. Quadriplegic patients with minimal neurological deficit may not need an orthosis; others may use an orthosis as a muscle-training

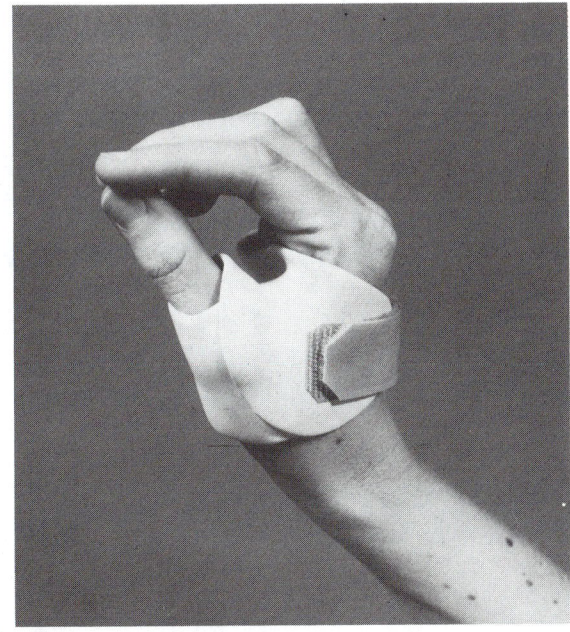

A

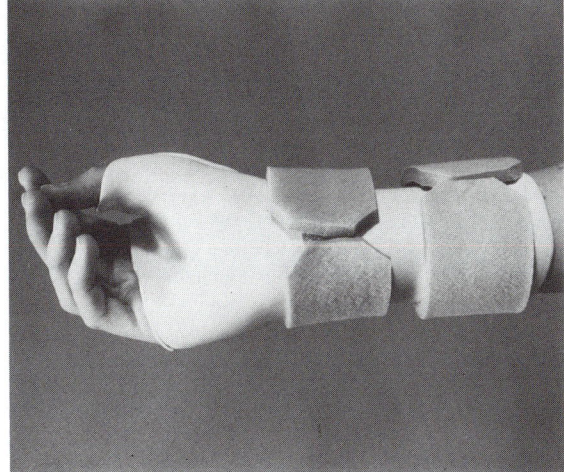

B

FIGURE 22–13 (**A**) A short opponens splint maintains the thumb in opposition to preserve a functional hand position. Good wrist movement is needed. (**B**) A long opponens splint is used for the same purpose when wrist movement is weak or absent.

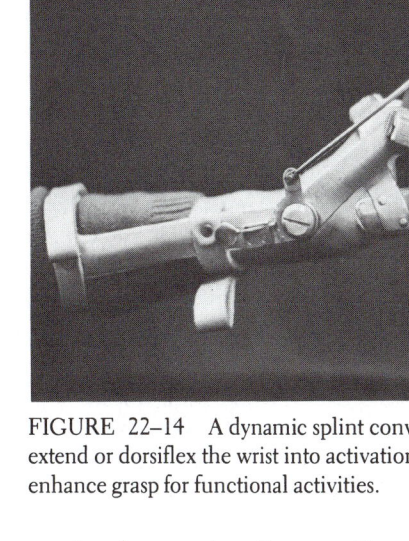

FIGURE 22–14 A dynamic splint converts the ability to extend or dorsiflex the wrist into activation of the splint to enhance grasp for functional activities.

or overhead suspension slings; see Figure 22–15. They can be used in conjunction with a variety of splints or clip-on utensils so the patient can perform self-care, DLS, or exercise activities.

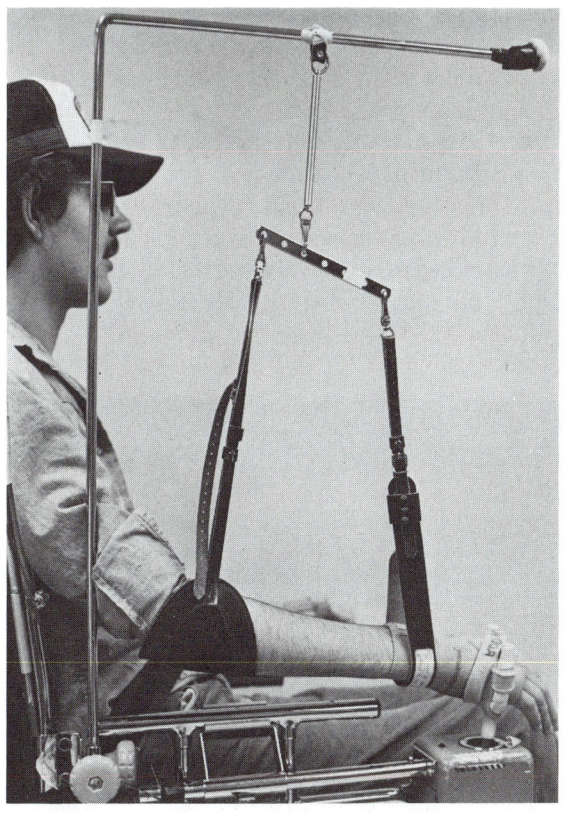

FIGURE 22–15 A quadriplegic man maneuvers an electric wheelchair with the aid of a mobile arm support. The nurse may be responsible for setting up this or similar devices when the patient uses them for such tasks as eating.

device and then remove it; some may need an orthosis as a permanent functional aid.

Mobile arm supports may be needed for patients who have weak elbow flexors and/or shoulder girdle musculature and cannot place their arms appropriately to allow upper extremity functions. Once trunk position and stability are achieved, antigravity support is provided to the shoulder and elbow. In other words the weight of the arm is counterbalanced in order to eliminate the effects of gravity, thereby enhancing the function of the upper extremity. Mobile arm supports may be metal structures attached to the wheelchair

Dynamic splints are applied during daily activities. They are not worn during the night.

Nurses or other care givers are often responsible for correct application, checking the underlying skin, and conveniently placing additional equipment, for example, adjusting table height, arranging meal tray, cutting food, and so on.

In addition, one commonly used aid is the universal cuff, into which an object such as a pencil or utensil may be inserted. A quadriplegic person may learn to apply this aid independently if it is appropriately adapted and the patient has adequate upper extremity function. See Figure 22–16.

The occupational therapist introduces any new orthosis to the patient and closely supervises its use until the patient becomes familiar with the new equipment. It is important for nurses to understand the benefits of orthoses to encourage and support patients' using them. Observe the patients' frustration levels or tolerance of orthoses used, and communicate any areas of concern to the occupational therapist.

Dressing

Dressing skills are complex and involve both fine and gross motor coordination. Complete dressing cannot be achieved until spinal stability occurs and the patient can bend the trunk adequately to reach the lower extremities.

Lower extremity dressing is a very difficult task. Often the patient cannot totally complete all the dressing skills and therefore needs help. See Figure 22–17.

Upper extremity dressing is possible as soon as thoracic or lumbar injured patients can comfortably roll from side to side. This eventually includes donning a brace. Lower extremity dressing can begin when long sitting is allowed. Dressing is then most easily achieved in bed. Long-handled adaptive aids such as a dressing stick, sock aid, or shoehorn may be needed.

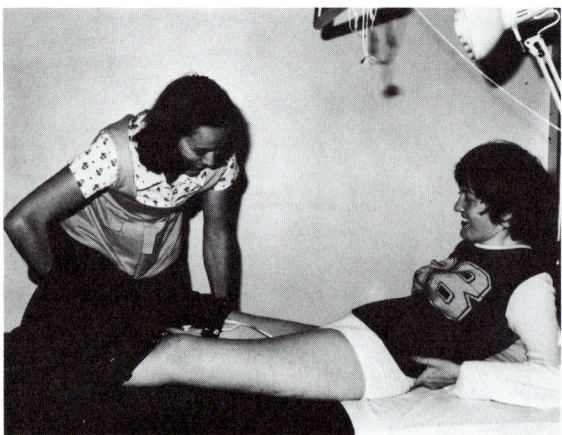

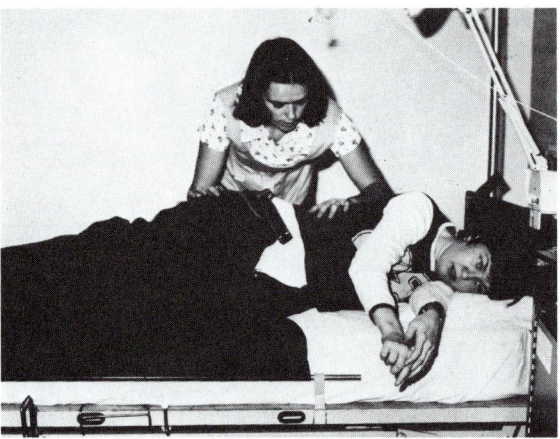

FIGURE 22–17   A nurse helps a quadriplegic woman with lower extremity dressing. Having the patient roll from side to side is the easiest way.

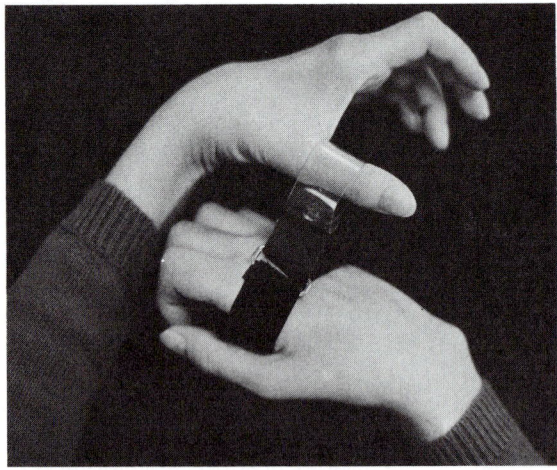

FIGURE 22–16   A quadriplegic woman applies her own utility cuff.

Upper extremity dressing for the cervical injured patient can begin when cervical orthotics provide stability or are removed altogether; lower extremity dressing can begin when patients can roll from side to side in bed and help with pulling on clothing. Mat activities in physical therapy help improve rolling ability and sitting balance before dressing skills are taught. When the patient improves with sitting balance during mat activities and progresses to long sitting in bed at a 90 degree angle of hip flexion, such activities as donning socks and shoes and pulling up clothing from feet can be introduced. The bed can eventually be progressively advanced to the usual flat position as dressing skills improve. Adaptive clothing and aids such as button hooks, zipper rings, and long-handled aids to reach feet may be needed. Overhead loops may also be necessary to assist in lifting body weight.

If the patient begins undressing in the wheelchair and uses a transfer board to return to bed, the board should be powdered lightly and covered with a towel to protect the bare skin.

Fashion is of interest to almost everyone. Ideas in clothing design and comfort for wheelchair users may be found in *Fashion-Able* (Rocky Hill, NY), the *Sears Roebuck and Co. Home Health Specialog*, or other resources. Velcro closures and pull-on loops are some adaptations. Tops, especially jackets, need to be short because sitting on them restricts shoulder movement. Often clothing—especially shoes—may have to be purchased in a larger size to avoid creating pressure areas and for ease in donning.

Coping with Spasticity and Pain

With the passing of spinal shock (explained in Chapter 6), *spasticity* can be anticipated following upper motor neuron damage with SCI. The average time for the appearance of spasticity is 6 to 10 weeks postinjury. Usually reflex excitability is at a maximum about 2 years after injury and may gradually diminish. Almost all patients with cervical cord injuries experience spasticity. Those with complete injuries often have more severe spasticity than those with incomplete SCI.

The three major approaches currently used singly or in combination to manage spasticity are physical, pharmacological, or surgical. Physical interventions dominate as the most practical and fruitful form of management. It is also very important to remain alert for an irritating focus below the level of SCI that will contribute to spasticity. The causes are most commonly related to the urinary system (infection, stones, and fistula); the intestinal system (flatus, impaction); and the integumentary system (wound infection, ingrown toenails, and pressure areas or sores).

Spasticity occurs in flexion or extension patterns. If spasms interfere with dressing, transfers, or bowel and bladder care, try to position the patient to break the pattern. For example, flex hips and knees to avoid extension or place the patient in a flexion position in the wheelchair to prevent back extension. Curl toes downward to stop the feet from jumping on the foot pedals of the wheelchair. Also avoid uneven pressure on limbs, such as pushing the foot hard against the footboard, which will cause clonus (jerking movements).

Always try to keep the patient calm, because spasticity increases with higher levels of anxiety. Fatigue and emotional exhaustion also aggravate this condition. It is important not to erroneously interpret spasticity as return of function. Be sure to explain the causes and difference between spasticity and voluntary movement.

Full range of motion exercises to joints twice daily will minimize the effects of spasticity. The therapist will combine these exercises with passive stretching of spastic muscles and, possibly, applications of hot or cold treatments. Collaborate with the therapist to select the exact passive exercises and frequency needed. Continually observe for contractures, joint damage, or stiffening and maintain correct positioning.

Common pharmacological agents used in both acute and chronic situations include baclofen, dantrolene sodium, and diazepam. Various other medication categories have been tried, but they have potentially greater side effects and substantially less efficacy.

In order to develop an effective intervention and education plan, observe the pattern and severity of spasticity, as well as the effectiveness of measures used to reduce it (Gardenhire 1985). Especially note the pattern and frequency that diazepam is requested because potential addiction can occur within 6 weeks.

A certain amount of spasticity can be helpful for performance of activities and for maintaining muscle tone, but excessive spasticity is associated with contractures and loss of functional abilities if unchecked. Chapter 27 addresses spasticity as a chronic problem.

Total loss of sensation below the level of injury is almost nonexistent and the sensations that do remain tend to follow bizarre patterns. Severe pain seems to be most troublesome for patients with cauda equina injuries. It is important to make sure that muscle or joint contractures are not the source of prolonged pain. Also late spinal instability is associated with pain. These conditions may be treated either conservatively, incorporating relaxation or biofeedback techniques, or surgically. Chronic intractable, incapacitating pain syndromes, sometimes associated with SCI, are very difficult to manage. See Chapter 28.

FUNCTIONAL ELECTRICAL STIMULATION (FES)*

The potential for helping the victims of SCI with electricity has long concerned health care professionals. After Galvani and Volta demonstrated in the late 1790s that electric current applied to either muscles or nerves stimulated muscle contractions, the intensity of research in the application of electricity has increased steadily. With the advent of computers, the hope of achieving a major breakthrough could be realized in the near future. With current technology, electrical neuromuscular stimulation effects muscle contractions, and now controlled, but limited, movement of paralyzed limbs, enabling the user to perform some functional activities like coming to standing, walking, and grasping. Products are already on the market that have great appeal to those who have lost so much with spinal injury (Benton, Baker, Bowman, and Waters 1981).

The pathology of SCI has a definite impact on what can or cannot be achieved with functional electrical stimulation (FES). In persons with traumatic SCI, a zone of injury extends up and down the spinal cord, the damage being greatest at the epicenter of injury. Microscopic study of the injured spinal cord shows destruction of the anterior horn cells that project nerve fibers to the skeletal muscles of the limbs. The net outcome of such damage is that several

---

*This section was contributed by Dennis M. Crowley, M.D.

nerve-muscle segments are denervated and no longer respond to safe levels of electric current. Although the denervated muscle of these motor units can be activated to contract, the amount of current needed to effect a response is so high that the subjects are at risk for electrical burns and tissue damage. Only the nerves of the undamaged but disconnected motor unit segments in the spinal cord below the level of injury are easily stimulated electrically. This physiological response explains why systems striving to restore hand function can only work with a select group of people with quadriplegia with injury at the C_{5-6} level. Candidates for electrically assisted ambulation must have a complete neurological level of injury above T_{11}. This limited responsiveness of denervated muscle to FES means that the technology does not apply to a large number of persons with SCI, most notably those with paraplegia with T_{12}, L_1, or L_2 fractures, as such injuries often destroy the anterior horn cells in the motor segments needed to provide pelvic and knee control critical to ambulation (Kralj, Bajd, Turk, Krajnik, and Benko 1983).

The goal of most researchers is to stimulate the human neuromuscular system, but the complexity of this challenge has resulted in different approaches in the application of electric current and its regulation. Most of the bioengineers in FES research use surface electrodes placed on key muscle groups and over the peroneal nerve, triggering a flexion spinal reflex response that facilitates steppage for the person. Most of these approaches also use assistive devices such as a reciprocating gait orthosis (long leg braces with a sophisticated cable-coupling system above the hips) and a walker. Some well-trained users can manage with forearm crutches (Kralj et al. 1983). In addition to enabling FES walking, bioengineers are also constantly working to improve the design and appearance of the assistive devices and other hardware in the system.

Another research approach with FES has been to insert electrodes percutaneously into the muscles. Many more muscles are stimulated using this approach: each subject has between 50 and 70 electrodes functioning at one time in an attempt to stimulate locomotion and to reduce the energy cost of ambulation. With this many muscles included in the system, the research team has been able to program 24 patterns of movement, most of which can be accomplished using short leg braces and forearm crutches (Marsolais and Kobetic 1988).

Both approaches have enabled individuals with complete SCI to walk for considerable distances. The most publicized examples have been Nan Davis walking up to the podium for her diploma at Wayne State University and Jan Smith walking 6.9 miles in the 1985 Honolulu Marathon.

The majority of the locomotion systems have been open systems of control, meaning that the stimulus intensity and pattern are all preprogrammed specifically for the user. The deficiency of this approach is that they lack gradation sensitivity and tend to overstimulate the involved muscle, thus leading to fatigue. The goal of most researchers is to develop

closed systems. This type of control entails the fixation of sensors and sophisticated computer technology to register angular changes and pressure changes. Current technology is far from providing this type of feedback, which forms the basis of ambulation, and manual activities.

Nowhere is this need for a closed system more apparent than with the application of FES to the restoration of upper extremity function and manual dexterity. Even though closed systems have not become functional for the upper extremity, both surface electrodes and intramuscular electrodes have provided some hand function to people with C_{5-6} quadriplegia since the mid-1970s. A stimulus control sensor is attached to the contralateral shoulder, and the user effects the desired movements in the dominant hand by proportional movements of the shoulder. A low profile, lightweight wrist splint provides wrist control. This system provides the user with a prehensile grasp for managing large objects and key pinch for small items. Studies have shown that the user is as good as an individual with a dynamic tenodesis splint, and in some ways more adept.

As good as this system is, it still falls short of functional restoration of manual skills for people with C_{5-6} quadriplegia because of the residual paralysis of the elbow extensors and the absence of controlled pronation and supination of the forearm. The lack of an integrated sensory feedback system also hampers the dexterity of the user. Research is ongoing to develop an electrosensing system via subcutaneous sensors in the C_5 dermatome and also by audio signal (Keith et al. 1988). See the Resources at the end of this text for more information on FES.

Although there has been considerable progress in the application of FES to the restoration of functional activities, the level of function is not as advanced and as easy as some researchers might project. The systems for ambulation are rather bulky and, even more important, still demand too much energy expenditure by the user to be functional. For most users, fatigue is the limiting factor. One other major problem is that the speed of ambulation (1.2 km/hr versus a normal speed of 6.4 km/hr) is too slow to be functional (Smith 1985).

Even though the application of FES sounds relatively simple, it demands a lot more of the user than simply getting hooked up and turned on. In fact, it can take 30 to 45 minutes just to don the orthoses and properly connect the wiring system. People who use FES have to make a major commitment of time and energy for training, practice, and research before they begin to experience any results. Any potential user must understand this reality before becoming too excited about the prospects of this technology.

Cost is also an important consideration. According to C. A. Phillips, the cost projections for an exercise program using commercially available electrical stimulators with five walking sessions per week for a year in physical therapy would amount to $25,000 for the year of therapy plus $8,600 to obtain the braces and the commercially available FES unit (Phillips 1989).

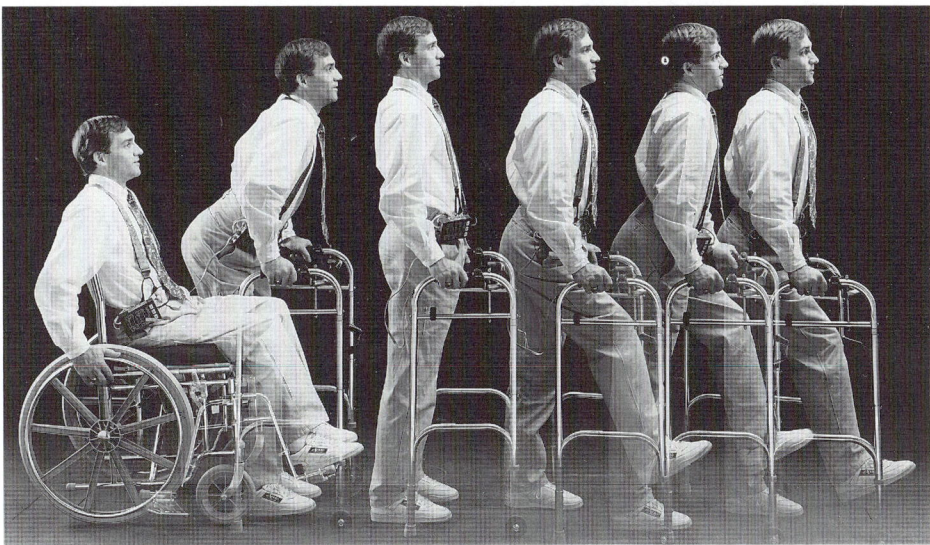

FIGURE 22–18   The Parastep System, designed and manufactured by Sigmedics, Inc.,
Northfield, IL, enables independent, unbraced standing and short distance walking by selected SCI
individuals. The technology provides users unprecedented mobility and an enhanced potential to
perform DLS.

    The Parastep System consists of a microcomputer-based neuromuscular electrical stimulator unit
that controls all standing and stepping functions. The user controls The Parastep System by
initiating commands to the microcomputer, a compact, lightweight unit clipped to the user's belt.
The microcomputer is powered by eight AA batteries housed in a lightweight battery pack and is
usually placed in the user's pocket. The control walker, designed with reciprocating stability,
completes the FES System.

Another reason why FES-enhanced activities are in the
research phase is that it is not known how much functional
electrical restoration will promote health. Although health
promotion is always cited as a benefit of FES, very little good
research supports the positive effects of FES on osteoporosis,
conditioning, and so on. Furthermore, the studies to date have
not had time to assess the long-term adverse outcomes.

To conclude, Yarkony and associates nicely summarize
the current state of functional neuromuscular stimulation
(FNS) as follows:

> FNS should be regarded as a potential adjunct to exist-
> ing methodologies which . . . can enhance the mobility
> and lifestyle of the user. However, since our research and
> that of others has been done on relatively small numbers
> of carefully selected patients, it is essential that investiga-
> tors in this field do not provide patients, laymen, and the
> mass media with expectations that exceed present knowl-
> edge or experience with FNS. [Yarkony, Jaeger, Roth,
> Kralj, and Quintern 1990]

DAILY LIVING SKILLS
(DLS)

Physical independence in daily life is something most people take for granted, and the loss of this freedom can be
devastating. Patients with SCI suffer this loss initially because of their lack of mobility and inability to take care
of their personal needs. This personal care, broadly described as daily living skills (DLS), includes all the things
people do every day for themselves. These include eating,
dressing, grooming, hygiene, attending to bowel and bladder needs, and communication skills, such as writing,
reading, or even typing. Functional living skills, then,
become one of the most important measures of effective
rehabilitation (Cichowski 1990; Data Management Service
1990). In fact, the entire health care team looks to these
levels of performance in helping the patient define goals
for the future. To survive in this hectic, independent
world, people with SCI must learn to get themselves up
and ready to face the world at school, work, and during
leisure hours.

Following assessment, therapists collaborate with the
patient to design a DLS program. In the beginning the goals
are most often the therapist's goals, because patients have
little specific idea of their potential. Expertise developed by
therapists has made it possible to outline functional expectations and establish realistic goals for groups of patients
with similar disabilities (Hill 1986; Nixon 1985). Table
22–7 summarizes expectations for potential functional status as related to the neurological level of injury sustained.
As the rehabilitation process evolves, goals are modified to

TABLE 22–7 Potential Functional Status as Correlated with Neurological Level of Injury

Neurological Status		
Neurological Level of Lesion[1]	Motor Ability	Sensory Appreciation[2]

Part A: Levels of Quadriplegia

Neurological Level of Lesion[1]	Motor Ability	Sensory Appreciation[2]
C_{1-2}	Limited movement of head and neck and ventilator dependent	Limited sensation to head, neck (C_{1-2}), and shoulder caps (C_{3-4}) 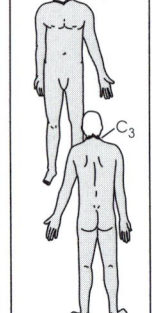
C_{3-4}	Good head and neck control; some diaphragm control and may require ventilator support part of the time	Full head, neck, and shoulder cap sensation *Add:* Upper chest and back and lateral aspect of upper arm)
C_5	Full head, neck, shoulder, and diaphragm control *Add:* Some elbow flexion	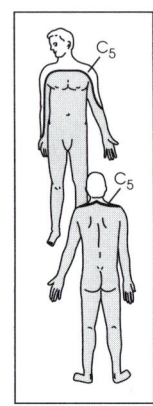
C_6	Strong elbow flexion *Add:* Some wrist extension (tenodesis)	*Add:* Sensation to the lateral aspects of forearm to include the thumb and first finger 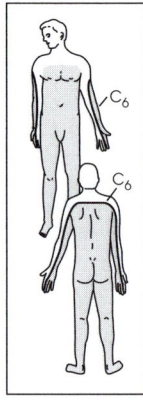
C_7	Full elbow flexion *Add:* Elbow extension, wrist flexion, and some finger control	*Add:* Sensation to the second finger
C_8-T_1	Moderate to full arm and wrist control *Add:* Moderate to full finger control	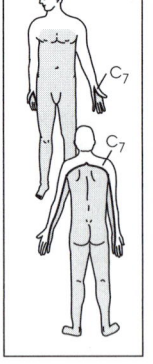 *Add:* Sensation to all the hand (C_8) and the medial aspects of the upper and lower arm (T_1) 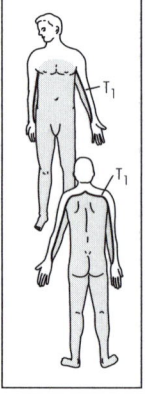

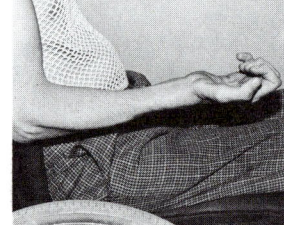
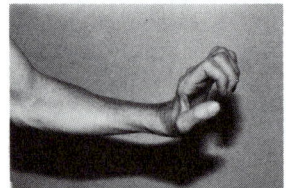
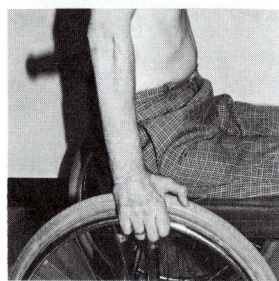
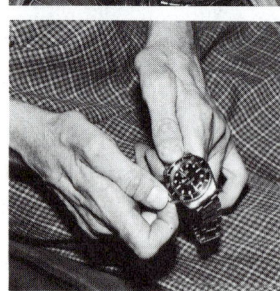
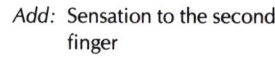

(Table continues)

TABLE 22–7 Potential Functional Status as Correlated with Neurological Level of Injury (continued)

Functional Ability[3]						
Eating and Grooming	Dressing	Bathing	Bowel and Bladder Care	Transfers	Mobility	Nonverbal Communication
Part A: Levels of Quadriplegia						
Dependent on an assistant	Dependent on assistant	Dependent on assistant	Dependent on assistant	Dependent on assistant	Requires electric wheelchair with breath, head, or shoulder controls. Likely dependent on a portable ventilatory support system all or part of the time	Independent with environmental controls[4]
Independent with aids[5] and setup[6]	Requires major assistance with aids	Requires wheelchair shower with major assistance	Requires major assistance with some aids and raised toilet seat	Major assistance required: variable with type of transfer	Requires electric wheelchair with adapted hand control and/or manual wheelchair wheel rim projections	Independent with aids and setup
Independent with aids	Requires minor assistance with aids	Independent in wheelchair shower with aids	Independent with aids and raised toilet seat	Minor assistance required: variable with type of transfer	Independent in manual wheelchair on level surfaces	Independent with aids
Independent with or without aids	Independent with aids	Independent in wheelchair shower or tub with bath board and aids	Independent with aids and raised toilet seat	Independent with aids in all transfers	Independent in manual wheelchair for most surfaces	Independent with or without aids
Independent	Independent	Independent in tub with bath board and aids	Independent with aids and raised toilet seat	Independent with or without aids	Independent in manual wheelchair	Independent

(Table continues)

TABLE 22–7   Potential Functional Status as Correlated with Neurological Level of Injury (continued)

	Neurological Status		
Neurological Level of Lesion[1]	Motor Ability	Sensory Appreciation[2]	

Part B: Levels of Paraplegia

T_{2-12}	Full upper extremity control *Add:* Limited to full (T_8–T_{12}) trunk control	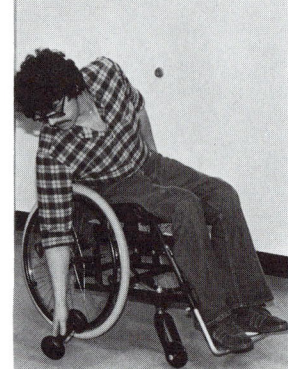	Full arm sensation *Add:* Partial trunk sensation to the level of the injury	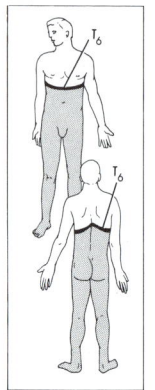
L_{1-5}	Full upper body control *Add:* Some hip (L_{1-3}), knee (L_{3-4}) and ankle (L_{4-5}) control and foot movement (L_5)	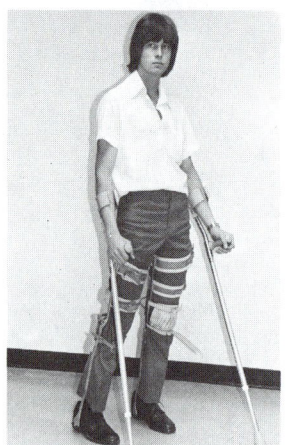	Full trunk sensation to the anterior upper leg (L_{1-3}), anterior/posterior and lateral aspects of the lower leg and dorsum of foot (L_{4-5})	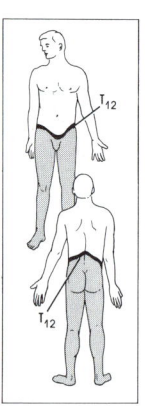
S_{1-5}	Moderate to full leg control *Add:* Some foot control (Disability can still be severe because of bowel, bladder, and sexual dysfunction)	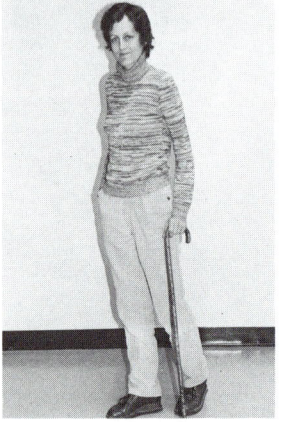	Sensation to the lateral aspect of the dorsum and the sole of foot (S_1); posterior aspect of the upper leg (S_2); sacral area (S_{2-5})	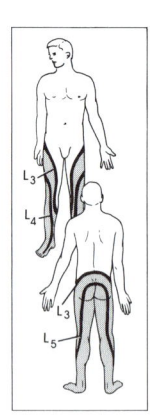

(Table continues)

[1]The neurological level of injury refers to the last normal functioning neurological level, not to the orthopedic fracture site: that is, a C_{5-6} level of injury means that the C_5 nerve root is normal and there is partial functioning of the C_6 nerve root. Many people with SCI will have a mixed neurological picture.
[2]For this chart *sensory* appreciation is defined as the ability to appreciate light touch, deep touch, pain, and temperature.
[3]*Functional ability* depends on many variables other than neurological status. The most significant ones are:
  • Motivation • Body build/strength/age • Sociocultural status • Preexisting medical condition(s)
  • Amount of motor and sensory sparing • Spasticity

TABLE 22–7 Potential Functional Status as Correlated with Neurological Level of Injury (continued)

Functional Ability[3]						
Eating and Grooming	Dressing	Bathing	Bowel and Bladder Care	Transfers	Mobility	Nonverbal Communication
Part B: Levels of Paraplegia						
Independent	Independent	Independent	Independent with aids and with or without raised toilet seat	Independent	Independent in manual wheelchair	Independent
Independent	Independent	Independent	Independent with or without aids	Independent	Optional use of knee-ankle-foot orthoses (KAFOs)	Independent
Independent	Independent	Independent	Independent with or without aids	Independent	Independent with or without ankle-foot orthoses (AFOs)	Independent

[4]*Environmental controls:* Technological equipment enabling a person to control various needs in the environment by the use of electrical devices and computer systems, for example, light, phone, television, and a door lock. A person accomplishes this by a single or dual control switch that can be adapted for use with different body parts such as the shoulder, head, chin, or tongue.
[5]*Aid:* A specially fabricated piece of adapted equipment or an altered version of an item already in use. Each aid is designed to meet the needs of an individual person and situation. Most aids are prescribed and fitted by the occupational therapist. (Examples are seen throughout the book.)
[6]*Setup:* Assembly or preparation of any or all of the items required by the person to accomplish a given task.

Prepared by Acute Spinal Cord Injury Unit, Shaughnessy Hospital, Vancouver, BC. Photography by G. F. Strong Rehabilitation Center.

become more specific to each individual. There is also a natural progression from simpler skills, such as eating and developing sitting balance, to more complex skills, such as dressing (Nawoczenski 1987). Therapists and nurses must continually assess and solve problems to meet individual needs.

The emphasis of self-care is on continual encouragement to learn and take responsibility for one's body and its new and different ways of functioning (Turney 1989). By virtue of their continual patient contact, nurses are in a unique position to reinforce all therapeutic activities (Heustis 1979) and make a valuable contribution to developing this independence. Nursing actions reflect the nurse's understanding of and commitment to the entire philosophy of rehabilitation, be it in the intensive care unit or on a recreational outing. However, this ideal is not always easy for nurses to put into practice. One conflict that must constantly be overcome is the urge to assist a struggling patient with a particular skill. This is contrary to the ingrained (but not always appropriate) image of the nurse as a "helper."

Another major conflict arises between nursing "efficiency" and patient goals. Obviously it takes longer to supervise a patient with an activity such as eating than it does to perform the task yourself. However, nothing can be more detrimental to patients than not letting them contribute to their care, regardless of how slowly it is accomplished. Sometimes we are not creative enough to allow patients these opportunities. Naturally in any given situation, each nurse must consider the constraints and limitations of time and other priorities of patient care that may interfere with patient goals. It is important to remember that these conflicts are not unique to nursing. Similar situations occur with all team members. Making therapists aware of problems may not only help solve them but also contribute to better interdisciplinary relationships.

To help the patient achieve potential functional living skills, the nurse must be familiar with general treatment programs; individual patient goals; adaptive equipment available; and the specific adaptations for each patient. This is important because the nurse must decide or inquire what assistance the patient may need. Detailed information must be readily available. Direct communication involving the patient, the nurse, and the therapist during daily activities facilitates thorough communication. Obviously this is not always possible. One efficient way to ensure continuity of care is the use of bedside charts that can be easily updated. An example is shown in Table 22–8. It is important that there be continuity regarding self-care activities into the evenings and weekends. Families often visit at these times. Their participation is essential, but they need education about the amount and kind of assistance that will reinforce independence.

People with Paraplegia

People with paraplegia are potentially physically capable of becoming independent in all self-care activities without the use of aids or specialized equipment. They can perform transfers independently, and selected patients with low paraplegia can master walking with the aid of leg braces and crutches and may achieve independence within a relatively short time, perhaps in 2 or 3 months.

People with Quadriplegia

The level of injury sustained dramatically affects the quadriplegic person's ability to perform functional living skills. For example, a person with quadriplegia at the C_4 level is totally dependent on others for all personal care needs, whereas a person with quadriplegia at the C_6 level can, by using adaptive aids, become independent with personal care and operate a regular wheelchair. This may mean the difference between requiring a personal attendant and living unassisted.

People with high quadriplegia with C_{1-4} neurological involvement are severely disabled. They are dependent for all personal care needs and will require a power wheelchair, environmental controls, and possibly ventilatory support all or part of the time. The unique problems associated with high quadriplegia are discussed in Chapters 23 and 29.

People with lower quadriplegia with C_{5-8} neurological involvement have suffered loss of hand function. With adaptive aids and teaching, however, they can become independent with many aspects of their personal care within a reasonable time frame (perhaps 3 to 6 months).

People with Incomplete Injury

People with incomplete injury at any level have some involvement that affects their level of functioning including personal care. Some incompletely injured persons can be severely disabled. For example, persons with a central cord injury may have no hand function but be able to walk. The length of time to achieve maximum potential varies.

LONG-TERM IMPLICATIONS

When assessing a person who has been paralyzed for some time, keep in mind that most active persons are at least relatively free from limited joint range of motion, muscle contractures, pain, and spasticity. Research also indicates that the majority of persons sustain, if not improve, the level

TABLE 22–8 Daily Living Skills (DLS) Status*

		OCCUPATIONAL THERAPIST:
		PHYSICAL THERAPIST:
NAME:		SPEECH PATHOLOGIST:
		DATE:
SPECIAL ATTENTION:		SPLINTING:
		BRACING:
		OTHER:

✓ DEPENDENT ✗ MAJOR ASSIST * MINOR ASSIST ☐ SUPERVISION ○ INDEPENDENT		
EATING		
GROOMING		
BATH/SHOWER		
DRESSING UPPER / LOWER		
TRANSFERS		
MOBILITY BED / W/C / WALK		
COMMUNICATION		

*This bedside chart has a plastic cover designed to be used with a grease pencil to facilitate continual updating.

of functional living skills reached during rehabilitation (Yarkony, Roth, and Heinemann 1988), with a few exceptions involving personal preference, such as channeling energies away from self-care activities into intellectual pursuits.

Throughout rehabilitation it is important to plan with the person's home situation and desires in mind. To begin with, architectural barriers in the home must be assessed. Physical alterations or the installation of equipment may be necessary to allow maximum wheelchair independence while minimizing effort and ensuring safety. Temporary adaptation is best when the person is going home only for short passes. Families must receive expert advice before initiating any costly permanent alterations. A quality resource with up-to-date general product information is the *Accent on Living Buyer's Guide*. Large manufacturers, such as the Whirlpool corporation, have information for installing and operating major appliances for easier use by disabled persons along with illustrated ideas for kitchen and laundry designs. See Resources. Community-based resources run for and by people with disabilities often provide practical and cost-efficient services to assist individu-

als, families, and professionals make the transition to home more smooth.

Next, the availability of all community resources must be explored. Sometimes geographical location is a problem, especially in rural areas, which are generally underserved. Families relocate because of alternative opportunities. Educational and employment background must also be considered. Can programs be modified to meet the patient's possible future requirements?

A most valuable asset is driver training for the disabled person. For convenience and safety a number of modifications can be made to regular vehicles that enable even the person with quadriplegia to drive. Hand controls are used to accelerate and brake, steering aids are available, and many vans can be equipped with electrical lifts for ease in entry. For many persons with paraplegia, driver training can commence within a few weeks after injury, thus enabling mobility, especially for outpatient services. The ability to drive safely enables the individual to enter the normal world for vocational, social, and recreational aspirations (Kent et al. 1979).

Community-based specialists must be able to comprehend the potential capabilities of clients to help them decide what they want to do and what they are capable of doing. Appropriate consultation and referral are often needed to differentiate between altered functional living skills as a personal choice and inactivity and decreased ability to care for oneself as a result of unresolved physical or psychological problems. The effects of aging must also be assessed.

Fitness, exercise, and physically active life-styles are virtually unexplored areas for many disabled people. Options and suggestions for involvement are introduced in Chapter 24.

REFERENCES

Adkins, H. V. 1985. *Spinal Cord Injury.* New York: Churchill Livingstone. *Primarily a physical therapy viewpoint focusing on practical and detailed application in the clinical setting.*

Benton, L. A. , Baker, L. L., Bowman, B. R., and Waters, R. L. 1981. *Functional Electrical Stimulation, a Practical Guide.* Downey, CA. Rancho Los Amigos Hospital.

Cichowski, K. (Ed.). 1990. *RIC-FAS—Rehabilitation Institute of Chicago Functional Assessment Scale.* Rev. Chicago: Rehabilitation Institute of Chicago.

Data Management Service of the Uniform Data System for Medical Rehabilitation and the Center for Functional Assessment Research. 1990. Guide for the Use of Uniform Data Set for Medical Rehabilitation. Version 3.0. Functional Inventory Measurement (FIM). Buffalo: State University of New York at Buffalo. *Computerized system of functional outcomes that may be assessed by various interdisciplinary team members at various intervals during the rehabilitation process. Results obtained are correlated with length of stay and compared with results of other participating centers. Results are designed for in-house use and program modification, and cannot be used for advertising purposes. Guidelines, instructional materials, and ongoing support available.*

Ford, J. 1980. *Wheelchair Handbook: A Guide to Selection, Cushion, Accessories and Maintenance.* G. F. Strong Rehabilitation Centre, Vancouver, BC, Canada. *A concise, liberally illustrated guide for rehabilitation professionals.*

Ford, J. R., and Duckworth, B. 1987. *Physical Management of the Quadriplegic Patient,* 2d ed. Philadelphia: F. A. Davis. *Filled with illustrations and guidelines to practice management of transfers and basic daily living skills and expanded to include information on housing, transportation, sexual management, and child care. Highly recommended.*

Gardenhire, M. 1985. In *Nursing Spinal Cord Injuries.* Ed. N. M. Woll. Totowa, NJ: Rowman & Allen Publishers. *Valuable text based on nurse practitioner program at the Veterans Administration Medical Center and California State University, Long Beach. Includes educational plan for individuals dealing with spasticity.*

Heustis, D. 1979. Physical therapy in rehabilitation. In *Current Perspectives in Rehabilitation Nursing.* Eds. R. Murray and J. Kijeck. St. Louis: C. V. Mosby, pp. 187–192. *Discusses the role of the physical therapist and approaches mobility and self-care.*

Hill, J. P. 1986. *A Guide to Functional Outcomes in Occupational Therapy.* Rockville, MD: Aspen Publishers.

Keith, M., Peckham, P., Thrope, G., Buckett, J., Stroh, K. and Menger, V. 1988. *Clinical Orthopaedics and Related Research.* (Aug.): 25–33.

Kent, H., et al. 1979. A driver training program for the disabled. *Archives of Physical Medicine and Rehabilitation* 60 (June): 273–276. *Report on results of a driver training program; includes recommendations for "van modifiers," eligibility requirements, and functional and general health assessment.*

Kralj, A. D., Bajd, T., Turk, R., Krajnik, J., and Benko. 1983. Gait restoration in paraplegics. *Journal of Rehabilitation Research and Development* 20: 3–20.

Marsolais, E. B., and Kobetic, R. 1988. *Clinical Orthopaedics and Related Research* 233 (Aug.): 64–74.

Nawoczenski, D. A. 1987. Physical management. In *Spinal Cord Injury: Concepts and Management.* Eds. L. E. Buchanan and D. A. Nawoczenski. Baltimore: Williams and Wilkins. *Well-illustrated chapter on key points of mobilization written by occupational and physical therapists.*

Nixon, V. 1985. *Spinal Cord Injury: A Guide to Functional Outcomes in Physical Therapy Management. Rehabilitation Institute of Chicago Procedure Manual.* Rockville, MD: Aspen Publishers. *Presents general evaluation, treatment, and outcomes, with specific descriptions on respirations, bed and wheelchair mobility, pressure relief, transfers, and self-range of motion among others. Functional electrical stimulation and other complications are also presented. Of interdisciplinary interest.*

Phillips, C. A. 1987. Medical criteria for active physical therapy. Physician guidelines for patient participation in a program of functional electrical stimulation. *American Journal of Physical Medicine* 66 (5): 269–286.

Phillips, C. A. 1989. Functional electrical stimulation and lower extremity bracing for ambulation exercise of the spinal cord injured individual: A medically prescribed system. *Physical Therapy* 60: 842–849.

Sargent, C., and Braun, M. A. 1986. Occupational therapy management of the acute spinal cord injured patient. *American Journal of Occupational Therapy* 40 (5): 333–337. *Describes program with guidelines for evaluation and treatment, orthotic selection and psychosocial considerations with the intent of implementing rehabilitation from the moment of injury.*

Schneider, F. 1981. Physical therapy assessment. In *Comprehensive Rehabilitation Nursing.* Eds. N. Martin, N. Holt, and D. Hicks. New York: McGraw-Hill, pp. 269–297. *Detailed musculoskeletal, neurological, cardiopulmonary, and functional assessment; includes numerous samples of charts and forms used in physical therapy.*

Smith, Jan. 1985. Personal observation in the Honolulu Marathon.

Turney, A. B. 1989. Toward Independence. Mobility Foundation, 8828 Stemmons Freeway, Suite 106, LB39, Dallas, TX 75247. *A series of seven videotape programs designed for patient education. Highlights bladder management, dressing for men and women, wheelchair seating, flexor hinge orthosis, and various transfers. Highly recommended by the American Association of Spinal Cord Injury Nurses.*

Yarkony, G. M., Jaeger, R. J., Roth, E., Kralj, A., and Quintern, J. 1990. Functional neuromuscular stimulation for standing after spinal cord injury. *Archives of Physical Medicine and Rehabilitation* 71: 201–206.

Yarkony, G. M., Roth, E. J., and Heinemann, A. 1988. Functional skills after spinal cord injury rehabilitation: Three-year longitudinal follow-up. *Archives of Physical Medicine and Rehabilitation* 69 (2): 111–114. Functional levels were maintained or improved during this time, which is consistent with previous but limited research.

Yarkony, G. M., Roth, E. J., Heinemann, A., Wu, Y., Katz, R., and Lovell, L. 1987. Benefits of rehabilitation for traumatic spinal cord injury. *Archives of Neurology* 44 (1): 93–96. *Study of 711 patients documents detailed functional improvement of patients with SCI who participated in comprehensive rehabilitation.*

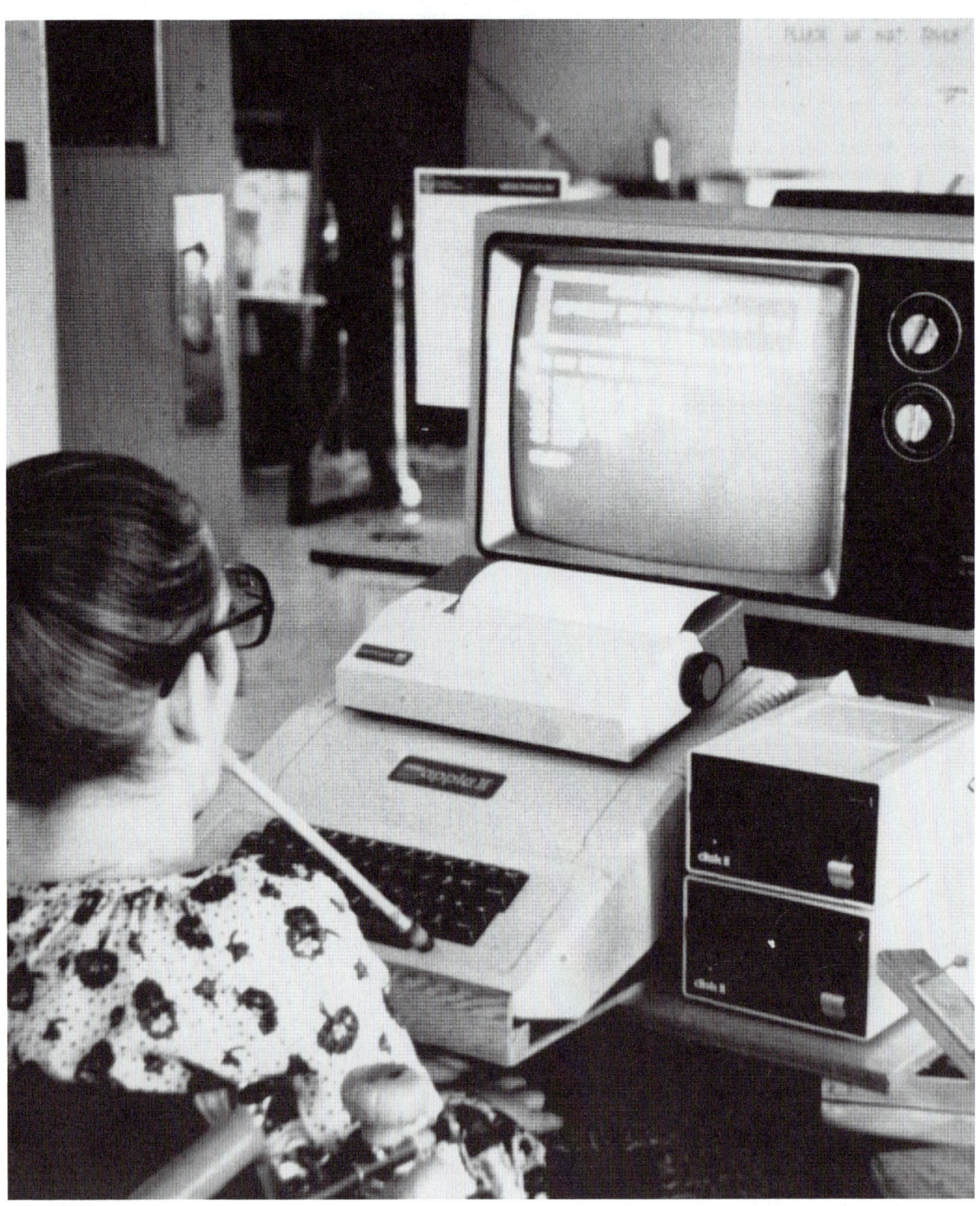

CHAPTER 23

Using Technology to Explore Options

Shayna Hornstein, P.T.
Katrina McKay, O.T.

Chapter Outline

Objectives of Technology Intervention

- To discuss the significant role that technology can play in allowing for independence in life-style for a person with high quadriplegia
- To provide an awareness of the use of technology in various environments and situations
- To highlight the need to identify and contact appropriate resources as required
- To develop a positive and encouraging attitude to the use of technology

We can assume that medical technology has been involved immediately following a high cervical spinal cord injury if survival is the outcome. In fact, advances in the application of medical and surgical technology can be credited directly for the increase in survival of persons with these injuries. The use of technology for independence in life-style, on the other hand, has not yet achieved the profile it deserves. In comparison, this technology is poorly developed, misunderstood, and in most cases, not adequately integrated into the mainstream of rehabilitation programs. In addition, people are quick to question the cost of this equipment without measuring its value.

In the past, independence for one who has a high spinal cord injury (SCI) has required significant attendant support, which in turn has demanded either abundant financial support or substantial dedication of time from family, friends, and volunteers. Today, however, with minimal investment and the clever use of well-established technology, people with severe physical disabilities have excellent opportunities to compete in and contribute to society. Environmental control systems, for example, reduce dependence on personal care assistance measured in hours of assistance per day.

The adaptation of technology is making the difference. Mobility is possible without legs to walk; writing can occur without functional hands; vocal ability is not necessary to create speech; written information can be searched and absorbed without eyes to see; a person with a high spinal cord injury can do complicated computer-aided design and drafting; a nonvocal person may work as a telephone receptionist—and we have only just begun using technology to open the doors for the future.

Preparing people for the change in life-style that they must assume with a high SCI is the ultimate challenge facing everyone in health care and related professions. Technology can be a very useful tool if the user is assessed appropriately, introduced skillfully, and trained in practical and interesting uses for their newly acquired skills. When planning programs that include technology, attend to the ongoing training needs of clients. Training funds are frequently neglected, resulting in underutilized technology. The technology remains only as good as the training provided in its use.

Factors to consider when applying technology to assist an individual attain greater independence include:

- Physical abilities
  - Head and neck control
  - Strength and endurance
  - Range of movement
  - Breathing capabilities
  - Swallowing abilities
  - General physical endurance (e.g., sitting tolerance)
- Psychosocial aspects
  - Work experience and history
  - Self-confidence
  - Judgment
  - Family and social dynamics
- Economic factors
  - Financial resources
  - Eligibility for financial support through various agencies
- Avocational and vocational interests and experience
  - Past work experiences and educational level
  - Personal interests, knowledge, and abilities
- Living environments
  - At home with family, institution, shared accommodation, and attendant care
  - Physical space for equipment and arrangements for assistance when required
- Existing medical equipment
  - Compatibility of existing equipment with technical devices (e.g., remote control for the computer linked up through the power wheelchair)
- Trial periods
  - Availability of technical equipment for trial in the environment in which it is to be used
- Reliable maintenance, servicing, and replacing of equipment

TECHNOLOGY FOR THE IMMEDIATE ENVIRONMENT

Calling for Help in the Acute Care Environment

The ability to call for help must be addressed immediately in the acute care environment. Individuals on ventilators need to make clicking sounds with their tongue, or similar audible sounds selected to attract attention of people nearby. A call bell system is also required, preferably with two levels of signal. One mode provides an emergency tone for immediate call for attention and a second mode with a normal tone for regular requests for assistance.

An accessible call bell system for a person with limited functional abilities should be mandatory if persons with this level of disability are to be accepted for treatment within a specific facility. These should be set up and working properly *before* the individual is admitted. There are several simple, commercially available switches to choose from, such as leaf, pillow, and tongue switches. Staff must be trained *always* to replace the call bell switch within reach of the user before leaving the individual's bedside. Compatibility with facility electrical wiring systems must be reviewed and approved.

Although elaborate equipment exists for augmentative communication, these systems are often not practical in the busy environment of an intensive care unit.

Direct Communication in the Acute Care Environment

When a cuffed-trach is in use, basic communication can be facilitated by teaching nonvocal patients some simple tricks to enable "silent" speech to be more easily understood. Dividing a sentence into smaller parts, enunciating, and spelling words out are helpful hints for facilitating basic communication in the early days. Communication boards can be homemade or purchased commercially. See Chapter 15, including Figure 15-9, for more information on nonverbal communication. These efforts should be coordinated with a speech pathologist who is familiar with ventilator-dependent quadriplegia.

MOBILITY

Power Wheelchairs

For an individual with high quadriplegia, easy mobility is essential. The possibility of independent mobility must be introduced as soon as the individual is able to tolerate sitting in a wheelchair.

The prescription and training in the use of a suitable power wheelchair are essential elements of the rehabilitation process. Demonstration wheelchairs should be made available by the medical equipment dealer for trial.

A specialized wheelchair is not merely a wheelchair with a variety of controls. It is a carefully selected, adjusted, and adapted system designed to suit each individual (see Tables 22–5 and 22–6). Proper selection requires the cooperative efforts of the user, the medical dealer, rehabilitation engineers, appropriate therapists, and other team members. The complete mobility system must be designed to give the person with a severe physical disability optimum freedom of movement and control over body positioning.

Selecting a specialized power wheelchair can be compared to buying an integrated stereo system. Both have "package systems" available but they may not be exactly what is wanted or needed. Choosing individual components can offer the required quality and diversity.

Most wheelchair manufacturing companies bundle different wheelchair components into complete systems or packages. The purchaser and user should be aware that they have a choice of what components can be selected to make the package complete. Electrical and mechanical compatibility of each component must be assured if the end product is to work efficiently.

It is important to discuss the options available with a nonbiased resource person who can provide informed recommendations. It is well worth the effort (and can be less expensive in the long run) to contact major rehabilitation centers and medical equipment supply companies across the country, particularly those with therapists on staff. Ask questions about their preferences when purchasing power mobility systems. These centers or companies frequently evaluate new wheelchair models and can offer information about how one system compares with others. They may also make referrals to other users of specific power wheelchair systems or other knowledgeable people.

Power Wheelchair Frame

There are two styles to consider:

- Standard power wheelchairs with belt drive that can be customized to accommodate commercially available ventilator trays, recline systems, and so on
- Module power-base wheelchairs that offer a choice of seating systems because the base is separate

The various components selected for a specialized power wheelchair system can be installed on the base and frame of most commercially manufactured power wheelchairs. Either the standard folding frame with motors or the solid power base frame from each manufacturer can be chosen. If a ventilator is being used, its mounting may alter the overall length and stability of the chair. If a recline and/or tilt mechanism is also in place, check whether the total range of recline and/or tilt is available with the ventilator mounted.

Also consider the type of vehicle transportation used. For example, if a van is used, can the recommended wheelchair be accommodated in the van using existing tie downs? Selection may be limited by what fits into the van. Access in and out of the van must also be checked.

Performance Features

Each manufacturer's wheelchair system has unique performance features—options that alter the performance of the chair. These options may be electronic, mechanical, or computerized. All medical equipment dealers should be able to discuss these features. Examples include:

- High/low speed controls
- Turning speed controls
- Acceleration/deceleration controls
- Braking systems
- Indoor/outdoor modes
- Tremor dampening and turning controls
- Latch and momentary mode controls

Control Options

A control interface system includes the control itself and the interface or way the user accesses the control. Today, control interface systems do more than just operate the wheelchair. They offer accessory control of a power recliner, remote control to compatible environmental control units, tape recorders, and door openers, all through a single actuating device. This offers new choices and sophisticated operation.

Proportional control is similar to an automobile accelerator: the farther the control is activated the more the speed increases.

- Joystick—hand, chin, head, foot, or mouthstick operated
- Mouth, tongue, lip, or head minijoystick control

Nonproportional (microswitch) control involves a switch control that is either on or off. An additional switch selector is usually available for changes in speed. Latched or momentary modes are available with some of these switches. Latch mode means that the commands are held active even though the driver may have released the control. A safety stop switch is essential. Momentary mode means that the drive commands are active only as long as the command is given.

- Chin (short throw)
- Cheek control
- Head rest control
- Pneumatic control—sip and puff
- Shoulder control
- Foot control
- Eyeblink control

Seating Options and Positioning Devices

Carefully assess wheelchair positioning devices to be sure that they provide a good postural appearance, prevent pressure sores, support a stable sitting position, and enable performance of functional activities. A stable pelvis is the first goal in achieving good posture. Positioning of the trunk, limbs, and head follow as emphasized in Chapter 22. Most positioning aids are custom designed or custom ordered to suit the individual.

Power Recline and Tilt Systems

Power recline and/or tilt systems are important and justifiable components to consider. Benefits of recline and tilt mechanisms include:

- *Pressure relief* from ischial tuberosities and sitting surfaces by shifting most of the direct pressure from the lower body to the back.
- *Increased sitting tolerance.* Both recline and tilt options offer a change in position when uncomfortable, tired, dizzy, or experiencing breathing or blood pressure difficulties.
- *Flexibility in transfers.* In some cases, power recline systems allow an easier transfer due to the wider range of positions available when the chair is reclined.

- *Ease with catheterizations.* The recline mechanism may facilitate intermittent catheterization procedures.
- *Body language.* Recline and tilt systems allow for body expression as active limb or trunk movement is often not possible.
- *Reduced need for attendant care.* Power recline and tilt systems allow clients to perform their own weight shifts.

Several choices are available. Most companies offer their own generic systems for both power recline and tilt. In addition, several independently manufactured power recline and tilt systems can be combined with most powered mobility bases.

A power recline system allows the user to recline independently from a seated upright posture to a full spine position, or any angle in between.

The power tilt feature allows for the back and seat of the chair to alter position in space without changing any of the fixed angles. The user can independently tip the chair back to relieve pressure without changing hip, knee, and ankle positions. This option offer several advantages. First, the person with poor sitting balance, pressure problems, or respiratory difficulties can receive the benefits of the reclined position, improving sitting balance and allowing intermittent pressure relief. Also, seating setups (that is, trunk supports, straps, cushions, and so on) can now remain fixed with a stable pelvic position.

When selecting a power recline or tilt system, a major consideration is the shear factor. This is the amount of frictional force placed on the skin when reclining. Shearing also wrinkles the person's clothing, which may lead to pressure problems. In addition, the body may shift during a recline, affecting the person's sitting balance and function. For example, a change in the sitting position may place a chin control out of reach.

Both the power recline and tilt mechanisms can be installed to function on the same power wheelchair. Careful consideration must be given to the location of the control for the recline and/or tilt feature.

Ventilator Trays

The ventilator tray carries the ventilator and batteries. It is usually housed underneath the wheelchair frame, protruding as little as possible behind the chair. It can also be mounted on the back posts of the chair if the chair does not have a recliner. Strong reinforcements to the back are necessary to hold the weight.

Be aware of the specific ventilator and battery dimensions when ordering the tray so that all of the parts fit securely. The controls of the ventilator (for instance, volume and rate) must be easily accessible.

Power base wheelchairs are not often used for persons requiring a mounted ventilator. The ventilator tray cannot be housed underneath the chair and must be either fitted on a tray on the back (which negates the use of a reclining system) or on a tray extending from the back (which changes the length and turning radius of the chair).

Service: Maintenance and Repair

Readily available maintenance and repair for a specialized power wheelchair is essential. Select a competent vendor, a medical dealer who is a reliable source for the latest equipment information and literature. The skilled medical dealer can solve problems and provide the necessary, special equipment.

When selecting a suitable, specialized power wheelchair system, investigate the company's service and maintenance policy.

When ordering, be sure that the company will initially set up the equipment and adjust it for the client's needs. Future costs of service calls should be specified at time of purchase.

Power mobility technology is changing rapidly. It is increasingly time consuming and difficult to maintain up-to-date knowledge and be familiar with each new product. People who purchase or prescribe these systems must consult people who specialize in these high tech resources to make certain that they are making the best choice. Contacting the nearest regional SCI unit or a community agency such as the Neil Squire Foundation that is familiar with this equipment is a good way to begin this complicated process.

Manual Wheelchair

A manual backup wheelchair must always be ordered for a person with high quadriplegia. It must accommodate the same positioning devices and components as used in the power wheelchair. The manual wheelchair does not require the same level of durability as the power wheelchair if it is to be used only as a backup, such as when the power wheelchair is not available or where a power wheelchair is not appropriate. Recline options for manual wheelchairs are available.

Consider custom modifications of quality, lightweight wheelchairs for the high quadriplegic user. With proper trunk and arm supports these lightweight chairs offer increased mobility for the user because they are lighter for the attendant.

Adapted Vans

A specially adapted, attendant-driven van is the most convenient transportation for someone who has high quadriplegia. There are many options of power lifts, interior designs, and other technology features. Contact a resource familiar with the latest features before making any expensive purchases. Most large rehabilitation centers have driving evaluation programs that can provide helpful guidelines for purchase. Considerations include:

- Will the power wheelchair fit on the lift?
- Where is the van to be parked?
- Will a side or a back entry be better?
- What height is desirable?
- Is visibility outside important?
- What tie-down system will be used?
- How will the user be positioned in the van for ease of maneuverability and visibility?

TECHNOLOGY FOR THE EXPANDED ENVIRONMENT

Microprocessor Tools and Accessories

Today, computer technology and its applications offer people with severe disabilities exciting new opportunities for academic, vocational, and recreational pursuits. Although it is unrealistic to attempt to keep up with all the latest devices, health care professionals must be aware of the general uses of this technology for persons with high quadriplegia as it has already improved the quality of many of their lives. Most important, care givers must know where to refer people for assistance.

One misconception is that computers are only useful to people with advanced education in computer-related fields. Not true! Most adults drive cars, but few have the comprehensive understanding of how cars work and how to fix them. The same applies to computers. Computer users are as varied a group of people as drivers are. People with a particular aptitude and interest in the workings of microprocessors can become computer programmers and technicians. Everyone else can use different variations of this tool at home, school, and in almost every occupation.

A comprehensive discussion of computers and software selection for persons with severe physical disabilities is beyond the scope of this chapter. However, several considerations remain consistent despite the rapid changes in technology.

Accessing the Keyboard

Access to the keyboard can be either very simple or extremely sophisticated. Many users begin using a mouthstick or hand splints with upper arm support for typing on the keyboard. However, less physically intensive methods of keyboard emulation are available. These include:

- Modified keyboards that provide assistance with holding down the operative keys (shift, control, alt) for single finger or mouthstick typists.
- Alternative keyboards—expanded, mini, or customized keyboards to meet the specific needs of the user.

PERSONAL VIEWPOINT

I am 30 years old, and I was injured (C$_4$) by a 5-foot fall from the front porch of an old-fashioned house in Victoria. Before this, I worked for 8 years in steel construction.

I am now finishing the last term of a 2-year accounting program at Vancouver Community College. Then I plan to take Certified General Accountant courses at night.

I also volunteer, doing part-time accounting work at the Neil Squire Foundation. I enjoy reading novels when I am not reading textbooks. For the last 4 years I have had season tickets for the BC Lions football games.

I was hospitalized for 2 years: 7 months in an acute care setting and 17 months at an extended care facility. I now live in the community and share a condo (and attendant care services) with several people with SCI.

Three weeks after my injury I was able to breathe on my own. I had not been able to talk out loud for a month because of intubation and a ventilator. The day the tube was removed from my lungs, an occupational therapist (who was making a brace for my neck) asked me if I was interested in computers. My immediate reply was "no."

However, 2 or 3 months later I heard of a computer course that teaches disabled students to operate computers and thereby become employable. At the time, I felt I would never be employed again, but the prospect of possible future employment made me become interested in computers. Although I am not pursuing a career in computers, I will use computers to compete in the job market. I type 36 words per minute, which I am assured is as fast, if not faster, than most accountants.

Because I cannot use my hands, I type using a computer program called ezMorse, which accesses the computer using a sip and puff switching mechanism and Morse code.

I would say to someone who has recently been injured, there are many opportunities for disabled persons. It may require additional training in whatever field you choose to pursue, but if you apply yourself there is not much you cannot do.

Don Danbrooke
Vancouver, BC

- Morse code, often operated by sipping and puffing on a straw, but can be used with any other dual switch. Many users have attained data entry rates of 30 words per minute using this method!
- Scanning, operated through a variety of input switches. The alphabet as well as the remainder of the keyboard are presented on the computer screen. Activation of the input switch selects the choice for input.
- Voice input, in which the user speaks to the computer.

In all of these methods, the computer responds as if someone has just pressed the key on the keyboard, when in fact the individual has just entered the Morse code, or has used a voice command for that character. Accuracy and efficiency are the most important factors when selecting an access via mouthstick is not the fastest or the easiest method available.

Accessing Software

Software written on floppy disks requires that the user be able to manipulate the disks, an often impossible task for the person with a high SCI. Therefore a computer should have a hard disk drive that can store the information of many floppy disks. The user can then move from file to file and program to program with ease. For an individual who cannot manipulate floppy disks, the hard disk drive allows hands-free or independent computing. Other software accessories that enhance efficiency are:

- On-line help that provides computerized access to a manual.
- User-friendly software—often a single keystroke command allows the user to move in and out of different applications easily. For instance, while writing a letter, one might need to answer the phone and jot down a number. The fewer keystrokes involved, the less fatigue.
- Keystroke savers and macros that allow users to type a few keystrokes to activate stored messages. For instance, striking "JS" might print "John Smith."

These examples illustrate how cleverly installed computer systems can enable a person with high quadriplegia to be an efficient, productive user who has quick access to the speed and power of the computer.

Computer Selection

Finding the appropriate computer for a person with high quadriplegia depends largely on the purpose for which it will be used. This question is often difficult to answer, particularly when the potential user has not had previous exposure to computers. Personal interests and career goals are important considerations. For example, an interest in graphics and design or music composition will often dictate particular computer systems to purchase as well as software requirements.

It is imperative to consult with knowledgeable sources before purchasing equipment. Local colleges and universities with applied computer science departments are a good general resource. In addition, several publications specifically address the needs of persons with disabilities. See Resources. Some guidelines to assist in the specific selection of equipment include:

- *Access.* As with all equipment purchased, efficiency, accuracy, and independence of access are critical.
- *Cost.* Although this is a big factor in any purchase, the consequence of a lower price tag on a computer usually means a lesser degree of independence is available (for instance, no hard disk drive, inadequate memory capabilities, and so on).
- *Growth and expansion.* A major concern of many purchasers is that the computer will be obsolete in 6 months. Technology improves constantly, and there will always be a computer with better capabilities and features and more power. Purchase a computer that meets the present needs of the user and that can be expanded or adapted to some of the new technology in the future. Make the most informed decision possible given up-do-date knowledge.

Computer Components

Monitors. Monitors are distinguished by whether they are monochrome or able to support different colors, and by their resolution (quality of picture). Watch for computer and monitor compatibility.

Modems. *MOdulator-DEModulators* are devices that allow the computer to communicate via the telephone line to other computers. The modem offers an exciting way to escape the isolation of one's disability and communicate with other people via the computer screen.

Printers. There are many models of printers, but three general kinds: dot matrix, daisy wheel, and laser printers. Although handling paper—such as tearing perforated paper—is not usually feasible for someone with high quadriplegia, the printer can be set up to allow for as much independence as possible. For example, software can often control the printer, or the printer's control buttons can be mounted within reach of a mouthstick.

Scanners. Scanners photocopy pages of typed text directly into the computer. Once stored, the user can then manipulate the text.

Facsimile. The facsimile or FAX transfers hard copies of information via telephone lines in seconds. FAXs can be built into computer systems, enabling access for a person with high quadriplegia.

Training

Training in the use of a computer and software is essential and is frequently overlooked when purchasing equipment. Training must be incorporated into the rehabilitation program. Local college and university computer science departments are valuable resources for developing training programs.

Environmental Control Systems (ECS)

With an environmental control system (ECS), a person with a severe physical disability can control virtually any electronic device without assistance. Following setup of the system, the person can independently control the on/off function of fans, lights, and radios, operate televisions and video cassette recorders, answer and initiate telephone calls, and unlock and open doors. The range of operations depends on the complexity of the system. An environmental control unit is usually set up as the person adapts to disability and is more medically stable.

Although ECS and a computer are usually separate devices at present, the trend is toward making the computer control the environment. Many ECSs have built-in computers. There is not yet agreement on whether the computer should control the environment or the environmental control system should turn on the computer. Many computers in the future will be able to control elements of the environment such as lights, temperature, appliances, and doors.

ECSs are introduced at different stages of rehabilitation in different centers depending on funding, space, technical expertise in selection, installation, maintenance, and general knowledge. The ECS is essential equipment for the person with high quadriplegia. Control of the environment is psychologically rewarding, reduces the need for assistance from others, and provides freedom to control things as one chooses. The complexity of the system varies depending on the financial and technical resources available, as well as the environment to be controlled.

The system that best meets the user's needs should be chosen, providing that it is safe and reliable. The ability of the system to expand to meet future needs should be considered. Determine available servicing and maintenance before purchase.

Input Method

Environmental control systems can be controlled in several different ways. These include:

1. Switch operation. Either a single or dual switch can activate an ECS. Switches come in many sizes and forms, but the most common ones used by people with high quadriplegia are pillow, pneumatic (sip and puff), leaf, and tongue switches. All ECSs using switch input operate on a scanning principle.

2. Keyboard (computer) operation. Some ECSs can be operated from a computer. Software enables the ECS to be operated without interfering with the computer application in use (for instance, word processing). The same method of access used to control the computer controls the ECS (for instance, Morse code).

3. Voice control. Voice control is relatively new for ECS. Consistency of speech is important for all systems. The noise from the ventilator, interrupted speech patterns, and low or irregular speech must be taken into account with the person with high quadriplegia. If lengthy conversations are tiring, voice input may not be appropriate.

4. Wheelchair control. Operation of an ECS from a wheelchair requires wireless remote control. If this input method will be used, it is important to outline this need at the onset of wheelchair selection.

The input method must be easy to use. Access methods that are complex, cumbersome, or frustrating to position correctly detract from the independence these systems intend to provide.

Central Processing Unit (CPU)

The central processing unit (CPU) contains the brains of the system. Most ECSs use a microprocessor or microcomputer as the CPU. This enables the complex ECS to be much smaller and compact than traditional ones. Switches usually plug into the CPU.

Feedback Information Display

The feedback information display tells the user the status of the system and consists of either auditory and/or visual signals. Tones and/or lights enable the user to know which channel is functioning once switches are activated. It is usually located on the front panel of the control box or on a remote display.

Appliances to Be Controlled

Virtually any appliance, from a bedside lamp or fan, to a telephone, or a stereo system can be controlled by an ECS. Initially following injury, this may only be a call bell, fan, and light. Later these would include a TV or radio. At home the telephone, curtains, and doors might be added to the appliance list.

Robotic Workstations

People with even the most severe disabilities can independently control many work and personal tasks with the new robotic workstation attendants appearing on the market.

In most systems, the robot arm can retrieve and return files, manuals, books, and letters, as well as manipulate paper, turn pages, and safely handle diskettes, telephone handsets, and even snacks. The robotic arm is typically controlled through any IBM PC/XT/AT or compatible computer. Success in its use depends largely on user attitude, accessibility, and system performance.

Home Automation

At the center of an automated home is a computer that can link up any number of kitchen appliances, security devices, and TV and stereo components. The computer can receive signals from telephones, hand-held controllers, or touch-sensitive video screens. The electrical wiring allows appliances to respond to one another. For example, when the telephone rings the stereo automatically lowers its volume. As someone moves into a room, the lights go on. If a visitor pushes the doorbell, his or her face is displayed on a TV screen. Thoughtful planning during the home renovations for an individual with a high SCI can take advantage of many of these technological advances, providing increased security and comfort.

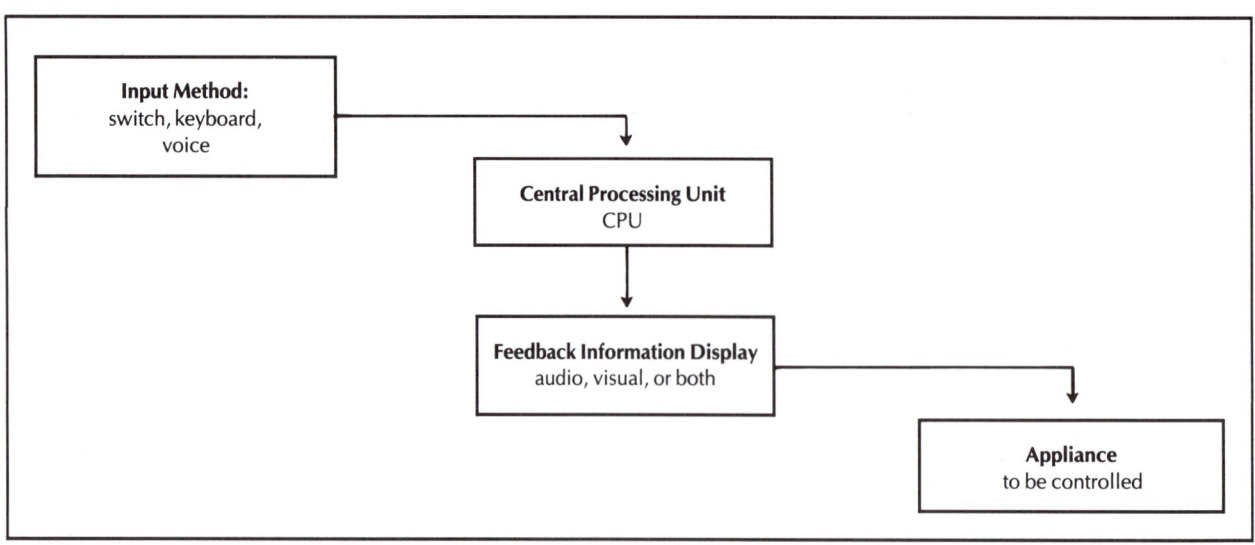

FIGURE 23–1 The four components of an ECS.

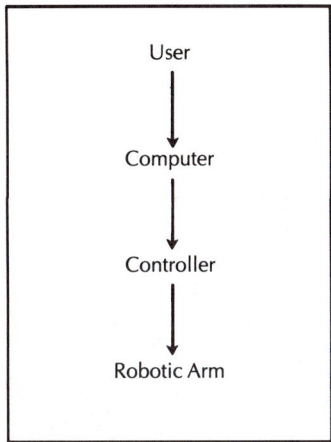

FIGURE 23–2 Control path
for operating a robotic arm.

CONCLUSIONS

Health care providers and rehabilitation professionals must continually ask the following questions when expanding programs:

- How can technology be integrated into the rehabilitation setting early so that control and independence are resumed by clients as quickly as possible?
- Can we justify *not* supporting the purchase of equipment costing a few thousand dollars when we *cannot* put a financial price tag on enhancing personal independence?
- Can we enable patients to take an active role in planning their return home by making phone calls, writing letters, and so on through the use of computers and other technical devices?
- How can we better prepare this new generation of people with high spinal cord injuries for return to work?
- Should we meet with employers to learn more about the workplace and how people with high SCI can be productive in these settings?
- Where can we meet other people who have survived these injuries and are back in society?
- How can we introduce these people to our staff and patients?

Staff expectations for people with high quadriplegia must change. Survival was questionable only a few years ago, but now these people have a good life expectancy. Professionals must now reexamine what quality life-style they can offer these individuals.

Individuals who can operate a telephone, control the environment, and operate a computer can resume control over many aspects of their lives. Planning, organizing, trouble-shooting, researching, directing, and communicating are facilitated by today's technology. Active participation in the rehabilitation process, and later in the community, thus become realistic for high quadriplegic individuals. By teaching people only the mechanics of the technology without giving them meaningful tasks to accomplish with these skills, the most important component of rehabilitation is lost. A mouthstick, a computer, and other technical aids are merely tools. If we train a person to hold a mouthstick without searching for a reason to use it, it will soon collect dust in a cupboard. The vast range of new tools provide new opportunities and require a reexamination of the quality of life possible after the devastation of high SCI.

The health care profession must encourage more studies of how to use this technology and how it impacts attendant-care, self-esteem, independence, and overall quality of life. Preliminary findings are encouraging. Government policies are beginning to accommodate this need, and more people recognize that technology is an essential component to living an independent life with a severe physical disability.

RESOURCES

At first glance, information is difficult to find regarding technical aids for people with disabilities. One way to keep updated with this ever-changing technology is to subscribe to a computer magazine. In addition, there are publications that are geared to the disabled population.

Local colleges, universities, and even high schools are good resources while in rehabilitation as well as when clients return to smaller communities. Communicating with computer science instructors may offer creative solutions for the provision of computer training for clients. Use the Resource section at the end of this book to find further information about adaptive technology.

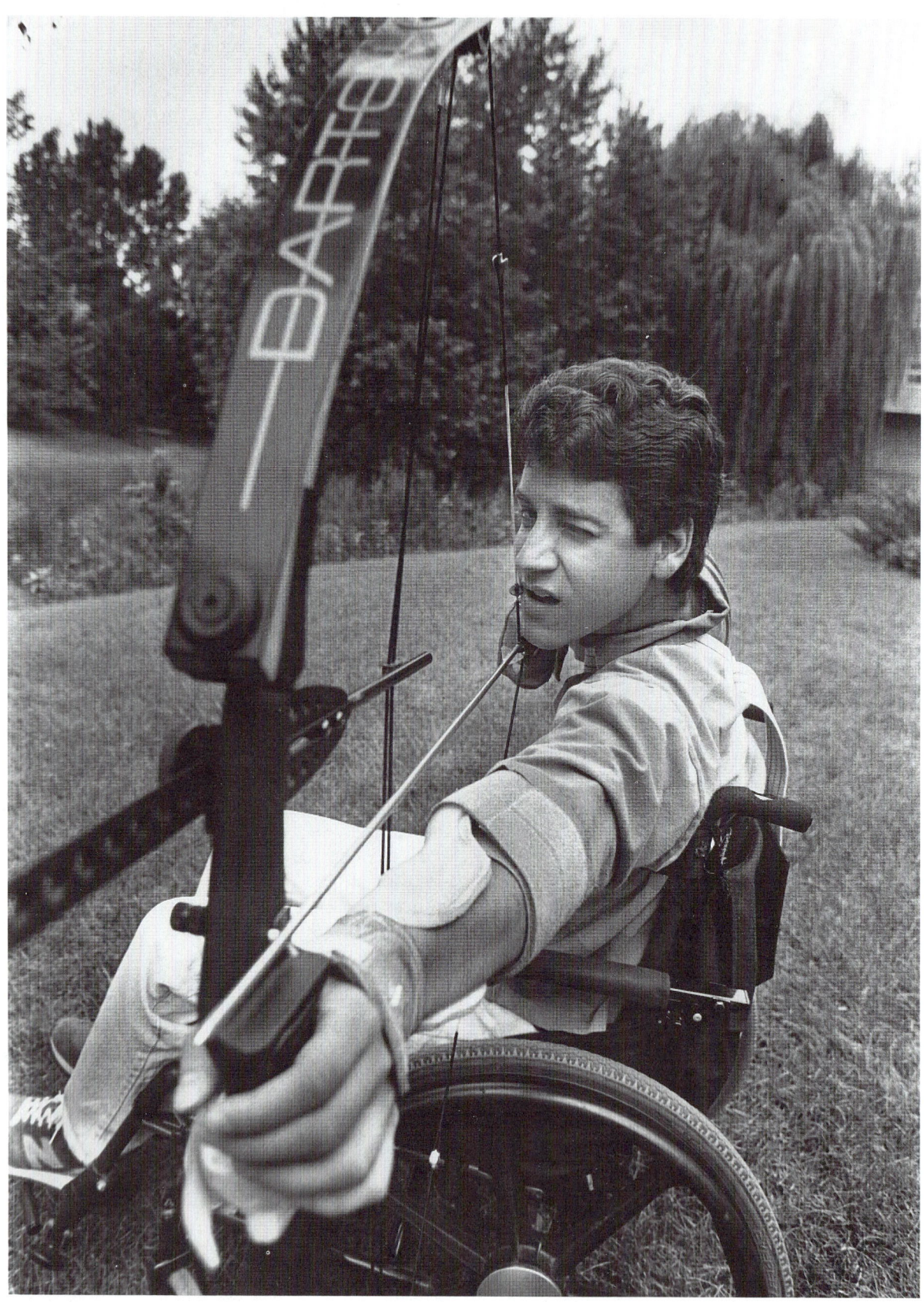

CHAPTER
— 24 —

Sports for Health, Recreation, and Competition

Julie G. Madorsky, M.D.
Arthur G. Madorsky, M.D.
Peter Eriksson, M. Sc.*

Chapter Outline

*The section Wheel into Fitness was contributed by Peter Eriksson.

Objectives of Fitness and Sport

- To provide perspectives on the value of sport and fitness for persons with disabilities
- To describe an approach to fitness for the everyday user and a more progressive approach for the elite athlete.
- To describe principles of adapting or modifying sports for persons with disabilities
- To inform and encourage health care professionals about integrating sport and fitness in rehabilitation programs

THE ROLE OF SPORTS IN REHABILITATION

Sporting and fitness activities create wonderful opportunities to get out, have fun, meet people with similar interests, and generally participate more fully in life. These activities are stimulating and exhilarating, and being part of a group often leads to new friendships and interests. Shared experiences have an equalizing effect because the focus is on a sport rather than on a disability. However, even though sports enhance rehabilitation, sports were a neglected therapeutic tool until recently.

Sporting and fitness activities complement other treatments in the rehabilitation of people with SCI. Through sports, it is possible to improve muscle force (strength), power (force/time/speed), coordination (skill/technique), balance, and reaction time. Cardiovascular disease is now the primary cause of death among people with SCI. Thus, it is crucial that the acute rehabilitation process include a broad range of activities that can enhance long-term physical fitness. Development of the cardiopulmonary system improves levels of fitness and endurance which, in turn, facilitate the achievement of health, functional, psychosocial, and vocational rehabilitation goals.

Sports also offer superb methods of testing the limits of ability, reaching beyond self-imposed and societally imposed boundaries to tap individual potential and harness the power of the champion within seemingly ordinary people. Whether the motivation is "going for the gold," improving one's personal best, or simply getting some exercise, achievement in sports by a person with SCI is often transforming. It develops self-assertiveness, a sense of competence, leadership, and self-esteem. Personal mastery experiences strengthen the conviction that one can be successful. Great accomplishments in one area tend to be broadly generalized to other situations in which performance may have been hurt by preoccupation with fears of personal inadequacies.

Wheelchair athletes become inspirational role models for us all. The achievements of even a few empower many—those who root for them on the sidelines, or watch proudly while they are featured on television.

Conservative Attitudes versus the Right to Risk

In the past it was rarely acknowledged that a physically disabled adult or child might gain as much enjoyment, benefit, and skill from athletic activity as a nondisabled person. The physically handicapped were spectators rather than participants. Well-meaning but impractical diversionary activities were developed for them, such as beanbag toss or balloon bounce, which hardly prepared them for normal competitive sports. Sanitized play experiences were engineered to ensure virtual success on the part of all partici-

---

PERSONAL VIEWPOINT

Rick Hansen became paraplegic at the age of 16 as a result of a motor vehicle accident. With determination and perseverance, Rick studied at the University of British Columbia and began serious training as a wheelchair athlete. In 1985, after graduating from UBC and becoming a World Class Marathon Wheeler, he set out on an around-the-world wheelchair trek, which was successfully completed in 2 years, 2 months, and 2 days. The trek covered more than 24,901 miles (40,000 km) through 34 countries. It was also a love story. Rick met and eventually married Amanda Reid, the physical therapist who accompanied the tour.

During the *Man-in-Motion World Tour*, Rick heightened the world's awareness of the abilities of disabled people and focused attention on the barriers that stand in the way of disabled people reaching their full potential. At the same time, his phenomenal journey raised $20 million. Annual research awards in the areas of SCI rehabilitation innovations and prevention are disbursed, mostly in Canada. (See also Man-in-

Motion Legacy Fund in Resources.) The book *Rick Hansen, Man in Motion*, and quality videotapes are available.

Rick Hansen was honored with the Companion Order of Canada, and represented Canada as Commissioner General at the World Expo '88 in Australia. He is a special consultant to the President's Office at the University of British Columbia with a mandate to establish a model center at the university that will completely open postsecondary education in Canada by promoting fully accessible, supportive environments for disabled persons. Rick is currently the first incumbent Fellow of a National Fellowship on Disability. Named Chairman of Independence '92, an international trade exposition and world congress on disability to be held in Canada in 1992, Rick resides in Vancouver with his wife, Amanda, and new daughter. Rick, with the assistance of a scientific advisory committee, continues to oversee the Man-in-Motion Legacy Fund.

pants, as if losing were tantamount to a pathology that had to be avoided at all cost. Such artificial situations, with few correlates in real life, denied physically disabled individuals the realistic experiences, hazards, and risks to which all people are entitled.

Principles of Sport for Persons with Disabilities

The wheelchair sports movement represents the desire of physically disabled individuals to have normal recreational and competitive athletic experiences and to reach their optimum level of physical fitness, skill, enjoyment, and satisfaction through sports events.

In both recreation and competition, the participants have insisted on departing as little as possible from the original version of each activity; for example, the baskets are not lowered for wheelchair basketball, and the game is played on the same high school and college courts across the country as everyone else uses. Wheelchair basketball is played according to regular National Collegiate Athletic Association (NCAA) basketball rules, with only a few changes made to accommodate the use of the wheelchair. Given the use of scoring handicaps, golf provides a good example of a recreational sport for playing with nondisabled competitors without modifying the game. Never compromising the challenges and risk factors basic to the sport is imperative (Kelley and Frieden 1989).

In most instances, the wheelchair is a common denominator for all participants and assumes the same significance in relation to activities as the polo player's horse, the hockey player's ice skates, and the track athlete's shoes. Its function accords it the status of athletic equipment, and the proficiency of its use becomes in part a measure of the athlete's ability. Sports wheelchairs bear little resemblance to the old-fashioned wheelchairs found in hospital corridors. They have evolved into sleek, low-to-the-ground, arm-powered go-carts, with numerous lightweight features.

INCORPORATING SPORTS INTO REHABILITATION

The Role of Health Care Professionals

Most newly disabled people are especially unaware of the positive opportunities for participation in sporting activities. This is true for family and friends also.* Health care professionals can encourage and inform them early to help physically disabled persons pursue an active lifestyle. Rehabilitation professionals can also educate other colleagues, administrators, legislators, and third-party payers regarding innovative methods that can optimize the health care and quality of life of disabled persons. Research suggests that postdischarge wheelchair athletes have fewer health complications than nonathletic persons with SCI (Stotts 1986).

Program Considerations

Ideal sport and fitness programs within rehabilitation make available:

- A variety of activities sufficiently broad to be attractive.
- Personnel sophisticated enough to produce rapid results that increase motivation
- A climate of expectation of lifelong commitment to fitness

The chances for successful involvement in sports are maximized by:

- An encouraging interdisciplinary team that recognizes the potential value of sport
- Early evaluation of interest and potential for involvement
- Opportunities to observe wheelchair sports
- Challenging role models
- Structured practice sessions during therapy time

Table 24–1 offers suggestions for establishing such a program.

Individual Considerations

Medical/Health Status
An individual must receive a physician's permission to exercise before participating in a physical activity program. This determines if a prescribed exercise program would be contraindicated by the participant's level of health or fitness. This protects people with SCI, who should not start training until previous injuries have properly healed. These injuries could be exacerbated by vigorous exercise, thereby negatively affecting daily living.

In order to be eligible to participate in competitive wheelchair sports, an individual must have a significant permanent physical disability of the lower extremities. Many participants can ambulate, but to be competitive in sports they need to use a wheelchair for mobility.

Regular medical examinations ensure the participant's ability to compete safely. Especially as established competitors become older, unrecognized medical conditions may complicate the known physical disability. Of particular concern are hypertension, cardiopulmonary and renal disease, diabetes mellitus, and anemia. Medical evaluation

---

*Go for It (Kelley and Frieden 1989) is an excellent introductory book, filled with easy reading and remarkable pictures. The Sports 'N Spokes magazine for wheelchair sports and recreation published by the Paralyzed Veterans' Association (Phoenix, AZ) is another excellent resource.

TABLE 24–1   Establishing a Basic Sports/Fitness Program

Needs assessment to assist in planning activities:

- Do patient numbers support initiation?
- What is the target disabled population?
- Are there more patients with quadriplegia or paraplegia?
- Are needs already being served by other organizations?
- Are linkages possible?
- Will community-based groups for people with disabilities be supportive?

Gain interdisciplinary momentum:

- Educate regarding values of sports/fitness
- Gain support of influential physicians and administrators
- Devise funding strategies

Determine and secure sources of funding:

- Will the facility fund start-up costs for the first year?
- Wheelchair sports programs are supported through and by fund raising. Work jointly with a foundation or development department for support.
- Consider events that could be used to generate funding such as tribute dinners, or golf or tennis tournaments.
- Consider formation of wheelchair sports board to raise revenue for program. Seek board members with wealth and influence who believe in the mission—most important!

Plan and implement the program:

- One full-time recreational therapist or individual with adaptive physical education or exercise physiology

training preferred. A wheelchair athlete is desirable but not mandatory.

Volunteers for program support.

Equipment and facilities:

- Identify equipment and facilities needed and available for the training program (such as resistance training equipment, lightweight racing wheelchairs, basketballs, uniforms, and tennis racquets and balls).
- Consider office space, storage space, and a small amount of clerical support.

Basic sports to consider for instruction, therapy, or competition:

- Basketball
- Table tennis
- Tennis
- Track
- Road racing
- Outdoor activities such as snow and water skiing, whitewater rafting, fishing

Public relations:

- Establish relationship with local media, newspaper, television, and radio, to maintain program and maintain high visibility.

Courtesy of David Kiley, B.S., R.T.R., Director, Wheelchair Sports Program, Casa Colina Hospital for Rehabilitative Medicine, Pomona, CA.

and management of these conditions usually allow the individual to participate in sports. Occasionally, a severe medical problem such as renal failure will be uncovered, which may preclude competition.

Stress Testing

Stress testing can evaluate cardiorespiratory fitness and develop parameters whereby maximally efficient training can occur. For individuals over age 35 who have been sedentary or who have a history of heart or blood pressure problems, a graded exercise test is essential. Arm ergometry, for example, can evaluate the response of the heart so that safe limits for training sessions can be established.

Contraindications

There may be specific medical factors to be considered and there may be specific contraindications for certain sports. For example, absolute contraindications to diving are pulmonary conditions that might result in trapping air, such as asthma, emphysema, or tuberculosis, which predispose to air embolism during scuba diving. Other conditions that preclude diving include coronary artery disease and convul-

sive disorders, because an attack while submerged is likely to be lethal.

Medical Classification

A system of medical classification has been refined so that disabled people can compete on equal terms with others. This system is similar to the categorization of competitors in general sports, such as boxing and weightlifting, in which body weight is accepted as the significant factor for equalizing competitive performance. In the case of wheelchair sports, the degree of disability becomes a critical factor in potential performance, so that a quadriplegic athlete with paralysis of the hands and the legs is not pitted against a person with below-knee amputation with normal upper extremities.

In addition to allowing individuals with a similar degree of disability to compete against each other, the classification system keeps physically stronger individuals from dominating the competition, encourages more severely disabled people to play, and in the case of group sports, facilitates balancing of disability levels of teams so that skill and expertise determine who will be the winner.

There are several systems for classification of wheelchair athletes. Muscle strength, the degree of sensory loss, spasticity, sitting balance, deformities, and the cooperation of the athlete during the examination are all evaluated. Training workshops are held periodically to certify physicians and therapists to perform medical classification.

Nutrition to Maximize Performance

A discussion of sports and athletics would be incomplete without reference to dietary recommendations. This subject is unusually haunted by mythology and folklore, contaminated by vitamin, drug, and steroid pushers, and self-styled nutrition specialists. Table 24–2 highlights some factual nutritional information.

WHEEL INTO FITNESS*

Personal Goals

Short- and long-term goals must be identified to ensure that the instructor or coach and participant are striving for the same outcomes (Figure 24–1). When they agree on realistic goals, commitment to activity is usually much greater and success is thus more likely. Short-term goals might be to lose weight, to wheel a mile without a break, or to do transfers to the floor from the wheelchair or vice versa. A long-term goal might be to become a recreational athlete or to wheel a longer distance without rest, for example, 10 miles of constant wheeling.

These goals may be affected by:

- Support of family and friends
- Preinjury sport and exercise history
- Availability of a training partner (Figure 24–2)
- Financial situation

The amount of time the participant is able to commit to exercise training must be determined. A minimum of three 30-minute workouts per week are required for positive training effects. Athletes must be prepared to devote at least 90 minutes of quality training per day in order to improve performance.

The participant's type and level of disability significantly affects expected levels of performance. Participants can maximize their potential by familiarizing themselves with the physiological abilities and limitations of disability. Consulting with the interdisciplinary rehabilitation team members and coach and reading available literature assist in this process. Figure 24–3 outlines a model for individual involvement.

*Wheel into Fitness was contributed by Peter Eriksson, M. Sc., Department of Physical Education and Sport Studies, University of Alberta, Edmonton.

TABLE 24–2 Nutrition to Maximize Performance

- The same diet that enhances health also maximizes performance.
- High-intensity effort during sporting activities demands extra energy.
- Athletes in high intensity training need up to 625 grams of carbohydrate in the daily diet (best obtained from grains, dried fruits, bread, and pasta).
- Muscle glycogen synthesis is maximized by starches instead of sugar.
- Athletes should be encouraged to force fluids at least one-third beyond desire. As little as a 2% drop in body weight due to water loss is associated with impaired performance.
- Athletes, especially women who are menstruating, should consume foods with high iron content. Some may benefit from iron supplementation.
- Athletes should not use vitamin or mineral supplements in amounts above the recommended daily dosages. A prudent diet provides more than adequate quantities of vitamins and minerals.
- Athletes obtain more than enough protein in their normal diets. There is no need for protein supplements.
- Extra fat may be harmful to health in the long term.
- A meal consisting of 500 to 800 calories of light, low-fiber starch is recommended 3 to 5 hours before an athletic event.
- During an endurance event, 400 ml of cold water every 30 minutes is helpful, with or without 250 mg/kg of glucose polymer.

Source: J. Madorsky and A. Madorsky.

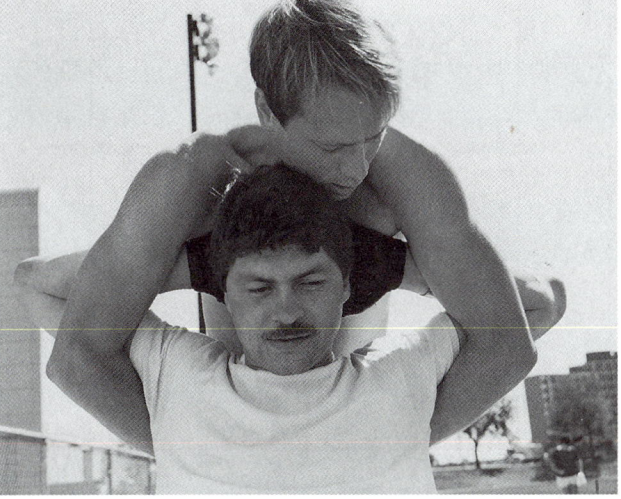

FIGURE 24–1 In the ideal situation, the participant has access to a qualified instructor/coach who can assess, prescribe, implement, and monitor physical activity programs to meet the participant's needs, interests, capabilities, and limitations.

Training Methods and Effects

The Training Year

Three *primary/macro* phases exist within the training year (Figure 24–4). These phases are further divided into *secondary/micro* periods. Thus, this system of subprograms prepares the participant for a greater level of fitness and/or peak athletic performances. By using micro periods, the participant also makes workouts more exciting.

Phase I: Weeks 1–6. The beginning fitness enthusiast first becomes familiar with different training methods and learns different weight-training techniques. For a track athlete, this period would normally occur from October to mid-November.

Essentially, it is an introductory period. Athletes and persons who have been active for more than a year often participate in different activities that develop strength and maintain their basic aerobic fitness levels, that is, take an *active* rest.

Phase II: Weeks 7–26. This phase may occur from about mid-November to the end of April. During Phase II, aerobic training predominates at first, followed by anaerobic activities. Development of a good recovery system also occurs at this time.

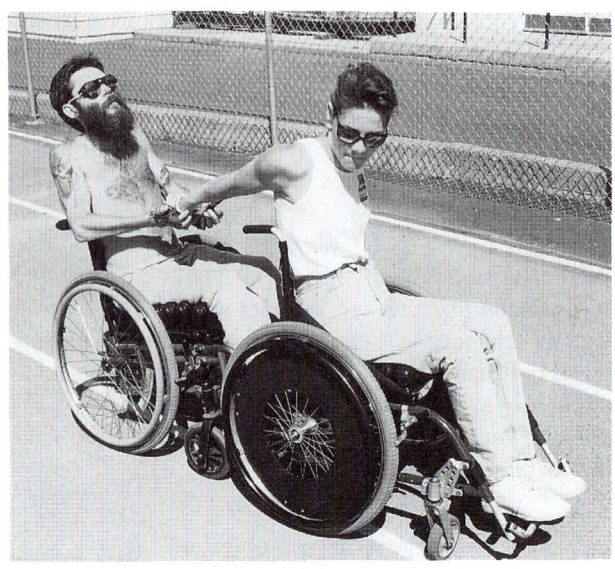

FIGURE 24–2 Training partners add to the fun and challenge of working out.

Phase III: Weeks 27 to the end of the competitive season. For the track athlete, this would normally continue from the beginning of May to the end of September. During Phase III, the athlete reaches peak performance and competes. Nonathletes measure progress or success by con-

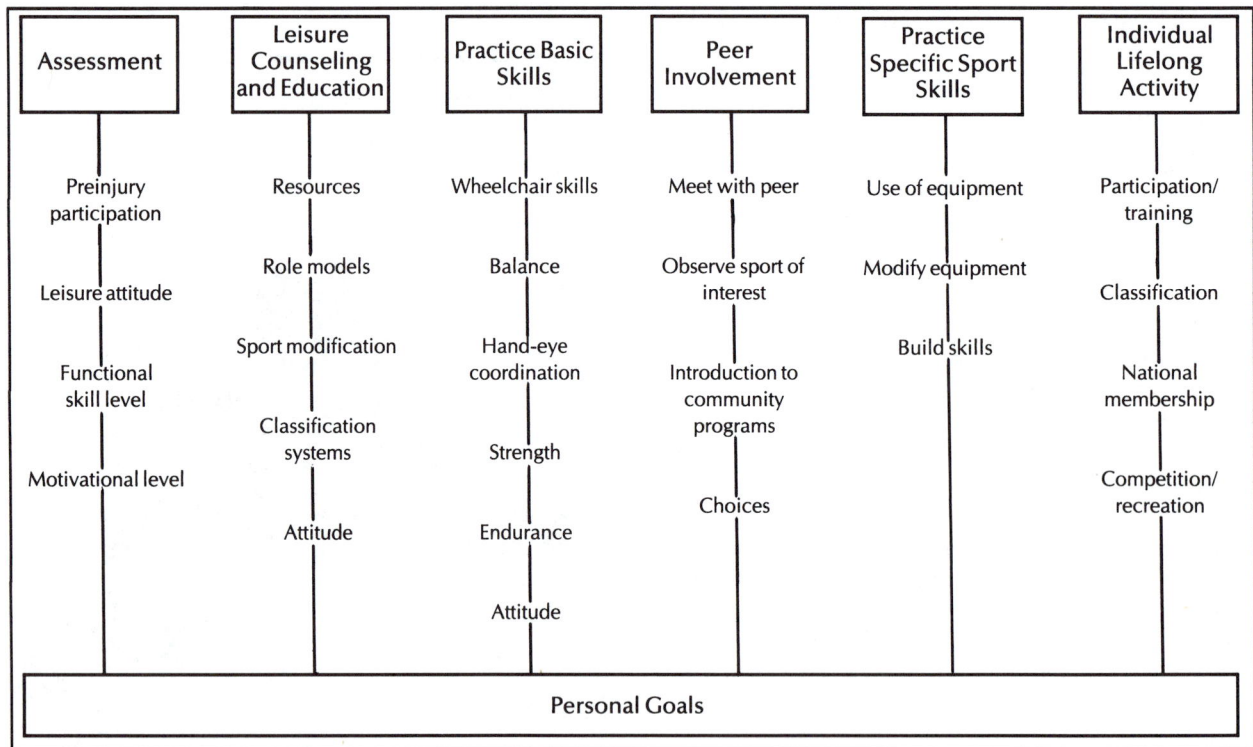

FIGURE 24–3 Model for involving spinal cord injured individuals in sports during acute rehabilitation. (Courtesy of Sherrie L. Burlo, B.S., Certified Therapeutic Recreation Specialist, Casa Colina Hospital for Rehabilitative Medicine)

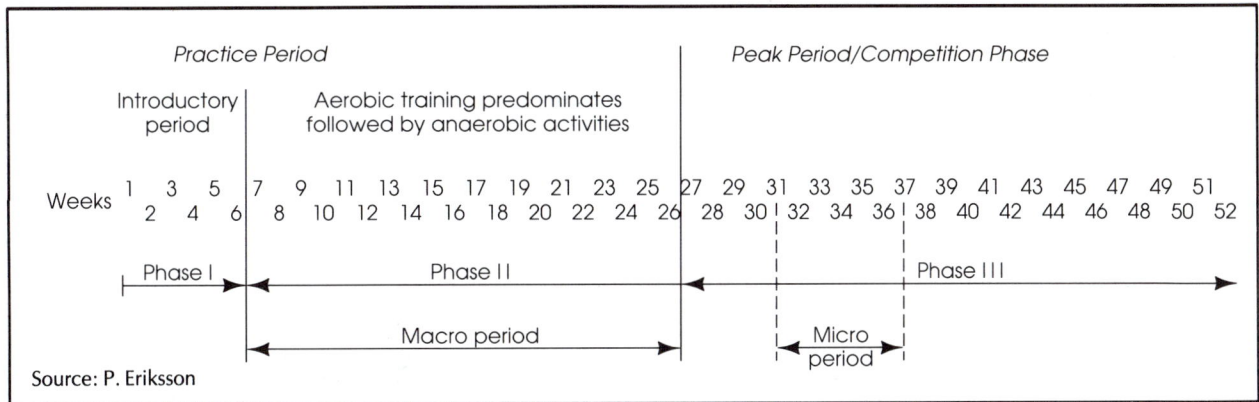

FIGURE 24–4 Division of training year into macro and micro periods.

ducting fitness and performance tests. They can also experience more intense workouts and introduce new activities for training variations.

It is important to maintain *training gains (overload)* throughout the year. During Phases I and II, workouts are geared to *quantity* of training volume increases while intensity remains low. The participant increases the duration of workouts progressively (that is, distance or time) while maintaining a relatively slow speed.

Phase III is spent performing *quality* training whereby speed and intensity are increased and volume is decreased. Because shorter distances comprise quality workouts, a natural increase in speed occurs (Figure 24–5).

The Principle of Supercompensation

Supercompensation is an underlying principle of training program design for today's participant. This method of exercising avoids overtraining and yet maximizes workout benefits. *The key to supercompensation is to allow adequate rest between subsequent workouts.* This rest period is important for the body to be able to replenish the working cells. (This principle is also applied to increasing gradually time periods spent off the mechanical ventilator. See Chapter 16). Supercompensation principles include:

1. The participant performs an initial workout.
2. During the workout the participant becomes exhausted.
3. The participant rests and recovers.
4. Performance *improves*.

The following occur when supercompensation is performed with an extended rest period.

1. The participant performs an initial workout.
2. During workout, participant becomes exhausted.
3. Participants have *too* long rest and recovery.
4. Performance *deteriorates*.

It is essential that balance between workload and rest be optimized to promote improved performance levels. If rest

periods are too long, there will not be an increase in performance levels. For example, if resistance training is conducted only once a week there would be too long a rest period between each training session and consequently no training effect from this type of training.

Figure 24–6 depicts several approaches to supercompensation. Each block may represent a single workout, a week of exercising, or a month of training. *Positive* approaches indicate a progressive increase in training quality, followed by a recovery period. *Negative* approach refers to a decrease in intensity followed by the recovery period. Recovery periods are not complete rests but instead are for *quality training*—and for *quantity training*—reduced duration for a more intense workout.

Supercompensation programs are usually highly individualized. Unfortunately, a trial and error system must be used to determine which approach is best for each participant.

It is easy for a participant to *overtrain*. Overtraining occurs when a person trains too frequently, or at an intensity beyond ability or fitness level without adequate rest between workouts. Thus, some experienced athletes who have been training three times per day for years may never improve.

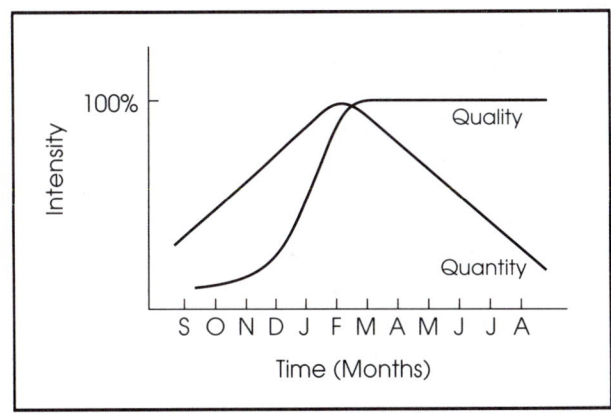

FIGURE 24–5 Changes in training intensity (quality) and volume (quantity) from September to August.

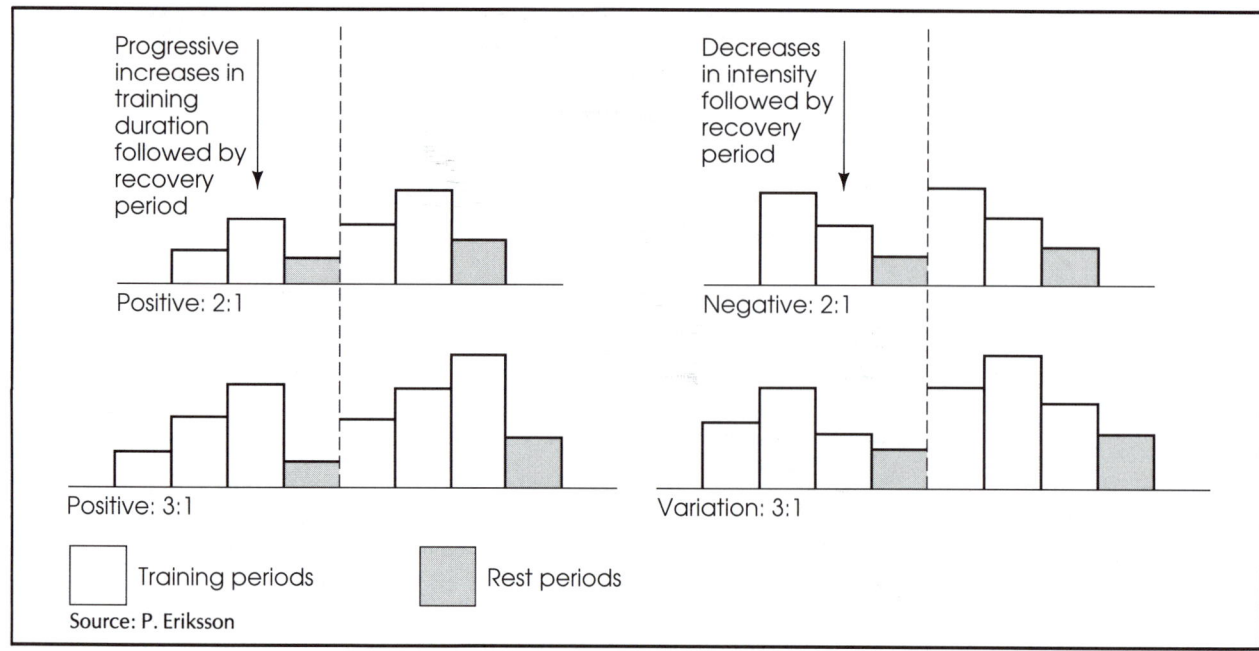

FIGURE 24–6 Four different approaches to supercompensation.

Instructors/coaches and participants must realize that during actual training workouts, the body becomes fatigued. Without the recovery phase, improvement *cannot* occur. Unfortunately, no exact rest schedule ensures that overtraining will not occur. Therefore, *remember to rest!*

General Training Methods

The type and intensity of recommended training depend on several factors, such as the person's level of fitness, scheduled competitive events, time of year, and purpose for training. The coach must keep these points in mind when identifying finer details of the workout.

Training *intensity* is monitored by observing the working heart rate and/or wheeling speed as indicated on a cyclocomputer. This monitoring is a precaution to minimize the risk of overtraining and can be carried out independently by the wheeler.

Determining workout intensity by monitoring the heart rate is effective for highly trained paraplegic athletes, but not accurate for those with quadriplegia (Eriksson 1988). Therefore, persons with quadriplegia benefit most from monitoring wheeling speed on the cyclocomputer. Consequently, each participant must match training intensity with chosen monitoring method by a *trial and error* system.

To understand the different types of training methods and their effects, become familiar with the terminology or language of fitness training (Table 24–3).

Distance Training

Distance training involves continuous work (without rest periods) of long duration. Therefore, total volume of work

is high. Short distance training involves wheeling between 5 and 15 km and long distance from 15 to 30 km. A single workout remains constant throughout. For example, a *new*

TABLE 24–3 Terminology Used in Fitness Training

Duration	Length of time athlete works without rest.
Frequency	Number of workouts per day, week, and so on.
Intensity	Degree of exertion (speed of wheeling, resistance of weights).
Periodization	A period when various training methods are recommended for use.
Repetition (Rep)	Number of times a specific exercise, routine, or event is repeated during a fixed part of the workout.
Rest Period	Length of time athlete is given to recover between work periods. These rest periods must often be determined on an individual basis.
Tempo	Variations in intensity and/or variations within components of a program.
Total Volume	Total time of work. If workout is one continuous effort, duration and volume are identical; if workout has periods of work and rest, volume is sum of the work times.
Volume per Set	Time athlete works for a series of reps or a single set.

Source: P. Eriksson

fitness enthusiast trains at low intensity and performs short distance workouts. Phase I training is usually geared to distance training.

Distance training promotes greater tolerance for endurance work at moderate intensity (submaximal work). For daily life this would enable participants to wheel for their own shopping or go for long walks without being dependent on another person's help.

Slow and long distance training has *local* effects on the capillaries and mitochondria of muscle groups. Fast and short distance training increases *central* capacity in the cardiorespiratory system.

Fartlek Training

Fartlek training also includes workouts of short and long duration. Short Fartlek training involves wheeling between 5 and 15 km, and long Fartlek from 15 to 30 km. During Fartlek training *tempo* changes frequently, which is the distinction between Fartlek and distance training workouts. Intensity for Fartlek training ranges between 40 and 95% of maximum. Shifts in intensity may be planned or may occur spontaneously, based on how the athlete feels or on type and nature of terrain.

Fartlek training combines the benefits of both distance and interval workouts. The following is an example of how to set up a Fartlek workout. The distance of this Fartlek example is 10 km. The average speed in a regular distance training session is 5 minutes per km. Total time for this Fartlek program would be 50 minutes. The program is outlined in Table 24–4 for close examination and understanding.

TABLE 24–4   A Sample Fartlek Workout of 10 km

Time	Exercise	% of Max. Speed	Total Time
5 min	Jog	50%	= 5 min
5 × 1 min	Interval	80%	= 5 min
	Rest (4 × 1 min)	60%	= 4 min
5 min	Jog	50%	= 5 min
2 × 5 min	15 sec work (90%) —15 sec rest	60%	= 10 min
3 min	Rest between set	50%	= 3 min
5 min	Jog	60%	= 5 min
3 × 2 min	Interval	75%	= 6 min
2 min	Rest (2 × 2 min)	60%	= 4 min
3 min	Jog	50%	= 3 min
		Total Time	= 50 min

Source: P. Eriksson

Interval Training

Interval training involves exercising for brief periods of time followed by *active rest* (easy wheeling). Intervals are either long, short, or shorter. Long intervals consist of 5 to 10 repetitions (reps) of 2 and 8 minutes of work (5 reps of 2-minute work bouts with 2 minutes of rest between repetitions). Short intervals require working for 60 to 90 seconds for 5 to 20 reps (for instance, 5 reps of work for 70 seconds, followed by 20 seconds of easy wheeling; allow 3 minutes of rest between sets; repeat sequence). Shorter intervals are 15 seconds in length and are repeated 8 to 40 times (15 seconds of work followed by 15 seconds of easy wheeling for a total of 5 minutes; allow a 3-minute rest; repeat sequence).

Interval training has a positive effect on the body's central capacity. It increases the participant's level of tolerance for short, fast work bouts. In daily life this can be related to pushing the wheelchair easier up a hill or having more power when pushing against a strong wind.

Resistance Training

Resistance training can be oriented to muscular strength, power, and endurance. Power resistance training is most important for wheelchair participants because they receive endurance training by carrying out daily tasks from a wheelchair and/or performing the wheelchair workouts. Participating in an additional endurance weight-training program increases the risk of overtraining and overuse injuries.

Ideally, resistance training is an integral part of the participant's rehabilitation program. When muscular strength is adequate, an individual is better able to transfer and propel up and down curbs, stairs, and hills. Benefits the athlete receives from regular participation in a power-oriented, strength-training program are many—faster starts, a kick during the home stretch, breaking away from the pack, and more efficient uphill propulsion.

A large variety of resistance-training equipment is available. Participants should use apparatus that allows them to carry out the program as independently as possible.

Resistance training activates more motor units in the exercising muscles and therefore, a greater muscle contraction occurs. The muscle also *learns* to contract faster.

The instructor/coach must be familiar with different types of training methods and how they can be appropriately incorporated into an exercise/fitness program. Participants with different levels of cord injury respond differently to various training regimens. Therefore, the coach must often experiment to determine an optimal exercise program.

To reach optimal improvement in a fitness training program, adhere to the following principles:

- Training has to be specific for each participant's needs.
- Training has to be consistent to give the expected result.

- Each activity in the training program has to have properly adjusted workloads organized in a progressive manner.
- Each period of training has to have the optimal resting time, before it repeats itself, to achieve on optimal effect.

Fitness is for everyone (Figure 24–7), but becoming more involved in elite sport requires greater structure and a greater time commitment for specific training (Figure 24–8).

Workout! Five Basic Steps

A basic structure for all physical activity workouts includes the following five components:

1. *Warm-up.* Wheel for 10 to 20 minutes (slow speed).
2. *Stretching.* While sitting in the regular or racing wheelchair, stretch all functional upper body muscles. Stretching routine lasts for 10 to 15 minutes and includes both dynamic (movement through full range of motion, such as arm circles) and static (stretch and hold) exercises. A partner is especially helpful to persons in racing chairs because the sitting position makes it difficult to

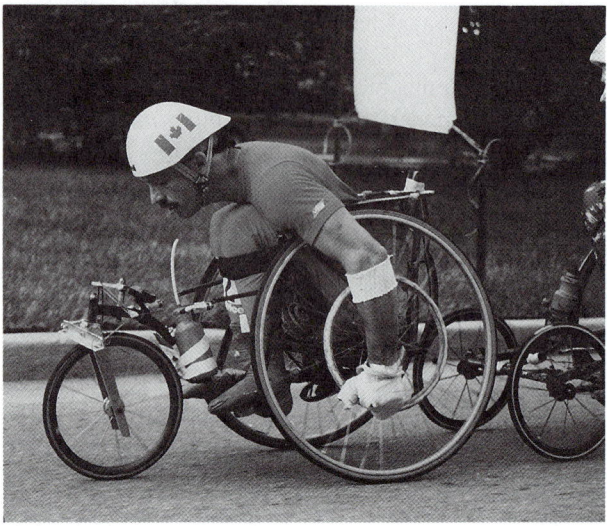

FIGURE 24–8 Elite athletic competition requires intense training.

perform some stretches. Warm-up and stretching components of the workout prepare participant for actual training session by:

- Increasing the body temperature by 1 degree C, which in turn provides a 10% increase in work efficiency
- Increasing the blood flow to the working muscle groups
- Stretching working muscles and ligaments

3. *Actual training session.* Work performed during this component is known as *training methods*, for example, Fartlek, long or short distance, or interval. Each training method has a specific purpose and, therefore, should be carefully selected.
4. *Cool-down.* Wheeling 10 to 20 minutes at a slow pace allows the metabolic waste products to be transported away thereby reducing the likelihood of muscle soreness and stiffness. The cool-down is as important as the warm-up procedure.
5. *Stretching.* This may be performed while still sitting in the racing wheelchair, but is better carried out while in the regular wheelchair because a greater range of motion is often attainable. Post-workout stretching should last from 10 to 15 minutes.

Exercise videotapes, specifically *Aerobics for Paraplegics* and *Aerobics for Quadriplegics*, available from National Handicapped Sports and Recreation Association, Washington, DC, are designed for nondisabled friends to sweat alongside. *Wheeling Skills*, available from the Department of Physical Education, University of Alberta, Edmonton, Alberta, offers a practical guide to daily training for persons with paraplegia.

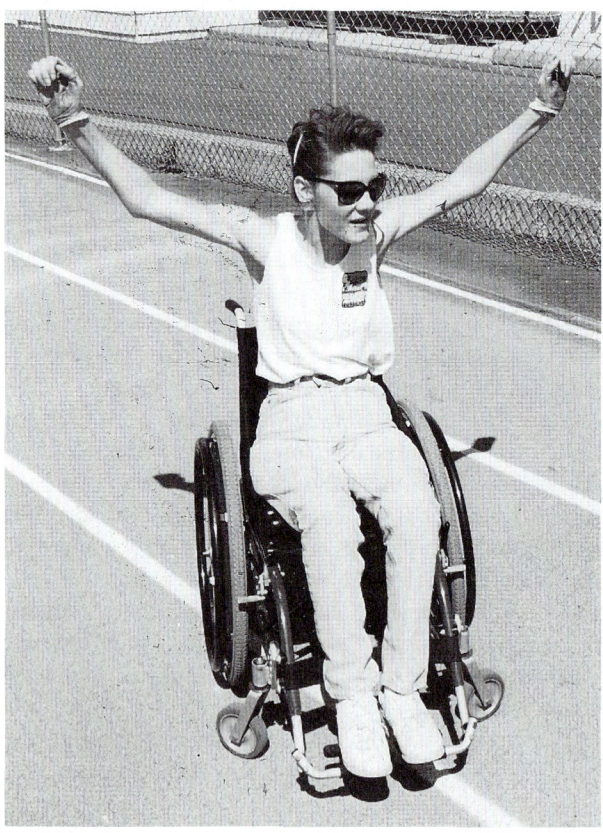

FIGURE 24–7 Working out has become part of America's life-style.

Specialized Training Methods

Long and Short Tempo Training

Long and short tempo training uses the *lactic acid* component of training and is used during different periods of Phases II and III (competition and precompetition). Lactic acid is used by the body as the main energy resource when the intensity is high and the circulatory system cannot provide the working muscle cells with oxygen. This method of training requires adding distance to the events in which the athlete participates or competes and varying the speed intensity.

Long tempo training includes distances from 300 m to 1000 m (for marathon wheelers even up to 2000 meters). Changes in speed may alternate between intense and less intense, progressing from low to high, or vice versa.

Example: 5 × 600 m = first 200 m in 75% of maximum speed, second 200 m in 85%, third 200 m in 95%.

This is a typical example from the competitive period of Phase III training.

Short tempo workouts incorporate distances from 100 m to 300 m, and the variation in speed is similar to long tempo training.

Example: 10 × 150 m = accelerate the speed up to 95% of maximum, with a long, active rest.

This example is typical of the competitive periods of Phase III as well.

Sprint Training (Lactic Acid/Alactic Acid Training)

Sprint training is designed to improve neuromuscular functioning and reaction time. This training is divided into two components:

- *Lactic acid training* (up to 120 m distance). In this type, lactic acid is produced and the body must efficiently eliminate it. Few repetitions and sets are performed at high intensity, and active rest periods are long. This training is used primarily in Phase III (competitive period).

    Example: 5 × 100 m in 95% of maximum speed with long active rest.

    This example can be used during competitive period of Phase III as well. Specific example as above should be used.

- *Alactic acid training* (up to 60 m distances). In this type of training, lactic acid is not produced in working muscles because working time for each repetition is very short and few sets are performed. This training is of very high intensity with long active rest periods.

    Example: 3 × 30 m with flying start in maximum speed, 2 × 80 m with flying start in high intensity, with long active rest (100% work in active, slow rest).

Both of these methods benefit the wheeler's speed and sprint endurance, that is, speed beyond the point of maximum acceleration. It is directed towards the improvement of anaerobic capacity.

Training during Phase I for sprint and middle distance athletes requires wheeling at low intensities for long durations. During this time, the majority of resistance training time is volume oriented (i.e., high reps and sets).

Phase II workouts continue to be *quantity* oriented. Training methods include long and short distance, Fartlek, long interval, long tempo, and strength training. In the second half of the Phase II schedule, the athlete begins to prepare for specific training and the competitive period. Therefore, volume of training begins to decrease while *quality* increases. Short tempo and sprint training are added to train the lactic acid system, while the Fartlek workouts are dropped.

Sprinters and middle distance racers must find the optimal combination of muscular strength, power (speed), and endurance. All of these components are important, and the training method should ensure maximum development of each.

Research indicates that 6 to 8 weeks of strength training without a change in the program will not result in significant improvement (Weinec and Langen 1983). Thus, it is important to change the resistance training program frequently and follow a periodization schedule. Muscular endurance improves as the athlete continues to wheel. Therefore, resistance training is directed toward strength and power components.

The training program must be adjusted to ensure an increase in wheeling speed. If a participant cannot maintain the desired speed due to exhaustion, the workout must be stopped. Training on asphalt provides optimal speed, which in turn produces positive effects. Continuous training on a rubberized track is slow due to high resistance, and the participant does not experience an increase in maximum speed. Every training session throughout the year includes some type of sprint training (for instance, 3 to 5 standing starts; 30 to 80 m accelerations to 90%).

Tempo training plays an important role in middle distance training. Coach and athlete must ensure that speed/tempo are progressively adjusted to different periods of the year. Today's middle distance racers change speeds frequently in races, and therefore athletes must be prepared to respond. For example, during Phase I, the 800 m distance can be performed as 400 m at 70% followed by 400 m at 85%. During Phase II, the 800 m distance can be reduced to 600 m and further divided to 200 m at 70%, 200 m at 80%, and 200 m at 90%. This variation in speed is called *ins and outs* or *split* work.

Endurance Training

Endurance training is the method used most frequently in wheelchair sport. If endurance is not adequately developed, negative effects can be experienced in other components of training, including recovery time. Coach and athlete must be well versed in energy systems, specifically anaerobic versus aerobic to be able to prescribe an ideal training schedule.

Aerobic Training

Aerobic training incorporates distance, Fartlek, and interval workouts; anaerobic training involves working close to actual racing speed by performing long and short tempo exercises. Goals for endurance training for long distance athletes and road racers are:

- To increase speed
- To increase length of time speed can be maintained
- To maintain or increase aerobic capacity (depending on the level of physical fitness)
- To maximize hill speed

Road racers incorporate hill training into their workout schedules, as well as longer total distance sessions. Lactic training is practiced during Phase III, once every 2 to 3 weeks, to enhance quality of training. Work time is 40 seconds to 90 seconds, performed 5 to 8 times. Rest periods between sets are long enough to ensure recovery. Uphill training sessions start on a flat surface to attain high speed. The hill cannot be too steep, because the athlete must be able to maintain high speed for the entire duration. The athlete also prepares for hills by performing Fartlek, distance, and interval routines. The coach and athlete must be aware, however, that many tactical and strategic movements occur during competition on the hills, therefore, it is important to master them.

Overspeed Training

Research from Finland pertaining to runners indicates that overspeed training enhanced maximal running speed. A positive effect has also been noted when wheelchair athletes use this technique during long or short tempo and short distance training. In this training, the athlete works at high intensity (close to maximal power output) at a speed that slightly exceeds maximum speed. For example, athletes perform 200 to 400 m short tempo distances at 90% to 95% of maximum power output with wind at their backs, or wheels on a slight downhill grade. The athlete ensures maintenance of high frequency pushes throughout this training. This training is only used during Phase III, especially during peak performance preparation. It also has a positive psychological effect on the athlete.

Wheelchair track and road racing athletes must specialize more in the future. Thus, each racer should train for and compete in only sprints and middle distances or only long distances and road racing. To be successful in racing, the athlete develops and maintains balance among muscular strength, power (speed), and endurance and must approach training in a very well-planned manner.

To maximize training for all groups of athletes, emphasize speed changes in the training program (*ins and outs/splits*) and develop speed with *overspeed* training on asphalt. Of course, an increase in the athlete's aerobic capacity and in length of time that speed can be maintained are also important.

With more education and information about work physiology, the athlete and coach can acquire greater understanding of how the body responds to training. This results in improved performances and avoids overtraining.

PREPARATION FOR CHOSEN SPORTS

When preparing for participation in a given sport, the training program should be tailored to the specific requirements of the sport. Training can be started in the hospital therapy departments, but there are advantages to early mainstreaming into community health clubs and athletic centers. Table 24–5 includes some tips for selection.

For both physiological and psychological reasons, it is important to emphasize strength, endurance, and skill training simultaneously. In developing increased strength the overload principle appears to be most important. A muscle will grow bigger and stronger only when it must respond to a demand that is not easily met. In fact, results are most consistent when a given muscle group is worked to the point of momentary failure.

For example, the trainee may select a resistance that will cause failure somewhere between 8 and 10 repetitions. The goal is to perform as many full repetitions as possible, but not to stop there. An attempt should be made to make

TABLE 24–5 Guidelines for SCI Individuals on Choosing a Fitness Center

- Shop around! Look for a fitness center that is accessible and convenient to your home or place of work.
- Look for a variety of equipment and activities so that you can work on various parts of your body without getting bored.
- Ask about the training of the attendants. Be certain they have training in exercise physiology or physical education.
- Find out if they are willing to cheerfully help you get on and off the machines if you need assistance.
- Find out if they require a health screening and if they will do a fitness evaluation, so that the intensity, duration, and frequency of your workout will be safe, as well as effective.
- Ask about their emergency policies, and if there is ready contact with an emergency medical service in case of injury.
- Look at the equipment. Is it clean and well maintained, and are the machines appropriate for your needs?

Source: J. Madorsky and A. Madorsky.

SPORTS RESOURCES

ARCHERY

Archery Sports Section, Sister Kenny Institute, 800 E. 28th at Chicago Ave., Minneapolis, MN 55407 (617–874–5712)

National Archery Association, 1750 E. Boulder St., Colorado Springs, CO 80909–5778 (303–578–4576)

BASKETBALL

National Wheelchair Basketball Association, 110 Seaton Bldg., University of Kentucky, Lexington, KY 40506 (606–257–1623)

BOWLING

American Wheelchair Bowling Association, N54W15858 Larkspur Lane, Menomonee Falls, WI 53051 (414–781–6876)

CYCLING

British Wheelchair Motorcycle Association (BWMA), 55 Lochinver, Birchhill, Bracknell, Berks, England RG12 4LD (Telephone 59796)

International Bicycle Tours, 12 Midplace, Chappaqua, NY 10514

FOOTBALL

Blister Bowl, P.O. Drawer P-P, Santa Barbara, CA 93102 (805–962–1474)

Supervisor of Recreation and Athletics, University of Illinois, Rehabilitation-Education Center, 1207 S. Oak Street, Champaign, IL 61820 (217–333–1970)

FLYING

International Wheelchair Aviators, 1117 Rising Hill, Escondido, CA 92025 (619–746–5018)

GOLF

Challenge Golf, P.O. Box 27283, Tempe, AZ 85282

HORSEBACK RIDING

Cheff Center for the Handicapped, P.O. Box 171, Augusta, MI 49012 (616–731–4471)

National Association of Sports for Cerebral Palsy, 66 East 34th Street, New York, NY 10016

North American Riding for the Handicapped Association, 111 E. Wacker Drive, Suite 600, Chicago, IL 60601 (312–644–6610)

MARTIAL ARTS

Stanley K. Gordon, M.D., VA Spinal Cord Injury Clinic, 5901 E. Seventh Avenue, Long Beach, CA 90822

Dennis Palumbo, 12028 F East Mississippi Avenue, Aurora, CO 80012 (303–671–7267)

Sifu Ron Rosen, 1510 York Street, Denver, CO 80207 (303–333–9977)

Ron Scanlon, Casa Colina Hospital, 255 E. Bonita Avenue, Pomona, CA 91767 (714–593–7521)

MOTORCYCLING

Wheelchair Motorcycle Association, 101 Torrey Street, Brockton, MA 02401 (617–583–8614)

NORDIC/CROSS-COUNTRY SKIING

Ski for Light, Inc., 1400 Carole Lane, Green Bay, WI 54313 (414–494–5572)

QUAD RUGBY

Manitoba Wheelchair Sports and Recreation Association, 1700 Ellice Avenue, Winnipeg, Manitoba, Canada R3H OB1 (204–786–5641)

United States Quad Rugby Association, 2418 West Fallcreek Court, Grand Forks, ND 58201 (701–772–1961)

RACQUETBALL

United States Wheelchair Racquet Sports Association, 1941 Viento Verano Drive, Diamond Bar, CA 91765 (714–861–7312)

ROAD RACING

International Wheelchair Road Racers Club, 30 Myano Lane, Stamford, CT 06902 (203–967–2231)

SAILING

American Wheelchair Sailing Association, 512 30th Street, Newport Beach, CA 92663 (714–675–5427)

Council for Disabled Sailors, American Sailing Association Foundation, 60 Padanaram Road, Unit 16, Danbury, CT 06810

SCUBA DIVING

Handicapped Scuba Diving Association, 1104 El Prado, San Clemente, CA 92672 (714–498–6128)

SHOOTING

National Wheelchair Shooting Federation, 545 Ridge Road, Wilbraham, MA 01095 (413–596–4407)

NWAA Air Gun Section Chairman, 296 Stony Hill Road, T–28 Wilbraham, MA 01095

SKIING

Breckenridge Outdoor Education Center (BOEC), P.O. Box 697, Breckenridge, CO 80424 (303–453–6422)

National Handicapped Sports and Recreation Association, Farragut Station, P.O. Box 33141, Washington, DC 20033 (301–652–7505)

(Box continues)

SPORTS RESOURCES   (continued)

SOFTBALL

National Wheelchair Softball Association, P.O. Box 22478, Minneapolis, MN 55422 (612–437–1792)

National Wheelchair Softball Association, P.O. Box 737, Sioux Falls, SD 57101

SWIMMING

Physically Challenged Swimmers of America, 22 Williams Street, Suite 225, South Glastonbury, CT 06073

United States Masters Swimming (USMS), 5 Piggott Lane, Avon, CT 06001

Wheel Aquatics, 1494 Marlborough Avenue, Los Altos, CA 94022 (415–967–7650)

TABLE TENNIS

American Wheelchair Table Tennis Association, 166 Haase Avenue, Paramus, NJ 07652

TENNIS

International Foundation for Wheelchair Tennis, 2203 Timerlouch Place, Suite 126, The Woodlands, Texas 77380

International Wheelchair Tennis Federation, 940 Calle Amanecer, Suite B, San Clemente, CA 92672 (714–361–6811)

TRACK AND FIELD

National Wheelchair Athletic Association, 1604 East Pikes Peak Avenue, Colorado Springs, CO 80909 (719–635–9300)

Wheelchair Athletics of America, 8114 Buffalo Speedway, Houston, TX 77025 (713–668–5376)

TRIATHLON

National Triathlon for the Physically Challenged, P.O. Box 1484, Cupertino, CA 95015 (408–255–8396)

WATER SKIING

American Water Ski Association, 681 Bailey Woods Road, Dacula, GA 30211

Mission Bay Aquatic Center, 1001 Santa Clara Point, San Diego, CA 92109 (619–488–1036)

WEIGHT LIFTING

United States Wheelchair Weight Lifting Federation, 39 Michael Place, Levittown, PA 19057 (215–945–1964)

WILDERNESS TRIPS

C. W. HOG, Idaho State University, Student Union, Box 8118, Pocatello, ID 83209 (208–236–3912)

Outdoors Program, Casa Colina Hospital, 255 E. Bonita Avenue, Pomona, CA 91767 (714–593–7521)

POINT (Paraplegics On Independent Nature Trips), 4101 Cummings, Bedford, TX 76021 (817–267–3029)

S'PLORE, 699 East-South Temple, Suite 120, Salt Lake City, UT 84102 (801–363–7130)

Wilderness Inquiry, 1313 Fifth Street SE, Suite 327A, Minneapolis, MN 55414 (612–379–3858)

MULTIPLE SPORTS

Canadian Wheelchair Sports Association, 333 River Road, Ottawa, Ontario, Canada K1L 8H9 (613–741–2463)

Courage Center, 3915 Golden Valley Road, Golden Valley, MN 55422 (612–588–0811)

International Sports Organization for the Disabled, Stoke Mandeville Sports Stadium, Harvey Road, Aylesbury, Bucks, England HP2 1PP

Shared Outdoor Adventure Recreation (SOAR), P.O. Box 14583, Portland, OR 97214 (503–238–1613)

The Sports Training/Research Institute for Disabled Athletes (STRIDA), 115 Wittich Hall, University of Wisconsin, La Crosse, WI 54601 (608–785–8695)

Vinland National Center, P.O. Box 308, Loretto, MN 55357 (612–479–3555)

Prepared by J. Madorsky and A. Madorsky

as many partial repetitions as possible until unable to move the resistance at all. One set of any given exercise, performed as noted above, is significantly more productive than any number of sets that are not performed to the point of failure.

Gradually increasing the exercise resistance as the muscle becomes stronger is termed progressive resistance. Let us take, for example, an exercise that requires two sets of 8 to 10 repetitions. With appropriate technique, 9 and finally 10 repetitions will be possible with that resistance since the muscle has increased in strength. When, as an example, 10 repetitions are possible on either two or three sets, five pounds is added to resistance. The resistance can be "tuned"

so that failure always occurs between 8 and 10 repetitions. Exercise myopathy, or overwork weakness, is virtually impossible under these circumstances: the last repetitions before failure are actually the safest from the standpoint of injury to muscle and joint because less tension and force are being produced by the muscle structure.

If the resistance is light so that failure occurs only after a relatively high number of repetitions have been performed, the training effect will be primarily an increase in muscular endurance, but if the resistance is heavy so that failure occurs after a relatively low number of repetitions have been performed, the training effect will be primarily an increase in muscle strength.

Individuals with SCI who use overload and heavy progressive resistance cannot tolerate daily training. In fact, due to the physiology of muscle, increase in muscle size and strength actually occurs during the rest period following exercise. It is recommended that at least 24 to 36 hours of rest from resistance training and endurance training be experienced to allow for recovery and allow for the training effects to establish themselves. Three training sessions per week appear to be reasonable for most patients with SCI, but for a significant number two workouts per week can be very effective.

NATIONAL WHEELCHAIR ATHLETIC ASSOCIATION (NWAA) EVENTS

The National Wheelchair Athletic Association (NWAA) uses a class system for organized competitions summarized in Table 24–6. Note athletes with comparable disabilities are included; other factors are considered and regulations are regularly reviewed.

Field Events

Conducted in accordance with National Collegiate Athletic Association (NCAA) rules, field events include distance, javelin, shotput, discus, and club throw, which is limited to Class IA athletes. These events are performed from the wheelchair in a stationary, stabilized position. Raising off the chair is a disqualifying maneuver.

Pentathlon

Pentathlon is a five-event competition open to all classes, which tests the athlete in a single day in the following events:

TABLE 24–6 NWAA Class System for Organized Competitions: A Summary

Class	Description
IA, IB, IC	Refers to athletes with complete and incomplete quadriplegia; triceps function is critical
II	Refers to complete and incomplete paraplegia; T_{1-5}; abdominal muscle and trunk control (sitting balance) is critical
III	Basically T_{6-10}
IV	Basically $T_{11}-L_2$
V	Below L_2
V, VI	For swimming events only

shotput, javelin or club throw (200 meter or 100 meter), discus, and distance (1500 meter or 800 meter). The winner of the pentathlon is the competitor who scores the highest number of points in all events.

Slalom

Slalom competition is a test of agility, strength, skill, and speed. The course is no longer than 100 meters. This event is held on a gymnasium floor or other smooth surface, and is defined by flags around which the athlete must maneuver the chair both forward and backward. In Classes II to V competition, obstacles are added that may include different sized ramps, platforms, slopes, hurdles, textured surfaces, low head clearances, and bridges. Missing any of the gates results in disqualification and each flag struck adds one second to the actual time. The slalom competitor becomes more acutely aware of ability to maneuver the wheelchair with agility, grace, and speed.

Swimming

The strokes used in competition are breast stroke, back stroke, freestyle, front style, and butterfly. Classes IA, IB and IC competitors swim 25 yards; Classes II and III swim 50 yards; and Classes IV, V, and VI swim 100 yards. The individual medley for Classes IA and IB is composed of 25 yards of back stroke and front freestyle. The individual medley for IC is composed of 25 yards of back stroke, breast stroke, and freestyle, in that order. Classes II and III swim 25 yards of the butterfly, back stroke, breast stroke, and front freestyle, in that order. Classes IV, V, and VI swim 50 yards of each stroke in that order. All swimming events start in the water. Many disabled swimmers have joined the United States Masters Swimming (USMS) program. They race against nondisabled swimmers, categorized by speed rather than age, sex, or disability.

Table Tennis

Table tennis is open to all competitors. Classes IA to IC are permitted to secure the paddle to their hand by tape or a brace. All competition is governed by the United States Table Tennis Association rules, with modifications as necessary to accommodate wheelchair movement. A single elimination system is used, which results in the loser of each match being eliminated from the competition and the winner advancing to the next round of play.

Table tennis is a keenly competitive indoor sport that requires little space. It is an ideal sport to start in the rehabilitation center and to continue at home. It is one of the sports that a person with a disability can play competitively against a nondisabled opponent. This is one of the few wheelchair sports in which a higher than usual wheelchair is acceptable. Some players keep such a chair especially for playing the sport; others use an extra-thick wheelchair cushion to raise themselves higher in the chair.

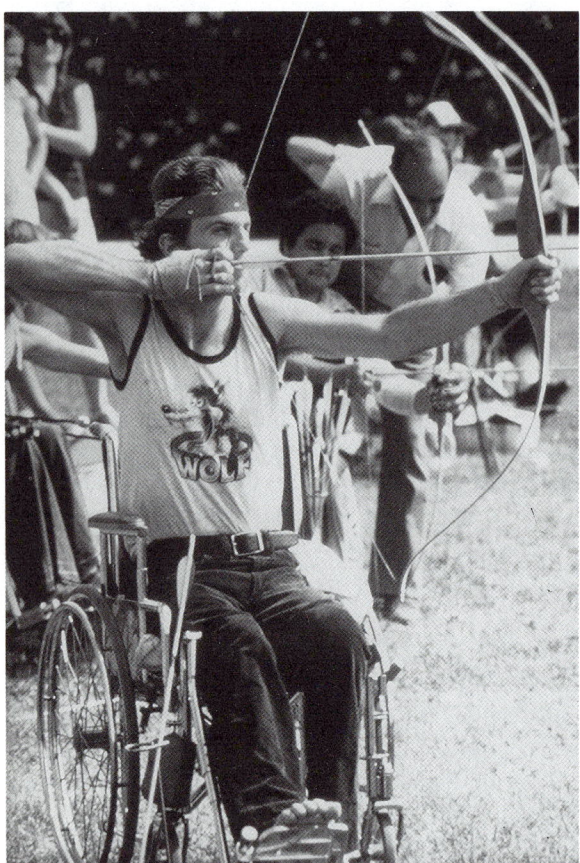

FIGURE 24–9 Archery is a favorite activity at many summer sports camps for spinal cord injured youth.

Target Archery

Target archery is conducted in accordance with international archery rules. It is not separated by class, except for the quadriplegic round in which special aids are used for shooting. Competitive rounds are novice round, short metric, and advanced metric for males and females. A spinal cord injured archer can compete not only in NWAA, but in any National Archery Association nondisabled meet.

Track

Events are run in preliminary heats and finals on a hard surface track with a minimum of six lanes. The front wheelchair castors constitute the starting and finishing points. Staying within National Wheelchair Athletic Association standards, the individual may modify the chair by canting the wheels for stability, adding eight-inch semi-pneumatic castors for a smoother ride and smaller push rims to achieve a greater number of revolutions per push. In all events except the 400-meter mixed relay, there is separate competition for males and females. See Table 24–7.

TABLE 24–7 Individual Track Events

Class	Dash	Distance	Relays
IA	60 M, 100 M	200 M , 400 M	400 M Mixed
IB	60 M, 100 M	200 M, 400 M	
IC	100 M	200 M, 440 M, 800 M	
III	100 M	200 M, 400 M, 800 M, 1500 M, 5000 M	400 M
V	100 M	200 M, 400 M, 800 M, 1500 M, 5000 M	800 M, 1600 M

Source: J. Madorsky and A. Madorsky

Weightlifting

This event is not classified like the other sports. Body weight alone determines the proper division for bench-pressing. The lifts achieved by people with paraplegia are phenomenal, in some cases above 500 pounds. The official body weights for the respective divisions are presented in Table 24–8.

OTHER SPORTS FOR RECREATION AND COMPETITION

Air Guns

Air rifle and pistol shooting competition requires shooting from three positions using a specially designed shooting table attached to the athlete's wheelchair. These positions are shot in accordance with the International Shooting Union rules.

TABLE 24–8 Weightlifting Divisions

Light featherweight	Up to 112–1/4 lb (51 kg)
Featherweight	Up to 125–1/2 lb (57 kg)
Lightweight	Up to 143–1/4 lb (65 kg)
Middleweight	Up to 165–1/4 lb (75 kg)
Middle heavyweight	Up to 209–1/4 lb (95 kg)
Heavyweight	Over 209–1/4 lb (95 kg)

Source: J. Madorsky and A. Madorsky

All-Terrain Vehicles

All-terrain vehicles include from three- to eight-wheel vehicles and provide opportunities for recreation in snow, water, sand, or on race tracks. The Wheelchair Motorcycle Association tests many of these vehicles and advises disabled ATVers, as well as the manufacturers, on modifications and accessories.

Basketball

Wheelchair basketball is the oldest competitive wheelchair sport and continues to be one of the most popular.

The National Wheelchair Basketball Association (NWBA) uses classification systems applicable to both incomplete and complete spinal cord injured individuals (NWBA 1979). Flexibility of approach needs to be exercised in difficult cases, such as incomplete SCI, poliomyelitis, and multiple sclerosis, keeping in mind that the whole purpose of the system is to allow fair competition.

To achieve proper team balance in wheelchair basketball, each classification is given a numerical value, as follows: Class 1—one value point; Class 2—two value points; and Class 3—three value points. At no time in a game can a team field five players with total value points greater than twelve.

The chair is considered a part of the player. General rules of contact in regular basketball, such as charging and blocking, apply to wheelchair basketball. For any jump-ball, jumpers must remain firmly seated in the wheelchair; that is, not lift buttocks off the seat by use of an arm or leg or force of movement, and must be in the jumping circle at the 45-degree angle to their own baskets. Offensive players cannot remain more than 5 seconds in the free-throw lane while their team is in possession of the ball in their particular court. A player may wheel the chair and bounce the ball simultaneously, just as a player may run and dribble the ball simultaneously in stand-up basketball. In addition, a player who possesses the ball can take no more than two consecutive pushes with one or both hands in either direction. If two pushes are taken, the player must shoot, pass, or bounce the ball one or more times before pushing again. The latter can be repeated without double dribble violation. Three or more consecutive pushes by a player who possesses the ball constitutes a traveling violation.

If a player in possession of the ball makes any physical contact with the floor, or tilts so far forward that the footrests touch the floor, or so far backward that the antitip castors touch the floor, it is a violation and the ball is awarded to the other team.

Players are considered out-of-bounds when they or any part of their wheelchairs touch the floor on or outside the boundary.

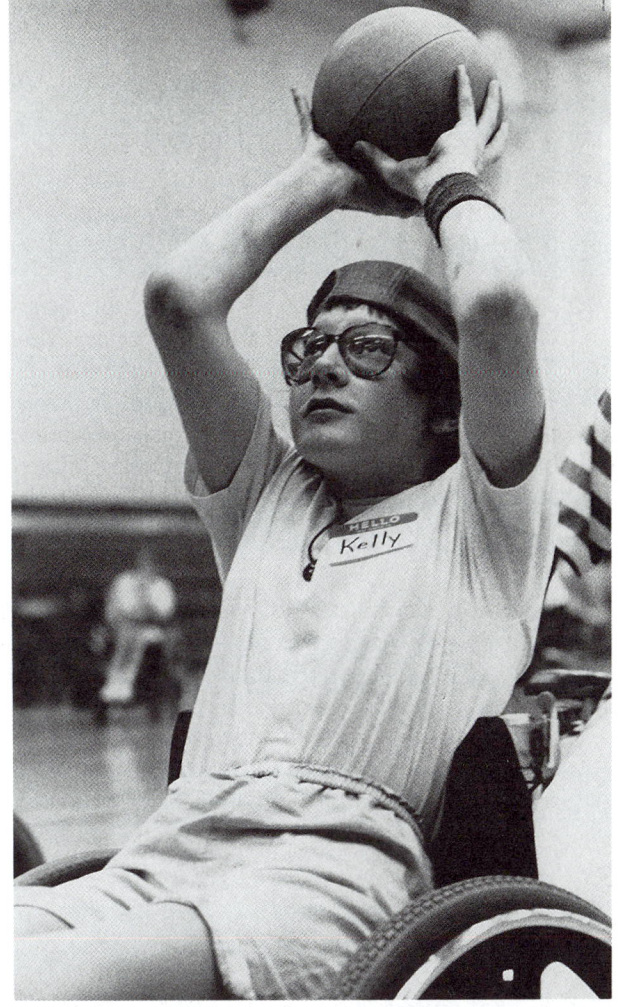

A

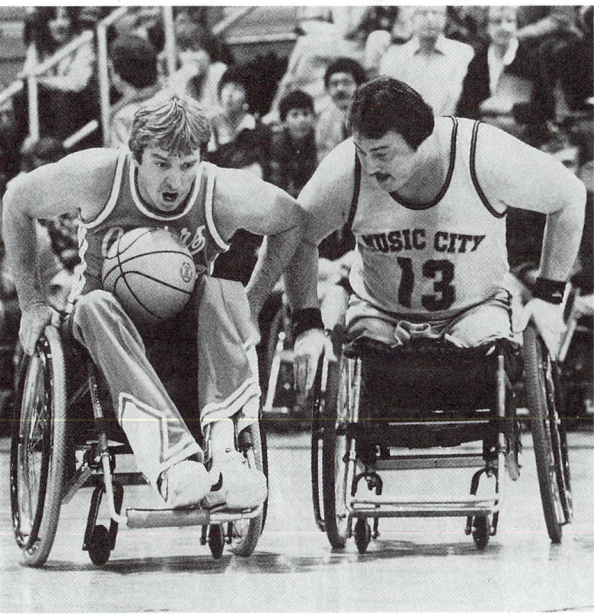

B

FIGURE 24–10 Wheelchair basketball is played at the recreational (**A**) as well as the competitive (**B**) level all over the world.

Basic rules are keeping firmly seated in the wheelchair at all times and not using a functional leg for physical advantage over an opponent. An infraction of this rule constitutes a physical advantage foul. Three such fouls disqualify a player from the game. A free-throw is awarded and the ball is given to the opposing team out-of-bounds.

A defensive player who commits a personal foul in the opponent's back court is charged with a back court foul. The offended player is awarded two free throws.

If a competitor falls from the wheelchair during play, the official will suspend play if there is any chance of danger to the fallen player. If not, the officials will withhold their whistles until the particular play in progress has been completed. If a player falls out of a chair to gain possession of the ball, or by falling keeps the opponents from gaining possession of the ball, the ball is awarded to the opposing team.

Bowling

Wheelchair bowling is regulated by the American Wheelchair Bowling Association (AWBA), which has been in existence for 27 years. Five hundred members take advantage of opportunities for local league play, as well as regional and national tournaments. Adaptive equipment is available, such as snap-handle balls and bowling sticks. Some people with quadriplegia use bowling ramps, although they are not sanctioned by the AWBA.

Cycling

Bicycling enables those with incomplete spinal cord syndromes and good balance to experience simultaneous workout of upper and lower limbs during an activity that provides speed and independence in mobility. The bicycle has been adapted to enable a person to use handpower to propel it. Some units attach to a wheelchair and others are self-contained cycles. Most individuals with lower extremity paralysis can ride a hand-powered tricycle. Standard handlebars are replaced by a hand-cranked chain and linkage attached to the front wheel to provide propulsion and a steering mechanism. Braking is achieved by back pedaling with the hands.

Another alternative for the wheelchair user is an attachable hand cycle unit. A single wheel and hand pedals are attached to the front of a manual wheelchair. Standard three-speed and five-speed models are available. The cyclist can travel at speeds of 10 to 15 miles per hour.

Indoor stationary bicycle exercisers for upper or lower extremities provide ideal preparation for cycling.

For those with upper neuron paralysis of the lower extremities, computerized functional electrical stimulation of the muscles of the legs allows for cycling a specially designed bicycle ergometer. Contractions of these muscles through the use of electrical stimulation can prevent or minimize disuse atrophy, increase muscle size and bulk, recondition the paralyzed or paretic lower extremities, and improve cardiopulmonary functioning.

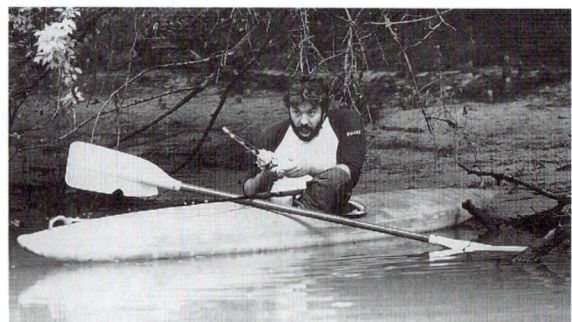

FIGURE 24–11 The great outdoors is for everyone. This spinal cord injured man is about to reel in a trout.

The computerized functional electrical stimulation protocol is divided into three phases:

- *Phase I: Leg Training.* Stimulation to quadriceps to assess tolerance to electrical stimulation and ability for strengthening through progressive-resistive exercises.
- *Phase II: Ergometry.* Stimulation of quadriceps, hamstrings, and gluteals to produce bicycling motion and physiological responses to exercises. This phase includes progressive treatment three times a week up to 30 minutes each time. When able to train 30 minutes without muscle fatigue, training frequency is dropped to twice per week.
- *Phase III: Community/home program.* Preprogrammed stimulation in the community or at home using custom-made garments with built-in electrodes. Programs of stimulation are encoded on computer cartridges that can be taken home or be used independently without the aid of professionals. Progress may be reevaluated every 3 months, with updating of the cartridge accordingly.

Fishing

Fishing is organized for recreation and competition on ocean, lake, and river trips. A variety of assistive devices are available for people with different disabilities: special switches, including sip and puff controls for reels, and casting devices that enable people with quadriplegia to toss the bait 40 feet or more.

Flying

The Federal Aviation Agency approves hand-controlled flying. Permanent and portable hand controls make it realistic for pilots with SCI to fly. Training and specially equipped aircraft are also available to those who wish to become sailplane pilots.

Football

Wheelchair football has been played for almost 40 years. Like stand-up football, the game tends to be rough. There are only

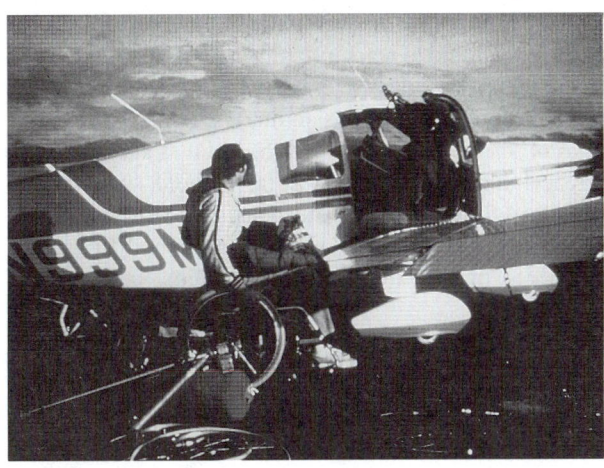

FIGURE 24–12 This pilot returned to flying after SCI. His plane has hand controls similar to, although somewhat more complex than, automobile hand controls.

a few changes from National Collegiate Athletic Association rules. A 60-yard hard surface playing field with eight-yard end zones, six-person teams, two-hand touch tackles, downfield throws to stimulate kicks and 15 yards for a first down include most of the modifications. Ramming or colliding chairs from the front is legal. Ramming from the rear or into the large wheels is clipping and results in a 15-yard penalty.

Football is played by either all-male or by co-ed teams. In the Blister Bowl, an annual wheelchair football tournament held in Santa Barbara, California, the rules stipulate that each team must have at least one woman or one person with quadriplegia on the field at all times.

Golf

Golf is another activity in which individuals with disabling conditions can participate with nondisabled partners. Many golfers with paraplegia play seated in either a manual wheelchair that has the arms removed, a three-wheeled scooter, or a motorized golf cart. Special seats that swing to the side permit the player to hit the ball from a quasi-standing position. People who can ambulate, with or without adaptive equipment, may play from the standing position.

Gymnastics

Gymnastics demands superb conditioning, strength, posture, and skill. Although no special competitive opportunities are provided for mobility-impaired individuals, individuals with paraparesis or cauda equina injuries compete successfully in high school and university championships.

Horseback Riding

Opportunities are available for individuals with SCI to participate in equestrian competitions through the National Association of Sports for Cerebral Palsy (NASCP). Competitors who have complete or incomplete cervical cord injury are catego-

rized as Class I; those who have complete or incomplete paraplegia below T_1 down to and including T_6 are Class II; and those with complete or incomplete paraplegia below T_6 down to and including T_{12} are Class III competitors. Class IV competitors are those who have paralysis between L_1 and L_3 levels; Class V competitors are paraparetic with L_{4-5} levels; and Class VI have S_1 through S_3 levels of paralysis.

All riders wear protective headgear with a full chin harness. Special adaptive tack, such as handholds, Devonshire boots, neck straps, saddle covers, and ladder reins may be used where appropriate. A ramped mounting area is made available for wheelchair users and an accessible staired block for ambulatory persons. Competition events include equitation on the flat obstacle course, relay race, and dressage.

Hunting

Hunting by either bow and arrow or gun is regulated by state laws. Many states allow disabled individuals to hunt from a vehicle and may issue free licenses. Information on state regulations may be obtained from each state's Wildlife Management Service.

Kayaking, Canoeing, and Rafting

Few modifications to the kayak are needed to accommodate most disabilities. Adjustments can be made to improve the seating system and back support, if needed.

Canoeing is available both as a recreational activity and for competitive races across lakes and down whitewater rapids. Though individuals with SCI who have good upper extremity and trunk function find canoeing an ideal sport, those with higher levels of injury may require adaptations, such as lowering the seat or replacing it with either a sling or a molded plastic seat to improve back support and stability. Most canoeists use their wheelchair cushions to provide skin protection while in the canoe. A paddle wheel has been developed for people who lack upper extremity strength and

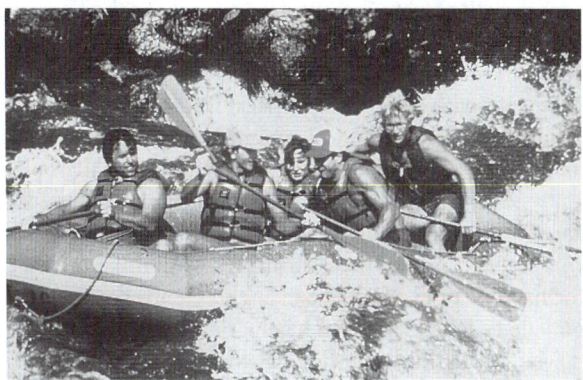

FIGURE 24–13 White water rafting is an exhilarating outdoor sport for the brave, whether nondisabled or disabled. It is, however, done under strict safety guidelines.

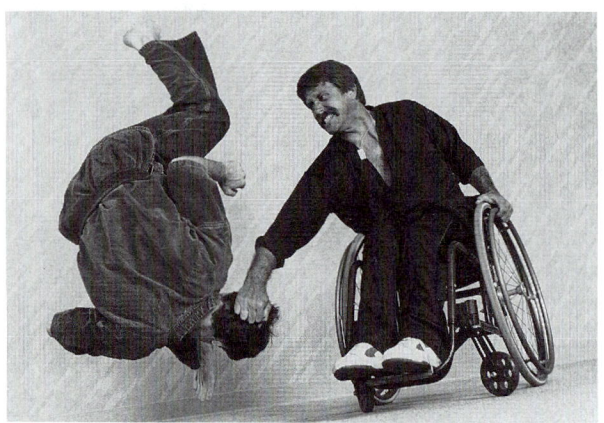

FIGURE 24–14 This 8th-degree black belt athlete studied martial arts *after* sustaining SCI. Martial arts provides excellent development of physical and mental skills. The ability to defend oneself is important to everyone.

endurance. It is used as on a hand-driven bicycle to provide power and balance.

Rafting is facilitated by seating individuals with SCI on several life preservers and their wheelchair cushions, which raises them high enough to lean over and paddle. A Velcro belt can also be hooked from the individual to the sides of the raft for increased stability.

Martial Arts

Today's wheelchair sports have correlates in real life and can be used as an effective means of developing the self-confidence and the physical skills needed to deal with real hazards and risks, thereby enhancing capability for survival (Madorsky, Scanlon, and Smith 1989). Since disabled persons are often perceived to be helpless and unable to protect themselves, they are seen as easy targets for violent crime, including homicide, assault, rape, and robbery. It is estimated that 100,000 disabled women were victims of rape in 1981.

Self-defense classes teach disabled persons a repertoire of coping skills to use when under physical attack. They also minimize the psychological handicaps of fear and vulnerability.

Persons with significant physical limitations need to develop an understanding of prevention, psychological defense, and assertive communication skills before attempting a physical defense. Underestimating one's capabilities is as dangerous as overestimating them. Current consensus favors preparation and practice for an assault situation so that the first one or two moves can be sufficiently devastating to provide time to escape, seek help, or sound an alarm.

Martial arts offer time-honored methods of self-protection for people who are physically disadvantaged. Kung Fu is also an effective method of training for self-protection and survival. It is based on techniques devised approximately 4,000 years ago by Chinese monks who sought to develop their

intelligence to outwit an opponent. Techniques of Kung Fu develop the mind to react instantly to any situation regardless of the practitioner's size, strength, or position in space (prone, supine, sitting, or standing). The practice of routines of offensive and defensive techniques also improves physical fitness, stability, accuracy, speed, and power, which culminates in automatic reactions to thwart a physical assault. Uechi-Ryu Okinawan Karate and Jujitsu are additional martial arts practiced by spinal cord injured individuals.

Mountaineering

Wheelchair mountaineering is a form of exercise, endurance, and survival training that is valuable in the long-term physical and emotional rehabilitation of selected individuals (Madorsky and Kiley 1984). Wheelchair users, like those who are handicapped, may rise to a challenge for no other reason than "because it is there."

Some of the incredible physical challenges that paraplegic climbers have overcome are exemplified by the 1982 climb of the 8,751-foot summit of Guadalupe Peak in Texas. Three members of the organization Paraplegics On Independent Nature Trails (POINT) completed this 5-day journey. The grueling climb was divided into three parts; the first involved traversing almost three miles of steep switchbacks with sheer dropoffs of more than 200 feet; the second part involved the trail, which wound about a mile from the crest through wooded mountainsides to a campsite three-quarters of a mile below the summit. The final day

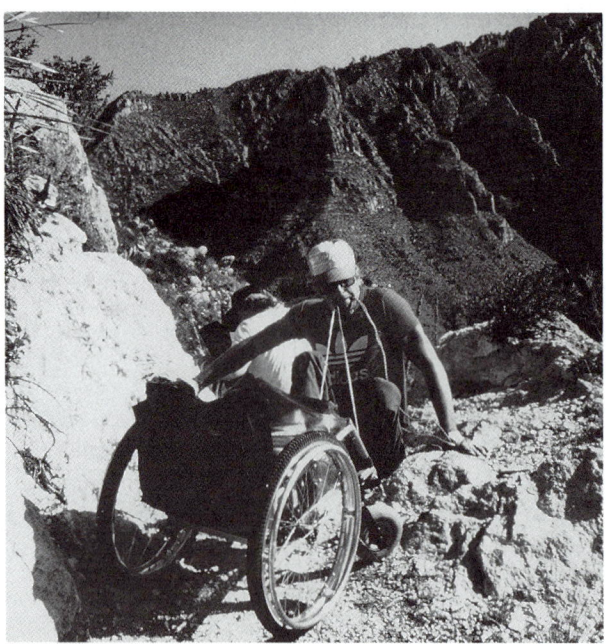

FIGURE 24–15 Mountain climbing is not for everyone, but this picture is a wonderful reminder of the high levels of physical conditioning that spinal cord injured people can and do achieve.

was spent climbing to the peak, where the angle of slope was 35 to 45 degrees. Slowed by intense midafternoon temperatures that neared 100°F, they crawled and clawed their way, and pulled their chairs up the last several hundred yards. The trail was so steep in parts that they had to get out of their wheelchairs and pull chairs and equipment along by ropes clenched between their teeth.

In 1989, a paraplegic climber ascended the 3,500 foot El Capitan by pulling himself up anchor ropes, the equivalent of 7,000 pull-ups. He used a **T**-bar, a special harness which allowed him to rest whenever he needed to, and well-padded pants that protected his paralyzed legs from being injured against the rock. An able-bodied partner provided assistance by anchoring ropes at each stage of the ascent.

Quad Rugby

Quad rugby is the only sport exclusively for persons with quadriplegia. Its aggressive roots are suggested by its original name, Murderball. Only manual wheelchairs are permitted; power chairs are not allowed.

The game is played with a volleyball on a basketball court, with two restricted zones about 5 feet deep by 24 feet long delineated on each end. Two teams of four players each attempt to score points by carrying the volleyball across the opposing team's end line.

As with wheelchair basketball, teams are balanced to allow players with different levels of quadriplegia to participate fairly. Players are classified according to the NWAA system. Players with the greatest levels of disability are assigned one point; those who are least disabled, three points. Each team's players must total no more than eight points on the court.

Up to three offensive players are allowed in the restricted zone for 10 seconds each. A fourth offensive player in the zone constitutes a violation. The ball handler is allowed unlimited pushes, but must bounce or pass the ball within 10 seconds. Zone defense focuses on physically taking the ball, forcing the offense to turn the ball over by boxing an offensive player in the zone for more than 10 seconds, or by pressuring a bad pass.

Racquetball

Racquetball is another exciting and fast-paced wheelchair sport that allows competition against stand-up players. Racquetball is played with a short-handled racquet and a hollow pressurized ball in an enclosed four-wall playing court. The game is played on regular racquetball courts. As in wheelchair tennis, two bounces of the ball are permitted for paraplegic players. Quadriplegic players, however, can continue to play the ball until it begins to roll. Serves must alternate to the left and right court, thus reducing the receiver's mobility disadvantage. Competitions at local, regional, and national levels are available through the American Amateur Racquetball Association (AARA). In 1986, for the first time, the wheeler's tournament was held in conjunction with the AARA's singles tournament.

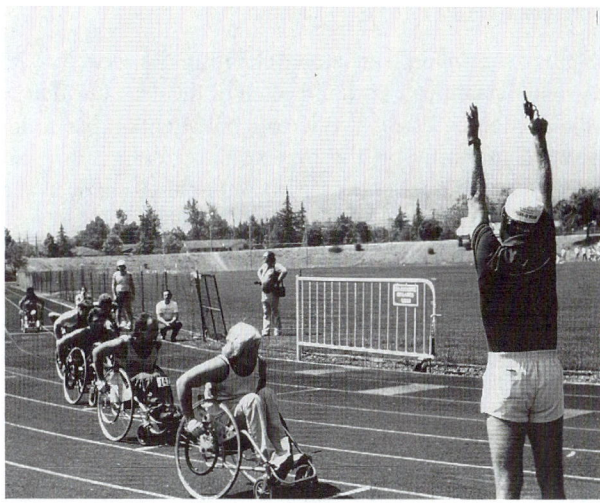

FIGURE 24–16   Road racing is done in lightweight wheelchairs as well as in special racing chairs.

Road Racing

Many track athletes prepare for regional and national wheelchair games by competing in 10 km races, as well as half and full 26.2-mile marathons. Wheelchair road racers compete alongside nondisabled runners. The record for the marathon distance by wheelchair athletes is faster than the world record time for a runner.

Wheelchair users also have an opportunity to shine in human-powered vehicle races on land, water, and in all-terrain vehicles (Madorsky and Madorsky 1983).

Rowing

Rowing for recreation and competition is gaining popularity due to the recent development of a monohull shell outfitted with outrigger pontoons, as well as the availability of a fixed-seat catamaran rowboat. Both are stable enough for operation by individuals with balance difficulties and permit transfers from a wheelchair. Shortened oars provide greater control. Disabled rowers now participate in national and international competition. Rowcycles are available to prepare athletes for the sport.

Sailing

New designs in sailboats allow paraplegic and quadriplegic sailors to participate in a full range of activities, including international competition. Some boats are especially adapted with a swivel seat to enable the sailor to remain seated while under sail. Others incorporate a slide hooked onto the main beam connecting the three hulls to ease transfer from wheelchair to cockpit. Yet other cockpits are adapted with pivoting helmsman and passenger seats. All sail handling and trim functions can be controlled from the cockpit. New designs in sailboats also allow sailors with disabilities to change sides within a boat without assistance.

Scuba Diving

Scuba diving offers recreational opportunities, as well as the psychological thrill of the freedom of the deep (Madorsky and Madorsky 1988). While national attention has so far focused primarily on the exploration of outer space, an increasing number of people are setting their sights in the opposite direction—to the exploration of inner space.

The Handicapped Scuba Association (HSA) provides three levels of certification, based on the degree of "buddy dependency" of the diver, as well as the ability to help a fellow diver in distress. This is assessed by evaluating the student's ability to master the HSA performance standards:

- Level A: Able to provide equal assistance to a fellow diver in case of an emergency. Qualified to dive with another certified diver, including a Level A diver.
- Level B: Able to care for self in case of an emergency, but cannot provide a fellow diver equal assistance in case of an emergency. Qualified to dive with two certified divers who may be Level A.
- Level C: Able to use scuba underwater safely, but unable to care for self or a fellow diver effectively in case of an emergency. Must dive with two certified divers, one of whom has been trained by a nationally recognized diver training agency in diver rescue.

In the gravity-free environment of the ocean floor, disabled divers use standard equipment: scuba tank, air regulator, buoyancy control device, weight belt, wetsuit, face mask, mouthpiece, and gloves. No equipment modifications are necessary. In case of urinary incontinence, their usual method of urinary collection suffices. Optional new equipment on the market can make diving easier and safer. A jacketlike buoyancy compensator holds the diver vertical while resting on the surface of the water. The octopus regulator enables a diver to share air supply with a buddy while keeping arms and hands free for propulsion through the water. A low-pressure inflator enables the diver to inflate the buoyancy compensator with the press of a button, again keeping the hands free and enabling a diver with paralyzed legs to continue to swim. Divers with weak leg muscles may benefit from the use of flexible vented fins. People who are unable to kick their feet may use a scooter, an electric propulsion vehicle.

Shooting

Shooting disciplines include trap and skeet shooting, silhouette shooting, air rifles, pistols, rifles, and hunting. Disabled and able-bodied people often practice and compete together. Orthotic adaptations are available for quadriplegic individuals. The sport demands great discipline, control, precision, and coordination.

Possible accommodations include special cloth or leather grips, special firing mechanisms, or help with loading the weapon and replacing targets.

Soccer

Soccer is played on a basketball or similar playing court, with a 13-inch playground ball. Each team consists of nine players, usually two goalies, two defensive players, and five offensive line persons. The rules of the game are similar to foot soccer except that the ball is passed, caught, dribbled, and thrown with the hands rather than kicked with the feet.

Softball

Wheelchair softball is played on any smooth, hard surface, such as a parking lot. First base is 30 × 15 inches, second and third bases are 15 inches square. A four-foot diameter circle is located around each base.

Competitive wheelchair softball is governed by the National Wheelchair Softball Association and is played under the official rules of 16-inch, slow pitch softball, as approved by the Amateur Softball Association. The defensive baseman has to have one or more wheels inside the circle, and the base runner must tag the base with one or more wheels, or with a hand, while seated in the chair.

NWBA Class I, II, and III players command one, two, and three points respectively. NWAA Quadriplegic Class IA, IB, and IC players count for one point. Players may total up to 22 points. At least one quadriplegic player must be included.

Tennis

Rules for tennis, as set forth by the International Tennis Federation, apply to wheelchair tennis with one major exception. The wheelchair tennis player is allowed two bounces of the ball. The first bounce must land inside the court boundaries; the second may land anywhere.

There are several men's and women's divisions in competitive wheelchair tennis, ranging from open, which is for the most advanced players, to the D Division for the novice player. People can play in any division they like when starting to play the sport; however, after winning two major

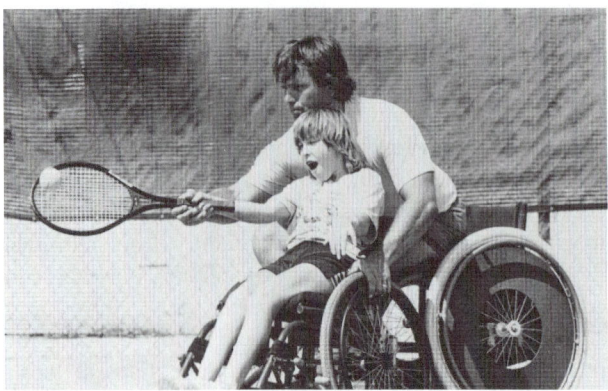

FIGURE 24–17 Wheelchair tennis at recreational and competitive levels has become one of the most popular sports for spinal cord injured individuals of all ages.

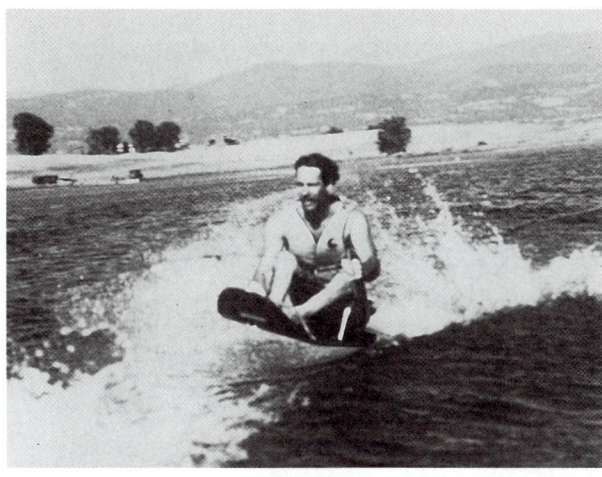

FIGURE 24–18 Water skiing for spinal cord injured people is no less exciting than for others.

tournaments in one year the player must advance to the next division. There is also a Junior Division for those under 18, and an E Division for people with quadriplegia, ambulatory quadriparesis, and those with impairment in at least three limbs. Also included in this division are power wheelchair users.

Mixed doubles have become an excellent way for a nondisabled and a wheelchair tennis player to compete against another nondisabled and wheelchair-using couple.

Water Skiing

The ski seat, a floating pair of skis with built-in bucket seat, handlebars, foot bindings, and foam flotation, makes water skiing possible for those who cannot ski standing up. Additional support can be built in for those with limited upper body strength and trunk balance. Ski gloves and Velcro strips enable people with quadriplegia to hold the handlebars.

A waterboard or waveski can be used for towing in a kneeling, sitting, or prone position.

A monoski is also available with a large surface area to increase stability.

Winter Sports

Alpine (downhill) and Nordic (cross-country) skiing, in monoskis or sitskis, provide opportunities for integrating able-bodied and disabled racers, as well as the chance to experience agility and breathtaking speed. The monoski is much more maneuverable, faster, and quicker than the sitski and better on ice. Ideally, it has a custom-molded seat, much like an amputee's prosthesis. Shortened ski poles, equipped with outrigger skis, are used for balance.

The monoski gives more control and speed than the sitski for those with good upper body control.

Ski competition for individuals with SCI is governed by the National Handicapped Sports and Recreation Association (NHSRA). Competitors are classified according to whether they have paralysis above or below T_{10}.

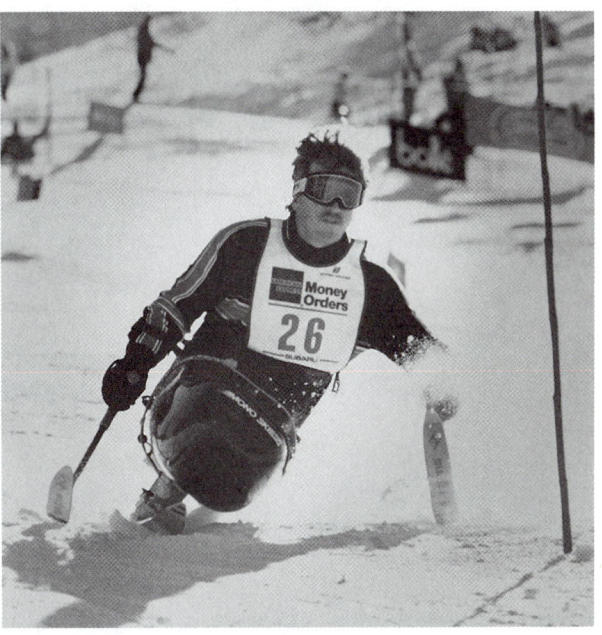

FIGURE 24–19 Snow skiing on the monoski, a new design, gives the skier speed and control comparable to the other skiers.

REFERENCES

Eriksson, P. 1988. Aerobic power during maximal exercise in untrained and well-trained quadri- and paraplegics. *Scandinavian Journal of Rehabilitation Medicine* 20: 141–147.

Kelley, J. D., and Frieden, L. 1989. *Go For It!* Orlando, FL: Harcourt Brace Jovanovich.

Madorsky, J., and Kiley, D. 1984. Wheel mountaineering. *Archives of Physical Medicine and Rehabilitation* 65: 490–492.

Madorsky, J., and Madorsky, A. 1983. Wheelchair racing: An important modality in acute rehabilitation after paraplegia. *Archives of Physical Medicine and Rehabilitation* 64: 186–187.

Madorsky, J., and Madorsky, A. 1988. Scuba diving: Taking the wheelchair out of wheelchair sports. *Archives of Physical Medicine and Rehabilitation* 69: 215–218.

Madorsky, J., Scanlon, J., and Smith, B. 1989. Kung fu: Synthesis of wheelchair sport and self-protection. *Archives of Physical Medicine and Rehabilitation* 70: 490–492.

National Wheelchair Basketball Association. 1979. *NWBA Physical Classification Handbook*. Lexington: University of Kentucky.

Stotts, K. M. 1986. Health maintenance: Paraplegic athletes and nonathletes. *Archives of Physical Medicine and Rehabilitation* 67 (2): 109–114.

Weinec, J., and Langen, E. R. 1983. Optimales Training, Leistung Physiologische Trainings Lehre.

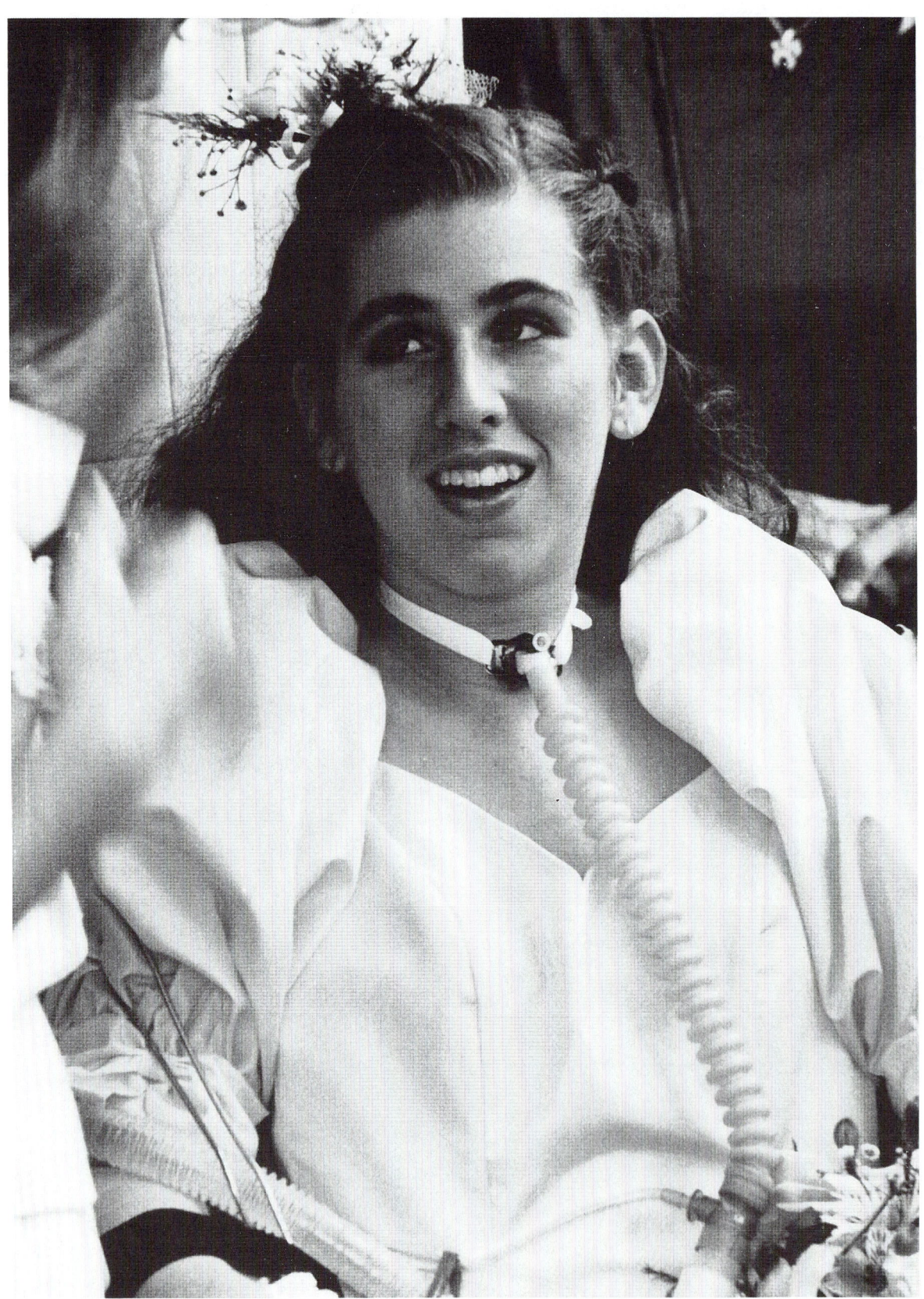

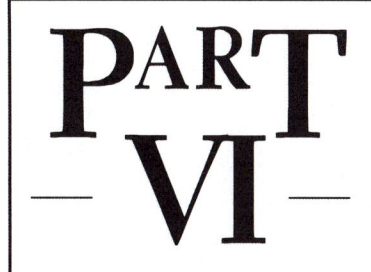

PART VI

SPECIAL CONSIDERATIONS

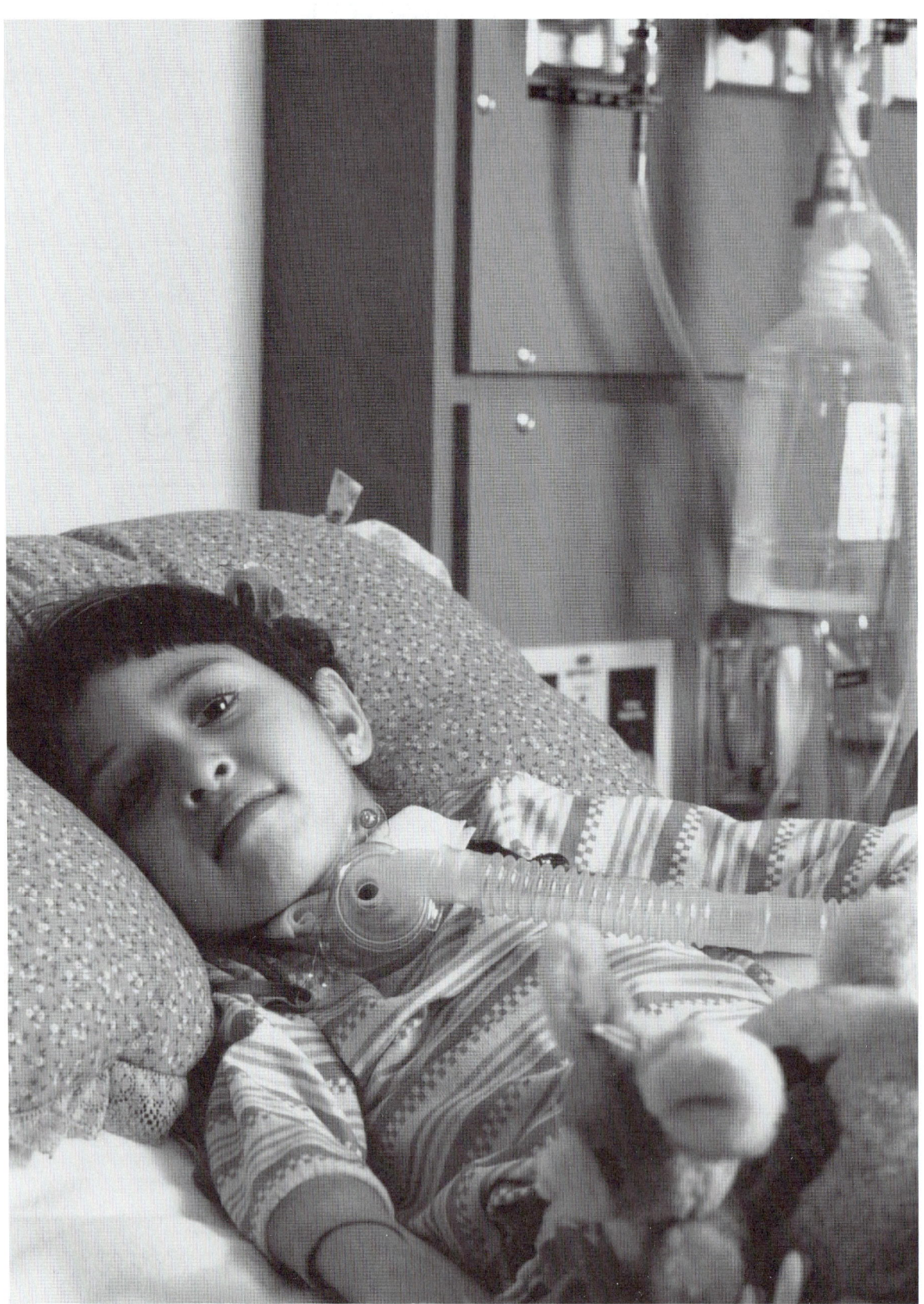

CHAPTER 25

Spinal Cord Injury in Children

Chapter Outline

Health Care Objectives

- To combine optimal SCI care with pediatric rehabilitation expertise
- To promote health and normal growth and development despite physical disability
- To link current resources and develop new ones to meet the health, educational, and social needs of children with SCI

*This section was contributed by James E. Wilberger, M.D., and Sarah Layman, C.N.R.N.
**These sections were developed with the assistance of Eileen Rosenfeld, R.N., and Michael Grossman, R.N., B.S.N.

Spinal cord injuries (SCI) with major neurological involvement are relatively uncommon in infants, children, and adolescents. Only 1% to 3% of all spinal injuries occur to people less than 15 years old (Gaufin and Goodman 1975). However, when spinal injuries do occur in this group, anatomical and developmental factors predispose the upper cervical spine to the most severe injuries. Children are thus more likely to suffer catastrophic neurological loss such as quadriplegia (Anderson and Schutt 1980; Babcok 1975; Burke 1970). Because SCI in infants, children, and adolescents is not common, information relative to the immediate care and management of the complications of spinal fractures, as well as rehabilitation and continuing care issues, are fragmented and incomplete. This chapter offers an overview of the unique problems associated with the spinal cord injured child.

EARLY ASSESSMENT AND MANAGEMENT OF THE SPINAL CORD INJURED CHILD

Injury to the spine or spinal cord should be suspected in any unconscious child with multiple injuries or a significant head injury. From 5% to 20% of all children with severe head injuries will have an associated cervical spine injury. If a cervical spine injury is present, there is a 10% to 15% incidence of associated thoracic and/or lumbar spine injury (Babcok 1975). Multitrauma coexists with SCI in approximately 75% of pediatric patients. Any awake, injured child who complains of numbness or weakness in the arms or legs or of pain in the back or neck should be considered to have a spine and/or spinal cord injury (SCI) until proven otherwise.

Adequate stabilization of the *entire* spine is essential. A backboard for transporting the child in the supine position provides stabilization. In small children, the neck can often be stabilized by taping the head to the backboard. Older children, particularly those who may be agitated secondary to head injury, are best stabilized by the use of rolled towels and generous taping of the head. Review Chapter 5. Various types of rigid cervical collars are also available in pediatric sizes. Vomiting is a frequent occurrence in injured children. Thus, if a child is to be transported in the supine position with the neck rigidly stabilized, insertion of a nasogastric tube is essential to prevent aspiration.

Once stabilization has been achieved and other life-threatening injuries dealt with, apply priorities and management techniques as presented in Chapter 5. First priority is to prevent the many complications that may occur acutely following SCI. The first week to 10 days following SCI are the most important, as life-threatening complications occur during this time. Especially try to detect and treat any complications that may occur as a result of pulmonary, cardiovascular, urinary tract, or gastrointestinal problems related to SCI. Similarly, attend carefully and early to the skin as well as to nutrition of the spinal cord injured child.

Pulmonary Complications

Pulmonary complications (as detailed in Chapter 15) are the single, most common cause of morbidity and mortality acutely following SCI. The higher the SCI, the greater the incidence of pulmonary problems; however, complications in children can occur even in conus-level injuries. Atelectasis and subsequent bronchopneumonia are common. Pulmonary embolism, a major complication in adult SCI, is rarely seen in children.

Be constantly vigilant to diagnose and treat the complication of pneumonia rapidly. The use of prophylactic antibiotics is not encouraged, even in children who require prolonged intubation or tracheostomy. Routine use significantly increases the occurrence of serious antibiotic-resistant pulmonary infections. Although pathogenic organisms are commonly found in routine tracheal cultures in such children, they most often represent bacterial colonization and not infection. If clinical evidence of pulmonary infection does develop, then it should be treated vigorously with appropriate antibiotics based on sensitivity studies from sputum and blood cultures.

Almost every child with a significant cervical spinal cord injury will require ventilatory assistance at some point during the acute stage of injury. An endotracheal tube with a soft cuff can be safely left in place for up to 10 to 14 days. Unless there is a cervical cord injury above the C_3 level or an associated severe head injury, the vast majority of children can be weaned from the respirator during this time and will not require a tracheostomy. However, if it appears that the respiratory insufficiency will be longer lasting—and certainly in the presence of a high cord injury in which the chance for recovery of independent respiratory function is small—then a tracheostomy should be performed sooner than the 10- to 14-day time period.

Another potential complication is that of *sleep apnea*. Automatic respiration is regulated by the reticulospinal system that lies in the anterior lateral column of the spinal cord from C_3. If these pathways are damaged significantly, then only voluntary respiration, which is dependent on consciousness, is possible, and cessation of breathing may occur during sleep. This syndrome should be carefully watched for in children with high level cervical spinal cord injuries and requires the use of an apnea monitor and/or pulse oximeter on a continuous basis for the first week to 10 days following injury.

Cardiovascular Care

Aside from spinal shock, several other complications associated with the cardiovascular system may be encountered in the initial care of the spinal cord injured child and require special attention. Bradycardia is not infrequently seen in association with cervical SCI. In the first 7 to 10 days following injury, bradycardia may be so pronounced as to produce hypotension and syncope. Bradycardia, if symptomatic, can be reversed with Atropine. All children with cervical SCI should be monitored electrocardiographically continuously for the first week following injury to watch for this complication.

Children are particularly sensitive to orthostatic hypotension, autonomic dysreflexia, and thermoregulatory dysfunction. These complications are detailed in Chapter 16.

Nutritional Care

Severe injury to the spinal cord, similar to other systemic insults and injuries, produces an immediate and often sustained catabolic response. The benefits of careful and early attention to nutritional status have been repeatedly shown. Children have a limited ability to tolerate prolonged periods of catabolism because of their intrinsically high basal metabolic rates and their small caloric reserve. The child will initially respond to catabolism by breaking down available protein stores to provide substrates for gluconeogenesis. The new glucose that is produced supplies obligatory needs of the central nervous system for glucose as an energy substrate. However, the breakdown of protein cannot continue indefinitely as the protein reserves of the body available for energy substrate are normally in the form of functioning enzymes, cellular building blocks, and muscles. Continued protein catabolism, therefore, represents a loss of essential biologic components. Starvation-related mortality results when one-third to one-half of body protein has been lost. At this low level of protein reserve, the general repair functions of the body are affected adversely by severe muscle wasting, ineffective coughing, pneumonia, impaired wound healing, poor resistance to infection, and diminished synthesis of enzymes and plasma proteins.

If the gastrointestinal tract is functional, it is by far the best means of supplying protein and calories. Use of a flexible, small-bore pediatric feeding tube prevents the possible complication of gastric irritation, gastroesophageal reflux, and aspiration. Various commercial products are available for enteral hyperalimentation. If a routine form cannot be used because of intestinal malabsorption, then use elemental formulas that contain amino acids, triglycerides, and simple sugars.

It is extremely important that proper nutrition be supplied early to children with SCI as protein catabolism begins several hours after the injury and continues throughout the period of relative starvation that follows. Complications during convalescence will worsen the protein breakdown process. Any attempts to reduce protein wasting and to provide adequate calories to counteract infection and stress and ultimately to induce tissue anabolism for wound repair, must be instituted vigorously at the earliest possible opportunity. Chapter 17 addresses special needs of SCI patients, which are different from other critically ill patients.

Children with SCI may also develop significant electrolyte imbalances. Profound *hyponatremia* may develop as a result of the syndrome of inappropriate anti-diuretic hormone secretion (SIADH). SIADH can occur with an insult to the nervous system and results in hyponatremia, excessive renal secretion of sodium, and hyperosmolar urine in the face of serum hypoosmolarity. If serum sodium drops too low, seizures may result. SIADH is corrected generally by fluid restriction until the hyponatremia is reversed. If fluid restriction is ineffective, or if the degree and duration of fluid restriction have significant adverse effects on the nutritional status of the child, consideration must be given to other modalities of treatment. If very low serum sodium associated with seizures occurs, more aggressive therapy is indicated. The use of loop diuretics in association with the replacement of fluid losses with 3% saline solution has proved to be extremely effective in rapidly returning serum sodium to normal in the face of SIADH.

Gastrointestinal Care

Paralytic ileus, a manifestation of generalized autonomic dysfunction, occurs almost universally in children with cervical and thoracic SCI. The development of a paralytic ileus, with subsequent abdominal distension, can result in respiratory compromise and also vomiting with a subsequent risk of pulmonary aspiration. As paralytic ileus can neither be prevented nor directly treated, primary treatment should consist of placement of a nasogastric tube to maintain constant aspiration of the gastric content. This will effectively prevent progressive abdominal distension and its associated complications. The nasogastric tube should be left in place until spinal shock subsides and peristaltic function returns, as evidenced by the return of active bowel sounds or the passage of flatus or stool.

Once the problem of paralytic ileus resolves, bowel retraining and regulation must be initiated and maintained to prevent severe constipation, impaction, and associated undesirable side effects. See Chapter 19. A *bowel regimen* should be initiated during the intensive care phase to provide for a daily bowel movement. The most effective bowel regimens to establish a daily routine make use of a combination of rectal suppositories and stool softeners. Many commercial preparations are useful and effective in adolescents. However, in small children, the dose and the mode of delivery may not be satisfactory. We have found that a combination of the stool softener, blond psyllium seed coatings (siblin) mixed with pureed prunes (lekvar) is most effective and acceptable. Mineral oil is contraindicated for routine use because it depletes the body of fat-soluble vitamins and its use often results in rectal seepage. Digital stimulation may be effective. However, it should be stressed that, whatever form of rectal stimulation is used, regular timing is necessary in order to achieve bowel retraining. If digital stimulation is not sufficient, one may proceed to the use of suppositories. It is best to start out with the mildest types such as glycerine suppositories and progress to a more stimulating agent such as bisacodyl suppository if necessary. Suppositories should be inserted on a regular schedule. Initially, the suppository can be used daily and then decreased to an alternate-day program. Daily defecation is not a necessity. Avoid enemas because of the potential problems of overstretching the bowel and the possibility of eliciting autonomic dysreflexia. Enemas may cause fluid and electrolyte imbalances, especially in the very young child with small fluid compartments. An ineffective bowel program can present in many ways. One must be alert to the subtle signs such as loss of appetite, abdominal distension, and general malaise. The more overt signs such as vomiting, abdominal pain, or cramping and diarrhea are less easily missed. It is important to differentiate true diarrhea from impaction. The diarrhea of obstruction is due to seepage around the impaction of stool and usually is accompanied by other signs that may have been overlooked. The child need not appear acutely ill. In the typical gastrointestinal viral or bacterial infection, the child may have fever and more frequent and explosive symptoms. When in doubt, impaction can always be ruled out by simple rectal examination.

More severe and life-threatening acute abdominal complications such as splenic rupture or liver lacerations, and chronic complications such as bowel obstruction or perforation, or other similar conditions, may be obscured because of a lack of pain perception in children with SCI. Occasionally, vague pain may be appreciated secondary to autonomic visceral afferents which are conducted into the spinal cord via the splanchnic, hypogastric, or pelvic nerves. Also, if the SCI is not above the C_5 level, referred pain secondary to diaphragmatic irritation may be felt in the shoulder region. Other signs of ongoing abdominal complications such as temperature elevation, elevated white blood cell count, or associated ileus are not reliable signs for the identification of abdominal disease in such patients. Similarly, clinical examination may be misleading as localized abdominal tenderness, muscle guarding, and rigidity will likely be absent even in the presence of severe peritonitis.

Thus, it must be recognized that children with SCI can develop such abdominal complications. Watch carefully for any indirect signs that may point to an ongoing abdominal problem.

Urinary Tract Care

The main source of systemic infection in acutely spinal cord injured children is the bladder. The bladder can also account for significant long-term disability secondary to associated renal damage if appropriate care is not begun early following SCI. The somatic musculature of the bladder is flaccid during spinal shock, although the bladder itself is not completely atonic because of a rich intramural autonomic network. Thus, during spinal shock, spontaneous voiding occurs only when the bladder overflows. In children, reflex micturition usually returns within a few days unless the sacral reflex center or the nerve roots supplying the bladder are destroyed.

The use of indwelling catheters in the acute spinal cord injured child has all but been abandoned except in cases of multiple associated injuries. Urinary output must be carefully monitored hourly with 1 cc/kg per hour being an acceptable rate of urine production. It is well known that infection will occur with 48 to 96 hours of the placement of an indwelling catheter. Aside from the acute problem of infection, the long-term use of indwelling catheters may be associated with significant urethral, bladder, and renal complications.

Regimens for bladder management are dependent on the age, sex, size, and weight of the child and the type of bladder. Fluid intake and output are crucial in establishing programs and schedules. In babies and toddlers, for whom the use of diapers is appropriate, one must assure adequate emptying of the bladder. With school age children, diapers are no longer appropriate and their continued use may be detrimental to the child's self-esteem and self-image. Clean intermittent catheterization (CIC) is an alternative and can be instituted at any age (Altchuler, Butz, and Meyer 1977).

The goal of CIC is not only to empty the bladder but also to prevent infection and retrain the bladder. In most cases, a catheter-free bladder with low residual and sterile urine should be achievable over a several-month period as detailed in Chapter 18. The CIC technique is relatively simple and can be taught to parents and patients. Children as young as 5 years of age have mastered this technique of self-catheterization (Carlson and Kass 1990; Hugh MacMillan Medical Centre 1988; Sullivan-Bolyai 1986). Children with quadriplegia will need detailed assistance with CIC. Also, very young children may be unable to perform the maneuvers necessary for CIC independently.

Medications may be a necessary adjunct to the bladder training program. Bethanecol chloride, a parasympathomimetic drug, may be used to help the bladder contract. Phenoxybenzamine hydrochloride, an alpha-adrenergic blocking agent, may be used to decrease sphincter resistance. Oxybutynin chloride and propantheline bromide anticholinergic drugs may be used to inhibit bladder spasticity. Imipramine hydrochloride, an antidepressant with anticholinergic properties, may be beneficial in decreasing the spontaneous emptying of the bladder.

Avoidance of overdistension and repeated urinary tract infection of the bladder are vitally important in maintaining normal bladder and renal function. The indwelling catheter should be removed as soon as possible and bladder retraining started. If infection occurs, it should be treated aggressively. Urinary asepsis may be helped by acidification of the urine with oral vitamin C and urinary antiseptic agents such as methenamine mandelate. Urolithiasis is a potential complication of persistent urinary tract infection (Tori and Kewalramani 1978–1979). This is more common in children than in adults and should be looked for if the urine cannot be kept free of infection. An intravenous pyelogram should be performed in the acute phase following SCI to establish a baseline and to rule out any abnormalities. Other bladder studies such as cystoscopy, cystometrogram, and renal scan may be obtained as clinically indicated. Regular urinalysis, regular urine cultures, and blood urea, nitrogen, and creatinine levels should be obtained for monitoring during bladder retraining programs.

Care of the Skin

Development of pressure areas is an undesirable complication of SCI in children. Immobility and a lack of sensation predispose to pressure necrosis of the skin and subsequent skin breakdowns. Pressure over the skin, particularly over the bony prominences, must be avoided as detailed in Chapter 21. The most common sites for the development of decubiti are the ischial, sacral, malleolar, trochanteric, and coccygeal prominences. In small children, the back of the head is particularly vulnerable to the development of an ulceration. Also, pressure points created by orthotic devices must be diligently checked, especially as children grow.

REHABILITATION ISSUES

SCI rehabilitation aims to facilitate maximum neurological recovery while helping the child to develop compensatory strategies for the neurological loss that has occurred. The rehabilitation goals for the young patient are similar to those for adults. However, children require considerable unstructured time and much of their learning occurs through play activity. The child is an important member of the family unit, and the family must be considered as an integral part of the treatment process. Grandparents and siblings are frequently involved in the outcome, although the mother usually bears the brunt of the long-term care of small children.

A model care plan for the child with SCI is presented in Table 25–1.

Collaboration to Provide Family-Centered Care

SCI not only has a devastating effect on the child, but also impacts and disrupts the family system as a whole. The injury may be viewed as a loss or a threat and perhaps, eventually, as a challenge. The psychosocial process of individuals and families learning to adapt to the disability has been described in Chapter 9. Children also need to develop self-esteem, control, and independence to cope with being disabled.

To promote adaptation of both the child and family to the varied consequences of SCI, early aggressive rehabilitation in a supportive environment is ideal (Deller and Gruydanus 1979; Nordan 1976). Table 25–2 outlines some activity guidelines. The key to the success of these activities lies not only in effectiveness on physical health, but also the extent to which functional capabilities enable children to move and play as freely as possible. Mobility and independence are essential to ensure access to everyday situations. Research suggests that children who are not freely mobile during their formative years are burdened with another handicap: poorly developed curiosity and initiative (Jaffe 1987). Children also desperately need continued opportunities to develop positive social skills to ensure access to the community at large later in life (Lehr 1986).

The rehabilitation process must begin during acute hospitalization. Erroneously, acute care professionals have, in the past, assumed that developmental progress can be safely postponed until the illness is overcome. But for children with SCI, this belief has been a major factor in the development of serious psychosocial implications including regression, dependency, delayed development, social deprivation, and, eventually, poor school attendance with lack of education and vocational goals. An acute care approach that concentrates solely on the scenario of medical and surgical interventions, therapies, and care, without realistically addressing continuing fears and future concerns, has the potential so to traumatize children and families that their preinjury drive may never be recovered (Sevorsky and Opas 1987).

Early collaboration among pediatric, SCI, and community-based professionals, including independent living specialists, is needed to blend expertise in health care services

TABLE 25–1 Care Plan for Quadriplegic Child (6 years old): Early Rehabilitation

Nursing diagnosis: Impaired physical mobility; alteration in elimination; alteration in comfort; disturbance in self-concept

Potential Problem	Pathophysiology	Expected Outcome	Intervention
Neurological deterioration	Spine instability due to hypermobility and laxity of ligaments causing cord compression Hypoxemia due to hypoventilation Hypotension due to loss of vasomotor tone and sympathetic innervation	Neurological stabilization Maintenance of bony alignment/spine stability Adequate ventilation Normotensive	Maintain traction or immobilization as indicated Log roll as needed, maintaining body alignment with head and neck well supported Preoperative and postoperative care as in Chapter 20 Provide care to promote optimal cardiopulmonary function (See Chapters 6, 15, and 16.)
Hypoxemia/ hypoventilation	Loss of diaphragmatic innervation with abdominal muscle fatigue (intercostals somewhat ineffective in normal child anyway) Statis of secretions Pneumonia Pulmonary embolism (rare)	Normal bilateral breath sounds present; adequate ventilation Absence of pneumonic process Absence of dyspnea, tachypnea (normal approximates adult) Diagnostic tests within normal limits for child	Monitor respirations hourly (minimum) Monitor arterial blood gases as indicated Use pulse oximeter as indicated Observe for signs of respiratory distress (check mucous membranes) Encourage use of incentive spirometry Deliver humidified O_2 at 3 l Turn including prone position every 2 hours and as indicated Suction as indicated, with pre- and postsuction oxygenation Keep endotracheal tube at bedside (age in years/+ 4 age = tube size as general guideline) Observe for signs of respiratory distress: agitation, restlessness, confusion, loss of color in mucous membranes, dyspnea, tachypnea; increased rate of rapid, shallow breathing Realize during acute stage that respiratory insufficiency due to fatigue is likely to progress Monitor hemoglobin and hematocrit Monitor vital capacity Place nasogastric tube Mobilize early
Hypotension	Loss of vasomotor tone with venous pooling Disruption of autonomic nervous system function	Normotensive Adequate urine output of approximately 0.5–2.0 cc/kg/hr	Use of compression stockings as indicated Vasopressors as ordered Accurate intake/output Monitor BP
Orthostatic hypotension	Venous pooling with loss of sympathetic innervation and vasomotor paralysis	Normotensive 80/60 Absence of lightheadedness and syncope	Gradual increase to upright position Use of tilt table as indicated Use of abdominal binder as indicated Return to horizontal position as needed Use of compression stockings Monitor BP when upright position is assumed
Peripheral edema	Venous stasis and pooling with loss of muscle tone	Reduction of edema (see Chapter 16)	Passive ROM exercises Elevate extremities Position change including prone and Trendelenburg every 2 hours Tensor wraps or compression stockings as indicated
Bradycardia	Loss of sympathetic outflow to heart with unopposed vagal stimulus	Absence of bradycardia (approximately 80 beats per minute normal)	Atropine as ordered Adequate oxygenation Monitor pulse Monitor arterial blood and pulmonary gas analysis

(Table continues)

TABLE 25–1 **Care Plan for Quadriplegic Child (6 years old): Early Rehabilitation (continued)**

Potential Problem	Pathophysiology	Expected Outcome	Intervention
Dysrhythmias	Hypothermia Hypokalemia	Normal sinus rhythm	Medicate as ordered Monitor EKG, temperature, and electrolytes
Autonomic dysreflexia	Autonomic nervous system dysfunction, associated with noxious stimuli below level of injury; occurs with SCI T_6 and above (see Chapter 16)	Normotensive Absence of associated sweating, flushing, chills, pilomotor erection, headaches, nasal congestion Resolution of noxious stimuli (cause)	Observe for rapid onset of symptoms Monitor BP Examine for cause (check Foley for block; check bladder distension; using topical anesthetic, check for fecal impaction) Eliminate stimulus as indicated Vasodilators as ordered Educate patient and family
Poikilothermia/ hypothermia	Vasomotor paralysis due to loss of sympathetic innervation	Normothermia (approximately 37.5°C in child)	Alter room temperature as indicated Use warm blankets as indicated keeping in mind that patient is insensate Hypothermia blanket as indicated Educate family in need for appropriate clothing and environmental temperature regulation as indicated
Pneumonia/atelectasis	Secretion statis due to paralysis of the muscles of breathing (inability to deep breathe and cough); decreased lung expansion with alveoli collapse Loss of diaphragmatic innervation Increased intraabdominal pressure	Afebrile Chest X ray without pneumonic process Bilateral breath sounds present and clear Normal arterial blood gases Absence of dyspnea, tachypnea	Monitor breath sounds and respirations hourly Observe for signs of respiratory distress (dyspnea, tachypnea, agitation, confusion) Monitor temperature every 4 hours Position change every 2 hours including prone and Trendelenburg position Bronchial hygiene techniques every 2 hours and as indicated Encourage use of incentive spirometry Suction as indicated with pre- and postoxygenation Administer antibiotics as ordered
Sleep apnea	Disruption of retriculospinal tract with high quadriplegia	Normal respirations during sleep	Observe quality and quantity of respirations during sleep Monitor respirations with apnea during sleep (usually during first 7 to 10 days) and when mechanical ventilation is discontinued
Paralytic ileus	Disruption of autonomic nervous system function (spinal shock). See Chapter 6	Absence of gastric distension Absence of vomiting Normal bowel sounds and passing of flatus	Place nasogastric tube to continuous low suction with antacid regime as ordered (see Chapter 6) Monitor presence and quality of bowel sounds Restrict oral intake until bowel sounds active
Threatened nutritional status	Decreased appetite Catabolic state Dysphagia	Good appetite Positive nitrogen balance Sufficient calorie intake Appropriate maintenance of weight for age and height (see Chapter 17)	Begin oral intake as soon as possible (consider total parenteral nutrition if unable to begin feedings within 48 hours) Make foods appealing to age Raise head of bed or place in upright position as indicated Realize child requires 80 kcal/kg with 30 g protein normally; calculate dietary needs appropriately Weigh daily
Impaction	Loss of voluntary control	Regular, predictable, reliable evacuation of stool Absence of gastric distension	Administer stool softener as indicated Initiate bowel regime Encourage fluid and fiber intake

(Table continues)

TABLE 25–1 Care Plan for Quadriplegic Child (6 years old): Early Rehabilitation (continued)

Potential Problem	Pathophysiology	Expected Outcome	Intervention
Impaction (continued)		Absence of autonomic dysreflexia (see Chapter 19)	Nutritional education Observe for signs of impaction (watery stool, ineffective bowel regime) Observe for signs of autonomic dysreflexia (sweating, flushing, pilomotor erection, headaches, chills) Use topical anesthetic with digital exam to prevent autonomic dysreflexic response
Incontinence of stool	Loss of voluntary control	Regular, predictable, reliable evacuation of stool without episodes of incontinence Absence of autonomic dysreflexia (see Chapter 16)	Initiate bowel regime as indicated Administer stool softeners as ordered Initiate bowel routine after meal to use gastrocolic reflex effectively Place in sitting or upright position to increase intraabdominal pressure Use topical anesthetic with digital stimulation to prevent autonomic dysreflexic response
Abdominal complications	Trauma Unopposed vagal stimulation with increased gastric secretions	Absence of life-threatening complications Absence of gastrointestinal hemorrhage (see Chapter 6)	Monitor gastric pH Administer antacids as indicated Guaiac test all stools Monitor daily hematocrit and hemoglobin Assess abdomen with percussion, palpation, and auscultation Observe for referred pain in shoulder region
Urinary retention	Overdistension of bladder	Maintenance of bladder tone Absence of infection Regular emptying Afebrile Absence of incontinence Absence of autonomic dysreflexia Absence of distension (see Chapter 18)	Anticipate urine output of 700 to 1000 cc daily Straight catheterization every 4 hours with #8 or #10 French catheter (if greater than 200 cc on two consecutive catheterizations, decrease time interval between catheterizations) Avoid fluid restriction Observe color and clarity of urine and check urinalysis, culture as indicated Use aseptic technique with catheterization Observe for signs of dysreflexia (sweating, flushing, pilomotor erection, chills) Monitor intake/output
Urinary incontinence	Overflow of bladder Reflex excitability return Loss of cerebral cortex control Infection Renal calculi	Absence of incontinence Regular emptying Absence of infection Afebrile (see Chapter 18)	Monitor intake/output Straight catheterization every 4 hours with #8 or #10 French catheter (adjust time interval if greater than 200 cc with two consecutive catheterizations or decrease in amount of urine obtained) Straight catheterization for residual after spontaneous void (increase times between straight catheterizations as residuals reduce) Encourage fluids Assist with triggering reflex voiding to promote bladder training with catheterizations Observe color and clarity, check urinalysis, and culture as indicated Observe for sedimentation in urine Mobilize early Place in sitting position for catheterizations to promote intraabdominal pressure and bladder emptying

(Table continues)

TABLE 25–1 Care Plan for Quadriplegic Child (6 years old): Early Rehabilitation (continued)

Potential Problem	Pathophysiology	Expected Outcome	Intervention
Urinary tract infection	Urine statis from incomplete emptying Introduction of bacteria via invasive procedures	Absence of infection Afebrile (see Chapter 18)	Encourage fluids Remove indwelling catheter Straight catheterization every 4 hours as indicated using aseptic techniques Observe color and clarity, check urinalysis, and culture as indicated Observe for incontinence Encourage fluids Mobilize early Administer antibiotics as ordered Straight catheterization for residual volumes
Pressure areas	Tissue pressure exceeds capillary filling pressure primarily over bony prominences Normal decreased body stores of fat in childhood Catabolic state Tissue sheering	Absence of pressure areas Absence of reddened areas Intact skin Control secondary factors contributing to pressure areas (see Chapter 21)	Inspect body surface with each turn Turn and position every 2 hours (minimum) Cushion areas of bony prominence Skin care with each turn Attention to areas under orthoses Nutritional education Keep skin clean and dry Place on water mattress or special apparatus as indicated Use draw sheet for lifts Position off areas of redness or breakdown Address secondary factors
Contractures	Fibrotic changes due to decreased circulation and shortening of collagen fibers Positioning difficulties due to spasticity and growth-related problems	Normal full ROM exercises of extremities Absence of contractures Tolerate prone position Achieve optimal position and control of spasticity (Chapters 20 and 27)	Position change every 2 hours, including prone position, and adequate support of extremities Maintain proper alignment ROM exercises with position change Physical therapy as indicated Splint as indicated Address spasticity and maintaining optimal position in bed and wheelchair
Thrombophlebitis (rare)	Venous stasis and pooling with paralysis	Absence of edema Absence of redness (pain, tenderness not sensed with SCI)	Passive ROM exercises with turning Assess size and color of extremities (measure at same level) Apply compression stockings or ace wraps Administer anticoagulants as ordered Position change every 2 hours including prone and Trendelenburg Mobilize early
*Decreased comprehension of problem	Lack of understanding of effects of disability Poor concept of time	Asks appropriate questions Voices basic understanding Behaves appropriately	Explain all care Begin early teaching, incorporating play and imagination Begin early training to encourage participation, independence (able to learn straight catheterization, weight change, skin evaluation, signs of autonomic dysreflexia)
*Decreased coping abilities	Reaction to injury Difficulty making decision Explosive behavior Loss of individuality Poor understanding of effects of SCI	Cooperates and participates in care planning Decreased explosive episodes Decreased verbal aggression	Provide structured activities; set limitations on acceptable behavior Allow for choice in daily routine where applicable Allow for change in plans, balance with free time

(Table continues)

TABLE 25–1 Care Plan for Quadriplegic Child (6 years old): Early Rehabilitation (continued)

Potential Problem	Pathophysiology	Expected Outcome	Intervention
*Interruption of emotional growth	Separation from family Decreased peer interaction Decreased independence Decreased ability to explore, be active	Family participation Peer interaction Maximize mobility and initiative School activities	Praise accomplishments Encourage contact with peers Encourage family participation in care Encourage preinjury routines where possible Social skills training Recreational/educational activities Complete educational plan Make referrals as necessary

*These potential problems are associated with disturbances in body image, self-esteem, and role performance related to change in body function. Achieving maximum control of body functions, encouraging expression of feelings, teaching self-care, assisting parents to promote independence, and discussing long-term plans with appropriate referrals applies to managing each potential problem in this care plan. Also interdisciplinary collaboration and patient and family health education are implied throughout.

Source: Sarah Lyman, C.R.N.P.

with educational and social opportunities to facilitate normal progression of growth and development. This is especially important if the child is cared for in an adult rehabilitation facility not geared to the child's ever-changing developmental needs. Conversely, in pediatric settings without expertise in SCI, cross-consultation is required to maximize potentials. The child must acquire both optimal functional gains specifically related to SCI *and* resume normal development, otherwise the outcome of treatment is limited.

Establish philosophy of care very early to encourage responsible participation of the child at an appropriate level. Children with SCI require both praise and discipline, as do all young people, but application should be tempered with an understanding of the many and frustrating demands placed on them. However, children with SCI must be helped to realize that unacceptable behavior remains unacceptable behavior despite physical disability. Overindulgence and overconcern place a child in a passive, dependent, overprotected role that will permeate the home environment and severely jeopardize future opportunities to live independently (Independent Living Research Utilization 1990). As children grow up and parents age, independent living abilities are the key to survival.

Parent participation during rehabilitation is often difficult due to extended periods of hospitalization, distance of travel to major facilities, and other family responsibilities that may prevent them from spending more time with the injured child. In some situations inappropriate parental input may actually inhibit a child's progress while the mutual needs between spouses and needs of other family members are not met. In fact, strained marital relationships

are not at all unusual. Sensitivity to ongoing family dynamics gives directions to interventions. Even the strongest families can become exhausted, functional families can become dysfunctional, and dysfunctional families will likely remain dysfunctional.

Expert assessment of multiple factors, as opposed to subjective impressions, best identifies pretraumatic capabilities on which to build. Professional impressions are influenced by personal perceptions and value systems. Ways to develop a positive attitude toward disability are integrated throughout this text. However, understanding parental values and beliefs, cultural responses, and altered perceptions due to the crisis of the child's injury and everyday stresses imposed on the family is essential. Chapter 9 addresses assessment and goal setting with the family further.

Families may not value independence and may be fulfilling their own needs by having their child more dependent on them for one reason or another. In these situations, expectations of the child to participate may be unrealistically high, but continued collaboration with parents to detail a care plan is helpful. Self-care assessment tools (Coley 1978; Shriners Hospital for Crippled Children 1989) and other measurement indices listed in Chapter 22 can provide a structure to promote sharing of viewpoints and to help visualize discrepancies. Assist the family to recognize the importance of the child's continual development of life skills, which includes as much physical independence as possible as well as chores, responsibilities, and interactions with peers and at school. The approach to problem solving in the rehabilitation environment will carry over into all aspects of the child's future.

TABLE 25–2 Comprehensive Rehabilitation Program for Children with Spinal Cord Injury

Level and Function Remaining	Treatment Guidelines	Functional Objective	Functional Equipment
C_4 Respiration Scapular elevation Neck movements	• Passive range of motion. • Improve head control and strengthen remaining neck and shoulder musculature. • Establish variety of positioning alternatives to prevent contractures, reduce spasticity, prevent pressure areas. • May require respiratory program including bronchial drainage, manual cough, diaphragm strengthening, change of position every two hours. A corset may be used to increase abdominal support. • Increase tolerance for upright position by increasing angle of and length of time on tilt table and in wheelchair (use cushion in chair to prevent pressure areas). • Train in use of adaptive equipment. • Explore alternatives for prevocational training. • Patient and family training in physical care, functional activities, use and maintenance of all equipment. • Provide home program.	• Tolerance for upright position • Safe bathing • Self-feeding usually not energy-efficient even with devices • Control of environment including lights, TV, radio, telephone • Electric wheelchair propulsion • Typing (about 5 words/min) • Return to school (adapted or special school placement may be necessary)	• Tilt table, manual or electric • Reclining wheelchair with cushion, elevating leg rests, and trunkal supports • Sling in bathtub or reclining shower chair • Cup with long straw, if placed appropriately, facilitates independent drinking • Touch-access environmental controls unit • Automatic dial telephone • Touch-access system, mouth-stick or sip 'n puff control • Electric wheelchair • Mouthstick or touch-access electric typewriter with power return button, self-correcting ribbon or other correcting mechanism, roll of paper • Angled tray or work surface • Adapted electric typewriter • Adapted tape recorder for note taking • Electric page turner for reading • Adapted computer
C_5 Shoulder elevation Shoulder abduction (partial) Scapular rotation and adduction Elbow flexion (partial)	• Passive range of motion. *Note:* Less than normal range is desirable in the finger flexors (for tenodesis grasp) and the back extensors (for sitting stability). • Strengthen all remaining musculature. • Establish positioning alternatives (see C_4). • Teach compensatory body management skills. • May require respiratory program (see C_4). • Increase tolerance of upright position (see C_4). • Teach assisted pressure relief techniques. • Train in use of adaptive equipment. • Explore alternatives for prevocational/vocational training • Patient and family training in physical care, functional activities, use and maintenance of all equipment. • Provide home program.	• Self-feeding (may not be energy-efficient for some patients) • Assist with hygiene (may not be energy efficient for some patients) • Other—see functional objectives under C_4	• Mobile arm support, ball bearing feeder, or bedside slings • Dynamic tenodesis splint, externally powered flexor hand splint, or universal cuff • Special feeding equipment may include: scoop dish or plate with plate guard, nonslip surface such as Dycem, nontip cup or long straw, built-up handles on silverware • Splints and equipment listed above • Electric razor • Electric toothbrush • Equipment remains as stated in C_4 but objectives are accomplished more efficiently
C_6 Shoulder flexion and extension Elbow flexion Supination Wrist extension Weak sensory function in hand	• Passive range of motion (teach self-range as indicated). *Note:* Less than normal range desirable in the finger flexors and back extensors. Greater than normal range is desirable in the hamstrings (for lower extremity dressing). Full range is desirable in elbow extension (for locking elbows for pressure relief and transfers). • Strengthen remaining musculature. • May require respiratory program (see C_4) and strengthening of accessory breathing musculature. • Establish positioning alternatives (see C_4).	• Relieve ischial pressure in wheelchair • Self-feeding • Assist with dressing • Assist with hygiene	• Arms of wheelchair used for sitting pushups • Wheelchair cushion • Universal cuff • Special feeding equipment including scoop dish or plate guard, nonslip surface such as Dycem, quad cup, rocker knife, spork, utensils with built-up handles • Dynamic tenodesis splint (when pinch is necessary) • Button hook • Velcro closures • Electric razor • Electric toothbrush

(Table continues)

TABLE 25–2 Comprehensive Rehabilitation Program for Children with Spinal Cord Injury (continued)

Level and Function Remaining	Treatment Guidelines	Functional Objective	Functional Equipment
C$_6$ (continued)	• Increase tolerance to upright position (see C$_4$). • Teach pressure relief techniques including wheelchair pushups and use of cushion. • Teach compensatory body management skills. • Teach activities of daily living (ADLs) including hygiene, dressing, feeding, bathing, skin care, and transfers. • Train in use of adaptive equipment. • Explore alternatives for prevocational/vocational training. • Patient and family training in physical care, functional activities, use and maintenance of all equipment. • Provide home program.	Assisted/independent transfers • Wheelchair propulsion • Tolerance for upright position • Self-bathing (may be independent except for transfers) • Writing • Typing (about 20 words per minute) • Using a telephone • Return to school (can be mainstreamed) • Driving a car (may be independent for some patients)	• Toileting devices including adaptations for catheter and leg bag, and suppository inserter • Mirror on gooseneck for skin inspection • Sliding board • Loops or trapeze for bed mobility • Grab bars • Electric or manual wheelchair with rim projections • Brake extensions • Tilt table (manual or electric) • Reclining wheelchair with cushion, elevating leg rests and trunkal supports. *Note:* Once tolerance for the upright position is achieved, standard wheelchair may be substituted for reclining wheelchair • Tub seat or shower chair • Hand-held spray attachment • Bath mitt with pocket for soap • Dynamic tenodesis splint • Pen/pencil holding device • Pencil or dowel in universal cuff or interlaced between fingers • Electric typewriter with automatic return • Touch-tone telephone • Pencil or dowel held in universal cuff or laced between fingers for dial telephone • Automatic dial telephone • Electric typewriter • Writing devices • Adapted tape recorder for note taking • Wheelchair bag for carrying supplies • Computer • Angled tray or work surface • Hand controls • Shoulder harness • Driving knob or cuff
C$_7$ Partial grasp and release (gross) Weak shoulder depression Active elbow extension Sensory function of hand	• Passive range of motion (teach self-range as indicated). *Note:* See passive range C$_6$. • Strengthen remaining musculature. • May require respiratory program and strengthening of accessory breathing musculature. • Establish positioning alternatives with increased emphasis on sitting and standing. • Teach compensatory body management skills. • Teach pressure relief techniques including wheelchair pushups and use of cushion. • Teach ADLs including hygiene, dressing, feeding, bathing, skin care, transfers, and homemaking skills. • Ambulation training for the younger patient (short distances only).	• Relieve ischial pressure in wheelchair • Independent self-feeding • Independent dressing (except for shoes) • Assist with hygiene • Independent transfers	• Arms of wheelchair used for sitting pushups • Wheelchair cushions • Utensils with built-up handle • Weave fork in fingers • Universal cuff • Button hook or Velcro closures • Zipper pulls • Pant loops • Sock aid • See C$_6$ • More energy-efficient • Hairbrush with large handle • Grab bars in bathroom, bedroom as needed • Sliding board

(Table continues)

TABLE 25–2 Comprehensive Rehabilitation Program for Children with Spinal Cord Injury (continued)

Level and Function Remaining	Treatment Guidelines	Functional Objective	Functional Equipment
C$_7$ (continued)	• Train for wheelchair mobility in the community. • Train in use of adaptive equipment. • Explore alternatives for prevocational/vocational training. • Patient and family training in physical care, functional activities, use and maintenance of all equipment. • Provide home program.	• Independent wheelchair propulsion • Tolerance for upright position • Assisted/independent bathing • Writing • Typing • Using a telephone • Cooking • Driving a car (with independent car transfer) • Return to school (can be mainstreamed)	• Rim projections if desired • Tilt table, manual or electric • Reclining wheelchair with cushion, elevating leg rests and trunkal supports. *Note:* See C$_6$ • Tub seat or shower chair • Hand-held spray • Bath mitt with pocket for soap • Pencil laced between fingers may be used • Built-up writing utensils • Felt-tipped pens • Pencil laced between fingers may be used • Electric typewriter • Pencil laced between fingers may be used • Touch-tone telephone • Automatic dial telephone • Wheelchair accessible work surfaces • Wheelchair accessible appliances • Other adaptive kitchen equipment as indicated • Hand controls • Steering knob or cuff • Electric typewriter • Wheelchair bag for carrying supplies • Tape recorder for taking notes • Computer
C$_8$ to T$_4$ Good to normal upper extremity function	• Passive range of motion (teach self-range). *Note:* Less than normal range is desirable in the back extensors. Greater than normal range is desirable in the hamstrings. • Strengthen remaining musculature. • Increase general endurance and conditioning. • Establish positioning alternatives (see C$_7$). • Teach compensatory body management skills. • Teach pressure relief techniques including wheelchair pushups and use of cushion. • Teach ADLs (see C$_7$). • Ambulation training for the younger patient. • Train for wheelchair mobility in the community. • Train in use of adaptive equipment. • Explore alternatives for prevocational/vocational training. • Patient and family training in physical care, functional activities, use and maintenance of all equipment. • Provide home program.	• Increase tolerance to upright position • Relieve ischial pressure • Independent skin inspection • Independent bathing • Independent transfers • Independent community mobility • Independent cooking • Independent light housekeeping (may not be energy efficient) • Return to school	• Tilt table, manual or electric • Reclining wheelchair with cushion, elevating leg rests and trunkal supports. *Note:* See C$_6$ • Arms of wheelchair used for sitting pushups • Wheelchair cushion • Mirror with or without gooseneck • Bath or shower chair • Sliding board may be used • Into wheelchair-accessible buildings • Sidewalk ramps • In wheelchair-accessible kitchen • In wheelchair-accessible house • Manual wheelchair with tray • Wheelchair bag for supplies

(Table continues)

562

TABLE 25–2   Comprehensive Rehabilitation Program for Children with Spinal Cord Injury (continued)

Level and Function Remaining	Treatment Guidelines	Functional Objective	Functional Equipment
T_5 to L_2 Partial to good trunk stability Increased endurance due to larger respiratory reserve	• Passive range of motion (teach self-range). *Note:* Greater than normal range is desirable in the hamstrings. • Strengthen remaining musculature. • Increase general endurance and conditioning. • Establish positioning alternatives (see C_7). • Teach compensatory body management skills. • Teach pressure relief techniques including wheelchair pushups and use of cushion. • Teach ADLs including hygiene, dressing, bathing, skin care, transfers, and homemaking skills. • Ambulation training (function and endurance will depend on level). • Train for community mobility (wheelchair or ambulation). • Train in the use of adaptive equipment. • Explore alternatives for prevocational/vocational training. • Patient and family training in physical care, functional activities, use and maintenance of all equipment. • Provide home program.	• Independent self-care • Wheelchair mobility • Ambulation (for short distances) • Independent housekeeping • Return to school	• Bathtub bench or shower chair • Mirror for skin inspection • Standard or low-backed wheelchair • Bilateral long leg braces with or without pelvic band • Crutches • In wheelchair-accessible house • Manual wheelchair with tray • Wheelchair bag for supplies
L_{3-4} Pelvic-trunk stabilizers Hip flexors, adductors, quadriceps	• Teach self-range if indicated. • Strengthen remaining musculature. • Increase general endurance and conditioning. • Teach compensatory body management skills. • Teach awareness of pressure areas. • Teach ADLs including hygiene, dressing, bathing, skin care, transfers, and homemaking skills. • Ambulation training. • Train for community mobility. • Train in the use and maintenance of braces/MAFOs if indicated. • Explore alternatives for prevocational/vocational training. • Patient and family training in physical care, functional activities, use and maintenance of all equipment. • Provide home program.	• Independent self-care • Independent ambulation • Independent housekeeping • Return to school	• No equipment necessary • Short leg braces or molded ankle/foot orthosis (MAFOs) • Crutches or canes may be used • No equipment necessary • Backpack for supplies if crutches or canes are used
L_5 to S_3 Hip extensors, abductors Knee flexors Ankle control	• Teach self-range if indicated. • Strengthen remaining musculature. • Increase general endurance and conditioning. • Teach compensatory body management skills. • Teach awareness of pressure areas.	• Independent self-care • Independent ambulation • Independent housekeeping • Return to school	• No equipment necessary • MAFOs may be used • Crutches or canes may be used • No equipment necessary • Backpack for supplies if crutches or canes are used

(Table continues)

TABLE 25–2 **Comprehensive Rehabilitation Program for Children with Spinal Cord Injury (continued)**

Level and Function Remaining	Treatment Guidelines	Functional Objective	Functional Equipment
L5 to S3 (continued)	• Teach ADLs including hygiene, dressing, bathing, skin care, transfers, and homemaking skills. • Ambulation training. • Train for community mobility. • Train in the use and maintenance of braces/MAFOs if indicated. • Explore alternatives for prevocational/vocational training. • Patient and family training in physical care, functional activities, use and maintenance of all equipment. • Provide home program.		

Source: Wilberger 1986: 212–221. Reprinted with permission of Futura Publishing Co., New York.

Going Home

Returning home can often be a most traumatic time. Familiar surroundings may no longer be comforting if getting around the house is a major task. Isolation from supportive professionals and other patients with similar conditions may have a negative impact. Physical care initially predominates. Peers, family, friends, and others in the community are often eager to help but do not know how. Careful planning and using problem solving skills will best support positive growth experiences and ease the transition. Take each problem, imagine the worst consequence, and make a plan for it. Tackle the barriers and keep breaking them down to a manageable size (Haw 1989).

Table 25–3 offers an organizational structure to assist families and professionals. Phase one is pivotal in determining parenting abilities, stamina, interest, and coping capacities to support care of their disabled child in the home. As the risk factors add up, community-based supports need to be strengthened. The issue of attendant care is a major factor and impacts the well-being not only of the child, but of the family. Lack of reliable care givers and of financial reimbursement for their services are widespread problems (addressed in Chapters 2 and 32). Creative planning to determine the amount of help needed and to locate and pay for services is often achieved to some degree, and most communities have some sort of network or information about state programs that may be of assistance. Alternatives, such as foster care, may have to be considered. Most often children do return home, but the lack of support services and mounting difficulties, as in the story of Johnny (see Box), may result in preventable deterioration in functional abilities and medical complications.

In Touch with Kids is a welcome versatile resource for both parents and children. This publication of the National SCI Association offers unique stories and resources, as well as actual networking opportunities.

Returning to School

Children with SCI usually wish to return to their preinjury schools. The 1968 Architecture Barrier Act and Public Law 90–480, Section 502 (Rehabilitation Act of 1973), have required compliance with new architectural and transportation standards. They mandate, for instance, that classrooms be accessible for wheelchairs and that the school must make architectural modifications. Personnel must be prepared to attend to personal care needs, transport, and help in the classroom.

Children with SCI are often fearful of how the other kids in the class will respond to them when they return to school. Health care professionals can often help by explaining what it means to have SCI. Kids on the Block, a powerful nationwide program of disabled puppets, began when a special education teacher realized how other classmates needed help to become comfortable with a disabled child returning to school. (See the box, Educational Resources, in this chapter for more information.)

At Play

Play is the work of children and is a critical factor in normal growth and development. While the child is in the hospital, recreational therapists and child-life specialists assist in identifying the child's interests and abilities and make recommendations on adaptive equipment that can assist the child in participating in a particular sport, such as archery, bowling, hunting, or fishing. See Chapter 24.

TABLE 25–3 System Care Plans: Chart of Phases, Roles, and Activities

Participant	Activity Acute Care to Stabilization Phase 1	Planning the Discharge and Home Care Phase 2	Implementing the Home Care Plan Phase 3
Parent Mother and/or father; legal guardian.	1. Helps determine if child can come home. 2. Evaluates and is evaluated on ability to give home care.	1. Helps develop Home Care Plan. 2. Requests training needed for Home Care Plan. 3. Helps identify needed services and supports. 4. Plans any necessary home modification. 5. Charts time required for ordinary domestic activities before child comes home.	1. Assumes major responsibility for care of child. 2. Evaluates and requests additional needed services. 3. Charts family activity after child comes home.
Care Manager Trained professional who devises, coordinates, and helps implement the Home Care Plan (see Chapter 14).	1. Serves as consultant to parent(s) and interdisciplinary team about community support systems.	1. Assumes overall responsibility for development of Home Care Plan. 2. Can participate with physician in developing Discharge Plan. 3. Works closely with parents and ensures availability of community support services.	1. Provides backup support to parents as they assume responsibility for care management. 2. Is available for periodic trouble-shooting.
Interdisciplinary Team Professionals from all disciplines (medical, nursing, social services, speech and hearing, educational, and often other parents) whose expertise comes from experience.	1. Serve as consultants about possibility of discharge to community. The hospital's nursing team provides information about levels of care, feeding, nutrition, and activity of the child.	1. Develop/consult/participate in Discharge Plan and Home Care Plan. 2. Help identify community resources. 3. Educate parents to prepare for child's placement at home: • Environmental changes • Confirmation of funding • Training	1. Serve as consultants as needed and provide ongoing support.
Community Support Services All resources, parent support groups, voluntary organizations, national organizations, vendors, and agencies ensuring the chlid's adjustment to the home.		1. Contacted by care manager, parents, or interdisciplinary team to check availability and provision of resources. 2. Consulted in Discharge Plan and Home Care Plan.	1. Deliver services.

Source: Bilotti 1984. Reprinted with permission of Georgetown University Child Development Center, Washington, DC.

Swimming is often enjoyed by children with SCI despite their physical limitations. Swimming is both recreational and therapeutic. The children can move freely in the water, and because of buoyancy can do things that they normally would have difficulty doing outside the water. Swimming also relieves spasticity.

Kids also enjoy going to the mall, movies, or just hanging out, and these activities make them feel as if they belong to the group. Children may also enjoy sleepovers and camping trips. Nothing is impossible!

As one mother of a preschool child with high quadriplegia explains, "Although our daughter understands on one level that she is unable to do many things, she believes on another level that she is actually performing those developmental tasks. We always search for imaginative toys, but tissues and rubber bands are favorites at our house" (Wicker in Johnson, Berry, Goldeen, and Wicker 1991: 18).

Safe, durable, innovative, low-cost products are hard to find. Adaptable toys that use batteries with safety controlled switches can provide lots of fun. Figure 25–1 pictures a disabled doll with a special purpose. Catalogues referenced in the box, Educational Resources, provide some resources.

FAMILY VIEWPOINT: THE NEED FOR ONGOING SUPPORT

Johnny is a 7-year-old boy who lives in a rural area of South Carolina with his father, mother and 3 older sisters. His father runs a small farm, and his mother works full time in a factory in town. Johnny is in second grade and is an average student. Johnny's jobs include feeding the farm animals and collecting eggs. During his free time, he enjoys activities with his father such as fishing, hunting, and an occasional camping trip. Financial resources are limited for this family. Farming is going through tough times.

Tragedy struck the family one July 4th weekend. While on a family camping trip, Johnny dove into a three-foot-deep creek, off of a 15-foot-high bridge. C_8 paraplegia resulted. A long acute period of hospitalization, complicated by respiratory arrest related to near drowning, followed. The rehabilitation period was difficult, but Johnny eventually became independent in his own care.

Johnny's parents' involvement in his care was limited because of their work schedule. They did visit every weekend. Once they were educated to care for a person with SCI, they began taking Johnny out on 6-hour passes. Recreational therapists met with the parents and taught them how to make adaptations so that Johnny could do the things he loved: hunting, fishing, and camping.

Johnny was almost ready for discharge. A home visit had been completed, and recommendations were made concerning accessibility of his home. Major changes to the home were almost impossible because of limited finances. Johnny's parents' private insurance ran out after the acute phase of his illness.

When a discharge date was agreed on, Johnny's mom took a week's vacation, which she spent with Johnny in the hospital's independent living center. They lived in a wheelchair-accessible apartment, away from the nursing unit. Mom provided all necessary assistance and followed Johnny's daily schedule. She reviewed information taught at previous education classes and also worked with members of the rehabilitation team to solve problems. After the week, Johnny went home.

Three months postdischarge Johnny developed a urinary tract infection that required hospitalization and intravenous antibiotics. This event frightened Johnny's mother so much that she began to do Johnny's catheterizations once he came home. When questioned about this, she felt that if she did his catheterizations Johnny would not get sick again.

Then, because Johnny had a small pressure sore, Mom began to do his skin checks every day, too. She and Johnny fought frequently about this because Johnny felt it was an invasion of his personal being. "Johnny is very slow in the morning to be independent in dressing. So I've been getting him dressed," she reported, "and also transferring him into his chair so that he gets off to school on time, and I get off to work on time." Mom felt Johnny cannot do his bowel program on his own because the bathroom is not accessible and he needs to do his bowel program in bed. She reported feeling exhausted most of the time. Johnny's dad was troubled but tended to withdraw. Family tension mounted, while Johnny's independence diminished.

Johnny and his family are trapped in a deteriorating situation. This story, and many others like it, reveal how vitally important it is to share preventive expertise with families and coordinate services between inpatient and outpatient services and between facilities and community services/resources. Chapter 33 describes other strategies to identify risks and minimize the stresses faced over time.

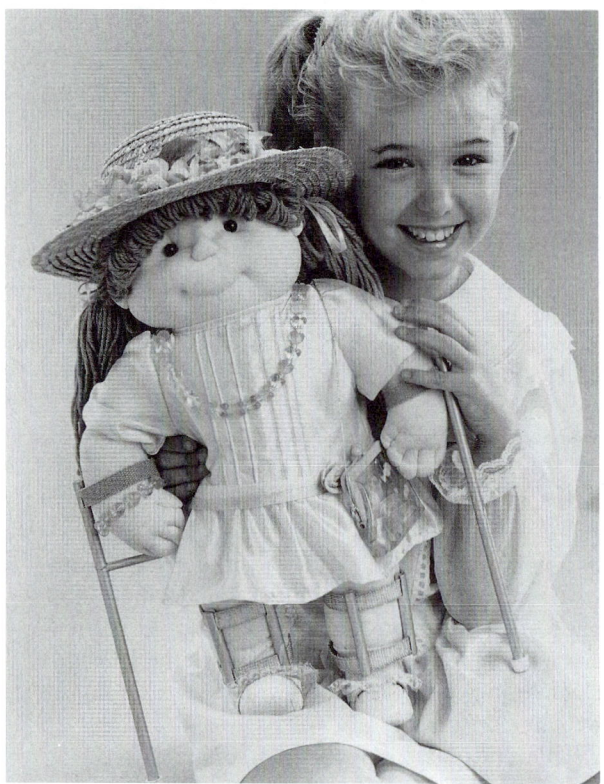

FIGURE 25–1 HAL'S PALS are designed to help children express feelings about their own disabilities or the disabilities of others.

PREVENTING SECONDARY DISABILITIES

Prevention of secondary disabilities is often generally described as prevention of secondary complications. Long-term implications and preventable consequences of SCI have been addressed throughout this text, and all the principles of management need to be applied. However, as children grow their needs constantly change, necessitating regular assessment and modification of care plans. Growing out of a wheelchair is the classic example!

Children especially must be constantly monitored and treated for marked skeletal system changes that occur with natural growth and development. *Scoliosis*, with an incidence reported as high as 98% following SCI in children (Betz 1989), is managed with placement of a thoracolumbar sacral orthosis (TLSO), which unfortunately, to be effective, must be worn all of the time when up in the wheelchair. Surgical intervention with fusions and/or spinal instrumentation may become necessary. Related care is outlined in Chapter 20. *Osteoporosis* also requires constant physician assessment and is particularly problematic during the formative years. Standing to bear weight, supported with

a frame, orthosis, or adapted wheelchair as in Figure 25–2, is believed to slow the process of calcium loss but is unable to reverse it. *Hip dislocation* is a recognized complication in children with SCI, but until recently it was not treated aggressively. Realizing how crucial positioning in the wheelchair is and the potential for ambulating with functional electrical stimulation have changed this approach. Abduction splinting or surgical intervention may be needed. Fortunately, *spasticity* seems less of a problem for young children, but if it does occur, treatment as outlined in Chapter 27 may be considered and modified.

Although this is not documented, an increase in preventable complications—primarily skin and urinary tract—has been noted by pediatric SCI specialists as children reach their teenage years. This increase seems to correlate with

---

EDUCATIONAL RESOURCES

Hals Pals, PO Box 3490, Winter Park, CO 80482. *Publishes a versatile* Power Kit *teaching guide to use in a classroom with a variety of disabled dolls, complete with wheelchairs and other aids, and coloring books.*

National Information Center for Children and Youth with Handicaps, P.O. Box 1492, Washington, D.C. 20013. *Operates clearinghouse, provides technical assistance, and responds to personal inquiries.*

National Spinal Cord Injury Association. *In Touch With Kids.* Woburn, MA: Author. *Regular column in National Publication with capacity for problem solving and sharing of experiences for parents and children. Welcome relief!*

Jesana Ltd., P.O. Box 17, Irvington, NY 10533. *A special catalogue filled with adaptive toys and creative ideas.*

Toys for Special Children, Inc., S. E. Kanor, Ph.D., 385 Warburton Ave., Hastings-on-Hudson, NY 10706

The Kids on the Block! 9385–C Gerwig Lane, Columbia, MD 21046. *An educational experience used successfully by teachers around the world in which children learn about disabilities through a one-to-one dialogue with puppets. Research studies found program to be effective in creating positive attitude changes among elementary school students toward their disabled peers. Colorful, imaginative use of disabled puppets is supported by props, scripts, audio cassettes, training guide, follow-up materials, and resource suggestions with ongoing support from the national company.*

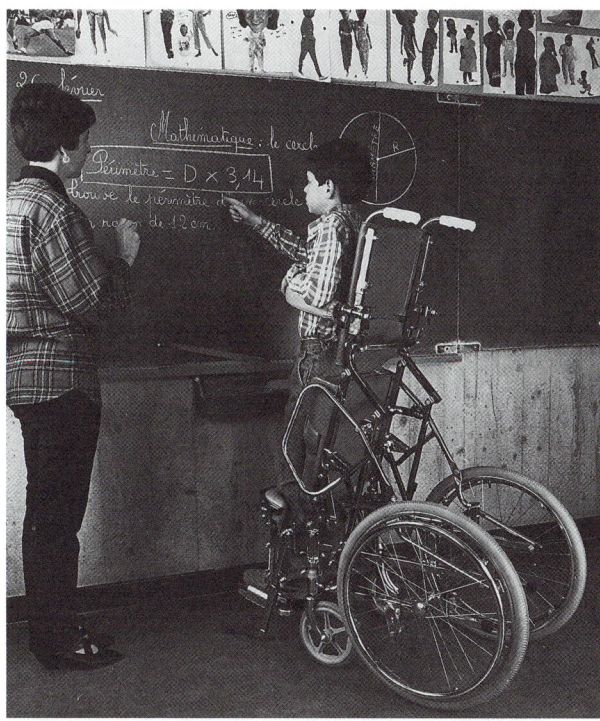

FIGURE 25–2 The "Lifestand" wheelchair offers convenience and independence (nonmotorized) in assuming the standing position in addition to use as a standard wheelchair. Available from I.D.C. Medical Equipment, Inc., Folcroft, PA.

the transition from parental supervision to the children's assuming greater responsibility for their personal care. It is important to approach any setbacks as learning opportunities rather than mistakes to be condemned.

Issues concerning sexuality naturally surface as children mature and may be particularly difficult for parents to discuss. Chapter 10 addresses these concerns and the necessity for access to information. Encourage parents to view sexuality issues in a broad sense. Concerns such as attractiveness and potential to become a romantic partner and parent impact self-image and esteem and therefore influence feelings of well-being in general.

Prevention of secondary disabilities is discussed further in Chapter 33.

FUTURE DIRECTIONS

Although most children and families do adapt, the road is long, helping hands are few, and costs are high. Society neglects disabled children (Hobbs and Perrin 1985). Johnson (1987) calls attention to the even more significant neglect of the family struggling with the traumatic consequences of SCI. Children and their parents particularly need help from well-qualified, nonparent care givers and relief from financial burdens. Political focus, legislative

collaboration, cooperative funding, and partnerships among professionals and families will also help.

One innovative model of services in British Columbia interrelates four major programs. They provide health-related support services under the joint jurisdictions of the Ministries of Health, Social Services, Housing, and Education, with assistance from parents' advisory committees:

1. *The At Home Program* is designed to help parents with the financial burden of caring for severely disabled children at home. It provides a benefit package of medical insurance, pharmacy coverage, supplies for health care needs, medically essential equipment including maintenance and repair, medical transportation, therapies, dental care, orthotics and prosthetics, and respite and relief care.

2. *The Associate Family Program* offers an alternative to families simply unable to cope, recognizes that the child's family is an integral part of the child's life, and family involvement is of utmost importance, even if the burden becomes too great to keep the child with the natural family. The child's parent(s) remain legal guardian(s) of the child and remain active in the child care planning and service delivery process, but the child lives with a selected "associate family." All community-based resources are coordinated and financial assistance is provided through the Ministry of Health. Ongoing monitoring and cost effectiveness and evaluation is the responsibility of the Ministry of Health.

3. *The Respite Program* recognizes the value and importance of community-based and flexible respite care to support and maintain family integrity. Medically fragile children, who include those with severe disabilities, are cared for by qualified nurses who participate in direct care, consultation, or supervisory roles. Care is provided by nurses, aides, attendants, or friends as needed, either in the home, at a day care center, or in a facility when a child needs to be readmitted for a variety of reasons. An interdisciplinary care team prepares for discharge by devising a master comprehensive community care plan and an individual care plan that connect all the medical, health, and equipment needs. Families' assessment of their own abilities and skills are included as well as safety assessment of the home. Plans must be detailed, individualized, integrated, responsive, and cost-effective to be of benefit. Joint care plans are distributed to families, primary care physicians, care givers, and agencies involved. Quality guidelines address verification of need, change in needs, determination of criteria to be assessed, management plans, and evaluation from a joint perspective.

4. *The At School Program* delineates support needed in the educational environment and coordinates and jointly funds a variety of care givers to provide services to severely disabled children so that they can participate in the mainstream public school system. This program closely resembles *Project School Care* designed by the

Boston Children's Hospital (with federal funding support) to integrate children with special medical needs into a school situation safely.

To overcome the disparate needs of children—both urban and rural, both rich and poor—umbrella plans need to be flexible, yet well enough defined, to ensure adequate linkages and quality of services. The Title V program in New York State is an example of such joint efforts, region by region, with a strong support from the American Academy of Pediatrics.

To this end, parents of children with SCI must be introduced to the following concepts during rehabilitation (Bilotti 1984):

- How to develop effective partnerships with professionals to maintain health and manage the effects of SCI in children

- How to become knowledgeable about benefits and entitlements and analyze financing of equipment and services needed
- How to participate in collaborative, commnunity-based teams to secure services for children with special needs
- Ultimately, how to assume additional roles as care givers, case managers, educational and social advocates, financial planners, and resource specialists

Whatever the structural or funding framework and the degree of government involvement, public and private leadership efforts, which vary widely from state to state, must cooperatively address the roles of health care professionals and their continuing education, parent-professional partnerships, the needs assessment and planning of responsive services for children and families, and reimbursement issues (Magrab 1987).

REFERENCES

Altchuler, A., Butz, M., and Meyer, J. 1977. Even children can learn to do clean self-catheterization. *American Journal of Nursing* 77: 97–101.

Anderson, J. M., and Schutt, A. H. 1980. Spinal injury in children: A review of the 156 cases seen from 1950–1978. *Mayo Clinic Proceedings* 55: 499–504.

Babcok, J. L. 1975. Spinal injuries in children. *Pediatric Clinics of North America* 22: 487–500.

Betz, R. 1989. Children with spinal cord injuries. Unpublished study, Shriners Hospital for Crippled Children. Philadelphia, PA.

Bilotti, G. 1984. *Getting Children Home: Hospital to Community.* Washington, DC: Georgetown University Child Development Center. *Describes phases of planning and identifies key roles of parents, interdisciplinary team, care managers, and those in community support services. Presents numerous worksheets and sample checklists, including sample letters to power companies and highway departments, for children with special needs. To minimize gaps, special section deals with organizational system of community resources.*

Burke, D. C. 1970. Spinal cord trauma in children. *Paraplegia* 10: 1–14.

Carlson, D. S., and Kass, E. J. 1990. *Clean Intermittent Catheterization: A Guide for Parents and Families.* Booklet available from Department of Pediatric Urology, Children's Hospital National Medical Center, 111 Michigan Avenue, NW, Washington, DC 20012.

Coley, J. L. 1978. *Pediatric Assessment of Self-Care Activities.* St. Louis: C. V. Mosby.

Deller, B., and Gruydanus, D. E. 1979. Psychological management of acute paraplegia in adolescents. *Pediatrics* 63 (4): 562–564.

Gaufin, L. M., and Goodman, S. J. 1975. Cervical spine injuries in infants. *Journal of Neurological Surgery* 42: 179–184.

Haw, N. 1989. *Keys to Freedom.* Booklet published by British Columbia Paraplegic Association and British Columbia Rehabilitation Society, Vancouver, BC, Canada.

Hobbs, N., and Perrin, J. M. 1985. *Issues in the Care of Children with Chronic Illness.* San Francisco: Jossey-Bass Publisher.

Independent Living Research Utilization, 1990. A *Message to Parents of Handicapped Youth.* Houston, TX: Author. *Discusses what the independent living movement can do for children. Includes issues such as teaching children with disabilities to be responsible, using available support systems; and identifying when to use attendant care. (ILRU has many other publications. Contact ILRU for more information.)*

Jaffe, K. M. 1987. *Childhood Power Mobility: Developmental, Technical and Clinical Perspectives.* Washington DC: RESNA Press.

Johnson, K., Berry, E., Goldeen, R., and Wicker, E. 1991. Growing up with a spinal cord injury. *SCI Nursing* 8 (1): 11–20.

Johnson, R. S. 1987. *Family Response to the Young Person with Chronic Illness: Two Case Studies.* Seattle: University of Washington Press.

Lehr, S. 1986. *Improving Social Behavior in Children in Order to Function in the Least Restrictive Environment Possible.* A *Summary of Conference Proceedings.* Prepared for the Georgetown University Child Development Center, National Center for Networking Community Based Services, Washington, DC.

Hugh MacMillan Medical Centre. 1988. *Clean Intermittent Catheterization for Children.* Toronto, Ontario: Author. *Excellent instructional videotape program for boys and girls.*

Magrab, P. R. 1987. *The Practicing Pediatrician and Family-Centered, Community-Based Health Care for Children with Chronic Illness and Disabling Conditions.* A *Summary of Conference Proceedings.* Prepared for the Georgetown University Child Development Center, National Center for Networking Community Based Services, Washington, DC. *Explores the Hawaii experience from perspectives of how to create change, interaction with the legislative process, the concept of* the "medical home," state child health plans, and a statewide inter-agency task force. Strategies and solutions for a national agenda are shared, and 26 state action summaries are presented. (Georgetown University Child Development Center also publishes an excellent workbook series to enable families to act as power brokers and case managers in their community.)

Nordan, R. 1976. The psychological reactions of children with neurological problems. *Child Psychology and Human Development* 6 (4): 214–223.

Sevorsky, J., and Opas, S. 1987. *Nursing Management of Children.* Boston: Jones and Bartlett Publishers. *An excellent text focusing on the promotion of health, growth, and development.*

Shriners Hospital for Crippled Children. 1989. *Spinal Cord Injury Self-Care Manual for Children.* San Francisco: Author.

Sullivan-Bolyai, S. 1986. Practical aspects of toilet training the child with a physical disability. *Comprehensive Pediatric Nursing* 9: 79–96.

Tori, J. A., and Kewalramani, L. S. 1978–1979. Urolithiasis in children with spinal cord injury. *Paraplegia* 16: 357–365.

Wilberger, J. E. 1986. *Spinal Cord Injuries in Children.* New York: Futura Publishing Company. *Focuses on the conservative and surgical management of the child with an injury to the immature spine. Multisystem assessment and treatments are explored throughout the early postinjury period and during rehabilitation.*

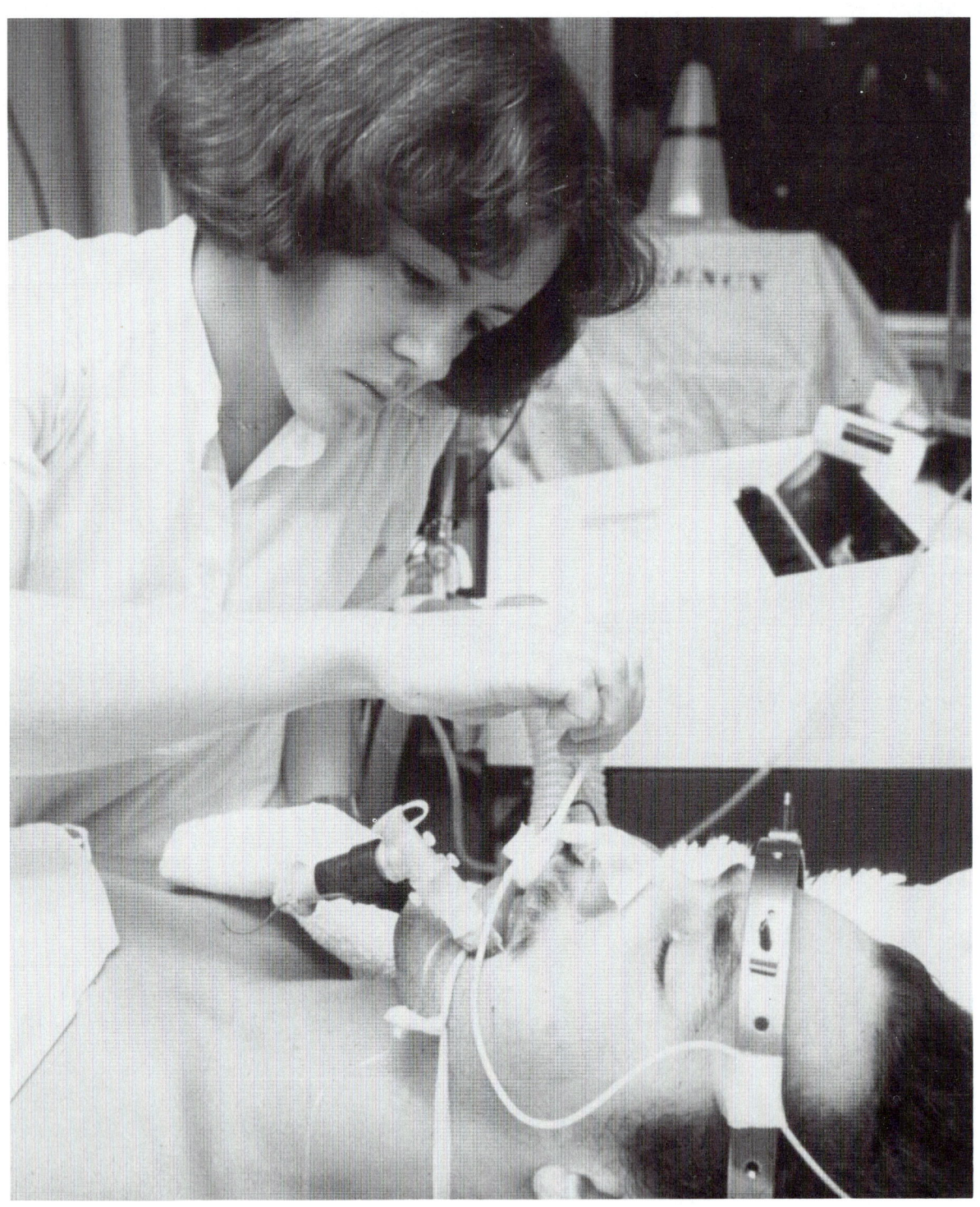

CHAPTER 26

The Combination Injury: Spinal Cord Injury with Concomitant Traumatic Brain Injury

Karen H. Hildebrand, R.N.
Alan H. Weintraub, M.D.

Chapter Outline

Health Care Objectives

- To review the incidence of combination spinal cord injury/traumatic brain injury.
- To describe a pathophysiological framework for understanding common cognitive deficits associated with traumatic brain injury.
- To describe issues related to assessment of these deficits in spinal cord injury rehabilitation.
- To understand the functional impact of brain injury on spinal cord injury rehabilitation programs.

The rapid acceleration/deceleration event following a motor vehicle accident or fall that results in spinal cord injury (SCI) can also result in concurrent traumatic brain injury (TBI). In fact, brain injury may be the most common associated injury occurring at the time of spinal cord trauma (Morris, Roth, and Davidoff 1985). The injury to the brain in these patients can vary in severity from mild (brief loss of consciousness) to severe (more prolonged loss of consciousness). Even though most concomitant brain injuries are mild (Wagner, Kopaniky, and Esposito 1983), the resultant sequelae can result in impairments of attention, concentration, memory, and other complex cognitive skills which in turn can profoundly affect the rehabilitation process and outcome of the spinal cord injured patient (Morris, Roth, and Davidoff 1985).

INCIDENCE

The effects of traumatic brain injury in a patient who has sustained SCI are often overshadowed by the more obvious physical sequelae of paralysis. Cognitive sequelae, which are often overlooked and underestimated, are frequently attributed to such likely phenomena as medication side effects, anxiety, depression, or preinjury personality traits. However, many spinal cord injured patients sustain concomitant brain injury at the time of initial injury, and

cognitive sequelae can be explained as such (Davidoff, Morris, and Roth 1985; Richards, Brown, Hagglund, Bua, and Reeder 1988; Rimel 1981; Wilmot et al. 1985).

In reviewing several studies, Morris and associates (1986) report that the incidence of concomitant brain injury in spinal cord injured patients ranges from 13% to 58%. This range varies depending on the assessment criteria used. Studies that report lower incidence tend to measure more obvious evidence of direct head trauma such as death from brain injury, skull fractures, intracerebral contusions, and hemorrhages as evidenced by cerebral scans. When using measures of loss of consciousness (LOC) and posttraumatic amnesia (PTA), which are more sensitive indicators of cerebral dysfunction, a higher incidence is found. Even brief loss of consciousness or posttraumatic amnesia without associated loss of consciousness may be associated with significant disturbances in cognitive, behavioral, and emotional functioning. Studies indicate that most brain injuries in this SCI population are mild, and surprisingly, there is no significant difference in incidence of TBI in people with quadriplegia when compared to people with paraplegia (Wagner, Kopaniky, and Esposito 1983).

OVERVIEW OF TRAUMATIC BRAIN INJURY

The Brain

The brain is a highly sophisticated, gelatinous structure made up of billions of nerve cells and fibers creating a *neuronal network* (Figure 26–1). This neuronal network functions like a computer by communicating impulses necessary to interpret sensory stimuli (sensation, smell, taste, vision, and hearing) as well as control and coordinate all body movements, thought processes, and emotions.

The three major parts of the brain are the cerebrum, the cerebellum, and the brainstem (Figure 26–2). The outer layers of the cerebrum or the *cerebral cortex* are divided into lobes that are responsible for higher-level functions of communication, perception, cognition, behavior, and emotions (Figure 26–3). Beneath the cortex are deeper structures (thalamus, hypothalamus, hippocampus, limbic areas) and pathways comprising the *subcortex*, which accounts for basic vital activities (blood pressure, heart rate, and body temperature) and states of wakefulness. Within the subcortex are long white matter pathways that transmit information between different centers and lobes within the brain. These subcortical pathways process information quickly and efficiently between the cerebral hemispheres. An intact neuronal network provides for each hemisphere

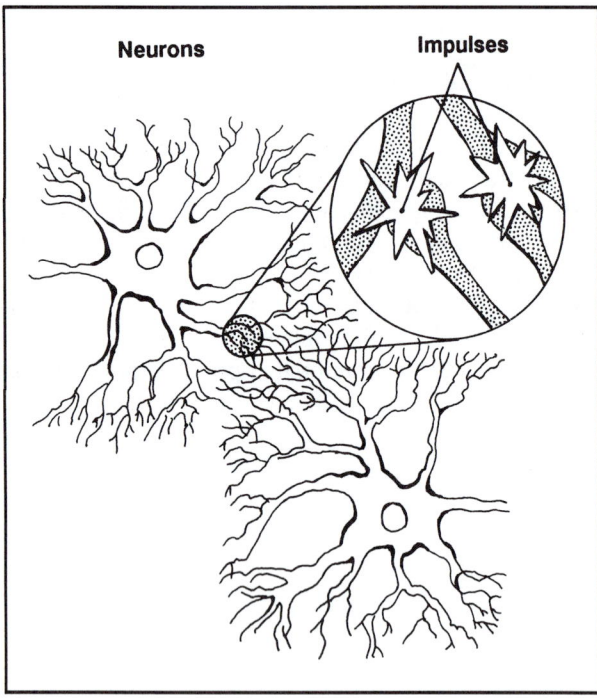

FIGURE 26–1 The neuronal network of the brain. From R. Ornstein and R. F. Thompson. 1984. *The Amazing Brain.* Ill. by David Macaulay. Boston: Houghton Mifflin Company.

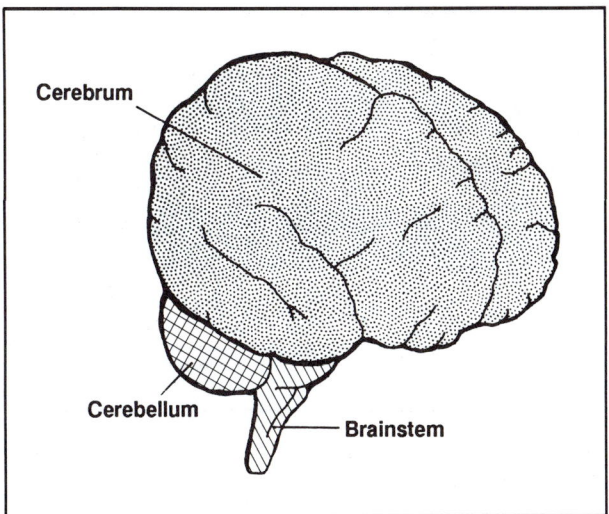

FIGURE 26–2 The three major parts of the brain. From R. Ornstein and R. F. Thompson. 1984. *The Amazing Brain*. Ill. by David Macaulay. Boston: Houghton Mifflin Company.

and each lobe with its own special functions to work together and enable a person to respond and function as an individual (review Figure 26–3).

The *cerebellum* controls and coordinates muscle movements and also plays a role in an individual's frame and equilibrium reactions. The *brainstem* is the final common pathway controlling movement necessary for verbal communication, swallowing, and extremity function. This

chapter's discussion is limited to injury affecting the cerebrum and its connecting pathways because correlative cognitive, behavioral, and emotional dysfunction may ensue.

Mechanisms of Injury

This complex brain is housed in and protected by the skull and is cushioned by a cerebrospinal fluid-filled system (Figure 26–4). Despite these protective structures, the brain is extremely vulnerable and can be easily injured or damaged. Acceleration/deceleration of the head such as occurs in motor vehicle accidents, falls, or even following a direct blow creates twisting wavelike forces within the brain that result in shearing, tearing, and injury to delicate nerve fibers (Figure 26-5). These mechanisms account for subsequent lesions within the brain that are either diffuse or focal in nature. Damaged areas not only vary in type but also severity and therefore contribute to various kinds of cognitive and neurobehavioral symptoms.

Diffuse Injury

Diffuse brain injury or diffuse axonal injury (DAI) is the shearing and tearing of a widespread distribution of nerve fibers that results from the rotational and wavelike forces generated within the brain following a rapid deceleration event (Figure 26–6). A significant injury of this nature not only disrupts the outer structures of the cerebral cortex or so-called cognitive integrative areas but injures deeper subcortical pathways resulting in loss of consciousness or di-

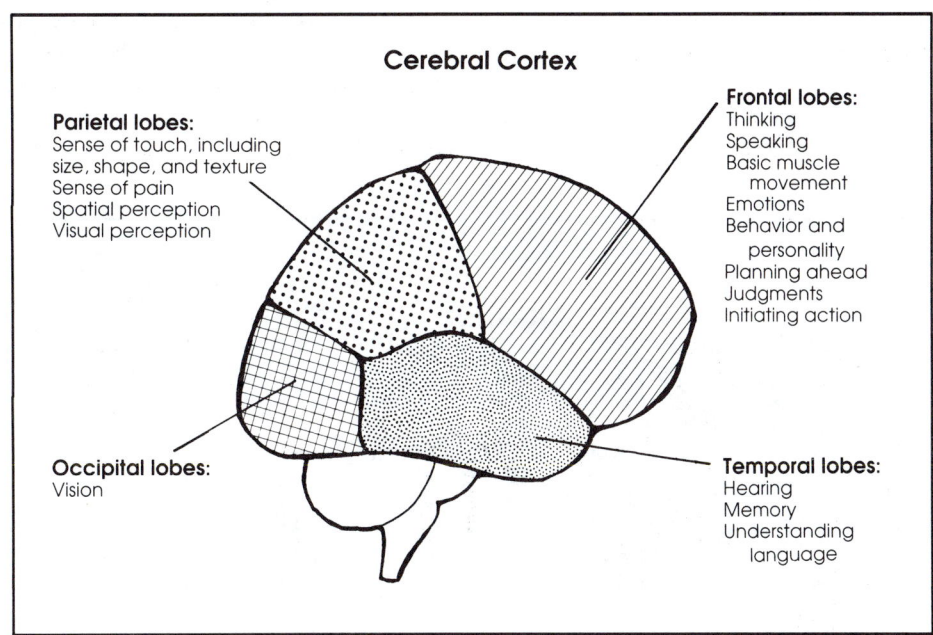

FIGURE 26–3 The cerebral cortex and higher levels of functions. From R. Ornstein and R. F. Thompson. 1984. *The Amazing Brain*. Ill. by David Macaulay. Boston: Houghton Mifflin Company.

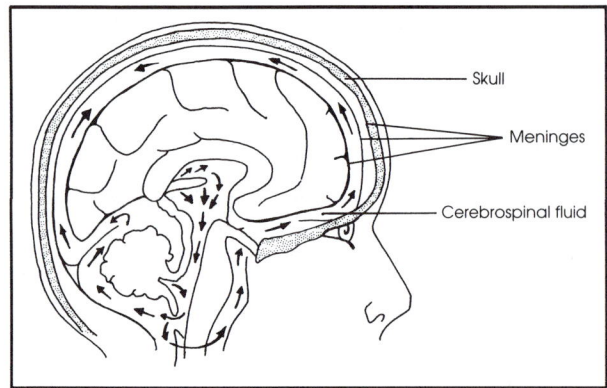

FIGURE 26–4 Protective coverings of the brain. (© Craig Hospital)

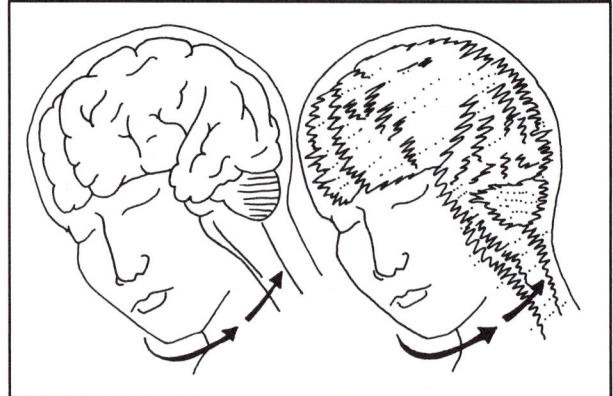

FIGURE 26–5 Acceleration/deceleration injury to the brain. (© Craig Hospital)

minished responsiveness or awareness. Unfortunately, the severity of diffuse injury is not easily demonstrated by cerebral scanning technology. Clinicians therefore rely on clinical parameters to understand injury severity and its coinciding recovery pattern. The length of time that the patient is unconscious can indicate the severity of diffuse brain injury and can last from seconds or minutes to weeks. The longer the period of unconsciousness, the more severe the injury and consequences.

As consciousness is regained, the patient generally experiences a period of confusion or inability to remember recent and present events. This phase of recovering consciousness is commonly called posttraumatic amnesia (Figure 26–7). As with coma, this anterograde amnestic period represents a total interval of disturbed consciousness that correlates with injury severity and sequelae (Table 26–1).

The familiar term, *concussion,* is really a mild diffuse brain injury. Therefore, in mild diffuse brain injury, loss of consciousness or posttraumatic amnesia may be brief or unnoticed. Nonetheless, these milder injuries may result in cognitive disturbances that cause future functional problems for the patient. Those cognitive disturbances may include impairments in attention, concentration, vigilance, and speed of information processing. A number of patients may even suffer from additional postconcussive symptoms including headaches, dizziness, irritability, fatigability, and depression (Barth et al. 1983). Generally, physical deficits have not been related to mild brain injury.

Patients sustaining moderate or severe diffuse injury will experience those aforementioned cognitive sequelae to a much greater degree and could have associated physical deficits (that is, superimposed hemiparesis). As a result, their functional outcomes will be even more significantly affected. Also, most likely, the acute postinjury course in these patients has been complicated by a more prolonged period of unconsciousness and posttraumatic amnesia.

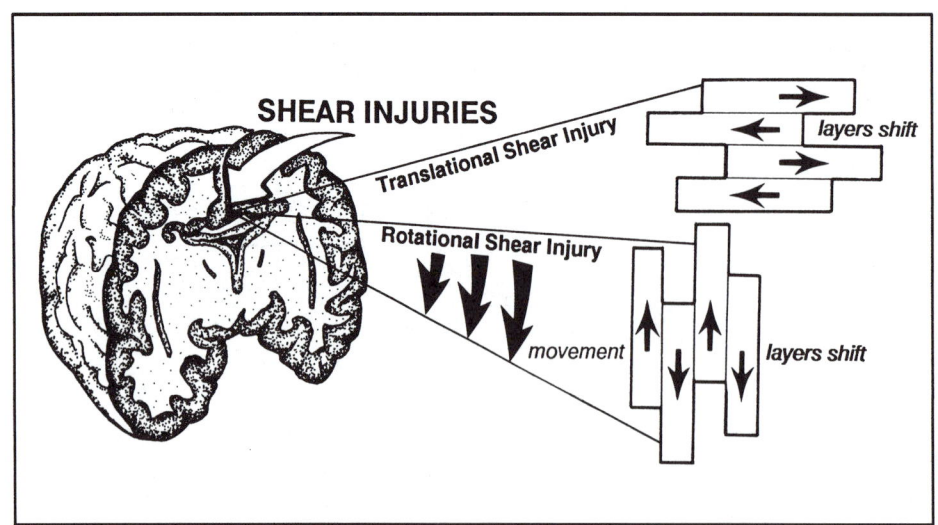

FIGURE 26–6 Shearing injuries to the brain following trauma. (© Craig Hospital)

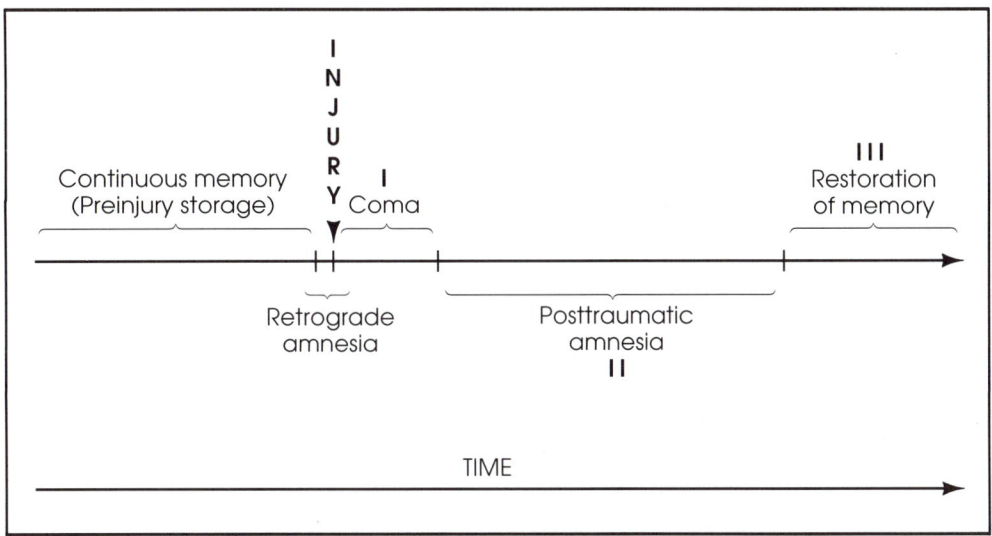

FIGURE 26–7   Early stages of recovery from closed head injury. Sequence of subacute disturbance of memory after closed head injury. The periods of coma (I) and posttraumatic amnesia (II) have been traditionally combined to yield a total interval of impaired consciousness that extends until continuous memory for ongoing events (III) is restored. From *Neurobehavioral Consequences of Closed Head Injury*, by H. S Levine, A. L. Benton, and R. G. Grossman. Oxford University Press, New York, © 1982. Reprinted with permission.

Consequently, brain injury becomes a major factor in care and treatment. These patients may benefit as well from a specialized brain injury treatment program.

Focal Injury

Focal brain injury predictably occurs in areas where inertial movement of the brain is directly opposed by bone or membrane. This leads to contusion (bruising) or lacerations of brain tissue by direct, sudden contact with the rough interior surface of the skull. These brain-injured areas typ-

TABLE 26–1   Duration of Posttraumatic Amnesia (PTA) and Severity of Injury

PTA Duration	Severity
Less than 5 minutes	Very mild
5 to 60 minutes	Mild
1 to 24 hours	Moderate
1 to 7 days	Severe
1 to 4 weeks	Very severe
More than 4 weeks	Extremely severe

Source: M. Rosenthal, E. Griffith, M. Bond, and J. D. Miller (eds): *Rehabilitation of the Head Injured Adult,* Philadelphia: F.A. Davis Co., 1983.

ically involve the anterior portion or frontal poles and inferolateral portions or temporal poles. Although these areas do not necessarily modulate consciousness, they are quite involved in other more specific intellectual and emotional actions (Figure 26–3). Thus, injury within frontal and/or temporal zones may not only contribute to difficulties in attention, concentration, and memory but also may cause the patient difficulties in reasoning, problem solving, planning, and judgment. These patients are often challenged in efforts to formulate, evaluate, modify, and execute a plan of action and display difficulties as well in the regulation of intellectual and emotional activity.

Less predictable areas of focal injury occur as a result of direct trauma to brain tissue from penetrating injuries (for instance, gunshot wounds or stab wounds), hemorrhage, contusions, or from depressed skull fractures in which pieces of skull are forced within the brain. The impairments that result from these focal injuries generally correlate with the function of the area of the brain that has been damaged. These injuries may be demonstrated by computerized tomography or magnetic resonance imaging. Examples of correlative focal deficits include aphasia, apraxia, hemianopsia, and hemiparesis.

Hypoxic Injury

Diffuse *hypoxic injury* may occur as a result of increased intracranial pressure in conjunction with systemic hypotension and/or acute ventilatory insufficiency. This may result in selective damage to highly sensitive areas within the brain that are oxygen dependent. Particularly susceptible to hypoxia are the hippocampus, hypothalamic/limbic areas, and cortical border zones between lobes within the brain. Therefore, if a patient has sustained a period of hypoxia associated with SCI, there may be correlative problems in memory functioning, retaining new information, and with emotionality. Sometimes when SCI is associated with cardiac or respiratory arrest, more significant hypoxia may occur. This would not only result in some of the memory problems previously mentioned but also may cause the patient difficulties related to a lack of blood flow and oxygen to borderline or watershed areas within the cerebral cortex. Correlative neurobehavioral disturbances may then be more severe and focal to include speech impairments (aphasia), perceptual impairments (apraxia), and inability to recognize familiar objects, surroundings (agnosia), and so on.

In summary, the type, location, and extent of injury within the brain are important predictors of cognitive sequelae. The deficits related to different types of TBI frequently occur in mixed patterns. Recovery patterns related to cognitive, behavioral, and social impairments can persist for many months into and beyond the rehabilitation process. Therefore, clinicians need to observe carefully even the most subtle cognitive and neurobehavioral disturbances that may impact a patient's ability to learn in the rehabilitation setting. These deficits can cause functional interference in areas varying from the simplest of daily living skills to higher levels of complex motor tasks. Ultimately, such deficits lead to significant impairment in independence and productivity.

ASSESSMENT

Because TBI results in an array of *cognitive disturbances* that affect the SCI rehabilitation process, it is important to recognize those patients early and set up appropriate intervention strategies. In addition to obtaining a specific medical and neurological history relative to concomitant brain injury (loss of consciousness and posttraumatic amnesia which at times is difficult to ascertain), identify other *preinjury personality variables*. Look for a history of drug/ethanol abuse, previous psychiatric intervention, behavioral disorders, or learning disability. Preinjury school records and vocational history are important components of the assessment process. Once preinjury personality and character variables are well established, then clinicians can better understand whether cognitive or behavioral observations are related to preinjury issues, an exaggeration of preinjury issues, the brain injury itself, or a combination of these factors.

Even following a mild diffuse brain injury, patients may experience difficulties with attention and concentration. In the rehabilitation setting, these patients may present with more than expected mental and physical fatigue. Their impairments in selective attention contribute to distractibility. They may display poor shifting of attention back and forth so that the patient frequently gets lost in a group conversation.

Disorders of initiation and planning of goal-directed activities are also common following diffuse injuries as well as more focal frontal/temporal injuries. These patients demonstrate an impairment in so-called abstract attitude. Patients thus frequently miss the point and can take information presented to them quite literally rather than symbolically. Additionally, they may have difficulties inhibiting actions before the desired action is required and present with impulsive and perseverative responses. Their overall initiation time is slowed. As a result, patients display confusion as to where to start and stop in solving a problem and consequently often use unrealistic problem-solving strategies. They may have difficulty ordering or sequencing more complex information. Because patients who have these difficulties also have trouble learning from their mistakes and successes, they may have difficulty in knowing when, where, and how to ask for help.

Disorders of judgment and perception are frequent following frontal/temporal and multifocal injuries. This may result in misperceiving or misinterpreting the actions or intentions of others. Patients may become easily confused by the presentation of multiple bits of information at one time. They may also be socially inappropriate in verbal communications. Usually, these patients have an unrealistic appraisal of self including their residual strengths and weaknesses.

Probably the hallmark of diffuse brain injury is disorder in speed of information processing. Thus, patients are extremely slow to react and in psychomotor activities (talking, writing, doing mechanical tasks, and so on). Processing time slowness frequently coincides with disorders of memory and new learning. It is important to understand that patients may experience specific, short-term memory deficits (verbal versus nonverbal information). Additionally, difficulties in organizing or processing important information affect learning new skills during SCI rehabilitation (weight shifts or catheterization schedule, for instance). These functional learning problems may affect future independent living and academic or vocational goals.

The Craig Hospital nursing staff and treating therapists use a screening tool called the *SCI/TBI Screening-Behavioral Checklist* (Table 26-2). This tool translates cognitive deficits in attention and concentration, speed of information processing, memory, new learning, judgment, and social appropriateness into concrete, observable behaviors within the SCI rehabilitation setting. Using medical demographic information, behavioral observations, and more formalized clinical neuropsychometric testing, clinicians are better able to determine those SCI patients with concomitant brain injury symptomatology and thereafter can plan their rehabilitation programs accordingly.

TABLE 26–2 SCI/TBI Screening—Behavior Checklist

A. Attention/Concentration

Description: The ability to attend to one stimulus or be engaged in one activity without being distracted by other stimuli.

Examples of how it might be demonstrated in the clinical setting:

1. No problems.

2. Mild problems—interferes occasionally, noted once or twice a week. The patient experiences a slight reduction in efficiency when engaged in an activity and exhibits some difficulty maintaining his focus on an activity or thought; seems mildly distractable; i.e., looks up from a task he is working on when others are passing by, talking in room.

3. Moderate problems—interferes frequently; 3 or more times per week. Patient has difficulty sustaining concentration (mental effort) on task at hand and is frequently distracted; requires frequent breaks in complex tasks. In verbalization patient may show frequent changes in topic. Patient may have difficulty selecting most important activity or topic to attend to. Requires redirection from others to return to desk. May be distracted by individuals carrying on a barely audible conversation across the room.

4. Severe problems—interferes constantly. Despite frequent breaks, the patient is unable to tolerate working for more than very short periods (i.e., 5 to 15 minutes). Patient is distracted by all types of environmental stimuli (i.e., phones; radio; looks out window, people walking, talking; items on table; pictures on wall). Cannot maintain a conversation on one topic, jumps from thought to thought. Perseveration may be noted; patient unable to switch thought or activity to something new. Poor ability for focusing attention on task at hand prevents the patient from completing tasks or learning new activities. Requires constant redirection.

B. Speed of Information Processing and Response

Description: The ability to complete activities or respond verbally within a reasonable amount of time.

Examples of how it might be demonstrated in the clinical setting:

1. No problems noted.

2. Mild problems—interferes occasionally—occasionally noted that patient seems somewhat slow in completing complex new tasks compared to other patients (i.e., once learned, how quickly transfer is completed, dressing, etc.). Noted once or twice per week.

3. Moderate problems—interferes frequently—patient seems slowed on most tasks (3 or more times per week). In group activities patient lags behind and can't keep up with change in activity or speed of repetitive movements. Ability to verbally formulate an answer may seem delayed; patient seems slow in initiating and following through once directions are given.

4. Severe problems—interferes constantly, in all areas of rehabilitation patient significantly slowed in ability to complete an assigned task, or respond verbally. Can be noted in activities such as menu selection, self-care activities, wheelchair skills. Delays in response time may create potential safety hazards (i.e., driving; wheelchair skills on rough terrain).

C. Memory

Description: The ability for acquiring and retaining new information; recall of day-to-day events.

Examples of how it might be demonstrated in the clinical setting:

1. No problems.

2. Mild problems—interferes occasionally. The patient needs some repetition of instructions. Occasional reminders are needed for schedule changes, keeping appointments.

3. Moderate problems—interferes frequently. The patient regularly fails to follow through on new assignments. The patient experiences frequent failures (3 times or more per week) to remember information from morning session to an afternoon session. Some trouble with staff names. At times disoriented to date; has difficulty finding way around the hospital. Needs reminders for weight shifts. Needs repetition to learn. Repeats questions frequently. May seem confused about day-to-day events.

4. Severe problems—interferes constantly. Needs much repetition, does not remember day-to-day events; morning to afternoon events; has difficulty keeping any scheduled appointments; remembering staff names. Can't find way to room; unable to remember to do weight shifts. Difficulty learning any SCI education, rehabilitation techniques. Can't remember visitors, phone calls; very confused about day-to-day activities.

D. New Learning

Descriptions: New learning refers to the patient's ability to process new information accurately and to incorporate the information into his ongoing program. This skill can be affected by such things as decreased memory, sequencing deficits, poor initiation, or organizational abilities. Problems with new learning may be noticed in functional skills such as dressing, transfers, chain loops, weight shifts, and skin care.

Examples of how it might be demonstrated in the clinical setting:

1. No problem.

2. Mild problem—interferes occasionally, noted once or twice per week. The patient has difficulty adjusting "behavior" or approaches from feedback given. Information or feedback has to be presented two or three times more than is customary. The patient may remember most of a sequence of a new task but occasionally misses details. Might seem slow in shifting from one task to another.

3. Moderate problem—interferes frequently, 3 or more times per week. Daily discussion is required for the patient to incorporate feedback. He may learn the task, but it is difficult for him to integrate tasks into ongoing "behavior" or newly learned skills. He doesn't generalize information well from one learning situation to other situations. He has considerable difficulty thinking of alternatives in solving problems. He is unable to analyze a situation from more than one perspective. Difficulty is noted in shifting from one task to another. Can show poor planning in day-to-day activities.

(Table continues)

TABLE 26–2 SCI/TBI Screening—Behavior Checklist (continued)

D. New Learning (continued)

4. Severe problem—the patient is unable to carry over tasks/information learned from one session to another. Does not respond to feedback as no change is observed. Information or instructions consistently need to be reviewed. Responds best to continued structure and direction; unable to learn new skills. Cannot problem-solve any difficulties encountered in rehabilitation program; unable to "plan ahead."

E. Judgment

Description: The ability to take into account the future consequences of one's actions. Requires ability to analyze a situation, utilize past knowledge and experience, process information, and respond appropriately and safely. Using good judgment also involves ability to generalize from one situation to the next. Impulsivity interferes with good judgment.

Examples of how it might be demonstrated in the clinical setting:

1. No problems.

2. Mild problems—interferes occasionally and noted one or two times per week. Patient might try and propel wheelchair with brakes on.

3. Moderate problems—interferes frequently; 3 or more times per week. A patient might attempt to go to the bathroom or toilet unaided when assistance is required. May verbally overestimate ability or skill level. Due to impulsivity (inability to stop and think through best response), patient frequently is unsafe in his actions. May be easily influenced by others' opinions.

4. Severe problems—interferes constantly. A patient is unsafe in his environment, might try to go down stairs in wheelchair. Constant supervision is required for safety if mobile. Poor ability to "judge" skill level in all activities. If impulsive, interferes daily. Verbally overestimates abilities (i.e., poor insight). May be highly accepting of opinions of others (or the total opposite).

F. Social Appropriateness

Description: The ability to relate to others, knowledge of one's self and effect on others; the ability to take another's perspective; to understand and respond verbally and nonverbally appropriate to the situation.

Examples of how it might be demonstrated in the clinical setting:

1. No problems.

2. Mild problems—interferes occasionally. One or more of the following behaviors might be noted once or twice per week: exaggerated emotional response to environmental events (i.e., room change, schedule change, staff change), can be shown through frustration, anger, or withdrawal; minor misunderstanding or misperceptions in social interaction with staff, other patients.

3. Moderate problems—interferes frequently, three or more times per week. Some of the following behaviors might be noted (include above described behaviors): off-color jokes inappropriate to situation; physically inappropriate (hugging, pinching, slapping); interrupts staff and can't "wait"; egocentric and self-centered in conversation; frequent misperception of social situation; doesn't pick up on nonverbal cues of staff; lacks sense of humor.

4. Severe problems—interferes constantly. Noted in all interactions, can include these examples (and all described above): seems childish and inappropriate; other patients don't like to be around this patient; he goes into detail about accident with anyone who asks; can use vile language; crude social/personal habits; chronically displeased with situation (being in hospital, staffing, etc.) and expresses at odd times; calling "supervisor" to complain; uses phone excessively; no ability to empathize; insensitive to other patients or staff needs; sexually inappropriate; asks many personal, inappropriate questions (i.e., "Will you marry me?" to any female).

Source: Craig Hospital 1987.

FUNCTIONAL IMPACT OF HEAD INJURY ON SPINAL CORD INJURY REHABILITATION PROGRAMMING: INTERDISCIPLINARY HEALTH CARE GOALS

Rehabilitation of the spinal cord injured person is a complex educational course geared toward development of a new life-style and new habits that will allow the patient a physically and emotionally fulfilling life. For the patient to learn those skills and routines that professionals take for granted requires every cognitive, emotional, and coping ability. When these skills and personal qualities have been impaired by an associated brain injury, no matter how mild, the patient's rehabilitation can be significantly affected (Morris, Roth, and Davidoff 1986).

It is imperative, then, to assess and understand the patient's cognitive and emotional status. Most important is a detailed neuropsychological assessment by an individual skilled in interpreting and translating the assessment into functional terms for the rehabilitation team. Understanding the best ways for a particular patient to learn new information can help the rehabilitation team structure education so that the patient can maximally profit from the program. (Of course, this is true for all patients with SCI, whether they have had TBI, preinjury learning disabilities, or just different ways of coping with trauma, change, and loss.) For example, in the assessment, the neuropsychologist might learn that a patient's memory problems are more impaired auditorily than visually. Therefore, the patient may not learn well from verbal instructions in catheterization techniques or transfer activities. The patient would be better able to learn these techniques or procedures if the nurse or therapist demonstrates or models these procedures a number of times after which the patient repeatedly practices under supervision. To expect the patient to learn a skill that is too challenging can frustrate the patient, and people with cognitive impairments may be less able to deal with frustration. Persistently challenging and frustrating the patient can cause subsequent emotional reactions that are ultimately unsatisfactory and nonproductive for the patient, family, and staff.

Table 26-3 lists some of the more common cognitive problems associated with mild head injury, functional affects that these problems have on the patient's rehabilitation program as well as home and community reentry, and some suggested strategies for managing and compensating for these problems. All patients do not have all these problems, and specific cognitive problems do not always result in the same functional issues or demand the same compensatory strategies. Every brain injury is different just as every person is an individual; mildly slowed speed of thinking or information processing will functionally affect an electrical engineering student more significantly and in different ways than it would affect a wall washer or a ditch digger.

Also consider the patient's family. Families often experience the same feelings of loss, sadness, and confusion as their spinal injured relative (Morris, Roth, and Davidoff 1986). A mild head injury raises many additional issues for the family. They know the patient's preinjury personality and cognitive abilities and may be able to identify changes of which team members are not aware that are interfering with the treatment program. Thus, the family must not only understand and learn to manage SCI, but also must deal with the concomitant head injury and the resulting cognitive and emotional sequelae. This will help them acknowledge and cope with the changes in their loved one and provide the structure, support, and assistance necessary for future functional independence (Morris, Roth, and Davidoff 1986).

Specific treatment of the cognitive impairments in mild TBI has not helped patients cope with or recover from these problems (Barth et al. 1983). Educating patients and families about these problems, providing a system of psychological support, and structuring routines in the environment to maximize function can be more effective ways of treating and compensating for these problems.

If the cognitive problems interfere too greatly with the rehabilitation program and the educational process, discharge from the rehabilitation setting may be necessary even though the patient has not reached maximum goals of independence. However, cognitive neurobehavioral symptoms evolve and often improve over a 1 to 2 year period. Initially, more physical and supervisory assistance at home may be required, but if they are provided for a time, cognitive abilities may improve such that the patient can return to the rehabilitation setting better able

TABLE 26–3 Functional Effects and Compensatory Strategies for Patients with SCI/TBI

Potential Problems	Functional Effects	Compensatory Strategies
Diminished attention and concentration	Difficulty with memory and learning new information	Shorten length of treatment times, including teaching sessions
		Present complete information when patient is rested and fresh
		Patient to take notes on difficult new material presented
		Patient should give feedback and retell or reteach to staff and others the information presented
		Develop a teaching "notebook" for the patient to use and keep track of important program goals
		Repeat information over several sessions

(Table continues)

TABLE 26–3 Functional Effects and Compensatory Strategies for Patients with SCI/TBI (continued)

Potential Problems	Functional Effects	Compensatory Strategies
Slowed speed of thinking or information processing	Difficulty with memory and new learning	As above
	Decreased mental and physical endurance contributing to altered performance	As above
	Added stress and may contribute to complaints of headache, fatigue, motivation, and apathy	Build breaks and rest times into patient's schedule Relaxation techniques
	Slowed physical reaction time	Delay teaching of high-level physical and wheelchair skills such as curbs, stairs and "wheelies"
	Driving may not be a consideration at this time	Psychological support for patient, family, and staff to work through frustrations and to understand consequences of the injury further
Decreased reasoning, sequencing and organizational skills	Reduced problem-solving abilities	Staff should be consistent, structured, and predictable
		Teach skills in steps and break them down into organized sequence for the patient both visually and verbally
	Difficulty assessing and solving problems that come up with skin, bowel, bladder, or health management—particularly an issue after discharge when facing these problems independently	May need supervision and assistance at home beyond what one would anticipate from a physical/functional aspect
		Work closely with support system, i.e., family/wife in longer term planning
		Needs an available resource (nurse or other health care professional) to assist in sorting out problematic situations
	Difficulty with decision making	Present patient only with a few of the most appropriate choices, such as in choosing equipment, etc.
		May need to address guardianship/ conservatorship if competency is a concern
Social inappropriateness	Tangential thought and verbal expansiveness related to impaired regulation, may appear disinhibited	Recreational therapy and group treatment to address social skills
	"Misperceives" social interaction leading to anger, depression and paranoia	Incorporate community-based programming to give patient feedback in practical, relevant new situations
	Alienation of relatives and friends with associated changes in work, marriage, and leisure activities	Consider a life skills trainer to help patient interface with employer, community, family
	Decreased insight to residual deficits	Videotape treatment sessions and group interactions, and use to give feedback to the patient
	Friends, relatives, etc. have unrealistic expectations because the patient frequently "looks so good"	Neuropsychological and clinical psychological support to further understand the personalities affected by the injury, i.e., patient, family, friends, employers
	Exaggerations of preexisting psychiatric disturbances which were "in-check" before injury	Educate and prepare family and patient for these issues
	Patient can become preoccupied with how life "used to be" leading to decreased anger control, frustration tolerance, and ultimate depression and suicidal ideation	Family and patient psychotherapy

Source: Craig Hospital.

to learn and profit from treatment (Morris, Roth, and Davidoff 1986).

IN CLOSING: FUTURE NEEDS AND CONSIDERATIONS ————

Awareness of traumatic brain injury in association with SCI is increasing. Studies related to the incidence of these combination injuries have shown a wide range of results likely due to inconsistent criteria and definitions of TBI. Research is needed to establish more clearly the incidence, functional ramifications, and long-term consequences of patients sustaining SCI with concomitant brain injury. Thereafter, rehabilitation professionals can explore innovative treat- ment methodologies, taking into account psychological needs, follow-up support, and economic considerations necessary to provide optimal, long-term functional outcomes.

REFERENCES ————

Barth, J., Macciocchi, N., Giordani, B., Rimel, R., Jane, J., and Boll, T. 1983. Neuropsychological sequelae of minor head injury. *Neurosurgery* 13 (5): 529–533. *A review of a number of minor head injured patients who demonstrate ongoing psychological and cognitive impairments, seemingly unrelated to LOC or PTA as indicators of severity of injury.*

Davidoff, G., Morris, J., and Roth, E., 1985. Cognitive dysfunction and mild closed head injury in traumatic spinal cord injury. *Archives of Physical Medicine and Rehabilitation* 66: 489-491. *A prospective study of 30 consecutive traumatic SCI patients to determine the incidence of associated closed head injury. Concludes that many traumatic SCI patients are at risk for cognitive dysfunction 8 weeks postinjury.*

Levine, H. S., Benton, A. L., and Grossman, R. G. 1982. *Neurobehavioral Consequences of Closed Head Injury.* New York: Oxford University Press. *A comprehensive text reviewing the nature of TBI including mechanisms of injury. A chapter format then discusses more specific neurobehavioral sequelae.*

Morris, J., Roth, E., and Davidoff, G. 1986. Mild closed head injury and cognitive deficits in spinal cord injured patients: Incidence and impact. *Journal of Head Trauma Rehabilitation.* 1:31-42. *A comparison of recent literature studying the incidence of associated head injury in spinal cord injury and a review of how cognitive and psychological sequelae of head injury can impact the SCI rehabilitation process.*

Ornstein, R., and Thompson, R. F. 1984. Macaulay, D., Ill. *The Amazing Brain.* Boston: Houghton Mifflin Co. *A fascinating text of anatomy and physiology of the human brain. Suitable introduction and foundation for further study of brain function.*

Richards, J., Brown, L., Hagglund, K., Bua, G., and Reeder, K. 1988. Spinal cord injury and concomitant traumatic brain injury: Results of a longitudinal investigation. *American Journal of Physical Medicine and Rehabilitation* 67 (5): 211-216. *A study of SCI patients evaluated neuropsychologically 7 weeks and 38 weeks postinjury. These patients showed cognitive improvement, suggesting initial problems were related to closed head injury as opposed to preinjury cognitive capabilities.*

Rimel, R. W. 1981. A prospective study of patients with central nervous system trauma. *Journal of Neurosurgical Nursing.* 13: 132-141. *A review of a study designed to provide information about the incidence, cause, and management of traumatic brain injury.*

Rosenthal, M., Griffith, E., Bond, M., and Miller, J. D. (Eds.). 1983. *Rehabilitation of the Head Injured Adult.* Philadelphia: F. A. Davis. *A comprehensive textbook on the treatment and rehabilitation of TBI by a variety of international contributors.*

Wagner, K. A., Kopaniky, D. R., and Esposito, L. 1983. Head and spinal cord injured patients: Impact of combined sequelae. *Archives of Physical Medicine and Rehabilitation* 64: 519. *Abstract of an article supporting the need for consultation between SCI and TBI treatment teams in order to provide optimum programming and outcome for these SCI/TBI patients.*

Wilmot, C. B., et al. 1985. Occult head injury: Its incidence in spinal cord injury. *Archives of Physical Medicine and Rehabilitation* 66: 227-231. *A study of 67 SCI patients to determine the incidence of concomitant undiagnosed head injury. Patients were studied cognitively using motor free evaluation tools, and by taking into consideration their premorbid academic history.*

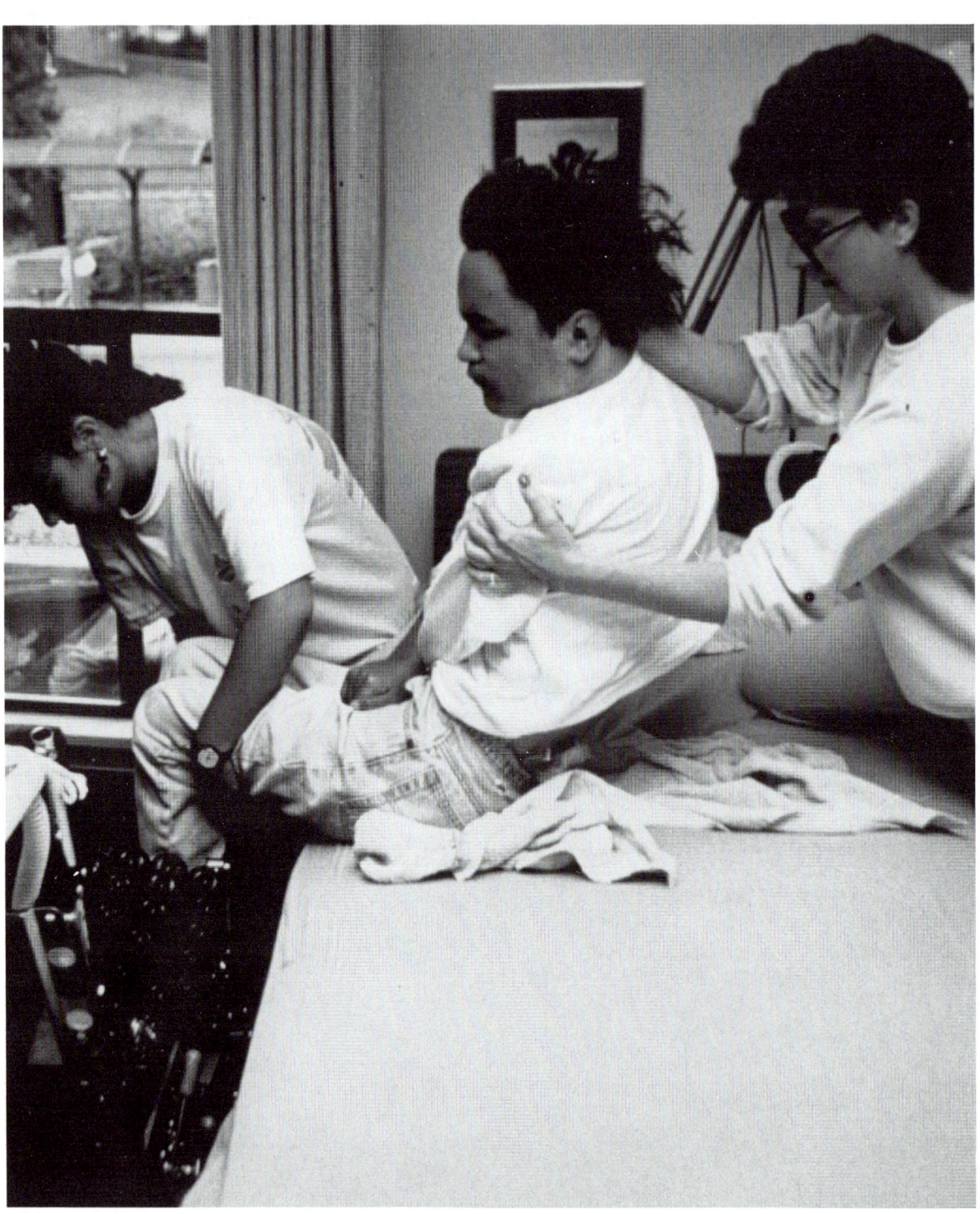

CHAPTER 27

Managing Spasticity

Daniel P. Lammertse, M.D.

Chapter Outline

Health Care Objectives

- To understand the anatomical and physiological basis and the functional consequences of spasticity
- To understand the basic elements of spasticity assessment and the options available for the treatment of spasticity
- To be able to identify complications stemming from spasticity

INTRODUCTION

Spasticity is a common accompaniment to the paralysis that occurs after traumatic spinal cord injury (SCI). It is commonly defined as a state of exaggerated muscular tone with increased tendon reflexes associated with an upper motor neuron lesion. See Chapter 4. In normal individuals, motor control function of the spinal cord is complex and includes both direct control of volitional movement via the pyramidal tracts as well as more obscure control of posture and muscular tone through other pathways. These neural control circuits include not only descending influences from suprasegmental centers but also integrative circuits within the spinal cord itself. Thus, when injury occurs in the spinal cord, the neurological consequences include not only the obvious loss of volitional control below the level of injury but also a disruption of suprasegmental influence on these circuits that control reflexes and tone.

In the early postinjury phase termed *spinal shock* (Chapter 6), these spinal cord level functions are suppressed, but with the passage of time they reappear and become autonomous because of the withdrawal of suprasegmental influence, which is generally inhibitory in nature. Thus, a state of increased spinal cord excitability generally evolves over a period of months, clinically manifested by spasticity. The stimulus for spastic muscle contraction may either be proprioceptive in the form of muscular stretching or it may be exteroceptive in the form of other cutaneous and nociceptive inputs to the cord. This second mechanism commonly produces the increase in spasticity associated with cutaneous stimulation, a distended bladder, or other nociceptive input from medical complications below the level of injury. The degree of spasticity typically evolves over the first year or two postinjury and thereafter tends to achieve stability which is influenced by the presence of medical complications. See Figure 27–1.

All patients suffering from paralysis associated with spine fractures will not have spasticity. A lower motor neuron injury, by injuring the final common pathway for motor function, results in a flaccid paralysis. This is most commonly seen with cauda equina injuries resulting from lumbar spine fractures in which the injury is to a peripheral nerve rather than the spinal cord. Even when the spinal cord has been the primary locus of injury, however, some lower motor neuron damage typically occurs because of anterior horn cell injury within the cord at the segmental level of injury. It is thus common for thoracolumbar or L_1 injuries to produce flaccid paralysis from injury to the conus medullaris, the lowest segments of the spinal cord. Although some spasticity at the ankle may be seen in patients with thoracolumbar junction injuries, spasticity of major clinical significance is most commonly found in patients injured above that level. See Figure 27–1.

Even though spasticity is an almost universal accompaniment to SCI paralysis above the thoracolumbar junction,

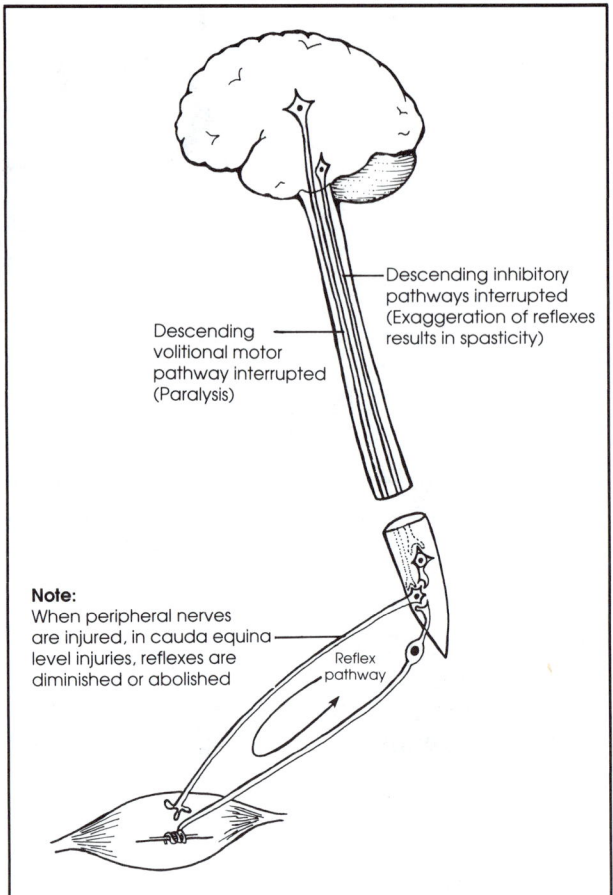

Note:
When peripheral nerves are injured, in cauda equina level injuries, reflexes are diminished or abolished

Descending inhibitory pathways interrupted (Exaggeration of reflexes results in spasticity)

Descending volitional motor pathway interrupted (Paralysis)

Reflex pathway

FIGURE 27–1   SCI involving upper motor neuron damage provides an anatomical and physiological basis of spasticity.

it should not be assumed that all spasticity is dysfunctional and requires specific treatment. To a certain extent, the return of muscular tone produces a beneficial postural effect. A certain degree of spasticity enhances postural stability at the hips and trunk. Unfortunately, as spasticity evolves over time, many patients do not stabilize at a beneficial level of tone but progress to an excessive and dysfunctional level. The health care team must develop effective and individualized treatment strategies for these patients.

INTERDISCIPLINARY GOALS OF THE HEALTH CARE TEAM

The consequences of spasticity that adversely affect treatment outcome can be classified as follows:

- Comfort
- Function
- Posture
- Safety

Spasms may be in and of themselves painful either directly, as in the case of patients with sensory incompleteness, or indirectly (and less dramatically) in patients with complete injuries. In this latter group, the postural consequences of spasticity may lead to muscular pain syndromes in sensory innervated volitional muscles. Spasticity also may significantly interfere with sleep, periodically awakening the individual with sudden uncontrolled movement.

Spasticity may be asymmetric and unevenly distributed across a given joint—flexors, for instance, are often more spastic than extensors. This may lead to *contractures*, which, if asymmetric, may lead to further *postural abnormalities* including scoliosis. Contractures can be a significant source of discomfort when vigorous passive ranging is required to maintain some semblance of functional range of motion and may also lead to skin complications because of postural consequences.

Spasticity has significant implications for safety, particularly in terms of mobility. Excessive spasticity may adversely affect the safety of transfers, not only the assisted transfers of people with quadriplegia but also in the most severe cases, the independent transfers of people with paraplegia. For patients with incomplete injuries in whom gaiting is feasible, spasticity may affect the safety of independent ambulation. The safety of adapted driving can also be adversely affected when strong spasms uncontrollably affect postural placement behind the wheel of a vehicle. The health care team, therefore, must develop treatment strategies to prevent these consequences of spasticity from having a significant impact on the individual's quality of life. Specific goals include:

- To assess the severity and functional consequences of the patient's spasticity
- To identify contributing sources of sensory input to the spinal cord that may provide opportunities for treatment
- To establish with the patient and family a practical home program of physical interventions to control spasticity
- To identify which patients may require pharmacological or surgical treatment based on an analysis of benefits and risks
- To educate the patient and family about the nature of spasticity and the rationale behind the treatment program

ASSESSMENT

History

Time from Injury
The pattern and severity of injury must be placed in the context of the time elapsed since injury. Patients whose spasticity has stabilized should not be expected to exhibit dramatic increases or decreases in spasticity unless related to complication. On the other hand, *in the first 1 to 2 years postinjury, patients commonly report a progressive increase in spasticity.* Significant changes in spasticity after stabilization should elicit a search for contributing sources such as medical complications.

Patterns of Spasticity
For patients who develop spasticity after spinal shock, *flexor* spasms tend to be the first to occur followed by *extensor* spasms (Guttmann 1976). Ultimately, most patients develop some degree of both flexor and extensor spasms depending on posture and the source of stimulus. The kind of spasm often has functional implications and should be explored when taking the history. For example, hip and back extensor spasms can seriously affect the security of seating posture in the wheelchair of a quadriplegic person and might result in the recommendation of a more substantial restraint system.

Association with Complications
When stable patients report a sudden change in spasticity, determine if there is an association with other medical complications. Urinary tract infections, a change in reflex voiding efficiency, a change in bowel program performance, the development of bleeding hemorrhoids, and pressure sores are some examples. In these individuals, although some specific spasticity treatment might be required in the short term, treatment should address the contributing source. *Changes in spasticity in a stable patient should always be considered as a potential indicator of a complication in another organ system.*

Functional Implications
In taking the history, always go beyond the issue of presence and severity of spasticity to assess the functional implications (Merritt 1981). Is the spasticity affecting the patient's sleep? Is the spasticity threatening the safety of transfers or ambulation? Is the spasticity causing pain? The appropriate treatment of spasticity should always address these issues.

Physical Assessment

The physical evaluation of spasticity must be performed within the context of the total neuromuscular examination. The motor and sensory examination should include evaluations of voluntary motor function in specific groups as well as the determination of the last normal level of segmental function. Note the degree of incompleteness of both motor and sensory function. Observe spontaneous involuntary movements and document the pattern of movement, whether flexor or extensor. Evaluate a response to physical stimuli including touch, pain, and passive muscle stretch. In patients with incomplete motor lesions, estimate the degree to which volition triggers spasm and conversely the degree to which patients can inhibit spasms. Deep tendon reflexes should be examined and the presence of clonus documented. Attempt to elicit the Babinski response, a pathological reflex characterized by extension of the great toe after cutaneous stimulation on the sole of the foot. *Range of motion* should be fully evaluated to determine the presence of contractures. *Posture* should be assessed both on the examining table and sitting in the wheelchair to determine the implications of asymmetric spasticity and contractures. The examination should also include a screening evaluation of other organ systems for possible contributing factors such as pressure sores, contractures, skeletal trauma, heterotopic ossification, hemorrhoids, constipation, and urinary tract infection.

Other Assessment Tools

Based on the history and physical examination, other radiographic and laboratory tests may be appropriate to further evaluate sources of change in spasticity stemming from complications in other organ systems. When the history and physical assessment show some deterioration of neurological function, the presence of posttraumatic cystic myelopathy as a cause of changing function should be entertained, and appropriate diagnostic testing such as magnetic resonance imaging should be performed.

GENERAL MANAGEMENT

Physical Treatment

Positioning
Proper positioning in bed is helpful because certain postures promote or inhibit certain reflex patterns (Young and Shahani 1986). The prone position tends to inhibit flexor spasms and promotes those of extension. In the supine and side-lying positions, reflex patterns tend to be more extensor in nature. In the standing position, extensor patterns are facilitated. By breaking up flexor synergy patterns, the standing posture may prove beneficial as a postural treatment of spasticity. Safety should be included in the assessment of posture and positioning. In this regard, interdisciplinary solutions to padding and belt restraints are sometimes required in cases of severe spasticity to maintain the position of the individual in the wheelchair or in bed.

Range of Motion
Passive range of motion exercises are beneficial not only for spastic muscles but also because they prevent contractures. Passive movement of affected joints through a full range should ideally be performed twice per day in severely spastic patients, or at least once per day in patients with a moderate degree of involvement. Note, however, that daily activity

provides for many patients an effective passive range to many critical joints. This is especially true if the patients stand or if they sleep in the prone position. Many patients, therefore, do not require formal, daily range of motion exercises to maintain adequate control of spasticity and avoid contractures. Standing is usually accomplished by means of a standing apparatus such as specially constructed bars, standing frames, or, alternatively, with long leg braces. Figure 25–2 illustrates a wheelchair option for standing. Patients whose spasticity is helped by standing usually stand for 30 minutes per session.

Other Physical Treatments
Spasms can also be treated by *heat and cold* (Young 1986). Cold applied locally in the form of ice massage or evaporative spray over a spastic muscle temporarily reduces hypertonicity. This technique is very localized, however, and it has not proven practical for most patients with SCI who typically have multiple spastic muscle groups. Alternatively, immersing a patient in a warm therapeutic pool tends to facilitate the effect of passive range of motion exercises and reduces spasticity. Another physical modality that may affect spasticity is *functional electrical stimulation* (FES). This technique, which induces contraction of spastic musculature through electrical stimulation of a peripheral nerve, is undergoing a resurgence of interest due to recent advances in technology. One clinically observed effect of such stimulation in some patients has been the temporary reduction of spasticity, perhaps by a fatigue mechanism. The exact nature of this phenomenon and its relationship to exercise parameters are not well understood. The technique can thus not be recommended purely for treatment of spasticity at this time. Chapter 22 presents further information on FES.

Pharmacological Treatment

When these conservative physical measures have failed to control spasticity adequately, the next step is typically to consider *antispasticity medications* (Young and Delwaide 1981; Davidoff 1985; Katz 1988). Many medications have been tried but only three drugs have gained wide acceptance: *baclofen, dantrolene,* and *diazepam* (Table 27–1). Of these three, baclofen is commonly the first drug to use for spasticity because although its efficacy is equal to the other two drugs, it has fewer potential adverse effects.

Baclofen is a derivative of the neurotransmitter gammaaminobutyric acid (GABA). Its theoretical mode of action is GABA-mediated interference with the release of excitatory neurotransmitters in the spinal cord. The usual starting dose is 5 mg three times a day increased by 5 mg every 3 days until an effective reduction in spasticity occurs or the patient reaches a total daily dose of 80 mg per day. Although sedation has been reported, this can often be

TABLE 27–1 Drug Treatment of Spasticity

Agent	Daily Dose	Typical Maximum Schedule	Clinical Considerations
Baclofen (Lioresal)*	5 to 80 mg	20 mg qid	First-line drug because of low toxicity and lack of abuse potential. Sudden withdrawal may produce hallucinations and seizures.
Dantrolene (Dantrium)	25 to 400 mg	100 mg qid	Risk of liver toxicity increased with daily dosage greater than 300 mg.
Diazepam (Valium)	5 to 40 mg	10 mg qid	More sedating than other options. Significant abuse potential. Physical dependence.

*Recently, intrathecal baclofen pumps have improved functional outcomes in some individuals with severe spasticity (Parke and Penn 1989).

avoided by beginning with a small total daily dose and gradually increasing until the desired effect is achieved. Patients should be told that a sudden large reduction or discontinuation of the drug can produce a rebound dramatic increase in severity of spasms as well as hallucinations and seizures. Therefore, instruct patients to taper the medication gradually when decreasing the dosage or discontinuing the drug. The health care team needs to be especially aware of this potential effect of abrupt withdrawal when patients are temporarily restricted from taking oral medications for medical reasons. For example, patients on chronic baclofen maintenance who experience a postoperative ileus longer than 24 to 48 hours may develop withdrawal symptoms. Either treat with an alternative medication such as diazepam or improvise an alternative route of administration such as a baclofen suppository.

Dantrolene acts directly on muscle itself by interfering with the action potential induced release of calcium ions from the muscle cell. Although drowsiness, dizziness, fatigue, and diarrhea can occur as adverse reactions to this medication, these effects are usually transient and occur early in the course of treatment. As with baclofen, adverse effects are also minimized by beginning with a low dosage and increasing gradually until the optimal regimen is established. Therapy is usually started at 25 mg per day and increased to a maximum of 400 mg per day in divided doses. Serious *hepatotoxicity* has been documented with the use of this medication, most commonly with dosages above 400 mg; this level should not be routinely exceeded.

Diazepam (Valium) acts at the spinal cord level by facilitating GABA-mediated presynaptic inhibition. Although it is probably equally as effective as baclofen and dantrolene, it tends to have more central side effects such as sedation than the other two drugs. Diazepam also can result in depression, which makes it a less attractive option in patients for whom emotional adjustment to disability is an ongoing concern.

All three medications can interact with alcohol and other central nervous system depressants, but diazepam is probably the most potent in that regard, requiring that patients be thoroughly educated about drug and alcohol interactions. Diazepam is also the only drug of these three with clear abuse potential and as such, this medication should be avoided in patients who have a history of substance abuse. Diazepam is usually initiated at a 2 mg dose once or twice per day and gradually increased until the desired effect is achieved or the patient develops untoward side effects. Rarely does an increase beyond 40 to 60 milligrams per day result in a significant decrease in spasticity without accompanying excessive side effects.

In discussing any of these antispasticity medications with patients, emphasize that the treatment regimen must be predicated on clearly defined functional goals. Patients should understand that spasticity cannot be eliminated through the use of medication, only reduced in severity. Encourage patients to attempt a gradual taper of medication every 3 to 6 months to ascertain its continued effectiveness. Many patients find that within the first several years postinjury, they acquire the body handling skills necessary to become drug free despite moderately severe spasticity.

Recently, *implanted intrathecal drug delivery systems* for baclofen and morphine have been tried experimentally for the control of spasticity (Penn and Kroin 1987; Erickson 1985). Preliminary reports on the effectiveness of this technique have been encouraging. Intrathecal delivery of antispasticity medication has the theoretical advantage of focusing the therapy at the site of pathology rather than giving the drug systemically. Whether this technique moves from experimental to general clinical practice awaits a more complete understanding of the risks and benefits based on trials currently under way.

SPASTICITY: A GLOSSARY

Ablative procedure	Procedure whose effect on spasticity is the result of a destruction or elimination of certain neural pathways.
Augmentative procedure	Procedure that affects spasticity by augmenting the neural inputs to motor circuits in the spinal cord by electrical stimulation.
Capsulotomy	A procedure often required in addition to tendon lengthenings to achieve adequate improvement in range of motion when the joint capsule has significantly contracted.
Cordectomy	The surgical removal of some portion of spinal cord tissue.
Cystic myelopathy	The formation of a cystic cavity within the spinal cord, which is a common localized occurrence at the site of injury. Less commonly, a localized cystic cavity will progressively enlarge and may cause loss of additional neurological function, increased spasticity, and other physiological manifestations.
Efficacy	Effectiveness.
Goniometric	Pertaining to the measurement of joint angles with a goniometer.
Intrathecal	Used to describe the location of drug delivery systems in the subarachnoid space.
Myelotomy	A procedure in which an incision is made in the spinal cord.
Neurectomy	A procedure in which a segment of the peripheral nerve is excised.
Neurolysis	A procedure in which peripheral nerve tissue is destroyed or dissolved by physical or chemical means. This is most commonly achieved either by creating a radio frequency heat lesion or by injection of phenol or alcohol.
Nociceptive	Used to describe neurons in the pain sensation pathways.
Rhizotomy	A procedure that interrupts or destroys spinal nerve roots.
Tendon lengthening	A procedure often used to treat spastic contractures of joints by achieving a lengthening of the musculotendinous unit.
Tenotomy	A surgical procedure in which a tendon is cut.

Surgical Treatment

When severe spasticity continues to be a source of additional disability despite attempts at conservative management, surgical approaches to treatment often must be considered. These options may be classified as ablative neurological procedures, augmentative neurological procedures, and orthopedic procedures.

Perhaps the simplest *ablative neurological procedures* commonly performed for the treatment of spasticity are *motor point blocks* and *nerve blocks* (Davis 1975). Most commonly, a 6% solution of phenol is injected into the motor point of a given muscle or alternatively, into a peripheral nerve causing neurolysis. This treatment is often only temporary, with spasticity returning within 3 to 6 months. Of these two options, motor point blocks have the advantage of being a pure motor procedure whereas most peripheral nerve blocks, being a procedure on a mixed motor and sensory nerve, produce both a motor and sensory deficit. In addition, painful dysesthesias may result in patients with sensory sparing who are subjected to a peripheral nerve block. The use of phenol peripheral neurolysis in patients with incomplete injuries is thus relatively contraindicated. One exception is the use of peripheral nerve blocks or surgical neurectomy for the obturator nerve that innervates hip adductors, the motors involved in the *scissoring* pattern of spasticity. Since the obturator nerve carries sensory afferents from only a very small cutaneous distribution over the medial aspect of the knee, obturator neurectomies are commonly performed to alleviate hip adductor spasm even in patients with incomplete sensory sparing. These injection techniques, however, are tedious to perform and often disappointing in their outcome.

Intrathecal alcohol or phenol injection is another ablative neurolysis that although once popular, is no longer in widespread use. This procedure commonly produced a gratifying reduction in spasticity but, unfortunately, also tended to result in areflexia of bowel, bladder, and sexual function as well. Intrathecal injections have thus given way to more discrete ablative procedures.

Rhizotomies, both ventral and dorsal, have been proposed for treatment of spasticity and generally have produced some beneficial effect (Foerster 1913). When done as an open procedure, however, these techniques require a considerable operation with a laminectomy exposure. The *percutaneous thermal rhizotomy* has more recently been developed as a means of treating spasticity without an open procedure (Herz et al. 1983; Kasdon and Lathi 1984). In this technique, radiofrequency electrodes are placed in the nerve root foramina under fluoroscopic guidance and a microwave heat lesion is generated on the dorsal root, preferentially lesioning the unmyelinated fibers carrying nociceptive input to the cord. This procedure is effective at reducing spasticity, and when properly performed, it rarely produces a flaccid paralysis but rather leaves the patient with some functional residual tone. Patients can experience a recurrence of dysfunctional spasticity, however, which may necessitate repeat procedures. The percutaneous thermal rhizotomy is not indicated for patients with significant pain sensation sparing because the heat lesions may result in painful dysesthesias.

Other surgical procedures to treat spasticity include *myelotomy* and *localized cordectomy*. The majority of these procedures are no longer in widespread use either because of lack of efficacy or because equally effective, less radical options have become available (Fogel et al. 1985).

As opposed to *ablative neurological approaches* wherein neurological tissue is destroyed to interrupt reflex arcs, *augmentative neurosurgical approaches* use electrical stimulation to attempt to achieve a reduction in spasticity. The technique is *epidural stimulation*. A variety of specific techniques have been proposed that all have in common electrical stimulation of the dorsal columns by an implanted epidural electrode (Barolat, Myklebust, and Wenninger 1988; Dimitrijevic 1986). The exact mechanism of this effect is not known but is in theory based on the presynaptic inhibition of nociceptive inputs to the spinal cord by electrical stimulation of afferent fibers in the dorsal columns. Although initially proposed for the treatment of chronic pain, epidural stimulation was found to have some effect on spasticity in a variety of disorders. This technique has remained controversial and, for that reason, has not gained general acceptance as a routine treatment for spasticity.

Orthopedic procedures for the treatment of spasticity are primarily tenotomy and tendon lengthening (Davis 1975). *Tenotomy* may be indicated when severe contractures have developed that cannot be adequately managed by stretching or splinting techniques. These procedures are sometimes combined with capsulotomies to achieve a functional range of motion. *Tendon lengthening* is most commonly performed on the Achilles tendon when shortening of the muscle-tendon unit has resulted in an equinus deformity. This may lead to difficulty in maintaining foot position on the wheelchair footrest or in fitting shoes. Also, by maintaining postural tension on the muscle-tendon unit, the equinus deformity tends to provoke clonus at the ankle, which may in turn elicit more generalized spasms. The Achilles tendon lengthening can often be performed percutaneously and is followed by only a brief period of postoperative immobilization. Once the patient is fully healed, stress adequate stretching exercises to avoid a recurrence.

SPECIFIC MANAGEMENT OF COMPLICATIONS

The most common secondary complications of spasticity are *contractures* and *skin ulcerations*. The health care team must closely follow the range of motion at all affected joints in patients with significant spasticity. This is best performed with periodic goniometric measurement of joint range. When a loss of range of motion is noted, the intensity and frequency of the program should be increased to regain the lost motion. Despite the best efforts of therapy and nursing staff, some patients exhibit such pronounced, unbalanced spasticity that the loss of range progresses. In these situations, consider casting and splinting techniques. When progressive loss of range continues despite these conservative measures, consider more aggressive management options. In patients within the first 6 to 12 months postinjury when more permanent procedures should be avoided if possible, motor point blocks may be a helpful temporary measure, giving the treatment team a chance to improve range of motion. In the most severe cases when contractures become fixed and pose a significant ongoing care problem, tenotomies or tendon lengthening and other related procedures may be needed. Severe contractures can lead to secondary skin complications, not only in intertriginous areas where maceration and superficial fungal infections can lead to skin ulceration, but also because of problems in maintaining adequate positioning of the contracted patient. Severe *flexion contractures of the lower extremities* commonly limit bed positioning options and predispose patients to develop pressure sores over the trochanters and sacrum. *Asymmetric contractures at the hips* can also result in an uneven distribution of sitting pressure over the ischial areas and lead to pressure ulceration. Thus, pay special attention to skin issues in spastic patients who may have developed contractures. The creative use of padding to relieve pressure over prominences is critical in these situations.

INDIVIDUAL AND FAMILY HEALTH EDUCATION

The ultimate measures of success in the rehabilitation team's management of spasticity are in the long-term maintenance of adequate control of spasms and in the avoidance of complications. This can only be accomplished through successful education and training of the patient and family. The disabled person and home care givers should be thoroughly trained in positioning and range of motion techniques before discharge from acute rehabilitation. If not already incorporated into the program, the person should be aware of other options such as standing. The disabled person and family should be thoroughly educated in the assessment of possible contributing factors in changes in spasticity. They should understand that not all increases in spasticity warrant an increase in antispasticity medications or consideration of antispasticity procedures but that in fact, spasticity improves when an underlying condition is treated. Persons who require pharmacological management should be fully informed of possible adverse effects of medications as well as drug and alcohol interactions. They should be advised regarding the consequences of abrupt withdrawal of medication or a too rapid increase in dosage. Educate

individuals who have more severe manifestations of spasticity regarding the risks and benefits of surgical options.

LONG-TERM IMPLICATIONS

Many clinicians feel that the long-term outlook for spasticity and related complications in a given individual is determined during the early course of management postinjury. If patients are properly positioned, receive proper range of motion, and can avoid medical complications, severe spasticity may be avoided. Nonetheless, despite the best efforts of the health care team, some persons will develop disabling spasticity that may require medications or in extreme cases, surgical intervention. If the long-term management approach is focused on the functional consequences of spasticity and the avoidance of complications, success can usually be achieved. Persons with SCI often report 1 or 2 years postinjury that their spasticity decreases or at least becomes more easily managed. This may be a result of the gradually reacquired sense of posture and body handling that patients develop over time. For this reason and because of the marginal efficacy of medications, patients with pharmacological management of spasticity should be encouraged to taper their dosage periodically to redefine their need level. Many people can thus become drug free, having used medications as a necessary crutch during relearning of body skills.

In summary, the long-term goal of spasticity management is to achieve adequate control of spasticity with minimum, necessary intervention to ensure maximal function, safety, comfort, and avoidance of secondary complications.

REFERENCES

Barolat, G., Myklebust, J., and Wenninger, W. 1988. Effects of spinal cord stimulation on spasticity and spasms secondary to myelopathy. *Applied Neurophysiology* 51: 29–44. *A report on a series of patients treated with spinal cord stimulation for spasticity with 5 of 16 patients showing some benefit at 1-year follow-up.*

Davidoff, R. A. 1985. Anti-spasticity drugs: Mechanisms of action. *Annals of Neurology* 17: 107–116. *An excellent review article on the mechanisms of action of the major antispasticity drugs.*

Davis, R. 1975. Spasticity following spinal cord injury. *Clinical Orthopedics and Related Research* 112: 66–75. *A review article that includes some discussion of positioning, range of motion, and older surgical techniques such as myelotomy that are no longer in widespread use.*

Dimitrijevic, M. M. 1986. Spinal cord stimulation for the control of spasticity in patients with chronic spinal cord injury: Clinical observations. *Central Nervous System Trauma.* 3 (2): 129–144. *A review of one center's experience with SCI stimulation, a still somewhat controversial topic.*

Erickson, D. L. 1985. Control of spasticity by implantable continuous flow morphine pump. *Neurosurgery.* 16 (2): 215–217. *A report of four cases evaluated for intrathecal morphine treatment of spasticity. Three patients were reported to have prolonged control of spasticity with this technique, which is still considered to be experimental.*

Foerster, O. 1913. On the indications and results of the excision of posterior spinal nerve roots in men. *Surgery, Gynecology and Obstetrics.* 26 (5): 463–475. *The classic article first describing the use of rhizotomy for the control of spasticity.*

Fogel, J. P., et al. 1985. Dorsal myelotomy for relief of spasticity in spinal injury patients. *Clinical Orthopedics and Related Research.* 192: 137–141. *An article reviewing the results of dorsal longitudinal myelotomy to relieve spasticity that concluded that the procedure is generally not successful.*

Guttmann, L. 1976. *Spinal Cord Injuries: Comprehensive Management and Research.* London: Blackwell Scientific Publications. *The classic text on spinal cord injury management written by one of the founders of spinal injury care. Chapter 23 deals with patterns of reflex disturbances, and chapter 32 discusses clinical management of spasticity with reviews of conservative as well as pharmacological and surgical options.*

Herz, D. A., et al. 1983. Percutaneous radiofrequency foramenal rhizot-omies. *Spine.* 8 (7): 729–732. *A review of 30 spinal cord injury pa-tients who received radiofrequency foramenal rhizotomies for spasticity.*

Kasdon, D. L., and Lathi, E. S. 1984. A prospective study of radiofre-quency rhizotomy in the treatment of post traumatic spasticity. *Neuro-surgery* 15 (4): 526–529. *A review of 25 patients treated with radiofrequency rhizotomy documenting a high success rate in the relief of spasms.*

Katz, R. T. 1988. Management of spasticity. *American Journal of Physi-cal Medicine and Rehabilitation* 67 (3): 108–116. *An excellent review of management concepts in spasticity with a lengthy bibliography.*

Merritt, J. L. 1981. Management of spasticity in spinal cord injury. *Mayo Clinic Proceedings* 56: 614–622. *A review of management issues in spasticity with emphasis on the hierarchy of interventions.*

Parke, B., and Penn, R. D. 1989. Functional outcome after delivery of intrathecal baclofen. *Archives of Physical Medicine and Rehabilitation* 70: 30–32. *A review of 21 patients who have received intrathecal bac-lofen pumps for spasticity. Results were encouraging with functional improvements being noted in most cases.*

Penn, R. D., and Kroin, J. S. 1987. Long-term intrathecal baclofen in-fusion for treatment of spasticity. *Journal of Neurosurgery* 66: 181–185. *An article, describing experience with seven patients using intrathecal baclofen, by the surgeon commonly recognized as the inven-tor of this technique.*

Young, R. R., and Delwaide, P. J. 1981. Drug therapy: Spasticity. *New England Journal of Medicine* 304 (1): 28–33, 96–99. *An excellent two-part review of medications available for the treatment of spasticity.*

Young, R. R., and Shahani, B. T. 1986. Spasticity in spinal cord in-jured patients. In *Management of Spinal Cord Injuries.* Eds. R. F. Bloch and M. Basbaum. Baltimore: Williams & Wilkins. *A compre-hensive text on the management of SCI that contains a thorough chap-ter on the physiology and management of spasticity.*

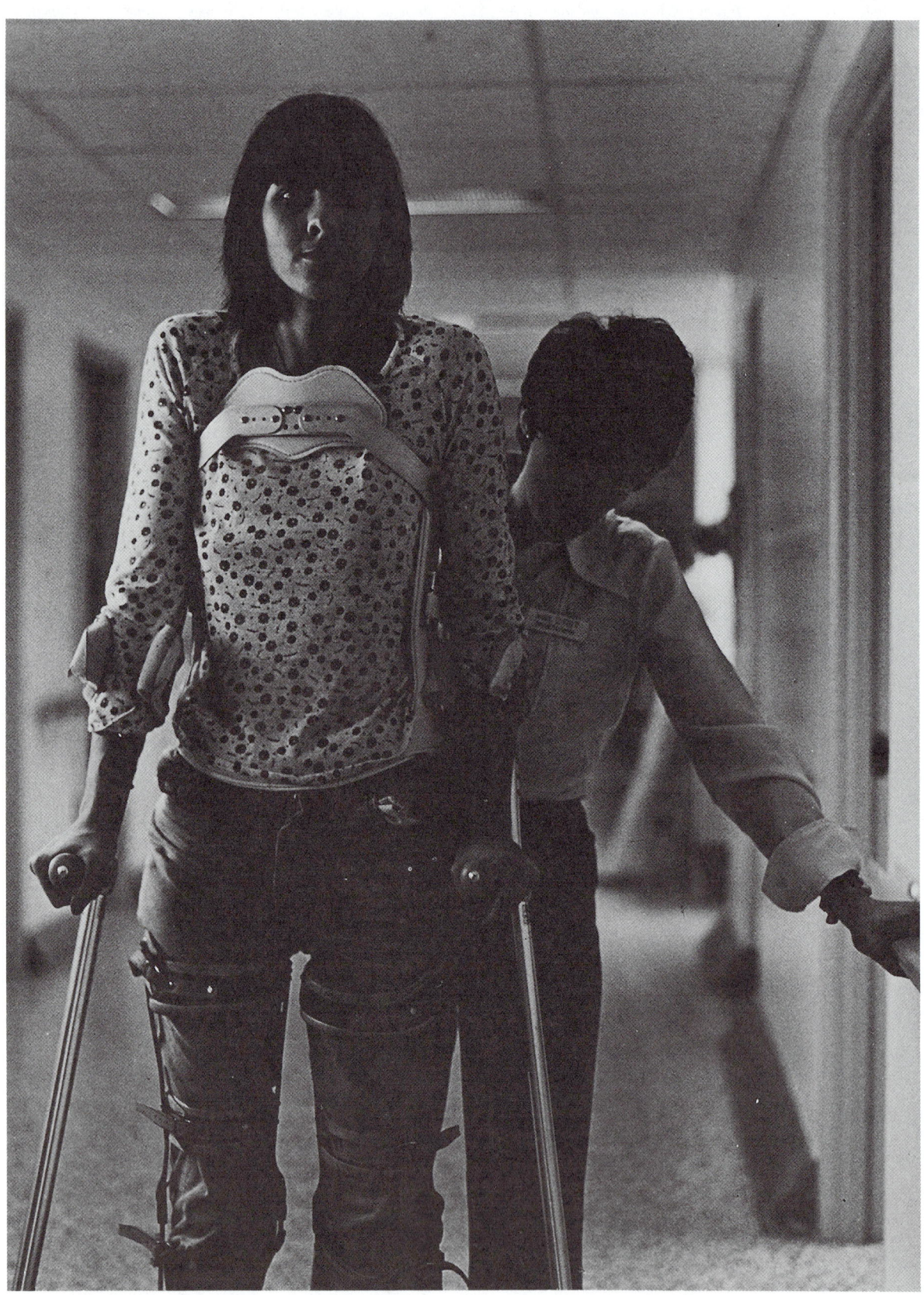

CHAPTER
– 28 –

Managing Pain

David Fairholm, M.D., F.R.C.S.C.

Chapter Outline

Health Care Objectives

- To recognize pain syndromes, including pathophysiology, that occur following spinal cord injury
- To understand that chronic pain is a condition with many factors in cause and management
- To outline individualized assessment and management approaches
- To encourage persons to live functional, productive lives despite an added disability of pain
- To prevent drug dependency
- To stress the importance of early recognition of syringomyelia and describe treatment options

INTRODUCTION

Every person who suffers a spinal cord injury (SCI) suffers pain. In the acute phase, pain arises from soft tissues such as ligaments, muscle, joint, and skin. Pain also arises from fracture dislocations of the bony elements. Acute pain syndromes often arise from nerve root or spinal cord damage which causes paresthetic pains in a segmental distribution. As the injured tissues heal, or neurological tissue is decompressed, most of the pain associated with the injury itself resolves. However, for many people, a *chronic pain syndrome* develops that can be severe and further disabling. Studies indicate that about 90% of people will have troublesome delayed pain following SCI. For two-thirds of these, the pain syndrome remains stable and is not disabling. These pain syndromes usually do not diminish with time, and in about 40% of the cases, the pain increases and contributes to disability.

Chronic pain syndromes may begin at the time of injury or, more commonly, may develop months or many years following the injury. Because of the aggressive nature of rehabilitation and reintegration, many people become functional in society before the debilitating effects of pain become evident. Despite this, there are still significant numbers of people whose lives are controlled and dominated by an unrelenting, chronic pain syndrome, most of which occurs within 6 months.

The nature and type of pain varies with the location of injury. Injuries of the *cauda equina* result in the highest probability of a pain syndrome, whereas those in the cervical cord are least likely to give rise to chronic pain. *Nerve root injuries* give quite a different pain syndrome from those affecting the spinal cord. Pain syndromes cause severe disability and are notoriously difficult to treat.

PAIN MECHANISMS

Chronic pain is a clinical syndrome that defies definition. Multiple factors are responsible for this unpleasant experience and its resultant psychological and sociological debility. See Figure 28–1. Therapeutic management must respond to the same multifactorial components.

Pain syndromes are usually produced by some type of tissue injury. A neurological mechanism generates and transmits impulses to the brain where there is a clinical perception called pain.

Significant advances have occurred in the understanding of pain-generating mechanisms with the general acceptance of the Gate Control theory of Melzak and Wall (1982). All pain of noncerebral origin is transmitted through the spinal cord. In the periphery, different receptor mechanisms respond to stimulation such as tissue damage, pressure, and heat. The generated impulse is electrically transmitted by nerves to the spinal cord. Myelinated nerves transmit rapidly, whereas small, unmyelinated nerves transmit slowly. Each group responds to a different stimulus an transmits a different type of sensation. All pain fibers terminate in a relay station within the *dorsal horn* of the spinal cord (in laminae I, II, and III) commonly referred to as the *substantia gelatinosa of Rolandi* (Figure 28–2).

The anatomy and physiology of the dorsal horn is extremely complex. The incoming impulse travels either directly to an end-organ cell or through a series of interneurons. The transmission across synaptic junctions (which is apparently chemical) may be accomplished by one of numerous neurotransmitters. The most common chemical transmitter for pain is probably substance P. The production and release of substance P is modulated in the dorsal horn by naturally occurring opiates called *encephalins*.

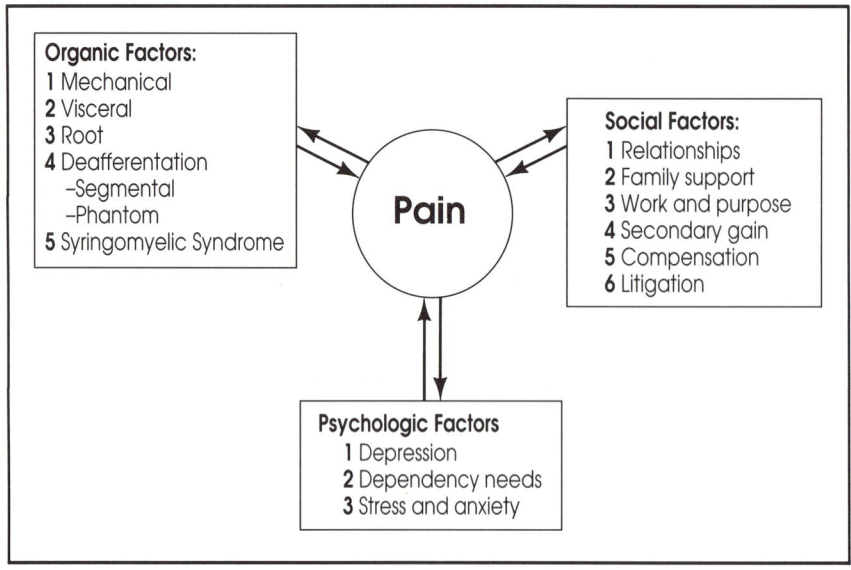

FIGURE 28–1   Factors influencing pain.

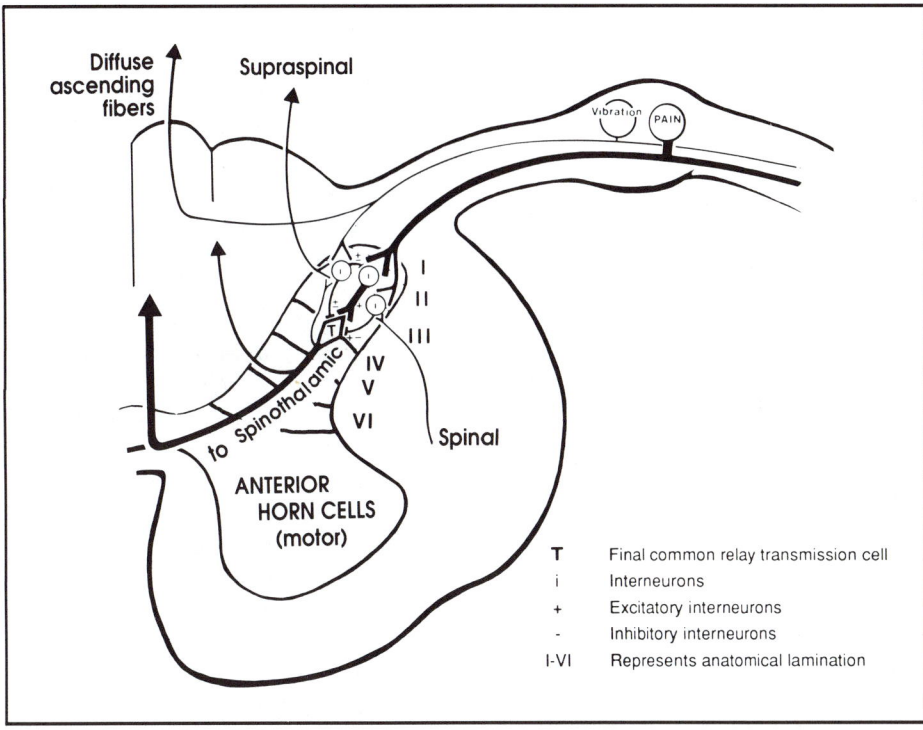

FIGURE 28–2 Schematic representation of pain relay in dorsal horn.

Numerous local, ascending and descending inputs influence the access of these stimuli to the final common nerve cell called the *T cell*, which relays the impulse upwards to the brain.

Within the substantia gelatinosa there are both excitatory and inhibitory influences (Figure 28–2). Large fibers in the peripheral nerve conducting deep touch pressure and vibration inhibit the relay station. There is increasing evidence that a complex brain stem inhibitory system projects back to the dorsal horn. This interplay of peripheral input, excitatory, and inhibitory modulation of impulses on the **T** cell is referred to as the *Gate Control* theory of pain. The **T** cell may transmit through several pathways to the thalamus of the brain. Most fast fibers that transmit sharp pain course upward within the spinothalamic tracts; however, unmyelinated fibers that transmit slow pain travel diffusely through the spinal cord before terminating on brain stem mechanisms. This understanding of the Gate Control mechanism of pain generation, relay, and transmission, and a developing understanding of the physiological mechanisms within the dorsal horn are opening up new options for pain management.

These neurological mechanisms generate and transmit impulses from the spinal cord into the thalamic areas of the brain and then project to cortical areas. At this level, pain becomes part of the conscious awareness of the person. Multiple factors interact to determine the interpretation, character, intensity, and response to this unpleasant sensation which we know as *pain*. Review Figure 28–1. Research over many years has determined great variation in individual pain thresholds, which are tremendously influenced by anxiety and attention, and psychological, cultural, and sociological factors.

Although there is now some understanding of the physiological mechanisms that produce pain, very little is known of the factors that determine the degree of disability resulting from pain. *Secondary disability* is the degree of incapacitation produced, and society is replete with examples of persons who are totally disabled by minor discomfort and of others who endure great agony to remain functional.

PAIN SYNDROMES OF SPINAL CORD INJURY

Pain syndromes following SCI have been classified into five types: mechanical, peripheral (nerve root in origin), visceral, central, or psychogenic.

Mechanical Pain

Mechanical pain of SCI usually occurs at the level of injury. It may originate in the surrounding damaged soft tissue and subsequent scar, but more commonly it originates from damaged facet joints or nonunion of a spinal fracture. It is often a dull, aching discomfort aggravated by movement and occurs later in the day following activities and mobilization. It may be associated with some focal tenderness in the paravertebral muscle. Such pain often responds to rest, immobilization, external orthoses, or simple analgesics. Another kind of mechanical pain is that of shoulder joint dysfunction secondary to either excess shoulder joint activities of wheelchair mobilization, or due to frozen shoulder of immobility. Soft tissue injury around the shoulder joint gives rise to a pain syndrome. Mechanical pain is usually recognized through careful history taking and appropriate examination. Routine and special radiological studies such as tomograms or CAT scans may show a treatable structural problem.

Mechanical pain of SCI is usually managed by muscle strengthening activities, relaxation techniques, simple analgesics, physical therapy, modified wheelchair seating, bed positioning, external orthoses, and reeducation in daily living skills (DLS). In some specific cases of nonunion, good results may be achieved following surgical fusion.

Peripheral (Segmental) Nerve Root Pain

Segmental nerve pain arises from damage to the peripheral nerve or radicular structures. This may occur at a foramen at the site of injury or, in the instance of spinal lumbar fractures, may be due to cauda equina injury. Pain is usually typically radicular, a sharp pain lasting several seconds, often stabbing or shooting in character, and usually follows the segmental distribution of the nerve root of origin. It may become continuous. In some situations it may be dysesthetic or causalgic, being aggravated by light touch or pressure on the skin. This latter is the result of slow conduction by small unmyelinated fibers. Management of radicular pain sometimes involves such local measures as protection from tactile stimulation or locally applied anesthetics. Simple surgical decompression of a nerve root may be effective. Chronic pain of nerve root injury, however, with its dysesthetic, causalgic pattern may be very difficult to treat. Medications are of limited success, and a variety of surgical procedures including sympathectomies, rhizotomies, and peripheral nerve block have been tried with limited success.

Visceral Pain

Visceral pain, which is uncommon, often has its origin in an abdominal viscus such as bowel or bladder. Its transmission is probably via sympathetic pathways to the high thoracic cord and is usually felt in the anterior chest, epigastrium, or suprapubic region. It is often precipitated by distension of the viscus and at times may be associated with autonomic dysreflexia. Comprehensive patient and family health education to encourage well-managed bowel and bladder programs, among others, are preventive measures.

Central (Deafferentation) Pain

Central pain arises from the spinal cord itself. Following SCI, there is a major disruption in the normal pain transmission pathways. As healing occurs in the spinal cord, there are attempts at regeneration of neurons and the axonal fibers. Axons sprout and make new neuronal connections, most of which are nonfunctional. There is reorganization of the interneuronal mechanisms in the dorsal horn such that the final pathway or T cell now receives input from many sources. Nonpain fibers, new interneuronal connections, recurrent fibers, and inhibitory mechanisms may all now become excitatory. As a result, the abnormal dorsal horn T cell responds to a variety of inputs causing abnormal, unpleasant sensations, or may ultimately become an autonomous cell, spontaneously generating pain. Because this has resulted from a loss of normal input into the T cell, this type of pain is called *deafferentation pain*. This is the common, severe pain experienced by persons with paraplegia. There are two varieties: *segmental* pain occurs at or about the level of injury; whereas *phantom* pain is perceived below the level of injury in the area of sensory loss. It is rarely seen in persons with cervical injury, not infrequently occurs in midthoracic injury, and is most commonly experienced by those with injuries at the thoracolumbar junction. The pain may be a variety of most unpleasant sensations. It is often described as burning, tingling, squeezing, gripping, constant, and intense, but may be sharp, shooting, stabbing, or occurring in waves. It is most commonly felt below the level of injury, in the torso, hips, and groin, but it may extend to legs, feet, and toes. The feet and toes may feel deformed or cramped. An uncommon variant may occur in the perineal area in which there is a sensation of large mass in the rectum or of sitting on a hot fire. The pain pattern is severe and unrelenting, with fluctuations in intensity. It may be aggravated by mobility and sitting in a chair, by distended bladder or bowel, or by urinary tract infection. Acute exacerbations are often precipitated by increases in spasticity or in conditions of pressure sores. Most often, however, it is continuous without aggravating or relieving factors. As in all pain, it is significantly affected by a person's emotional state.

If phantom sensations predominate, they are often shooting, jabbing waves of unpleasant sensation into the legs, accompanied by a cramping, distorted, twisted sense of position. These may be aggravated by cutaneous stimulation at or about the level of injury. Only recently, with the understanding of pain mechanisms in the dorsal horn, has a satisfactory surgical treatment been developed.

Psychogenic Pain

Psychogenic pain is uncommonly experienced following SCI as there is usually some clear organic component to the pain syndrome. However, as in all pain syndromes, emotional, psychological, social, and cultural factors significantly affect functional abilities and must be assessed.

SYRINGOMYELIA

A specific pain pattern following SCI is caused by *cystic degeneration* of the spinal cord. At the site of injury, numerous small microcysts that develop in the reparative process coalesce to form a central, cystic, fluid-filled cavity at the site of injury. In a small percentage of these, the cyst enlarges and is called a *syrinx* (Figure 28–3). Although there is considerable controversy about the mechanisms of development, it is thought that there is a dissociation of pressure between the intracranial compartment, the spinal subarachnoid space, and the fluid collection within the central spinal cord. During day-to-day activities or during extreme exertion, the fluid within the spinal cord progressively dissects through the cord tissue causing an enlarging cavitation up and down the spinal cord. This occurs first in the dorsal horns, the weakest areas of the spinal cord, and produces pain. As the syrinx slowly rises, the central part of the spinal cord is progressively destroyed resulting in a slowly rising neurological deficit. Pain and temperature fibers that cross within the center of the cord are preferentially affected. As more of the cervical cord is affected, the anterior horn cells in the gray matter are destroyed, resulting in progressive wasting, weakness, and loss of reflexes in the hands and upper extremities.

Because the primary area of dissection is the dorsal horn, a pain syndrome is present in virtually all persons with *syringomyelia*. The pain is present above the level of the original injury, often into the upper back, shoulder blades, shoulders, and into the arms. Initially it may be a shooting, sharp, lancinating pain associated with exertion, but this gives way to constant, severe pain across the back of the shoulders, neck, and arms. The character and distribution of the pain slowly change over time as more relay neurons in the dorsal horn are destroyed. Because syringomyelia is a progressive condition following SCI, it is extremely important that the syndrome of rising neurological deficit and pain above the level of injury be recognized early and appropriate management carried out. Anyone suspected of developing syringomyelia requires magnetic resonance imaging to provide immediate, accurate diagnosis (Figure 28–4).

PREVENTIVE AND RESTORATIVE MANAGEMENT

Because the production of pain is such a multifactorial problem, the management of chronic pain syndromes of SCI must likewise be multifaceted (Figure 28–5) and interdisciplinary in approach. Table 28–1 summarizes factors to consider for assessment of pain.

D	Dorsal horn
A	Anerior horn
c	Cortical spinal cervical long tract fibers
t	thoracic
i	lumbar
s	sacral

FIGURE 28–3 Schematic diagram of a syrinx.

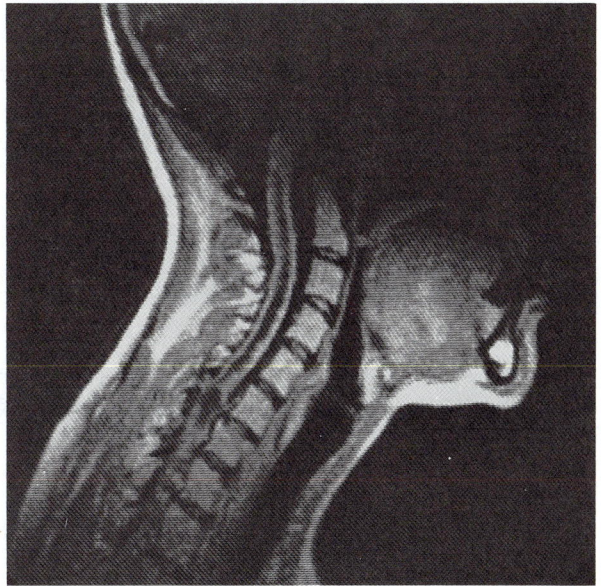

FIGURE 28–4 Magnetic resonance image of posttraumatic syrinx, injury level C$_{6-7}$.

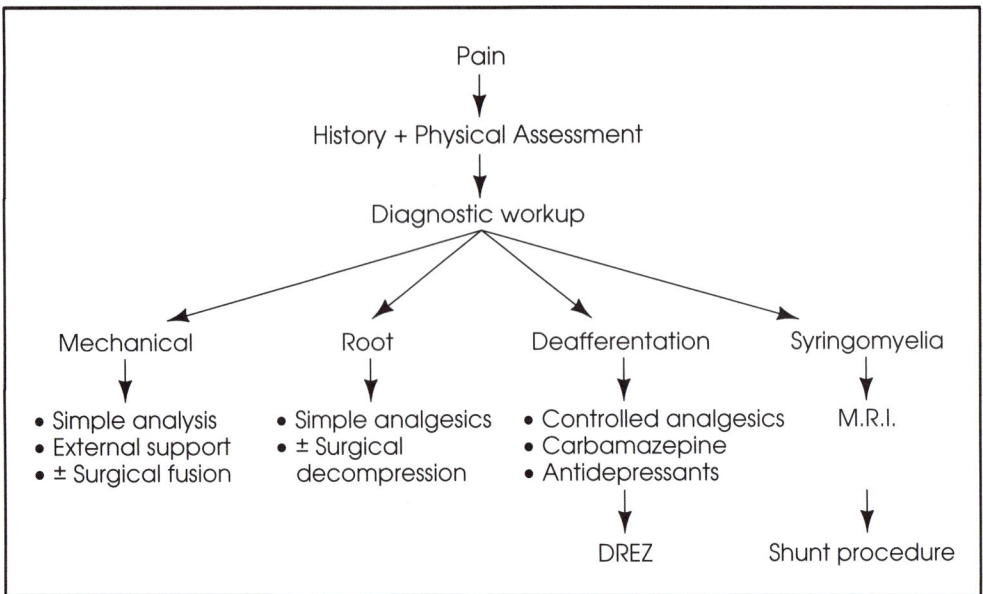

FIGURE 28–5   Flow sheet for pain management.

Promoting Health and Independence

Participatory planning is a key factor in successful pain management. Persons with SCI must be involved in goal setting, selecting approaches to meet those goals, and actively involved in recordkeeping to monitor when goals are met. Encouraging their ability to manage themselves (independence) and to monitor their own bodies' reactions is effective in the management of chronic pain associated with SCI (Ozer 1988). Individual, family, group, and peer counseling support services have this ultimate goal.

In conjunction with other treatments, attend to comprehensive plans for improving general health and updating functional abilities if indicated. Reeducation in self-care, bowel and bladder retraining, and nutrition are some prime examples. Exploring new educational and vocational opportunities as well as leisure activities are also major elements of comprehensive pain management.

Psychosocial Aspects of Pain

Every person with chronic pain changes drastically in psychological response and sociological environment. Psychosocial adaptations are an integral part of the rehabilitation process, and factors such as interpersonal relationships, family integrity, employment, productivity, and the secondary gain factors of litigation and compensation, are major determinants of the functional state of the person with chronic pain. Support and counseling to develop coping and corrective mechanisms are important. Hypnosis, biofeedback, and relaxation techniques are examples of psychobehavioral interventions.

Many factors can augment pain, including others' disbelief that the pain is real, or fear or monotony. Care givers and families may help by practicing distracting techniques such as slow breathing, massage, and active listening. Contralateral stimulation (rubbing one leg when the other one hurts) can sometimes help, or sharing pleasant experiences and encouraging persons to describe the sights, smells, and sounds imagined (imaging). Relaxation techniques reduce anxiety, ease muscle tension, help the person disassociate from the pain, promote rest and sleep, and combat depression (McCaffery 1989). For persons with SCI, these techniques may enhance other treatment modalities.

Pharmacological Management

Analgesics

Simple analgesics such as ASA or acetaminophen may be effective for mechanical variants of chronic pain. Analgesics are seldom effective in the control of central pains or pains of nerve root origin. The issue of analgesic use in benign chronic pain is extremely important. The tendency is for gradually increasing amounts of medication and a gradual shift to stronger and more potent drugs. This commonly results in drug dependency and addiction. Particularly addictive drugs are pentazocine (Talwin), oxycodone (Percodan, Percocet), anileridine (Leritine), as well as the usual narcotics, meperidine, and morphine sulfate. If analgesics are used for a long term, this should be done cautiously. Simple analgesics such as acetaminophin, salicylic acid, Fiorinal, and codeine should only be used in the lowest effective dosage and in a rotating manner every 3 to

TABLE 28–1 Factors to Consider for Interdisciplinary Assessment of Pain

History

Pain history includes (Kozier and Erb 1991):
- History of SCI
- Onset and duration
- Location (segmental versus diffuse)
- Intensity
- Quality
- Precipitating factors
- Associated symptoms
- Effect on DLS (review functional abilities)
- Measures taken to relieve pain
- Analgesics and other medication history
- Other treatments used

Modulators of pain (factors that increase or decrease perception of pain) include (ASIA 1989):
- Posture in wheelchair (see also Chapter 20)
- Positioning in bed
- Activity level (rest, exercise)
- Sleeping patterns
- Smoking/alcohol/drug abuse
- Stress and coping abilities
- Management of the effects of disability, primarily bowel and bladder elimination, skin care, spasticity, and autonomic dysfunction
- Medications taken
- Other treatments used

General health history includes:
- Health problems
- Ability to maintain optimal health and manage the effects of disability
- Nutritional history
- Change in patterns of functional abilities
- Psychosocial aspects including preinjury profile and ability to cope with life; present resources and abilities to cope with stress; degree of stress in present situation; present eating and sleeping patterns; educational background; employment history; leisure activities

Physical Assessment
- Physical status of all body systems
- Detailed neurological examination focusing on the area of pain, including responses to different sensory stimulants (dysesthesia or causalgia patterns) and mechanical factors

Diagnostic Tests
- Radiological studies, tomography, CAT scanning (structural changes)
- MRI for central causes (syringomyelia)

Source: Cynthia Perry Zejdlik.

TIPS FOR SIMPLE ANALGESICS

- Monitor response to analgesics with detailed recordkeeping. Flow sheets are helpful for noting the medication(s), exact time of taking, and effect—for instance, described on a scale of 1 to 10.
- Assess response to analgesics. Note duration and degree of relief. The intervals between medications may be too short or too long.
- Analgesics work better if taken on a *regular* schedule rather than as needed. Oral analgesics take an hour or so to work, and pain may be experienced for a long time before the effects are felt.
- Take *before* pain is felt, or *as soon as the pain starts* to return, for maximum effect. Higher doses are needed to relieve, rather than prevent, pain.
- Beware of so called *potentiators* of pain, such as muscle relaxants, perhaps alcohol.
- Plan activities at peak periods of pain relief.
- Know when to rest to avoid fatigue, which tends to make pain worse.
- Know side effects and watch for them. For example, codeine is very constipating and may result not only in bowel program problems but autonomic dysreflexia.

(Source: Cynthia Perry Zejdlik)

---

4 weeks. More recent development of long-acting opiates with less propensity to addiction such as buprenorphine and sustained-release morphine, taken judiciously, may give some relief with an acceptable risk of drug dependency. Addiction is extremely detrimental because of the associated negative side effects of dependency, depression, apathy, and emotional distress with ensuing complications related to physical care.

Psychotropic Drugs

One of the most effective medical regimes for chronic pain is the use of psychotropic drugs, which are particularly helpful in pain syndromes following neurological injury. The use of antidepressants such as amitriptyline, and the antipsychotics such as fluphenazine, either singularly or in combination, may effectively alleviate depression and reduce debility from pain syndromes. Drugs should be started at a low dosage, gradually increasing to maximum therapeutic doses. Because these are effective through a re-

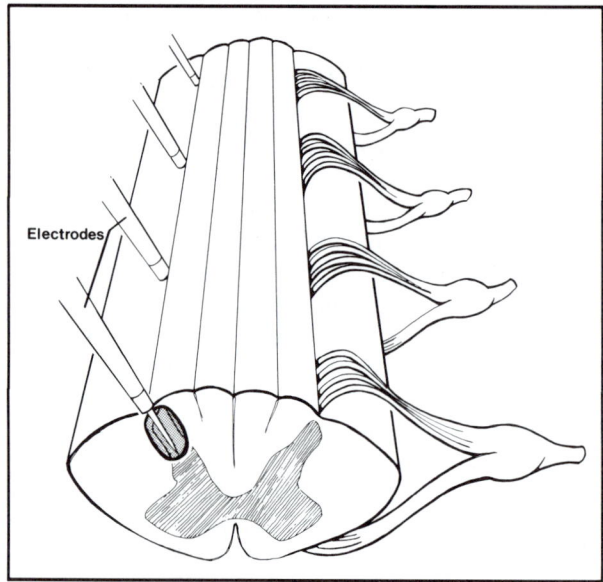

FIGURE 28–6 Schematic diagram demonstrating the production of a DREZ lesion.

arrangement of brain chemistry, several weeks are required before evaluation is possible.

Antispasticity Drugs

Control of *spasticity* is often a major factor in the control of pain syndromes. Benzodiazapines are often a first line. Drugs such as baclophen and Dantrium commonly reduce spasticity and are effective in relieving pains. See Chapter 27.

From time to time some persons may respond to anticonvulsant medications. Drugs such as carbamazepine, valproate sodium, or phenytoin alleviate some of the central pains and neuralgias.

Electrical Stimulation Procedures

With a broader understanding of the pain mechanisms as proposed by the Gate Control theory, it is known that stimulating large A-Delta fibers can inhibit pain transmission. The simplest method for this is TENS—Transcutaneous Electrical Nerve Stimulation—which may be effective for transient or prolonged relief of pain. Numerous studies have shown some conflicting results in effectiveness, and pain relief is often achieved by a trial and error method of electrode placement and changes in stimulus parameters. There are occasional reports of epidural or direct stimulation applied to the dorsal column of the spinal cord, but this is also controversial. These procedures are no longer in widespread use.

Surgical Treatment

Numerous surgical procedures have been devised, but to treat the pain of paraplegia unfortunately most of them have been ineffective. Most important, standard cordotomies, and even local cord excision, do not give lasting relief of this benign pain and may themselves produce a chronic central pain syndrome. All types of peripheral procedures such as neurectomies or rhizotomies have been singularly ineffective. In recent years, with the increased understanding of the importance of dorsal horns of the spinal cord in pain production, selective destruction of this area by a radiofrequency dorsal root entry zone (DREZ) lesion (Figure 28–6) has shown some promise in relief of central pain of spinal cord origin. Numerous reports in the literature now claim 60% to 80% effectiveness in long-term pain relief with this procedure. It seems not to be effective for pain syndromes arising from the cervical area and is of only limited effectiveness in pain syndromes arising from the midthoracic area, or where rectal and perineal pain is a feature. Its primary effectiveness is in thoracolumbar-level injuries

EXPERIENCING DEAFFERENTATION PAIN

John, a 35-year-old man, suffered a T_{11-12} fracture dislocation with complete sensory and motor paraplegia. He underwent Harrington rod fusion and proceeded with rehabilitation. Two months following injury John began to have pain into his feet. This slowly began to rise in both feet, up the back of both legs, posterior thighs, and hips. It was described as a burning, intense, crushing sensation, a feeling that his feet were about to "explode in fire balls." Waves of painful sensation would shoot up and down his legs. The most intense pain was in the feet and lower legs. The pain has gradually become a constant, severe, dull, continuous ache. Simple analgesics and narcotics such as baclofen, diazepam, carbamazepine, and amitriptyline have been used for more than 4 years without relief. He was clearly addicted to oxycodone. Despite his severe pain, John remained remarkably functional, doing maintenance work around his farm.

His examination shows a transition sensory level at T_{11-12} bilaterally with a flaccid lower extremity paraplegia, a typical deafferentation pain of paraplegia at the thoracolumbar region. He was admitted to the hospital and underwent a thoracolumbar laminectomy and a DREZ lesion, T_{10} to L_1, which dramatically relieved his pain. John readmitted himself to the hospital 2 months later for treatment of his addiction, and he is now fully employed and is on no medications.

A DREZ lesion is the treatment of choice for pain syndromes in persons with paraplegia with segmental and phantom pains primarily arising from the thoracolumbar area.

Treatment of Syringomyelia

One of the treatable causes of pain in SCI is syringomyelia. Because this condition is *progressive*, early diagnosis and management are crucial. The only recognized, effective treatment is surgical decompression of the cyst cavity. Current surgical therapy involves one of two surgical procedures:

- The *syringo-subarachnoid shunt* is placed to equate pressures between the syrinx and the subarachnoid space. This is most suitable where a large cyst has progressed into the cervical cord and usually involves only a single-level cervical laminectomy.
- The *syringo-peritoneal shunt* drains or collapses the cyst, usually into the peritoneal cavity.

Although syringo-peritoneal shunts are the most common, drainage into the pleura has been done. A laminectomy where the cyst is largest allows the safest entry into the cord, and connection is made by subcutaneous catheter into the abdominal cavity. A surgical procedure is effective in more than 80% of cases for pain relief and arrest of neurological progression. There may often be significant neurological recovery.

SUMMARY

Chronic pain experienced by persons following SCI is a devastating and debilitating complication. Although it affects approximately two-thirds of all patients with SCI, it causes severe debility infrequently. Management of pain must be multifactorial, considering mechanical, neurological, psychological, and sociological factors. Simple analgesics and the comprehensive treatment of depression are the major medical aspects of management. The recently developed DREZ operation holds promise and is now considered the treatment of choice for persons with severe deafferentation pain associated with SCI. *Syringomyelia* is a unique and common treatable cause of postinjury pain.

EXPERIENCING SYRINGOMYELIA

Karen, a 23-year-old woman, suffered a C_6 quadriplegia from a tobogganing accident. About 2 months following her injury, she began to have pain in the right index finger and thumb. Initially it was shooting and throbbing, but it became increasingly severe and continuous. Gradually the pain spread into the biceps region, the elbow, the triceps, and then into the shoulder and scapula. At about the same time she noted increasing weakness of both upper extremities—more so on the left. She had increasing difficulty pushing her wheelchair due to loss of strength in the triceps.

Karen's examination showed a right Horner's syndrome. She had normal sensation on the right upper extremity above the C_6 level and impaired pinprick sensation over the C_5, C_6, and C_7 dermatomes on the left. She had loss of temperature on the left up to the angle of the jaw and absent reflexes in the left upper extremity.

The history of delayed onset of a pain syndrome, characterized by a changing character of the pain pattern and associated with a rising neurological deficit, gave a clinical diagnosis of *posttraumatic syringomyelia*. An MRI examination demonstrated a large central syrinx in the cervical cord.

This woman underwent a C_5 laminectomy and insertion of a syringo-subarachnoid shunt. Postoperatively she had a dramatic improvement of the pain in the right upper extremity and significant improvement in the strength of the arms, such that she could push her wheelchair.

---

with segmental or phantom pains into the legs. The surgical procedure requires exposure of the spinal cord at and above the level of injury. Very selective lesions are made by radiofrequency generation in the root entry zone at and up to about 5 cm above the level of cord injury. If effective, pain relief occurs almost immediately and appears to be long lasting.

REFERENCES

American Spinal Injury Association (ASIA). 1989. *Instructional Course: Pain in SCI: Epidemiology, Neurophysiology, and Clinical Management.* Ann Arbor: University of Michigan Medical Center.

Kozier, B., and Erb, G. 1991. *Fundamentals of Nursing Concepts and Procedures.* Menlo Park, CA: Addison-Wesley.

McCaffery, M. 1989. *Nursing Management of the Patient with Pain.* 3d ed. Philadelphia: Lippincott.

Ozer, M. 1988. *The Management of Persons with SCI.* New York: Demos Publications.

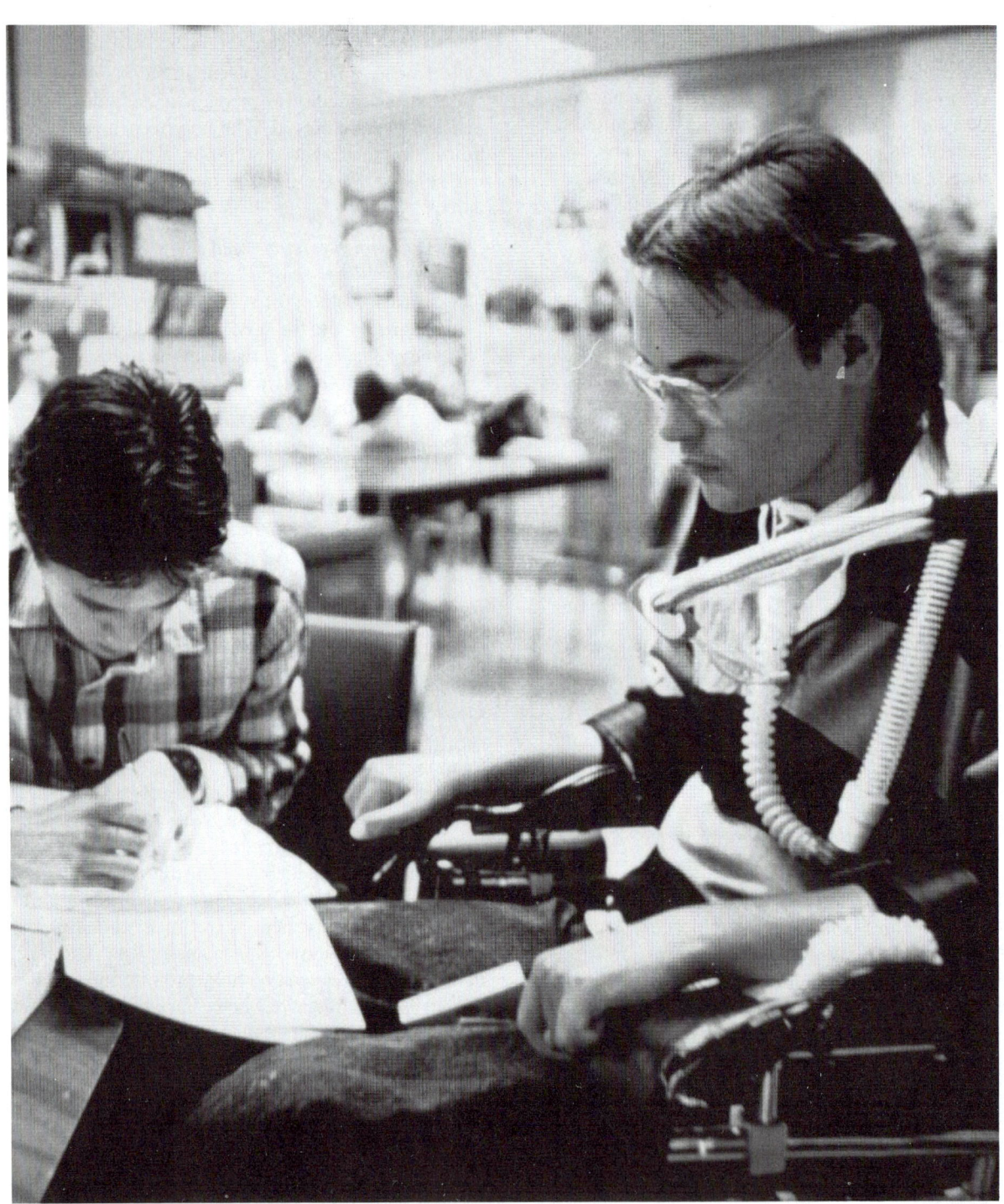

CHAPTER 29

Living with High Quadriplegia*

Chapter Outline

Health Care Objectives

- To increase awareness of the remarkable potential for adaptation to high quadriplegia
- To increase sensitivity toward individual responses to severe disability
- To understand the significant role of the family, health care professionals, and society in relation to the person with high quadriplegia
- To increase opportunities for personal growth and choice through expanded rehabilitation services and alternatives
- To appreciate related bioethical issues and describe assessment and resolution of areas of conflict
- To look beyond the formal rehabilitation period toward enhancing life goals and plans for persons with high quadriplegia

*This chapter was developed with the assistance of L. Butt, Ph.D.; F. C. Jimenez, R.N., M.Ed.; L. McNutt, M.S.W., and K. DeSilva, J.D.

In the recent past a severe injury at the high cervical cord level was invariably fatal, but this is no longer true. People with high quadriplegia are surviving, and the severity of residual disability poses awesome challenges to the individual, the family, the health care profession, and society as a whole.

CONSEQUENCES OF HIGH QUADRIPLEGIA

A Physical Definition

Persons with high quadriplegia (SCI at the C_4 level and above) experience variable losses of movement and sensation of the head and neck area. To understand clearly the diagnosis and potential functional abilities, it is important to remember how terminology is used to describe the level of injury. If a person is diagnosed as having a C_3 quadriplegia, this means the C_3 neurological level of the third cervical cord segment and root is *intact*, while the fourth is not. In other words, C_3 is the last neurological level to function normally.

The spinal respiratory center is located primarily at the C_4 level of the cord but receives some innervation from C_3 and C_5. See Chapter 15. Through the phrenic nerve outflow the spinal respiratory center innervates the diaphragm, the main muscle of breathing. When the diaphragm is nonfunctional, the person will need permanent respiratory support. The accessory muscles of breathing are also innervated by the cervical cord (C_{2-7}) and refer to the sternocleidomastoid, which also receives innervation from the spinal accessory (cranial) nerve, and scalene muscles located in the neck and upper chest. By strengthening and retraining these muscles, some people can achieve some periods off the ventilator.

Following traumatic cervical cord injury a person with C_4 quadriplegia is expected to establish voluntary control of breathing, albeit at a subnormal capacity. However, if the injury is higher (and complete), this is not possible.

A person who has a C_2 or C_3 functional level will have full sensation of the head and upper neck and some neck control. This eventually enables balance of the head, which helps maintain an upright position in the wheelchair and allows various mouthstick activities. Most important, partial preservation of the accessory muscles of breathing offers potential to develop tolerance for being off the ventilator for a few hours. Little or no sensation or motor control of the head and neck is preserved except for the "face mask" area when a person has a C_1 functional level. Without neck control, people have difficulty with balance of the head and difficulty maintaining an upright position in the wheelchair without external support. Without some accessory muscles

of breathing, there is little or no potential for developing tolerance for being off the ventilator.

Most cord injuries extend several segments above and below the main traumatic area, and therefore damage may extend into the brain stem where the nuclei of the lower cranial nerves are located. This can cause sensory and motor impairment of the face and most important, the swallowing muscles. This type of deficit may be temporary—particularly if caused by cord edema—or permanent. Assessment and treatment then become highly individualized to prevent aspiration and to provide nutritional requirements. See Chapter 17.

Maintaining physical functions for persons with high quadriplegia incorporates the same principles of promoting health and managing the effects of disability for other persons with SCI as described throughout this text. For example, optimal bowel and bladder elimination requires the specific skills outlined to manage dysfunctions caused by upper motor neuron lesions.

An Individual Perspective

The person with high quadriplegia has a myriad of issues with which to contend for a successful outcome. These issues encompass physical, psychological, and social areas. For example, in the *physical domain*, the person with high quadriplegia must contend with respiratory compromise and almost total loss of body movement and sensation. Within the *psychological domain*, the person faces an altered self/body image, role changes, dependence on others for the most basic needs, and dependence on substantial equipment, including the ventilator. In the *social sphere*, the person with high quadriplegia must acquire predictable and reliable attendant help, deal with educational and vocational ambiguity, and face uncertain financial stability. The constant need to secure multiple support systems is coupled with constant effort to overcome personal and social disadvantages.

Yet despite these obstacles many people adapt remarkably well to this severe disability. The process of adapting to this catastrophic injury is dynamic rather than static and involves an ever-changing array of pressures. Each phase of rehabilitation presents unique stressors. Throughout the rehabilitation process and beyond, stresses (including the misconception of others as to what those stresses are) wax and wane in terms of impact on the individual and the family.

A Societal View

It is apparent that adaptation to high quadriplegia is not the responsibility of the person and family alone, for society as a whole helps create the problems to which the individual must adapt. As many disabled people emphasize, much of the disability associated with physical impairment is a result

RESPIRATORY QUADRIPLEGIA: SOME REFLECTION ON ITS MEANING

FROM THE INJURED PERSON'S POINT OF VIEW

I am a person with respiratory quadriplegia. I am this way against my will, for the risks I took in life did not prepare me for this. Perhaps nothing could.

So here I am, I cannot move my arms or legs. I cannot dress or feed myself. I cannot talk with my hands anymore, and I can no longer run in joy or anger. I have lost the pleasure of feeling someone touch my body or being able to reach out to hold another with my arms. Please forgive my anger; it is not always directed at you.

A machine helps me breathe and orders me to measure my speech to its respirations. I hate the machine, for it reminds me of what I have, but I need the machine, for it reminds me that I am.

I will learn to change from my previous life-style, but it does take time. It takes so long even to read again. Jog five miles and you know how I feel after turning pages with a mouthstick. Sometimes I need to be pushed a little or encouraged to try new things, but I must be able to feel some control, for I have already lost so much.

Let me talk a little about my fears and my exhaustion as well as about my goals. Sometimes I need to cry. This is a risk. And sometimes I need to laugh and see others laugh. Always I need to teach others about myself; at times I am very tired of it all.

So here I am. I am alive. I laugh and cry just like you. I am not ill but a person with a disability. Just like you I have good days, bad days, feelings, and ideas. I also have dreams and hopes. This bed and chair is not my life. Most of my body's numb, but I can still feel my heart, my hair, my face, perhaps my neck. I have not lost the pleasure of feeling someone stroke my face or of offering pleasure to another with my lips, my face. In a way I'm born again. I'm learning new ways to talk and do, for myself and for others. With practice I am not so tired, and new tasks soon become routine.

And so, here I am. It is not something I can ever accept completely, but I can acknowledge myself in this situation and learn to cope. And I must always have hope. Please remember that.

FROM ANOTHER'S POINT OF VIEW

I know someone who has respiratory quadriplegia. At first I am afraid that this could happen to me. How would I cope, what would I do? I'm not sure how to act or what to say. I feel sorry for you and am afraid of my pity, for I suspect you do not need it.

I must learn to listen to a sentence often interrupted by a machine and wonder if I say the right or the wrong thing. But is there a right or wrong thing, maybe I should just talk? This machine, it doesn't talk, yet it means so much. I need to know about it, so I need not feel so afraid.

Sometimes I forget the energy it takes to read or get out of bed and I grow impatient. When I am tired or have many things to do it is easy to forget to show a willingness for little things. I forget you cannot use your arms and legs as I can and that you probably still remember when you could. Sometimes I forget how much you risk when you explore new things and I need to remember my own fears and how I cope.

Feeding and dressing an alert adult is, at first, strange to me. I'm not sure how to make it a comfortable experience. Perhaps my own awkward feelings make it the same for you. Thank you when you gently let me know how you feel.

I am confused when you are angry and I'm not sure why. How can I make myself remember that it may not be me you are angry at but your situation? Maybe we can talk about it, or perhaps you just need to be left alone for a while.

After a time I see beyond your disability, for you are just a person after all. In many ways you manage your life and I needn't try to tell you now. You have the same rights to privacy and respect as any other person I know. We can, perhaps, share our ideas and perceptions. Doing so, I must watch you struggle to find your balance between dependence and independence and wonder when to speak my mind or to step aside. Later we can laugh, when it's a little easier. Above all I must remember that just because you require so much care it does not mean you are ill.

How much you have taught me about life and about myself. Your struggles and failures teach me about my own. I think now that there are no such things as failures but only experiences to build on. Thank you for that.

Compiled from a series of encounters by Linda MacNutt, M.S.W. Vancouver, BC

of social conditions and values rather than limitations imposed by physical incapacities (Mechanic 1961). Spinal cord injury is the disability: social barriers are the handicap.

The individual, the family, and health care professionals are all part of society, and general values and beliefs in society define each group's attitudes toward disability. For instance, one value or norm that defines disability as a problem for society is the concept of beauty (Goffman 1961). One criterion for beauty is physical wholeness, and thus the severely disabled are not viewed as beautiful but as pitiable or even contemptible.

Another important value held by society is that of independence or self-reliance. This emphasis may make injured people less inclined to want or accept help. But people with high quadriplegia have no choices in this regard. They depend on help in all aspects of daily care and must try to seek self-reliance in other things. It is important to remember that their need for help does not mean they are sick or not self-directing.

Society also values productivity. Visible contributions, particularly work, are interpreted as accomplishment, and who people are (self-concept) is often measured by what they can do. People who do not contribute are often viewed as a burden to society, for their maintenance is a great financial cost, and often the disabled person is relegated to second-class citizenship. The "disabled" role is transformed into the "useless" role. Society continually wrestles with justifying substantial financial expenditures to gain limited results. One cannot deny that the constant care required by people with high quadriplegia is costly. Unfortunately such a cost-benefit analysis does not measure the accomplishments of the individual and the need to ensure a high quality for the life that is saved.

Severely disabled people may be encouraged to act "normal," but they face social contradictions. Stigma, limited employment opportunities, lack of technological aids, lack of transportation, and architectural barriers are some examples (Rogers 1989).

These factors isolate the severely disabled person, which limits stimulating contact with other human beings and minimizes the potential for enhancing inner personal resources. High quadriplegia therefore is a problem that cannot be separated from society. Adaptation to disability is a joint responsibility because society as a whole helps define disability.

PSYCHOSOCIAL ASPECTS OF HIGH QUADRIPLEGIA

Although advancements in early care have evolved rapidly, solutions for the continuing issues surrounding the quality of life have not. The magnitude of challenges has rendered the traditional medical model of care inadequate to meet these unique needs. As a result, providing direct psychosocial support encompasses some very broad issues and is complicated by lack of widespread rehabilitation opportunities for people with high quadriplegia.

The onset of injury resulting in quadriplegia may be defined as a *crisis*. See Chapter 9. It is a traumatic event that requires solutions, invariably new, in relation to the individual's previous life experience. Consequently there is severe disruption of living patterns accompanied by tension and distress that results in a reorganization of the life situation. In the case of the person with high quadriplegia, the crisis revolves around extreme and traumatic physical injury with subsequent implications for the individual, family, health care, and community systems.

The Injured Person

It must be emphasized that psychosocial adaptation to the crisis of high quadriplegia usually occurs over a very long time. It is unrealistic to expect that vast identity changes imposed by severe disability be incorporated too quickly, especially considering that the concept of self begins to develop in early childhood. Burnham and Werner (1979) describe disturbances in formal thought or cognition caused by the traumatic physical and emotional injury as significant factors in slowing the adjustment process. For the person with quadriplegia, it is also logical that the inability to communicate (when a cuffed tracheostomy tube is necessary during the early months) may retard the expression of emotional factors inherent in the adjustment process.

As time progresses the impact of severe disability is realized. Major consequences include changes in body image, methods of communication, locus of control, and personal roles, factors further described in Chapter 9.

Self/Body Image

Persons with high quadriplegia must develop new body images, for they can no longer define themselves in pre-injury terms. Some people feel success in life is due to physical prowess in sports and have difficulty thinking of what to do to feel good about themselves again. One person described feeling that her head and body were split. She thought of herself only as a head and felt disgust with her paralyzed limbs.

People must also adapt their body images to include mechanical aids. Reidentification in this existential sense is difficult indeed. The power wheelchair and the ventilator become extensions of the self in relation to mobility and life itself. There is often inner turmoil in the relationship between the individual and machines (Burnham and Werner 1979).

The "half-person, half-machine" self-image presents a unique set of problems. The idiosyncratic meaning of the ventilator for each person must be understood to assist in the immense transition from illness to wellness. Persons

PERSONAL VIEWPOINT

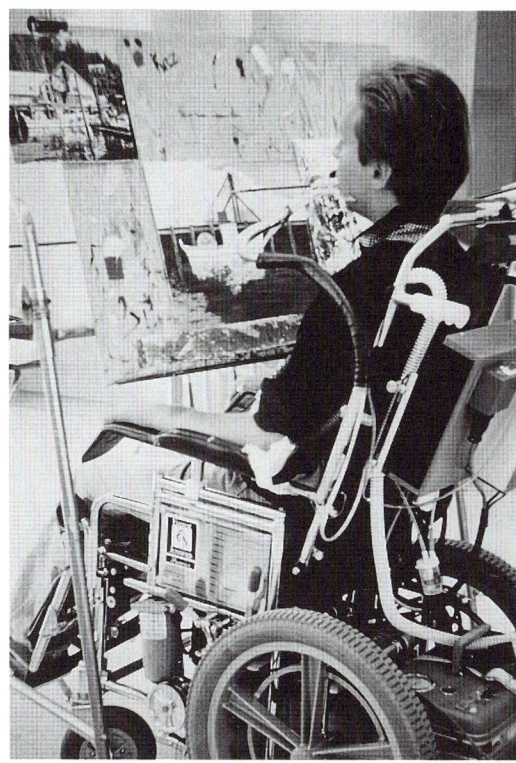

After many years in a long-term care facility, I now share a beautiful apartment with several other ventilator-dependent persons. This has given us complete control of our lives.

Eleven years ago I was injured when some friends and I decided to celebrate the first days of summer on a neighborhood balcony which gave way. I fell 30 feet, resulting in a complete C_2 quadriplegia. The journey from a life dominated by physical activity to finding value in other pursuits occurred much sooner than I expected. My life is very full, satisfying and happy. I took up mouth painting out of sheer boredom only to find that my creativity resulted in selling most of what I paint! Employment in the federal Spinal Cord Injury Prevention Program and resultant national opportunities for travel and speaking engagements, offers a challenge to me.

When I was first injured, I remember that the emotional dependence on nurses was overwhelming. Not many nonnursing professionals recognize this. Initially, it was very difficult to adjust. Even when hearts are in the right place, the "I know what is best for you" attitude came creeping through. It was bad enough living for 7 years in an 8-by-8 foot stall, surrounded only by curtains, without having to contend with insensitive staff invading my privacy at any time.

Involving the person in care, strengthening that special bond, contributes so much to a harmonious atmosphere. All levels of nursing would run smoother if teamwork included the injured person. It is important that nurses help each other emotionally, as well as physically; attitudes, sensitivity, and communication are of utmost importance.

Personally, I would like to see nurses fight for much more input into the course of rehabilitation rather than the physician-dominated model. Physicians told my family and me what they thought we wanted to hear. They were seldom around when issues arose, and we felt so bothersome and rushed when the doctors were there, especially during the acute stage.

I credit much of what I have accomplished to the superb care I continue to receive that keeps me in optimal health, enabling me to do what I want to do. The support of family and friends and the ever-growing community understanding has contributed vastly to my present life-style.

Robb Dunnfield
Vancouver, BC

---

who have had to relinquish life-sustaining breathing ability to a machine must adapt to this dependency.

Methods of Communication

Persons with high-level injuries must discard many methods of communication. They can no longer use their hands to express themselves in speech, or touch another when words are not enough. Instead, they must master the skill of controlling speech while on the ventilator. They must now describe rather than point out objects, find new releases for powerful emotions, and try to find words instead of the actions previously used for communication.

Locus of Control

Locus of control refers to the amount of perceived control over life events. Persons with internal locus of control perceive themselves as primary directors of their own lives. This contrasts with external locus of control individuals, who believe in the prominence of luck, fate, or chance. Early studies in the concept of control in nondisabled individuals have correlated internal locus of control to a myriad of positive psychological characteristics.

Consequently, shifting to a belief that control is external, or reinforcing a previous belief to that effect, would present major barriers to an individual's struggle toward life goals.

Despite difficulties that persons with high quadriplegia may have maintaining control over the immediate environment—especially the most basic functions, such as eating or dressing—general control over the rewards and satisfactions of life does not necessarily change.

Therefore, to promote a positive adaptation process, people must become sensitive to the importance of choices. Even small choices become significant because they reestablish some measure of control. Being able to decide what to eat first (peas or carrots) or what time to bathe are important to physically dependent persons even if they seem mundane or inconvenient to others. Eliminating choices in daily life contributes to developing an undesirable external source of control.

As one person with ventilator-dependent quadriplegia explains, "Looking back over the years, which were spent mostly in a long-term care facility, I think some of my worst memories were the constant battles over the ground rules and policies. For me that battle was worth it because giving in would have meant I had become *institutionalized*, what everyone fears in a similar situation to mine."

Personal Roles

The process of identification with new roles is probably influenced by the individual's perception of the sick and disabled roles. Due to the initial life-and-death situation in acute care, injured people are indeed ill. But there is danger of stabilizing in the sick role on a long-term basis. Illness may be preferable to disability as it may sustain a belief in cure and lack of acknowledgment of the disability. One person stated that he half believed he would be cured when transferred from acute care, simply because leaving the hospital *should* have meant that he was cured.

Persons also have to reexamine educational and vocational pursuits and reassess dreams or ideals within the limitations of severe disability. After injury, recreational pastimes change from the more concrete (action oriented) to the more abstract (watching television, listening to the radio, reading, or perhaps artwork using a mouthstick). Such activities often require the use of electronic environmental controls. Ironically, although intellectual or abstract pursuits are gradually emphasized, access to life experiences is reduced.

Self-Concept

Self-concept is a particularly important variable in the outcome of this profound disability. The impact of devalued status in society for disabled individuals affects how newly disabled persons feel about themselves. When ventilator-dependent quadriplegic persons incorporate this negative image, a compromised self-image will result.

However, compromised self-esteem may not be a natural consequence of SCI. In one study, Green, Pratt, and Grigsby (1984) found that despite lower scores in physical areas, indices of personal, moral-ethical, and social areas were significantly above the scaled norms. Persons who live independently, provide their own transportation, and manage their care attendants tend to have positive self-images. In living productive lives, identities are rebuilt, and in the process, individuals may actually develop better self-images than before. See Chapter 9 for further information. Many of the current studies and beliefs do not focus on persons with higher levels of injury; thus it is only speculation that these self-image issues are greater for ventilator-dependent quadriplegia in that the sequelae are more pronounced.

The Family

Psychosocial implications for the family as a whole as well as for each member of that system are closely related to those experienced by the injured member. As time progresses family members, too, begin to understand the injury's full consequences. See Chapter 9.

Perceptions of the Disabled Family Member

Dreams, hopes, and expectations for a child, sibling, or spouse are not changed easily. It is difficult to perceive a person as incapable of walking or even eating without assistance again. In addition, the person's inability to breathe without a respirator can generate fear of death, fear of the machine, and fear of inability to handle potential emergencies.

Family Roles

High quadriplegia forces extensive changes in the typical roles of every family member. The family is an interdependent system, and thus an alteration in the disabled individual's capabilities necessitates concomitant behavioral changes for other family members. Any change in the family system has a cascading, rippling impact. Disability can prove problematic in that not only are preinjury roles often rendered impossible, but also there is ambiguity or uncertainty regarding new roles the disabled individual may play within the family. These role changes are—understandably—highly disconcerting to the family.

With regard to family power structures, the disabled individual may be viewed as developing into a power figure due to the mechanistic tasks of personal care and all the attention that it requires. Power can also be centered around the individual's ability to manipulate the family's well-being. For example, a depressed attitude can affect the family mood and motivate people to meet the disabled person's idiosyncratic needs. Role strain through such task reorganization is common. For example, conflict arises when a parent tries to help a son or daughter toward independence while the demands of physical care almost force overprotective relationships.

Each family reacts uniquely to these role changes. Staff must understand that the disabled individual cannot be

---

PERSONAL VIEWPOINT

I was injured in a diving accident 4 years ago. My family all reacted in different ways, each coinciding with their various personalities. Dad was the strongest one holding the family together, always being positive around me, but breaking down many times outside the hospital—I found out months later. However, I believe it was a healthy and necessary reaction at the time. Mom and my two sisters reacted in a similar way by showing compassion, understanding, and patience throughout my good and bad times. My oldest brother, then and now, finds it harder to cope and adjust to my situation—always waiting to wake up and find things back to normal. My youngest brother was affected the least because of his age and easy-going nature.

Some of my closest friends stood by me and handled the situation as well as could be expected, maybe a little awkwardly at first. Others I never did see again. Some of the ones I least expected to come in have become my closest friends. You sure learn who your friends are. Without my family and friends there is no predicting what might have been.

---

rehabilitated in a vacuum. The mutual interdependencies and role interactions within each family are crucial in the rehabilitation process.

Health Care Professionals

Caring for a person with high quadriplegia is stressful because professional and personal attitudes and values become important factors in the therapeutic environment.

All practitioners experience another's disability only indirectly, and their perceptions are filtered by personal and professional attitudes. Inevitably a question asked when faced with the realities of respiratory quadriplegia is, "Could I live as Joe must live now?" Severe disability is often questioned because people identify with the injured person and have difficulty anticipating any quality of life remaining. How often have staff said, "If this ever happens to me, someone pull the plug"? But as one injured person explains, "The shock of being told I would never move again was devastating. I wanted to die, and if I could have reached my ventilator hose I would have pulled it out. Now, although I feel it sometimes doesn't matter one way or the other, when my air goes off, I fight for it."

Be reassured that most people with respiratory quadriplegia and their families eventually can cope and do enjoy life.

The several personal viewpoints throughout this chapter reveal that life still offers purpose. As Burnham and Werner (1979) describe, eventually low moments do not seem to override the will to live for people with respiratory quadriplegia. Private definitions of personal purpose, such as fulfilling the responsibilities of parenthood, reflect a driving force much stronger than the search for physical sustenance. Too often we underestimate the resilience of the human race.

Individuals and families rely on health care professionals to look objectively beyond the crisis at hand. Consequently, it is important to view the family over a long period of time so as not to take on their feelings of crisis and devastation in the immediate situation. Rather than dwell on "if this happened to me," look instead to people who successfully cope with high quadriplegia for a vision of what is possible. The interdisciplinary team must assume the varied roles of expert practitioner, counselors, advocates, educators, coordinators, and planners to ensure as many opportunities as possible for a full and positive future for people with respiratory quadriplegia and their families. See Chapter 1.

A PROCESS TO PROMOTE PSYCHOSOCIAL ADAPTATION

Assessment and Goal Setting

To promote psychological health when contending with high quadriplegia, it is highly important to acquire a thorough psychosocial profile. Issues related to a person's pretraumatic personality, ego strength, family dynamics, prior exposure to losses and concomitant coping strategies, age and developmental timing of the trauma, educational and vocational history, cultural background, interpersonal and financial supports, and avocational outlets are aspects of a sound psychosocial assessment.

Accommodation to this monumental trauma is a dynamic process; as such, continued assessment is likewise a dynamic process. An essential aspect in forming a positive alliance with injured persons and families is the staff's appreciation of the highly individualized, subjective interpretation of the disability. Consequently, staff must try to minimize clinical inference, conjecture, bias, supposition, and prejudice. It is imperative, given the family system, to address the psychological, educational, medical, financial, and social needs of family members, including the children.

It is necessary to work out realistic rehabilitation goals. If individuals—or perhaps more often, families—believe that the severity of disability is temporary, it usually indicates massive anxiety and a present inability to integrate the implications of SCI fully. All too often, staff confront their "denial" to dismantle it. This response unnecessarily creates an adversarial relationship that is not therapeutic and diminishes the rehabilitation outcome. However, with time, a supportive staff, and a sound rehabilitative and educational foundation, an appreciation of the injury and its sequelae is gradually gained: the injury can be managed and tolerated. Then goals can be formulated and refined to ensure success. Additionally, individuals and families must learn to make the transition from illness to wellness, actively participating in the rehabilitation process. Significant partnerships in goal setting, care, and decision making gradually develop.

If distance among the individual, family, or staff develops, quick therapeutic responses are essential to diminish defensive withdrawal and misunderstandings. Regularly scheduled individual-family-staff conferences to ensure congruence among goals, expectations, and plans encourage constructive expression, provide positive outlets, foster personal control, and make possible a satisfying life. Staff-only conferences are usually necessary to clarify psychosocial needs and to provide consistent, supportive, behavioral direction that is helpful for everyone.

Promoting Physical Well-Being

To promote psychosocial adaptation it is fundamental to apply the concept that basic physical needs must be met before psychological growth can flourish. It is profoundly important to become comfortable with the needed specialized equipment to help create a relaxed environment conducive to meaningful communication. In reality, preparation of numerous staff members just to meet the exceptional *physical* needs and minimize associated fears of the high quadriplegic person is frequently a major problem.

Consistency and *predictability* promote better rehabilitation outcomes. Education and training for staff must focus not only on the technical aspects of care, but also on the relationship between the individual and all the necessary equipment. Despite the complexity of support measures needed, care for the *person* is paramount.

To allay fears related to physical well-being:

- Always approach the person first, the equipment second. For example, explain ventilator settings and necessary changes *before* making adjustments.
- Use *early* interdisciplinary collaboration to secure a way for the individual to communicate while on mechanical ventilation. Meaningful communication must be maximized early because inability to communicate is one of the most problematic stressors and interferes with working through feelings and concerns.

- Become competent with related care and equipment. See Chapters 15 and 23 for detailed explanations of related respiratory care and mobility equipment. Include explanations and reinforce, as necessary, the safety features (alarm systems) of the ventilator and other equipment.
- Discuss beforehand all procedures and care routines and the rationale for selection.
- Assess concerns and permit emotional expression, giving support and empathy. Staff who can do this are valuable role models for others. Share information about progress. Many people appreciate the ability to read and contribute directly to the chart.
- Maximize continuity of care each shift by preparing oncoming staff together.

Dealing with Loss Associated with Severe Disability

Adaptation to high quadriplegia is highly individualized, affecting how a person deals with loss. As detailed in Chapter 9, background and personal characteristics, illness-related factors, and features of the physical and social environment determine the nature of outcome, *not* a predictable psychological progression through specified stages. Securing peer counselors/consultants with high quadriplegia is of great value in interpreting fears and concerns, which results in finding practical, workable solutions.

To increase the quality of care delivery to the individual and family, staff should:

- Understand the frequently observed responses to high quadriplegia, the distinction between anticipated mourning/grief reaction versus reactive depression, and the potential value in the expression of anger and related affects
- Know the major adaptive tasks confronting the individual and family, and also understand constructive or destructive coping strategies
- Understand how background and milieu contribute to successful coping
- Reflect a positive inner attitude developed by gaining a firsthand awareness of life-styles now possible.

As the life-threatening impact of trauma subsides, expression of feelings such as "Why did they save me? I'm of no use to myself or anyone else. Let me die" are often heard. Several people with high quadriplegia explain that these and similar statements are expressions of the desperate fear of the unknown future.

They were seeking *reassurance* and needed to know that life would improve.

How to respond? The need to respond positively, but realistically without false hope, was emphasized. Be reassured that a warm, caring, and honest relationship provides a sound baseline, despite probable feelings of personal helplessness. Sit down and encourage the patient to talk about feelings and past and present experiences; perhaps share some of your own. Guard against responses that block communication. When talking about a death wish, statements such as, "What a ridiculous thing to say," or "I know how you feel" communicate a lack of sensitivity and tend to cause further alienation.

False hope prolongs recovery and aggravates suffering. To be optimistic and realistic, at the same time, try to focus on how a particular part of the present situation will improve. Perhaps it means removal of a stomach tube, ability to sit up, a portable ventilator, a new wheelchair, or ability to take a college course. This approach is in keeping with the here and now, rather than overconcern with interpretation of theory.

It is surprising how an awkward response can be interpreted as false hope. For example, a young boy with high quadriplegia and his parents were discussing his return to school in time for graduation. When they looked to the nurse for approval, the nurse "simply didn't have the heart" to initiate a discussion on why this activity would not be possible. Instead the nurse quickly left the room. Avoiding the subject created more uncertainty, which allowed unrealistic expectations to grow. Sometimes it may not be appropriate to explore a subject further, but be sure to refer concerns to counseling professionals of the health team. Do not hesitate to seek guidance and support from them.

The adaptation process is lengthy and progress is slow. It is important to keep expectations realistic and compatible with the person's preinjury personality. A person's failure to achieve goals can lead to many unresolved frustrations and discouragement for all concerned.

Providing Health Education

Health education facilitates the process of adaptation. The general educational approach described in Chapter 11 acquaints the person and family with the extent and meaning of the disability and encourages them to assume an active role in the management of disability and maintenance of optimal health. Understandably, they may not be fully ready to learn care measures for some time.

In addition to the physical tasks at hand, the individual and possibly the family must develop an effective approach for directing others in various aspects of personal care. Incorporating the expertise of counseling professionals into educational programs helps to develop skills in supervising and relating to others, in essence, assuming a new role as educators themselves. See Chapter 32. If this concept is successfully introduced and if all concerned view the intro-

duction of new staff members as an opportunity to enact these new roles, rehabilitation becomes more flexible and less stressful.

When individuals begin to apply their knowledge and take initiative in participating or supervising their daily care they demonstrate an acceptance of responsibility for their bodies and daily lives (Burnham and Werner 1979). Regulating fluid and dietary intake, or supervising inspection and implementation of measures to prevent skin breakdown are some examples of such responsibilities.

Long-term planning can help persons exercise control over the environment, thereby enhancing feelings of self-worth. Involvement in making business and financial decisions, planning modifications to the home environment, and beginning to resume the role of a parent or son or daughter are good opportunities.

The physical dependency created by high quadriplegia places a great deal of responsibility on the family. Therefore, it is extremely important to develop a sensitivity to the family's needs and reactions that can block learning. To gain the fullest benefits, the adaptation level of the family must complement that of the individual.

The following situation was described by a 23-year-old woman with high quadriplegia.

> My mother became increasingly silent after my accident. Her usual reaction was to internalize feelings about problems. Later on she wouldn't have anything to do with my care, such as emptying my leg bag, tipping my chair back, or even moving my limbs to a more comfortable position. As far as she was concerned the health professionals were there to do that sort of thing. I finally perceived the source of the problem, and with many misgivings, rightly or wrongly, our roles were temporarily reversed. I confronted her with the reality that she had a daughter who was permanently disabled, and if she wanted to keep her she must accept the fact there would be times when we would be alone together. The discussion was a turning point that cleared the air. Slowly she was able to learn about my care.

In this situation, opportunities for professional intervention were clearly missed. Closer liaison with counseling professionals could have helped alert the nurse to the ways in which family members dealt with problems and the kinds of behavior that would indicate the mother was having difficulty. Meanwhile, many afternoons had been wasted trying to force the mother to learn various activities. The mother's angry reactions and demanding requests were confusing and frustrating to the staff, especially when the patient was coping so well. Finally the patient and her mother could have benefited from counseling support to explore their feelings and enhance the mother-daughter relationship. If the underlying problems had been recognized, professional intervention could have helped resolve these conflicts much sooner and made the educational process more effective.

Planning for Transition to Less Acute Settings

Critical care issues such as fears of death, pain, and disability; sleep deprivation; isolation; fear of strangers caring for them; and fear of transportation must be resolved before a person can move to the next stage. The person must be not only physically ready but also psychologically confident to transfer to a portable ventilator and relocate to a less acute setting. This transition is a major hurdle in the rehabilitation process.

Relocation or transfer from one unit to another or one facility to another is a crisis for the patient and the family, second only to the major crisis of the physical injury. The relocation process, then, can have a significant impact on psychosocial adjustment. The change in environments is usually great, with new staff, a new physical environment, new patients, and new programs. Difficult changes most frequently mentioned in this regard are decreases in staff, different physical environment, and difficulty of separation from former primary care nurses.

Emotional Reactions

Relocation may arouse many emotional reactions such as anxiety, uncertainty, and confusion, as well as loss of control. Separation from primary care nurses is difficult, and a sense of loss may be increased when there is no opportunity to discuss these feelings.

The effect of relocation can also be very positive. The need to move on is very pressing for most people. They feel ready to leave the more acute care settings despite leaving familiar and caring people. They are, perhaps, eager to relinquish the sick role in favor of increasing freedom to come and go in a new, less structured environment.

In terms of crisis theory, if people helping to restructure a life situation emphasize succumbing features, the injured person will probably be filled with bitterness and despair, but if the possibilities for growth are emphasized, adaptation should be characterized by hope, confidence, and personality growth (see Chapter 9). Relocation, then, can serve as a catalyst to maximize positive cycles of adaptation.

Continuity of Care

Planning for continuity of care is a major factor in determining how well the individual and family are able to handle the move. Although the value of interdisciplinary, even interagency, conferences is recognized more and more, the content—not to mention the practicality of actually having them—needs to be addressed.

As an example, let us examine the preparation and follow-up care for a patient transferring from a critical care unit to a ward setting. Typically the stay in the unit has been long, and the move is suddenly necessary because patients with more acute illnesses take priority. Often a detailed nursing care plan does accompany the patient, but it is difficult for the receiving nurse to welcome the patient; prepare the bedside environment; and select, communicate, and transcribe appropriate information all at the same time. Meanwhile, the slightest difference in a suctioning technique or a change in visiting hours can balloon into a major, unpleasant issue, and the difficulties begin.

How can this situation be improved? If the nursing service as a whole, including nursing leaders and the nurses who are transferring and receiving the patient, understand the long-term goals and the magnitude of potential problems, the approach will be more unified and supportive, yet flexible. This will involve taking measures to ensure adequate information and communication with nurses at the bedside.

For example, when sharing information about individual needs, be prepared to explore even the seemingly direct statements. It is not sufficient, for example, to note that the patient requires suctioning about every 2 hours. Can the patient communicate the need to be suctioned? How will the suction setup differ? Are the catheters the same? Does the procedure differ? Who will be doing it? A registered nurse or a nursing assistant?

The issue of what category of staff perform what procedures is frequently complicated. Although suctioning a tracheostomy is not generally considered a nursing assistant's responsibility, the person with respiratory quadriplegia has unique needs. If a nursing assistant cannot perform this procedure, is it likely that opportunities for rehabilitation will be limited? For example, will outings off the ward be limited, perhaps just to sit outside? Such limitations can significantly prolong hospitalization.

If all members of the nursing care team are not allowed to meet the patient's basic needs, what messages are sent to the family? What implications does this have for the nursing assistant trying to manage daily bedside care? After all, family and even friends are expected to learn these procedures eventually.

These kinds of decisions affect policy making, implications of which may extend outside the health care facility to licensing bodies. However, if individualized needs are to be met, these questions must be addressed well ahead of time for adequate planning.

Preparing the Individual and the Family

When the team judges the person to be medically and emotionally capable, initiate discussion of the potential transfer. At this point the social worker and primary nurse, in view of their daily contact, may be the appropriate persons to meet with the patient. The formal discussion should provide individuals the opportunity for full expression of thoughts and feelings (positive and negative) about the move.

Most patients find it difficult to be flexible at this point. If so, do not let the patient's rigid expectations and preferences prevent approaching the subject. This is also the time to begin termination of the primary care relationship (if the process has not already begun) and create opportunities for expression of feelings about this separation.

Discussion of goals and of probable length of stay in the new environment will help minimize vague expectations and uncertainty associated with increasing stress. *Above all, emphasize that the improvement in the patient's general state of health is making the move necessary.* This improvement dictates changes in care requirements, but unless the individual and family are well prepared, the new nurse's approach is often perceived as incompetent.

The acute care team must help the person and family view the anticipated changes as a positive step in the transition period toward a more homelike situation. The receiving staff must be alert for potential problems and be prepared to demonstrate immediate confidence despite different ways of doing things. It is also helpful if the individuals, family, and new staff can be open to the new role of the injured person as educator in terms of individual needs.

It is reassuring for the individual and family to know that there will be a formal opportunity for discussion following relocation. It is also helpful if the original social worker or clinical nurse specialist can maintain contact during the transition period to enhance continuity.

Participating in the Choice of an Appropriate Setting

Selecting the most appropriate setting following the acute phase is difficult. Providing safe and detailed care while increasing opportunities for independence and rehabilitation is a serious problem.

Caring for ventilator-dependent persons on a general ward is often an isolated experience for a facility. Therefore, staff are often inexperienced in this kind of care. In-depth staff education is necessary but not always feasible. As a result, persons with high quadriplegia often experience detrimental, costly, and prolonged stays in critical care areas. When relocation does occur, it may be to a setting in which rehabilitation is not the primary focus and the risk of severe complications is high. These factors emphasize the need for development of specialized, integrated, rehabilitative services.

PROVIDING REHABILITATION OPPORTUNITIES*

A good program for persons with high quadriplegia must be based on excellent health management by an interdisciplinary team who are both knowledgeable and experienced.

*This section was developed with assistance from Kathleen De Silva.

Besides maintaining physical integrity and increasing mobility, consistently emphasize psychosocial and education and vocational rehabilitative services. Educational goals and carer opportunities are vital because persons with high quadriplegia must maximize their mental abilities.

The following elements may be integrated into a rehabilitative program to provide a person with high quadriplegia varied experiences:

1. *Physical exercise programs.* Alterations in body image threaten self-esteem. Physical exercise programs, such as physical therapy mat programs, aquatics, or hydrotherapy programs, help persons combat the feeling that the mind and body are split. The experience of rolling and of being touched may deemphasize the feeling of physical and psychological fragility and allow persons to see their bodies move again. In addition, they can consider themselves "touchable," which contributes to feelings of emotional well-being.

2. *Breathing program.* A breathing program, or ventilatory muscle training, may be considered successful even if the person can manage only a few minutes off the ventilator at a time. This provides a safety margin in the event of a mechanical breakdown, building confidence and improving self-image and self-esteem. Techniques are fully described in Chapter 15.

3. *Adaptive equipment.* Adaptive equipment is vital to maximize the potential independent functioning of a person with high quadriplegia. Such items include motorized wheelchairs with chin, mouth, or voice control; computers with adaptive keyboards or voice activation; devices such as mouthsticks, page turners, and reading racks; accessible desks and other modified work stations; telephones operable from bed or wheelchair; and environmental control units with various options. Chapter 23 explores technology further.

4. A *mix of peer and professional counseling.* A variety of personal and family issues, social comfort, sexual concerns, and many other topics can be explored through individual and group counseling. The opportunity to share and express feelings and to exchange practical information with others familiar with the situation can reduce tension and feelings of isolation and develop strengths and ways of coping.

Stress management might help increase social effectiveness. A stress management course developed by Garrison (1978) focuses on the teaching of relaxation to cope with undesirable responses to stress. Garrison suggests that paralyzed people imagine tensing and relaxing ineffective muscles.

5. *Social skills.* New social communication and behavior skills can be learned and practiced. See Chapter 31. Individuals can learn to have some control in their interactions with others through verbal skills. This training could also help people make the transition from a concrete to a more abstract form of thinking. The individual may also lack

PERSONAL VIEWPOINT

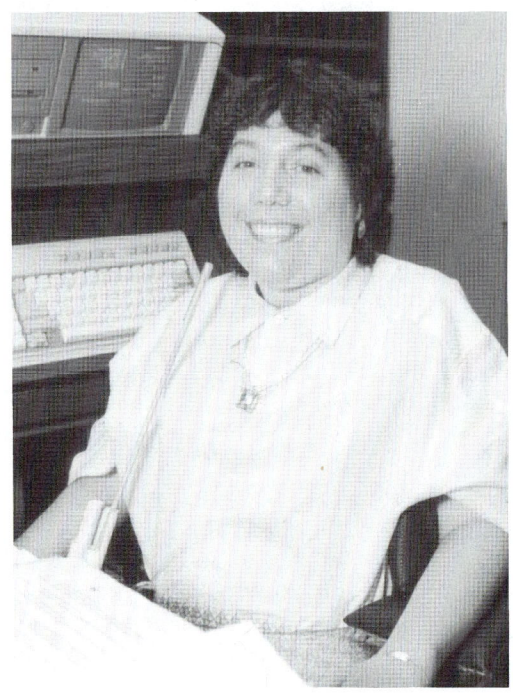

I was injured on the uneven parallel bars while practicing for the gymnastics team one day after school. I was 16 years old at the time and a sophomore in high school. Shortly thereafter, my family moved to Houston, Texas, so that I could go to The Texas Institute for Rehabilitation and Research (TIRR). (We had been living in Shreveport, Louisiana.) Since I was a C_{1-2} injury, a respirator had been required at all times. At first, I was on an MA-1. The first side of my phrenic pacemaker was implanted in December 1970—about 2 years after my injury, which occurred in April 1968. The following year, the other side was implanted, and I began to gain time using them.

My mother took care of me while I lived at home with help from my younger brothers and sisters who would do such things as turn pages, wash my face and hair, and change television channels. Both my parents attended class with me. I stayed in a room that was built on to the house. Then we moved to a new house where the study was my bedroom.

When my mother had her seventh child, we hired someone to come in part-time during the day. Otherwise, my parents did all my care. (I have a wonderful family and consider myself very fortunate in this respect.)

The events leading to my moving out were very sudden and unexpected. My mother died in 1974 when the baby was a year and a half old. I went into TIRR for back surgery and during the months of recuperation, my father and I decided that the best thing was for me to find a private attendant and move into my own apartment. My parents and I had discussed this before, but now it was almost a necessity.

I advertised and interviewed for 2 months and finally hired a young woman in her twenties just before Christmas. She trained at TIRR for about 2 weeks and then we moved into an apartment. It was quite a memorable experience! I have been living in the community ever since.

I graduated from the University of Houston College of Law in 1980 and passed the Bar Exam that same year. Shortly afterward, I opened a small women's store with a friend of mine.

I have worked as in-house counsel at TIRR for more than 7 years. As the hospital attorney, I handle corporate matters, contracts, leases, medical staff issues, real estate, tax, and risk management. I also serve as assistant secretary to the Board of Trustees and handle a variety of other administrative functions.

In 1984, I was deeply saddened by the loss of my father who died suddenly of cancer. That same year, I was married to a wonderful person named Peter Simmons. He is an ex-sailor who worked as the ship's chief engineer and has a degree in marine science. Peter is also in a wheelchair and now works as a house husband and as president and executive director of Independent Life Styles (ILS), a nonprofit organization that provides shared, in-home attendant services to physically disabled persons. I assist him as vice president, so we are both actively involved in fundraising and running a small business. ILS is unique in that it is managed entirely by persons with disabilities.

Shortly after my father's death, I established a foundation in memory of both of my parents. The foundation's purpose is to support alternative living arrangements for persons with disabilities, and I serve as the foundation's president.

For the past 2 years, I have also served as president of the homeowners' association where I live. In addition, I am the chairperson of the MetroLift Advisory Committee which reviews and oversees the local paratransit system, and I participate on a special task

(Box continues)

PERSONAL VIEWPOINT *(continued)*

force that is in charge of implementing the new lift-equipped mainline bus system in Houston.

Being married to Peter has been the happiest time of my life! We have a nice, comfortable townhome with two dogs, two aquariums and various antiques that we collect.

I have taken interesting trips. When Peter and I were married, we flew to upstate New York to visit his parents who lived in a small town in the Catskill Mountains. As we were boarding the plane, the crew insisted that we had to sit on different aisles for some rather vague "safety reason." Since this was supposed to be our honeymoon, we explained that we wanted to sit together, so they finally agreed that we could sit on the same aisle as long as our attendant sat between us! Just before we landed, they told me that my wheelchair had been mistakenly left in Houston and would be arriving on the next plane. So we waited in the airport lobby at midnight on a Saturday night, tired and frustrated, until it got there. Our destination was still 2 hours away, and we had rented a so-called "luxurious" stationwagon for the drive. However, we were told that the rental booth was located at a different airport so our attendant had to ride a shuttle bus to get the car. Then, we enlisted the services of two strangers to help lift us into the car because our foot pedals would not even fit close to the door. Somehow, we managed to fit three people, two wheelchairs and luggage for three into that compact car! When we finally arrived at Peter's parents, the local fire department came and helped carry us into my new in-laws' house! Needless to say, the whole trip was quite an experience!

I also traveled to Washington, DC, to attend a seminar for hospital in-house attorneys. This past year, Peter and I flew to Vail, Colorado, for a seminar on high quadriplegia at which I was a speaker and panelist. There was some concern about the effect the altitude would have on my breathing, but I adjusted quickly to the cool, dry climate. We were driven by van from Denver to Vail and the scenery was breathtaking! On the way back to the Denver airport, we rode with some friends from the seminar and we all had a great time!

Peter and I have also made several trips in our own van to visit my grandmother in Louisiana. The van has been customized for two wheelchairs with a tiedown for each and hand controls for Peter to use. Of course, we frequently go out on weekends to various restaurants, shopping centers, museums, parks, and other leisure activities, such as visiting family and friends.

I have received two very special honors over the last few years. I was featured in *Esquire Magazine*'s 1984 Register, "The Best of the New Generation—Men and Women Under Forty Who are Changing America." In 1988, I was selected by Texas Executive Women and *The Houston Post* as one of Houston's 10 "Women on the Move." These tributes have meant a great deal to me, and I am honored to be recognized for achievements that I view as part of my everyday life.

Kathleen De Silva, J.D.
Houston, TX

personal goals, knowledge of how to master tasks, and a sense of meaning or purpose to life. A task-centered approach to the development of realistic life goals can provide a feeling of purpose and accomplishment.

6. *Management and attendant training.* During the rehabilitation process, the individual should participate in attendant training and management classes and, if possible, practice living independently in a supervised setting at the rehabilitation facility as well as practicing at home when on day and weekend passes. Of course, family members and other care givers must undergo intensive, hands-on training before the person leaves the hospital.

7. *Recreational activities.* During hospitalization, it is important to provide as many evening and weekend activities as possible, usually through therapeutic recreation. This might include card games, bingo, dominoes, board games, home movies, outdoor barbeques, and other activities. Field trips can be coordinated to sports events, museums, the zoo, shopping centers, restaurants, theaters, parks,

and other events away from the facility. It is also extremely valuable to visit the homes and work environments of other persons with similar disabilities to see how they function.

Recreational activities can help prevent social and intellectual isolation. Programs that help individuals learn how to play and develop hobbies or interests in accord with their physical limitations improve the quality of life.

8. *Educational/vocational assessment and career planning.* Consulting professionals must have a knowledge of the individual's skills, personal goals, and education to offer concrete, useful, and innovative program suggestions. It should be emphasized, though, that the person with high quadriplegia may not be ready for training and education for some time. Individuals consistently mention the need for time to adapt to the new situation and master small tasks such as using a mouthstick before exploring vocational goals.

However, the staff should be familiar with the person's particular interests and capabilities. They should be able to

*This section was contributed by Lester Butt.

PERSONAL VIEWPOINT

It is an art to make people feel comfortable around you. When my family and friends visited me they gradually performed little tasks for me. As they became more confident, and I was able to react calmly, it was easy to teach them about my ventilator and my care.

In terms of helping family and friends learn how to help a disabled person, it is extremely important that individuals learn as much as they can about their own care, including the equipment they depend on. It is essential that disabled persons are aware of the problems they can encounter in day-to-day living and be prepared for those exigencies. In the case of ventilator-dependent persons, understand the equipment, know what can go wrong with it, and know what to do when something does go wrong. This is much easier to do if individuals are not totally dependent, but can breathe on their own for a little while. It is even more important for the person who has no breathing to make sure that people know what to do in an emergency. Disabled people should make sure that the people around them know what to do when the occasion arises. Even if individuals are living in an institution it is important that they accept some responsibility for personal care.

inform the individual about various schools, colleges, and trade or vocational programs and should also be aware of accessible campuses and the availability of dormitories with student/attendant placement. Although the respiratory needs of a person with high quadriplegia may require intensive personal care by family providers or private attendants, it is always beneficial to know about all available options. Financial information, such as scholarships and funding through state vocational rehabilitation services, should also be provided. It is also helpful to learn about a variety of useful study techniques, for example, note-taking can be accomplished by photocopying fellow students' notes or by using a tape recorder.

9. *Independent living skills.* Trends toward deinstitutionalization continue, along with an increase in consumer participation in services. In the United States today, staggering medical costs often necessitate returning to live at home. However, options are limited if the home situation is not stable, if community support systems are not adequate, or if a young person desires to free aging parents from care burdens. Independent living skills and resources to overcome personal, social, and economic barriers are addressed in Chapter 30.

DILEMMAS IN REHABILITATION: BIOETHICAL CONCERNS*

One can readily observe the proliferation of important actions and case law concerning bioethics (Dine 1988). In 1960, long-term dialysis was made possible, but the high cost of treatment and the shortage of machines resulted in the formation of a selections committee at the University Hospital in Seattle. Patients who were not selected died. The controversy focused nationwide attention on the concept of bioethics. Several years later the Hastings Center, an ethics think tank in Briarcliff Manor, NY, and the Kennedy Institute of Ethics at Georgetown University in Washington, DC, were founded. The centers regularly publish materials about ethics, develop model legislation, and provide advice on landmark ethics cases.

Models of Health Care

Increasingly, rehabilitation has been confronted with bioethical dilemmas. However, bioethics was not based on the rehabilitation model of health care, but rather on acute care models, the ultimate health goal of which is cure. Typically, patient relationships with health care professionals are discrete, finite, and episodic, which is in marked contrast to rehabilitation. Again, this is in contrast to the rehabilitation model of care. Given these distinctions, the Hastings Center issued a landmark special supplement to bridge the gap between the traditional medical model and the rehabilitation model of care (Caplan, Callahan, and Haas 1987).

Whereas cure is inherent in the traditional model, rehabilitation and continuing care goals are often broader and more expansive. Disability by definition is mostly chronic and irreversible. Individuals play a crucial role in their own care. They inform the health care team of the extent to which any impairments produce dysfunction or disability (Caplan, Callahan, and Haas 1987). In rehabilitation, patients are not passive; on the contrary, they are active partners in the rehabilitation process. They assist in determining goals to regain emotional stability, preserve residual function, prevent further disabling complications, and develop compensatory functional capacities for day-to-day survival.

In rehabilitation, values and quality of life are also markedly important. The rehabilitation team, the individual, and often the family must find shared values and a shared vision of quality of life so that they can establish mutual goals.

However, the most salient difference between the traditional and the rehabilitation model revolves around the

BRIEF INTERPRETATIONS

BIOETHICS

Bioethics involves the moral rules, principles and values that guide relationships between health care providers and their patients. Within the general purview of bioethics, two distinct principles dominate and often conflict with one another: *paternalism* and *autonomy*.

PATERNALISM

Paternalism, in the context of the health care delivery system, refers to the relegation of decision-making authority to health care professionals. This principle assumes that, given training and expertise, professionals can most effectively and accurately make decisions in the patient's best interests.

AUTONOMY

Autonomy is the principle of self-determination or self-governance. The practices of informed consent and the right to refuse treatment involve autonomy. Recently, respect for the patient's autonomy has acquired a distinctive primary role in the health care delivery system, allowing competent adults to make decisions for themselves. The right of persons to control their own bodies is a basic societal concept that has been long recognized under law. All citizens have a fundamental right to be free from unwarranted intrusion into their private lives, guaranteed by the Bill of Rights, specifically the first, third, fourth, fifth and ninth amendments.

INFORMED CONSENT

Informed consent implies that all competent patients have the right to be informed regarding potential treatments, potential risks and benefits, and the context of the particular modality in the broader scope of the person's health care. This process, of necessity, must not be coercive and must be accurately objective.

Informed consent is predicated on the patient's ability to accept or reject the proposed treatment (competency). The concept of informed consent creates many dilemmas because it tries to balance different values—specifically, on one side, *beneficence* (health or well-being, usually defined by the health care professionals) and, on the other, *autonomy* or *self-determination*. (Caplan 1988)

More and more frequently, clinical questions arise about the capacity or *competence* of a specific patient to give an informed consent. If the patient is not competent, then patient consent does not constitute an authorization to treat. If incompetent, the individual does not inherently possess the right to refuse treatment (Drane 1985). However, it is not always easy to determine competency because no commonly accepted definition of competency exists and a variety of parameters are used to make this judgment.

COMPETENCY

Evidencing a choice, factual understanding of issues, rational manipulation of information, and appreciation of the nature of the situation (Appelbaum and Roth 1982) are four possible standards for judging *competency*. In 1982, the President's Commission for the Study of Ethical Problems in Medicine and Biomedical and Behavioral Research defined competency, or decisional capacity, as based on the possession of a set of values and goals, the ability to communicate and understand information, and the ability to reason and deliberate.

To assess competency, Appelbaum and Grisso (1988) have identified the following factors:

- *Communicating choices.* The patient not only possesses choices, but requires the consistency and communication of stable choices for prolonged periods.
- *Understanding relevant information.* This includes memory, reception, storage, and retrieval of information; and comprehension of the nature of the treatment and appreciation of risks and benefits. Obviously, deficits in attention span, intelligence, or magnitude of stress can impact this dimension.
- *Appreciating the situation and its consequences.* Persons may comprehend certain information, yet fail to grasp what it means for them; that is, a person lacks understanding about specific implications for the future.
- *Manipulating information rationally.* This involves the ability to use logical processes to compare the benefits and risks of various treatment options and weigh information to reach a decision. Appelbaum and Grisso (1988) point out that rational manipulation involves arrival at conclusions consistent with initial premises.

(Box continues)

BRIEF INTERPRETATIONS *(continued)*

THE LIVING WILL AND DURABLE POWER OF ATTORNEY FOR HEALTH CARE (ADVANCE DIRECTIVES)

The *Living Will* is a directive that indicates the individual's preferences regarding types of treatment considered heroic or extraordinary. The legal difficulties with the Living Will are that the form is often vague and nonspecific. These points of confusion are circumvented in the *Durable Power of Attorney for Health Care*. In this document, the competent individual appoints a medical surrogate decision maker, called the *attorney-in-fact*, in the event the individual is rendered incompetent. If incompetency occurs, the attorney-in-fact has the legal sanction to act in the patient's best interests regarding medical decisions. Inherent within this arrangement is the appreciation of the incompetent individual's values by the surrogate decision maker, thus assuring the patient's best interests are served.

provider-patient relationship. The traditional model of care delivery is characterized by *paternalism*. Health professionals, primarily physicians, traditionally make decisions autonomously regarding care and treatments. Guided by principles of beneficence and nonmaleficence to provide care that only benefits the patient, does no harm, or keeps patients from harm, professionals are bound to assist patients in need. Additionally, professionals are not obliged to disclose information either to the patient or family that the physician considers would have a detrimental impact. The physician thus assumes the role of the authoritative expert, although this stance is now challenged by many consumers.

A second model of provider-patient relationships is the *contractual model*: care is provided, but only such care as is desired or requested by individuals. Respect for the *autonomy* of the patient dominates. Patients may, if they choose, reject care that is beneficial as long as such refusals are based on voluntary, informed choice. If principles conflict, patients have a right to know and providers have obligations to tell the truth (Caplan, Callahan, and Haas 1987).

There are inherent difficulties in the application of the contractual model to rehabilitation. Often informed consent is obtained early in treatment; however, despite the protracted nature of rehabilitation, frequently no further attempts are made to update informed consent as rehabilitation progresses. Additionally, the contractual model of informed consent occurs in the context of the physician-patient relationship. However, the norm in rehabilitation is that a patient does not relate solely to one doctor. More frequently, there is an entire rehabilitation team, as well as several physicians and consultants, with whom to contend. Last, this model assumes that the patient is competent to enter into this egalitarian relationship. However, patient competency during the acute rehabilitation phase is often questioned by the treating professionals. Caplan, Callahan, and Haas (1987) ascribe this to the following issues:

- Rehabilitation professionals believe that patients do not immediately appreciate the risks and benefits of rehabilitative care. This realization develops over a prolonged period.

- Often rehabilitation professionals will *not* honor a patient's request to refuse treatment in the acute phase because they believe that the initial phase of a disability poses a most arduous accommodation that takes time to assimilate successfully.

Ackerman (1982) describes autonomous behavior as having two primary features: behavior governed by plans of actions formulated through deliberation or reflection, and behavior based on intentional and voluntary choices harmonious with personal life plans. However, in a disease or disability physical, cognitive, psychological, and social constraints can prohibit truly autonomous behavior. Furthermore, denial, depression, guilt, and fear inevitably compromise autonomy. Patients may therefore make choices that may not be in harmony with their life plans. Furthermore, many patients with quadriplegia sustain secondary occult head injuries with the initial SCI (Chapter 26), which constitutes potential cognitive and emotional constraints that may be difficult to assess.

Given the inherent problems for rehabilitation in the traditional (paternal) and contractual (autonomous) models of care, Caplan, Callahan, and Haas (1987) advocate a third option, a hybrid: the *educational model*. In this schema, the clinicians have more latitude in terms of paternalism during the initial phases of rehabilitation. The interdisciplinary team has freedom to overrule the patient's and family's wishes because the team has a more comprehensive understanding of the rehabilitation process. The team's actions are sanctioned in order to restore autonomy to the patient. As understanding of the disability increases, the team gradually restores autonomy to the patient. The educational model requires close monitoring of the patient's increasing level of understanding and capacity for competency and awareness.

Assessment must be ongoing and zealous; once it is clear that patients have had the opportunity to accommodate to the realities of their functional impairments and have overcome other constraints, their right to control the direction and composition of their rehabilitative care will be restored to them (Caplan, Callahan, and Haas 1987).

The three types of provider-patient relationships (traditional, rehabilitative, and educational) all have inherent theoretical flaws. It is impossible to categorize people with high quadriplegia generically; that is analogous to stating that all humans possess identical personality traits. The desirable model is the model that matches the individual person. Rehabilitative literature has yet to reflect that widespread professional practice finely appreciates the nature of individual personality differences. All too often, the magnitude of the physical trauma overshadows personality uniqueness. An appreciation of the person, together with the appropriate provider-patient relationship, maximizes the possibilities of favorable outcomes in rehabilitation.

Many issues for people with high quadriplegia (or SCI in general for that matter) have ethical overtones (Haddad 1986). Refusal of patients to be turned when pressure areas exist, for example, represent real, confusing, and very time-consuming problems for patients and direct care providers. Frequently, these situations are not addressed adequately or in a timely fashion, from an ethical standpoint. These dilemmas are best addressed by an interdisciplinary team (Purtilo 1988). Care givers must understand the rationale for the chosen approaches because they will often be the ones who carry out those decisions. To this end, interdisciplinary hospital and community-based ethics committees are increasingly seen. Although some committees educate their members, each profession should take responsibility for providing educational opportunities to prepare care givers for future increasingly complex situations.

However, the most salient aspect of bioethics for persons with ventilator dependency is the ventilator itself. Advanced health care technology has made the ventilator both friend and foe: it saves and sustains life but at great cost in both human and economic terms. Once turned on, the machine seems to become autonomous, as in the much publicized case of Karen Quinlan (Dine 1988).

The Right to Die

Quality of Life

The most important area of bioethical concern for people with ventilator-dependent quadriplegia is quality of life. Quality of life almost escapes definition because it varies so widely from one person to another. As many disabled people attest, life is to be cherished despite disabilities and handicaps. However defined, the difficulty is whether the person, the physician, the treatment team, or the family make the judgment. The physician's assessment of the quality of the patient's life often is the basis for judgment. The assessment involves value-laden assumptions about the relative desirability of certain kinds of existence (Purtilo 1986). Health care professionals need to recognize and reduce their own preconceptions so that they can provide objective assessment. Efforts to measure quality of life objectively are generally more advanced for people with men-

tal impairments (National Rehabilitation Research Center 1990). Works by Shalock, Keith, and Hoffman (1990), for example, provide excellent assessment guidelines that could apply to the general population as well as for people with physical disabilities. Given these variances as to what constitutes quality of life, informed consent guarantees to competent adults the right to answer this question for themselves.

Economic Concerns

Purtilo (1986) describes two central ethical aspects in the treatment of ventilator-dependent persons: the cost of using the ventilator vis-à-vis general allocation of available resources and the issue of quality of life for the ventilator-dependent individual. The concern for cost expenditure relative to health care is well justified. In the United States $1.25 billion a day is expended for health care, which represents approximately 11% of the GNP (Veatch 1988).

Both Purtilo and Veatch advocate clearer criteria for determining when ventilators actually benefit the individual.

Requests to Discontinue Mechanical Ventilation

The most problematic situation confronting the rehabilitation team is when the acutely injured, ventilator-dependent person with quadriplegia wishes the ventilator discontinued and desires death over life. Rehabilitation professionals often believe that competent decisions are inconceivable in the acute postinjury phase. However, advance directives, such as the *Living Will* or *Durable Power of Attorney for Health Care*, add authenticity and credibility to the acutely injured patient's right to die. See Brief Interpretations Box. Despite the recognition in many states of advance directives, however, most disabled people do not have such documents.

Without advance directives, the rehabilitation team must deal with a request to discontinue ventilator support through accurate, deliberate, and protracted *assessment*, a process requiring a collaborative effort by the patient, the family, and the rehabilitation team. There should be predictable and frequent contacts with the patient and family. Difficulties tend to occur if communication is minimal. Despite the natural tendency to avoid these highly stressful situations communication is imperative.

Maynard and Muth (1987) describe the degree and type of understanding, sensitivity, analysis, and complexity involved in allowing a patient to die by discontinuing the ventilator, a process that lasted 25 months postinjury.

Rehabilitation professionals must be familiar with the evaluation of mental status and be aware of the psychological and cognitive impact of the person's particular illness, disease, or disability. The information shared with the patient must be presented in a readily comprehensible manner. The evaluation must acknowledge medication effects, fatigue, stress, and cognitive deficits. In order to gather the most accurate and objective feedback, it is imperative to interview the patient *over time* in a variety of situations. Socioeconomic, educational, and cultural issues can markedly affect the individual's presentation; consequently, an appreciation of these variables is most important. Additionally, it is important to understand that competency is not an easily defined state. Individuals are not necessarily totally competent or incompetent. Possibly a better evaluation question is, "Competent for what or in what area?" The definition of competency is obviously problematic, but of necessity, this issue must be directly approached when making highly important management decisions.

Ascertain whether there is *any* evidence of ambivalence manifested by the ventilator-dependent patient. The evaluation must discover what motivates the patient's desire to die. For example, does the wish to die represent a transient, depressive episode? Is the patient's request predicated on fear and misconceptions? Is the patient's request a symbolic attempt to gain control? Many possible underlying motivations can masquerade as death wishes. The team must be sensitive to these issues to serve the patient and family well.

If disagreements persist about the direction of treatment or nontreatment, consider other options. A bioethics committee in the facility can provide a forum for potential resolution. Typically, committees do not make decisions but attempt resolution of treatment differences. If these measures fail, courts serve as the final option. If competency is an issue, the court can appoint experts to evaluate this. If the ventilator-dependent individual is judged to be incompetent, and if no attorney-in-fact has been designated, the court can appoint a responsible family member or a guardian ad litem. A *guardian ad litem* is a third party chosen by the court to make decisions in the patient's best interest. Traditionally, the court weighs a patient's proclaimed desire to die against the state's interests in preservation of life, the need to protect innocent third parties, the duty to prevent suicide, and the requirement to help maintain the ethical integrity of professional practice.

As technology and health care progress and the survival rate of people with ventilator-dependent quadriplegia increases, there will, of necessity, be more appreciation of bioethical dilemmas. There exists a delicate balance between the rights of the individual to become autonomous and the expertise of the rehabilitation team with its tendency toward paternalism. As Menter and Maddox (1989) note, most problems in ethics arise out of disagreement as to which principle—paternalism or autonomy—should govern a situation. By promoting the goals of independence in rehabilitation, the team minimizes adversarial postures and promotes the most desirable outcomes, as measured by patients and their families.

THE LIFE PLAN: A HEALTH CARE FOCUS*

The continuum of health care available to the person with high quadriplegia can best be described as a *life plan*. In its broadest definition, the life plan implies both a philosophy of care and a range of services. The philosophy of care focuses on the independent living concept. This concept is explored more completely in Chapter 30. Its role in the enhancement of the disabled person's quality of life cannot be overemphasized. Support services encompassed in this life plan may include community-based and hospital-based services for the purpose of maintaining optimal functional stability while the person enjoys life and pursues personal goals and needs from the home environment. Generally costs are substantially less for ventilator-dependent individuals living at home than for those living in institutions (Banaszak, Travens, and Frasier 1981; Feldman and Tuteur 1982; Sivak 1983; Canadian Paraplegic Association 1987). More recently, a comparison of management options and costs for long-term, ventilator-assisted persons showed that home care, versus living in an extended-care facility, reduced cost by two-thirds (Loma Linda University Medical Center 1989).

Personal Goals and Alternatives

In past decades persons with ventilator-dependent quadriplegia needing lifetime care often had few, if any, alternatives to institutional-based care; however, effective services developed by demonstration projects in the 1980s have enabled more people with quadriplegia to set personal goals and make choices. The evidence is growing that these persons will benefit from community-based care and can pursue independent living styles. Other promising signs include increasing political support for home-based, long-term care in general, and for financial reimbursement for home-based care including community support services.

The independent living concept for disabled individuals in the community emphasizes consumer control and involvement to increase self-determination and minimize unnecessary dependence on others. Chapter 30 presents the tenets of the independent living philosophy instrumental in helping spinal injured individuals readapt to the mainstream. Today even people with high spinal injuries who need ventilator support can lead meaningful lives in their communities. Independent living for them is now a reality (West 1988).

As ventilator-dependent quadriplegic persons return to live in their communities, the need for support systems in the community becomes greater. Community resources

---

*This section was contributed by Fina Canave Jimenez.

PERSONAL VIEWPOINT

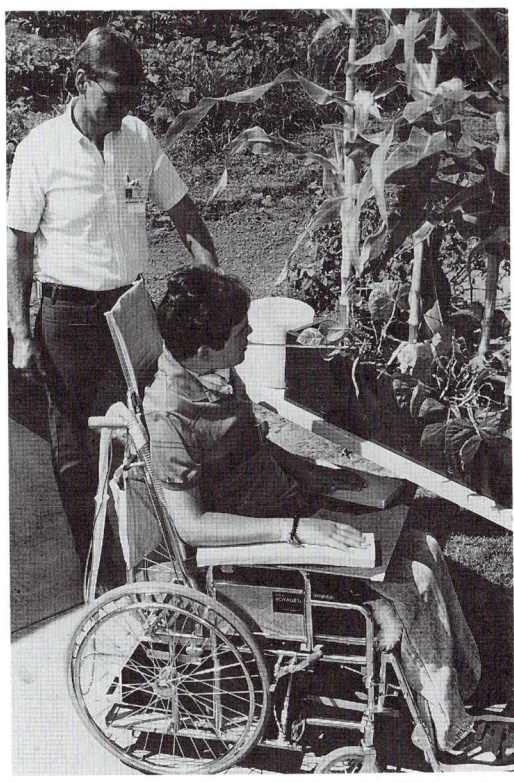

Larry Harned explains, "I drive under the planter so I can reach with my mouthstick to plant the seeds and then cover them with dirt. Then I use a straw for watering."

I am 23 years old and was injured by a gunshot wound to the neck which left me with a complete C_3 quadriplegia. During high school I liked fishing, hunting, swimming, and hiking in the mountains. I also enjoyed gardening. I pursued these interests in the Army while a mortar man supporting an armored batallion in Fort Hood, TX.

Now I love to work in the garden here on the VA grounds, planting seeds with my bird-beak mouthstick (others prepare the soil and the planter) and watering with a straw. The wonderful reward is seeing the corn, tomatoes, and beans grow from start to finish after all my hard work. Also I feel closer to God seeing the miracles of growth in the garden. We are fortunate to have an accessible greenhouse so I run all around the garden.

The American Horticultural Therapy Association makes possible this pleasant natural environment so that I can get out of the concrete environment. The incentive, motivation and productivity that culminates in tangible results go beyond therapeutic benefits. Many people enjoy and learn as they cooperate with each other in the design, care, and nurturing of the project.

Health is God's gift, and, after near-death experiences wracked with the complications and subsequent infections secondary to spinal cord injury, I encourage all people with SCI to enjoy the times when they are not sick.

The little outings, special dinners, barbeques, an Abilities Expo where potential equipment to help disabled people was shown, Wheelchair Olympic Games (where I won a silver medal in ramp bowling) are valuable activities that make it pretty nice to live here.

Restrictions that prevent me from using my computer at my bedside, or even on the ward are frustrating. I must use the computer in a class or during O.T. I love writing to my family and friends, even though we are so far apart, and could finish letters much sooner, if allowed.

For recently injured people, I and others cannot stress enough that learning the care requirements is a key to freedom for spending time enjoyably. Try to be as independent as possible because it makes you feel proud again. Stay busy. I like to read, often the Bible, and I enjoy magazines (turning the pages with my mouthstick) and music, too. Don't give up on your dreams and don't forget to say your prayers—maybe even try a little gardening!

Larry Harned
VA Center
Long Beach, CA

such as health, social service, and educational and vocational agencies and their personnel must enable them to attain and maintain quality of life. For example, for individuals who live with their families, daily stresses that affect the whole family structure and family dynamics must be addressed. Reliable *respite* care services for the family must be available to give family care givers some relief for a short period of time.

Initiatives from the public and private sectors, as well as disabled persons themselves, have recently led to development of cooperative housing arrangements, another viable alternative to institutional care (British Columbia Rehabilitation Society 1990). Implementation of the concept can vary, although it is primarily a communal living arrangement, whereby independent living units, attendant care, and other support services are shared.

CREEKVIEW 202: AN IMPOSSIBLE DREAM COME TRUE

Creekview 202, which gets its name simply from the number on the door, is home for seven individuals with high quadriplegia, six of whom require ventilators. In 1983, the Creekview Housing Cooperative, funded by Canada Mortgage and Housing Corporation and identified by Inner City Housing (a nonprofit agency), developed a 100-unit apartment complex. When approached by the 7 young men and the British Columbia Paraplegic Association (BCPA), supported by the British Columbia Rehabilitation Society, Creekview Housing welcomed this group of disabled persons and allocated 4,700 square feet (equivalent to nine single apartments) for their requirements. Located in the popular False Creek area of Vancouver, desirable for its favored ambiance and amenities, Creekview 202 is both beautiful and functional. The condominium incorporates individual bed-sitting rooms and wrap-around balconies with views of the bustling Granville market below as well as the North Shore Mountains. The spacious living room, dining room, kitchen, and computer and art center are shared, and a private room for live-in attendants is also provided—a sharp contrast to the ward in a long-term care facility (Pearson Centre, a member facility of the British Columbia Rehabilitation Society) where these disabled individuals lived for up to 13 years.

Independent living, enabling the integration of persons with severe disabilities into the mainstream of life, is the essence of this project. The demonstration project is a community-living alternative to institutional living that is cost effective—less than half the cost of institutionalized care, approximately $100.00 per day per person cheaper as reported by independent health care consultants (British Columbia Rehabilitation Society 1990)—not to mention the quality of life issues for those who enjoy living there despite the severe outcomes of physical disability. Also, this same report documented that health status and quality of care have been maintained or improved.

Creekview 202 is a major step forward in alternative housing not only because it was a first in North America but also because for 5 years, all levels of government, as well as community and professional organizations, contributed to its development. From the momentum gained by the innovative administration and staff at Pearson Centre, to the $12,000 stretcher-bathtub donated by the patrons of the Princeton Pub in East Vancouver, to the responsive Ministry of Health, every aspect of this project fell into place, putting British Columbia at the forefront of social change, philosophically and practically ahead of other provinces and countries.

Recognizing the importance of a coordinated approach, the BCPA, Pearson Centre, representatives of Government and the tenants formed a planning committee to address architectural design, finances, support services, policy and procedure manuals, medical equipment needs, staff training, health and medical care, co-op member education, group dynamics, promotional packages, furnishings, technical aids, and emergency systems. The six residents acted as co-chairpersons on each of 13 committees.

The Legal Services Branch of the Ministry of the Attorney General established that Creekview 202 did not come under the Community Care Facility Licensing Act; therefore the operation of the apartment is the responsibility of the disabled tenants.

Creekview 202 is a model for the next undertaking, Noble House, which will be several self-contained apartments grouped together for the purposes of linking 24-hour attendant and other care needs. This venture will be a model for other disabled persons and seniors who may have similar needs.

This project began because of the dedication of peer counselors for several persons with high quadriplegia who remained in an institution after formal rehabilitation. As expressed by Norman Haw, Director of Rehabilitation Services for the BCPA, "It was really hard for me, as a rehabilitation counselor, to deal with a ventilator-dependent client whose only option was to live in an institution. But when several clients repeatedly expressed a sincere desire to move back into the community, the BCPA called a planning meeting to flush out ideas that would eventually become the philosophy and building blocks of the project."

Funding was of course the first major issue but beyond that, Norman Haw, who himself has quadriplegia, explains that attitudes of health professionals and the lay community alike were the most difficult barriers to overcome (British Columbia Rehabilitation Society 1990). However, by deliberately attacking all potential problems and preparing for the worst possible consequences, they discovered that continually break-

(Box continues)

CREEKVIEW 202   (continued)

ing issues down into manageable portions was the best method to provide solutions and avoid panic.

The education of the tenants in everyday aspects of care and community life became central to the viability and stability of the project. The services of a rehabilitation counselor, psychologist, and social worker, who were chosen on the basis of their personal communication skills, facilitated this process. However, the tenants learned much more about communicating with people and about conflict resolution by working through the committees. Bringing out other people's ideas, not always in agreement with one's own, and learning about listening and compromise were the best preparation. When the project was operating, everyday situations such as, "I want chicken for dinner but someone else wants spaghetti," became real challenges that demanded a positive, family-style, decision-making process which minimized professional intervention. Resolving small issues before they became large and unmanageable was emphasized.

With increasing recognition of the importance of community resources and the subsequent development of such support services, the quality of life for people saved from catastrophic injury is gradually enhanced. Of paramount importance is the collective expertise needed to develop comprehensive services, without duplications and gaps. But coordination among hospitals, community-based resources, payers, government agencies, and the disabled community is plagued by various difficulties and is rarely a reality. As technology and advances in health care continue to save people with greater and greater degrees of disability, there has never been a greater need to overcome the universal barriers imposed by personalities, perceived professional territories, and other private kingdoms to benefit disabled survivors, families, and communities at large.

Norman Haw, Director, Rehabilitation Services, BCPA
W. Fraser, President, B.C. Rehabilitation Society,
Vancouver, BC.

When home-based or independent-living settings are not available for ventilator-dependent quadriplegic persons, alternatives, such as extended care hospitals, skilled nursing facilities, or nursing homes must be explored. High technology service traditionally provided only in the acute care hospital setting, such as ventilator care, are now available in these facilities.

Institutionalized settings are still major providers of lifetime care for ventilator-dependent persons in communities that lack resources and technologies for continuing care. However, one of the most encouraging results of the National Regional SCI Systems Project was the low number (3.1%) of spinal cord injured people that were placed in nursing homes (Stover and Fine 1986: 47). Forty years ago, few people succeeded in getting out of a hospital. The experiences of the past decade reveal that only a small percentage, about 5% to 6%, require custodial care in nursing homes, and only a few of those were full-time residents.

Long-term institutional care of the ventilator-dependent quadriplegic person is neither cost effective nor appropriate in human terms. During the 1980s, changing approaches and conditions in these settings have helped improve services and care. For instance, care is now more likely provided in a homelike milieu. However, institutional settings must always remain an option to avoid crisis when home care is no longer feasible or the best option for the individual, family, community, and funding agencies. Care at home

RISK

To laugh is to risk appearing the fool.
To weep is to risk being called sentimental.
To reach out to another is to risk involvement.
To expose feelings is to risk showing your true self.
To place your ideas and dreams before the crowd
    is to risk being called naive.
To love is to risk not being loved in return.
To live is to risk dying.
To hope is to risk disappointment.
To try is to risk failure.
But risks must be taken,
    because the greatest risk in life is to risk nothing.
The people who risk nothing do nothing,
    have nothing, are nothing, and become nothing;
They may avoid suffering and sorrow,
    but they simply cannot learn to feel,
    and change, and grow, and love, and live . . .
Chained by their servitude, they are slaves;
    they've forfeited their freedom.
Only the people who risk are truly free.

Author Unknown

is not the best alternative for every ventilator-dependent quadriplegic person.

Planning and Implementation

Independent living is concerned with the disabled person's quality of life and ability to make decisions about that life—even if it means taking *risks*—having control and choices as well as comfort and enjoyment. The conceptual model presented in Figure 29–1 provides a framework for planning and moving severely disabled individuals to integrated, independent, community living. The following process is adapted from the Creekview project (British Columbia Rehabilitation Society 1990), which has demonstrated a viable model for successful living alternatives for high quadriplegic persons and ventilator-dependent individuals.

1. *Ensuring client control.* Client control is *central* to planning for independent living. The client's needs are considered in the housing design, type of care required, development of client and attendant training, procurement of equipment, and planning for support and leisure services. The client assumes the role of *care manager* from the initial phases of planning to implementation.

2. *Working with health care professionals.* Discharge of a ventilator-dependent client requires an interdisciplinary team. Collaboration and effective communication involving the disabled person, the family, health care professionals, and community resources can smooth the transition to successful community living. The roles of all the professionals involved should be specified and integrated into the total plan.

3. *Providing client and family education.* The process of client and family education is discussed in Chapter 11. The educational program presents the knowledge and skills clients and care givers need in the home or other

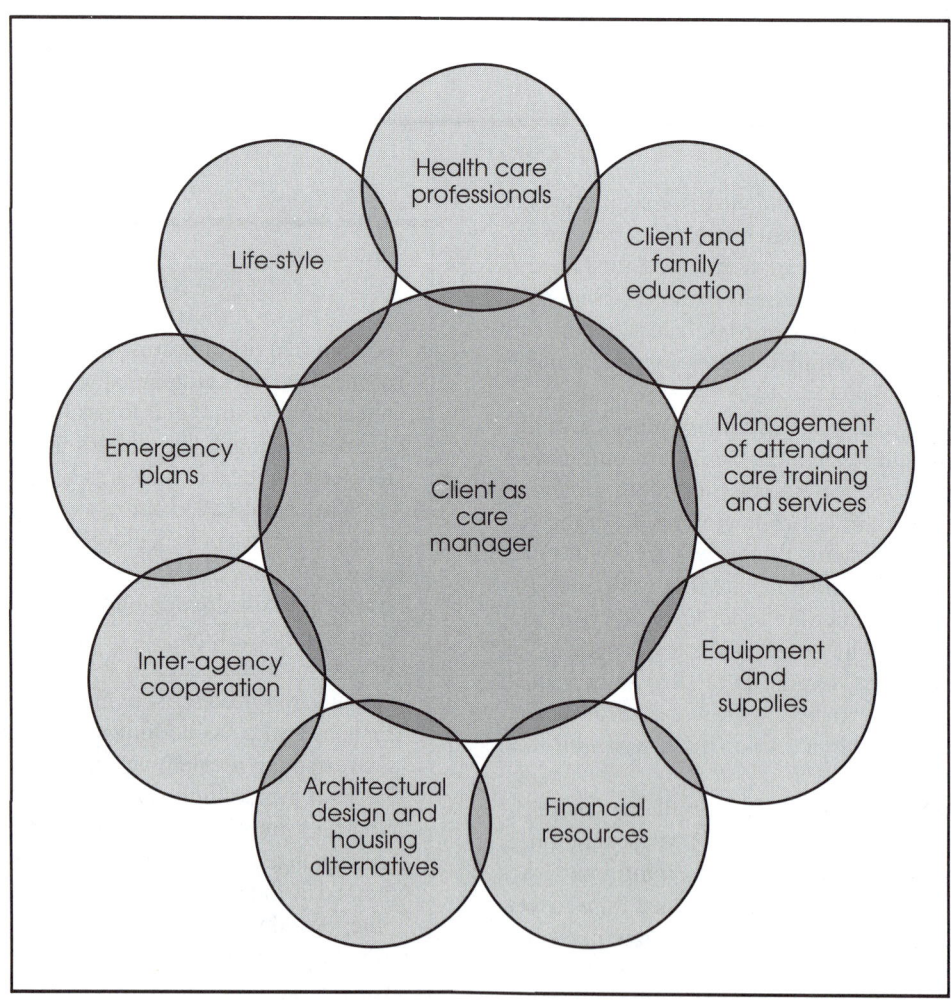

FIGURE 29–1 Conceptual framework for planning and implementation of community living for ventilator-dependent quadriplegic clients. (From Fraser, Haw, and Jimenez 1989. Adapted with permission.)

community settings. Table 29–1 gives an example of an attendant-training program. Clients are responsible for ongoing management.

In addition, client education should also include life skills training as needed in order to take control of their lives. Other training could be in supervisory skills, decision making, conflict resolution, budgeting, home management, and role training as co-op member and employer. Chapter 1 describes general issues that independent living specialists and rehabilitation professionals identify as necessary for community living.

4. *Planning and managing attendant care services.* Attendant care is a major expense for persons with high quadriplegia. Attendant care services are provided by families, friends, and hired attendants. Inadequate attendant care often makes home or community-based living more diffi-

TABLE 29–1 Sample Attendent-Training Program for Clients with Ventilator-Dependent Quadriplegia. Program designed in modular format; theory class and clinical experience supervised by client.

Program Schedule		Content
Block 1	Theory = 12 hours Clinical = 28 hours	Introduction and overview of psychosocial interactions and communication skills; personal hygiene, mobility, nutrition and elimination needs; clean and aseptic techniques.
Block 2	Theory = 6 hours Clinical = 34 hours	Client-related respiratory care (trach care, bronchial hygiene techniques, including suctioning); ventilators and breathing circuit.
Block 3	Theory = 6 hours Clinical = 34 hours	Equipment-related care (sterilization, disinfection); malfunctions (troubleshooting); power wheelchair management; care of environmental control systems; and other technical aids.
Block 4	Theory = 6 hours Clinical = 34 hours	Management of airway patency, respiratory emergencies, and other selected clinical problems such as infection and autonomic dysreflexia.

Total hours over 4-week period

Source: George Pearson Centre, *Attendant Training Manual: Care of the Ventilator-Dependent Quadriplegic Client.* Vancouver, BC: 1985, p. 20. Adapted with permission.

cult, if not impossible. Determination of required attendant hours and services is critical to the success of community-based care. Ultimately, how well the disabled person can manage personal care providers determines the quality of assistance received.

5. *Securing equipment and supplies.* The ventilator-dependent quadriplegic person needs help in itemizing, evaluating, and securing prescribed durable medical equipment and supplies. Today, high-technology home equipment, such as ventilators and circuiting, are better, safer, and more portable. Monitoring has become more dependable, less invasive, less hazardous, and permits a more humane type of care. Community agencies provide resource guides that outline how to identify local, regional, and national resources, criteria for evaluating home care equipment vendors, support services for equipment maintenance, and strategies for resolving problems. Examples of these guides are in the Resources at the end of the book.

6. *Accessing financial resources.* Funding comes from several sources and varies from state to state and province to province. Fundings may come from private insurance companies, federal and state or province programs, private foundations and organizations, and charitable contributions. Each of these sources can have different criteria for disbursement, eligibility, and service coverage.

Health care professionals, whether hospital or community based, are primary resource persons who help the ventilator-dependent quadriplegic person access cost-effective financial resources. Attorneys also may help overcome difficulties with payment sources.

7. *Exploring architectural design and housing alternatives.* Specific considerations on architectural design and housing for the ventilator-dependent quadriplegic person include home and environmental assessment. Accessibility, maximal space and mobility, heating, environmental control and communication systems are examples that contribute to a physical environment in which the person can function as independently as possible.

8. *Linking with community services and interagency collaboration.* Access to the full range of community health, social support, educational, and recreational services must be available to serve the long-term needs of the ventilator-dependent quadriplegic person. The quality of services provided is contingent on the existing resources and relationships among the various agencies. Three important factors influence interagency relationships: hospital discharge planning, coordination of care, and communication among health care professionals. These are facilitated through regular interagency meetings, community-hospital councils, and joint ventures such as collaboration on training, client evaluation, family conferences, and project development. However, involved independent living specialists are vital to successful outcomes.

9. *Outlining emergency plans.* A plan must outline backup emergency and contingency details. Community-

based support services must be arranged with the fire and police departments, utility companies, emergency transport, and hospital emergency departments to establish protocols. A list of required emergency and backup equipment must be in place before discharge including all emergency phone numbers.

10. *Looking at life-styles.* Boredom, social isolation, and decreased opportunities in employment, recreational and leisure activities are also major life-style disadvantages facing the ventilator-dependent person. To facilitate planning, assist the person to assess how time is spent in a typical day, and degree of satisfaction with current life-style activity level and diversity. Interest inventories can be helpful. How to compensate and attain new skills can be taught as part of the person's life plan. Access to peer consultants and referral to recreational therapists are recommended. See Resources for further information.

In addition to educational and vocational training, ventilator-dependent persons need access to community-based programs that help promote healthy life-styles; the latter may include weight reduction, smoking cessation, and stress reduction programs. Involvement in these activities among high quadriplegic persons is likely to have a positive influence on reducing age-related problems and premature death.

Evaluation

Criteria for evaluating the effectiveness of health care planning and management for life must be based on the individual assessed personal goals and life-styles of each ventilator-dependent quadriplegic person. The concept most applicable for establishing broad evaluation guidelines is best described by McLane (1987) and McConnell (1988). A life plan requires a safe, growth-promoting immediate environment in which physiological and psychological needs can be met. This environment has two parts: the physical environment and the social, or interpersonal, environment.

The following questions should be included in an evaluation:

1. Is the ventilator-dependent quadriplegic person living in the environment of choice according to preferred life-style? If not, have all the acceptable alternatives been explored? Is the living arrangement appropriate and realistic? The primary objective is to help individuals pursue personal goals and choices.
2. Is the ventilator-dependent quadriplegic person safe in the present living arrangement? Lifetime care and management require knowledge of risk factors and systems to address them.
3. Does the ventilator-dependent quadriplegic person accept responsibility for the ongoing maintenance and management of the plan? Is the life plan consistent with the person's wishes and expectations?

Mobilizing the huge array of resources necessary to promote a satisfying life-style requires comprehensive care and planning by a team of rehabilitation professionals with specific expertise in high quadriplegia. Equally important are people involved in community-based services, who must also be expert and resourceful in providing safe, ongoing, and reliable assistance. Although it is certainly possible to develop such an approach, achievement in practice is still severely limited. Books such as *The Management of High Quadriplegia* (Whiteneck et al. 1989) help health care professionals and others develop more specialized services and encourage an active, meaningful life. An interdisciplinary focus on care from the moment of injury through acute and rehabilitative care, preparing for discharge, and life in the real world is explored. The complexities surrounding the person with high quadriplegia are emphasized not only by the health care team but by input from consumers, researchers, case managers, third party payers, attorneys, and ethicists.

REFERENCES

Ackerman, T. 1982. Why doctors should intervene. *The Hastings Report* (Aug.).

Appelbaum, P., and Grisso, T. 1988. Assessing patient's capacities to consent to treatment. *New England Journal of Medicine* 319 (95).

Appelbaum, P., and Roth, L. 1982. Clinical issues in the assessment of competency. *American Journal of Psychiatry* 138: 1462–1467.

Banaszak, E. F., Travens, F., and Frasier, H. 1981. Home ventilator care. *Respiratory Care* 26 (12): 1262–1268.

British Columbia Rehabilitation Society and British Columbia Paraplegic Association. 1990. *Keys to Freedom*. Vancouver, BC: authors. Describes development of Creekview 202 so that this independent living project can be replicated. Videotape. *Life of Independence*, also available.

Burnham, L., and Werner, G. 1979. The high level tetraplegic: Psychosocial survival and adjustment. *International Journal of Paraplegia* 16: 184–192.

Canadian Paraplegic Association, BC Division. 1987 (May). Creekview 202 Project Evaluation Report, p. 21.

Caplan, A. 1988. Informed consent and provider-patient relationships in rehabilitation medicine. *Archives of Physical Medicine and Rehabilitation* 69 (May).

Caplan, A., Callahan, D., and Haas, J. 1987 (Aug.). Ethical and policy issues in rehabilitation medicine. A *Hastings Center Report Special Supplement*.

Dine, D. 1988. Ethics. *Modern Health Care* 14 (Oct.).

Drane, J. 1985 (Apr.). The many faces of competency. *The Hastings Center Report.*

Feldman, J. and Tuteur, P. G. 1982. Mechanical ventilation from hospital intensive care to home. *Heart and Lung* 11 (2): 162–165.

Fraser, W., Haw, N., and Jimenez, F. C. 1989. Community living—Alternatives for ventilator-dependent quadriplegics. *Canadian Congress of Rehabilitation Proceedings,* Toronto.

Garrison, I. 1978. Stress management training for the handicapped. *Archives of Physical Medicine and Rehabilitation* 59: 580–585.

Green, B., Pratt, C., and Grigsby, T. 1984. Self-concept among persons with long-term SCI. *Archives of Physical Medicine and Rehabilitation* 65: 751–754.

Goffman, E. 1961. *Asylums* New York: Anchor Books.

Haddad, A. 1986. Ethical issues in long-term home care for ventilator-dependent clients. *Pride Institute Journal* 5 (2).

Loma Linda University Medical Center. 1989. *Management Options and Cost Comparisons for the Long-Term Ventilator-Assisted Patient,* Loma Linda, CA: author.

McConnell, E. S., and Matteson, M. A. 1986. *Gerentological Nursing: Concepts and Practice.* Philadelphia: W. B. Saunders.

McLane, A. 1987. *Classification of Nursing Diagnosis: Proceedings of the Seventh Conference.* St. Louis: C. V. Mosby.

Mechanic, D. 1961. The concept of illness behavior. *Journal of Chronic Disability* 15: 189–194.

Menter, R., and Maddox, S. 1989. Ethics. In *The Management of High Quadriplegia.* Ed. G. Whiteneck. New York: Demos Publications.

Maynard, F., and Muth, A. 1987. The choice to end life as a ventilator-dependent quadriplegic. *Archives of Physical Medicine and Rehabilitation* 68 (Dec.).

National Rehabilitation Research Center. 1990. *Proceedings: National Invitational Conference on Developing a Comprehensive Health Ser-vices Research Capacity in Physical Disability and Rehabilitation,* Sept. 26–27.

George Pearson Centre. 1985. *Attendant Training Manual: Care of the Ventilator-Dependent Quadriplegic Client.* Vancouver, BC: Author.

The President's Commission for the Study of Ethical Problems in Medicine and Biomedical and Behavioral Research. 1982. *Making Health Care Decisions.* Vol. 1. Washington, DC: U. S. Government Printing Office.

Purtilo, R. 1986. Ethical issues in the treatment of chronic ventilator-dependent patients. *Archives of Physical Medicine and Rehabilitation* 67 (Oct.).

—. 1988. Ethical issues in teamwork: The context of rehabilitation. *Archives of Physical Medicine and Rehabilitation* 69 (May).

Rogers, M. 1989. More than wheelchairs. *Newsweek* (Apr. 24): 66–67.

Shalock, R. S., Keith, K. D., and Hoffman, K. 1990. *Quality of Life Questionnaire: Overview and Standardization Information Manual.* Mid-Nebraska Mental Retardation Services, Inc. P.O. Box 1146, Hastings, NE 68901.

Sivak, E. D. 1983. Pulmonary mechanical ventilation at home: A reasonable and less expensive alternative. *Respiratory Care* 28 (1): 42–49.

Stover, S., and Fine, P. 1986. *Spinal Cord Injury: The Facts and Figures.* Birmingham, AL: National Spinal Cord Injury Research Data Center, University of Alabama.

Veatch, R. 1988 (Aug./Sept.). Justice and the economics of terminal illness: A dilemma for hospitals and physicians. *The Hastings Center Report.*

West, S. 1988. The Independents. *Hippocrates* (Nov./Dec.): 80–86.

Whiteneck, G., et al. 1989. *Management of High Quadriplegia.* New York: Demo Publications. *The authors represent three outstanding centers for treating persons with high quadriplegia: Craig Hospital in Colorado, the Santa Clara Medical Center in California; and the Institution for Rehabilitation and Research in Texas.*

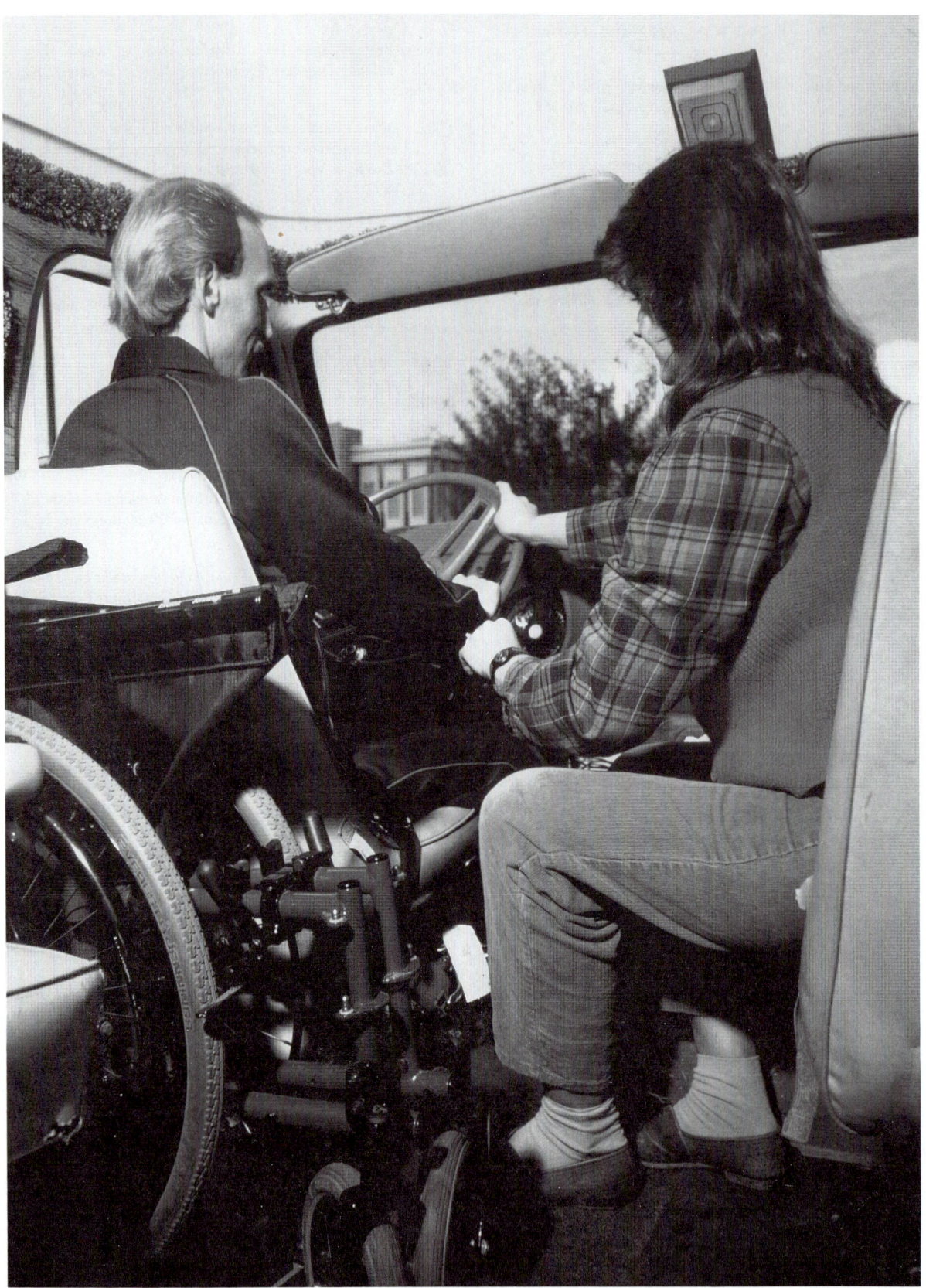

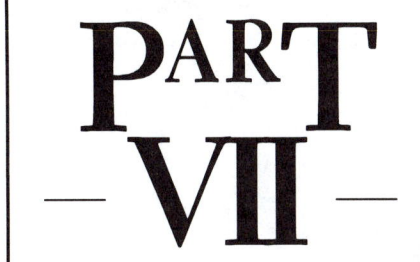

PART VII

TOWARD INDEPENDENCE

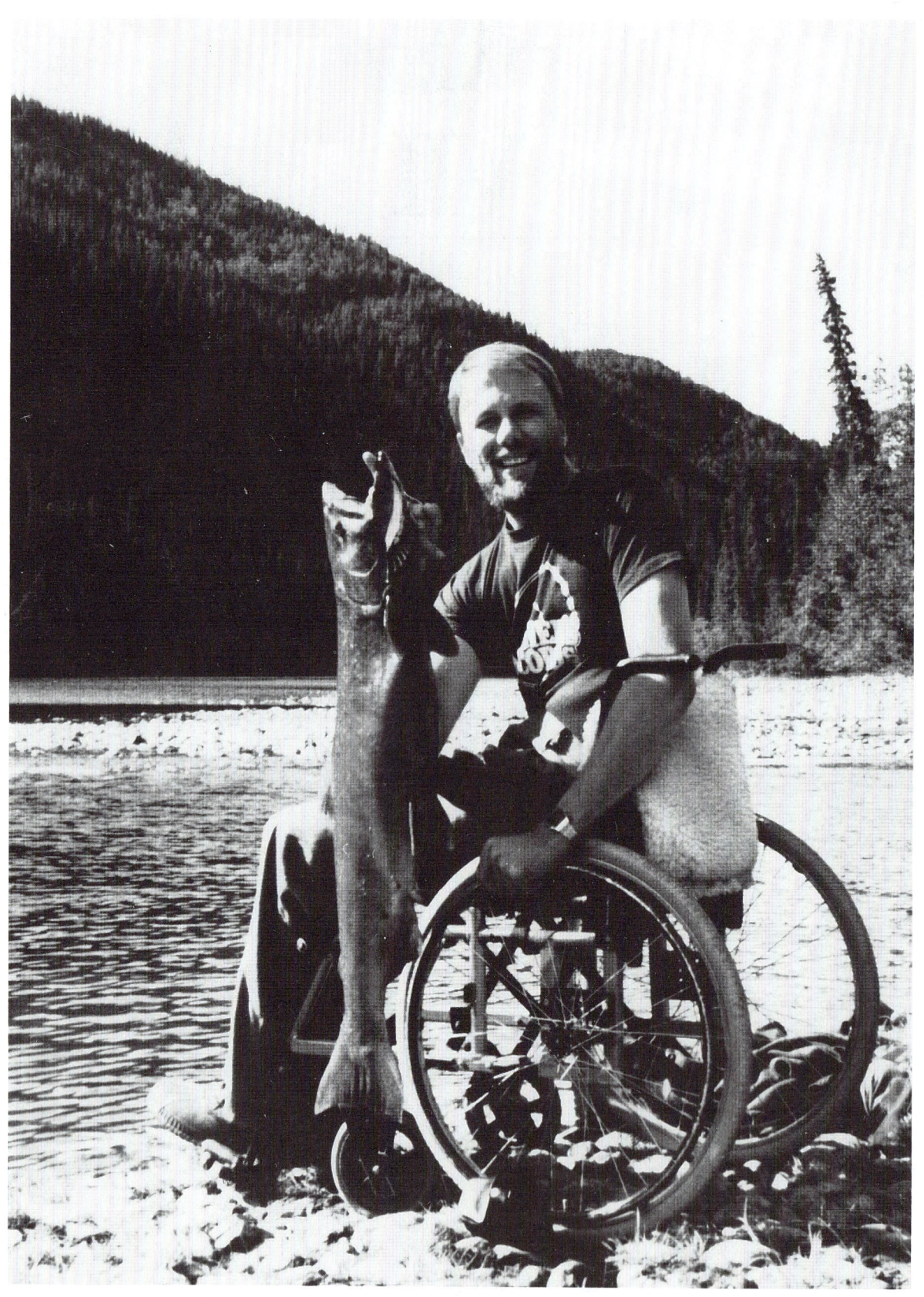

CHAPTER 30

Is There Life after Rehabilitation?

Lex Frieden, M.A.

Chapter Outline

Objectives

- To provide perspective on the positive outcomes of rehabilitation
- To present some ways, in addition to providing optimal professional care, in which the health care team can promote positive outcomes for people with SCI

LIFE GOALS

Whether they express it or not, people with spinal cord injuries (SCI) begin to wonder about the outcome of their predicament almost from the point of injury. Their expectations of the future and the goals they set for themselves are shaped by a wide range of variables. First impressions may be affected by the extent and nature of information they are given about their injury, the reactions of family members, and previous experiences with and attitudes toward persons with similar injuries.

In most cases, the first questions people deal with are those of survival: Yes, no, and, if yes, how? Patients continue to ask these questions, if only of themselves, long after they begin the rehabilitation process. The answers they give themselves may change many times during the course of rehabilitation, and their answers are largely determined by what they learn and how they are treated.

Early patient expectations of outcome may be unrealistic and extreme. They may range from the fear of forever being a "vegetable," confined to bed, and in need of 24-hour professional care, to a belief in complete recovery with no serious consequences. Patients develop more realistic expectations as individual circumstances become known and as the educational function of rehabilitation takes effect. Patients who are treated as adults, given responsibility, and taught to manage their own care are likely not only to be more realistic about their disabilities, but also to experience a significantly higher quality of life following rehabilitation.

The expectations, hopes, and goals of people with SCI often change following discharge from the hospital or rehabilitation center. These changes occur for at least several reasons. Individuals may experience some functional return, gain additional strength in residual muscle function, increase their stamina and tolerance, make personal and environmental adaptations, learn new ways of doing things, and acquire new adaptive equipment.

Some changes may lead to reestablishment of a positive self-image and expanded options for living. Other changes effected by life beyond the protective walls of the hospital may damage self-image, narrow expectations, and restrict options. Old friends may stop by once and never come again. Other friends and family members may pamper, patronize, and pity. The realities of economic and environmental barriers may be overwhelming. People with SCI may have physical setbacks and complications. Bowel and bladder accidents, pressure sores, and infections that persist may become overbearing.

All the changes that occur following discharge necessitate constant reassessment of individual options, expectations, and goals. For this reason, many centers have established follow-up programs to keep in touch with patients after discharge and to provide support during the crucial stages of adjustment and readaptation to community life. Although these programs are generally limited by insufficient funding, they constitute an important part of the overall rehabilitation process.

The question is often asked, "What are the long-term goals of individuals with spinal cord injuries?" More than likely, the answer is that their goals are generally the same as anyone else's. Most people want to have a family, a home, a job, a car, and social and recreational opportunities. The Australian approach, the Comcare System, described in Chapter 1, focuses on the importance of integrating injured workers back into the workplace.

Some professionals, friends, and family members have, in the past, discouraged people with SCI from adopting or seeking these goals. Many injured people have been led to believe that these were impossible, unrealistic goals and that they should be satisfied and happy just to be alive. In fact, the general public's expectations of life for people with SCI were weighed on a different scale of normality from their own. What was considered a normal life-style for the general population was not considered normal for people with SCI. As a result of these attitudes, many people with SCI restricted their goals and lowered their expectations. Sometimes hope for a better life was buried so deeply that it disappeared.

THE CONCEPT OF INDEPENDENT LIVING

During the late 1960s and early 1970s, a new concept of rehabilitation began to be expressed by people with SCI and other disabilities. This concept, called *independent living*, focuses on quality of life issues. It was at first a sort of reaction to repression. Some disabled people felt their lives were unnecessarily restricted by their disabilities. They acknowledged that barriers to independence were increased by disability, but they believed that these barriers could be overcome. They felt that supportive programs could be established and environmental accommodations could be made that would allow them to seek the same goals that were open to the general public. They rejected the assumptions that they should be confined to institutional care, that they had fewer rights than nondisabled people, and that the government's obligation to them was limited because of their disability.

These people began to assert themselves in public forums. They formed lobbying groups; they claimed equal rights as citizens to public services like transportation, housing, education, and employment; and they claimed the right to vote. Although most of these rights were not denied intentionally or directly, they were denied by virtue of the fact that public transportation, housing, schools, businesses, public offices, and polling places were generally inaccessible.

INDEPENDENT LIVING: A DEFINITION

Independent living involves control over one's life based on the choice of acceptable options that minimize reliance on others in making decisions and in performing everyday activities. This includes managing one's affairs, participating in day-to-day life in the community, fulfilling a range of social roles, and making decisions that lead to self-determination and the minimization of physical or psychological dependence on others.

Independence is a relative concept that each individual defines personally. Similarly, the concept of independent living is quite broad, subsuming many levels of functional independence.

Some severely disabled people view these varying levels of functioning as important distinctions of independence. For instance, certain activities not central to personal control of one's destiny or the day-to-day management of one's life are considered to be the essence of living independently. Some individuals perceive physical activities such as dressing oneself to be important examples of their ability to live independently. On the other hand, others view any extra time and energy spent dressing themselves as time and energy that could be spent more profitably at work. In fact, whether one performs these particular activities oneself or relies on the assistance of others has little to do with the amount of control one exercises over one's own life.

Independent living is not dependent on programs that foster functional independence. Instead it is based on the individual's ability to choose and achieve a desired life-style and to function freely in society.

It should be stressed that not every person will be capable of achieving total independence in the sense described here. Some persons may not be able to or may not choose to exercise self-determination in certain matters. In such cases, the person may opt for or be restricted to a kind of modified independent living, limited independent living, or semi-independent living.

The *independent living movement* is the process of translating into reality the theory that, given appropriate supportive services, accessible environments, and pertinent information and skills, severely disabled individuals may actively participate in all aspects of society.

From the concept of independence, a movement emerged to address barriers to a higher quality of life for disabled people. This movement included disabled people, family members, friends, neighbors, and people throughout society, as well as health care professionals, politicians, and policy makers. The movement led to:

- New laws asserting the equality of disabled people and protecting their rights
- New or adapted accommodations making housing, transportation, public places, schools, and job sites accessible to people with disabilities
- More positive attitudes by the general public toward people with disabilities and by disabled people toward themselves
- Perhaps most important, new opportunities for severely disabled people, including those with SCI, to seek independence, to enjoy the benefits of their labors, and to enjoy the quality of life that society offers

As a result of the independent living movement and changes that have occurred during the past few years, people with SCI may now realistically seek goals that once were limited to people without disabilities. In fact, limits imposed by SCI may be less important in determining successful achievement of goals than certain other demographic and socioeconomic variables that are not related to disability. Many patients now go directly from the rehabilitation center to independent living arrangements in the community; others do so after a temporary stay with their families; and still others do so after participating in extended vocational rehabilitation or transitional living programs.

BARRIERS TO INDEPENDENCE

There are three principal barriers to achieving goals of independence for people with SCI:

1. *Environmental barriers* that are beyond the immediate control of the individual. They are exemplified by curbs, steps, and narrow doorways.

2. *Personal barriers* that are directly related to and controlled by the individual. Personal barriers are negative attitudes, low self-esteem, poor self-image, feelings of dependence, unreasonable insecurity, unwillingness to take risks, preoccupation with cure, lack of ability to organize and plan, and unnecessarily limited expectations and goals.

3. *Economic barriers* that are related to inability to purchase needed equipment, supplies, and services. Economic barriers may restrict the possible solutions to both environmental and personal barriers.

Ways to Overcome Barriers

There are now more ways to overcome the barriers to independence than ever before. To overcome environmental barriers, one may purchase or make adaptive equipment and devices. For example, people with high quadriplegia may purchase electrically powered wheelchairs controlled by slight movements of the chin or by sipping and puffing into a straw. Also available are sophisticated remote control devices and primitive robots. In addition to customized, individual solutions, there are solutions of a broader, more systematic scale. These include mass transportation vehicles made accessible by widening doorways, expanding seating areas, and installing ramps or lifts, and communitywide efforts to install ramps on curbs and to provide access to both public and private buildings. These innovations are now wide-

spread, and continued advocacy efforts are leading to more solutions of this nature each day.

There are also several possible solutions to personal barriers. Rehabilitation counselors, psychologists, social workers, and other professionals can help a person analyze and overcome personal barriers. Peer counselors may share information, serve as role models, and provide necessary support. Family members and friends can give encouragement and help. Finally, self-determination, self-encouragement, self-control, and simply the passage of time may help the disabled person overcome personal barriers. On a broader scale, constructive attitudes and expectations of the general public and positive portrayals of disabled people by the media may also help overcome personal barriers.

Economic barriers may be the most difficult to overcome and the most important because they can affect solutions to the other two types of barriers. Most people depend on private and public insurance, private and public aid, or their own ability to earn money in order to overcome economic barriers. For people with SCI, however, independence costs more than it does for nondisabled people. This is because in addition to the normal expenses of housing, transportation, food, clothing, and routine medical care, people with

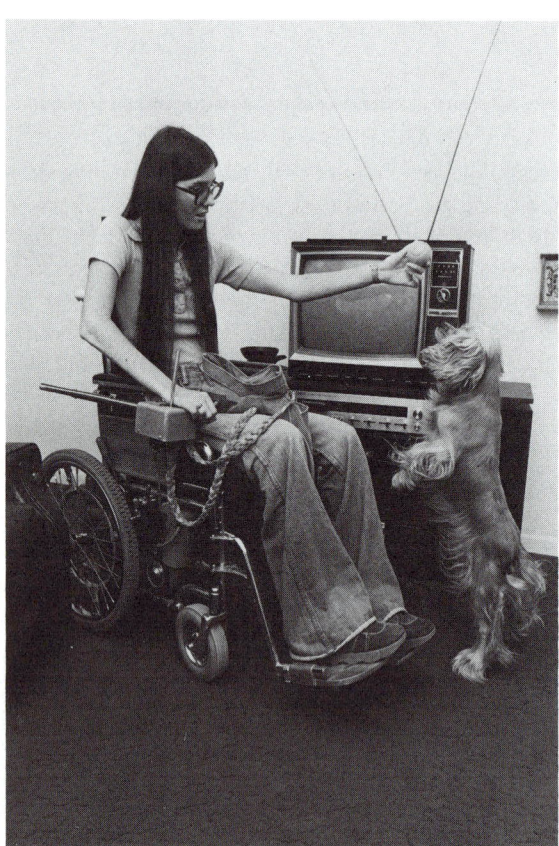
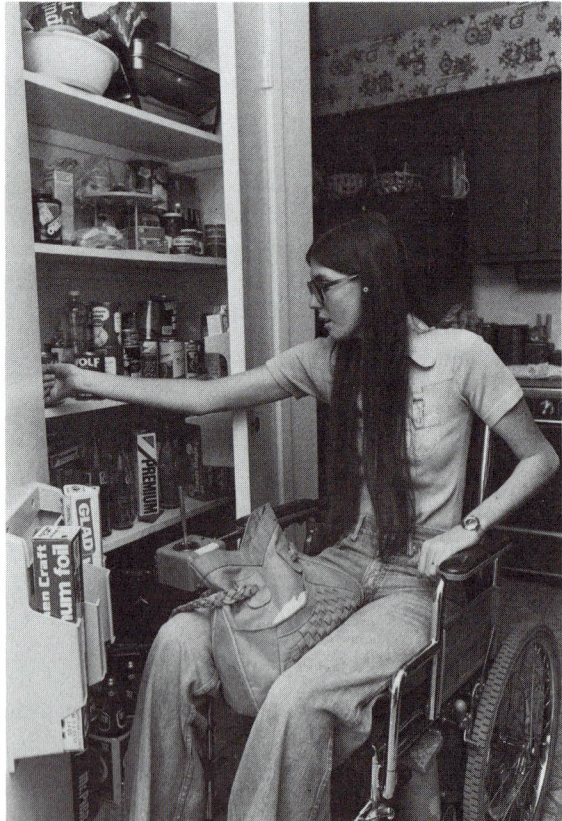

FIGURE 30–1 Adapting: Terry Ensign participated in a transitional living program, which provides a homelike environment in which to apply rehabilitative skills. Terry is now married and has her own home and two children.

SCI often have expenses for adaptive equipment, medical supplies, and personal assistance services (attendant care). The economic barriers to their independence are also frequently complicated by the fact that to be independent, one needs a job, but to have a job, one needs to be reasonably independent.

Individual solutions to economic barriers are typified by a person who receives housing subsidies to help pay for housing, vocational rehabilitation agency grants or subsidies to help pay for educational or work-related expenses, welfare or human service agency subsidies to help pay for personal assistance expenses, and work income or Social Security disability insurance payments to cover other expenses. More general solutions to overcoming economic barriers may be legislated in the form of a nationalized health insurance program, a nationwide personal assistance service or home health care program, or establishment of a nationwide system for purchase and distribution of equipment and devices for disabled people.

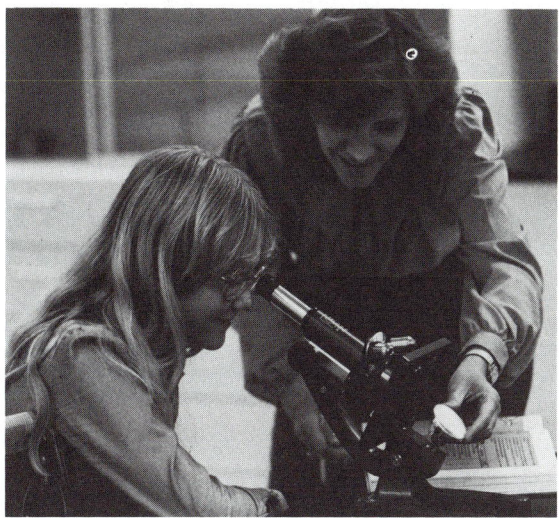

FIGURE 30–2   Learning: Stacy Norman, a wheelchair user, resumes her high school education.

Independent Living Programs

The independent living movement called for a new method of service delivery in which needed services would be provided in a way that would encourage people with disabilities to make their own decisions and to be responsible for their own lives. Thus, independent living centers came into existence. These centers are unique, with very specific characteristics including:

- *Consumer control.* A center's board of directors and staff positions are at least 51% people with disabilities
- *Core services.* A center's array of services must include peer counseling, independent living skills training, advocacy, and information and referral about housing, personal assistance services, and goods and services available from other agencies; other services a center may provide are transportation, equipment repair, and recreational events
- *Cross-disability services.* A center offers services to persons with different types of disabilities rather than focusing on services to a specific disability group

Today there are more than 170 independent living centers, with at least one in each state and U.S. territory. There are also approximately 200 additional programs that have an independent living focus. Although not comprehensive, consumer-controlled, independent living centers, these programs provide services that assist people with disabilities to live independently. See the Resources at the end of this text for additional information.

A particular type of independent living program, the *transitional living program*, has proven to be exceptionally effective in helping people with SCI acquire the knowledge and skills they need in order to establish an independent life-style following rehabilitation. Transitional programs include support services to provide opportunities for practi-

cal application of newly acquired skills in such areas as personal and attendant care, health care, homemaking, financial management, getting around in the community, seeking accommodations and employment, time management, interpersonal development, and so on. Most important, these programs encourage individuals to make their own decisions and be responsible for their own lives.

Community Support Services

There are many community agencies, organizations, and groups working to help overcome the barriers to independence posed by disability. A system of vocational rehabilitation agencies exists throughout the United States. These agencies, funded principally by the federal government, provide educational and vocational counseling and other services to assist disabled people in finding, getting, and keeping employment. They pay for some medical treatment, education and training, equipment, supplies, transportation, attendant care, and other services for eligible clients. Located in every state, these agencies have counselors working in most rehabilitation centers and most large communities.

In addition to the networks of vocational rehabilitation and independent living centers, many other public and private service organizations throughout the United States provide vital primary care and support services to aid disabled people in their communities. These organizations include medical and vocational rehabilitation centers, voluntary organizations such as Goodwill and Easter Seal societies, and home health care agencies like the Visiting Nurses Association. Parallel development of similar organizations exist in Canada and most other Western countries.

Perhaps more important to those who are well adjusted to living in the community are advocacy organizations and social and recreational groups.

TABLE 30–1 Independent Living Programs: Four Primary Variations

Conceptually, *an independent living program* is generic—the most broadly defined term relating to organizations working with disabled individuals who wish to live independently. Several different kinds of programs providing services that foster independent living have been identified: independent living center, independent living residential program, and independent living transitional program.

The kinds of features an independent living program has depends on the needs of the clients served, the availability of existing community resources, the physical and social makeup of the community, and the goals of the program itself.

Independent Living Program	Independent Living Center	Independent Living Residential Program	Independent Living Transitional Program
Community based	Community based	Community based	Community based
Consumer involved	Consumer controlled	Consumer involved	Consumer involved
	Nonresidential		Goal oriented
	Nonprofit		Time linked
Provides/coordinates:	Provides/coordinates:	Provides/coordinates:	Provides/coordinates:
Housing	Housing	Housing	Skills training in independent living
Attendant Care	Attendant care	Shared attendent services	Other services
Information	Peer counseling	Transportation	
Other services	Financial/legal advocacy	Other services	
	Community awareness and barrier removal programs		
	Other services		

Reprinted from Lex Frieden, Laurel Richards, Jean Cole, and David Bailey, "A glossary for independent living." *ILRU Sourcebook: A Technical Assistance Manual on Independent Living.* Houston: The Institute for Rehabilitation and Research (TIRR), 1979.

Advocacy Organizations

Advocacy organizations assist people with disabilities in two principal ways:

1. They may function as case advocates, representing and advising an individual on matters related to specific benefits, programs, or civil rights.
2. They may function as class or systems advocates, representing the needs and interests of all people with SCI or other disabilities or any other specifically defined group.

Advocacy organizations play an important role in our sociopolitical system by representing people who either cannot or choose not to represent themselves.

In the United States, the national advocacy organizations that seem to be most effective in representing disabled people are those with memberships made up mostly of disabled people. These include the National Council on Independent Living, the Paralyzed Veterans of America, and the National Spinal Cord Injury Association. The latter two focus on issues affecting people with SCI. In addition to their advocacy work, these organizations provide other services such as counseling, information, and referral. Be-

sides their national offices, each of these groups has chapters organized at state and local levels.

In addition to these consumer-oriented groups, several organizations of professionals in the field of rehabilitation are active advocates. These groups include the American Congress of Rehabilitation Medicine, Association of Rehabilitation Nurses, American Rehabilitation Counseling Association, National Rehabilitation Counselor Association, and the American Spinal Injury Association. Each of these organizations has been effective in lobbying for progressive legislation to benefit disabled people and in speaking out for improvements in the health care, social service, and rehabilitation systems at many levels. In particular, the American Spinal Injury Association has begun to provide an important forum for the exchange of information and ideas related to the care and treatment of people with SCI.

Social and Recreational Groups

Besides advocacy organizations, social and recreational groups may provide valuable peer support and opportunities for meaningful involvement with other disabled and non-

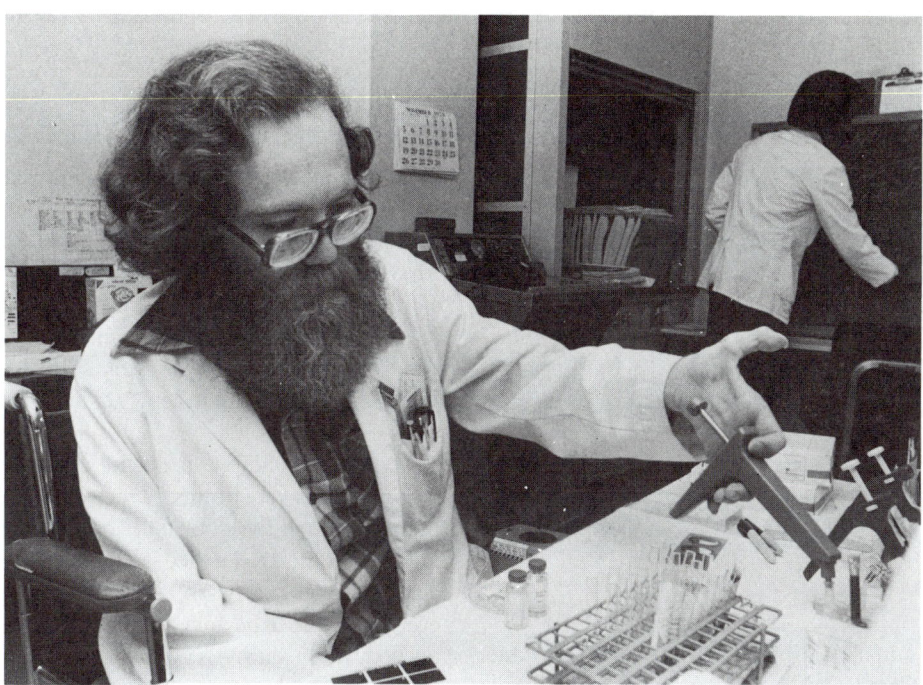

FIGURE 30–3   Working: Bob Henry works as a laboratory technician.

disabled people. These groups are usually locally organized according to the interests of people in their own communities. They may focus on such diverse activities as handicrafts, square dancing, sailing, hunting, basketball, and tennis. In the last few years, national organizations, such as Wilderness Inquiry II and Vinland National Center, which provide opportunities for such rigorous outdoor recreational activities as canoeing, backpacking, camping, and skiing, have experienced a great increase in demand for their programs. See Chapter 24. Also national sports organizations have become popular. The National Wheelchair Basketball Association, National Wheelchair Tennis Association, and the National Wheelchair Pilots Association among others organize local, regional, and national competitions and exhibitions to match skills and promote positive attitudes toward their associations and the people they represent. Wheelchair events for people with disabilities have been featured in the 1984 and 1988 Olympic Games.

Besides finding needed support and camaraderie among organizations of and for disabled people, people with SCI often discover that they are accepted into community groups such as civic clubs, garden clubs, and neighborhood circles. Many disabled people feel that their participation in such organizations fosters better understanding and attitudes of the general public toward people with disabilities. They believe that these groups may be just as supportive and, perhaps, more effective in breaking down barriers to independence than those made up mostly of people with disabilities.

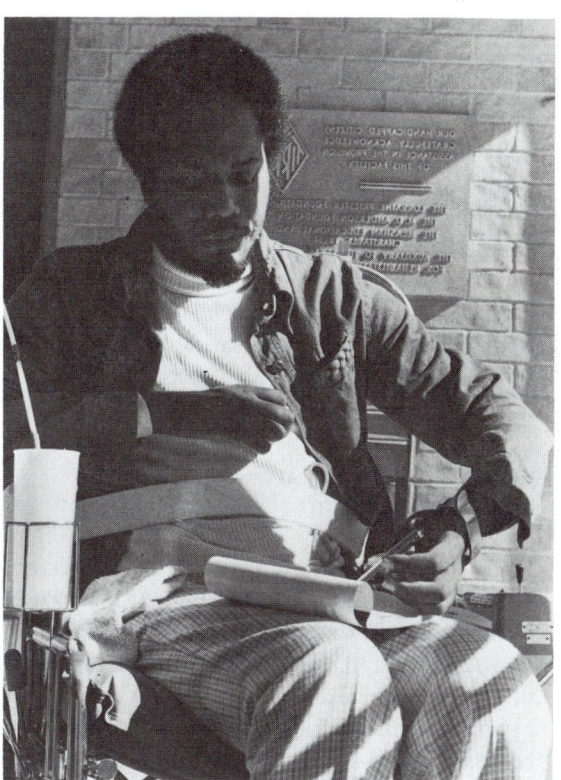

FIGURE 30–4   Helping: Charles Harrison participates in community activities.

PERSONAL VIEWPOINT

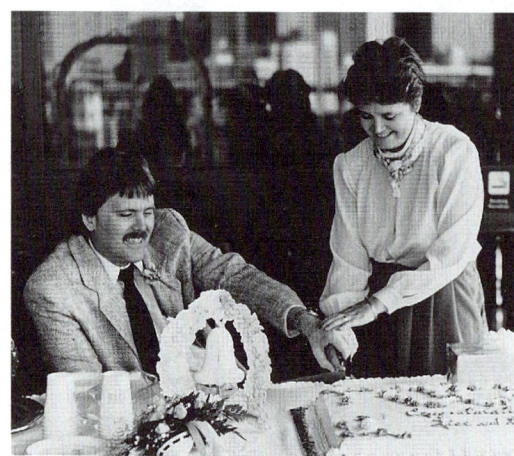

I live in Tampa, Florida with my wife, Lise Jane McMullen Casady, and our dog, Sara Jane. Our home is modified slightly for wheelchair accessibility by having level entranceways and widened bathroom doors. One of the nicest features of our home is a screened patio where we do a lot of our entertaining. The patio has a built-in jacuzzi constructed so I can transfer myself in and out unassisted, which has given me a renewed sense of independence.

I fit the typical profile of a spinal cord injured person. I had no idea at the time that I was at so great a risk. I had my crash on July 14, 1976, after a hard day of work in a summer job. A buddy and I went out looking for fun. I purchased a twelve-pack of beer with an altered driver's license and both of us popped open a can while we drove around. One beer followed another, and after a quick swim at a swimming hole, I could feel the buzz from that beer. Instead of playing it safe and letting someone else drive my car, I insisted on being the driver. My friend tried to convince me to let him drive, but I refused and jumped into my 1972 Camaro for the quick trip into town.

My car was going about 75 to 80 miles an hour when we approached a sharp left curve in the highway. My friend yelled something but it was too late: I lost control of the car. Whenever I hear that phrase, "lost control of the car," it always reminds me of my crash. That six-pack of beer that I had put away earlier had subtly impaired my reflexes and alertness. I fractured my cervical vertebrae at the C_{5-6} level causing a spinal cord contusion. This injury left me with incomplete quadriplegia with some sensory function intact. Over time, some motor function has returned to about the C_{6-7} level, which has allowed me greater independence.

Just before my injury, I had completed my first year of college and had joined an agriculturally oriented fraternity, where I began to test my independence. I had a close association with the Future Farmers of America. I had been an officer and was selected to be a FFA State Farmer. I had also served as a junior deacon in my church. I was going with a beautiful young lady and, at age 19, seemed to have a bright future. Nothing could stop me from reaching my goals—or so I thought.

My view of the world during those first 5 weeks postinjury was very limited. I viewed the ceiling for 4 hours and then the floor for 4 hours. Boredom took hold very quickly. I relied on someone to feed me, clean up after me, wash me, shave me—just about everything had to be done for me. I felt as if control of my body had been given up to strangers and could only hope that they knew what they were doing. I lost my girlfriend when I couldn't face having her see me completely helpless.

I was transferred to Howard Rusk Rehabilitation Center in Columbia, Missouri, after 7 weeks and spent the next 6 months learning how to live with my disability. I began planning to go back to college. Finally, 8 months after discharge, I felt confident enough to be able to take care of myself and reentered college on my own.

Living on my own after my injury was incredibly frightening. I found a totally accessible apartment complex that met my needs but segregated the "gimps" from the other students. I excelled in college, graduating with honors and receiving a B.S. in Agricultural Economics. I was selected to be in an honorary scholastic fraternity and was named in Who's Who Among Students In American Universities and Colleges in 1980.

After numerous interviews, I joined Cargill, Inc., a giant agribusiness conglomerate, as a junior grain merchant. I spent 3 years there and I thank that company for transferring me to Tampa, Florida where I have lived since 1981. I dabbled in retail sales and eventually decided to reapply for Social Security Disability Insurance until I could find a career doing something of which I could be proud. I began doing volunteer work regarding disability issues, and eventually found my niche in helping other persons deal with their disabilities.

Since May 1989, I have worked with Self-Reliance, Inc., a center for independent living, where I serve as the community outreach coordinator. This center is instrumental in assisting disabled individuals achieve independent living objectives and minimize their reli-

(Box continues)

PERSONAL VIEWPOINT (continued)

ance on other persons. A major function of my job is to research and write grants to finance existing and future programs. The increase in self-confidence and self-esteem I received from a fulfilling place of employment is one of the most important things in my life.

I am currently a member of Tampa General's quad rugby team, the only quad rugby team in Florida. I enjoy movies, photography, videotaping, swimming, music, playing "Jeopardy!," and spending time with my wife, my friends, and my dog.

Other activities include serving as president of the local chapter of the National Spinal Cord Injury Association; serving on the governor-appointed State of Florida Spinal Cord Injury Advisory Council; being spokesman for the statewide DUI Prevention Program, "Cruisin' Without Boozin'," which is cosponsored by Tampa General Hospital and the Circle K Corporation; working in a prevention program, "It's A Break For Life," which aims to prevent spinal cord and head injuries in the teenage population; and serving on the Mayor's Alliance for the Handicapped in Tampa, which seeks to improve the quality of life for residents with any type of disability.

In retrospect, I can now see that during my rehabilitation, I had several unhelpful experiences. There was insufficient informative material to read about SCI, which delayed my fully understanding the ramifications of my particular injury. Most of what I have learned concerning accessibility, sexuality, fertility, advocacy, and research has come through my own efforts since discharge. Professionals who treated me indifferently only added to my already low self-esteem. Their hesitancy to discuss sexuality compounded my fears about the future and women. The lack of anybody to talk to who had a disability during the first 5 weeks of acute care contributed to an overwhelming fear of the unknown future. Last, being told that I would be dependent on someone for the rest of my life (which was not true) added to the already immense pressures in dealing with the injury and its resulting disability.

I would tell recently injured people that *life is not over!* As with anything else, you have to make the best of what you have. People never expect this to happen to them, but it's up to individuals as to whether they rise above the challenge or give up and be defeated by their handicaps. People with SCI may lose the ability to walk but they don't lose the ability to think, to dream, to care, to love, to have fun, to want the best out of life. Strive for as much independence in life as possible because this gives improved self-image and self-confidence that enhances success in life. Even if people cannot do certain things for themselves, being able to have the control and ability to direct how those things

are done will enable people to take responsibility for their lives and be proud of what they accomplish. Never relinquish the basic rights of freedom of choice and self-determination. The warehousing of young spinal cord injured persons in institutions such as nursing homes is probably a greater tragedy than the injury itself. Nothing kills hopes and dreams faster than being confined to a place where everyone else has already given up.

I encourage families to remain supportive through those first trying months or years after the injury. The stages one goes through are crucial to being able finally to accept the disability. Do not give up hope of recovery, but also do not expect the person with SCI to walk again. The disappointment felt when people realize that they will never walk again could be overwhelmingly devastating if someone they care about continues to expect the impossible. Also don't make it more difficult for the person with SCI by being overly demanding or critical of the staff when they are doing their best. Listen carefully and ask questions if you don't understand procedures, but don't overprotect the person with SCI and criticize the care they receive.

Make prevention programs a high priority for this country's young people. Conduct research and find out what works in a prevention program, and model that program for nationwide use.

Because I work in the independent living movement myself, I see the need to shift away from the medical model of rehabilitation for spinal cord injured persons in which they rely on someone else to determine what they can do and move toward an independent living model of care that gives these individuals responsibility to take control of their own lives.

Danny Joe Casady

POSTSCRIPT

As a nurse in the field of SCI, and the wife of Dan, I feel that it is extremely important to avoid labeling patients—for instance, "a C_{5-6} will be able to do XYZ, and *no more.*" The truth is that no one knows what particular patients will be able to do, or when they will be able to do it.

Always give patients reasonable goals to work toward, however small. The ability to accomplish even the smallest tasks is very rewarding to patients at this time of their lives. Try to arrange for the patient to speak with someone as early as possible, who has been through it. Above all, try to understand the feelings your patient is having: fear, confusion, humiliation, anger, depression, and more. Be kind; you are that person's lifeline.

Lise Casady

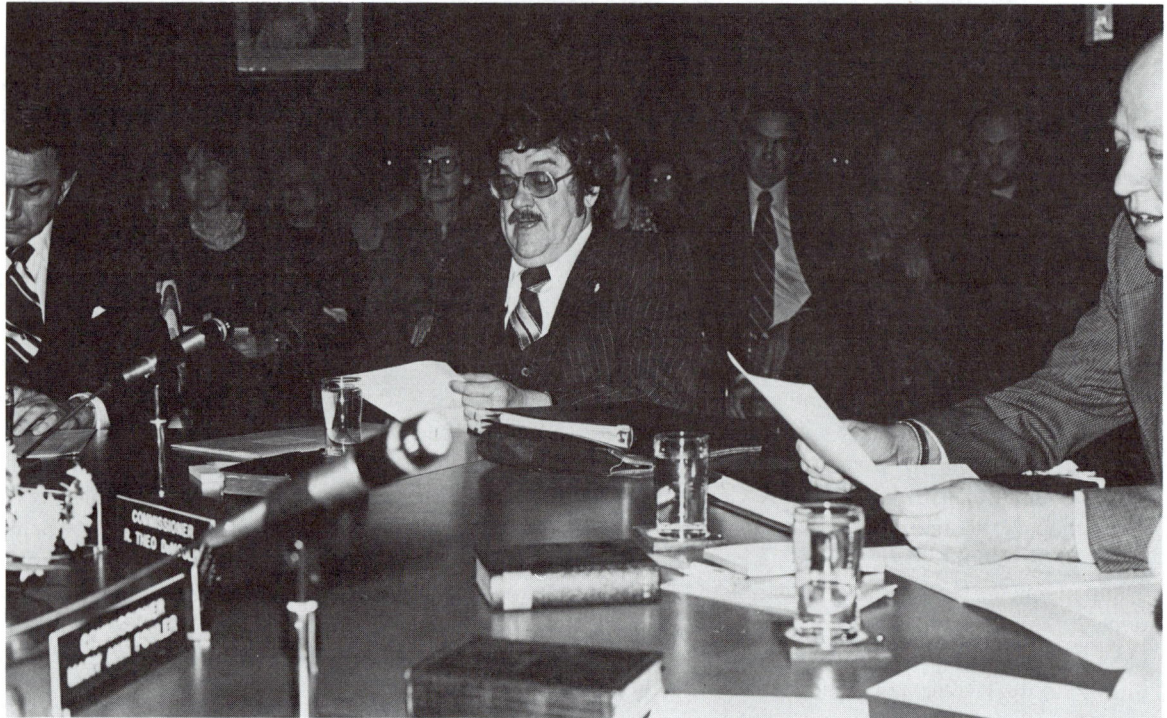

FIGURE 30–5   Leading: Wheelchair user Doug Mowat, an elected official, conducts a public forum.

THE NURSE'S ROLE*

At this point, it is appropriate to consider the nurse's role in life after rehabilitation. Actually, this begins during the early stages of comprehensive rehabilitation. The extent to which a person has a good outcome following rehabilitation directly depends on the quality of care provided during the entire rehabilitation process and on the expectations, attitudes, and self-image shaped during this initial stage of life after injury. The nurse is one of the first persons encountered by the newly disabled person, and, as such, makes a huge impression on the individual's perception of disability.

Following discharge from the rehabilitation center, the individual may require in-home follow-up, occasional outpatient clinic visits, and routine checkups. Obviously, nurses may be involved in each of these activities, and in this way, may be instrumental in helping the individual readapt to life in the mainstream. Even beyond the point of direct contact with the individual, nurses may be helpful in promoting more positive attitudes toward people with disabilities.

There are many important ways by which nurses can affect the quality of life of people with SCI in addition to those involving direct care:

* They can help prevent SCI by developing pragmatic educational and legislative programs to make driving, sports, and other activities safer.
* They can participate in research on minimizing the effects of SCI.
* They can lobby for improved health care for disabled people, for more and better rehabilitation facilities and programs, for improved follow-up and home care programs, and for more comprehensive payment mechanisms to meet the additional expenses caused by disability.
* They can join consumer groups or professional organizations to work toward more access for people with disabilities and for laws preventing discrimination and in appropriate institutionalization.
* They can support the development of new independent living centers by advocating funding for these programs at local, state, and national levels.
* They can actively initiate and support opportunities for peer counselors and consultants to participate formally in established rehabilitation programs.
* They can request national professional organizations to address strategies to encourage people with disabilities to seek careers in their professions and to reduce barriers that would discourage, restrict, or impede disabled people from a career in the health care field.

*The nurse's role is similar to the role of other health care professionals in securing independent living potentials for disabled people.

CONCLUSION

Because most nurses and other health care professionals see people with SCI at their most vulnerable, soon after the injury is incurred, and only infrequently after the person has established an independent way of life, it may be difficult for them to realize that people with SCI are capable of living productive, rewarding lives despite the severity of their disabilities. Today people with SCI can lead comparatively normal lives in their communities following rehabilitation and may, in fact, be just as productive and just as active after their injuries as they were before. People with SCI are now doing things they were not expected to do a few years ago, such as having children, working as farmers, being auto mechanics, and holding elective offices. Even the biggest barriers—lack of knowledge and negative attitudes—have begun to disappear. Independence for these people is a realistic, achievable goal.

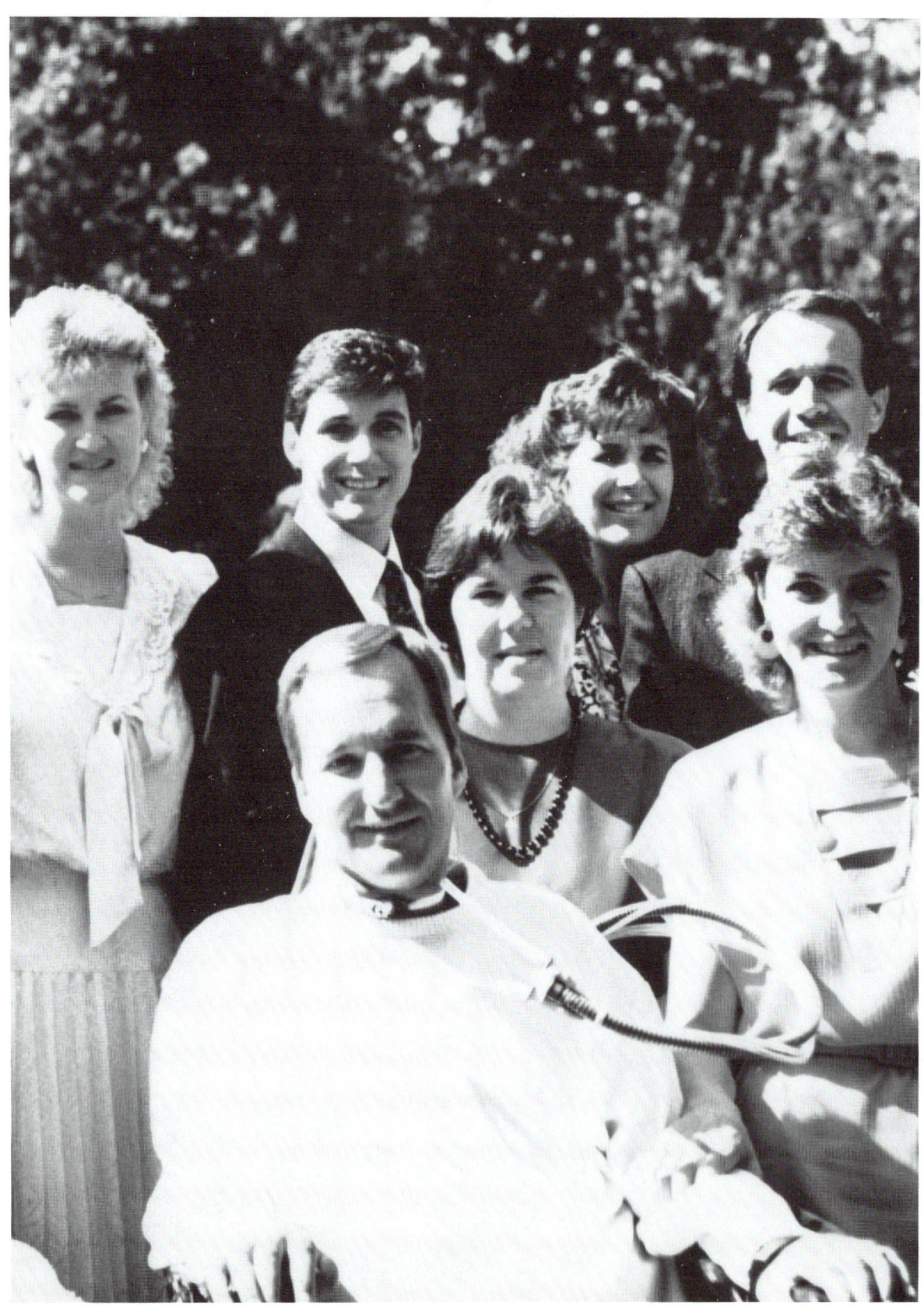

CHAPTER
— 31 —

Social Relationships and Interpersonal Skills: A Guide for People with Sensory and Physical Limitations*

Michael Dunn, Ph.D.

Chapter Outline

*This chapter was developed with the assistance of Carolyn Vash, Ph.D., and reprinted with the permission of Elizabeth Pan, Ph.D., and the Institute for Information Studies.

Objectives

- To increase awareness of the social consequences of spinal cord injury (SCI)
- To illustrate why intervention is necessary and how it can be accomplished to promote social skills of disabled patients

A spinal cord injured person shares a common experience of people with sensory and physical limitations:

> "Ever since my injury people don't seem to treat me the same as before. When I make a mistake, people are too embarrassed to tell me, and when I do my regular job, people act like I'm a genius or something. What's going on, anyway?"

Disability has extensive social and interpersonal implications as well as the obvious physical ones. This chapter explores these implications in detail and suggests alternative ways of dealing with well-recognized, but only recently studied, problems.

Interpersonal relationships are often difficult for many people but may be even more difficult for those with disability. However, general and disability-specific social skills for establishing and maintaining relationships can be learned in many ways.

The person with a disability might ask, "Why do I need information on this subject? Aren't things the same as always? Am I not the same person?" On the one hand, it is true that the person has not changed but many people, whether or not they have disabilities, need education in interpersonal relationships, too.

On the other hand, because of disability, people are, in some ways, different, if only because they are often treated as if they were. In addition, when people become disabled, new situations arise, such as falling out of the wheelchair. It is helpful to learn to manage these occurrences effectively and with social comfort, as well as relationships with others.

General social skills are not taught in school; people are expected to learn them on their own. However, this does not always happen. The demand for education in these areas has been so great that courses on social communication and interpersonal relationships are continually being added to college curricula. Many self-help books for the general public are available.

Films have the advantage of *showing* good and bad examples of behavior. Popular films such as *Coming Home* and *Born on the Fourth of July* serve as consciousness-raising devices, even though some may be too dramatic or overdone for "real life." Such films do, however, show how disabilities can affect the social aspects of living. Educational films and tapes are also available (Schachtel and Dunn 1990; Rakos and Schroeder 1980).

Some suggestions may seem very concrete and specific, but they may not appeal to everyone. Many of these ideas have been developed from the personal and clinical experience of persons with SCI. Individuals should try these suggestions for themselves and evaluate their usefulness in their own environments.

THE SOCIAL ENVIRONMENT OF PEOPLE WITH SCI

Many disabled people are aware of problems arising from different ways that people treat them and conclude that they are personally responsible because of something they are doing wrong. They do not realize that many of these problems are commonly encountered by disabled people simply because of others' attitudes toward disability.

Various research studies have shown that disabled people are perceived by the public as different from nondisabled people; for example, they are seen as less socially skilled, more dependent, more politically conservative, or more personally good. It has also been shown that experience alone does not change the public's attitudes about disabled people. However, when disabled and nondisabled people relate on an equal basis, attitudes do become more favorable.

The public also holds contradictory views of people with disabilities. For example, someone may say to a beautiful woman who is blind, "When I heard you were blind, I didn't expect someone so attractive." In other words, people do not expect that a "beautiful" person could be disabled. Sometimes a disabled person is also assumed to be fragile and easily hurt, emotionally or physically.

These are all forms of stereotyping. The tendency of one group to stereotype another stems from a number of factors: fears that disablement could happen to them; uncertainty about how to respond to an ambiguous situation; anxiety about saying the wrong thing; fear of causing embarrassment or hurt feelings; lack of contact and experience with disabled people; a generalized tendency to devalue disabled individuals; assumption, in some cultures, that disabled people or their families have done wrong and are being punished for it; general ignorance about disability; and generalizations about disabled people based on a few experiences.

Such negative attitudes conflict with cultural values requiring us to be kind, compassionate, and helpful to people with disabilities. These conflicts can create discomfort, anxiety, emotional arousal, ambivalence, and condescension. Fear of revealing unacceptable feelings may lead nondisabled people to become more formal and controlled in their behavior at first, and later to form overly favorable or unfavorable opinions about a disabled person.

One result of these conflicting attitudes and behaviors is that disabled people may receive less criticism and more praise than deserved. Therefore, they may learn to ignore praise and pay closer attention to criticism. A side effect of this loss of honest feedback may sometimes be aggressiveness and/or passive behavior on the part of the person with the disability.

Other results of society's conflicting attitudes and behavior are social isolation and lack of social mobility for disabled people. At parties or other social events where people haven't previously met, disabled individuals may have fewer social contacts, especially from nondisabled people in the group. This is particularly so when the disabled person has reduced communication ability or mobility. Numerous surveys have shown that people with disabilities tend to be less active socially than people in general. Activities such as shopping; going out to movies, restaurants, or other forms of public entertainment; attending PTA, lodge meetings, or other social or political group meetings; doing volunteer work; and attending school or vocational training classes tend to be reduced. Additionally, only a small percentage appear to know about groups by and for disabled people, which are potential sources of support, information, and encouragement.

Finally, such poor health behavior as allowing pressure sores, genitourinary infections, and emotionally influenced illness to develop, may be partially the result of poor self-esteem, feelings of loss of control, and desire to hide the disability. Many such feelings can arise from inadequate social relationships.

One conclusion to be drawn is that persons may be seen as members of a minority group. When performance is above average they are said to be "a credit to their disability." When they perform below average, they are, after all, "disabled and not to be blamed or censured."

The ensuing problems may seem insurmountable, but many disabled people have learned to manage them and are very comfortable and effective in their interpersonal relationships.

MANAGING PROBLEMS ————

Listening

Listening skills allow people not only to listen to and understand what other people are saying but, more important, to let others know that they are listening and that they understand. Many social and interpersonal problems result from poor listening skills.

Passive listening is shown by head nodding, eye contact, and by not doing other things while a person speaks (like reading or thinking about what to say next).

Listening can also be indicated by *verbal following*, a technique of repeating the other person's key words and saying "Uh, huh."

Active listening conveys understanding by paraphrasing the person's comments. One way to do this is to define terms

by saying "Is what you mean . . .?" Also, one can summarize the individual's statements by saying, "We seem to be getting to the point where . . ." The functions of active listening are to:

- Clarify what has actually been said and meant.
- Encourage the expression of emotions.
- Establish a relationship with the individual.
- Show acceptance of what the individual is saying without judging it.
- Encourage the person to explain further.
- Check out the accuracy of one's own perceptions and assumptions.

Sometimes people discover they did not understand what a person really meant to say. By paraphrasing, or by checking out perceptions of what the person was trying to communicate, they can often clarify with the individual what was actually meant.

Asserting Oneself

One's degree of assertiveness strongly influences interpersonal communication. The major alternatives to assertiveness are to be passive-submissive, or to be aggressive. Individuals always have a choice. They may decide under what circumstances they will be passive, assertive, and aggressive.

Table 31–1 compares these three types of behavior. It describes them in terms of their major characteristics and consequences. For example, passivity permits others to infringe on one's rights, and it is self-denying. Assertion is an emotionally honest, direct expression of feelings and is self-enhancing. Aggression is overly direct, hostile, and self-aggrandizing, and it imposes one person's choices on others. Review of the total table leaves little doubt that choosing the assertive option over either the passive-submissive or aggressive options will enhance the quality of social relationships.

Many people with disabilities find that placing special emphasis on the nonverbal aspects of assertiveness helps to compensate, to some extent, for the effects of negative public attitudes and behavior. For example, if disability permits, good posture, eye contact, firm voice, calmness, and avoidance of nervous mannerisms or tics, can facilitate social interaction greatly. Remember, however, to use social feedback to regulate behavior. People who act socially "crippled" are likely to be treated accordingly.

Expressing Negative Feelings

The expression of negative feelings is a problem for many people. They tend to hold back criticisms, complaints, and unhappy feelings—in a passive-submissive way—to avoid

TABLE 31–1   Comparison of Social Behavior Styles

	Passive-Submissive	Assertive	Aggressive
Behavior	• Ignores; does not express own true rights, needs, desires, feelings • Emotionally dishonest, indirect, inhibited, manipulative • Self-denying	• Appropriately emotionally honest, direct, expressive • Expresses and asserts own needs, rights, desires, feelings • Self-enhancing	• Inappropriately emotionally honest, direct, expressive (overreacts, hostile, angry) • Expresses conceived rights at expense of others • Self-aggrandizing
Verbal communications	• Rarely thinks through long-term goals for self • Apologetic, uncertain words, veiled or indirect meanings • Operates from unstated assumptions; does not say what is meant; hedging, ramblings • "You know"; "I mean"; "that is"; "er . . . ah"	• Recognition of inner needs, wants; focuses on long-term goals • Uses objective words; communications are polite but firm, simple and clear • Direct, honest statement of feelings and needs, gives opportunity to others for same • "I think"; "I feel"; "I'm beginning to believe"; and so on; says "no" initially if refusing a request	• Knows what one wants (short term) and intends to get it no matter what • Tends to use subjective, emotional, imperious words, long explanations • Direct statements, often sharp and accusatory, or cuts others short; puts down others • "Your fault"; "you made me"; "you better . . . or"; "everyone thinks"
Nonverbal communications	• The other must guess or intuit what one wants • Appears not to mean what is said, sometimes shy, or sly • Voice often hesitant, sometimes wavering, even whiny • Eyes averted or downcast, sometimes pleading or teary • Often leans for support, twisted stance, or sagging posture; fidgety	• Attentive listening behavior; thinks before speaking • Words, facial expression match assured manner; communicates caring and strength • Voice firm, relaxed, well modulated, fluent • Eyes open, frank, direct with eye-to-eye contact • Usually well-balanced, erect, but relaxed posture; smooth gestures, no foot shuffling or hand wringing	• Exaggerated show of strength, may be flippant, sarcastic, bullying, grouchy, picky • Demanding manner, authoritative, superior style • Voice often shrill, loud, or very quiet with lips compressed • Eyes sometimes direct, coldly appraising; narrow, not really "seeing" • Aggressive, defiant or threatening posture, rigid body; sharp abrupt gestures
Outcome or consequences	• Permits others to infringe on one's rights • Rarely, if ever, achieves desired goals • Future limited to unspoken (and understood) bargain • Allows others to choose for self	• Stands up for legitimate right so that the rights of others are not violated • Often, but not always, achieves desired goals • Future open • Chooses for self	• Assumes illegitimate rights; intent is to hurt, humiliate, or to get even • Usually achieves desired goals by hurting others • Retribution may follow long-range block • Chooses for others
How you feel	• Smug if manipulative, usually disappointed in self at time • Anxious, tense, hurt, and possibly angry later	• Feels good about self at time • Confident and self-respecting	• Angry, righteous, and superior at the time • Possibly guilty, self-critical, or remorseful later
How others feel toward you	• Presumptive, irritated, disgusted • Possibly pity or disregard	• Generally trustful • Generally respectful	• Unfriendly, untrusting, cautious • Possibly angry and vengeful
How others feel toward self	• Superior • Possibly guilty, or angry toward self if manipulated	• Treated as equal • Valued, respected	• Hurt, humiliated • Possibly frightened
Psychological costs or payoff	• Unpleasant and risky situations, conflict, and confrontations are avoided, but self-value diminishes • Needs are not met • Over time, depression and anger accumulate	• Feel good, less inner conflict; goals clearly thought out; self-esteem and confidence increase • Needs usually (but not always) met • Freer and more honest relationships with others	• Must justify emotional outbursts by inflating ego ro saving up resentment • Those one has hurt are wary; alienates others • Encourages dishonesty in others

Adapted and modified from Alberti and Emmons (1974) and Jakubowski-Specter (1973).

hurting or alienating others. Then, when they can no longer hold the negative feelings back, they are apt to explode emotionally—in a very aggressive way—and hurt or alienate the other person anyway. The problem is, they hurt themselves by doing this. Assertiveness can stop this vicious cycle. Table 31–2 lists some clues that indicate that assertive behavior is necessary.

Many people also find it difficult to reject help that another offers, even though it is unneeded and unwanted. The content of what one says is important. Say "no" early in the refusal and be firm. Saying "no" is more effective, and kinder, when an alternative is suggested. How poised one sounds and looks is also very important. Whether one says "no," and how one says it, are often functions of the relationship with the person offering help.

Disclosing Oneself

Self-disclosure, an important component of assertiveness, means verbal communication of one's feelings or desired behaviors. Name your feelings—for example, "I feel embarrassed"; use similes such as, "I feel like a tiny frog in a big pond"; or express an urge to action; for example, "I'd like to hug you." These are ways of expressing emotions—how one is feeling right now. Note that these expressions use the word *I* and not *you*. For example, saying, "You're making me angry," is not self-disclosure; it is an accusation. It implies that the other person is to blame and usually provokes a defensive reaction. However, stating, "I'm feeling angry in response to what you're saying," is taking responsibility for one's own emotions and simply sharing them, not implying that they are the other person's fault. In general, use of I-statements facilitates all communication about feelings.

Encouraging assertiveness in others is also an important interpersonal skill. People may need reassurance that deserved criticism is genuinely desired. Afterward, say something like, "Thanks, I'm really glad you told me; I didn't know I was coming across like that." It is often useful for disabled people to make implicit, or hidden, feelings more open, direct, and explicit; this is a way of making people more comfortable with being assertive and giving criticism. Say something like, "A lot of people have difficulty expressing negative emotions to disabled people because they are afraid they are going to hurt the disabled person's feelings. I really want to hear criticism from you if you feel it because that's the only way I can learn where I need to improve."

Communicating positive emotions is an aspect of assertiveness that needs to be emphasized as well. It is important to tell people when one feels good, to compliment them, and to express positive emotions, particularly in close relationships.

First, *warmth* and respect are essential to communicating a willingness to listen. This may involve maintaining eye

TABLE 31–2   Clues that Assertive Behavior Is Needed

- Having pent-up feelings of frustration and anger or unreturned love; constantly engaging in thoughts about a certain person or situation
- Steering clear of situations to avoid meeting someone, especially when feeling anxious or resentful
- Withdrawing from an interpersonal situation, and then feeling anxious or resentful
- Creating problems for others to gain some satisfaction, to get even, or to protect one's rights; for example, "forgetting" to run an errand or "accidentally" blocking someone's way
- Using indirect hints to get a message across, and expecting the other person to understand them
- Making excuses to justify one's behavior, especially when feeling uneasy; feeling the need to smile and apologize
- Feeling continued resentment toward another person
- Putting oneself down relative to another person; for example, thinking, "I'm not as good"; "He must be right"; "I can't compete with him"
- Denying oneself and one's feelings relative to another person; for example, thinking: "My needs are not that important anyway"; "I'm not going to worry about it"; "They might get angry and disapprove of me"; "I want to be a 'nice guy' about this"; "I mustn't take a chance on hurting someone's feelings no matter what"
- Acting aggressive by showing a lack of consideration for others' needs and feelings in verbal or physical ways.

Adapted from Rakos and Schroeder (1980)

contact, a relaxed posture, and leaning toward or sitting closer to the person. Communicate interest and help people tell their own stories by using head nods, avoiding interruptions, repeating key words, asking open-ended questions, and paraphrasing what has been said. Open-ended questions help elicit more information about a particular subject from the person. These questions cannot be answered "yes" or "no." They allow the person to expand, to give you more detail, and to express things the way they feel them. Examples of open-ended questions are, "What do you think about . . . ? Would you tell me about . . . ? How do you feel about . . . ?" communicate warmth, and respect the person's worth, integrity, and abilities by using nonevaluative language, using the person's name, and making positive statements about the person.

Second, communicating positive emotions involves the expression of *empathy*, showing understanding of the individuals' feelings as well as the events or the facts about which they speak. In other words, when someone says, "That fink gave me an F on my exam," reflect the feelings by saying, "Gee, you must really feel bad about that." The response, "Oh, in what course did he give you an F?" would show concern with facts, not feelings. In general, empathy reflects feelings, particularly those expressed nonverbally. Try to make statements rather than ask questions; for instance, beginning "I'm sensing"; "I'm hearing"; "It sounds like." It also helps to acknowledge how difficult it is to express feelings if an individual is having trouble doing so. Also communicate empathy nonverbally, through the intensity of the response, tone of voice, and the pace and volume of speech. The degree of body tension shown usually communicates involvement—sitting close, leaning forward, or occasionally touching the person.

The third aspect of communicating positive emotions is to demonstrate *genuineness*. This is a matter of admitting lack of understanding, asking for clarification, and acknowledging limitations as well as any potential for helping an individual. Try to communicate a willingness to look at one's own feelings and reactions in an honest way.

Receiving Compliments

Many people find it difficult to accept compliments. When they are complimented, they may challenge the person's judgment by saying, for example, "Oh no, it's just an old dress I threw on." Such refusal to accept compliments suggests false modesty. Sometimes people throw a compliment back when they feel embarrassed about accepting it. They may say, "Thanks, you look great, too." This can make the person who made the compliment feel uncomfortable, as if the person was suspected of fishing for a compliment. It is generally best to assume that people are expressing sincere, straightforward appreciation, and simply thank them for that. Say, for instance, "Thanks, it really feels good to hear you say that." Such honest responses please the person who pays a compliment.

Confronting Others

Confrontation is a social skill that involves pointing out apparent inconsistencies between another's verbal and nonverbal behavior. An example of a confronting statement is, "You say you really hate that guy, but you are saying it with a smile, so I really don't understand what you're trying to say." It is a difficult skill for many people to master because they fear it may lead to rejection. However, when properly done, it can strengthen a relationship rather than weaken it. Because it calls for much caring and involvement, it may sometimes be better to delay confrontation until ready to deal with an issue. Say something to the effect, "I'm really too tired right now; may we talk in about an hour, after I get a little bit of rest?" When delaying confrontation, one should set a specific time for dealing with the particular situation. When the time comes, confrontation can be made easier for both parties by applying principles of constructive feedback. See the section headed Close Relationships in this chapter.

Conversation

The techniques of initiating conversation depend on whether the goal is small talk or a serious discussion. Initiating enjoyable small talk in social situations is the more difficult task for many people. In a serious discussion, the urgency of the topic tends to take over; there is less need for techniques. This provides a clue as to what makes small talk successful: the person actually cares about the topics chosen. Often, conversation begins with an attempt to draw other people out, to encourage them to share an opinion or a bit of personal (but not *too* personal) information.

Whether the goal is small talk or a serious discussion, maintaining a productive or enjoyable conversation requires active listening skills. When changing the subject, try to mention the other's point and then explain the change. For example, "I understand what you're saying, but . . . ." Also use bridging statements to make a connection between the two topics. For example, "Your last point reminds me of . . . ." When trying to end a conversation, try to find a natural pause, make less eye contact, and simply say, "I've enjoyed talking with you," followed by an appropriate way of excusing oneself (for instance, "I want to catch Sally before she leaves").

Some disabled people often have difficulty letting a conversation be focused on their own disabilities. People are often curious, but if one prefers not to let the disability become the focal point of the conversation, try to deal with that early in the interaction.

Touching

Physical contact is an important aspect of being close to another person and expressing positive emotions. Touching functions as a greeting, communicates warmth, gets attention, and communicates sexuality. Touching is not used as much in our society as in some others; moreover, many people are somewhat anxious about touching people who have disabilities. However, initiating the touching in appropriate circumstances may make them more comfortable with returning such gestures. If motion limitations or prosthetic devices make touching complicated or impossible, it becomes important to educate the other person verbally with such statements as, "Gee, I'd hug you for that if I could." This lets other people know that physical contact would be pleasing, and they can decide whether they wish to initiate it.

Maximizing Physical Attractiveness

Physical attractiveness is important in our society. Good grooming, nice clothing, and cleanliness are the basic elements. Research has shown that good-looking people "are seen as more responsible for good deeds and less responsible for bad ones; their evaluations of others have more potent impact; their performances are upgraded; others are more socially responsive to them, more ready to provide them with help, and more willing to work hard to please them" (Huston and Levinger 1978: 122). In other words, physically attractive people have many social advantages. Although no research has demonstrated it, general experience indicates that disabled people who are attractive enjoy many benefits, make friends more easily, and get better and faster service from agencies. When a disability impairs attractiveness in some ways, it is even more crucial to compensate by doing everything possible to increase it.

Meeting New People

Good social skills will not do any good if one does not know where to find people with whom to relate. A technique that works places the individual in situations where compatible people are found. To choose the best places for meeting like-minded individuals, one must first know oneself—one's interests, values, abilities, and preferences for certain types of companions. This self-knowledge forms the basis for deciding whether to join a social club, a political or religious organization, or a community group; take an adult education class; put a personal advertisement in a particular newspaper or magazine; go to art shows, museums, or flea markets; or ask friends or acquaintances about their favorite local "hot spots." One advantage of special-interest clubs and classes is that they allow people to get to know others as like-minded persons first, rather than as people for whom disability is their most obvious characteristic.

HANDLING COMMON DISABILITY-RELATED ISSUES

This section describes ways to deal with social situations that cause anxiety, discomfort, or potential embarrassment relating to disabling conditions of many kinds. Some of the suggested approaches may be used in one-to-one interactions, and others are suitable for use in public education programs.

Acknowledging One's Disability

This technique makes nondisabled people more comfortable, even if it makes the disabled person a little anxious or uncomfortable. The payoff comes later: disabled people feel more comfortable once others feel more comfortable. Curiosity is normal, and self-disclosure helps to satisfy this curiosity and get the subject of disability out of the way. It involves brief explanations of sensory or physical limita-

tions. Without the understanding that a brief explanation can provide, another person may be afraid of saying something stupid, hurtful, or embarrassing, and such fears can wreck a conversation. Disclosure etiquette involves describing your disability in calm, matter-of-fact ways and assuming that the listener can accept the description in an equally matter-of-fact manner. Able-bodied people are often unaware of what disabled people can and cannot do. Try to find a natural time in the conversation to give such information. Self-disclosure gives an excellent opportunity to show that one can take disability in stride, which encourages others to take it in stride, too.

Using Humor

Humor is a powerful technique for putting people at ease in difficult or sensitive situations. Humor can show that a person is not experiencing disability as an overpowering problem and can appreciate its comic aspects. Satire points out ironies, but it is not bitter. Bitterness is never funny.

Telling stories on oneself, or giving joking answers to thoughtless questions, usually helps people feel more comfortable if done with a smile. The first step is to develop the ability to see the humor in the situation. Next, learn to express it in a unique style. Bear in mind, however, that any skill can be overused or misused, and humor is no exception. If it dominates communication or is used unkindly or hostilely, its effectiveness will be weakened.

Making the Implicit Explicit

This technique is used mainly in close relationships, but it can also help acquaintances deal with their feelings of discomfort. Try to reflect any discomfort that a person feels by saying something like, "It's really hard for many people to talk about my disability, even though they have questions they feel a need to ask. If I were in your place, I think I would want to know that . . ." is often a good start for giving information without embarrassing the other person.

Asking for Help

Asking for help is difficult for many people, but it may be more difficult for disabled people because they often need more help. Two basic ground rules for successfully obtaining help are:

- Try to make eye contact with people to facilitate interaction
- Be very specific in the request.

These rules help build self-confidence and also improve the probability of success. These techniques also help people to assist, which is not always easy to do. Specific directions must virtually always be given to strangers. For example, a wheelchair user asking for help up a curb will need to show or tell the person where to hold, and what to do, and where to stop. Use your best posture and a firm voice in asking; this helps avoid appearing to be in an inferior position. If one takes a passive approach in asking for help, the helper may act oversolicitous or condescending. If one uses an aggressive approach, there may be an aggressive counterreaction. Finally, thank the helper for helping. People generally feel good about helping, and thanking them gives an even greater reward.

Refusing Undesired Help

This is difficult for many disabled people for two closely related reasons: fears of discouraging potential sources of help that might be needed later, and the rationalization that it makes people feel good even if the help is not necessary. Refusing unwanted help in an appropriate, assertive manner, however, can make everyone feel good about the interchange. In addition, it can help people realize that they are not here to make people feel good. Visibility of a disability often makes people try to help when help is not wanted or needed. To counteract this try not to make eye contact because its absence discourages others from approaching. For example, when trying to put the wheelchair into the car, ignore the people passing by, which can reduce the probability that they will attempt to give unwanted help. Appearing competent and remaining calm, however hard one has to struggle, also discourages offers of help. When offers are made, simply look at the person, refuse politely, and continue with the task. Make a quick response, because if one stammers, some people will not believe help is not needed and may continue to offer unneeded assistance. When this occurs, politely, but assertively, thank the person for *not* helping. A very effective standard response is, "I prefer to do it myself, but thank you *very* much for asking." This conveys "no" immediately and clearly and, at the same time, shows appreciation of the helping motive. It does not discourage the person from approaching others who might want and need help in the future, and it rewards the person for kindness even though no help was supplied. Everyone wins.

Handling Unwelcome Social Advances

Many disabled persons have experienced unwelcome social advances that seem to be related to their disabilities. Some people assume that disabled persons will have more sympathy for their problems. Others want to tell about remedies they believe will work. Still others may be drunk or simply hoping for a captive audience who cannot quickly get away. Control these situations by using techniques opposite to those used for encouraging social interaction. Make no eye contact; try to do other things; pay attention to someone or something else; make no verbal comments that could encourage communication; if you can, move away; if you cannot, ignore, or use firm refusals, if an individual persists. Be firm but polite; an aggressive response may lead to counteraggression particularly if the individual is drunk. A last caution: accepting an offer of a drink may obligate one to listen to a long story!

Dealing with Staring and Questions

Being stared at becomes a problem for some disabled people because of what they tell themselves about the staring. When people think they are being stared at because a person sees them as freaks or weirdos, they are bound to feel uncomfortable. On the other hand, if they believe they are being stared at because a person is surprised at seeing such good-looking people using wheelchairs, they probably will not mind it at all. For most people, the truth probably lies in between these extremes. People are naturally curious and will look at whatever is new to them. Realistically, a disabled person may present an unusual experience to many nondisabled people. Aggressive staring back or saying, "What's the matter, never seen a cripple before?" only embarrasses the other person. If it is upsetting, it is usually best to take no notice and ignore it. People who are socially extroverted and self-confident enough can simply enjoy it. After all, most people want to be unique; disabled people *are*. Be a good model, smile, and have a good time. This is an opportunity to let people know that disabled people are "regular" people who engage in many ordinary activities and enjoy life. It is important to be oneself because people are sensitive and quickly pick up on false bravado or enjoyment. It may help one to know that one has done one's best to be an attractive person who conveys a sense of self-respect and self-liking.

Questions, like stares, are seen as insulting by some disabled people. However, they can also be viewed as good opportunities to do spontaneous public education. Assuming the questioner has been polite, if there is time, try to answer the question. If people care enough to ask, they might care enough to share accurate information with others. Curiosity management is very important in close relationships, where often it is better to explain some aspect of disability before questions arise. This is especially true in matters of sexuality. See Chapter 10.

DISABILITY-SPECIFIC SOCIAL SKILLS

In addition to the shared interpersonal problems that disabled people encounter, a few situations arise that are specific to particular types of disabilities. These include situations that are embarrassing, cause difficulties, or in other ways decrease a person's desire to be out in public. The major tactic for dealing with these situations is to *stay calm*, because it will be easier to manage the second time around. Often, anxiety about dealing with certain situations presents the greatest problem. However, unless people are willing to take the risk of putting themselves in the feared situation, they cannot learn to deal with it; experience helps to lessen anxiety.

Bowel and Bladder Problems

Bowel and bladder accidents are acutely embarrassing because of early training and cultural prohibitions about soiling oneself. Loss of bowel or bladder control is viewed as childlike and stirs up strong negative emotions. Unavoidable accidents do happen. The best way to handle such situations is to disclose the problem to the extent that is comfortable and excuse oneself. Try to stay relaxed. If one takes it in stride, others can, too. Some people feel more at ease by just saying they have had some problems and must leave. Others may want to say, "I am having problems with my bowels and must leave." It is usually best to excuse oneself because if one stays, anxiety may make things worse. If an accident occurs during an important event such as a job interview or meeting, try to schedule a new appointment before leaving. If uncomfortable about delaying departure for the few moments this will take, simply say, "I will call later to reschedule." One also might want to disclose the frequency of occurrence and briefly explain why such accidents occur among people with SCI, depending on the closeness or importance of the relationship.

It may be reassuring to know that many people with SCI or other disabilities that predispose them to bowel and bladder accidents tell stories on themselves about having had accidents on their first dates with their husbands or wives. Because they eventually married these individuals, accidents obviously do not automatically alienate other people. What *can* turn them off is a display of emotionality.

Communication Problems

For people with all types of disabilities, words such as *see*, *walk*, and *hear*, when used by some nondisabled people, may cause some communication difficulties, because their discomfort or embarrassment may sidetrack the conversation. Some people talk to disabled people through their companions, so it may be necessary to ask people to speak directly instead. To solve communication problems, the first step is to communicate that a problem exists. Then, when someone talks too loudly, talks about disabled people in their presence as if they were not there, or gets upset about saying "see" or "walk," take these good opportunities to give helpful feedback and make people more comfortable. Confidence in effective communication is gained gradually.

Socialization Problems

Being born with a disability or acquiring one early in life can present a special set of problems because initial socialization may be lacking. Parents of disabled children often feel forced to be overprotective and may have more conflict in their marriages. The bonding that ordinarily takes place between parents and children may be impaired. Disabled children may not be allowed to make decisions or explore the environment as much as other children. Also, they may be isolated at home and not get to see disabled and nondisabled children interacting. In other words, disabled children need models of social behavior, which they may not receive.

Members of a peer group (people with whom one identifies and feels close) play important roles in helping children learn about both cooperative and competitive behavior. They allow expressions of aggression; reward independent behavior; permit different social roles to be tried in the safe context of the group; and offer confirmation or disconfirmation of self-judgments about competency and self-esteem. Peer groups also share information and experiences regarding disability. Thus, disabled children need not feel theirs are unique personal problems, and nondisabled children can learn to accept disabilities.

One way of compensating for the lack of such early socialization experiences is to join disability-related groups that offer ready-made peer groups relative to disability. There are good models and poor models, ways of dealing with situations that can be adopted and ways that should be avoided. Peers tend to give more honest feedback than others who fear hurting a disabled person's feelings.

Parents can help their disabled children by recognizing the problems that poor socialization creates and by giving their children honest feedback. Also, when parents move to new neighborhoods they can invite the neighbors and children in to get acquainted and help start peer relationships. It is often useful to join or start parent support groups in which the difficulties encountered in raising physically limited children can be shared. Frustrations can be reduced when parents support each other.

Reactions to Deformity and Disfigurement

The human tendency to be prejudiced against people with different skin colors reflects a low tolerance for people whose appearance is notably different from what is considered "right" or "average." Consequently, if one's face is disfigured or body deformed as a result of a disability, one may as well expect some negative reactions. The problem usually solves itself, given a little time, opportunity for continued contact, and the disabled person's willingness to wait and understand, without feeling insulted.

Many people who have had seriously disfiguring accidents say that failing to prepare others in advance about their unusual appearances may lead to fear, surprise, and embarrassment for all concerned. When they cannot prepare others in advance, they prefer to stand in the shadows or at a greater distance than usual at their first meeting to let other persons slowly become used to them. Learning to manage being stared at or intentionally ignored will ease social interaction regardless of the degree of disfigurement or deformity that disability may entail. Remember that looks do not matter, but rather how one feels about them. People can become so preoccupied with a minor facial or figure flaw that they make themselves miserable imagining everyone is staring at it. At the same time, a number of severely deformed or disfigured people have developed highly successful careers in the public eye and also have rewarding social and love lives. The key is the high degree of esteem they feel for themselves. They communicate this self-respect to others and, as a result, their deformities and disfigurements seem to disappear, simply blotted out by the beauty from within.

Reactions to Wheelchairs

The wheelchair appears to be a powerful social stimulus. Its visibility and association with so-called invalidism often provoke inappropriate responses from others: attempts to reassure, encourage, cure or bless you, for example. It is important to realize that one is not personally responsible for these reactions. Dealing with them assertively will slowly help to break down the negative connotations of disability that evoke such behavior by others. Remember, not every comment—however inappropriate—must be met with confrontation. If a remark appears well meant and the person shows no signs of intruding further on one's privacy, simply accept it. If unwanted follow-up seems likely, however, one can assertively end the conversation. For example, say, "I appreciate your interest, but I'm well informed about my disability and intend to follow a different course of action."

Wheelchair problems are more difficult to manage because safety may be at stake. When disabled people fall out of the wheelchair, lose a crucial part of it, or need help up a curb, they must give the people who are helping specific directions on what to do. If they do not, inexperienced helpers may injure them or make an embarrassing scene. Whether it is easier to solve the problem oneself or to ask for help is the disabled person's own decision, based on capabilities and emotional needs.

Managing discussions concerning wheelchairs is also an important ability. Ideally the focus of conversation ought to be on the individual as a person and not as the contents of a wheelchair. If allowing others to talk about the wheelchair too much seems to be a dehumanizing interpersonal experience, briefly explain or comment and change the subject.

SPECIAL SITUATIONS: SPECIAL SKILLS

Individuals behave differently in different situations. The skills needed for relating to others sometimes depend on the nature of the relationship and the purposes for interacting. Many people are encountered daily not because of who they are but because of the positions they hold. Interaction may be brief, or longer-term relationships may develop, as with one's car mechanic, doctor, or welfare worker. In a sense, the jobs they hold and the need for their services make them special. Children are also special, because how people relate to them will influence whether they develop healthy or unhealthy attitudes about disability and people with disabilities. Finally, the most special people are loved ones, with whom there is a close or intimate relationship.

Brief Encounters

Superficial relationships with people such as salespersons, waiters, and passing acquaintances are usually the easiest to handle assertively and require less risk. However, some people have such poor self-concepts that they feel they must try to please everyone. Disability may increase this tendency in some people. When one wants to say "no" to a persistent salesperson, reject unwanted attention from a stranger, or gain the attention of an inattentive waiter, use a firm voice, eye contact, and few, if any explanations. Although it is important to be courteous, such superficial encounters are not the times to be concerned about being liked.

Dealing with clerks and salespersons is facilitated by using a moderately loud voice when making a request, and by making eye contact or facing the person. People in wheelchairs may not be seen because of their lower height. Occasionally, clerks and salespersons may be anxious about talking to them or may expect them to be with a helper who will make any purchases.

Quietly initiating a request for a table from a restaurant host, asking a waiter for information about a menu, or initiating a food order can prevent the waiter from asking one's companion for the disabled person's order. When it does occur, simply respond as if the question had been appropriately addressed directly to the disabled person. Many disabled individuals coach their regular dining companions to respond politely, "I don't know," allowing the disabled person to answer.

People encountered at parties, meetings, or in casual social situations may respond to disability with more emotion than the disabled person feels. When an opportunity arises, briefly and calmly reassure them. Point out that the disability occurred a while ago and disabled people are much less affected by disability than are people to whom it is new.

Children, with their natural curiosity, deserve answers to their sometimes surprising questions. The openness and honesty of children should be returned. Reassure their parents that it is all right for them to ask questions. This offers a good opportunity to explain disability and help people feel less nervous about it. Say something like, "It's okay for him to ask questions. I think it's important for people to find out about disabilities to help kids be more comfortable." Educate the parents as well as the child.

Repeated Interactions

Ongoing relationships involve more risk, anxiety, and sometimes guilt, and require more understanding, more explanations, and demands for compromise. To illustrate this, a car mechanic may have to know why the car is needed so soon, and the disabled person may have to reflect the mechanic's concerns and show understanding of the mechanic's position.

Ongoing Contact with Health Professionals

People who work in the helping professions such as medicine, nursing, social work, and psychology, may know a lot about disability, but they often only see people who are having difficulties. Therefore, they may not have realistic attitudes about disabled people living in the community and may expect them to be less capable and happy than they are.

They need accurate information on how disabled people function in the community so that they can help more effectively. Also, they need appreciation; that is one of the reasons they chose their professions. Therefore, express appreciation and support to them for their understanding and help.

In medical situations, one often has to ask for explanations and diagnoses, express a lack of understanding, or suggest alternatives and compromises. People who tend to forget questions they want to ask in anxiety-arousing situations can list them beforehand. When health professionals are asked what they want patients to do in their own medical care, they say, "Learn about your body so you can assume responsibility for it." They want people to learn, so do not be offended when they seem hurried and unwilling to answer questions. Insist on answers; it will benefit everyone.

When consulting a health professional, be specific about complaints and symptoms. However, do not assume the doctor or nurse knows everything and can fix everything. They have limitations, and clients need to know what they can and cannot do. The role of most rehabilitation professionals is to *teach* people, not to do for them, even though it might be more efficient to do certain tasks themselves. Use the medical experts' knowledge and skills, but make sure to become well-informed in order to make decisions about rehabilitation.

Teachers

Like others in our society, teachers often know little about the actual capabilities and limitations of disabled people. Therefore, be able to explain limitations and suggest workable compromises or alternatives that will permit effective functioning in school settings. A few people may resist changes to meet course requirements in nonstandard ways.

Employers

The job market is a difficult situation with which to deal. The relationship between a worker with a disability and an employer is complicated by ambivalent feelings and by current federal regulations on hiring disabled people. In general, employers may feel they *should* hire disabled people because of public pressures and because of possible legal and financial consequences if they do not. Therefore, when they do hire them, they may overidealize them and hold unrealistic expectations of their abilities. In other words, to overcome conflicts about hiring a worker with a disability, employers may have to make disabled people look better than they are to compensate for the anxieties associated with hiring them.

Early in employment, try to define the limits of one's ability and let the employer know this, as related to the disability and to the job performance preparation. Later on, if a task must be refused because of insufficient experience or physical limitations, show understanding of the employer's position and feelings and explain clearly.

Other people may assume that disabled people are more preoccupied with disability-related matters than they actually are. One way of dealing with this is to disclose some of one's concerns that are unrelated to disability. In other words, talk about meeting the mortgage, being tired from a late night, or other ordinary human problems. This helps people realize that disabled people are human beings with concerns, strengths, and weaknesses similar to their own.

When employers want to fire disabled workers, they sometimes become overly critical and excessively blaming. This helps them justify an action that they regret having to take. Again, reflect the criticism and thereby let the person indicate understanding of what they are saying. Then ask for the specific behavioral changes the employer wants. Emphasize a desire to do well. Individuals should let the employer know that despite mistakes, they are committed to the job, want to learn, and will try to meet standards (even though it may be hard to agree with parts of the criticism). Perhaps indicate understanding of how difficult it must be for an employer to deal with fair employment practice regulations when they appear to interfere with making a profit. This serves several purposes: it makes the implicit issue of fairness explicit; brings it into an open discussion; and provides an opportunity to explain how the disabled person can best help the company earn a profit. Think this through in advance and perhaps role play with a friend to develop a clear, brief presentation (Jackson 1989).

In general, conflicts appear to be lessening as more disabled people get jobs. Nondisabled employers and co-workers are learning from personal experience that people with disabilities are pretty much like themselves. However, it is important to be assertive when such situations do arise.

Service Providers

People with disabilities may need attendants, readers, drivers, interpreters, notetakers, and perhaps, other personal support providers. The interpersonal skills required in hiring, training, supervising, and terminating the employment of personal service providers are discussed in Chapter 32.

Dealing with bureaucracies can be very difficult for anyone. Knowing how the agency operates, showing patience, making specific requests, participating actively, and working toward compromises can be effective. Just as clients want agency workers to understand their needs, it is important for clients to understand agency workers' situations and limitations, too. This requires learning about the agency— its rules and procedures—and practicing patience and tact. Also, the ability to state needs and requests accurately and simply is vital. Many bureaucratic snags arise from confusion over what an applicant or client really wants.

Disabled people need to take the lead in the helping process. The skills described in the section, Asserting Oneself, can be applied here. For instance, carry papers personally from one office to another, because waiting for the interoffice mail causes delays. The persistent person keeps paperwork moving on people's desks! Do not hesitate to suggest ways to help the agency be helpful. New ideas offered in a spirit of cooperation and shared responsibility are usually welcomed.

Close Relationships

Close relationships are generally riskier and require more attention to empathy, giving explanations, and making compromises. Negotiation skills are often needed in close relationships. Negotiating simply means bargaining about what each person is willing to give in exchange for something from the other. For example, a disabled person may want or need to negotiate for help. However, one's partner may get resentful. To avoid asking for help too often, it is often a good idea to negotiate the frequency of those requests and agree to a trade-off. The trade-off might be as simple to do as not getting angry when one's partner does something annoying. It is not necessary to trade a physical task for a physical task. A by-product of negotiating is learning what really matters to another person.

Another way to negotiate involves constructive feedback to keep communications open and honest. This includes letting other persons know they are doing or saying something that could cause anger or unhappiness and, perhaps,

limit or end the relationship. Because such feedback often involves criticism, it must be done tactfully and fairly. Chapter 13 on team functioning offers tips on how to give constructive feedback to another person in ways that help the relationship and are not perceived as attacks.

Parents of disabled people often overprotect them. The techniques of constructive feedback can help children teach parents how much more they could help if they protected less. Encourage parents to give feedback on how the child's actions affect them. Then, both parents and child can anticipate and acknowledge each other's feelings; give brief, honest explanations; and seek mutually acceptable compromises.

This last topic may be a problem more people would like to have. An unexpected, large increase in income— through settlement of a suit or the granting of service-connected benefits to a veteran—may strain relationships with relatives. People who are not experienced in handling large sums of money sometimes try to buy love and affection. They may try to impress people with the amount of income they have. At the same time, they may think that nobody loves them except for their money. These kinds of situations can disrupt family relationships. If someone wants to give people money, make sure everyone understands the giver's reasons. Generally, money should not be used as a reward or punishment with loved ones. If there are strings attached, the relationship may be headed for trouble.

ACQUIRING INTERPERSONAL SKILLS

Settings

1. *Hospitals.* Trieschmann (1988) has pointed out that acute care hospitals are rarely good places to learn interpersonal skills. Too often, the so-called patient is seen as a passive recipient of instructions and guidelines from hospital staff. Thus, few opportunities to test alternative ideas may be given. When staffing is low, passive-submissive behavior may be rewarded so that duties are accomplished, and assertiveness may be treated as a personality problem! Rehabilitation hospital personnel are becoming aware of the problems this creates for their patients later on, however, and are trying to correct their errors. Some facilities are now offering assertiveness skill training to inpatients and outpatients.

2. *Rehabilitation centers.* Rehabilitation centers for people with sensory and physical disabilities usually have the advantages of larger staffs and large peer groups that give opportunities to see different kinds of models, both good and bad. Also, a large psychosocial staff may be available. Still, the emphasis is on physical or sensory retraining. The ability to use available sensory and physical skills to their

greatest advantage helps in dealing with people interpersonally. However, specific training in interpersonal skills and social relationships is also needed, and in most rehabilitation centers, little is offered. A few outstanding exceptions include the Palo Alto Veterans Administration Medical Center, which has social skills training programs for blind, brain injured, and spinal cord injured people; Presbyterian Hospital in New York City; Craig Rehabilitation Center in Englewood, Colorado; and The Institute of Rehabilitation and Research in Houston, Texas. This situation will probably change in the next few years as rehabilitation centers recognize the importance of good interpersonal relationships for disabled people.

3. *Independent living centers*. These facilities offer good opportunities for peer relationships, a wide variety of good models, and the most opportunity for practice in the real world. They typically use peer counselors, people who are personally familiar with the social disadvantages of disability, and who also may be trained in social relationships, community reentry, and interpersonal skills.

Sharing feelings about the social implications of disability, trying out suggestions such as those given in this book, getting feedback, and changing approaches to situations can be facilitated by the support given in these centers. Being coached by an individual who has dealt with similar situations before makes people less anxious and, therefore, more successful in their own efforts. Independent living centers have also developed programs that offer learning modules covering practical aspects of independent living such as money management, social skills, sexuality, using community resources, consumer affairs, activities of daily living, housing arrangements, time management, and vocational opportunities. The most useful programs teach factual knowledge plus interpersonal skills.

4. *The community*. Most disabled people are not involved in independent living centers, hospitals, or rehabilitation centers but instead live in the so-called natural environment of the community, which can be a haphazard or counterproductive training ground. See Cogswell (1968) for more on the natural environment of spinal cord injured people. However, real-life situations do make the best training experiences. People respond in their normal ways and give beneficial feedback.

Exercises

Certain exercises can strengthen and improve social and interpersonal skills. It should be emphasized that these exercises are growth experiences; they are not panaceas or cure-alls. Strengthening social skills through such exercises helps people deal with the social environment but will not, by themselves, resolve social problems. It may also be necessary to change certain attitudes about social behavior, or to change specific behaviors. These exercises may also help people learn how to accomplish these goals.

Exercises to Do by Oneself

These exercises are designed to help people increase comfort and decrease anxiety in difficult situations. They are also designed to increase one's own motivation and involvement in learning social skills. They develop ways to practice interpersonal skills mentally, to rehearse them, and to imagine how to deal with troublesome situations.

Relaxation. Relaxation is a difficult skill for many people. Society is a stressful environment, and some people respond to stress by tensing their muscles or becoming emotionally upset, which may cause excessively rapid breathing, poor blood circulation, or stomach acid secretions. To reduce these troublesome physiological responses which may occur in new situations, learn to relax by using these exercises.

First, find a quiet place where there will be no interruptions. Then, get into a comfortable position. Sit or lie down, and try to become aware of particular muscles. Notice where the tension is, then tense and relax each of the major muscle groups starting with the facial muscles (a very important group) and working downward. If a muscle group is paralyzed, imagine tensing it. While tensing the muscle for a few seconds, be sure to inhale; then exhale when relaxing the muscle. As the muscle relaxes, think the work *relax*, and imagine a calm, peaceful scene that gives a sense of happiness and comfort. This may be the seashore or mountains, or even a favorite room. Practice this exercise twice a day for 2 or 3 weeks until it becomes automatic. Then use this technique to relax in difficult situations or when attempting new things.

Another relaxation technique is deep regular breathing. Practice filling the lungs to a count of four (or any other number that is comfortable), hold it in for half that count; then use the full count to exhale all of the breath. The more this is practiced at home, the more effective it will be when used in social emergencies such as feeling afraid to speak in class or before a group. Breath control is a very important part of relaxation. Even if one's vital capacity for breathing is seriously impaired by disability, it is still possible to control the *regularity* of breathing. This is almost as calming as breathing more *deeply*. Add half a dozen (or more) of these breathing cycles to the daily exercise program.

Mental rehearsal. Mental rehearsal involves trying out a behavior or response in the mind. Imagine a situation and how to handle it. This is not a substitute for action; it is an aid to action. It is being used more and more by athletes, and is a good way to reduce anxiety in new situations. Some people may have the needed assertiveness skills but still feel anxious about trying them. Mental rehearsal may help such individuals anticipate their own feelings and examine any irrational ideas that might hold them back before making an assertive response.

Table 31–3 gives a series of rational statements to repeat to oneself while imagining being in a different social situation. These statements can help people deal with the anxiety they feel about entering the situation.

Table 31–4 presents a series of statements to use in a similar way for coping in the actual situation. Saying these statements to oneself when one is anxious helps to reduce anxiety. When combining mental rehearsal with relaxation techniques, it is most effective to say these statements to oneself after becoming relaxed.

Self-reinforcement. *Self-reinforcement* means strengthening the ability to perform an activity by rewarding oneself for making gains. Some people take an all-or-none approach to reaching goals. If they do not succeed completely, they do not take any credit for the gains they did make. It is much more effective to set small, step-by-step goals for oneself. Each time one of these small goals or steps is reached, give a small reward. Instead of promising oneself a long vacation after reaching the final goal it is better to reward oneself with a movie or a dinner out for having accomplished the small goal. The reinforcement depends on what one considers to be a reward.

Some people make lists of specific things they would like to have or do and use those for self-rewards. This may call for a little self-discipline. For example, a person who enjoys watching football games might watch a particular game only after accomplishing a small goal that has often been postponed. Sometimes, self-reinforcement can take the form of simply saying to oneself, "You did a good job there" or "You're making fine progress." The good feelings that come from self-reinforcement can help increase a person's self-esteem and increase involvement and motivation to continue with any desired behavioral change program.

TABLE 31–3   Rational Statements to Reduce Worry about Situations that Have Not Yet Happened

- I will never be able to please everyone all the time no matter how hard I try.
- I have the right to stand up for myself no matter how well known another person is.
- If I make a mistake, I am only proving that I am human.
- If this goes wrong it is unfortunate, but it's not awful; it's not a catastrophe.
- All human beings make mistakes no matter how much they try to avoid them; mistakes may be unfortunate, but they are not terrible.
- I will learn from the mistakes I make. Not everyone is going to like what I do all the time, and it is not logical for me to expect them to.
- I am important and want to stand up for myself.
- If I lose someone's approval by asserting myself, I will onlyprove that I can't please everyone all the time.
- I will learn to cope with occasional rejection from others.

Adapted from Rakos and Schroeder (1980)

TABLE 31–4   Rational Statements to Reduce Anxiety in Difficult Situations

- Take a deep breath and relax. Stay calm!
- I'm in control—stay calm!
- This anxiety will eventually disappear as I gain experience.
- Here is a good situation to try assertion in. It will be over shortly.
- Keep calm and look right at them. This is a good learning situation, so I will go through with it.
- I'm not going to do this perfectly, but that's to be expected.
- Nothing terrible will happen if this fails.
- I am going to stand up for myself this time.
- I am probably anxious over nothing. They will probably respect what I have to say.

Adapted from Rakos and Schroeder (1980)

Using role models. Using role models simply means observing how others deal with similar situations. It is a way of learning from the experience of others—from both their mistakes as well as their successes. Role models can be found everywhere: in books and films, and by watching people in everyday life. Consumer-operated, independent living centers are particularly good places to find socially successful disabled role models; so are associations of blind, deaf, or physically disabled citizens. Try watching how successful disabled people deal with problematic situations. Concentrate on the components of assertiveness. Pay attention to the consequences of these approaches. Watch what happens to the person who uses a particular approach and see if it is a desirable consequence. In this way, one can often learn as much from bad examples as from good ones.

Behavior rehearsal. Behavior rehearsal is like mental rehearsal except that one actually tries out the behaviors and evaluates them in private. Use a tape recorder to practice speaking loudly, firmly, and fluently. Use a full-length mirror to get feedback on posture and to encourage making eye contact. A videotape recording of the rehearsal could give the best information on both the auditory and visual aspects of the performance. It allows one to see oneself as others do.

Few individuals can afford such a luxury, but a few rehabilitation centers provide social skills training using videotape feedback. Act out social situations many people find difficult. Imagine the other person responding, watch the mirror, and then replay the audiotapes. Compare your response to the guidelines presented in Table 31–1. Is it too passive or submissive? Is it overly aggressive? Or is it appropriately assertive and likely to be effective?

Exercises to Try with the Help of Others
Even though self-exercises are helpful, their disadvantage is that there is no person to try things out with and to give

actual social interaction experiences. Therefore, it is often very useful to develop and maintain a *support group* that can give honest feedback, encouragement, moral support, and social rewards. These should be people one can trust and be honest with: friends, relatives, peers from an independent living center, attendants, readers, interpreters, or agency workers and professionals one particularly likes. Relatives sometimes have difficulty giving critical feedback and often need reassurance that even if their comments cause temporary hurt feelings, they are appreciated because the person wants to know how to relate to other people better.

For different reasons, one's personal employees may also hesitate to be honestly critical. However, if the relationship is a fairly trusting one for both people, the personal service provider may be a very good source of feedback.

When asking for feedback from members of a support group or other people, one might say something like, "How do you think I did in that situation?" or "I'm trying to work on refusing unreasonable requests, did I say 'no' firmly enough?" or, "Would you listen to how I say this and see if I'm convincing?" and, sometimes, "I'm trying to change, and I really want your honest opinion." Such statements and questions demonstrate that a person needs and wants honest feedback. Be careful to thank people for their honesty and equally careful not to strike back when a comment stings encourages more constructive feedback.

Rehearsing ways of handling situations with supportive people can reduce anxiety and embarrassment later when trying the response in a real situation. Use two other people, one to role play and one as an observer. It is very difficult to look at one's own behavior while engaged in the situation. An observer is often helpful in behavior rehearsal exercises. Also, these support people can switch roles so each one takes a turn as the observer. Tables 31–5 and 31–6 give some exercises to try.

It may also be useful to create situations based on problems actually encountered. To do this:

- Rate the situations for how much difficulty they cause. Start with the easier situations.
- Try a way of handling each situation for a few minutes, and then get feedback from the other person who is role playing and from the observer. Try again and get feedback until everyone is satisfied with the performance. Specific feedback is most helpful. Remember, however, that other people are not the final judges. An individual does not have to agree with the recommendations of the support group.
- Also reverse roles; that is, the disabled person can take the role of a salesperson. Try to "be" that person and observe how the support person responds.
- Try interacting more aggressively, assertively, or passively, and see how the other person's responses change with different types of approaches.

TABLE 31–5   Disability-Specific Situations for Role Playing

Narrator:	You see a person pulling into a parking space reserved for handicapped drivers. It has a wheelchair sign over it. The driver rolls down the window and says:
Man:	"Will it be okay if I park here? I'll just be a minute or so."
Narrator:	You have not seen a friend since you were injured. You meet on the street and she says,
Friend:	"Oh, no! I didn't know that you were paralyzed. How did it happen? How long is it going to last?"
Narrator:	You are in a hallway looking for a telephone. You finally see one but realize it is too high for you to reach the coin slot; you'll need to get some help with the phone. You look around and see someone coming down the hall. He looks your way and says:
Passer-by:	"Hey, how ya' doin' today?"
Narrator:	You are in a favorite restaurant with your date. She has just finished giving her order to the waitress. The waitress looks at your date and asks her:
Waitress:	"And what will *he* have?"
Narrator:	You are at a party, and you discover that your external catheter has popped. Another guest notices the wet spot on your slacks:
Guest:	"Did you spill something?"
Narrator:	You are shopping downtown. A woman comes up to you, puts her hand on your shoulder and says:
Woman:	"Will you pray with me to the Lord and be saved, so you can be whole once again?"

Adapted from Dunn and Herman 1982

- Try having the other person in the interaction act as a successively harder and harder person with whom to deal. For example, instruct the person to use aggressive intimidation to make responding more difficult.
- Finally, try the approach that seems to work best in the natural environment. If someone else can observe one's response, all the better. If that is not possible, the actual consequences can provide feedback on how one did in the situation. If an approach works, makes a person feel better, more comfortable, and less anxious, and if the outcome is good, then probably that situation is being managed adequately.

Resources

If the suggestions presented in this chapter do not help, one's problems seem too serious for self-help, or one's friends

TABLE 31–6 Practice Examples for Behavior Rehearsals

Narrator:	You are in a restaurant with some friends. You order a very rare steak. The waiter brings steak to the table which is so well done it looks charred.
Waiter:	"I hope you enjoy your dinner."
Narrator:	You bring your car to a service station to have a grease job and the oil changed. The mechanic tells you that your car will be ready in an hour. When you return to the station, you find that in addition to the oil change and the grease job, they have given your car a major tune-up. You tell the guy at the front desk your name and ask for the keys.
Clerk:	"Will that be cash or charge? That comes to $215.00."
Narrator:	You have just come home from work, and as you settle down to read the newspaper, you discover that your spouse has cut out an important article to save what is on the reverse side. You really like to read the whole newspaper.
Spouse:	"You don't mind? I just wanted to cut this out before I forgot about it."
Narrator:	You are at home alone watching an exciting event on TV when someone knocks at your front door. When you open the door you find a man who says he is selling vacuum cleaners.
Salesperson:	"Let me come in and demonstrate our latest model. It will take only fifteen minutes of your time."
Narrator:	You are having lunch with a friend who suddenly asks if you would lend him $30.00 until payday. You have the money.
Friend:	"Please lend me the money; I'll pay you back next week."
Narrator:	You are in a crowded grocery store and are in a hurry. You have picked up one small item and get in line to pay for it when another shopper with a cart full of groceries cuts in line, right in front of you.
Shopper:	"Do you mind if I cut in here? I'm late for an appointment."

Adapted from Eisler, Miller, and Herson (1973)

cannot give enough objective feedback, consider using expert help.

Assertiveness courses are offered at many community colleges and other state-supported schools, and often the costs are low. These courses emphasize general social skills and rarely deal with disability-related issues.

Group counseling or therapy offers another possibility. It provides opportunities for practicing social interactions, a good source of feedback from others, and more support from a trained leader. People should choose a group that is working on problems they want to manage and that has a style that will help them learn. Ask a nearby rehabilitation, independent living, or college counseling center for recommended groups. When trying outside help, do not hesitate to drop out if it does not seem to suit one's needs. It is best, however, to consult the group leader about decisions like this to get feedback about whether the desire to leave the group is related to getting close to issues that are emotionally upsetting. Perhaps one should stay, despite temporary discomfort, to learn what is needed.

Mental health workers in rehabilitation hospitals or in private practice are a valuable resource if problems require individual professional help. Rehabilitation psychologists and social workers realize that disabled people are often so concerned about their bodily problems that it is difficult to admit that they may also have interpersonal difficulties. Yet disabilities may create interpersonal problems, which are as important to solve as the physical problems.

State vocational rehabilitation agencies typically provide training in job-finding skills, which include teaching how to conduct oneself on job interviews and to deal with employers. These services are very useful. The skills learned can help in many relationships even though they are designed to aid, specifically, in relations with employers. The ability to be assertive with employers will carry over to other situations.

Many books are available on assertiveness in general social situations. In addition, for general assertiveness, a home study course is available on audiotape (Rakos and Schroeder 1980).

IN CLOSING

This chapter has presented a number of situations that are difficult to manage. It has shown reasons why, in the real world, these situations are difficult; it has suggested exercises for learning how to deal with these situations; and it has attempted to encourage individuals to examine their social skills and change those aspects with which they are not satisfied. Change is difficult and does not always proceed in a regular pattern. There will be ups and downs, mistakes and successes. Treasure the mistakes! They offer excellent and important learning experiences. Study them to find more effective approaches.

REFERENCES

Alberti, F. and Emmons, F. L. 1974. *Your Perfect Right: A Guide to Assertive Behavior*. San Luis Obispo, CA: Impact Publishing.

Cogswell, B. D. 1968. Self-socialization: Readjustment of paraplegics in the community. *Journal of Rehabilitation* 34: 11–13.

Dunn, M. and Herman, S. 1982. In *Behavioral Psychology in Medicine Assessment and Training Strategies*. Ed. D. Doley. New York: Plenum Press.

Eisler, R., Miller, P., and Herson, M. 1973. Components of assertive behavior. *Journal of Clinical Psychology* 29: 295–299.

Huston, T. L., and Levinger, G. 1978. Interpersonal attraction and relationships. *Annual Review in Psychology*, 115–156.

Jackson, T. 1989. *Guerrilla Tactics in the Job Market*. New York: Bantam Books.

Jakubowski-Specter, P. 1973. *An Introduction to Assertive Procedures for Women*. Washington, DC: American Personnel and Guidance Association.

Rakos, R. F., and Schroeder, H. E. 1980. *Self-Directed Assertiveness Training*. BMA Audio Cassettes, 200 Park Avenue S., New York, NY 10003.

Schachtel, D., and Dunn, M. 1990. *Social Skills in the '90s—Coping with SCI in Social Situations*. Videotape. Atlanta, GA: Shepherd Spinal Center.

Trieschmann, R. 1988. *Spinal Cord Injuries: Psychological, Social and Vocational Adjustment*. 2d ed. New York: Demos Publications.

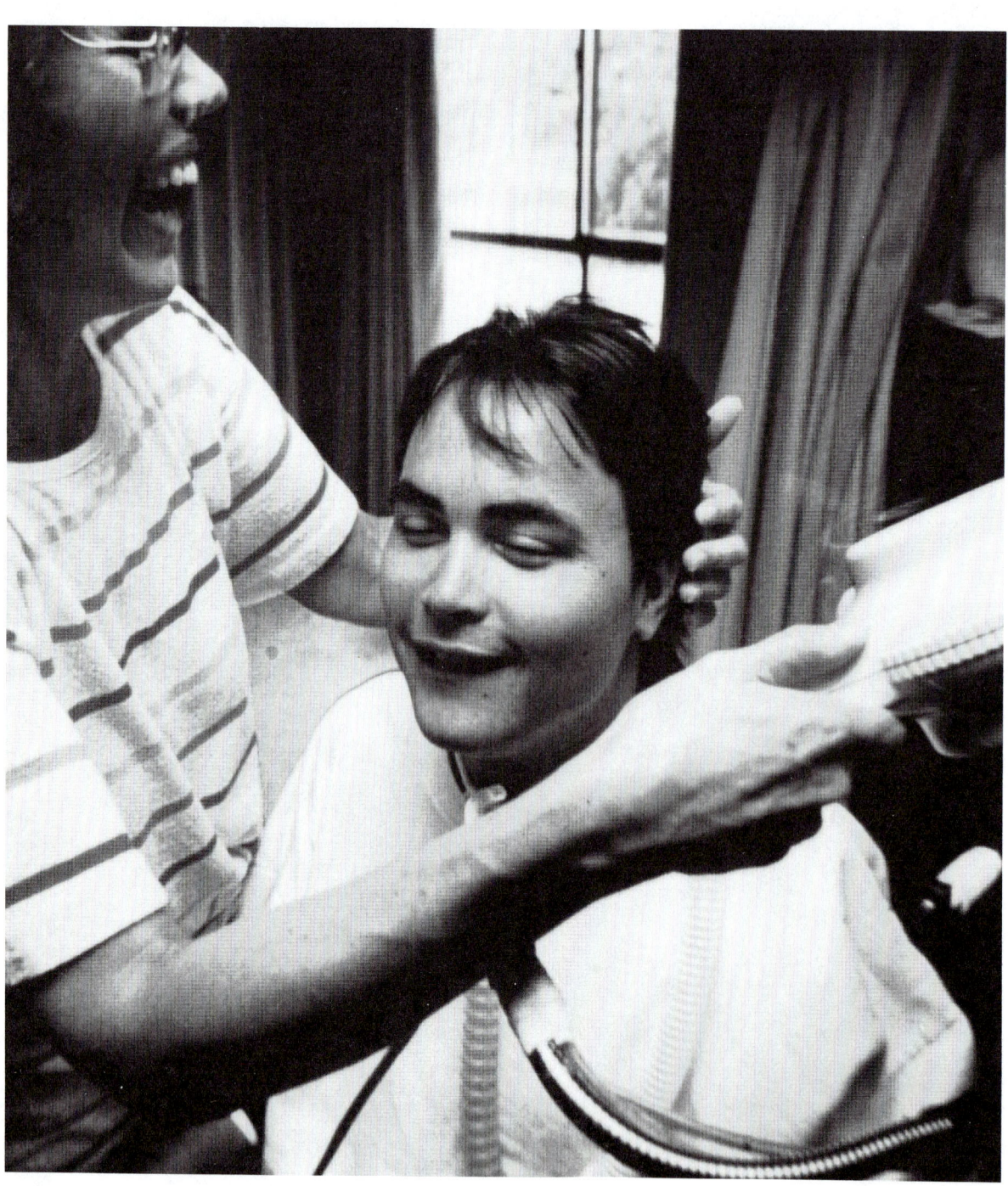

CHAPTER 32

Teaching Attendant Management Skills

Alfred H. DeGraff, M.S., S.E.A.

Chapter Outline

Objectives

- To describe the advantages of the direct management of attendants by people who receive assistance
- To review the growing need for health care facilities to establish programs that teach patients attendant management skills
- To propose a program model to best prepare individuals

> Give me a fish and I eat for a day—Teach me to fish and I eat for a lifetime!

Many people with physical limitations imposed as a result of spinal cord injury (SCI) require physical assistance throughout life. Some people require extensive help each day; others need only occasional help either weekly or for special projects.

Needs can include assistance with personal hygiene, bathing, toileting, grooming, dressing, wheelchair transfers, eating, cooking, shopping, laundry, housekeeping, transportation, and maintaining medical equipment. This assistance enables people with SCI to pursue education, employment, religious interests, sports, leisure, recreational pursuits, and travel.

Typically these services are provided by a person hired to be an *attendant*. Traditionally, attendants were trained and supervised by an outside agency. However, for disabled people living independently, this approach is frequently not workable and is very costly. The independent living movement is based on the idea that people with disabilities (consumers) should be in control of the support services they use and purchase. Consumer control means rights, responsibilities, and *choices* (DeGraff 1988; Ulicny, Adler, Kennedy, and Jones 1987).

LIFE GOALS

Whether physical assistance is needed hourly, weekly, or monthly, an individual with SCI needs certain skills. The overall goal of these skills is to acquire and maintain dependable and quality assistance on a schedule that accommodates the person's life-style.

Even for the most simple request, a variety of skills is needed to:

- Identify the need for assistance
- Decide how to communicate the request in a clear, effective, often assertive manner
- Organize the tasks at hand
- Receive the help
- Provide feedback

More extensive skills include finding, interviewing, training, evaluating, paying, and even firing help providers.

In essence, these skills are *management* skills and are vital regardless of whether aides are acquired from agencies or from direct, personal recruitment. Even the best trained, most experienced aide must be oriented to specific duties and informed of personal needs and preferences. Everyone who receives help must provide initial instruction as well as maintain a smooth, ongoing working relationship. The level of person-to-person management skills attained usually determines the level of success in using attendants and, therefore, the degree of success in meeting personal objectives each day.

DILEMMAS IN ATTENDANT CARE

Ideally, the frequency and type of assistance would vary in direct proportion to level of physical abilities and desired amount of independence, that is, the individual's preference as to when and how to spend time and energy on various daily living activities (conserving strength for more important activities such as school or work and other interests). Realistically, however, services are severely limited by lack of funding sources; lack of availability of reliable attendants (often related to low wages); and a widespread lack of recognition of the types and severity of problems encountered by disabled people.

Another problem is that not all attendants are worthy and honest. Consumer exploitation in the form of robbery or physical abuse, for example, is widespread. Increasing awareness of this problem and introducing steps to decrease its likelihood must be explored long before discharge from a rehabilitation center.

Currently, there is not a coherent system of attendant care. Philosophies and definitions vary from state to state and one location to another. Even if a payment source is secured, confusion reigns over who is allowed to do what, especially concerning invasive procedures such as catheterizations. In acute care settings such procedures may only be performed by nurses, but as people with greater and greater degrees of physical disabilities survive and technology becomes part of their daily lives, some of these restrictive practices must give way to new rules, even if risks are involved.

Just a few years ago, no one envisioned a student dependent on a mechanical ventilator in a classroom. Constant, reliable support services are needed behind the scenes to make this happen. The only alternative is a life without access to attendant services, filled with barriers that result in human tragedy and high economic cost. Health care professionals must continue to support people with disabilities beyond the critical care period, through research and political and social action (see Chapter 2).

THE CONCEPT OF CONSUMER MANAGEMENT OF ATTENDANT SERVICES

There are two primary sources for attendant services: agencies or direct personal employment. An agency recruits, interviews, trains, pays, and otherwise manages aides for each client who requires services. Agency services are essential to anyone who lacks either the ability or desire to employ their own aide directly. Using agency personnel seems to provide some assurance that someone will always be there, but actually this is frequently not the case. Most agencies acknowledge there is an increasing demand for qualified aides while there is a shrinking supply of aides willing to work for agencies. Consequently, agencies find it difficult, if not impossible in many areas, to meet client needs and schedules. In major cities, waiting lists of 300 clients are not uncommon, not to mention the dry periods such as weekends and holidays when help is simply not available. Increasing numbers of disabled people, who can bring financial resources together and have mastered adequate management skills, are thus opting to employ aides directly.

Research strongly supports the use of consumer-directed models of attendant services management, as well as long-term, large-scale demonstration projects (Ulicny et al. 1987). Projects demonstrating cost containment and a means to provide flexibility in attendant duties stimulate appropriate client training programs in rehabilitation centers to best prepare clients for successful independent living.

From an ethical viewpoint, when examining the rationale for teaching and learning management skills, it is important to understand the numerous ways in which attendants affect personal life-styles. People who learn to manage the assistance they use have certain advantages, or *freedoms* (DeGraff 1988). See Table 32–1.

Program planners must make decisions about effective approaches to attendant instruction and whether to train aides or the consumers who manage the aides. Too often, programs have fostered dependence rather than the desired independence. Obviously both clients and attendants need appropriate instruction to ensure a safe transition to the community. Attendants must be trained to assist ventilator-dependent persons, for example, but the focus must remain on consumer control to prepare for lifetime needs.

For the predominantly young SCI population, instruction that teaches independent management is most important, especially when assistants are willing to work but have no related previous experience. The skills of managing personal attendant assistance allow maximum control; the mere feeling of being in control contributes significantly to feelings of competency and assertive actions essential to living independently.

BARRIERS TO INDEPENDENCE: CONSIDERATIONS FOR ESTABLISHING AN INSTRUCTIONAL PROGRAM

In the past, there has been confusion because of the mistaken beliefs that all requests for physical assistance can be met by a local agency that trains and manages attendants,

and that necessary management skills develop from common sense and self-instruction.

As already noted, the agencies have significant difficulty filling client requests. However, clients who have learned adequate management skills can usually directly recruit a sufficient number of aides who wish to avoid agencies and work directly for an individual.

Furthermore, very few people can learn the wide variety of management skills by mere common sense. The trial-and-error approach is time consuming and costly. For many people who initially rely on family help after hospital discharge, this experiential learning usually creates unnecessary stress for family members. When outside aides are initially employed, there is often one aide crisis after another and, consequently, a high rate of turnover. For these physically dependent people without adequate management skills, the inability to find and maintain quality help is often the most frequent source of frustration, depression, and the loss of optimism and motivation. Formal instruction in attendant home health aides management can significantly minimize these common problems.

Most health care facilities find that establishing an instructional program in attendant management is not an overwhelming task, especially once a program model is identified that can be used in whole or with modifications.

SHOULD A PROGRAM BE ESTABLISHED? ASSESSING THE NEEDS OF THE CLIENT CONSTITUENCY

Few rehabilitation programs provide adequate instruction in teaching people how to plan their needs for physical assistance, and then directly manage others in providing that help. However, most health care programs include the objective of preparing people with physical limitations to cope with everyday life and should assess appropriate instruction in attendant management. In planning a program of appropriate instruction, the facility or agency should first assess the needs of its client constituency.

Patients or clients who have physical limitations and need some level of assistance usually can be grouped into three primary categories (DeGraff 1988).

The first category includes people who want to manage their assistance and have adequate psychological and physical abilities to do so. These people are the most important ones to instruct according to individual needs. For instance, people who will require extensive physical assistance for a lifetime should be able to choose the most comprehensive level of instruction, and high-functioning people or individuals with a short-term need for assistance will probably choose briefer, less comprehensive instruction.

TABLE 32–1   Freedoms

Freedom from having to use parents or relatives as attendants

Many people would like to relocate on their own but hesitate to do so because they are unsure of whether they could find help as reliable as that which their parents currently provide. Or maybe *they* are confident that they could find other help, but their *parents* lack that same confidence and consequently pressure them to stay home.

In other situations, problems occur between parents and children because of role confusion. Traditionally, a parent raises a child for eventual independence, and the child looks forward to leaving home. When SCI occurs to either party, frustration and depression can be realized by both parties because this traditional goal seems to be gone forever. The goal of freedom has been replaced by the initial impression that the injured party will always be physically dependent on the other party. Indeed, the ability to manage outside sources of assistance can restore the dream of independence for both parent and child.

Many people with disabilities currently reside at home with attendant help provided entirely by parents or relatives. For some

people, this is a very satisfactory living situation. For others, there is a wish either to continue to live with one's folks but to supplement the attendant help they provide with some outside help, or to actually move out of the household to the independence of a new location across the neighborhood or across the country.

There are many justifiable reasons for wishing to relocate. They include the desire to pursue training at a college, university, or vocational school, or to pursue a career. Other people who require assistance simply yearn for the privacy and independence of living on their own. Maybe they have their sights set on a potential relationship.

Regardless of the reason, almost everyone who needs assistance must recognize that the time will come when parents or relatives will no longer be able to provide assistance. Parents will either become too old to help physically, or brothers and sisters will someday move out on their own.

Freedom from having to use a spouse or lover as an attendant or sole attendant

Whether someone has a lover or spouse or hopes to find one, both persons should know that there are alternatives to having a partner automatically assume all attendant needs. Understandably, to gain as much privacy as possible, the first inclination for a new couple is often to do away with outside attendants. The partner therefore begins to assume all attendant responsibilities, which perhaps had formerly been divided each day between two or more attendants. Those responsibilities were divided because they were probably too extensive for one person to handle. Fatigue can result in a frequent turnover of overworked attendants, and it certainly should be prevented from happening in a relationship planned for a lifetime.

In a romantic relationship visual contact and touching is part of sexual attraction. When one partner relies on the other for assistance with toileting, for example, these activities can become associated with very unromantic feelings which can become detrimental or even fatal to a couple's sex life. Because of these unromantic

associations, sexual interest can diminish, and contact and touching may no longer result in sexual arousal for the spouse who assumes attendant duties. Meanwhile, the partner may be frustrated in trying to retain an original set of associations and interest. This does not happen to everyone but many people need to consider this carefully.

A desire to hire outside help need not be a sign of a mate's rejection or of an unstable relationship. On the contrary, it can prevent problems, or at least minimize their occurrence. Judicious choices should be made when deciding which attendant needs will be assigned to outside help. A high priority might be given to certain duties, possibly because of their heavy physical nature (such as lifting) or their routine occurrence when a mate would like to be doing something else. On the other hand, it is unwise to schedule outside help that would interrupt valuable private time, when both could sleep in or stay up late, for example.

Freedom to directly control the type, quality, and schedule of attendants—and to change attendants—whenever necessary

If a person owned a fancy restaurant that had a posh reputation, the owner would certainly want direct control over hiring waiters. If a restaurant owner would insist on direct control over waiters who serve other people, then why should people who require assistance for personal needs settle for anything less?

Yet many attendant referral programs in home health agencies, college campuses, and independent living centers do manage personal care attendants for individuals who need assistance in this way. Many programs recruit, screen, interview, attempt to train, and even supervise the salaries of attendants, instead of helping people who require assistance to acquire these skills for their own management and direct control.

Of course some people are either unable or unwilling to directly instruct and manage the help they use. For them, the use of an agency or attendant coordination program to instruct and manage is essential. However, for others who are capable of managing, there is little reason not to learn management skills, and therefore be free from the limitations which come with using many coordinating services.

Even with the best coordinating services, when people who require assistance are assigned aides, many times they are quite limited in

the type and quality of aides they are given each day. In addition, many people find that they must start and end their daily personal activities not according to their own schedule, but according to when their assigned aide shows up. In many instances, the agency schedules the same aide among several service recipients each day. If one of these "clients" on an attendant's morning list takes a bit longer to help than expected, or if the attendant is late getting to even the first morning client, then the attendant's arrival at every subsequent client is often delayed and each individual's personal schedule is affected unexpectedly. The preventive measure taken by some agencies against these delays from occurring is to strictly limit the amount of time that an aide can spend with a client to the exact amount of scheduled time; consequently, any unexpected accidents or other personal needs of a client simply cannot be accommodated!

The answer to avoiding these problems, for those capable of managing the assistance they use, is to take a bit of time to learn how to take direct control over hiring and firing of the aides who are personally used . . . direct control over their type, quality, and schedule. Management skills make it possible to control these factors and to change attendants whenever necessary.

(Table continues)

TABLE 32–1 Freedoms (continued)

Freedom from being dependent on aide pools or referral agency lists, and the consequent ability to relocate wherever and whenever necessary

Many agency services maintain a pool or listing of people who are willing to provide aide help. An aide pool can be quite helpful to individuals who have either just moved into a new area or who have not yet developed skills for recruiting aides on their own. First, newcomers usually need aide help immediately on arrival to the new area, before (it would seem) personal recruiting could take place. Second, the newcomer may not be familiar right away with resources for personally recruiting aides in the new city or college campus.

Although a home health aide agency or an attendant pool is helpful to many such newcomers, it is not essential. Very competent attendants can be hired, sight unseen, from a thousand miles away. Surely, not every individual who requires assistance and who has moved to a new section of the country has either convinced an old attendant to move with them or chosen their new home only according to where there was another attendant pool!

Furthermore, people who need assistance can become detrimentally dependent on a local, handy attendant pool. Even after becoming well established at a community or college campus, one naturally finds that using the pool is sometimes easier than doing one's own

recruiting. In fact, many individuals never even bother to learn how to recruit because they have become so comfortably dependent on using the pool as their only means to finding new attendants. This dependence—like any other—can lead to losing control of one's life-style and to limiting personal freedom and independence.

If attendant pools used by referral agencies always met one's needs adequately, or if they existed everywhere, then there certainly would be no objection to becoming comfortably dependent on them. But there are actually many problems with pools. A constant supply of aides may not be available through agencies due to their recruiting problems. The service's inability to supply aides may be temporary or prolonged. Several hours might elapse before a replacement can be recruited by the agency, or the delay might last several days.

Furthermore, sooner or later, almost everyone finds the need to move away from the local pool of an agency, campus, or independent living center. Being able to manage one's own attendant help provides maximum flexibility to relocate one's residence wherever and whenever necessary.

Freedom from having to use agency or college campus attendant training services

In addition to maintaining attendant pools, many professional agencies, college campuses, and independent living centers provide attendant training services. However, these programs usually attempt to hire and train attendants *for* the individuals who require assistance. The actual services vary, but they can include recruiting, interviewing, screening, conveying an awareness of the appropriate role of an attendant, training in the delivery of a wide variety of personal care services, assigning an attendant to an individual (or the same one to several individuals), and possibly even supervising an attendant's time sheets and salary payments.

An attendant training program that performs all or part of these functions can be a benefit to someone who has not yet learned how to be independent in managing that help. Pretrained aides are also essential to those who are themselves unable or unwilling to train and manage assistance. However, for those capable of managing, an attendant training program, like a constantly available attendant pool, has the detrimental potential to postpone one's eventual need to learn these management skills. People who rely on these services too many times do not bother to learn how to perform these procedures independently. Consequently, when they inevitably move, they are suddenly faced with the need to learn the

management procedures. Ironically, the individual would already have developed the self-sufficient skills if the "helpful" attendant training program had not existed!

In addition, regardless of how poorly or how well a training program works, people who need assistance must inevitably provide the final details of instruction to each aide about their own particular needs. A program usually teaches a group of prospective aides in the generic types of help that they *might* be asked to deliver, because the program cannot predict the specific needs of each individual whom each attendant will be helping, and therefore which specific services each attendant should learn. When a person who needs assistance initially meets even the best trained, most experienced aide, that aide is certain to make the key request, "Please instruct me as to what specific needs you have and the manner and schedule in which you would prefer your particular duties performed."

Consequently, a college campus or independent living center program that is truly interested in helping people prepare for self-sufficient, independent living should offer first a well-structured program to train *those who use assistance,* and possibly second a program to train *those who provide assistance.*

Freedom from having to pay the high hourly administrative rates to professional home health aide agencies, if one is not eligible for third-party funding

A primary professional source for finding aides or attendants in many communities is a home health aide agency. The agency recruits, trains, schedules, pays, and otherwise manages aides for the client. These services are very important to many people, especially people who are new to a locale and unsure where to find attendants on their own, have brief impairments or illnesses, people for whom attendant services are funded and the funding source requires the use of agency-supplied aides, and people who are unable or unwilling to manage their own attendant assistance.

First, there is some inflexibility in not being able to change a personal schedule quickly once an aide on a set schedule has been

assigned. There is also a lack of full freedom to change aides if problems occur. In addition, a replacement aide might not be readily available from the agency's pool in case a regular aide does not arrive as scheduled.

Furthermore, the agency aides who provide help are often restricted by the agency in the amount of time that they can spend with a client, which is unfortunate if unpredictable accidents happen. In addition, agencies often restrict aides in the types of work they can perform, as contrasted with the numerous types of work that an individual can request directly employed attendants to perform.

(Table continues)

TABLE 32–1   Freedoms (continued)

A further issue is monetary. The agency charges administrative fees for its management services as well as other overhead expenses, in addition to the hourly salary that it actually pays the home health aides employed for the client. The total of these agency fees is often as much as four to eight times the aide's salary. For example, if an aide is paid $6 an hour, the total fee charged by the professional agency could range from $25 to $50 per hour of provided assistance. Agencies are paid primarily by third-party funding sources, such as government agencies and insurance companies. Many gainfully employed, private citizens are not eligible for long-term, third-party funding and cannot afford agency rates on their own.

In the second category are people who want to manage and have the psychological ability to do so, but who lack one or more physical abilities required for managing. These management abilities can include adequate verbal or audible communication as well as the abilities to maintain paper or computer records for personnel, salaries, and taxes.

It has often been assumed that this individual cannot manage any of the help received, and that this "helpless, totally dependent person" must be "cared for." In truth, the person simply cannot perform a few physical tasks related to management. The solution lies in maintaining complete managerial control while assigning certain training or clerical duties to one of the aides. As an example, a person with high quadriplegia probably would have extensive needs and use more than one part-time aide. A family member or senior aide who best knows the person's routine could act as an attendant coordinator and verbally assist the person during the training of new aides. During this training, the trainee would be reminded that the person with SCI remains the ultimate manager to whom the new aide will be accountable.

The third category of people requiring physical assistance lacks the cognitive abilities to manage or for whatever reason has no desire to do so. For these people, management instruction is probably not appropriate. Instead, the health care program should maintain an adequate list of area attendant agencies for referral. These agencies usually assume responsibility for coordinating and managing a dependent patient's needs. Agency services may not be required when the need for physical assistance seems to be short term and family members seem willing to provide assistance. If family members will be assisted by outside aides, some management instruction for the family is often helpful. However, even in these situations, the list of agencies should be kept available in case the family care is short lived or not adequate.

Having made this assessment of client needs, ask two basic questions:

- Do we serve a significant population of clients or family members who could benefit from an instructional program?
- If so, what program model could be used in structuring our particular program?

THE THREE-SIDED PROGRAM MODEL

Once a facility determines that a significant population would benefit from an instructional program, a program structure should be formulated. A three-sided program model (Figure 32–1) integrates elements of instruction, support, and practice opportunities.

Instruction

Instruction can range from a simple, informal, one-to-one advisory session between a patient and a professional to a structured, formal course of several classes. Whatever the form, initial instruction for the person with SCI should begin as soon after the injury as possible. Even in the acute care setting, encourage patients to be responsible for:

- Beginning to learn which daily living skills (DLS) qualify for self-care and which ones validly require assistance from others
- Learning the safe and efficient methods both for providing self-care and instructing others to provide assistance
- Encouraging self-advocacy when the patient's needs are not reasonably met or poor quality help is provided
- Teaching how to state assertively many of their needs for physical assistance
- Preparing to learn a set of attendant management skills that are appropriately comprehensive to one's high level of need

During rehabilitation, the interdisciplinary staff should first educate patients of their responsibility to learn which personal needs qualify for self-care and which ones validly require assistance from others. Three categories of activities qualify for requesting assistance:

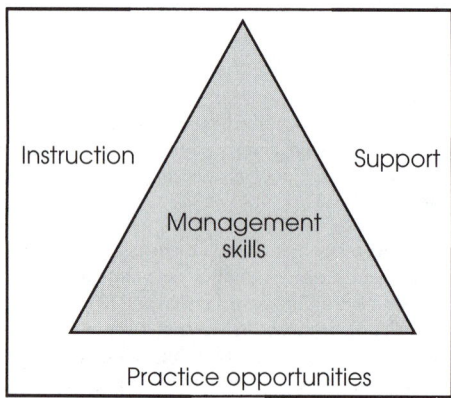

FIGURE 32–1   A three-sided program model.

- Activities, or parts of activities, that are truly beyond one's physical abilities
- Activities that, because of physical limitations and not laziness, take too long or use too much personal energy if attempted independently
- Activities that might jeopardize one's health or safety if attempted independently

Second, the interdisciplinary staff should help the patient learn safe and efficient methods both for providing self-care as well as instructing others to provide assistance. During treatments the patient should not passively receive care, but instead should know what care is being provided, how it is being provided, and why it is being provided in that manner. If a treatment occurs routinely, the patient should be encouraged to self-advocate regarding the quality of care received. The patient should be reminded that poor care will result in poor health, and that monitoring the quality of care is the patient's responsibility for a lifetime. Patients enter into these activities at different rates; to accept responsibility is to accept the disability, to some degree.

With regard to stating needs for assistance assertively, patients should be taught not to adopt a passive, dependent role in which they expect that routine DLS needs will be automatically cared for by health professionals. Preparation for hospital and rehabilitation discharge should begin the first day, no matter how many months ahead actual discharge might be. The well-established passive, dependent mind set of an inpatient is poor preparation for the assertive, self-caring mind set essential for success in the mainstream of society.

Too often staff involved in the discharge process begin to instill the self-care mind set during the last week of an inpatient stay. By then, the passive mind set is too well established. The patient arrives at home expecting the hospital care to continue from relatives and family. Many outpatients come to the confusing, sudden realization that their relatives, family, or even attendants are not 'round-the-clock nurses. Suddenly, the outpatient has a new role of stating needs for personal assistance and then instructing the available help in the best ways to provide that assistance.

The next stage of instruction in the acute care or rehabilitation setting can best be implemented by health professionals and peers who have experience in using attendants. The patient must learn a set of attendant management skills: strategies for finding, interviewing, training, paying, and otherwise keeping happy the people who will provide physical assistance. Each patient who will be using physical assistance should learn management skills that are appropriately comprehensive for the degree of help that will be needed.

Based on the results of the client need assessment and the resources of the rehabilitation facility, attendant management instruction will usually assume one or more of three forms:

1. *Individualized counseling* This is the least structured and most frequently provided method of instruction. Typically, an individual with attendant management concerns approaches a nurse, social worker, counselor, other health professional, or a peer who already uses attendants. Usually a particular topic is raised. Often the two best resources for information are the experience of peers who use attendants and a comprehensive, well-indexed reference text. When health professionals notice that they are answering an increasing number of attendant questions, it is often time to begin group instruction.

2. *A series of meetings on various topics* When a small group of people with common concerns is identified, more structured instructional meetings might be warranted.

Identify and list the common topics of concern. A group may decide to meet just once or twice and address several topics in each meeting; if the available information is more extensive and time permits, schedule several meetings on one or two topics each.

To maximize meeting attendance, distribute the schedule of topics in advance to participants. Encourage participants to share their positive and negative experiences as well as questions on each topic. If a comprehensive text is available or if someone has personal experience of a topic, the meetings can be centered around a lecture. In any case, total group involvement through discussion and role play should be encouraged.

3. *A formal course* The series approach can evolve into a formal course of several classes when:

- An instructor or several instructors knowledgeable about several management topics are skilled and interested in teaching a course
- A group of people are interested in pursuing a course
- An appropriate schedule of class times and meeting place are available

Perhaps the element that most separates a series of meetings from formal courses is the existence of an instructor who is willing to outline and structure each topic in a manner suitable for classroom teaching and has the ability to teach the class and involve the students in an interesting manner. The instructor is usually a health professional or a peer with experience in using attendants. Sometimes several instructors, each with specialty topics, can join to teach a course. With several instructors, however, there must still be a coordinator to administer the course.

The Box, A Listing of Topics for a Comprehensive Course, suggests the content of an attendant management course. Approximately 15 classes should be scheduled to cover such a list adequately; fewer classes can be used for a less comprehensive approach. Classes should be a maximum of 30 to 45 minutes and be held two to three times per week. A class held just once each week lacks continuity; students forget material and lose interest between once-a-week classes.

A suggested structure for each 45-minute class is as follows:

- 3–5 minutes of review of the main topics covered in the previous class, a refresher to reinforce learning
- A 1-minute introduction to the topic for the current class
- 10 to 15 minutes of lecture

A LISTING OF TOPICS FOR A COMPREHENSIVE COURSE

The following list (DeGraff 1988) suggests topics for a formal course for people who have extensive needs for physical assistance from others. An abbreviated list of topics should be used for briefer forms of instruction and when the clients need for assistance is not as extensive.

Introduction

Why this course is unique and important

Definition of terms to be used: nurse, aide, nursing assistant, nurse's aide, home health aide, personal care aide or attendant, homemaker, housekeeper, household maintenance, domestic cook, sitter, companion, transportation driver

Section I: Why Learn Management Skills?

1. Rights for disabled person and the attendant
2. Two approaches to aide/attendant instruction and manuals
   - Training the aides for those who receive assistance
   - Training those who require assistance to be able to independently manage the aides whom they use
3. Why learn management skills?
   The 6 freedoms:
   - Freedom to directly control the type, quality, and schedule of aides—and to change aides—whenever necessary
   - Freedom from being dependent upon aide pools or referral-agency lists, and the consequent ability to relocate wherever and whenever necessary
   - Freedom from having to use agency or college campus aide/attendant training services
   - Freedom from having to pay the high hourly administrative rates to professional home health aide agencies if one is not eligible for third-party funding
   - Freedom from having to use parents or relatives as aides
   - Freedom from having to use a spouse as an aide, or sole aide
4. The three management situations: Which one applies to you?
   - You have all the abilities required for managing those who provide you assistance
   - You have the emotional and mental abilities; however, you lack physical, visual, or verbal abilities for some management tasks
   - You are not able or willing to manage those who provide you assistance

Section II: Strategies for Being a Good Manager

5. The top 10 reasons why attendants quit and are fired

6. Settings in which you use help
   - Acute care hospital
   - Rehabilitation hospital
   - Transitional and residential independent living center
   - Nursing home or infirmary
   - Private housing
   - College residence hall or vocational-technical campus area housing
   - Day or evening travel
   - Overnight travel
7. Types of help and the services that each provider performs
   - Health professionals working at institutions
   - Agency-provided health professionals in your home
   - Health professionals whom you employ in your home
   - Comparisons: Should you use agency-provided or personally recruited help in your home?
8. Qualities and strategies of a good manager
9. Passive, aggressive, and assertive: Which style is best for stating needs?
10. Job expectations
    - The attendant's expectations of you
    - Your expectations of the attendant
11. The favorable physical work environment
    - A clean and pleasant work area
    - An efficient layout of each work area
    - A sufficient inventory of supplies
    - Prescription medical equipment: Stocking the supplies and tools of preventive maintenance

Section III: Identifying and Dividing Needs for Assistance

12. Abusing help with inappropriate requests
13. Three types of activities that qualify for attendant help
    - Request primarily physical assistance
    - 4 ways to request help from attendants
14. Making a master list of your needs for assistance
    - Advantages to making a list
    - Steps to follow in making your list
    - An example
15. Dividing needs with more than one attendant
    - Advantages to dividing
    - When dividing is wise and unwise
    - Strategies for dividing your needs

Section IV: Paying Salaries and Taxes

16. Methods for paying attendants
    - Volunteer attendant help: Don't overuse it or rely on it

(Box continues)

A LISTING OF TOPICS FOR A COMPREHENSIVE COURSE (continued)

- Paying attendants with appreciation and salary: Strategies for expressing appreciation
17. Salaries: Determining salary rates and merit increases
    - 3 options for using starting salaries and merit increases
    - Starting salary rates
    - Merit increase rates and schedules
18. Monetary salaries: Cash, noncash, or both
    - Cash salaries
    - Personal-budget funding for cash salaries
    - Third-party funding for cash salaries
    - Noncash salaries
19. Tax obligations for attendant employer (Caution: Changes from year to year)
    - Kinds of employees whom you directly employ
    - Knowing your obligations when paying cash wages
    - Knowing your obligations when paying noncash wages
    - Recordkeeping strategies
20. Medical deductions and credits for attendant employers
    - Deducting attendant cash and noncash salaries
    - Tax credits for attendant services
    - Services as medical or business-related deductions
21. A list of IRS tax publications for attendant employers

Section V: Recruiting, Interviewing, Training, and Parting with Help
22. Creating a job description for attendants
    - The importance of a job description
    - Parts of a job description
    - Job description examples
23. Residence locations for an attendant
    - As a roommate
    - In the same living area
    - In the same building
    - Within the nearby neighborhood
    - Using a variety of attendants to advantage
24. Sources for recruiting attendants
    - Referrals from current attendants
    - Previous attendant applicants or employees

- Home health aide agencies
- Nearby college campus
- Surrounding community
- Local medical facilities
- Disability organizations in a campus or community
- Employment agency
25. Methods for recruiting attendants
    - Some secrets of advertising
    - Newspaper ads and newsletter notices
    - Posters and index card notices
    - Expressing the attendant position by word-of-mouth or by telephone
26. Interviewing, screening, and hiring prospective attendants
    - Objectives for interviewing and screening
    - Applicant traits to favor and avoid
    - Interview observation skills from Sherlock Holmes
    - Step-by-step procedure
27. Training and ongoing management
    - Adopting the qualities of a good manager
    - Becoming organized
    - Providing clear instruction to attendants
    - Providing good ongoing management to attendants
28. Predicting, recognizing, and resolving attendant problems
    - Correcting simple performance problems
    - Signs of a healthy job relationship
    - Symptoms of an unhealthy job relationship
    - Possible reasons behind negative symptoms
    - Steps in resolving these and other problems
    - When attendant problems cannot be resolved, prepare to part ways
29. Parting ways from an attendant
    - Depression about a departing attendant is common
    - The simple facts behind an attendant's departure
    - Steps to accepting the resignation from an attendant
    - Steps to firing an attendant
30. 10 top guidelines for maximum independent living

- 10 to 15 minutes of discussion and role play
- 5 to 10 minutes of questions relating to the current class topic or any other attendant issue
- A 1- or 2-minute introduction to the next class topic, plus a homework assignment that either reinforces the current class topic or stimulates thinking about the next class topic

In such settings as an independent living center, the students are part of an overall program in which being respon-

sible to a schedule, meeting goals, and increasing maturity are emphasized. If the setting is appropriate, it is suggested that participants be graded during the course in preparation for receiving a certificate of satisfactory completion.

Classroom exams are not necessary for determining each student's course grade. A passing grade can be based on simple factors such as the student's participation in the following ways:

- Being present for the roll call at the beginning and end of each class meeting

- Taking an active part in the participation and discussion of each class (in the overall opinion of the instructor)
- Attending at least 80% of the class meetings (a missed beginning or end roll call is considered an absence)

Everyone appreciates recognition, and a certificate of satisfactory course completion can be a powerful incentive for many people to attend classes regularly, participate, and learn more. The grading factors should be announced on the first day of class and each roll call should be obvious.

Support

The need for support services is common within various medical, social, and psychological program models. These services are often essential to many programs as a bridge between textbook skills instruction and the problems and questions that arise during the everyday practice of those skills.

Support services fulfill ongoing, long-term objectives by providing information and counseling regarding:

1. *Safe and efficient personal care methods.* One of the roles of an inpatient in rehabilitation is that of student. During an inpatient stay, individuals who foresee being eventually discharged with physical limitations should learn everything possible about functional abilities and safe and efficient methods for providing their own personal care. Inpatient resources include physicians, nurses, and therapists. Role playing, developing checklists, videos and manuals are good training materials. However, questions and problems will arise after hospital discharge. Often this same hospital staff can still provide information, as can health professionals in the community. Regardless of the specific sources, this ongoing support service is essential for periodic consultations.

2. *Management of attendants.* A formal period of instruction in attendant management skills is merely a starting point to the lifelong process of learning skills through practice. Long after the formal instruction has ended, attendant users will periodically have questions and problems and need advice. They may say, "I don't know why, but . . . my last three aides suddenly quit," "I am having trouble with tax authorities in deducting my aide salaries," or "My current aide is abusing me and I don't know what to do." Typical sources for management advice of this type will probably not include hospital staff, but might be peers who use attendants, nurses in the community, social workers, a SCI community group, or a counselor at a local independent living center. Then the formal rehabilitation setting needs to be informed to help minimize recurrence.

3. *Sources for finding attendants.* Probably the most frequent question about using attendants concerns how to find dependable aides who will provide high-quality service. Because this question is also among the most difficult to answer, the issue merits being a separate objective for support services. Attendants are generally available both from agencies and through direct employment. Agency sources vary in their ability to supply aides to fill specific client needs and schedules. Sources for direct, personal employment vary according to each residential area and the time of the year. Support resources for finding aides in a community can include peers who use attendants, nurses in the community, a SCI community group, local independent living center, college campus disability office, medical facility, or employment agency. A comprehensive reference for managing attendants can be consulted for using these resources as well as for directly recruiting from the general community with newspaper ads and other public notices.

4. *Coping with attendants.* People who use attendants sometimes have trouble coping with managing aides as well as being constantly dependent on their assistance. Those who use attendants must learn to cope with many emotional concerns, which can require a support system.

The people who can provide support services for the different objectives include physicians, nurse practitioners, nurses, home-visit nurses, nursing assistants, attendants, peers who use attendants and social workers and counselors. The settings where support can be found include acute care hospitals, rehabilitation centers, outpatient support clinics, SCI community organizations, public health departments, the disability office at a college campus, and independent living centers.

Overall, the most knowledgeable resource in many communities is the peer who has experience using attendants. An increasing number of communities are forming specialized peer support groups from volunteers who have been coping successfully with their own disability for several years. Some organizations sponsor periodic discussion meetings between groups of experienced peers and the recently injured; other groups have also formed mentoring structures where recently injured people can request a one-to-one peer advisor who can be approached as necessary about individual concerns. Sunnyview Hospital, Schenectady, New York, has used SCI peer-support groups as well as a one-on-one mentoring system.

Whatever the specific support source for a situation, a policy should guide the supporter in providing assistance. In the spirit of promoting independent living, advice, counsel, and information should be provided when requested. Support rarely involves assuming responsibilities and implementing duties on behalf of someone and is not given unless requested. This approach promotes learning new management skills, improves coping ability and develops independence.

In summary, support services are an integral part of the three-sided program model. Whatever the source or specific objective of a support in a particular situation, the role of the support should be to advise and provide skill-promoting information. Some of the best resources are experienced peers who have a disability.

Practice Opportunities

An important element in many instructional programs is providing practice opportunity. In each learning situation, lectures and textbook information are reinforced by the opportunity to practice and experiment. To be effective, the practice opportunities that a student has with an attendant should have at least the following features:

- Practice regarding a specific skill should follow a clear, well-organized instruction session
- The instruction session should clearly encourage or even require practice of a specific skill on which instruction has focused
- The opportunity to practice should permit the student to make and benefit from mistakes without the threat of overwhelmingly negative consequences
- The opportunity should be supported with an adequate and responsive system

1. *Practice should follow instruction.* Before one can practice a technique of attendant management, one needs clear instruction in that technique. The instruction must clearly define a skill to be practiced.

2. *Instruction should encourage or require practice with the nurse acting as the attendant in the patient's room.* Only the sharpest, most eager students will practice specific skills without at least some encouragement to do so. As shown previously, an element of any form of instruction should be to encourage or even require practice in specific skills between instructional sessions. Often this encouragement can come in the form of a homework assignment from the instructor:

"Each time you request some help, take a second to evaluate your communication and see whether your aide reacts favorably toward assertive requests. Be prepared in the next session to comment briefly on your experiences." The staff need to be encouraged to give feedback: "Yes, you really explained that clearly."

3. *Practice should permit mistakes without punishment.* The setting for practicing skills with an aide varies: hospital, health care facility, home, college campus dormitory, career or vacation setting, or independent living center. In any residential setting, the student should be permitted to make mistakes and benefit from them. Some settings especially promote independent living, such as a residential center. In these situations, it is sometimes possible to integrate the attendants used at the center with the instructional team.

Regardless of the setting, aides, relatives, spouses, and friends who supply assistance are often encouraged to attend the management classes with the student. In this way, the aide understands the management techniques and can pos-

itively reinforce the student during between-class practices. Do not let a relative, spouse, or other aide strongly discourage the individual from being assertive and practicing skills. Some dominating family members and traditional, medical-model aides and nurses resent receiving instructions from the person receiving their assistance. Consequently, these people actually punish those in their care with negative, passive-aggressive attitudes and actions.

An excellent opportunity for an inpatient to practice management skills in a real-life setting is to spend time at home in preparation for hospital discharge. Mistakes made during each pass can be reviewed by the patient with hospital staff after returning. It is a shame that several insurance companies are no longer permitting these beneficial overnight stays.

4. *Supplement practice opportunities with responsive support.* During practice sessions, mistakes need discussion, individual questions require answers, and negative experiences simply need soothing. The ready availability of support encourages people to practice, experiment, and learn; without the comfort of available support, many students resist taking risks.

IN CLOSING

Even when formal program implementation is agreed on in principle, additional problems surrounding the issue of when to introduce formal instruction remain. Clients may not be fully ready for such training before they leave in-house rehabilitation programs; efforts may thus need to be continued in an outpatient setting. Patients progress from informed observers, to active participants, to experts over varying degrees of time, and with varying degrees of ability. However, if plans for such outpatient programs are not secured and provisions for the transition period are inadequate, attendant training issues will probably be neglected and rehabilitation outcomes will not be optimal.

Funding sources should be thoroughly and creatively explored by professionals with expertise, starting with sound legal advice obtained in the early postinjury period and including social service and case management interventions. Rehabilitation professionals are realizing more fully that successful outcomes are measured *after* formal rehabilitation has come to a close. By listening and then responding to people who actually live constantly with a disability, professionals can initiate programs geared toward better management of continuing care over the years.

REFERENCES

DeGraff, A. H. 1988. *Home Health Aides: How to Manage the People Who Help You.* Clifton Park, NY: Saratoga Access Publications.

Ulicny, G., Adler, A., Kennedy, S., and Jones, M. 1987. *A Step-by-Step Guide to Training and Managing Personal Attendants.* Part One: *Consumer Guide.* Part Two: *Agency Guide. (Contains checklists).*

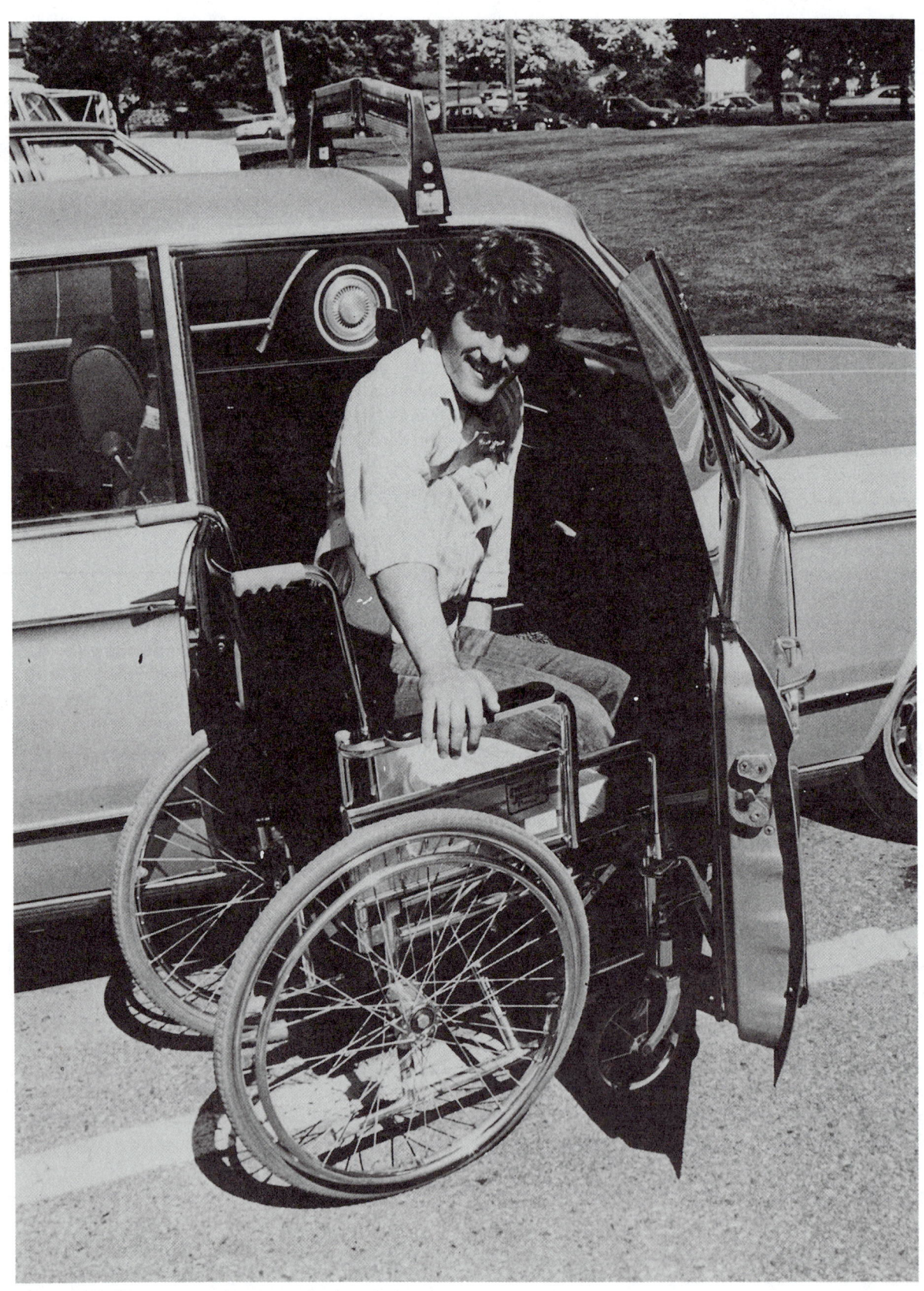

CHAPTER
— 33 —

A Health Care Focus on Life Planning: Preparing for Continuing Needs*

Chapter Outline

Health Care Objectives

- To understand the significance of the discharge process and factors that give direction to planning
- To secure quality short- and long-term delivery of continuing care services
- To understand the effects of aging with SCI and apply perspectives to appropriate services and interventions

*This chapter was developed with the assistance of George Richardson, M.R.C., Robert Menter, M.D., and J. Little, R.N., Vancouver, BC.

GOALS OF TRAUMA REHABILITATION

Rehabilitation is defined by the National Council on Rehabilitation as "the restoration of the individual to the fullest physical, mental, social, vocational and economic capacity of which each is capable." Individuals must learn the physical skills necessary for functional mobility; many must engage in altered occupational training or retraining; and most must learn new social skills necessary to relate successfully in the community at large. Some of these skills may be acquired easily, while some will require more effort and time, and others may never be performed independently, depending on the extent of injury and such factors as the extent that each desires.

Establishing a system of early notification and identification of newly injured people provides each injured person an opportunity to talk with professionals who have knowledge of the problems, issues, and resources faced by people with SCI. Accessing expertise, coordinating resources, and maximizing rehabilitation dollars spent is of ultimate concern to everyone. The Box, SCI Program Management, details considerations in management of a SCI system of care.

Rehabilitation of people with SCI is a longitudinal process of recovery and adaptation. This process begins at the time of injury and extends well beyond rehabilitation. All efforts of care and support from prehospital services, through the acute care hospital and rehabilitation center, play a key role in each injured person's life and ultimately, a part in the outcome after SCI.

After completion of the rehabilitation program, people practice and implement the information they have learned. Putting their lives back on course emotionally, physically, socially, and financially is a priority. The discharge from rehabilitation is not the end, but rather the beginning for the spinal cord injured person who must now cope with the realities of life. Specialized and coordinated continuing care services after discharge are recognized as increasingly important in helping injured individuals and their families maintain optimal health and achieve maximum autonomy, independence, and enjoyment from life.

THE DISCHARGE PROCESS

During the rehabilitation process goals are set, attained, and refined and new ones are initiated. In this evolving cycle, the rehabilitation process reaches its potential value or capacity, the therapeutic environment is no longer therapeutic, and the discharge process actively begins.

The discharge process is the final step in the formal rehabilitation process. It includes preparation to maintain health, to manage the effects of disability, and to reintegrate into community life. The discharge process is of intrinsic importance because it is a pivotal point on which to capitalize on the entire rehabilitation process.

Rehabilitative goals are determined not only by physical abilities, but also by social, psychological, and vocational adaptation. In order to provide for appropriate support services, joint evaluation of progress in all aspects of rehabilitation is essential.

Involving the individual, the family, health care professionals, and community resources in comprehensive discharge planning and preparation can smooth transition to successful community living. Fragmented discharge planning and preparation can hinder or even prevent this transition.

Factors That Affect the Discharge Process

The discharge process is affected by both positive and negative factors, including those directly related to the abilities of the individual and family and those that depend more on the environment. Consideration of several interrelated variables helps determine the kinds of problems people have when discharged and the approaches that will be most effective (MacLean 1981). Important variables include the individual, the family, the environment following discharge, the rehabilitation program, and community services. The crucial question is, Does the person have the resources and capacity to be safely sustained in the community? (Brown, Judd, and Unger 1987)

The Disabled Person

Factors that influence individual concerns and responses are related to self-concept and self-esteem, time since injury, physical health, and functional skills.

Psychosocial adjustment. In the aftermath of SCI, individuals' self-concept and self-esteem are particularly vulnerable. Extensive research concludes that successfully living with a disability depends on the value or worth (self-concept and self-esteem) people place on themselves. Psychosocial adaptation then, rather than intellectual abilities or level and completeness of injury, is the critical factor in determining rehabilitation success (Trieschmann 1988).

Although physical rehabilitation may be complete at the time of discharge, mental, social, and vocational adjustments are probably not. Good physical restoration does not guarantee good emotional adjustment. As a result, individuals being discharged have different problems and require different approaches, largely depending on psychosocial adjustment to injury. Furthermore, although discharge may be timely, there tends to be an intensity and anxiety that accompanies fear of the unknown indicating that postdischarge services are required. (Upton 1990)

SCI PROGRAM MANAGEMENT

Program management is the comprehensive management of resources spent for program results. It concerns quality of service, staff productivity, functional outcome (benefit), program market share (niche), reimbursement resources, and public expectations.

WHY:

- To maximize resources spent on spinal cord injury rehabilitation.

HOW:

- Implementing a cost-to-revenue/cost-to-benefit accounting system to evaluate the current delivery of services.
- Clearly assess program content:
  1. Goal of the program (purpose)
  2. Clinical team involved (personnel resources)
  3. Environment and equipment (resources)
  4. Definition of service delivered (output)
     - average amount of therapy per patient per day
     - average length of stay
  5. Method of program evaluation (outcomes)
- Assess
  1. What are all the *costs* in running this program?
  2. Is it as effective as it could be?
  3. What can be done to make it better?
  4. How do you anticipate change and plan for it?
  If no one has the time or information to answer these questions, then the program cannot be effectively managed.
- Prepare a budget
  In hospital-based programs, financial departments have previously been reluctant to share financial information outside of the boardroom.
  Instead they would project an annual program budget by adding a 5% to 10% increase for inflation and for capital equipment requested by clinicians.

The current trend is toward clear justification of every dollar budgeted (zero-line cost accounting). Financial departments more frequently provide clinicians with department cost reports and give them increased responsibility in the decisions.

Together they first project expected use:

1. What was last year's average daily census, average visits per day/week? Do you anticipate increase this year? (Is it a new program that is still expanding?)
2. What are relevant outside factors? For instance, are there changes in funding resources (Medicare DRGs or increase in Medicaid days)?

3. Changes in inside factors? New director, new marketing ideas that may enhance utilization, change in clinical expertise?
4. Competition—what are other organizations doing today and planning for tomorrow?

After establishing a list of assumptions that are mutually acceptable by clinicians and administration, it is possible to project utilization. It is important as you construct a budget to write down the assumptions. With the assumptions visible through the budget process, contingencies can also be developed.

If a new service is planned, anticipate increases in staff and supplies. Review monthly and adjust as necessary.

Although many factors—from changes in governmental funding, to breakthroughs in research—affect a program's viability, it is essential to tailor a program to meet existing needs. Flexibility in delivery of service is the key to program survival.

WHO:

The ideal, a clinician with a degree in business management, is becoming more abundant. An administrator/program director with clinical expertise can both balance the clinical composition of the program and manage financial matters professionally.

If the program is small, a clinician frequently can function both as a part-time nurse or therapist and as program manager.

Persons skilled in market concepts, accounting, budget development, and human resource management will be successful program managers.

PERSONAL INSIGHT

I was first hired as a program manager because of my nursing expertise (BSN), although what was really required were business administration skills (MBA).

The four new program managers hired with me were all clinicians, but I was the only one with education in marketing concepts, budget development and productivity analysis.

Throughout this 3-year experience, upper management asked why was I the only one who asked budget questions and was concerned with productivity and marketing ideas. I was respected for being a forerunner, while truly I was the only one prepared for the position.

Sinclair Sheridan, R.N., B.S.N., M.B.A.
Administrator, New Medico Neurological Program
Hardee Memorial Hospital
Wauchula, FL

Physical health and functional abilities. A current assessment is necessary to determine physical health and functional readiness. The discharge decision requires a global view of each person's situation in addition to demonstrated progress in specific areas. Team members with individuals and families work together closely to evaluate the skills, knowledge, and attitudes that are necessary to manage the implications of disability.

Principles of management of all body systems and how needs have changed following SCI are addressed throughout this text. This information provides the knowledge necessary to teach the person and family what they need to know, including how to minimize risk factors, prevent complications, perform or supervise personal care, care for equipment, obtain supplies, and respond appropriately to problem situations. Sections on potential complications, self-care, and long-term implications in the previous chapters are relevant.

Comprehensive assessment cannot be completed in isolation from psychological considerations. Poor mental health will lower resistance to physical stress. For example, if depression is manifested in poor nutritional habits or drug or alcohol abuse, the details of physical care quickly become dangerously neglected. Thus, comprehensive joint assessment, with identification of risk factors, is a crucial step in the discharge process.

The Family

The impact of disability on families and on family roles is an important variable influencing discharge planning. Immediately following SCI, an individual is sick, and the rules and norms of the "sick role" apply. Generally families are supportive during this period, and problems do not become clear until the extent of the disability is known. Families grieve, and at the same time they must assess and reorganize family objectives and goals to accommodate a disabled family member. Role conflicts may arise if expectations of the disabled person differ among family members. A common conflict can be seen when, for example, a capable husband and father returns home after being in the hospital for a long time. His wife, now used to managing the household in general, may have difficulty in resharing that role. Failure to return to preinjury roles and responsibilities, or at least similar ones, can be devastating for the injured person. Family attitudes and capabilities related to managing the effects of disability are of paramount importance. Care tasks can significantly interfere with the quality of relationships over time. To minimize future problems, it is vital to assess both individual and family concerns during discharge planning with insight.

The Environment Following Discharge

Ideally the environment the disabled person chooses following injury is an essential consideration when planning discharge. It must be the most comfortable and easiest place for adaptation possible. This is where the person will come to "get away from it all," to relax and be happy, to live.

Good preparation for living in that setting is essential. Poor or nonexistent renovations and adaptations in the home can cause tremendous stress at a time when the person is going through one of the most difficult periods of adaptation to injury.

Significant others play an important role in the discharge setting selected. For the most part families must be involved in discharge preparations. The strength and desire on the part of individual and family to make discharge living arrangements helps determine how actively the health care team must be involved. For some people, the issues concerning attendant care are essential to create a desirable discharge environment. Often people with SCI have never been employers, and they need to learn still another new role to cope with unfamiliar living arrangements (see Chapter 32).

The Rehabilitation Program

The rehabilitation environment is important throughout the entire program. It must be an environment where individuals are active participants in making decisions about their care to the extent they are able and are encouraged to solve problems for themselves. It must also be one where individuals are allowed to grieve their loss, and where they can learn how to stop being patients and start being real people again.

In relation to the discharge process, it helps immensely if staff members have a comfortable attitude of encouraging learning and fostering independence and autonomy. Professionals in the rehabilitation setting must strive toward a good knowledge and understanding of all the aspects that influence and assist individuals and families in good rehabilitation and thus preparation for discharge.

Rehabilitation concepts that promote readiness for discharge include:

- Early referral to specialized facilities.
- A consistent rehabilitation environment conducive to developing autonomy.
- Early determination of individual and family goals and how best to achieve them.
- Early understanding by the individual and family of the program offered—its capabilities and limitations.
- A focus on psychosocial support, in addition to promotion of physical health and functional capabilities.
- A proper mix of professional and peer counseling resources.
- Comprehensive educational services including preparation for accessing and using community-based resources including housing, transport, and employment services, for example. See Chapter 1 for a joint program offered by independent living specialists and

health care professionals. This includes provision of independent living situations on the ward and transitional living situations when facilities permit.

- Good communication and working relationships with community-based services and resources to facilitate planning and coordination of continuing care services.
- Encouragement to participate in activities outside the rehabilitation center.

Therapeutic excursions and leaves.

Adjustment to living with the stresses imposed by spinal cord injury requires a gradual exposure to community situations outside the spinal cord injury care unit. Therapeutic passes and excursions into the community, prior to discharge, are considered an essential element of a total management program. [*Guidelines* 1981:11]

Experiencing early reintegration into the community enhances readiness for discharge and minimizes fears of the outside world. Valuable opportunities for resocialization have been facilitated by the advent of day and weekend passes. With careful planning soon after admission, an excursion into the community may be possible within 2 to 4 weeks after injury.

It is important to set goals for these therapeutic adventures and evaluate experiences on return. Initially the team plans for success by careful consideration of all details. As the disabled person becomes more confident and capable, the team disengages.

Evaluation. Evaluation following passes might deal with practical questions such as:

- Was the person able to instruct others when unable to do something?
- How did the family respond to the person's new role or to their new role as attendants?
- What precautions were taken against incontinence when on pass, and how was it dealt with if it did occur?
- Did the individual take the initiative to check the accessibility of a building before going there?
- How did the person deal with social barriers in the community?

Be sensitive to the person's response on return from a pass. Patients experience the realities of disability outside the rehabilitation environment, and thus emotional reactions, particularly behavioral outbursts, typically occur when they return. The team must look beyond the behavior at hand and explore the cause if their interventions are to be both timely and meaningful.

It is necessary to encourage these experiences, otherwise patients are not exposed to real-life situations and do not have opportunities to find out what they can or cannot cope with. Passes frequently provide an incentive for learning based on the concept that adults tend to view education as a means to overcome a problem at hand (Knowles 1972).

For example, incontinence in the rehabilitation center is one thing, when a quick change of the track suit will solve the not so obvious problem; it is quite another if good clothes become obviously wet in front of friends. The situation may encourage the individuals to learn more about drinking patterns and bladder control or condom application. If this situation is not experienced until after discharge, however, the person will not have access to the same resources to solve the problem. Unfortunately, the situation is more likely to cause social isolation; the person may simply be too afraid to risk going out.

Especially note the effect of physical care tasks on family relationships. For example, a middle-aged quadriplegic man returned home having his wife perform his bowel care every other day. Both partners disliked this experience but coped with it at first. After a while they found they argued a lot on bowel care days and soon found themselves not speaking to each other on those days at all. Eventually the couple separated and the wife revealed that the "distasteful event" of bowel care was a major causative factor.

Evaluation of this situation and others like it suggests that more sensitivity in discharge planning or follow-up care might have prevented such a drastic outcome. The team must look beyond the procedure at hand and examine role implications. In this situation, was there a role conflict when the wife was expected to be an attendant and partner at the same time? Could the wife have managed bowel care with less offense if aides were used? Would attendant care have relieved the source of stress and helped preserve the relationship?

Access to Community Resources and Services

Related resources and services for disabled people in the community aid in the discharge process. Although tremendous progress has been made in the past decade with development of these resources, today more people with greater degrees of disability survive SCI, and more people return to the community sooner after injury. This trend creates the need for and emphasizes the lack of appropriate ongoing health service systems in most communities. This situation is not unique to people with SCI; it is part of a major health and economic concern: How best to develop resources to meet the ever-increasing needs of people who require long-term health care.

Existing health care services and related personal care assistance are available in the community from a variety of sources. However, unless supported by specialized liaison and educational activities, referrals are less than ideal. While health care professionals in the community may lack expertise in recognizing and dealing with the uniqueness and severity of the problems encountered by people with SCI, those in rehabilitation centers may have little or no idea of the problems faced in the community. This situation is especially pronounced when the rehabilitation center is in a large city and the individual is from a distant rural community.

Vocational Planning*

When people with disabilities make the decision to go to work, they are, in most cases, eligible to receive support through a *state vocational rehabilitation service* funded by a combination of state and federal dollars. For people with SCI this decision is usually made sometime during or shortly after their rehabilitation program. Early referral is thus encouraged.

Federal monies available to support vocational services are distributed on a formula basis, according to the population of the state. The state vocational rehabilitation agency has responsibility for delivering vocational rehabilitation services to people who meet eligibility requirements. Any person who has a medically definable physical or mental disability that constitutes a handicap to employment and can benefit from services in terms of employability is eligible to receive services from a state vocational rehabilitation agency.

Services that might be provided to an eligible person with a disability include evaluation and diagnostic services; counseling and guidance, including vocational counseling and personal adjustment counseling and referral; physical and mental restoration services; vocational and training services including vocational adjustment materials, tools, tuition and fees, and books; maintenance and transportation to support participation in vocational rehabilitation programs; interpreter services for the deaf; reader services; telecommunications; rehabilitation engineering services; and other services that would assist the person to obtain and maintain gainful employment.

Persons with disabilities may be referred to a state vocational rehabilitation office by a physician or other medical personnel, a social service agency, a private rehabilitation or insurance company, an educational institution, a friend or acquaintance, or self-referral. The state vocational rehabilitation agency might first place a person in an extended evaluation program to determine the existence of vocational potential. When the person is severely disabled, this evaluation process allows for some services to be purchased so that a more effective determination of employability can be made. Persons determined to be eligible might then receive services.

Severely disabled persons who are ineligible for state vocational rehabilitation services may be referred to the state independent living program, funded by the federal and state governments within the state vocational rehabilitation agency. To be eligible under this program, the person must be severely disabled, and the services provided must improve independent functioning in some way.

THE DISCHARGE PLANNING PROCESS

It is logical that psychological and social adaptation are not complete when persons are discharged from a rehabilitation center. They continue to need help in accepting an altered reality, learning new roles, and coping with the many tasks necessary to manage the effects of disability. To help ensure that positive adjustments continue after discharge, use a process to include assessing progress at intervals throughout the patients' and families' rehabilitation process, determining readiness for discharge, identifying problems as persons prepare for discharge, and planning and evaluating interventions to meet changing needs.

It is important to have established criteria to detect risk factors (Davidoff et al. 1990) and *assess* progress through the rehabilitation process to determine:

- How well persons understand their condition
- How well they cope and solve problems
- How well they perform daily living skills or, when appropriate, instruct others to perform them
- How much responsibility persons demonstrate in maintaining health and managing the effects of disability
- Whether they are ready to learn new roles
- How well they manage their skills both in the rehabilitation setting and on excursions and leaves
- How they interact with peers, professionals, and family
- How they teach others to assist with their care
- How much interest they take in various aspects of their rehabilitation
- What plans they have for the future

Assessments of readiness for discharge may be enhanced by using various functional outcome measurement indices (see Chapter 22). Self-directed checklists are great for individuals to chart their progress; when negative or uncertain responses become positive, readiness for discharge is indicated (Gardenhire and Fields 1987).

Goal setting is a progressive or building step, but in relation to discharge planning it is more a *reassessment* and *refining* of long-term goals. The long-term goals set on admission are largely based on professionals' knowledge of physical potentials related to the level and extent of injury and on the person's plans for the future. These goals may

*This section was contributed by Laura Williams, Deputy Project Director Improving Service Systems for People with Disabilities Independent Living Research Utilization/Robert Wood Johnson Foundation Houston, TX.

need some adjustment. For example, a young quadriplegic woman planned to return home to live with her family. When she realized how independent she could be with some attendant care, however, she decided to share accommodations with a friend. Unfortunately, conflicts arose among family members. Timely reassessment of both individual and family goals during discharge planning can help prevent such problems.

During preparation for discharge, *interventions* relate to assessment and to reassessed and refined goals and, of necessity, vary. Skilled interventions help persons and families reduce the uncertainties faced in returning to the community and promote healthful living.

Intervention that ease transition to home and community life include:

- Encouraging active involvement in the rehabilitation program.
- Encouraging early and frequent community excursions and passes.
- Assisting in modification of care tasks and equipment-related needs for home use. Gathering equipment and supplies; predicting how long supplies will last and where and how to get more; and arranging personal contact with vendors are helpful activities.
- Focusing on educational and vocational opportunities.
- Assisting in home renovations or other housing alternatives.
- Completing individual and family health education including provision of written materials for future reference; reviewing access to community resources and services; and communicating with the primary care physician and health care providers as appropriate.

Whenever possible, community-based care givers and resource persons should participate with newly disabled persons while they are in the rehabilitation setting in how best to plan for returning to the community. It is important to be aware of and link services to address potential health and social problems, many of which are related to inactivity. Often people with paraplegia, who are capable of independence with personal care and mobility and therefore do not require physical assistance from others, become more isolated than those with quadriplegia. As a preventive measure, health care professionals promote activity for all people with SCI.

As options increase, it is important to be aware of the type, quality, and availability of continuing care resources. Knowledge of current resources profoundly affects the discharge decision. Participate with the disabled person, family, and other health care professionals to determine the degree of risk to the person and relate this risk factor to the intensity of continuing services required.

PERSONAL VIEWPOINT

A 32-year-old, self-employed, quadriplegic businessman is preparing for discharge from the rehabilitation center. He understands his disability and how to care for himself and takes responsibility for the care he must get. He can afford and wishes to live in an apartment of his own. He will need an attendant for most of his personal care, housecleaning, and meal preparation. Unfortunately he is a difficult man to care for, and since most nurses dislike doing so, there is a real possibility that he may not be able to survive in the community.

To help him prepare for living in the setting he chooses, interdisciplinary interventions in the discharge process may include:

- Helping him understand the present and, possibly, future problem
- Explaining the difficulty in finding good attendants and providing guidelines on securing and retaining them
- Encouraging him to learn to work with nurses who will act as attendants in the rehabilitation setting and developing his ability to accept constructive criticism from health care professionals
- Helping him find, hire, and train an attendant while he is still in the rehabilitation setting (Nosek 1991) (Chapter 32)

Needs will vary, but most persons will require some assistance. Those who are having difficulty with adaptation will require help commensurate with their ability to be responsible for their own care. Those who have developed more adaptive behaviors may require help in learning new roles.

Knowledge of the ways that people learn new roles provides direction for planning interventions that facilitate successful enactment of the new roles. Planning appropriate sequencing of activities of increasing social difficulty and contact with a peer and professional counselor may help provide support through this phase of psychosocial adaptation. Developing assertive versus aggressive skills makes surviving easier.

Evaluation is essential to determine the effectiveness of predischarge assessment and planning. The outcome of rehabilitation is eventually determined by disabled persons' ability to maintain optimal health, manage the effects of disability, adapt to an altered reality, and develop skills that will allow them to live in the community.

Follow-up services are used for evaluation, not only to assist the individual patient and family, but also to incorporate feedback mechanisms to give future directions to the discharge process. Evaluation methods currently in use include home visits, telephone contact, questionnaires, comparison of discharge summary forms to current status, follow-up clinics, and liaison activities.

The sharing of expertise between rehabilitation and community professionals promotes a system of continuing services with a preventive, rather than a crisis intervention, focus. It is realized that an informed resources person close at hand is in a better position to prevent a problem situation from becoming a crisis situation (Trieschmann 1988).

CONTINUING CARE SERVICES*

Discharge from rehabilitation is not the end of adjustment for people with SCI, but a beginning in the real world where they must continue their adaptations and recovery. During this time of trying to put their lives on a positive course, many people need the services and support from the rehabilitation center staff, their family and local community. Optimally, this support should be provided in a timely and structured manner, particularly during the first year after discharge.

Components of Continuing Care Services

Many people with SCI find themselves trapped in complex and inadequate situations that do not meet their health or related care needs. Chapter 2 has addressed the need for a health care services research capacity in SCI to improve this national dilemma.

The Model SCI Systems recognize *follow-up* services as an integral component of the rehabilitation process. See Chapter 1. Follow-up programs generally refer to the specialized services provided by a rehabilitation center. These services interact with other components of the health delivery system which provide an array of services to assist people with SCI to fulfill their roles and participate actively in their families and communities.

Each rehabilitation center must develop follow-up services based on the unique needs of the SCI people it serves; the qualities and resources of the facility; and its programs in relation to the availability and quality of community services. Services should promote wellness in the context of a health care systems approach rather than a sickness treatment model (Trieschmann 1988). These two approaches are compared in Table 33–1.

*This section was contributed by George Richardson, M.R.C.

TABLE 33–1 Comparison of Two Service Models

Health Care Systems Approach	Sickness Treatment Model
Acute and chronic orientation	Acute orientation
Synthesis of parts into whole	Analysis into parts
Systems approach	Fragmented approach
Objective and subjective data	Objective data only
Problem prevention and crisis intervention	Crisis intervention
Professional and disabled person are both sources of knowledge	Professional is source of knowledge
Person is active participant in health process	Person is passive recipient of services
Psychosocial component considered to be normal	Psychosocial component considered abnormal
Services coordinated by a case manager	Little coordination of services
Equal access to a variety of services	Physician is gatekeeper to all services
Community focus	Hospital and clinic focus
Focus on personal, physical (organic), environmental interaction	Focus on physical (organic) variables almost exclusively

Adapted from Trieschmann (1988)

Essential principles for providing specialized follow-up services include:

- Follow-up services are an integral part of the rehabilitation process, because people with SCI will encounter problems and new experiences after discharge that affect their ability to continue progress.
- A clearly defined entity must have programmatic responsibility to develop both short- and long-term follow-up services.
- A staff should be able to evaluate a broad range of concerns that include, but are not limited to, health issues and services, housing, attendant care, financial concerns, psychosocial issues, equipment, home modifications and drug and alcohol treatment.
- Case management services should coordinate existing resources to ensure appropriate and continuing care for individuals on a case by case basis (White 1988). The case manager assumes responsibility for identifying needs, planning, arranging service delivery, and

monitoring service provision and outcome. This service function should be accomplished in collaboration with individuals and their families to be effective. See Chapter 14.

Phases of Continuing Care Services

The inpatient rehabilitation program is a critical link that sets the stage for the provision of short-term postdischarge and long-term follow-up support services. A comprehensive discharge plan clearly outlines the issues that impact a person's return to family, home, and community. The plan should contain sufficient detail to provide a firm basis for follow-up services.

The staff member responsible for coordinating the discharge plan and helping identify areas of concern after discharge can provide immediate postdischarge services to the individual. This staff member should be responsible for bringing together all the issues jointly worked on during the rehabilitation process.

Ideally, the staff member responsible for the discharge plan should also provide the short-term follow-up services on a proactive basis for at least 6 months postdischarge. Clients with SCI require this time to make a more stable adjustment. Initially services are provided as an extension of the inpatient program. Because the long-term support and community resources needs of individuals change over time, and given that the professionals responsible for helping implement the discharge plan usually have other inpatient responsibilities, it is important for rehabilitation facilities to designate other staff case manager/coordinator positions to provide longer term follow-up services and support.

In order to address the health care systems model of treatment adequately, as described by Trieschmann (1988), persons should periodically have the opportunity for reevaluations at the rehabilitation center. This provides a definitive method for support to disabled persons and their families and an opportunity to reinforce the information provided during the inpatient program. These reevaluations should, at a minimum, occur at 6 months post-discharge, or sooner if needs should arise. Reevaluation will enable persons to receive full and thorough review by the treating team in order to assess changes and recommend problem-solving strategies that will assist in their continued adaptation.

To provide continued support for longer term issues, persons returning as outpatients to the center should be assigned a specific case manager/coordinator who will provide assistance by providing longer term follow-up support. It is vital that injured persons understand the total range of options available before discharge in order to participate fully in determining future plans. What follows generally depends on the will, concentration, and courage of each person. The follow-up staff who provide both short- and long-term services and support are primary resource persons in the adaptation period.

The final phase of follow-up, which varies from individual to individual, establishes a supportive environment for persons as needs arise. The proactive follow-up services should last approximately 1 year postdischarge and move toward a maintenance phase. This maintenance phase, with ongoing support and services available from the treating facility, enables persons to take increasing responsibility for determining their quality of life. It is probably best supported by an outpatient team, a specific staff of professionals available on an ongoing basis.

Approaches

One way of providing ongoing assistance in a health care system approach is to offer *outreach clinics* within certain areas. These areas are determined by the distance from the rehabilitation facility because disabled persons who cannot return due to distance or transportation restrictions are likely to delay seeking services for problems until they become a crisis.

The purposes of the clinics may vary, but they generally include:

- Access to physicians, nurses, occupational and physical therapists, counselors, and a clinic coordinator
- Various health assessments with diagnostic tests and a course of action outlined
- Assessment of functional capabilities and psychosocial issues
- Family services
- Consultation with and support to local health care professionals who offer services to spinal cord injured persons
- Education and information on the effects of spinal cord injury and disability-related concerns to persons, families, and service providers

Professionals in the home community provide varied continuing support services. These professionals may include, but are not limited to, physicians, social workers, and staff of organizations such as local support groups, self-help organizations, spinal injury associations, and other public health professionals.

Despite the best physical and emotional health of individuals with SCI, medical, functional, and psychosocial issues develop with age. Professionals responsible for this long-term follow-up support must also begin to understand more clearly the nature of the aging process and decline as it relates to SCI. Close collaboration with individuals and families is needed to consider and decide what services will meet increasing needs.

THE A. ESTIN COMARR SPINAL INJURY CLINIC
RANCHO LOS AMIGOS MEDICAL CENTER
DOWNEY, CALIFORNIA

Rancho Los Amigos Medical Center is a 735-bed, publicly funded facility that cares for persons of all ages with severe disability and chronic illness. It is part of the Los Angeles County hospital system and has provided care for spinal injured persons since 1956.

The majority of its clients are funded by MediCal and Medicare programs. Historically, few community-based physicians would accept these clients following inpatient rehabilitation. The complexity of care required, the physician's lack of specialized knowledge of SCI, the lack of physically accessible community health services, and limited financial resources resulted in these clients' returning to Rancho's outpatient clinics for follow-up. The need for continuity between discharge and follow-up became evident.

A 1968 study to determine the kind of nursing service delivery that would improve the care of severely disabled individuals led to the concept of a *liaison nurse*. The liaison nurse meets continuing care needs and links the client to a myriad of community resources. It should be noted that the current role reflects many of the facets of the intrafacility nursing case management role being described now in the nursing literature.

During the early 1970s lengths of stay and frequency of passes enabled individuals to resolve most home and community issues while still inpatients, but by the late 1970s, changing health care financing led to decreased lengths of stay and limited numbers of passes. People began to experience more postdischarge problems and physical complications. Consequently, the liaison nurses focused on the needs exhibited in the outpatient clinic services. A liaison nurse, nurse manager, and staff nurse returned to school and became certified nurse practitioners. They developed and managed the *Continuity of Care Clinic*, which opened in 1979. The clinic has demonstrated cost-effective care, a decrease in inpatient readmissions, increased compliance with treatment programs, and improved client satisfaction. Because of these positive outcomes, the nurse practitioner clinic expanded in 1983, and in 1989, moved into new and larger quarters. The clinic was renamed in honor of Dr. A. Estin Comarr.

Clinic services include health education and reeducation, prevention of complications, reinforcement of the client's self-management skills, psychosocial support, occupational and physical therapy services, equipment reassessment, and driver's training. Individuals also require access to internal and external resources, continuity from inpatient through outpatient services into the community, verification of disability for outside agencies, and prevocational counseling. As a part of a larger organization the clinic personnel also assist with follow-up program evaluation and interface with the Spinal Injury Model System Program. The availability of these clinic services reduces use of more expensive Los Angeles County Health Care services and decreases both the rate of complications and the cost of lifetime care.

Certified nurse practitioners continue to provide primary care to all clients of the spinal injury clinic. The approach is holistic, with each nurse practitioner managing an individual case load of primary clients.

Nurse practitioners deliver patient care in collaboration with and under the supervision of the clinic physician and in accordance with client management protocols. Referrals to other clinics, specialties, or community agencies are made in consultation with the clinic physician and liaison nurse.

Client services continue to evolve as more needs are identified. Future plans include expanded hours and times, potential for lifetime care programs, satellite or mobile clinics, and expanded capability to meet the needs of this population as they age. Services to meet the growth needs of professionals working with the spinal injured population include professional education, research opportunities, and community education programs.

Because it is a publicly funded organization, the continued growth of the clinic and the availability of its services are dependent on the public's awareness, willingness, and ability to meet funding needs.

M. Murphy, M.S.N., R.N., C.A.N.P.
M. Pires, M.S., C.R.R.N.
J. Vance, B.S.N., C.Q.A., C.R.R.N.
N. Willis-Sukosky, M.N., C.R.R.N., C.N.A.
K. Wunch, M.S., C.R.R.N.

AGING IN SPINAL CORD INJURY*

Aging encompasses at least three major lifelong, overlapping, yet distinctly different developmental processes:

- Physiological changes
- Societal changes
- Self-realization issues

Consequently, the subject of aging may be approached from quite different perspectives. Physiological change includes loss of muscle mass that results in decreased strength, a decrease in range of motion and osteoarthritis leading to pain and decreased function, an increase in occurrence of urologic and bowel problems, and so on. Societal changes include growth and development as a child, leaving the home, marriage and parenting, loss of one's parents, loss of a spouse. Self-realization involves such issues as growth and development to young adult, development of ethics and morality, spiritual discovery, and finding meaning in life.

Perhaps one of the most distinctive features of aging is the increasing uniqueness and differentiation of each individual. For instance, a group of 20-year-old, C_6 quadriplegic people would have a similar profile of functional abilities, health impairment, and organ system reserves. This same group 30 years later would vary tremendously in terms of obesity, range of motion, cardiac reserve, strength and functional ability.

Because aging in SCI is such a new field and so little is known, much of what is discussed is speculative, with some tentative solutions, rather than tried and proven specifics, of which there are none.

*This section was contributed by Robert R. Menter, M.D.

The Aging Model Related to People with SCI

Physiological aging is the steady erosion of the reserve built into each organ system of the body. As the reserve is gradually diminished, the vulnerability to disruption of normal function of that system increases. Research has shown typical aging patterns in all systems of the body. In any given individual, the particular pattern of aging varies. In one individual with severe asthma, the reserve within the pulmonary system may be used at an early age, incapacitating the overall function of the body. In a person with rheumatoid arthritis, the pattern of aging may be expressed in decreasing range of motion and increasing pain, leading to decreasing function of the body as a whole. An individual with SCI undergoes dramatic changes in many systems such as skin sensitivity, bladder function, and bowel function, which interfere with the overall mobility and health of the system. Because there is a tremendous amount of reserve built into each organ system, and a complex system of adaptation (rehabilitation), most people continue to function but at reduced capacity.

A conceptual model of how aging may impact the total function following the onset of a spinal injury may be described in three phases (See Figure 33–1):

- Acute restoration
- Maintenance
- Decline

Acute restoration is the process by which an individual goes from no function immediately following injury to the maximum amount of function consistent with the level of neurological injury modified by variables such as motiva-

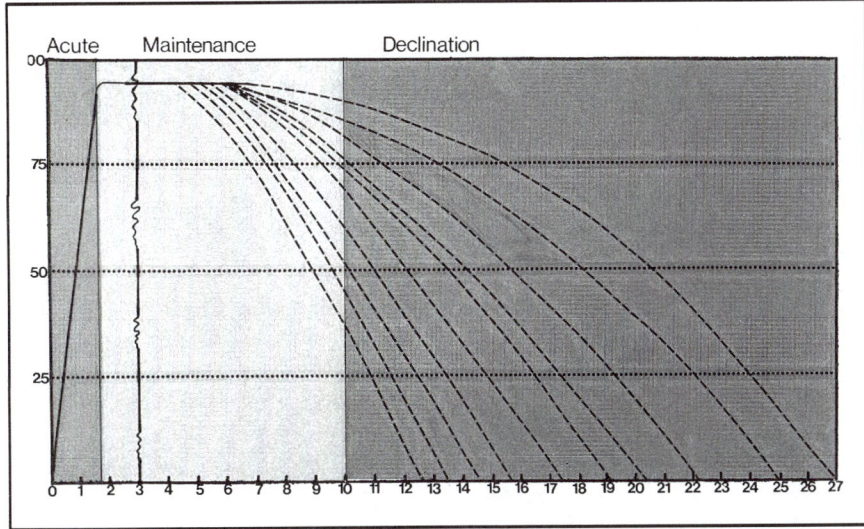

FIGURE 33–1 Influence of physical disability on aging.

tion. Usually, the acute rehabilitation phase is completed within 2 years following the injury.

The next phase, *maintenance*, is an indefinite and lengthy phase in which the person maintains that level of function established following injury.

The last phase, *decline*, occurs when the gradual onset of the physiological aging process interferes with the individual's function. Whether it be in muscle strength, range of motion of the joints, decreasing respiratory or cardiovascular capacity, or more frequent skin breakdown, problems interfere with and decrease the overall function of the body. As this steady erosion of reserve occurs, the individual gradually decreases in function. Little is known about this phase. The pattern of decline may vary greatly or have some consistent patterns. The goal is to understand the patterns so that individuals may try to control or prevent some of the consequences.

Some insight is provided by other disabilities in various phases of the aging model. The survivors of the polio epidemic, for example, are in the phase of decline. This population is now approaching some 40 years after onset. In the early 1980s, the polio survivors began to experience significant changes for which they were unprepared, and thus have had to alter their life-style significantly. Some of the changes included increasing pain, increasing weakness, increasing fatigue, all in excess of what had been expected for their age. These changes require their using more physical aids and limiting their physical activities. One overriding concern is what they can do now to preserve as much function and activity for the future as possible.

The SCI population, now in the acute restoration and maintenance phases, may anticipate similar changes in the future. However, each individual has a unique pattern of aging based on physiological age, societal interaction, self-realization, anatomical or neurological level of injury, and length of time postinjury.

Factors That Affect the Aging Process

The following major components determine the aging process:

- Genetic
- Trauma
- Life-style
- Stress adaptation
- Sociological roles

Of these factors, genetic characteristics are the only ones beyond control. How people choose to live determines trauma risk factors, life-style, adaptation to stress, and sociological roles. Four of the five major determinants of aging can be controlled; thus, many of the consequences of aging can be prevented or postponed.

Studies of longevity have shown the following determinants to be significant:

- Diet
- Exercise
- Smoking
- Work and retirement
- Marital status
- Social activities

In each area an optimal balance enhances good health.

An important factor in the aging process is the cumulative effect of life-style circumstances such as smoking, exercise, nutrition, and economic support, which may substantially alter system reserves and functional abilities.

Stress and how it is managed is a significant factor in aging. Unmanaged stress may lead to such diverse problems as hypertension, heart disease, obesity, peptic ulcer disease, and respiratory disease. Each of these medical conditions can significantly interfere with an individual's life-style. Good health requires effective stress management so that stress does not focus on any target organ but is dissipated in a more constructive manner.

Wellness is the concept that best encompasses the principles of controlling the consequences of aging and achieving longevity with as high a quality of life as possible. Wellness is defined as a life-style for achieving good health, and with good health, one's highest potential. Key components of wellness programs involve nutrition, physical awareness, stress reduction, and self-responsibility. Although most information relating to wellness has been developed in the nondisabled population, these same principles hold true for the disabled population as well.

Society and individuals with SCI are becoming increasingly interested in the problems of aging as greater numbers live into the phase of decline. Some spinal injured individuals have lived 30 to 40 years since the onset of paralysis. Although few in number, these individuals appear to have distinctly different problems from those of able-bodied people of the same age.

The following are examples of normal changes of aging by system and some of the concerns they create in SCI people. The normal skeletal system aging is reflected in *osteoarthritis* with associated decrease in range of motion and increased pain. Another normal aging change is *osteoporosis* and its associated increased risk of fractures. These normal aging changes, when imposed on an individual with SCI who already has decreased range of motion, pain, and osteoporosis, may produce an accelerated aging pattern with consequences noted at a much earlier age than in the general population.

The normal muscular system is known to age with resultant *decrease in strength*. This additional loss of strength of aging may in SCI significantly change the ability of individuals to be independent and care for themselves.

PERSONAL VIEWPOINT

I was injured (C$_8$) in a skiing accident in 1961. At the time I was a high school senior and was on the ski patrol. I enjoyed all sports. After high school and rehabilitation, I graduated from a technological institute with a degree in mechanical engineering.

My first job was in industrial sales. I enjoyed helping customers solve mechanical problems. After 3 years I was approached by the Canadian Paraplegic Association (CPA) to work with them as a rehabilitation counselor. This required additional courses, but my personal experience made the course material especially interesting and I have worked for CPA ever since. Establishing close relationships, not only with the newly injured but with the various treatment professionals, is very rewarding.

When I learned to drive with hand controls, I discovered a freedom of movement that made me equal to other drivers on the highway. Before this, my mobility was restricted to slow and awkward wheelchair movement or relying on other people to drive me. This love of driving led me to become involved in car rallying. I joined the Volvo car club and spent several years as a competitor on weekend rallies throughout the back country of British Columbia.

In 1970 I wanted to buy my own sailboat, a 17-foot dinghy. My mother in her wisdom, suggested I should see if I could still swim. I wasn't a great swimmer before my injury so I heartily agreed. The prospect of capsizing the sailboat was not too appealing. I was introduced to Stan Stronge who agreed to teach me to swim. I didn't know at the time that he was the national swim coach for the Canadian Wheelchair Sports Association. Before I knew it I was swimming for Canada in Jamaica at the Pan American Games in 1971. Swimming gave me a marvelous sense of freedom as it eliminated the burden of limbs that didn't work and the encumbrance of the wheelchair.

The coach was a long time "para" who had been involved in rehabilitation counseling for many years. To encourage new swimmers to come out to practice (I discovered later that it was no accident), his volunteer swim helpers were attractive young ladies. I wasn't the only swimmer who worked extra hard and attended every practice with more on my mind than swimming!

I have been very involved in wheelchair sports since then and have competed on many international teams representing Canada. In my days, I've tried tennis, racquet ball, table tennis and murder ball (quad rugby).

My appreciation of murder ball changed after I fractured my pelvis in 1985 as the result of a rather energetic game! This revealed my extreme osteoporosis. I also fractured my tibia-fibula in a very suspect manner only one year later. I was entering a swimming pool from my wheelchair as I had frequently done and when I came out of the water, my lower leg was at a funny angle. This is a major physical consequence of being in a wheelchair for over 25 years.

Following 5 years of marriage that ended in divorce, I met the most wonderful woman in the world. Patricia introduced me to tenting and camping. I had always loved the outdoors but could not believe that I could manage in a tent. I wasn't entirely wrong. However, the mutual ignorance of difficulties and good humor combined with practicality permitted us to enjoy a wonderful introduction to camping on Orcas Island in the Pacific Northwest. The fact that the tent was a pup tent gave rise to amusement when I tried to sit up and get dressed. Anyone looking from the outside would think that the tent had taken on a life of its own as I thrashed about inside. We also learned that wheelchair-accessible designation for campgrounds was useful only as a general indication, and personal inspection was required before setting up camp. Skills learned in rehabilitation need continual modification!

Once bitten by the camping bug, we decided to wander further afield. We drove to Disneyland along the Pacific Coastal route and camped along the way. Although we didn't camp every evening, we did find some good campgrounds and enjoyed the beauty of the coast. Disneyland is a "magic kingdom" designed for young and the young at heart. Being in the latter category we had a great time going on as many rides as possible but also taking time to just sit and watch people. Everyone was so happy and in such a good mood there. I must say I wasn't too disappointed that I wouldn't be able to ride "Space Mountain," but just sitting near the exit door, I could vicariously experience the thrills and chills of the ride as people staggered out, gasping about how thankful they were to be on solid ground again. One benefit of being in a chair is that we could proceed to the head of the line. We enjoyed such rides as the Pirates of the Caribbean, It's a Small World, and the Matterhorn.

Now that we're living in Alberta, we are looking forward to camping near Rocky Mountain House, which was the western destination of the historic voyagers.

(Box continues)

PERSONAL VIEWPOINT (continued)

Because of these shared experiences, we are able to apply our problem solving skills and good humored approach to life and have developed a strong and loving relationship.

Some time ago my interest in kayaking resulted in locating a swimming pool where canoe and kayak lessons were held. Minor modification to seating and lots of practice in the warm pool encouraged me to try some bigger waters. Patricia was a "chicken" when it came to rolling in the kayak so I had to find another paddle partner. An energetic physical therapist friend agreed to come to the pool and try the boats. I gave her some rudimentary lessons from the deck and we were

off to try the Pacific—at least a sheltered portion of it—False Creek in Vancouver harbor. It was wonderful to experience a new form of freedom on the water. We were able to paddle amongst the wharves and the yachts that sail to the corners of the earth. I still get a particularly good feeling when I hear her tell another therapist that she has been kayaking and mentions that she was taught by a quadriplegic friend!

Tom Parker
Executive Director
Alberta Paraplegic Association
Edmonton, Alberta, Canada

The normal gastrointestinal system ages with decreased volumes of saliva, acid, bile, and pancreatic juice, along with decreased peristalsis and constipation. These normal changes, when superimposed on preexisting problems of decreased peristalsis and constipation of SCI, may produce *accelerated refractory bowel dysfunction.*

The normal skin ages with a thinning of the skin and dermis along with loss of subcutaneous fat. These changes in neurotopic skin with loss of protective sensation and body control may present increased difficulty for people with SCI in maintaining sitting time and tolerance.

A Research Perspective

Little is known about the effects of aging in SCI. Most current information is anecdotal and limited to the perspective of the individual affected. Survival of people with SCI has evolved through a series of steps, so that most of the survivors of the 1940s and 1950s have low-level and mid-level paraplegia. Not until the 1960s and 1970s did people with low-level quadriplegia (C_7 and C_8) and then finally people with mid-level quadriplegia (C_5 and C_6) survive in significant numbers. In the 1980s the emergence of prehospital and critical care systems has allowed people with high-level quadriplegia (C_1 through C_4) to survive. When studying problems associated with aging in SCI, remember that people with paraplegia are now approaching 30 to 40 years of cumulative aging; whereas those with low quadriplegia are, for the most part, approximately 20 years postinjury; and those with high quadriplegia, as a group, 10 years postinjury.

Further complicating the study of aging with SCI is the problem of differing goals of rehabilitation prevalent in the different decades. In the 1950s rehabilitation was defined as survival, and goals were merely to get home to a sedentary existence. Sedentary life-styles have their own set of complications such as obesity, increased cardiovascular disease,

and increased smoking, among others. In contrast, in the 1970s and 1980s rehabilitation goals were active life-styles with involvement in the community and as much independence as possible. These goals may contribute to entirely different patterns of aging, such as overuse syndromes, wearing out joints and muscles, as well as increased stress in trying to compete in the community. Because of the differing goals of rehabilitation, the individuals injured in the 1950s and 1960s may have different patterns of aging from those injured in the 1970s and 1980s.

Last, there is a clear difference in aging patterns depending on the age of onset of SCI. Youth is the common factor. As the aging of America continues, more and more people live into their 70s and 80s and develop degenerative changes of the cervical spine with associated spinal stenosis. Significant numbers of individuals now experience SCI at an elderly onset as opposed to the usual youthful onset. Initial studies indicate these older individuals have quite different clinical courses after injury than their younger counterparts.

It is essential, therefore, to establish effective data bases to track and identify the various patterns of aging so that programs to inform individuals and help them control, postpone, and prevent some of these changes can be developed.

In 1982, Dr. George Hohmann, Ph.D., a paraplegic survivor of World War II, spoke at Craig Hospital on issues of aging in SCI. Dr. Hohmann was 40 years postinjury. The problems he identified among his fellow survivors of spinal cord injury were grouped into six categories:

- Orthopedic complications
- Neurological complications
- Medical infections
- Obesity
- Family challenges
- Psychosocial issues

Orthopedic problems include increasing pain and restricted range of motion particularly in the arms, shoulders, and neck which are thought to be overuse syndromes as a result of using the arms and shoulders to perform tasks they were not designed to perform. Equally significant was the increasing incidence of fractures of osteoporotic lower extremities. Less understood, but a more frightening problem, was the collapse of the spine at or below the level of the injury as a result of developing joint changes below the level of paralysis.

Neurological complications refer to the development of a significantly higher incidence of carpal tunnel syndrome and ulnar nerve atrophy than in the normal population. This is perhaps related to the trauma on the palms and wrists secondary to using crutches and wheelchairs and the pressure on the elbows associated with armrests on the wheelchairs or supporting the body with their elbows while sitting at a table. Other individuals suffered from mysterious loss of neurological function above the level of their injury, which is now understood to be posttraumatic cyst myelopathy (syringomyelia described in Chapter 28).

Medical infection refers to the apparent decreasing resistance to overwhelming infections. Individuals who seem to deal with infections effectively for 20 to 30 years appear to lose their resistance and abilities to deal with infection.

Obesity, a secondary complication of a sedentary lifestyle, became a significant problem. Individuals became so fat that neither they, nor their spouses, could provide their care such as doing a bowel program or transfers. In many instances, individuals were forced to move to nursing homes as a result of their obesity.

Family challenges were reflected in the long-term effects of spouses providing care in addition to all of their other responsibilities. With age, the demands on spouses become greater rather than less, at a time when the spouse is less able to provide that care. Changes in life-style for the disabled spinal injured person occurred earlier than their nondisabled partner, who had yet to feel the onset of aging, and was not ready for changes in their life-style.

Psychosocial issues were reflected in withdrawal from life without overt depression. This may be a sense of helplessness and loss of control over life. Accompanying this is a loss of interest in sexuality, self-esteem, and hope.

To the problems identified by Dr. Hohmann, add the problem of *bowel dysfunction*. Very common are problems of bowel constipation and impaction in spinal cord individuals whose bowels seem to have been functioning well for many years. Often these individuals have been on bowel programs every 3 to 5 days and describe having results each time but increasing difficulty with indigestion and bloating and gas. On X ray the entire colon is packed with firm stool and in some cases the appearance of megacolon. The explanation seems to be that, although the individuals are having results each time they do their program, they are not emptying out the entire amount that they have accumulated during the interval between bowel programs. An example would be shoveling sand into a funnel. If three scoops of sand go in each day and only two scoops come out, there is a gradual backing up and filling up even though the sand continues to come out.

CHANGING ROLES OF HEALTH CARE PROFESSIONALS IN RELATION TO PEOPLE WITH DISABILITIES

Direct Professional Services

Immediately following SCI, health care professionals are considered the experts, and of necessity, injured persons and their families largely experience a one-sided relationship as recipients of knowledge and expertise. But in planning continuing care needs for life, specifically dealing with the aging issues, there are no experts. It is imperative that health care professionals recognize personal limitations and be open to relationships based on a shared exploration of new frontiers (Trieschmann 1987). This requires empathy and emphasis on listening, analysis, and problem solving.

In the development of the discharge plan and in future services, it is vital that the injured person and family members take an active part in the decision-making process. Wright (1960) stresses that inner strength and self-respect grow when people feel they have an important role in planning life and when what the injured person says and feels is regarded as important. As an active participant in the discharge and follow-up process, the individual's motivation and self-esteem increase chances to do well in the world in general.

Florence Strobel Kahn, a nurse who has quadriplegia, explains that one of her biggest hurdles to overcome about being disabled was her negative attitude about people with disabilities. "I had them before I was injured and they were inside of me after! Attitudes hindered me. How much do they hinder other health care professionals?" See her Personal Viewpoint in Chapter 9.

Throughout this text, the reader is urged to look inwardly, to personal values and beliefs, and also outwardly, to those who are living with SCI for that unique insight into the real world beyond the centers where professionals work. It is impossible to reach the fullest professional potential without learning from people with disabilities. They provide a vision of what is possible and help to identify the most helpful approaches.

Injured people often speak of rehabilitation as a journey, a terrifying journey without a map, where health professionals are seen as guides or bridges. Ms. Kahn sees three bridges:

- Have a vision for me, even before we meet.
- Talk to me, and not my disability. Wherever I am in this journey, respect me.
- Educate me. It took years for me to understand the changes in my body and its weird signals and then to problem solve each situation . . . and I am a nurse!

Personal introspection and growth increase our professional value and naturally extend a comfort zone to injured persons and their families. Perhaps there are not so many mistakes in interactions with injured persons and their families as experiences from which to learn. Promoting self-esteem during the rehabilitation process and beyond is built in small steps. Health care professionals can positively and powerfully influence the rebuilding of self-esteem and the lives of catastrophically injured people—one moment at a time.

Additional Roles

Beyond direct professional services to people with SCI, health care professionals are increasingly and actively seeking input from consumers regarding various research projects and direct planning of future services. The Model SCI Systems conduct various long-term studies (Apple and Hudson 1990), and consumer surveys or questionnaires are common. For example, quality of life issues may be thought of in terms of life satisfaction, competence and productivity, empowerment and independence, and community integration issues (Schalock, Keith, and Hoffman 1990). Although hard to define, quality of life is believed to impact health, but SCI-specific studies are barely documented although they are currently being sought (Zejdlik 1991).

Sharing the concerns of a rapidly growing, aging population, Perry (1991) suggests that limitations faced by people with SCI are similar to limitations in function experienced by older people. Neurological research to restore function is critical to caring for all people in both human terms and staggering economic costs. Provision of long-term care is

also a common concern and offers a logical base for concerted action (Zola 1990).

Innovative planning in continuing care services focuses on integrated services that seek alternatives to reduce dependency on institutional care and respond more flexibly to local needs. The Victoria Health Project (1990) is a unique example of a wellness approach to care for frail elderly and chronically ill persons in the community. New approaches to feeling good are offered through wellness centers, quick response teams (composed of nurses, therapists, and social workers) to address sudden changes in health status at home, outreach services, seniors for seniors volunteer forces, care givers' support network, and home support training courses offered at local colleges.

Secondary disabilities have a substantial impact on people with SCI (Berczeller and Bezkor 1986; Bedbrooke 1984; Green 1990). Current prevention strategies and interventions are now being addressed on a national level by representatives of health, rehabilitation, and consumer communities. The Centers for Disease Control (CDC), the National Council on Disability, the Association of State and Territorial Health Officials, the National Institute on Disability and Rehabilitation Research, the National Academy of Sciences/Institute of Medicine, and the American Spinal Injury Association (ASIA) have cosponsored a conference that identified five general types of SCI complications: cardiovascular-cardiopulmonary, genitourinary and bowel, neuromusculoskeletal, skin, and psychosocial. Their collective efforts are very promising. Recommendations included the need for uniformity in definitions, shared research and data collecting techniques and strategies, and implications for both public and professional education to promote wellness (Graitcer and Maynard 1990). The inclusion of public health expertise is particularly exciting because this will potentiate badly needed services (National Council on Disability, Minority Health Professions Foundation, Centers for Disease Control 1991).

There is much to learn and coordinate in order to improve situations for people with disabilities. Health care professionals are expanding their roles and aligning themselves more closely with people with SCI to help secure enjoyable, productive lives for those in need of trauma rehabilitation.

REFERENCES

Apple, D., and Hudson, L. (Eds.). 1990. The SCI model: Lessons learned and new applications. *Proceedings of the National Consensus Conference on Catastrophic Illness and Injury.* The Georgia Regional SCI Care System, Shepherd Center for Spinal Injuries, Atlanta, GA.

Bedbrooke, G. 1984. *Lifetime Care of the Paraplegic Patient.* White Plains, NY: Longman.

Berczeller, P. and Bezkor, M. 1986. *Medical Complications of Quadriplegia.* Chicago: Year Book Medical Publisher.

Brown, D., Judd, F., and Unger, G. 1987. Continuing care of the spinal cord injured. *Paraplegia* 25(3): 296–300.

Davidoff, G. et al. 1990. Rehospitalization after rehabilitation of acute SCI: Incidence and risk factors. *Archives of Physical Medicine Rehabilitation* 71: 121–124.

Gardenhire, M., and Fields, C. 1987. Preparing the SCI patient/caregiver for discharge—A helpful tool. *SCI Nursing*: 38–42.

Graitcer, P., and Maynard, F. 1990. *Preventing Secondary Disabilities among People with Spinal Cord Injuries.* Atlanta, GA: Centers for Disease Control, U.S. Dept. of Health and Human Services, Public Health Service.

Green, D. 1990. *Medical Management of Long-Term Disability.* Rockville, MD: Aspen.

Guidelines for Facility Categorization and Standards of Care: Spinal Cord Injury. 1981. American Spinal Injury Association and American Spinal Injury Foundation. Chicago: Author. *Clearly presents purposes and requirements of the major components of care: emergency medical services, trauma centers, specialized acute care and rehabilitation facilities, and follow-up community care.*

Knowles, M. 1972. *The Modern Practice of Adult Education.* New York: Association Press. *Classic text on principles and methods of adult learning.*

McLean, S. 1981. The discharge process and spinal cord injured patients. Unpublished material. University of British Columbia, Vancouver, BC.

National Council on Disability, Minority Health Professions Foundation, Centers for Disease Control. 1991. *National Conference on the Prevention of Primary and Secondary Disabilities: Proceedings.* Atlanta, GA.

Nosek, P. 1991. *Personal Attendant Management* (audiovisual training series). Houston, TX: Independent Living Research Utilization (ILRU).

Perry, D. 1991. Long-term care and aging: Alliance for aging research. In *NCCSCI Dialogue.* Washington, DC: National Coordinating Council on SCI (Feb.): 6.

Schalock, R., Keith, K., and Hoffman, K. 1990. *Quality of life questionnaire, overview and standardization of information.* Hastings, NE: Mid-Nebraska Mental Retardation Services.

Trieschmann, R. 1987. *Aging with a Disability.* New York: Demos Publications.

—. 1988. *Spinal Cord Injuries: Psychological, Social, and Vocational Adjustment.* New York: Demos Publications.

Upton, V. 1990. *Perceptions of People with Quadriplegia on Readiness for Discharge from a Rehabilitation Centre.* Vancouver: British Columbia Rehabilitation Society. Unpublished study.

Victoria Health Project. 1990. *A Joint Effort of the Greater Victoria Hospital Society, the Capital Regional District and the Ministry of Health, Province of British Columbia, Canada.* Victoria, B.C.: Ministry of Health.

White, M. 1988. *Case Management: What Is It? Discharge Planning Update.* American Hospital Association.

Wright, B. 1960. *Physical Disability—A Psychological Approach.* New York: Harper & Row Publishers.

Zejdlik, C. 1991. *Lifetime Needs of People with SCI* British Columbia Rehabilitation Society, Vancouver. Unpublished material.

Zola, I. 1990. Aging, disability and the home care revolution. *Archives of Physical Medicine and Rehabilitation* 71:93–96.

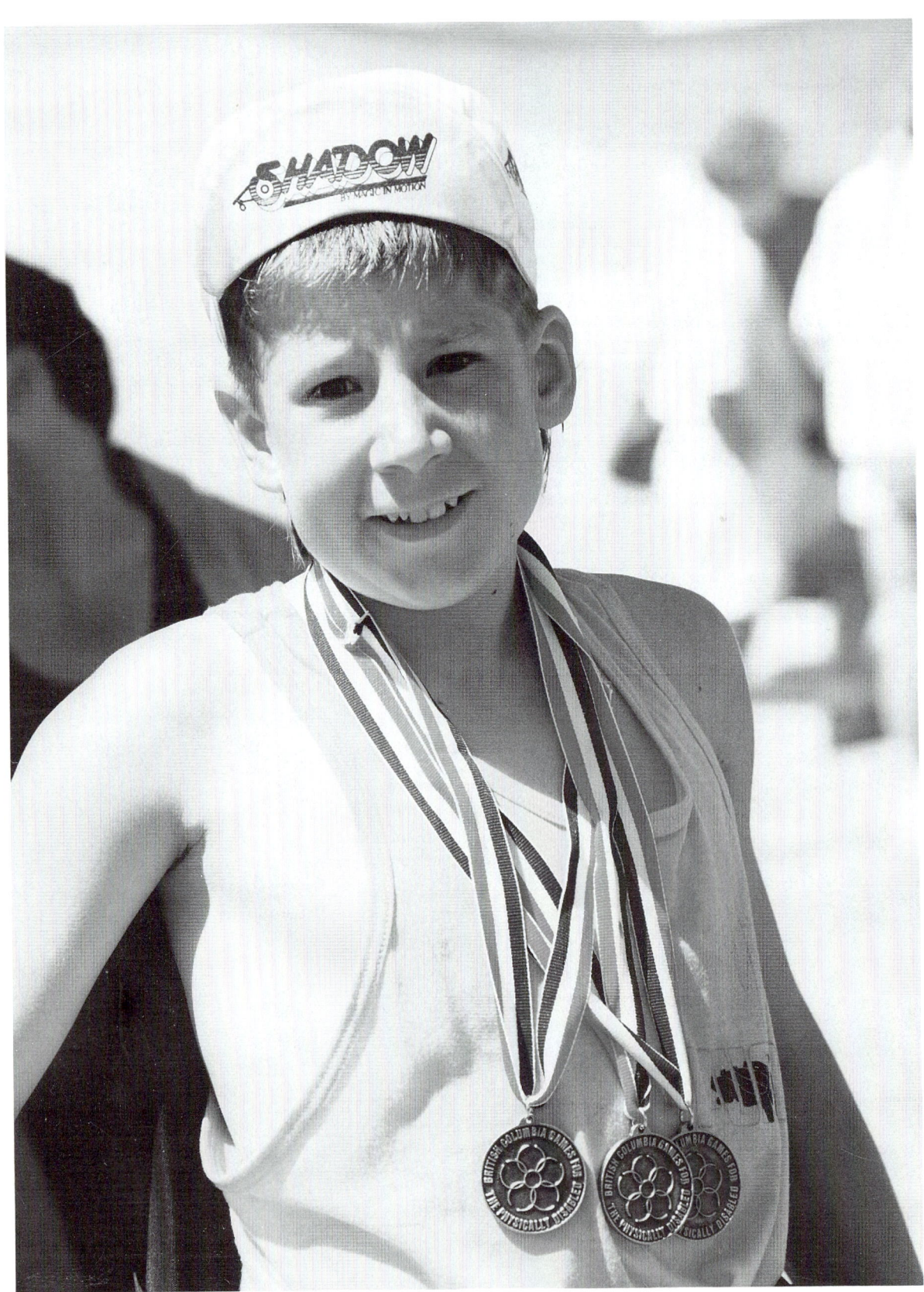

EPILOGUE

And the Future
of Spinal Cord Injury?

Sam Maddox

What lies ahead in the unique world of spinal cord injury?

An understanding of both the past and of the present permits some informed guesses.

Things are rapidly changing in the health care world. How many "case managers" were there 15 years ago? Or DRGs or HMOs or MRIs? Remember when hospitals or clinics considered it tacky to advertise or promote their services in the news media?

Patients are now demanding to be called clients or consumers, and they question or challenge authority as never before, putting the provider in an adversarial role—a major change from the old days when a patient was patient. Medicine is not the father-knows-best field it used to be; what some would term the medical priesthood has been well-bashed by the consumer movement, which sees medicine not as an art but as a commodity. An offshoot of this high-expectation consumerism is litigation—anything short of medical perfection becomes legally actionable. Simultaneously, hospital marketing staffs spent $1.3 billion in 1988 to simulate the illusion of having cured all diseases and fixed all disabilities.

Every health care specialty has become more specialized and is prone to flux. In some fields speculation on the coming years might be depressing. The dentist is hardly the brontosaurus of medical professionals but with all those years of preaching about fluoride and flossing and watching between-meal snacks, most people have indeed avoided lots of office visits. Dentists joke about putting themselves out of business, but it may not be funny. Several major dental schools recently announced closings.

This is not to imply that paralysis is destined to become as obsolete as tooth decay. But the notion of putting rehabilitation medicine out of business is not imaginary. There are two facets to SCI extinction. The first, addressed in Chapter 7 on biomedical research, is very promising: some

sort of procedure or treatment will come along to return some function in people with damaged spinal cords. "Cure" in the usual sense of "take this pill or get this transplant and be the same as you were before" probably will not be the case, but for many people with SCI, some restoration will be possible. Even the people who do not read all the neuroscience literature agree that it is not *if* but *when*.

"Walking again" is dramatically appealing, but it is such a remote possibility at this point that it cannot be predicted for sure. The initial research payoff may come slowly and without the hoopla that results from the mass media's appetite for miracles. For a person limited by severe spasticity or pain, or for a quadriplegic person unable to manipulate a knife and fork, today's research will have a profound impact.

Prevention will also reduce the incidence of SCI (note Chapter 3). Many programs urge people to play it safe, buckle seat belts, jump in feet first. There is concern whether all the good intentions translate into fewer accidents, but there is evidence that after participating in school-based programs, some people get hurt less often. For example, the "Feet First First Time" program has apparently been effective in reducing diving-related injuries in Florida. In Southern California's surfer culture, "Project Wipe Out" has the same goal. In Tampa, a snappy "Cruisin' Without Boozin' " program gets the attention of a young, at-risk audience and may get the desired results.

The momentum to galvanize United States public opinion about prevention of paralysis has been boosted by the Foundation for Spinal Cord Injury Prevention, which coordinates the many varieties of prevention programs and supports those efforts with advertising, a speakers bureau, and so on. Moreover, the Centers for Disease Control in Atlanta is pushing states to adopt mandatory reporting laws to improve SCI statistics; better stats, the thinking goes, will

THE KENT WALDREP STORY

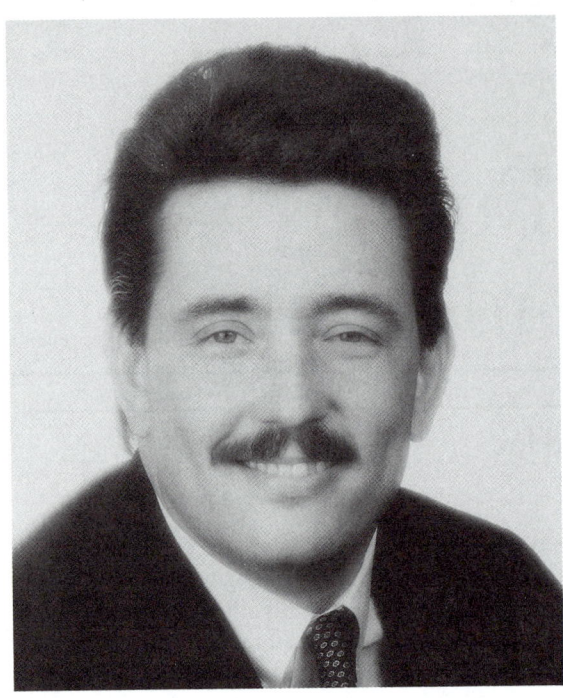

In 1974, Kent Waldrep lay in a Birmingham, Alabama hospital. A junior running back for Texas Christian University, he had suffered a broken neck during a football game against Alabama. The medical diagnosis: quadriplegia.

After the injury, Waldrep vowed to walk again, and searched for research developments that could improve his mobility. He still remembers, with some bitterness, his early hospital experiences with negative rehabilitation attitudes.

Waldrep worked hard at physical therapy and in 1978 went to the Soviet Union for specialized treatments. His trip drew reactions from the U.S. medical establishment but excited the paralysis community through the news media, which covered the trip extensively.

Upon his return, Waldrep founded and was president of the Kent Waldrep International Spinal Cord Research Foundation (which evolved into the American Paralysis Association in 1982). Waldrep built the largest charity in America focusing on paralysis research that captured the coveted Silver Anvil and Silver Spur Awards from the National Public Relations Society of America.

In June 1985, Waldrep left the APA to broaden his efforts in pursuing a cure. The Kent Waldrep National Paralysis Foundation was formed to intensify fund raising and public education efforts in the private sector for paralysis research. Waldrep also wanted to implement a financial assistance program whereby help could be provided to paralysis victims in need of medical equipment or transportation (see Resources).

Kent Waldrep was named one of the Ten Outstanding Young Men of America in 1985 by the United States Jaycees. His many other awards include an appointment to the National Council on the Handicapped by President Reagan in 1982 and reappointment in 1983 and 1986. He was named Outstanding Professional Fund Raiser of the Year in 1982 by the Dallas Chapter of the national Society of Fund Raising Executives. In 1979, the Southern Baptist Radio and TV Commission produced a documentary on Waldrep as part of their series entitled "The Athletes."

He has lectured about SCI and disability at college campuses, high schools, secondary schools, churches, civic clubs and banquets across the country. Waldrep has also been featured in national media publications such as *People Magazine, Time, Look, Newsweek* and *USA Today*. Television appearances have included the Today Show, Good Morning America, the NBC Nightly News, Cable News Network, and dozens of local affiliate interviews across the country.

Building a national consciousness for the problem of paralysis is Waldrep's constant priority. "This country has yet to realize the magnitude of this epidemic," Waldrep firmly states. "The economics alone are staggering! Our national government spends $4.5 billion annually on health maintenance programs to subsidize spinal cord injury victims alone! It costs private health insurance carriers an additional $4 billion a year. Yet, less than $25 million is currently being spent by federal and private sector agencies on medical research to cure paralysis and eliminate much of these costs; and you can't even calculate the savings in human suffering.

"Paralysis is a tragic circumstance that can touch any family in this country at any moment of any day. There are no warning signals and there are no preventive measures other than education.

"I will one day walk again because of the effort of this foundation and many other individuals dedicated to solving this problem," Waldrep strongly predicts. "But when I walk away from my wheelchair, I plan to take a lot of others with me."

enable better identification of high-risk people. The goal is to use information on injury incidence to prevent injury.

It is impossible, however, to legislate or enforce safety. In Colorado, motorcyclists lobbied lawmakers to vote down a mandatory helmet law, but not based on the usual "it's my brain and I'll bash it on the pavement if I want to" personal freedom argument. Although statistics prove that riders are far safer in a crash if using a helmet, cyclists in Colorado made a case for the *danger* of helmets—citing a United States Navy case involving a "hangman's fracture" in a single soldier injured in a parachute accident. The force of the helmet and strap assembly supposedly caused the man's cervical injury; experts, however, say motorcyclists are at virtually no risk from injuries associated with helmets.

However, to some extent laws and education programs do matter. The "unseen banana peel" theory of risk will always apply—people can be careful to the point of paranoia but they cannot ever be perfectly immune to the randomness of life.

Still, demographics may be working against the continued growth in the acute neurotrauma business—there will be fewer 19-year-old males in coming years, 19 being the most common age of a newly spinal cord injured person. Also, long-term trends in reduced alcohol consumption will most likely continue, which in turn may limit the injudicious behavior that so often precipitates injury. And safety is being better engineered, too; airbags, which are finally available on most automobiles sold in the United States, will save lots of fragile nervous systems.

People are not going to stop breaking their backs; the spinal community will grow. In fact, the community will grow old. This becomes the new frontier, and another new challenge for health care professionals. There has never before been a population who have lived a long time with paralysis. As pointed out in Chapter 33, many folks are approaching 50 years of wheelchair life and are apparently developing a whole new constellation of health care needs. Using the model of the post-polio population, it appears the aging process is accelerated after many years of disability. The message that might emerge from this is that the commonly prescribed superactive life-style may not be such a good idea. Are significant shoulder problems later on worth the fun and games today for wheelchair athletes? What are the psychological ramifications of people who have always pushed their own chairs having to depend on a power chair?

The aging issue is looming over all of health care. Undoubtedly, professionals in the SCI field, especially nurses and others involved in direct care, will always have lots of work.

Actually, the major issue facing SCI care in the early 1990s might well be that there is just too much work. At the time of writing, there are not nearly enough nurses in the field to take care of the present SCI population. Based on what nurses tell of the situation in the United States and Canada, there is about one nurse vacancy for every three or four working. Some speculate the ratio might worsen by the end of the century to the drastic level of one missing for every one working. The good news is that there will be jobs. The not so good news is that the workload will not get any lighter.

Spinal cord injury is a tough business, physically and emotionally. It is tough on everybody—the injured, the families, the care givers. It is especially tough on the injured person; typically young, male, and very often streetwise and impulsive. The forced dependency of the rehabilitation setting is difficult to accept. Many people are injured because of substance abuse and continue to seek some substance to abuse. In the big cities, more people than ever are being injured by acts of violence. In a major rehabilitation unit in Detroit, six of ten SCI involve people with a history of substance abuse, four of ten involve interpersonal violence.

The volatile mixture of a nonconforming personality with the rigidity of the ward can lead patients to reject the whole process. They have to take their frustrations out on someone. The nurse, who is the authority figure most often present, is the easiest target. The result is usually either confrontation or appeasement, one leading to fight and resentment, the other flight and guilt, both leading to helplessness and ineffective rehabilitation.

Anger and guilt are powerful emotions; either can drive people away from the high ideals that brought them into nursing and drive people out of the profession. Are there ways to defuse the high tension on the rehabilitation ward?

Nurses who hope to survive this often abusive patient relationship will be forced to deal with it head on—with open lines of communication, limits on what is acceptable behavior, and perhaps with a Toughlove attitude. This is a sort of "controlled crisis" approach to patients who act out, which is addressed in Chapter 9. Behavior in this context is a matter of choice; misbehavior is an option that can be eliminated.

Toughlove was developed in 1978 by Phyllis and David York to deal with behavior problems of their teenagers. They often felt helpless, confused, and guilty about their role as parents; the Toughlove philosophy enabled the Yorks to find support, set goals, be consistent and therefore become empowered. Books, tapes, and personal appearances spread the word, helping many in homes, classrooms, and communities to take a stand and confront unacceptable behavior.

Phyllis York broke her neck in a fall in 1983 and has quadriplegia. The Yorks became aware of the complex dynamics of the rehabilitation setting and of the sudden life change involved in disability; they have recently expanded the program to help families and care givers of people with disabilities. One evolution of the Toughlove concept deals directly with the hostility directed toward nurses from spinal cord injured patients.

Working in a trauma unit or rehabilitation hospital has never been easy. People come into the system at their worst; staff attempt to patch them up, put them back in charge of their lives, send them out to the world, fill the bed with another case, ad infinitum. Because there is so much hurt and pain in this work, it is perhaps a normal tendency to deal with each incoming patient as impersonally as possible. People become cases; Joe Doe becomes the C_5 in bed 12. Impersonal may not be the same as uncaring but some insulation may be necessary; it is not productive to take the caseload home.

However, as injured people move into the world again, they survive, they thrive, they live lives that are good and bad, happy and sad, with very little surrendered to their limitations in mobility. For the rehabilitation team, it is essential to know that arriving broken does not predict a broken life.

Since the attitude of the professional is critical for the effectiveness of the care, it seems only natural that the attitude should be based not on hopelessness and despair but on success. That is not always the case, though. Many say the longer some of their colleagues are in the business the less optimistic they become. Care givers have the important role of motivation and optimism, reassuring people in crisis with the upbeat message that they are not alone, that the outcome of rehabilitation is worth it. One should not have to take this upbeat message on faith. Success outside the world of the rehabilitation unit is much more likely than failure.

Trauma medicine does many things very well. Rehabilitation centers report the numbers of so-called complete SCI are declining because of quicker and better emergency management. This is a striking example of the need for specialization. Many communities now have well-planned triage systems to get injuries involving the brain or spinal cord to appropriate hospitals.

People are staying in hospitals shorter times after SCI. People with high-level quadriplegia, including those who use mechanical ventilation, are surviving and living with a level of independence unknown 15 years ago. Many spinal cord injured men are becoming fathers now, due to fertility techniques that were inconceivable 10 years ago! Thanks in large part to the integrated rehabilitation team approach, many more injured people are coming back into their communities better prepared for life with a disability.

Good health and even psychological care does not mean every SCI person gets a good job and a nice home, or that many communities are any better prepared to welcome people with disabilities. But 20 years of civil rights activism has forced better accommodation of citizens with disabilities. Subtle changes in social awareness have served to demystify the differentness of disability, which translates into less pity and devaluation. Of course, people with disabilities are still prejudged. Yet, as those with disabilities often remind us, no one is more than "temporarily able-bodied" (TAB), and the day may come when disability emerges as a socially acceptable way of life.

The disabled community was not noticeably politicized a decade or so ago. Today, voices of protest are raised more frequently. They do not demand curb cuts and bus lifts, though. This movement has been more than the symbolic change of some people only wanting to be called "physically challenged" rather than "handicapped." The civil rights agenda maintains that the root problem of disability is not physical limitation but society's limiting attitudes. The message is that dignity and humanness cannot be masked or denied by disability.

The consumer empowerment idea came to the SCI community very early, at the instigation of veterans of World War II: in 1945 by the Canadian Paraplegic Association (CPA), in 1947 by the Paralyzed Veterans of America (PVA). Both spent their first two decades working in advocacy, referral, accessibility, and recreation. CPA is not specifically veteran-oriented today; PVA, although it limits its membership to veterans, nevertheless serves the entire SCI community. In recent years PVA has been active in legislative lobbying, barrier-free design, accessible transit, and health care and spinal cord regeneration research.

Nonveteran persons with paraplegia in the United States formed the National Paraplegia Foundation in 1984; now known as the National Spinal Cord Injury Association (NSCIA), the group works mostly in the area of information and referral, with chapters all over the country.

Consumer-based advocacy took on a new attitude in the 1970s when medical researchers finally turned from the age-old dogma that SCI was unfixable. Spurred on by the lack of government support for "cure," groups including the Spinal Cord Society, the American Paralysis Association, PVA, CPA and NSCIA began funding researchers directly. More recently, the Miami Project to Cure Paralysis has received much attention for its "Apollo Project" approach to research. Miami has recruited a large critical mass of scientists to work under one roof specifically on the problem of paralysis, but strength lies with international commitment and communication.

Government science programs in the United States, Canada, Europe, and Japan, for example, still pay for the bulk of neuroscience research, but the consumer movement has been willing to put up seed money recognizing innovation and front-line research the federal research bureaucracies pass over in favor of more certain payoffs.

More recently, the consumers have been joined by what might be called the self-responsibility movement of the late 1980s, including those of new-age sensibility who no longer consent to handing over control for their health to the abstract impersonality of machines, drugs, or neurotechnocrats.

Related to this is the wellness model for health care, based on the rediscovery of the obvious: what people do to themselves affects their health. Many people who must frequently deal with the traditional, allopathic medical business, as those with SCI certainly do, become very well informed about their own care and assume full responsibility for what happens to their bodies. This forms the basis of holistic health, the aim of which is to treat the whole person and the related causes of problems, not just the problems in isolation.

Holistic health care has much appeal for many people in rehabilitation because the goal of rehabilitation is first and foremost to return autonomy to the person seeking care. This approach holds that the more responsibility the care givers *take* from the person, the more that will have to be given back. So, the more a person demands to be self-determined in relation to health providers, the better.

There are aspects of the holistic or alternative health care movement that may take some time to settle into the mainstream of care. The therapeutic value of nutrition or massage may be easy to accept, but is the power of naturopathy or metaphysical healing ready for the local trauma unit? Probably not, but there is a trend in technical medicine to rediscover the power of the body to heal itself.

This change in people's relationships to health care services can be disconcerting to those people who have always done it by the book, but it should not be seen as a bad thing. A little humility is long overdue. Providers are being reacquainted with the art side of their science- and technology-based decision making. This humanism in health care apparently is not instinctual; it is being taught in medical and nursing school curricula now. One wonders if empathy and patience, or humor, can be taught in a pressurized academic environment of detached analysis and prescriptive treatment. The professions are paying attention as the consumer movement and the civil rights movement merge on the issue of dignity: people want respect.

Economics, the persistent distraction of what it all means to the bottom line, represents another major change in the way health care is conducted these days. Who pays for it? Who can afford it? Where are our priorities, as a society, for providing the best care? Will health care resources be so thinly stretched that care and treatment will be rationed?

Many health care insurance policies now include a pre-care clause. Before doctors can do anything short of emergency life-saving procedures, they first have to get approval from the insurance carrier. This is intended to hold costs down but it is now a fact of medical life that third parties have a major role in treatment, even though they never step onto the ward.

In rehabilitation, the role of the case manager appears to be increasing, adding a new level of oversight—and perhaps bureaucracy—to the process. Medicare guidelines further restrict what the rehabilitation team can do, leaving an obvious worry that the best care will be available only to rich people.

There is another economic factor in SCI and rehabilitation medicine. Because the U.S. government reimburses for rehabilitation beds more open-endedly than, for instance, gall bladder operations, which are set as a fixed diagnostic related group cost, many hospitals have entered the trauma and rehabilitation business. Some critics suggest the term, spinal cord injury unit, has been stretched to the limits of credibility. This *de factor* decentralization of expertise may turn out to be a gripe from the old-line facilities that are losing beds to the upstarts. Or it may mean quality of care has been diluted. No one is quite sure yet.

From a nurse's perspective, several key areas of change have redefined the profession. Yet medicine is still adrift in change. Technology races ahead as clinical application tries to keep pace; information is overwhelmingly specialized; health care costs continue to escalate. Medicine of high tech is shifting to one of high touch. The paternalism of the medical model is evolving into the partnership of the education model—the health care professional doesn't do the healing; the professional makes information and treatment available so the client does the healing.

Change is either a threatening scenario or it is an intriguing opportunity. People who resist change are consumed by it. The ones who embrace the future are empowered by it.

So where does this leave the nurse and the people with SCI who need a good nurse?

There will be fewer nurses on the spinal unit but they will have more job satisfaction than nurses today have. Nurses who survive the early 1990s will be elevated in status. They will earn more money and be given more responsibility and more footing with doctors in patient care. The many chores nurses have always done will be handled by ancillaries, and it will be a fact of life in medicine that the lower-level positions will be hard to keep filled.

On the whole, SCI nurses will perform tasks tomorrow much as they did 10 and 20 years ago. The nurse has been and will continue to be the primary contact person between injured persons, their families, and the rest of the rehabilitation team. The spinal unit nursing staff will always have all the medical management aspects of sudden, catastrophic injury to deal with—vertebral stability, respiration, skin integrity, bowel and bladder function, and so on—in both the acute stabilization phase and the rehabilitation life-adaptation phase.

It is likely the nurse will have even more to deal with in aspects of trauma care, in particular, resource identification, and patient education. The sheer volume of information available to the full range of practitioners in physical medicine is overwhelming; information itself does not equal knowledge. The nurse, as the pivotal member of the team, will have the added responsibility of linking patients to usable information—resources—that help them reclaim their self-reliance. This means the nursing profession itself must be committed to a vigorous, never-ending process of self-education and information transfer.

What have been the biggest changes in rehabilitation in the last 10 to 20 years, especially from the perspective of the nurse practitioner? This book clearly attests to the establishment and acceptance of specialized trauma rehabilitation and the integrated team approach to treating SCI. The technology available to rehabilitation practitioners and to the person with SCI have made great leaps forward.

All of this together means nurses will become even more important to the success of tomorrow's rehabilitation process. Nurses will be highly trained and highly valued members of the spinal injury recovery team, using new tools and new ways of thinking to do their jobs better, which is to say, to put people who have undergone dramatic life changes back in charge of their lives.

Resources

AUDIOVISUAL AIDS

Only a few videotapes, audiotapes, and films are cited in this text. Contact TIRR for professional/public SCI database. Free access. 1-800-44-REHAB.

HOTLINE AND NETWORK

National Spinal Cord Injury Hotline (NSCIHL)

24-HOUR TOLL-FREE NUMBERS: NATIONAL: 1-800-526-3456; IN MD: 1–800–638–1733

Gives specific information and referrals concerning acute and rehabilitative care, research, local contacts, and SCI organizations. Endorsed by the NSCIA, the National Study Center for Emergency Medical Systems, the ATS, the National Research Institute for Neural Injury, and the Stifle Foundation. Cooperation and support has been established with the APA and the PVA.

Spinal Network

California Spinal Cord Injury Network, 3911 Princeton Dr., Santa Rosa, CA 95405. *Focuses on education, legal, and family resources.*

Sam Maddox, Publisher. Box 4162, Boulder, CO 80306. *A true network and fine resource designed to connect persons with SCI to ideals, experiences, and resources in the SCI community and to become aware of the variety of choices open to reach personal goals. Publishes the book Spinal Network (1987), and Spinal Network Extra. (quarterly magazine). Essential reading. Full of resources, connections, book reviews news, and commentary.*

MODEL SCI DEMONSTRATION PROJECTS

Model demonstration projects (in 1990) included: Spain Rehabilitation Center, University of Alabama, Birmingham, AL; Rancho Los Ami-gos Medical Center, Downey, CA; Rocky Mountain Spinal Cord Injury Center, Craig Hospital, Englewood, CO; Georgia Regional Spinal Cord Injury Center, Shepherd Spinal Center, Atlanta, GA; Midwest Regional Spinal Cord Injury Center, Northwestern Memorial Hospital, Chicago, IL; New England Regional Spinal Cord Injury Center, University Hospital, Boston, MA; Southeastern Michigan Regional Spinal Cord Injury Center, Rehabilitation Institute of Detroit, Detroit, MI; University of Michigan Regional Spinal Cord Injury Center, University of Michigan Hospitals, Ann Arbor, MI; New York University Medical Center, Institute of Rehabilitation Medicine, New York, NY; Strong Memorial Hospital, University of Rochester, Rochester, NY; Regional Spinal Cord Injury Center of Delaware Valley, Thomas Jefferson University, Philadelphia, PA; Texas Regional Spinal Cord Injury Center, The Institute for Rehabilitation and Research, Houston, TX; and University of Virginia Medical Center, Charlottesville, VA.

ORGANIZATIONS

Most organizations mentioned in this text are listed here. See also Chemical (Drug/Alcohol) Dependency under Psychosocial Adaptation in the Supplemental Reading Section of these Resources; Table 3–3 for organizations interested in safety issues, and the Sports Resources box in Chapter 24.

Australia

There is no national organization for persons with SCI: all are state based. The following have branches throughout Australia:

Australian Quadriplegic Association, 1 Jennifer St., Little Bay, New South Wales, Australia 2063. *Publishes the journal, Quad Wrangle.*

Comcare, 393–397 Swanston St., Melbourne, Vic. Australia 3000.

Disability Advisory Council of Australia, G.P.O. Box 9848, Canberra, Australian Capital Territory, Australia 2606.

Industrial Rehabilitation Services, 60 Margaret St., Sydney, New South Wales, Australia 2000.

Paraplegic and Quadriplegic Association of New South Wales, 33–35 Burlington Rd., Homebush, New South Wales, Australia 2140. *Publishes the journal Paraquad News.*

Paraplegic and Quadriplegic Association of Queensland, Horan St., Brisbane, Queensland, Australia 4104.

Spinal Injuries Postgraduate Course, N.S.W. College of Nursing, Locked Bag No. 5, Glebe, N.S.W. Australia 2037.

Canada

British Columbia Paraplegic Association (BCPA), 780 S.W. Marine Dr., Vancouver, BC, Canada V6P 5Y7.

Canadian Paraplegic Association (CPA), National Office, 1500 Don Mills Rd., Don Mills, Ontario, M3B 3K4. 416–391–0203. *Established in 1945 by returning veterans, and now offers services in every province. Extensive information and referral services provided by rehabilitation counselors (most of whom are spinal cord injured). Provides regional consultants, prevention programs, and a disabled speaker's bureau, and maintains a new injuries registry. Has initiated important innovations in housing for persons with high quadriplegia, and in programs concerning acute care, sport, high quadriplegia, and care for life time needs. Publishes the Caliper (national monthly journal) and numerous brochures, bulletins, and newsletters.*

Canadian Rehabilitation Council for the Disabled (CRCD) One Yonge St., #2110, Toronto, Ontario, M5E 1E5. *Provides a national network for disabled individuals, professionals, and organizations. Publishes Rehabilitation Digest Journal, Access (newsletter), and films.*

Rick Hansen Man-in-Motion Society, 780 S.W. Marine Dr., Vancouver, BC, V6P 5Y7. *Legacy Fund totals more than $20 million dollars. Annual Awards are granted in fellowships, scholarships, and rehabilitation in support of SCI research, rehabilitation, prevention, and wheelchair sport. See Chapter 24 for Rick's personal story.*

Hugh MacMillan Centre, Toronto, Ontario. Technology aids.

Neil Squire Foundation, 4381 Gallant Ave., North Vancouver, BC, V7G 1L1 Canada. 604-929-2414. *Nonprofit organization that specializes in development and training in the use of adaptive equipment for increasing the independence and return to community living for persons with severe physical disabilities. Publishes a quarterly newsletter with practical hints and applications of technology for this population. Promotes a network of communication and information sharing.*

Great Britain

International Medical Society of Paraplegia, National Spinal Injuries Centre, Stoke Mandeville Hospital, Aylesbury, Bucks., England HP21 8AL. *Primarily a scientific organization of physicians and researchers, conducting annual conventions and other educational sessions. Publishes Paraplegia Journal.*

Royal Association for Disability and Rehabilitation (RADAR), 25 Mortimer Street, London, England W1N8AB.

Spinal Injuries Association (SIA), Yeoman House, 76 St. James's La., London, England N103DF. *Provides information, advocacy, and numerous services for individuals and families.*

United States

Alliance for Technology Access (ATA). 1307 Solano Ave., Albany, CA 94706. *Offers a nonprofit nationwide network for hands-on experience opportunities.*

American Association of Neuroscience Nurses (AANN), 218 North Jefferson, Suite 204, Chicago, IL 60606. *Fosters the health, welfare, and education of the general public, sets high standards in the practice of neuroscience nursing, and promotes the growth of nursing as a profession. Publishes Journal of Neuroscience Nursing, Synapse Newsletter, and Neuroscience Nursing.*

American Association of Spinal Cord Injury Nurses (AASCIN), 75–20 Astoria Blvd., Jackson Heights, NY 11370–1178. *Established in 1983. Promotes education for excellence in clinical practice and nursing research related to nursing care of persons with SCI. Encourages nurses to conduct research to improve quality of care. Holds annual conferences that offer a forum for nurses to network and share strategies. Publishes the journal, SCI Nursing (quarterly), with submissions from staff nurses as well as nursing researchers and other leaders; and Education Guide for Spinal Cord Injury Nurses: A Manual for Teaching Patients, Families and Caregivers (1990).*

American Association of Spinal Cord Injury Psychologists and Social Workers (AASCIPSW), 75–20 Astoria Blvd., Jackson Heights, NY 11370–1178. *Strives to improve its members' skills and techniques and promotes research to improve the overall quality of care. Sponsors annual meetings.*

American Congress of Rehabilitation Medicine, 130 South Michigan Ave., Suite 1310, Chicago, IL 60603–6110. *The only rehabilitation association dedicated to coordinating all the disciplines in rehabilitation medicine. Publishes Archives of Physical Medicine and Rehabilitation.*

American Paralysis Association (APA), 500 Morris Ave., Springfield, NJ 07081. *Dedicated to find a cure for paralysis with a focus on SCI. APA's mission is worldwide with programs that support neural regeneration and recovery research with priority for applied research on chronic paralysis. Operates national HOTLINE (NSCIHL). Facilitates the search for support and resources for research, rehabilitation, statistics, literature, accessibility, advocacy, and equipment.*

American Paraplegia Society (APS), 75–20 Astoria Blvd., Jackson Heights, NY 11370–1178. *A physician-oriented organization dedicated to improving the quality of medical care for individuals with SCI. Publishes Journal of American Paraplegia Society.*

American Rehabilitation Counseling Association, 5999 Stevenson Ave., Alexandria, VA 22304. 703–823–9800.

American Spinal Injury Association (ASIA), 250 East Superior St., Room 619, Chicago, IL 60611. *Primarily physician oriented. Pursues excellence in SCI care with a strong focus on interdisciplinary education. Publishes ASIA Bulletin (semiannual) and ASIA Meeting Proceedings (from 1972 to the present).*

American Spinal Injury Foundation, 250 East Superior St., Room 619, Chicago, IL 60611. *Established in 1982 with the assistance of ASIA to link research with charitable funding sources. Publications related to nursing education and long-term implications of SCI.*

American Trauma Society (ATS), 1400 Mercantile La., Suite 188, Landover, MD 20785.

Ann Arbor Center for Independent Living. (See University of Michigan.)

Apple Computer, Office of Special Education and Rehabilitation, 20525 Mariani Ave., MS 43-S, Cupertino, CA 95014. *Maintains database and works with educators and organizations.*

Architectural and Transportation Barriers Compliance Board (ATBCB), 1111 18th St., NW, Fifth Floor, Washington DC 20036–3894. *Publishes Access America: The Architectural Barriers Compliance Act and*

You; Access America: Laws Concerning the ATCB; Access Travel: Airports; Aircraft Stowage Procedures for Battery Powered Wheelchairs.

Association of Rehabilitation Nurses (ARN), P.O. Box 1014, Skokie, IL 60077. *Growing international membership reflects the interest in rehabilitation nursing as a specialty. Sponsors annual conferences and regional activities including certification course in rehabilitation. Publishes Rehabilitation Nursing Journal and newsletters.*

Coordinating Center for Home and Community Care (CCHC), P.O. Box 613, Millersville, MD 21108.

Clearinghouse on Disability Information, Office of Special Education and Rehabilitative Services (OSERS), U.S. Dept. of Education, Room 3132, Switzer Bldg., Washington DC 20202-2524. 202-732-1241. *Created by the Rehabilitation Act of 1973. Responds to inquiries, research, and documents related to disability information operations. Especially helpful regarding federal legislation and programs that aid disabled people. Publishes OSERS News in Print and newsletter about federal activities. Provides a wealth of information on education, employment, architecture and transportation accessibility, research updates, legislation and law enforcement, housing (rights and practical access information), health insurance, statistics, directories, bibliographies, newsletters, magazines, and other federally supported clearinghouses.*

Closing the Gap, P.O. Box 68, Henderson, MN 56044. 612-248-3294. *Publishes bimonthly newspaper Closing the Gap, the largest single information source available. Also sponsors an annual conference.*

Eastern Paralyzed Veterans of America (EPVA), 432 Park Ave. New York, NY 10016. *Largest chapter of the PVA. Extremely active in both cure and care research, interdisciplinary education, and supportive services to benefit all persons with SCI. Supports AASCIN, AASCIPSW, and APS.*

Functional Electrical Stimulation (F.E.S.) Information Center, 25100 Euclid Ave., Suite 105, Cleveland, OH 44117. 1-800-666-2353. *Affiliated with Case Western Reserve University and Services for Independent Living, Inc. Supported by NIDRR. Aims to increase national awareness of F.E.S., and to facilitate the exchange of information among researchers, manufacturers, professionals, and consumers. Offers information and referral services.*

Higher Education and the Handicapped (HEATH) Resource Center, One Dupont Circle, NW, Washington, DC 20036. 1-800-54-HEATH. *Provides information and referral to students and professionals on issues ranging from opportunities to legal aid.*

Independent Living Research Utilization (ILRU), 2323 South Shepherd, Suite 1000, Houston, TX 77019.

Institute for Information Studies. Formerly PSI.

IBM National Support Center for Persons with Disabilities, P.O. Box 2150 (A06S1), Atlanta, GA 30055. 404-364-2500. *Publishes Guide to Resources for Persons with Disabilities, which includes listing of resource groups (primarily U.S.) for various disabilities, as well as hardware adaptations.*

Job Accommodation Network (JAN). Morgantown, WV 26506-6122.

Robert Wood Johnson Foundation, College Rd., P.O. Box 2316, Princeton, NJ 08543-2316.

Loma Linda University Medical Center, Pulmonary Rehabilitation, 25455 Barton Rd., Suite 207A, Loma Linda, CA 92354.

Miami Project to Cure Paralysis, 1501 NW 9th Ave., Miami, FL 33136. *Perhaps the most visible SCI research effort. Focuses on cure, and F.E.S., and related research. Newsletter available.*

National Association of Rehabilitation Facilities (NARF), P.O. Box 17675, Washington DC 20041. *Members include more than 750 rehabilitation facilities serving some 500,000 persons with disabilities. Promotes excellence in management, advises on financial and reimbursement issues, and assists in research and program development for persons with physical disabilities, mental impairments, and those experiencing social or vocational barriers. Publishes Rehabilitation Review (weekly), Daily Review.*

National Association of Rehabilitation Professionals in the Private Sector, P.O. Box 708, Twin Peaks, CA 92391. 714-337-0745.

National Coordinating Council on Spinal Cord Injury (NCCSCI), 801 Eighteenth St., NW, Washington, DC. *An association of organizations, institutions, and individuals dedicated to stimulating, coordinating, and supporting cure and care research, public education, and professional training programs. Publishes DIALOGUE (bimonthly newsletter).*

National Council on Independent Living, 310 S. Peoria St., Suite 201, Chicago, IL 60607.

National Council on the Aging, 600 Maryland Ave., West Wing 100, Washington, DC 20024. 202-479-1200. *Brochures, publication lists and Current Literature on Aging Catalogue; Network information on community-based, long-term care; employment; family as care givers; senior citizen's housing; and rural activities.*

National Council on the Handicapped, 800 Independence Ave., SW, Suite 814, Washington, DC 20591. *Established as an advisory body by Congress in 1973. Now a federal agency that deals with federal laws, policies, and programs for disabled people. Numerous publications.*

National Easter Seal Society, 70 East Lake St., Chicago, IL 60601. *Serves more than 1 million people with disabilities annually (approximately 60% children).*

National Head and Spinal Cord Injury Prevention Program (NHSCIP), 22 South Washington St., Park Ridge, IL 60068.

National Head Injury Foundation (NHIF), 333 Turnpike Rd., Southborough, MA 01772. Family Help Line 1-800-444-NHIF.

National Institute on Disability Research and Rehabilitation (NIDRR), U.S. Dept. of Education/OSERS, 400 Maryland Avenue, SW, Washington, DC 20202-2646. *Supports the Model Spinal Cord Injury Systems and related research efforts. Publishes Rehab Briefs (monthly newsletters); NIDRR Program Directory (lists activities by state); NIDRR Grants, Contracts and Cooperative Agreements (fact sheet).*

National Institutes of Health (NIH), Bldg. 31, Room 8A-06, Bethesda, MD 20895. *Largest medical research funder in the United States. Technical information related to regeneration research and skin and urological problems are relevant to SCI. Rehabilitation issues are a newer focus.*

National Rehabilitation Counselor Association, 633 South Washington St., Alexandria, VA 22314. 703-836-7677.

National Rehabilitation Information Center (NARIC), 8455 Colesville Rd., Suite 385, Silver Spring, MD 20910-3319. 1-800-346-2742 or 301-588-9284 (V/TDD). *Disseminates research and technological in-*

formation for the rapidly evolving disability and rehabilitation field. Sponsored by NIDRR and currently administered by Macro Systems. For persons with disabilities, families, health care professionals, researchers, students, policy makers, the media, and the general public, offers continually updated services from its REHABDATA data base, which lists more than 25,000 publications on the total rehabilitation process. Publishes NARIC Quarterly (newsletter on disability and rehabilitation resources); Spinal Cord Injury: A NARIC Resource Guide for People with Spinal Cord Injury and Their Families (1990).

National Spinal Cord Injury Association (NSCIA), 600 West Cummings Park, Suite 2000, Woburn, MA 01801. 1–800–962–9629. *Founded in 1948 by PVA as a civilian response to the health and social problems resulting from SCI. Has local chapters and national offices to serve individuals, families, and health care and other related professionals in overcoming the problems associated with SCI. Sponsors prevention programs and research efforts to minimize cord damage and associated complications during acute care. Overall health maintenance a focus of a growing network of local chapters. Provides national educational and research conferences, information and referral, and advocacy and information exchange by members. Publishes* Spinal Cord Injury LIFE *(quarterly),* National Resource Directory, OPTIONS, *and specialized facts sheets.*

National Spinal Cord Injury Statistical Center, Spain Rehabilitation Center, Room 522, University Station, Birmingham, AL 35924.

OSERS. (See Clearinghouse on Disability Information.)

Paralyzed Veterans of America (PVA), 801 18th St., NW, Washington, DC 20006. *Organizes and ensures quality health care and rehabilitation for veterans with SCI and job opportunities and civil rights for all veterans and all Americans with a handicap. Supports legislation and advances in health care and technology to improve life for all persons with SCI. Sponsors special programs: Medical and Research Affairs Dept.; National Advocacy Program; National Legislation Program; National Barrier-Free Design Program; National Service Program; and National Sports and Recreation Program. Publishes brochures and the magazines,* Sports 'n Spokes *and* Paraplegia News. *PVA Publications, 5201 North 19th Avenue, Suite 111, Phoenix, AZ 85015.*

President's Committee on Employment of Persons with Disabilities (PCEPD), 111 20th St., SW, Room 636, Washington, DC 20036. *Publications:* Black Adults with Disabilities: A Statistical Report Drawn from Census Bureau Data; College Freshmen with Disabilities: Preparing for Employment; Data on Disability for the National Health Interview Survey; Disabled Adults of Hispanic Origin: A Statistical Report Drawn from Census Bureau Data; Disabled Women in America: A Statistical Report Drawn from Census Bureau Data.

Public Services Information (PSI) International, 510 North Washington St., Falls Church, VA 22046.

Rehabilitation Institute of Chicago, Education and Training Center, 345 East Superior St., Chicago, IL. *Send for course registration information and order books, materials, and training packages, many of which are SCI specific.*

Rehabilitation International, 25 East 21 St., New York, NY 10010. *Founded in 1922. Has more than 135 member groups in 77 countries. Holds quadrennial world congresses and other educational and research-oriented meetings to address global concerns; provides technical assistance, particularly in developing countries, and maintains official relations with UNESCO, WHO and many other national entities. Publishes* International Rehabilitation Review, International Journal of Rehabilitation Research, *and* Rehabilitation *(in Spanish).*

RESNA, Dept. 4813, Washington, DC 20016–4813. (Formerly the Rehabilitation Engineering Society of North America.) *An interdisciplinary association for the advancement of rehabilitation and assistive technologies, with a focus on linking appropriate technology with disabled individuals. Publishes* Rehabilitation Technology Review *(quarterly), and a newsletter.*

Rehabilitation Services Administration (RSA), 400 Maryland Ave., SW, Washington, DC 20202. *Funds state vocational rehabilitation programs and independent living centers.*

Rehabilitation Services Administration, Office of Independent Living, 330 C St., SW, Switzer Bldg., Washington, DC 20202. 202–732–1400. *Information on locating Independent Living Centers.*

Research and Training Center on Independent Living (RTC/IL), University of Kansas, BCR/348 Haworth, Lawrence, KS 66045–2930.

Rural Institute on Disabilities (Network), 52 Corbin Hall, Univ. of Montana, Missoula, MT 59812.

Social Security Administration (SSA), Office of Information, Room 4J–10 West High Rise Bldg., 6401 Security Blvd., Baltimore, MD 21235. *Publishes booklets:* Disability *(1988), 22 pp., a general overview of the SSA disability program; and* Supplemental Security Income *(1988) 11 pp.*

Spinal Cord Society (SCS), Wendell Rd., Fergus Falls, MN 56537. *C. E. Carson, Ph.D., President, states "SCS is a citizen advocacy organization devoted to goal-oriented research and treatment aimed at an eventual cure capability for both old and new spinal cord injuries. Since its beginning in 1978, the SCS has grown to over 200 chapters with members in over 30 countries and has initiated sister organizations in Canada, New Zealand, Holland, Ireland, and Switzerland. The SCS pioneered computerized walking therapy, which has triggered a revolution in the rehabilitation field, for which it was commended by President Reagan in the State of the Union Address in 1984. It has also pioneered regeneration and reactivation research, and both animal and human clinical trials with various drugs, electrical and molecular surgery treatments which show great promise of a solution to the problems of spinal cord injury paralysis within this decade."*

Trace Research and Development Center, S151 Waisman Center, 1500 Highland Ave., University of Wisconsin, Madison, WI 53705. 608–262–6966. *Publishes a three-book series that provides an excellent resource on communication aids, switches and environmental control units, and computer access.*

Virginia Spinal Cord Injury System, University of Virginia Center, and Virginia Dept. of Rehabilitation Services, Woodrow Wilson Rehabilitation Center, Box W–279, Fisherville, VA 22939.

Health Care Financing Administration (HCFA), U.S. Dept. of Health and Human Services, 6325 Security Blvd., Baltimore, MD 21207. *Publishes* Guide to Insurance for People with Medicare *(1988), 19 pp. (#02110);* Medicare *(1988). 14 pp.; and* Your Medicare Handbook: A Comprehensive Guide to Your Medicare Hospital and Medical Insurance Benefits *(1989) (#10050).*

University of Michigan Medical Center, Dept. of Physical Medicine and Rehabilitation, Model Spinal Cord Injury Care Center 300 N. Ingalls Bldg., Ann Arbor, MI 48109–0491.

Kent Waldrep National Paralysis Foundation, 14651 Dallas Parkway, Suite 136, Dallas, TX 75240. *Committed to the easiest possible cure for SCI. Primarily raises funds for research but also provides care and financial assistance. Publication:* Spinal Victory *(See personal story of Kent Waldrep in Epilogue.)*

World Institute on Disability (WID), Suite 4, 1720 Oregon St., Berkeley, CA 94703. *Clearinghouse and advocacy center, promoting an independent living philosophy and personal attendant issues. Skilled surveyors and interpreters to a variety of individuals and local, state, and national organizations. Offers valuable consultation services.*

SELECTED CONSUMER-ORIENTED PERIODICALS

Achievement: The National Voice of the Disabled. C. J. Lampos, Editor, Boosters of Achievement, 925 N. E. 122nd St., N. Miami, FL 33161.

Accent on Living. Raymond C. Cheever, Editor and Publisher, Cheever Publishing, Gillum Rd. and High Dr., P.O. Box 700, Bloomington, IL 61701.

Mainstream. 2973 Beech St., San Diego, CA 92102 (Cyndi Jones, publisher).

Rehabilitation Gazette: International Journal of Independent Living for the Disabled. Gini and Joe Laurie, Editors, 4502 Maryland Ave., St. Louis, MO 63108.

SUPPLEMENTAL READINGS

Acute Care

All acronyms are of organizations listed in these Resources.

Collins, W. F., Piepmeier, J., and Ogle, E. 1986. The spinal cord injury problem—A review. *Central Nervous System Trauma* 3 (4): 317–331. *A research focus on the importance of minimizing the secondary effects of initial cord injury.*

Dietz, J. M., et al. 1986. Reflections on the intensive care of 106 acute cervical spinal cord injury patients in the resuscitation unit of a general traumatology center. *Paraplegia* 24 (6): 343–349.

Guin, P. 1990. Standardized nursing care plans for acute spinal cord injury: Improved documentation. *Spinal Cord Injury Nursing* 7(1). *Plan to integrate computerized nursing care plans to facilitate documentation and quality assurance with future capacity to identify staffing and scheduling needs. Cooperative initiative among 10 spinal cord injured centers in Florida.*

Kiwerski, J. 1986. The results of early conservative and surgical treatment of cervical spinal cord injured patients. *Central Nervous System Trauma* 3 (4): 317–331. *Large review study of 1180 patients concludes that results to a large extent depend on when special treatment begins rather than on conservative versus surgical management.*

Meyer, P. R., and Gireesan, G. T. 1987. Management of acute spinal cord injured patients by the Midwest Regional Spinal Cord Injury Care System. *Topics in Acute Care Trauma Rehabilitation* 1 (3): 1–31. *Describes cardiopulmonary functions and support. Excellent, concise overview of initial trauma care.*

Sargant, C., and Braun, M. A. 1986. Occupation therapy management of the acute spinal cord injured patient. *American Journal of Occupational Therapy* 40 (5): 335–337. *Describes program with guidelines for* evaluation and treatment, orthotic selection, and psychosocial considerations with the intent of implementing rehabilitation from the moment of injury.

Aging with Spinal Cord Injury

American Association of Retired Persons (AARP), 3200 E. Carson St., Lakewood, CA 90712. *Powerful resource. Provides inexpensive current information on health care policies and research interpretation.*

Bayley, J. C., Cochran, T. P., and Sledge, C. B. 1987. The weight-bearing shoulder. *Journal of Bone and Joint Surgery*, 69A (5): 676–678.

Bortz, W. Disuse and aging. 1982. *JAMA* 248 (10): 1203–1208.

Brady, S. 1988. Implications of aging in spinal cord injury. *SCI Nursing* (4): 4344.

Brenes, G., LaPorte, R. E., and Collins, E. 1986. High density lipoprotein cholesterol concentrations in physically active and sedentary spinal cord injured patients. *Archives of Physical Medicine and Rehabilitation* 67: 445–450.

Callahan, D. 1988. Families as caregivers: The limits of morality. *Archives of Physical Medicine and Rehabilitation* (69): 323–328.

Coe, R. G., 1982. 22 years a tetraplegic. *Lancet*.

Corbet, B. 1987. The options group: Perspectives on aging with spinal cord injury. North Am. Reinsurance Corp.

DeJong, G. 1986. Evaluating housing and in-home service alternatives for persons aging with a physical disability. A Symposium Presentation made at the Annual Meeting of the American Congress of Rehabilitative Medicine.

DeVivo, et al. 1987. Seven-year survival following Spinal Cord Injury. *Archives of Neurology* (8): 872–5.

Dychtwald, K. 1989. *Age Wave: The Challenges and Opportunities of an Aging America.* Los Angeles: Tarcher Publisher.

Hohmann, G. 1982. Aging in SCI survivors WWII. Craig Hosp. 5th Annual John S. Young Lectureship.

Hohmann, G., Corbet, B., and Trieschmann, R. Getting older now. *The Spinal Network.* Boulder: Sam Maddox, Publisher.

Hooker, E. Problems of veterans spinal cord injured after age 55: Nursing implication. *Journal of Neuroscience Nursing* (4): 188–195.

Mather, J. H. 1986. A philosophy of caring for the elderly. *Paraplegia News* 18–22.

Menter, R. R. Aging and spinal cord injury: Is decline accelerated? *The Spinal Network.* Boulder: Sam Maddox Publisher.

Menter, R. R., Trieshmann, R., and Corbet, B. 1987. Aging in spinal cord injury. Review course 13th Annual ASIA Meeting, Boston, MA.

Ohry, A., Shemesh, Y., and Rozin, R. Are chronic spinal cord injured patients (SCIP) prone to premature aging? *Medical Hypotheses* (11): 467–469.

Shock, N. W. 1984. *Normal Human Aging: The Baltimore Longitudinal Study of Aging.* NIH Publication #84–2450. Washington, DC: U.S. Dept. of Health and Human Services.

Silver, J., et al. 1987. *Personal and Social Implications of SCI. A Retrospective Study.* London: Thames Polytechnic.

Smith, E. L., and Serafass, R. C. 1981. Exercise and aging, *The Scientific Basin*. New Jersey: Enslow. 45–57, 167–178.

Subbarao, J. V., et al. 1987. Spinal cord dysfunction in older patients– rehabilitation outcomes. *Journal of American Paraplegia Society*. (2): 30–35.

Szasz, G. 1989. Sexuality in persons with severe physical disability: A guide to the physician. *Canadian Family Physician*. 35: 345–361. *Outlines the principles of assessment and management of sexual problems in the family physician's office.*

Whiteneck, G. G., Menter, R. R., and Manley, S. 1988. Status of SCI persons more than ten years post injury. *Implication of Long-Term Follow-up of the SCI Population*. Chicago: American Spinal Injury Association, pp. 59–83.

Williams, M. E. 1984. Clinical implications of aging physiology. *American Journal of Medicine* (76): 1049–1054.

Williams, T. F. 1984. *Rehabilitation in the Aging: Philosophy and Approaches*. New York: Raven Press.

Wylie, E. J., and Chakera, T. M. H. 1988. Degenerative joint abnormalities with paraplegia of duration greater than 20 years. *Paraplegia* (26): 101–106.

Yarkony, G. M., et al. 1988. SCI rehabilitation outcome: The impact of aging. *Journal of Clinical Epidemiology* (2): 173–77.

Brain Injury

Binder, L. 1986. Persisting symptoms after mild head injury: A review of the post concussive syndrome. *Journal of Clinical and Experimental Neuropsychology*. 8 (4): 323–346. *Summarizes the neuropsychological effects of mild head injury and in addition reviews neurophysiological evidence of brain damage in those situations. Additionally reviews the literature discussing preexisting emotional problems and posttraumatic emotional reactions. The effects of compensation and litigation on the postconcussive syndrome are also discussed.*

Blair, C. D., and Lanyon, R. I. 1987. Retraining social and adaptive living skills in severely head injured adults. *Archives of Clinical Neuropsychology* 2: 33–44. *A paradigm is presented worth considering in a social skills retraining program.*

Dahlberg, C., Lammertse, D., Schraa, J., et al. 1988. Identification of head trauma in spinal cord injured patients: A complex issue. *Scientific Paper Presentation, American Academy of Rehabilitation Medicine*, Seattle, WA, October 1988. *An overview including a validated assessment tool for identifying patients who have sustained concomitant TBI in an SCI setting.*

Davidoff, G., Thomas, P., Johnson, M., Berrent, S., Dijkers, M., and Doljanac, R. 1988. Closed head injury in acute traumatic spinal cord injury: Incidence and risk factors. *Archives of Physical Medicine and Rehabilitation* 69: 869–872. *This study was to determine the incidence and duration of loss of consciousness and posttraumatic amnesia and to establish various risk factors for combined CHI and SCI.*

Davidoff, G., Roth, E., Morris, J., Blyburg, J., and Meyer, P. 1986. Assessment of closed head injury in trauma-related spinal cord injury. *Paraplegia*. 24: 97–104. *Medical records reviewed were in 122 patients sustaining traumatic SCI to determine the frequency of emergency room assessments for loss of consciousness and posttraumatic amnesia. It was determined that early recognition of craniocerebral trauma is an important component of the acute management of SCI patients.*

Davidoff, G., Morris, J., Roth, E., and Blyburg, J. 1985. Closed head injury in spinal cord injured patients: Retrospective study of loss of consciousness and posttraumatic amnesia. *Archives of Physical Medicine and Rehabilitation*. 66: 41–43. *A review of medical records in 101 SCI patients. Again, incidence was identified using criteria of loss of consciousness and posttraumatic amnesia.*

Diller, L., and Gordon, W. A. 1981. Interventions for cognitive deficits in brain-injured adults. *Journal Consult Clinical Psychology* 49: 822–834. *Suggestions regarding the remediation of specific cognitive sequelae in adults who have sustained TBI.*

Gennarelli, T. A. 1986. Mechanisms and pathophysiology of cerebral concussion. *Journal of Head Trauma Rehabilitation*. 1: 23–29. *A review article discussing the underlying mechanisms and pathophysiology within the brain following a cerebral concussive event. A spectrum of severity is described with clinical and pathophysiological correlation.*

Gentilini, M., Nichelli, P., et al. 1985. Neuropsychological evaluation of mild head injury. *Journal of Neurology, Neurosurgery and Psychiatry*. 48: 137–140. *An Italian-based study intended on tracking the natural course of individuals sustaining mild head injury. It was concluded that cognitive impairments one month after trauma significantly improved although one would raise questions as to the methodology.*

Levin, H., Mattis, S., Ruff, R., et al. 1987. Neurobehavioral outcome following minor head injury: A three center study. *Journal of Neurosurgery* 66: 234–243. *This was a multicenter study intended to follow the natural course of patients after minor head injury. The data suggested that patients improve by the third month postinjury and thereafter there are no permanent disabling neurobehavioral impairments in the great majority of patients who are free of preexisting psychiatric disturbance or substance abuse.*

Prigatano, G. 1986. *Neuropsychological Rehabilitation after Brain Injury*. Baltimore, Johns Hopkins University Press. *A text describing various approaches to neuropsychological sequelae following TBI. These approaches are placed in the context of treatment and functional outcome.*

Silver, J. R., Morris, W. R., and Otfurionski, J. S. 1981. Associated injuries in patients with spinal cord injury. *Injury* 12: 219–224. *Discusses a variety of associated injuries in patients who have sustained SCI. It is noted TBI is among the most prevalent associated injuries.*

Case Management

Major professional organizations and certifying organizations to which rehabilitation case managers may belong include American Congress of Rehabilitation Medicine, American Rehabilitation Counseling Association, Association of Rehabilitation Nurses, National Association of Rehabilitation, and National Rehabilitation Counselor Association. See Organizations, U.S., for addresses. For certification of insurance rehabilitation specialists and certified rehabilitation counselors, contact Board for Rehabilitation Certification, 1156 Shore Drive, Suite 350, Arlington Heights, IL 60004. 312-394-2104.

Clinical Issues

AANN. 1984. *Core Curriculum for Neuroscience Nursing* 1 Chicago: AANN.

Bowe, F. G. 1978. *Handicapping America*. New York: Harper & Row.

Carlson, C. E., Griggs, W. T., and King, R. B. 1989. *Rehabilitation Nursing Procedure Manual*. Rockville, MD: Aspen Publishers.

Cole, J. A., Sperry, J. C., Board, M. A., and Frieden, L. 1979. *New Options*. Houston: TIRR.

Crewe, N., and Zola, I. 1984. *Independent Living in America*. San Francisco: Jossey-Bass.

Dittmar, S. 1989. *Rehabilitation Nursing: Process and Application*. St. Louis: C. V. Mosby.

Gliedman, J., and Roth, W. 1983. *The Unexpected Minority: Handicapped Children in America*. New York: Harcourt Brace Jovanovich.

Hanak, M., and Scott, A. 1983. *Spinal Cord Injury: An Illustrated Guide for Health Care Professionals*. New York: Springer Publishing. *Outstanding integrated guide with rehabilitative focus.*

Hixon, A. K. 1990. Implementation of standards of practice: A spinal cord injury program. *Spinal Cord Injury Nursing* 7 (1). *Describes successful approach to developing and implementing standards of SCI care. Enhancement of methods for staff to monitor care showed evidence of improved outcomes.*

McQuat, F. L. 1989. Ethical dilemma: The spinal cord injured patient with acquired immunodeficiency syndrome. *Spinal Cord Injury Nursing* 6 (4): 75–76. *Presents areas of conflict during rehabilitation, especially from an economic viewpoint.*

Meythaler, J. M., and Cross, L. L. 1988. Traumatic spinal cord injury complicated by the AIDS related complex. *Archives of Physical Medicine and Rehabilitation* 69 (3, Pt 1): 219–222. *Using a case example, points to the necessity of health care professionals in the rehabilitation setting to become familiar with AIDS as they will likely be involved increasingly in the future. Because the life expectancy can still be quite long, AIDS patients warrant rehabilitation.*

Pearson, L. 1989. Ethics and rehabilitation—How to develop your ethical awareness. *Spinal Cord Injury Nursing* 6 (3): 48–51. *Focuses on unique dilemmas encountered in rehabilitation, the nurse's role, and future challenges.*

Rehabilitation Nursing Foundation. 1987. *Rehabilitation Nursing: Concepts and Practice—A Core Curriculum*. 2d ed. Skokie, IL: Author. *An easy-to-read package capturing the role of the nurse in the rehabilitation process. Clinical guidelines are accompanied by nontraditional activities necessary for interdisciplinary functioning, community reintegration, and advocacy.*

Resenbogen, V. S., et al. 1986. Cervical spinal cord injuries in patients with cervical spondylosis. *American Journal of Rehabilitation* 146 (2): 277–284. *Examines incidence and cites cervical spondylosis, which narrows the spinal canal and makes the cord more susceptible to injury, as a major factor in older patients.*

Roberts, C. A., and Burke, S. O. 1989. *Nursing Research: A Quantitative and Qualitative Approach* Boston/Monterey: Jones and Bartlett. *Provides a basis for understanding nursing research, and evaluating and applying findings to clinical practice. This comprehensive guide includes an extensive glossary.*

Williams, J. and Kay, T. 1991. *Head Injury: A Family Matter*. Baltimore: Paul H. Brooks Pub. Co. *A wonderful guide to supporting families; applicable to SCI trauma.*

Economic Consequences and Implications

APS. 1989. *The Economic Consequences of Spinal Cord Injury* Research Briefs (Issues #3-#6). *Topics include definitions of SCI, classification, incidence, and prevalence; dissemination survey; measuring the costs of medical care; estimates of SCI prevalence; traumatic SCI demography and etiology; and direct costs of SCI.*

Bureau of Economic Research, Rutgers University. 1986. *Economic Consequences of Severe Disability*. New Brunswick, NJ: Author. *Supported by a grant from the PVA SCI Research Foundation, Project No. NAO–467.*

Bureau of Economic Research, Rutgers University. 1985. *Economic Consequences of Spinal Cord Injury*. New Brunswick, NJ: Author. *Supported by a grant from the PVA SCI Research Foundation, Project No. NAO–384.*

MacKenzie, E. 1989. *Cost of Injury in the United States: Report to Congress*. Baltimore: Rice and Associates. *A staggering and sobering report on the real and hidden costs of injury in today's society.*

Federal Help, Legislation, and Disability Rights

AASCIN. 1990. *Communicating Effectively with Legislators*. *A practical booklet designed to help nurses become more vocal about their roles in the health care system.*

Goldman, C. D. 1987. *DISABILITY RIGHTS GUIDE Practical Solutions to Problems Affecting People with Disabilities*. Media Publishing, 2440 "0" St., Suite 202, Lincoln, NE 68510-1125. *Winner of the 1988 Book Award from the President's Commission on Employment of the Handicapped. Discusses accessibility, housing, employment, education, and transportation. Relevant laws are presented with state and federal contacts.*

Pocket Guide to Federal Help for Individuals with Disabilities. 1987. Washington, DC: Clearinghouse on the Handicapped, U. S. Department of Education *Contains information on education and employment, financial and medical assistance, civil rights, tax benefits and transportation.*

Health Services Research

Robert Wood Johnson Foundation. 1990. *Improving Service Systems for People with Disabilities*. Princeton, NJ: Author.

National Rehabilitation Hospital. 1990. *National Invitational Conference on Developing a Comprehensive Health Services Research Capacity in Physical Disability and Rehabilitation, Proceedings. Emphasis on four major areas of concern: trauma care, rehabilitation services (organization and financing), attendant care and personal assistance, and long-term institutional care. Given the severely limited funding resources, the area of relevance of research in relation to practical application is paramount.*

High Quadriplegia

Audiovisual Learning Aids

American College of Chest Physicians and Travenol Laboratories. 1986. *Videotape program on hospital to home transition of a young man partially dependent on a ventilator. Contact ACCP, 911 Buse Hwy., Park Ridge, IL 60068.*

Loma Linda University Medical Center. 1989. *The Ventilator Assisted Patient: Preparing for Home. Videotape.*

TIRR. 1981. *Portrait: Kim Enbey. Kim, a 16-year-old girl with apneic quadriplegia, is shown during a day experiencing various educational and rehabilitative activities. Presents an insightful look at her personality and reactions during her 2-year rehabilitation period. Videotape.*

TIRR. *Proceedings from the Multidisciplinary Care of High Quads C4 and up: Second Multi-Center Conference: An Audiovisual Report. Eight audio tapes, photographic reproductions of more than 400 slides, and accompanying handouts.*

Equipment and Supplies

Barrington Publications. 1984. *Rx Home Care. 1984 Buyer's Guide.* Los Angeles.

Daedalus Enterprises, Inc. 1984. *Cardio-Respiratory Care Equipment and Supplies Buyer's Guide (For Hospitals and Homes),* Dallas.

Spencer, G. T. *Guidelines for Ventilator-Users in Europe.* Phipps Respiratory Unit, South Western Hospital, London, SW9, England. *Provides information on lodging and technical services such as available equipment for loan, during travel (transformers, adapters, receptacles).*

General

Groher, M. E. 1984. *Dysphagia: Diagnosis and Management.* Boston: Butterworth Publisher. *Examines the pathophysiology of evaluation and management of swallowing disorders. Chapter 6 explores prefeeding management, training, and the use of adaptive equipment applicable to those with high quadriplegia.*

Harper, R. W. 1981. *A Guide to Respiratory Care: Physiology and Clinical Applications.* Toronto: J. B. Lippincott.

Kirby, N. A. 1989. The individual with high quadriplegia. *Nursing Clinics of North America* 24 (1): 179–91. *Overview addresses respiratory support, aided communication and environmental controls.*

Kochansky, M. T. 1986. Oximetry, technology, and the medicare guidelines. *Respiratory Care* 31 (12): 1185–1187.

TIRR. 1985. *Nursing Care of "High Risk" Ventilator Dependent Quadriplegics. Manual includes topics related to staffing plans; patient classification tools for planning care; direct care guidelines; specific protocols, policies, and procedures; and equipment guidelines. Assessment criteria for development of the nursing care plan and patient and family teaching guidelines are also included. 97 pp.*

Home Care Perspectives

Aday, L. A., Aitken, M., and Wegener, D. 1988. *Pediatric home care: Results of a national evaluation of programs for ventilator-assisted children.* University of Chicago, Center for Health Care Administration Studies. Chicago: Plurions Press. *Methods of evaluation and appreciation of the impact of severe disability on the home front. Has wide application for adults also.*

Brownlee, S., and Williams, S. J. 1987. Physiotherapy in the respiratory care of patients with high spinal cord injury. *Physiotherapy* 73 (3): 148–152.

Bruhn, J. G. 1977. Effects of chronic illness on the family. *Journal of Family Practice* 4 (6): 1057–1060.

Continuing care of the ventilator-dependent patient (postgraduate course). 1986. *Respiratory Care* 31: 265–337.

Coordinating Center for Home and Community Care (CCHCC). *A Nurse in Your Home.* Undated Publication. Millersville, MD: Author.

Frank, J. I., and Walker, N. 1984. Experience with a prolonged respiratory care unit—Revisited. *Chest* 86 (4): 616–620.

Frye, B., and Hilton, T. 1988. Preparing the caregiver to manage ventilator-dependent patient at home. *Rehabilitation Nursing* 13 (1): 38–42.

Goldberg, A. I. 1984. The regional approach to home care for life supported persons. *Chest* 86 (3): 345–346.

Goldberg, A. I. et al. 1984. Home care for life supported persons: An approach to program development. *The Journal of Pediatrics* May: 785–795.

Haddad, A. 1986. Ethical considerations in long-term home care for ventilator-dependent clients. *Pride Institute Journal of Long-Term Home Health Care* 5 (2): 3–7.

Kopacz, M. A., and Moriarty-Wright, R. 198. Multidisciplinary approach for the patient on a home ventilator. *Heart and Lung* 13 (3): 255–262.

Lee, M. Y., et al. 1989. Rehabilitation of quadriplegic patients with phrenic nerve pacers. *Archives of Physical Medicine and Rehabilitation* 70: 549–552. *Through four case studies presents considerations for establishing and safely maintaining phrenic stimulation, including community support services to enhance independence.*

Levine, S. P., et al. 1987. Independently activated talking tracheostomy systems for quadriplegic patients. *Archives of Physical Medicine and Rehabilitation* 68 (Sept.): 571–573.

Massachusetts Dept. of Public Health. Home care for children on respirators. *New England Journal of Medicine* 309 (21): 1319–1323.

O'Ryan, J. A. 1986. An overview of mechanical ventilation in the home. *Rx Home Care* (Dec.): 45–49.

Posch, C. M., and Edwards, P. 1988. The ventilator-dependent child: Challenge and opportunity. *Rehabilitation Nursing* 13 (1): 15–18.

Purtilo, R. B. 1986. Ethical issues in the treatment of chronic ventilator-dependent patients. *Archives of Physical Medicine and Rehabilitation* 67: 718–721.

Report of the surgeon general's workshop on children with handicaps and their families. 1982. U. S. Dept. of Health and Human Services. *Focus on ventilator-dependent children.*

Sivak, E. D., et al. 1983. Pulmonary mechanical ventilation at home: A reasonable and less expensive alternative. *Respiratory Care* 28 (1): 42–49.

Independent Living

Accent on Living's Buyers Guide, Box 700, Bloomington, IL 61701. *Quality magazine with up-to-date general product information.*

de Balcazar, Y. S., Bradford, B., and Fawcett, S. B. 1989. *Common Concerns of Disabled Americans: Issues and Options.* Lawrence, KS: RTC/IL.

DeJong, G. 1985. *Economics and Independent Living.* RTC/IL Monographs on Independent Living. Lawrence, KS. RTC/IL.

Heinemann, A. W., Billeter, J., and Betts, H. 1988. Prospective payment for acute care: Impact of rehabilitation hospitals. *Archives of Physical Medicine and Rehabilitation* 69 (Aug.): 614–618.

Heinemann, A. W., et al. 1989. Functional outcome following spinal cord injury: A comparison of specialized spinal cord center versus general hospital short-term care. *Archives of Neurology* 46 (Oct.): 1098–1102.

ILRU. *An Orientation to Independent Living Centers*. Houston TX: Author. *ILRU also publishes a directory of centers and other programs providing independent living services in the United States. The RSA's Office of Independent Living can also provide information about IL centers.*

Levy, C. W. 1988. *A People's History of the Independent Living Movement*. Lawrence, KS: RTC/IL. *Warm reading to introduce the visionaries who helped to create the Independent Living Movement. Recommended to gain insight into the struggles and barriers experienced by persons with disabilities.*

Litvak, I. and Heumann, J. 1987. *Attending to America*. Berkeley, CA: World Institute on Disability.

Quality of Life. 1990. Berkeley, CA: World Institute on Disability. *Agenda for enhancing quality of life of people with disabilities. Highly recommended.*

Tools for Independent Living. Whirlpool Corporation, Appliance Information Service, Benton Harbor, MI 49002.

Nutrition

Glanz, K. 1985. Nutrition education for risk factor reduction and patient education: A review. *Preventive Medicine* 14: 721–752. *Examines the use of behavioral and biological measures of nutritional education for managing various diets and reports on the types and effectiveness of various strategies. Includes suggestions for the advances in practice, theory, and research in patient education.*

Goldfarb, I. W., and Yates, A. P. 1980. *Total Parenteral Nutrition Concepts and Methods*. Pittsburgh: Synapse Publications. *Cornerstone text on providing nutritional support.*

Kirshblum, S., and Zafonte, R. 1989. Dangers of elastic bandage immobilization in the spinal cord injury patient. *Abstracts Digest, Annual Meeting, American Spinal Injury Association*, Las Vegas, p. 34.

Kiwerski, J. 1986. Bleeding from the alimentary canal during the management of spinal cord injury patients. *Paraplegia* 24 (2): 92–96. *Among 2000 patients with SCI (admitted to a facility over a 14-year period), describes 52 patients that experienced severe hemorrhage for the alimentary canal. Bleeding most often occurred in patients with complete cervical cord injuries during the early postinjury period. Anticoagulants and steroids add to the risk, but severe disturbance of the autonomic nervous system appears to be the basic factor. Diagnostic difficulties must be overcome to establish early and appropriate intervention.*

Klinger, J. (comp.). 1978. *Mealtime Manual for People with Disabilities and the Aging*. 2d ed. Published by Campbell Soup Co., Box (MM) 56, Camden, NJ 08101. *Directed toward disabled homemakers; includes meal-planning and kitchen-tested techniques and recipes, current supplies, prices, and other information. Specific sections for the homemaker who uses a wheelchair, has upper extremity weakness, or lacks sensation. Very useful.*

Kuric, J. 1989. Nutritional Support: A prophylaxis against stress bleeding after spinal cord injury. *Paraplegia* 27: 140–145. *Research indicates that a nutritional regimen that meets total energy requirements decreases the likelihood of peptic complications after SCI.*

Richards, C. 1988. Nutritional support of the mechanically ventilated patient. Unpublished material, University Hospital, Vancouver, BC. *Interpretation prepared for Physical and Rehabilitation Services.*

Segal, J. L., Milne, N., Brunnemann, S. R., and Lyons, K. P. 1987. Metoclopramide-induced normalization of impaired gastric emptying in spinal cord injury. *American Journal of Gastroenterology* 82 (11): 1143–1148. *Concludes that impaired gastric emptying due to SCI may be pharmacologically modified to resemble normal emptying. May be of help to therapeutic efficacy of orally administered medications when drug absorption is dependent on gastric mobility or emptying.*

Walters, K., and Silver, J. R. 1986. Gastrointestinal bleeding in patients with acute spinal injuries. *International Rehabilitative Medicine* 8 (1): 44–47. *Reviews incidence and presentation of symptoms. Large study over 11-year period documented mean occurrence was 22.5 days postinjury.*

Patient and Family Education

Schachtel, D. 1989. *Education: The Key to Independence*. Atlanta: Shepherd Spinal Center.

Virginia Spinal Cord Injury Care and Teaching Manual. 1988. Fisherville, VA: Virginia Spinal Cord Injury System. *Soft-cover workbook designed for personalized patient and family use, for example, What is the level of your injury? What type of bladder do you have, and what are the possible goals for management of your bladder? Also includes numerous opportunities for patients to enter information, such as current medications, dosages, side effects, precautions. A list of questions and a teaching/evaluation checklist are included at the end of each comprehensive section. Includes helpful section on psychosocial-sexual factors. A valuable teaching and resource aid.*

Yasenchak, P. and Bridle, M. 1988. *Your Skin: An Owner's Manual*. Fisherville, VA: Virginia SCI System. *An excellent practical guide, especially for high-risk individuals postdischarge.*

Prehospital Care

Barrett, A. S. 1984. A guide to airway management. *Emergency Medical Services* 13 (5): 40–60.

Butman, A. M., and McSwain, N. E. 1984. Emergency patient removal. *Journal of Prehospital Care* 3: 23–26.

Campbell, J. E. 1985. *Basic Trauma Life Support Manual*. Bowie, MD: Brady Communications.

Committee on Trauma, American College of Surgeons. 1985. *Advanced Trauma Life Support Manual*. Chicago: American College of Surgeons.

Committee on Trauma, American College of Surgeons. 1986. *Prehospital Advanced Trauma Life Support Manual*. Chicago: American College of Surgeons.

Iserson, K. V. 1981 Blind nasotracheal intubation. *Annals of Emergency Medicine* 10: 486–171.

Jacobs, L. M., Berrizbeitia, L. D., Bennett, B., et al. 1983. Endotracheal intubation in the prehospital phase of emergency medical care. *Journal of the American Medical Association* 250: 2175–2177.

Kossuth, L. C. 1967. The initial movement of the injured. *Military Medicine* 132 (1): 18–21.

McGuire, R. A. 1987. Spinal instability and the log-rolling maneuver. *Journal of Trauma* 27 (5): 525–531.

Morse, T. S. 1969. Transportation of critically ill or injured children. *Pediatric Clinics of North America* 16 (3): 565–571.

Podoisky, S., et al. 1983. Efficacy of cervical spine immobilization methods. *Journal of Trauma*. 23: 461.

Shimazu, S., et al. 1983. Outcomes of trauma patients with no vital signs on hospital admission. *Journal of Trauma* 23: 213.

Smith, M., Bourn, S., and Larmon, B. 1989. Ties that bind: Immobilizing the injured spine. *Journal of Emergency Medical Services* 14 (4): 28–35.

Toscano, J. 1988. Prevention of neurological deterioration before admission to a spinal cord injury unit. *Paraplegia* 26 (3): 143–150.

Prevention

Audiovisual

See Chapter 3 for other audiovisual resources.

Disabled Forestry Workers. 1988. *Every Twelve Seconds*. Videotape. *A 1-hour documentary that deals with safety and disability issues from the perspective of an injured worker.*

Mathews, R. M., White, G. W., and Fawcett, S. B. Undated Publication. Slide Show Presentations: A Vehicle for Community Support. Available through Lawrence, KS: RTC/IL University of Kansas.

Readings

McGinnis, J. National priorities in disease prevention. *Issues in Science and Technology* Winter: 1988–1989.

National Center for Statistics and Analysis, National Traffic Safety Administration. 1989. *Occupant Protection Facts*. Washington, DC: Author.

National Safety Council. 1988. *Accident Facts*. Chicago: Author.

Refshauge, W. 1987. Towards prevention of spinal cord injury (Technical Report Number One–1987). Melbourne, Australia: The Menzies Foundation. *An Australian perspective on prevention.*

Psychosocial Adaptation

Audiovisual

Corbet, B. 1989. *Survivors* (Videotape). Access, Inc., 177 South Lookout Mountain Rd., Golden, CO 80401 303-526-7209.

TIRR. 1982. *Attitudes toward Persons with Spinal Cord Injury*. Houston: TIRR. *A 6-hour videotape series on attitudes toward people with disabilities as reflected by public outlook and policies. Aims to increase awareness of attitudes and offer a forum where viewers can examine their own attitudes and behaviors.*

TIRR. 1983. *Mended Dreams*. Houston: TIRR. *Videotape program especially helpful to persons with new disabilities who are confronted with questions about themselves and their future. Valuable for attitude awareness for professionals and families also. Intertwines scenes of persons at work and during leisure with personal interviews to describe their attitudes about their work, families, friends, and themselves.*

TIRR. 1988. *Prescription Medications, Alcohol, and the Person with Spinal Cord Injury*. Houston: TIRR. *Videotape program provides information about alcohol and medication use to decrease problems with mixing. Encourages communication about alcohol habits and increases awareness of the potential abuse for alcohol in persons with SCI. Message emphasized by personal interview and intended for patient and family education.*

TIRR. 1988. *Recreational Drugs and Medications and the Person with Spinal Cord Injury*. Houston: TIRR. *Videotape program presents facts and potential for abuse. Message presented through personal interview with a disabled person who abused drugs and mixed recreational drugs with medications. Intended for patient and family education.*

General

Apple, D. 1989. *Hysterical paralysis. Abstracts Digest, Annual Meeting, American Spinal Injury Association, Las Vegas* p. 40. *Presents an updated overview of assessment and treatment of this response.*

Bishop, D. S. 1980. *Behavioral Problems and the Disabled, Assessment and Management*. Baltimore, MD: Williams and Wilkins. *Deals clearly with behavioral problems; addresses the problems of sleep and pain; provides an overview of problems unique to the disabled child; and describes staff interaction in various settings. Specific chapters are devoted to crisis intervention techniques, to SCI, and to the relationship between alcohol and drug abuse and physical medicine and rehabilitation.*

Crewe, N. M., and Krause, J. S. 1988. Marital relationships and spinal cord injury. *Archives of Physical Medicine and Rehabilitation* 69 (6): 435–438. *Compares marriages of persons married before and after onset of SCI. Those married after injury reported a greater degree of satisfaction and tended to be working and socially active outside their homes.*

Dunn, M. 1975. Psychological intervention in a spinal cord injury center: An introduction. *Rehabilitation Psychology* 22 (4): 165–178. *Describes emotional responses, physical, social, and sexual adaptation and examines some staff responsibilities in terms of giving feedback to prepare patients for life in the community again.*

English, R. W. 1983. *The Role of the Family in Rehabilitation*. NARIC Research Contract No. 3–83-0006 from the National Institute of Handicapped Research, U.S. Dept. of Education, Washington, DC. *Presents analytical synopsis, description of principles, and annotated reference materials.*

Gibbons, F. X. 1985. *A Social and Psychological Perspective*. Monographs in Independent Living. Lawrence, KS: RTC/IL.

Harriman, M., and Garfunkel, M. 1981. The value of self-help groups in spinal cord injury rehabilitation. *Model Systems' Spinal Cord Injury Digest* 3 (Fall): 26–33. *Advocates the formation and integration of self-help groups within rehabilitation programs. Four types of self-help groups are proposed. Self-help groups emphasize matuality and interdependence and provide an opportunity to share feelings and information.*

Hart, G. 1981. Spinal cord injury: Impact on clients' significant others. *Rehabilitation Nursing*, Jan.–Feb. 11–15. *Findings from interviews, beginning within hours after injury, suggest significant others have many needs, including: to feel adequately informed, to feel helpful to the client, and to feel the client is getting good care. To benefit the client, the nurse must listen and react to the concerns and needs of significant others as part of the rehabilitation approach.*

Killen, J. M. 1990. Role stabilization in families after spinal cord injury. *Rehabilitation Nursing* 15 (1): 19–21. *Study investigated 215 family members and describes how role changes demanded of the spouse are the greatest. Implications for nursing interventions are described.*

Lawson, N. C. 1978. Significant events in the rehabilitation process: The spinal cord patient's point of view. *Archives of Physical Medicine and Rehabilitation* 59 (Dec.): 573–579. *Report of a research study using tape-recorded daily logs, hospital staff ratings, behavioral measure of verbal output, and an endocrine measure to determine significant events during hospitalization. Results suggest that prolonged depression is counterproductive to the rehabilitation process and that important people in the patient's life exert a most significant influence. Discusses programmatic implications.*

Pittman, J. L., and Mathews, R. M. *Peer Counseling: Four Exemplary Programs.* Monograph 35. Lawrence, KS: RTC/IL.

Rogers, J. C., and Figone, J. J. 1979. Psychosocial parameters in treating the person with quadriplegia. *American Journal of Occupational Therapy* 33 (7): 432–439. *The development of a more flexible, comprehensive treatment model that gives priority to developmental status, changing life goals, interpersonal relationships, and social roles. Highly recommended.*

Rohrer, K., et al. 1980. Rehabilitation in spinal cord injury: Use of a patient-family group. *Archives of Physical Medicine and Rehabilitation* 61 (5): 225–229. *A report on a program of one-day workshops held for patients with SCI and their families. Stresses education, as well as a therapeutic sharing of feelings.*

Romano, M. D. 1976. Social skills training with the newly handicapped. *Archives of Physical Medicine and Rehabilitation* 57 (June): 302–303. *Describes the premise that restoring an individual's social competence maximizes the probability of success of the physical rehabilitation process.*

Turnbull, A. P., Summers, J. A., and Brotherson, J. A. 1984. *Working with Families with Disabled Members.* Lawrence, KS: RTC/IL.

van den Bout, J., et al. 1988. Attributional cognitions, coping behaviors and self-esteem in inpatients with spinal cord injuries. *Archives of Clinical Psychology* 44 (1): 17–22. *Observations by a nurse, physician, and psychologist are described and comparisons made between patients recently injured and those who have had SCI for a longer term.*

Wiley, L. 1979. Realistic goals don't mean failure. *Nursing* 9 (5): 55–58. *Nurses explore personal feelings when limit setting, consistency, and reality confrontation do not always achieve the optimal outcome for a patient with a self-destructive, sociopathic personality.*

Chemical (Drug/Alcohol) Dependency Organizations

The following organizations can provide names of other groups concerned with this issue.

Addiction Intervention with the Disabled, Sociology Department, Kent State University, Kent, OH 44242. 216-672-2440. Publishes quarterly newsletter.

AL-ANON Family Group Headquarters, P. O. Box 862 Midtown Station, New York, NY 10063. 212-302-7240. Al-Anon, Alateen information catalogs of pamphlets and books.

American Council for Drug Education, 204 Monroe St., Rockville, MD 20850. 301-924-0600. Publishes books on health hazards of marijuana and cocaine; films, videos, kits, books, brochures, research; assists parents and industry leaders in effort to address drug use.

National Clearinghouse for Alcohol and Drug Information, P.O. Box 2345, Rockville, MD 20852. 301-468-2600. Reference, literature and data base searches.

National Drug Abuse Treatment Referral and Information Services, 332 Springfield Ave. Summit, NJ 97901. 1-800-COCAINE. Brochures and posters. *Public service of Psychiatric Institutes of America.*

Office for Substance Abuse Prevention, Division of Communication Programs, Room 13A54, 5600 Fishers La. Rockville, MD 20857. 301-443-0373. *Publishes newsletter with information of new programs, publications, and so on.*

Rehabilitation

Fine, P. R., Stover, S. L., and DeVivo, M. J. 1987. A methodology for predicting lengths of stay for spinal cord injured patients. *Inquiry* 24 (summer): 147–156. Blue Cross Blue Shield Association. *A predictive model that showed a 45% variance in length of hospital stays and adjusted hospital charges in a large study (2,169 patients) of seven diagnostic groups of patients with SCI requiring extensive rehabilitation services after acute care. Strategies for alternative methods of payment to ensure better payment delivery systems throughout the life span are presented.*

Halstead, L., et al. 1986. The innovative rehabilitation team: An experiment in team building. *Archives of Physical Medicine and Rehabilitation* 67 (6): 357–361. *Describes an effort to create innovative approaches to team care and presents practical guidelines to increase patient participation and to develop a rounds coordinator role and a structured format with integration of research findings. Other tools are included. Group evaluation demonstrated less physician involvement, increased patient and interdisciplinary staff participation. Offers a comprehensive review toward making lasting interdisciplinary changes and makes a plea for other teams to continue exploring to bring out latent creativity and resources in their team memberships.*

University of Michigan, Dept. of Physical Medicine and Rehabilitation and Ann Arbor Center for Independent Living. 1989. *Hospital to Community: A Collaborative Program for Independent Living and Medical Rehabilitation. This is a model program designed to assist persons with SCI in achieving and acquiring maximum independence and control over their lives following injury. Highly recommended for interdisciplinary teams.*

Sports and Leisure

Exercise Equipment

Flexaciser, C. P. M. II. Rehabilitative Health Products, 3950 Atlantic Ave., Suite 59, Long Beach, CA 90807. *Offers a continuous passive motion machine that operates on the principle of cross-lateral patterning (like walking) to maintain movement of both upper and lower extremities.*

Freedom Machine. Olympic Enterprizes, Inc., 2323 W. Encanto Blvd., Phoenix, AZ 85009. *Designed for training the competitive athlete. Allows access to wheelchair users for rehabilitative exercise. Innovative features allow 30 exercises using a variety of muscle conditioning apparatuses, pulleys, military and bench press units. Accommodates up to 4 persons at a time.*

Saratoga Cycle. Saratoga Access and Fitness, Inc., P.O. Box 1427, Fort Collins, CO 80522-1427. *Adaptable and fun accessories available. Chosen by several top rehabilitation centers and universities, such as the Miami Project.*

Supplemental Readings

Corcoran, P., Goldman, R., Hoerner, E., et al. 1980. Sports medicine and the physiology of wheelchair marathon racing. *Orthopaedic Clinics of North America* 11: 697–716.

Curtis, K. A. 1982. Wheelchair sports medicine. Part IV: Athletic injuries. *Sports 'N Spokes* 7: 20–24.

Rick Hansen, Man-in-Motion Legacy Fund. See Organizations, Canada.

Labanowich, S. 1978. The psychology of wheelchair sports. *Therapeutic Recreation Journal* 12: 11–17.

Madorsky, J., and Curtis, K. 1984. Wheelchair sports medicine. *American Journal of Sports Medicine* 12 (2): 128–132.

National Association of Sports for Cerebral Palsy. 1983. *Classification and Sport Rules Manual.* United Cerebral Associations, New York, NY.

Palaestra Challenge Publications, Ltd., P.O. Box 508, Macomb, IL 61455.

PVA. n.d. *Wheelchair Sports: Competitive and Recreational.* Phoenix, AZ PVA Publications.

PVA. *Recreational and Competitive Wheelchair Sports.* Brochure.

Sports 'N Spokes. Magazine for wheelchair sports and recreation. PVA Publications.

Travel Guidebooks. Free lists of guidebooks published by the Royal Association for Disability and Rehabilitation, London, and by Rehabilitation International USA. See Organizations for addresses.

Technology

Dickey, R. 1986. Electronic technical aids for persons with high level spinal cord injury. *Central Nervous System Trauma* 3 (1): 93–110.

Dickey, R., and Shealey, S. 1987. Using technology to control the environment. *American Journal of Occupational Therapy* 41 (11): 717–721.

Garber, S., Lathemm, P., and Gregorio, T. 1988. *Specialized Occupational Therapy for Persons with High Level Quadriplegia.* Houston, TX: TIRR.

Hornstein, S., Steer, J. E., McKay, K. S., Hurley, M., and Cameron, W. M. 1987. Neil Squire Foundation computer comfort program for high-lesion quadriplegics and other severely disabled adults. *Abstracts Digest, ASIA:* 51–56.

Hurley, M., and Kinnee, A. 1989. Microcomputers and the disabled. Unpublished Manuscript, *Neil Squire Foundation*, N. Vancouver, BC. *Manual designed to complement a 2-day workshop on computers for adults with severe physical disabilities. Reviews hardware, software, adaptive devices.*

Kinnee, A. 1988. Environmental control systems. *Neil Squire Foundation Newsletter*, Fall, 5–8. *Review of commercially available environmental control units.*

Locker, D., and Kaufert, J. 1987. The impact of changing technology. *Rehabilitation Digest:* 9–10.

McKay, K. 1989. Specialized power wheelchair systems for people with severe physical disabilities. *Neil Squire Foundation Newsletter*, Winter 5–8.

McDonald, D., Boyle, M., and Schumann, T. 1989. Environmental control unit utilization by high-level spinal cord injured patients. *Archives of Physical Medicine and Rehabilitation* 70: 621–623.

RESNA 1989. *Assistive Technology Sourcebook.* Washington, DC: Author. *Provides a comprehensive guide to assistive technology and resources. Explains emerging trends and resources to help locate information, including training aids and funding sources.*

Sloane, E. *Sloane Report.* Bimonthly written by Eydie Sloane, PhD., who directs the Exceptional Technology Laboratory for Dade County, FL. *Examines the different microcomputer companies and offers good advice to anyone exploring the field of technology for people with disabilities.* Dr. Eydie Sloane, P.O. Box 561689, Miami, FL. 305–251–2199.

Symington, D., Lynwood, D., Lawson, J., and MacLean, J. 1986. Environmental control systems in chronic care hospitals and nursing homes. *Archives of Physical Medicine and Rehabilitation* 67: 322–325.

Trauma Coding

TRI-CODE. Tri-Analytics, Inc., 23 Ellendale St., Suite A, Bel Air, MD 21014. *Computer program developed to satisfy critical injury coding needs. Designed by trauma nurse coordinator and coding experts and researchers. Jointly offered with the Association for the Advancement of Automotive Medicine (AAAM). Consistent ICD–9–CM codes and AIS–85 severity values.*

INDEX